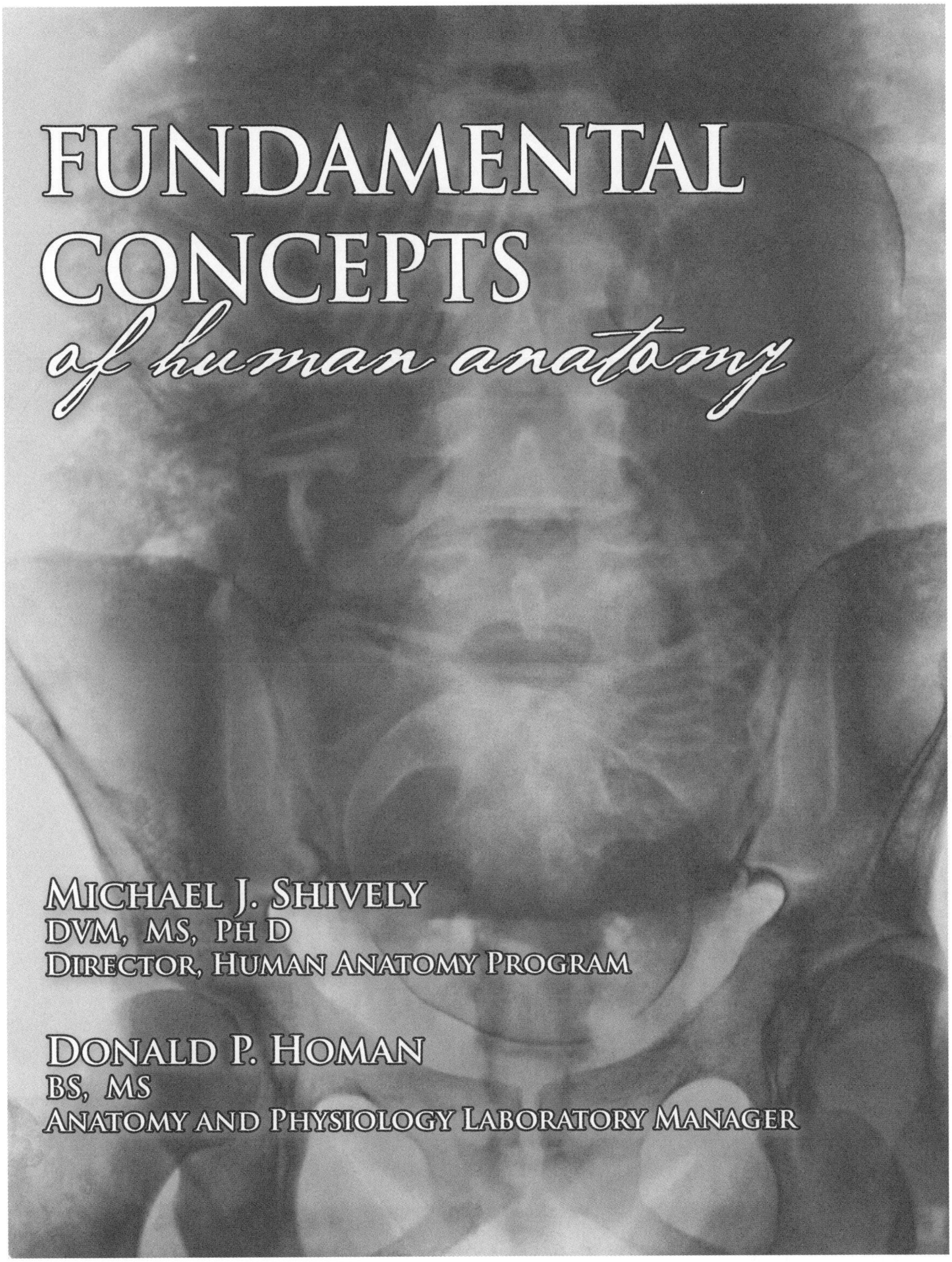

Utah Valley University
Orem, Utah

bluedoor
small publishing done big™

President: Jon K. Earl

Executive Publisher: Lucas Tomasso
Publisher: Dawn Earl
Publisher: Paul Raymond
Marketing Manager: Stacey Martin

Senior Production Editor: Harry Beckwith
Senior Production Editor: Connie Dayton
Senior Production Editor: Amy Schneider
Production Editor: Stephanie Larson
Production Editor: Peggy Li

Consulting Editors: Bruce D. Wingerd, Edison State College
Suzanne F. Frucht, Ph.D.
Gary Shin, California State Universiy — Long Beach
John F. Wiginton, University of Mississippi

Cover Design: Stephanie Larson

ISBN-13: 978-1-59984-064-2
ISBN-10: 1-59984-064-2

Published by bluedoor, LLC
6595 Edenvale Boulevard, Suite 150
Eden Prairie, MN 55346
800-979-1624
www.bluedoorpublishing.com

This book was previously published by Pearson Education, Inc.

Printed in the United States of America.
10 9 8 7 6 5

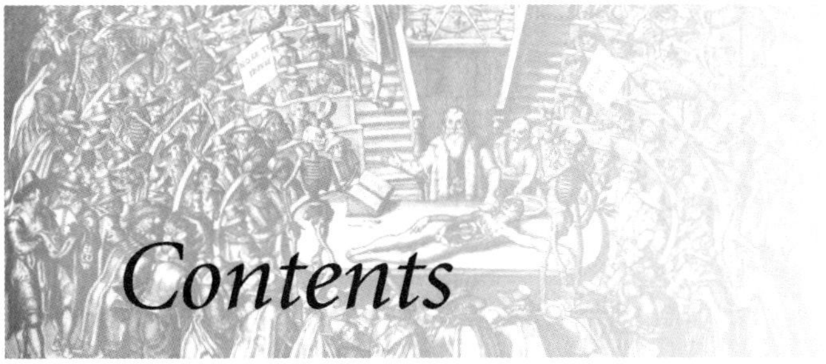

Contents

	Preface	iii
	Acknowledgements	v
	How to Use this Book	vii

Chapter

1	Introduction to Human Anatomy	1
2	Cytology	31
3	Histology	57
4	Integumentary System	91
5	Basic and Appendicular Osteology	113
6	Axial and Developmental Osteology	151
7	Arthrology	189
8	Skeletal Myology/Muscular System	225
9	Introduction to Nervous System and CNS	285
10	Peripheral Nervous System	323
11	Autonomic Nervous System	375
12	Eye	401
13	Ear	431
14	Endocrine System	459
15	Cardiovascular System	491
16	Lymphatic System	559
17	Digestive System	587
18	Respiratory System	635
19	Urinary System	671
20	Male Reproductive System	697
21	Female Reproductive System	725
22	Human Development	751

Appendices

I	Skeletal Muscles	779
II	Summary of the Special Muscles of the Digits of the Hand	793
III	Cranial Nerve Facts and Learning Aids	795
	Index	797

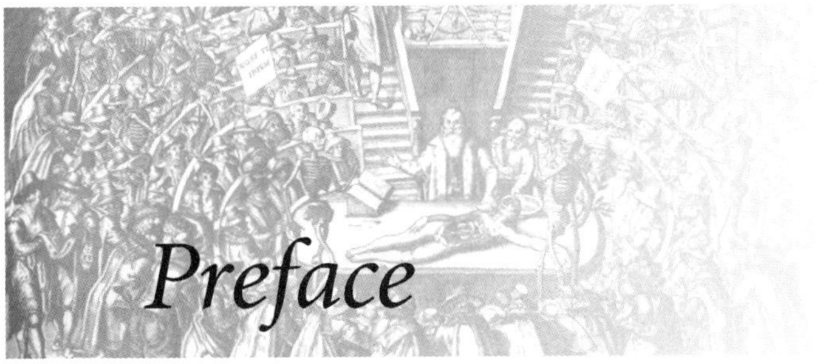

Preface

In the fall of 1992, we were given departmental responsibility for revising and upgrading the Human Anatomy course at Utah Valley State College (then Utah Valley Community College). It was in a sad state of disarray—taught by several different lecture instructors and a whole host of lab instructors whose collective experience in the field of anatomy was (pardon the pun) grossly deficient. We began by writing a lab guide to replace the unadorned term list which had been used to direct student laboratory study, incorporated proper nomenclature, and started instructional sessions for our laboratory teachers and student teaching assistants.

When we began reviewing several potential texts for the course, we were uniformly impressed by the quality of the illustrations, but were disappointed in the accuracy of the textual material. Even the basic anatomic facts were often misstated and clouded by a smokescreen of half-truths and blatant inaccuracy. The nomenclature used was heavily laced with slang, obsolete, and inventive terminology. Finally, the illustrations, while beautiful, were often mislabeled or misrepresented actual anatomy. When we took a couple of presentations to a meeting of anatomy and physiology teachers a few years ago, we discovered the problem. The authors (and instructional consumers) of most introductory anatomy texts are not formally trained anatomists. Indeed, when we queried the convention attendees about their backgrounds in gross anatomy, less than half a dozen had an MS or a PhD in gross anatomy. Authors of three of the texts we had reviewed attended this meeting. Only one of them was trained in gross anatomy.

We returned from this experience with a greater understanding of why anatomical textual inaccuracies exist. We also began to realize that many of the consumers of these texts are not overly concerned about accuracy. Nonetheless, we felt an obligation, as two of a dying breed of biological scientists who *do* have a formal background in gross anatomy, to contribute, hopefully in a positively useful manner, to the literature of human gross anatomy. Our collective cadaver experience totals sixty-one years. The total number of cadavers that we have totally or partially dissected numbers in the hundreds. We have taught human and veterinary anatomy at the undergraduate, professional, advanced, and graduate levels as well as basic biology, histology, physiology, comparative vertebrate biology, radiology, and surgery.

With this background and experience, we decided to write our own summary of human gross anatomy guided by two specific objectives: brevity and accuracy. The nomenclature that we used corresponds to that listed in the *Nomina Anatomica* (Sixth Edition). Slang, archaic, and inventive terms have either been omitted, or in cases where their continued use in medical science so justifies, have been mated with proper terms and set apart by the use of quotes. For the last nine years, rough drafts of this work have been used by anatomy students at our institution and their feedback has been invaluable as we have revised and refined the material.

We hope that our colleagues who teach gross anatomy at the introductory/undergraduate level will find our efforts useful. More importantly, we hope that our students will gain an appreciation and wonderment for the marvelous structure of the human body.

M.J. Shively
D.P. Homan
Orem, Utah

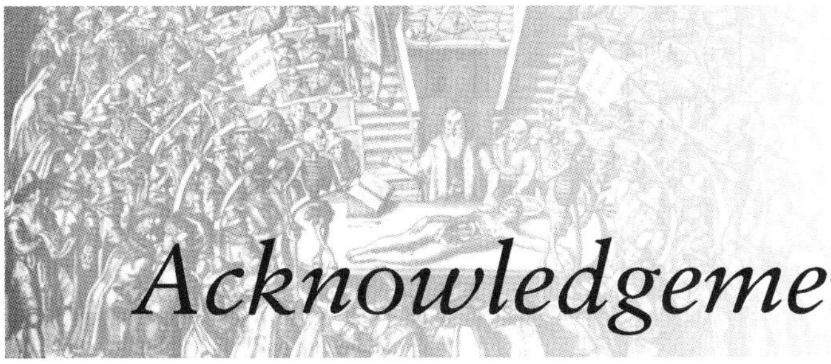

Acknowledgements

We would like to express appreciation to a number of individuals who have directly or indirectly influenced our anatomical and professional lives. Major professorial guidance includes John Stump and David Van Sickle of Purdue University and Lamont Smith of Brigham Young University. Department Chairs Gordon Garrett, Bruce Parker, Renée Van Buren and Mark Bracken; and Deans J.D. Davidson, James Harris, and Sam Rushforth have encouraged our work (or at least not sabotaged it).

Several authors of existing anatomy texts have contributed in various ways. The late Kent Van deGraaff was a personal friend, and his work set a standard for us to try to emulate. Ron Seeley and the late Sandy Grabowski were interested in and intrigued by our concern for accuracy. We were flattered when Rick Martini valued our observations enough to suggest that we contact individual authors with our critiques and suggestions. Dr. Catherine Hurlbut (FCCJ-Deerwood) proofed our manuscript in its entirety, and offered numerous valuable suggestions.

Our students have been a valuable resource as reviewers and editors. Ms. Eva (Howes) Beauregard, one of an elite few who have scored better than 100% in our course (due to built-in bonus points on tests) has been especially helpful in the final revisions leading up to publication. Ms. Sue Pawlowski, another outstanding ex-student, has helped us at numerous times with word processing rough drafts. In addition, our appreciation goes out to the several generations of department secretaries and administrative assistants including Kerri Howlett, Katie Valentine, Marci Beck, Kolene Mills, Erin Falgoust, Kristie Dockstader and others.

Finally, we are indebted to our wives and children for their generous support. There have been many nights and weekends that they have temporarily released us from our more important duties as husbands and fathers so that we could pursue this project.

MJS and DPH

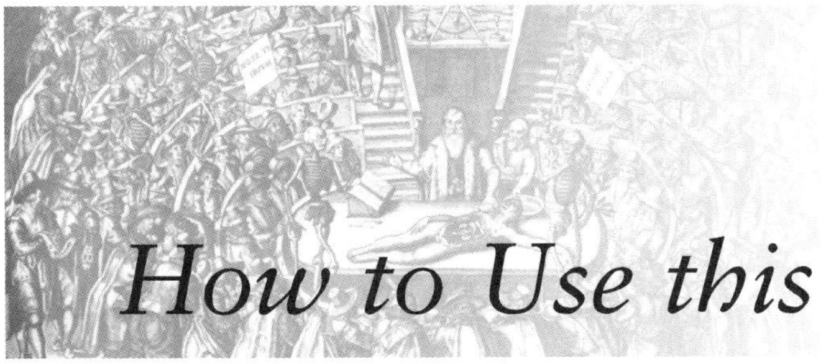

How to Use this Book

We've always been a bit taken aback by the parts of textbooks that are devoted to instructions on how to use them. But we did grow up in an era where students actually read their textbooks, and we are told (and have personally observed) that students don't necessarily do that today. So, to get the most out of this book: **READ IT!**

1. Read each **Chapter Outline** before (and after) reading the chapter. Notice the subheadings which indicate how the chapter material is organized. The outlines summarize the major points in the chapter and are composed of complete sentences to increase their instructional value.

2. Look at the **Etymology** to gain some appreciation of the derivational meaning of the nomenclature. This does not need to be memorized, but it will aid your study. The parenthetical G or L after each root indicates its derivation (Greek or Latin).

3. Digest each section of the chapter by writing the answers to the **Written Objectives** found in the chapters. There are three good reasons that these should be written out in your own words. First, it insures that you have a full understanding of the material. Second, these objectives cover the major points that you should know for tests and quizzes. And third, writing them out creates hard copy that can be quickly reviewed next week, next month, or at the end of the term.

4. Read through the **Clinical Case Studies** at the end of the chapter. Don't expect to *know* the answers when you read through the explanations for the first time. However, try to remember them when you review them the second or third time.

5. Study the **Points to Ponder** as a means to gain a different perspective on the chapter material. These brief essays contain a mix of factual and tongue-in-cheek observations designed to stimulate thought (and occasional smiles).

6. Learn the proper names for each of the **Slang and Obsolete Terms** listed at the end of the chapter. The Latin from the *Nomina Anatomica* is given only to show that the English terms are afforded correct translation.

7. Circle your answers to the 10 multiple-choice **Review Questions** as though you are actually taking a quiz on chapter material. Check your answers against those given. A score of eight or above indicates that you have a fundamental grasp of the material. Analyze the questions that you miss in detail. Why did you miss each one? Does the correct answer make logical sense? Knowing why each incorrect response to a multiple choice question is *not* the answer is just as

important as knowing *why* the answer *is* the answer. (We know you think you understand what you thought you just read, but do you realize that is *exactly* what we meant?)

8. Work through the 20 **Thought Questions**. You should *not* expect to *know* the answers to all of these questions outright – but once you see the written answers and explanations, you should think—"yes, I can agree with that!" Group discussions are encouraged.

9. Re-read the Chapter Outline.

10. Repeat items 3, 4, 7, and 8 with higher expectations than the first time you did them. When you can repeat all four of these items from memory with a high degree of proficiency, you have developed a reasonable understanding of the material and you are fully prepared for lecture quizzes and tests on that information. Welcome to the world of gross anatomy. May the planes and directional terms (and, of course, the force) be with you!

11. Note that abbreviations were often used in the text—especially in the labels of illustrations. These include:

		(plural)
artery	a.	aa.
bone	b.	bb.
joint	jt.	jts.
ligament	lig.	ligg.
micron	μ	μ
muscle	m.	mm.
nerve	n.	nn.
vein	v.	vv.

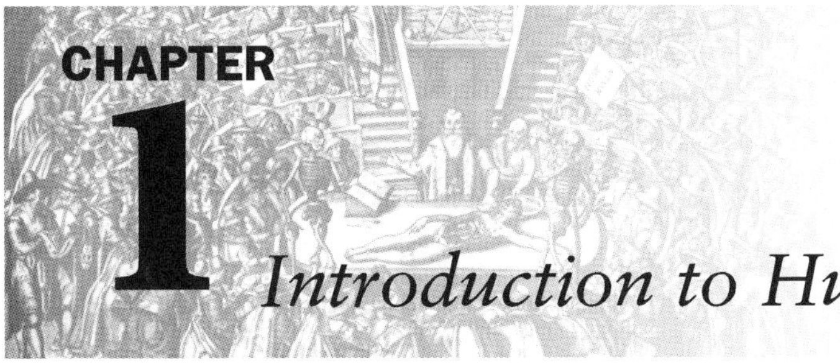

CHAPTER 1 Introduction to Human Anatomy

Chapter Outline and Key Concepts

INTRODUCTION

Anatomy (= morphology) is the science of body structure (*vs. physiology*, the study of function).

Anatomy is derived from word roots that mean "to cut apart."

There are many subtypes of anatomy (gross, radiographic, clinical, *etc.*)

TECHNIQUES OF ANATOMICAL STUDY

Observation and palpation are noninvasive and inexpensive.

Significant anatomic information is gained during surgical procedures.

Diagnostic imaging techniques include MRI, ultrasonography, radiographic procedures, and radionuclide imaging.

Dissection remains one of the very best methods of anatomic study.

ANATOMIC NOMENCLATURE

Official Latin names for anatomic structures are listed in the *Nomina Anatomica.*

The Latin names or their translated versions (into any modern language) are official nomenclature—all other names are unofficial (slang, obsolete, inventive).

Official names are selected based on their descriptive/instructional value.

TAXONOMY OF MANKIND

Human beings bear the scientific name *Homo sapiens* (genus/species).

Taxonomically, humans are animals, chordates, vertebrates, mammals, primates, and hominids.

HUMAN ANATOMIC CHARACTERISTICS

Mankind has the largest brain/body size ratio in the animal kingdom.

Structural features characteristic of (but not limited to) humans include bipedal posture, opposable thumbs, stereoscopic vision, crooked teeth, and a well-developed vocal organ.

LEVELS OF ORGANIZATION

Ten levels of structural organization can be identified in the human body from subatomic particles and waves to body systems.

Only structures at the last three (largest) levels (tissues, organs, systems) can be studied grossly.

There are four basic kinds of tissue in the body (epithelium, muscle tissue, nervous tissue, and connective tissue) and numerous specific subtypes.

Organs are structures formed by two or more (usually several specific) types of tissue.

Organs are grouped into five visceral systems and seven somatic systems.

MAJOR PARTS OF THE BODY

Gross subdivisions include the head, neck, trunk, superior limbs, and inferior limbs.

The head can be divided into the face and cranium.

The trunk has four divisions: back, thorax, abdomen, and pelvis.

Subparts of a superior limb include the shoulder, arm, elbow, forearm, and hand (wrist, metacarpus, digits).

Subparts of an inferior limb include the hip, thigh, knee, leg, and foot (ankle, metatarsus, digits).

BASIC PRINCIPLES OF MORPHOLOGY

The body has five generalized structural features:

Stratification—layering as found in skin and the intestinal wall.

Tubulation—cylindrical design exhibited by vessels, spinal cord, and intestine.

Zygomorphism—bilateral symmetry or right and left versions of various body parts.

Metamerism—linear sequencing exemplified by the vertebrae and ribs.
Cavitation—hollow spaces within the head and trunk occupied by various organs.

ANATOMIC PLANES

A single median (midsagittal) plane divides the body into right and left halves.
Sagittal planes are parallel to the median plane.
Frontal (coronal) planes are vertically oriented planes (perpendicular to sagittal planes) that divide the body into front/back portions.
Transverse planes are horizontally oriented and divide the body into superior and inferior parts.

DIRECTIONAL TERMS

Orientational terms, many of them paired, are used to describe positional interrelationships.
The three major pairs of directional terms are anterior/posterior, superior/inferior, and medial/lateral.
For descriptive purposes, the body is assumed to be in a standard (normal anatomical) position.

CLINICAL CONSIDERATIONS

A physical examination, performed by a medical practitioner, is done to detect abnormalities that may relate to disease.
Organs of some systems can be visually evaluated (skin).
Many organs/systems require special instrumentation or procedures to evaluate.

Selected Definitions

Anatomic nomenclature—the terms used to name body components. Proper nomenclature listed in the *Nomina Anatomica* is often compromised by the continued use of slang, obsolete, and inventive terms.

Anatomy—the science of body structure. It is essentially synonymous with morphology (the study of form) and is divided into numerous subtypes.

Auscultation—evaluation of body structures based on the noises that they produce. Auscultation is of limited value anatomically because most organs do not produce sounds.

Biological macromolecules—large organic molecules that are synthesized from smaller organic components by living organisms. The four main groups of them are proteins, lipids, polysaccharides, and nucleic acids.

Cell—a unit of living matter surrounded by a semi-permeable membrane and capable of reproduction in an environment devoid of other living things. There are dozens of different kinds of cells in the body.

Diagnostic imaging—the various techniques used to demonstrate the relationships of body components without physically invading the body. These include several forms of radiography, ultrasonography, magnetic resonance imaging (MRI), and radionuclide imaging.

Dissection—the process of methodically cutting the body apart in order to study its individual components and their relationships. Dissection was the first means of anatomic study and remains the best single technique today.

Lumen—the hollow space within a tubular organ. Many body organs have such a design including most of the organs of the visceral body systems as well as the heart, vessels, and even the brain and spinal cord.

Mucous membrane (mucosa)—the lining layer of the tubular organs of the visceral body systems. Mucous membranes contain epithelium and connective tissue (as do serous membranes) and typically include muscle tissue as well.

Normal anatomic position (NAP)—a standardized body position used when comparing positional relationships of body components. In the NAP, the body is standing erect with the head and feet forward, the superior limbs hanging straight down at the sides of the trunk, the palms to the front, and the fingers straightened and directed downward.

Organ—a body structure composed of at least two different tissues. Most organs contain several kinds of tissue and they vary from small, simple entities like capillaries to large complex structures such as the heart and brain.

Organelle—a structural subcomponent of a cell composed of various combinations of biological macromolecules. Organelles play strictly defined functional roles and include the nucleus, endoplasmic reticulum, ribosomes, lysosomes, and mitochondria, as well as several others.

Palpation—the identification and study of body parts by touch and feel. A significantly large percentage of body structures can be identified in this manner, but patience and practice are required.

Parenchyma—the functional part of an organ (*vs.* the structural portion which is called the stroma). In a gland, for example, the secretory cells form the parenchyma and the connective tissue framework that supports the secretory cells comprises the stroma.

Plane—a flat surface virtually passed through the body for the purpose of comparing positional relationships. Vertical planes divide the body into right/left parts (sagittal planes) or into front/back parts (coronal planes). Transverse planes (horizontally oriented) divide the body into upper and lower portions.

Principles of morphology—the structural design features of the body. They include tubulation (hollowness that continues from organ to organ), stratification (layering), zygomorphism (bilateral symmetry), metamerism (linear sequencing), and cavitation (space between organs).

Serous membrane (serosa)—the thin, transparent membrane formed of epithelium and connective tissue that lines the closed body cavities. Serous membranes are variously named pleura, pericardium, and peritoneum to distinguish those into which lungs, heart, and abdominal organs are invaginated (respectively).

System—a group of organs that fulfills a specific function. Depending on one's organizational scheme, body organs are grouped into eight to twelve systems which are divided into two categories: visceral systems and somatic systems.

Taxonomy—the science of classifying and naming plants and animals. The major taxa (categories) within the animal kingdom are phylum, class, order, family, genus, and species. For mankind these are Chordata, Mammalia, Primates, Hominidae, *Homo*, and *sapiens*, respectively.

Tissue—a group of similar cells and their extracellular products. There are four *basic* tissues in the body (muscle tissue, epithelial tissue, connective tissue, nervous tissue), and these are subdivided into numerous *specific* tissue types.

Viscus (plural = viscera)—any organ that belongs to one of the visceral body systems. Such systems have a tubular design, a mucous membrane lining and one or more openings at the body surface.

Etymology *Qui docet discit*—**"He who teaches, learns."**

ana (G), *up, apart*—anatomy
chord (G), *a string*—chordates
sect (L), *to cut*—dissection
hetero (G), *other, different*—heterotrophy
homo (L), *man*—*Homo sapiens*
meros (G), *part*—monomer
meta (L), *between, after*—metamerism
mono (G), *single, alone*—monomorphic
morph (G), *shape*—morphology
noto (G), *back*—notochord
logo (G), *discourse*—splanchnology
palp (L), *touch, feel*—palpation
peri (G), *around*—peripheral
physis (G), *nature*—physiology
poly (G), *many*—polysaccharide
sagitta (L), *arrow*—sagittal
sapiens (L), *knowing, wise*—*Homo sapiens*
serum (L), *whey*—serous membrane
sonus (L), *sound*—ultrasonography
stereo (G), *three-dimensional*—stereoscopic
sub (L), *under, below*—subatomic
tome (G), *cut*—anatomy
trophein (G), *to nourish*—autotrophic
ultra (L), *beyond, excessive*—ultrastructural
zygon (G), *a yoke*—zygomorphic

Introduction

The term **anatomy** was derived from Greek and Latin word roots which literally mean *to cut apart.* This describes the major technique (dissection) used to study the body and its parts. Anatomy encompasses all aspects of the science of body structure versus **physiology** which is concerned primarily with body function. Anatomy is essentially synonymous with **morphology** (morph = *form*, ology = *the study of*). More than thirty specific anatomical subdivisions have been recognized. Some of these and the subject matter that they encompass are summarized in Table 1-1. Note that the first three (gross anatomy, microscopic anatomy, and ultrastructural anatomy) are distinguished from each other by the sizes of the items under consideration. The remaining subdivisions of anatomy are concerned with various other aspects of the science of body structure. Some of them overlap to varying degrees.

Table 1-1 Major Subdivisions of Anatomical Science

Subdivisions	*Subject Matter*
Gross Anatomy	Body structures large enough to study without magnification.
Microscopic Anatomy	Structures requiring magnification up to about 1000 times.
Ultrastructural Anatomy	Structures studied with magnification of over one thousand times.
Developmental Anatomy	Structural changes from fertilization to maturity.
Radiological Anatomy	Images of body structures using x-ray techniques.
Functional Anatomy	The interrelationships and mechanics of body parts.
Clinical Anatomy	Anatomy applied to diagnosis and treatment of diseases.
Regional Anatomy	Specific regional parts of the body (head, thorax, limbs, *etc.*)
Systemic Anatomy	Anatomy of the body divided into its organ systems.
Comparative Anatomy	Homologous structures of different animal species.
Pathological Anatomy	Structural changes that occur during disease.
Surgical Anatomy	Body structure related to surgical procedures.
Topographic Anatomy	Positional interrelationships of body structures.
Surface Anatomy	The form and markings of the surface of the body and the relationship of the surface features to deeper structures.

Objectives

1. Define: anatomy, physiology, and morphology.
2. Differentiate common subdivisions of anatomy from each other based on the specific subject matter including the three subtypes which are distinguished by the size of the structures studied.

Techniques of Anatomical Study

Historically, the first method used to study body structure was **observation** of wounds. **Dissection** followed observation as man began to investigate beyond the observable wounds of the injured and deceased. There is evidence from several ancient cultures (including the Egyptians) that a number of anatomical relationships were established several thousand years ago by dissection (simply opening the body and observing its structure). This practice was suppressed at different times, however, due to religious taboos. Today, dissection is one of the most practical, least expensive, and most efficient

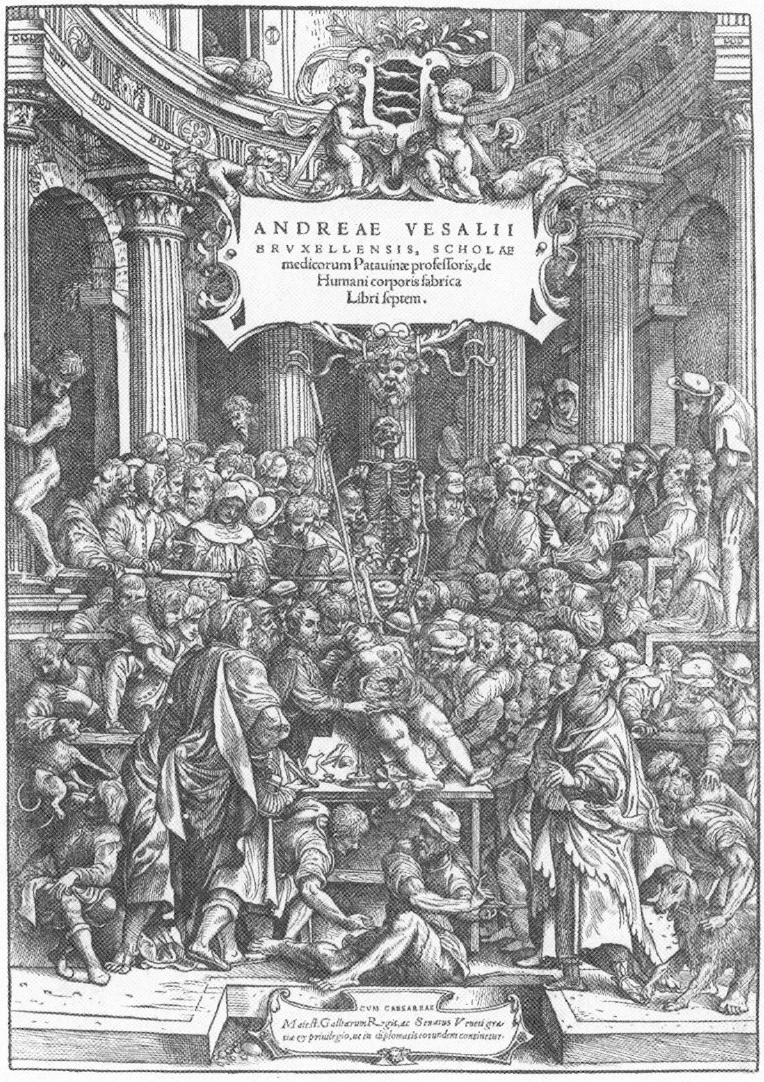

Figure 1-1

Dissection Performed by Andreas Vesalius in 1543

Dissection is one of the earliest techniques devised for anatomical study and it remains one of the most efficient. Lack of embalming/preservation techniques made dissection considerably less pleasant in previous centuries than it is today.

tools of anatomical science (Figure 1-1). Modern medical science recognizes anatomy as the cornerstone of a medical education, and dissection of human cadavers is part of essentially every professional medical curriculum. There is no better way to study most aspects of human gross anatomy than directly from a cadaver. Videotapes, models, and dissection/study of lower vertebrates (cat, rabbit, fetal pig, *etc.*) can never totally match the insights gained from *hands on* study of human anatomic structures.

Palpation involves the identification and study of body parts by touch and feel. A surprisingly large number of body structures can be studied (at least to some extent) in this manner. Good palpation skills require some time and practice to develop. However, some body structures, especially skeletal components, are quite readily palpable even by novices. Essentially everyone can find their own kneecap [patella] and the large bony prominences on each side of their ankles [medial malleolus of the tibia, lateral malleolus of the fibula]. The bony prominence forming the point of the elbow is the olecranon of the ulna. Those on each side of the elbow region are the medial and lateral epicondyles of the humerus. Palpation is not limited to the skeletal system. Many muscle bellies and tendons, some vessels and nerves, and a few other organs can be evaluated by palpation. Significant advantages of palpation include the facts that it is non-invasive and is physiologically harmless to the individual.

Surgery involves the removal, rearrangement, and/or remodeling of anatomic structures. It not only makes use of anatomical knowledge but contributes significantly to the anatomical knowledge pool. In fact, surgeons are among the best anatomists. Obviously, surgery is not a primary method of anatomical study (there are relatively few subjects who volunteer), but anatomical knowledge still remains a major by-product of surgical science.

Radiography is the science of using x-rays to produce photograph-like images (**radiographs**). It is one of the major tools for studying body structures in living subjects. It is painless and non-invasive, but x-rays have been shown to be carcinogenic (cancer producing). There are a number of specialized radiographic techniques that are used in certain situations including contrast radiography, tomography, and computerized axial tomography (CAT-scan).

Magnetic resonance imaging (**MRI**) is a relatively new body imaging technique which uses powerful magnetic fields to energize (excite) the electrons in certain chemical components of the body. The energy given off by these electrons can be *captured* and displayed on cathode ray tubes (CRT's). MRI has the advantages of radiography (painless and non-invasive) and seems to have no deleterious side effects. It is, however, quite costly.

Ultrasonography uses relatively low energy vibrations (ultrasound) to image body parts. The vibrations are produced by a special machine and are directed into the body at the skin surface where they differentially bounce off (echo from) various internal organs. As these sound waves return to the body surface they are collected and displayed on a screen. The resulting images are called **sonograms**. Ultrasonography has been used for many years to study fetuses *in utero*. It is painless, non-invasive, and harmless but its images do not have high resolution (*i.e.,* they lack detail).

There are several other techniques used to gain anatomical knowledge. Some of these include the highly sophisticated imaging method called positron emission tomography (PET-scan). This involves the injection of radionuclides (radioactive isotopes) into the bloodstream and measurement of metabolic activity by monitoring the radioactivity in different parts of the body using gamma ray counting devices and/or gamma cameras. Other, less sophisticated anatomical techniques include injecting plastic resin into hollow organs and then immersing the structures into corrosive chemicals to dissolve away the tissues (**injection/maceration**). This leaves a plastic cast for subsequent study. Dermestid beetles are sometimes used for skeletal preparations because they eat most body tissues except bone tissue, cartilage, and ligaments. **Percussion** is a variation of palpation involving tapping on the body surface and listening to the sounds (normal/abnormal) produced. **Auscultation** involves listening to the sounds that various body structures make (most of them, incidentally, do not make any sounds at all). All of these anatomical and clinical techniques have a common goal: to demonstrate details of structure and function that are otherwise not accessible.

Objectives

3. Define each technique used to study anatomy and indicate if it (1) invades the body, (2) is potentially harmful, and (3) produces permanent (hard copy) images.

Anatomic Nomenclature

Because of continuing religious sanctions against dissection of the human body, much of the anatomical study in recent centuries was done in secret. Lack of communication between the various investigators led to a confusing array of anatomical names for identical structures. In 1895 an attempt to unify the nomenclature began in Basel, Switzerland and a basic list of five hundred terms was assembled. Since that time, periodic meetings of the International Congress of Anatomists have updated and added to this list to produce the official world standard of anatomic nomenclature (sixth edition) known as the ***Nomina Anatomica* (NA)**. This book is an official list of the several thousand anatomic structures which have been identified (the brain alone has over 1000 named parts). The official (proper) anatomic names are listed in Latin but anatomists are free to translate those terms into any modern language. The major advantage of a standardized nomenclature is to reduce the confusion inherent in the use of anatomical "slang." The latter still remains one of the major stumbling blocks to the advancement of anatomical knowledge and many modern texts are still full of archaic and unofficial terms.

When anatomists serving on the International Committee of Anatomic Nomenclature select proper anatomic names, they do so with several criteria in mind:

1. The terms should be relatively short and simple, but should also have inherent instructional and descriptive value. For example, *left atrioventricular valve* (of the heart) tells exactly where the structure is located. *Trapezius muscle* describes the shape of that structure.
2. Terms derived from proper names (eponyms) should not be used (because they lack descriptive value). This concept was the beginning of the end for *fallopian* tube, *eustachian* tube, *malpighian* corpuscle, *Achilles* tendon, *etc.*
3. Every structure should have a name and a given name should be used for only one structure. This does not preclude the use of related names for analogous structures (styloid process of the radius, styloid process of the ulna, styloid process of the temporal bone).
4. Differentiating adjectives should be opposites wherever possible. For example, *superficial* digital flexor muscle, *deep* digital flexor muscle, *medial* epicondyle of the humerus, and *lateral* epicondyle of the humerus.
5. Structures that are topographically related should have similar names: *femoral* artery, *femoral* vein, *femoral* nerve, *etc.*

Objectives

4. Explain why eponyms are not used in proper anatomic nomenclature and why some structures are given names that may seem unnecessarily long.

Taxonomy of Mankind

Human beings belong to the **Animal Kingdom** which includes the living, multicellular organisms that are **aerobic** (require oxygen) and **heterotrophic** (use carbon-based organic compounds for energy). The Animal Kingdom has been subdivided into several smaller groups called **phyla**.

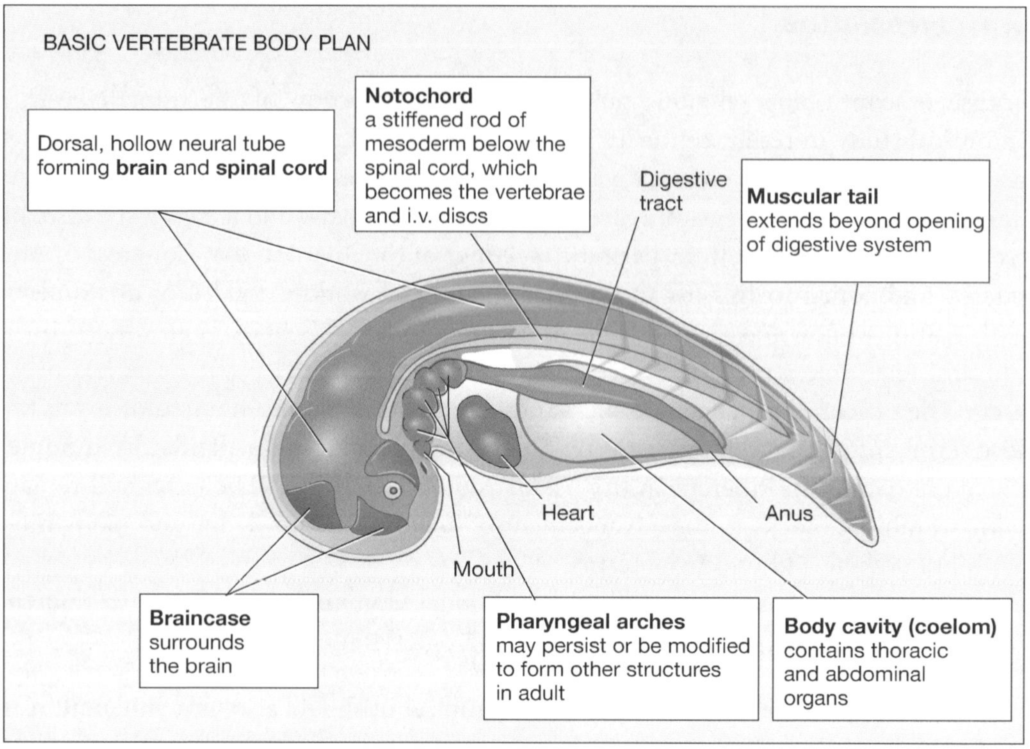

Figure 1-2

Schematic Diagram of a Chordate Embryo

This drawing illustrates several chordate anatomic features. The most significant of these are the dorsal hollow neural tube, notochord, and pharyngeal arches.

Mankind belongs to the phylum **Chordata** which includes the animals that developmentally possess a dorsal hollow neural tube, a notochord, and pharyngeal pouches (Figure 1-2). The dorsal hollow **neural tube** becomes the definitive brain and spinal cord. The **notochord** differentiates into the bodies of the vertebrae and the intervertebral discs. The **pharyngeal pouches** differentiate into the tympanic membrane, palatine tonsils, thymus, and the parathyroid glands. There are several subgroups (**subphyla**) of chordates: Hemichordates, Urochordates, Cephalochordates, and **Vertebrates**. The latter includes all animals possessing a vertebral column and is divided into several major **classes**: mammals, birds, reptiles, amphibians, and three groups of fish (Figure 1-3). **Mammals** are vertebrates characterized anatomically by hair, mammary glands, three pairs of auditory ossicles, and most of them have four limbs. They are divided into about twenty groups called **orders**. Man, monkeys, and lemurs belong to the most highly advanced order (**Primates**) and have prehensile limbs and large brain mass/body mass ratios. Primates are subdivided into several **families** and mankind is the only living member of the family **Hominidae**. The **genus** (***Homo***) and **species** (***sapiens***) designations form the two word **binomial nomenclature system** for living organisms developed in the 1700's by Carolus Linnaeus. Genus must always start with a capital letter and species is always lower cased. Both genus and species are either underlined or italicized. Each level of biological classification (phylum, class, order, *etc.*) is called a **taxon** and includes groups of related organisms which have common anatomical characteristics. The major taxons for mankind (summarized in Table 1-2) are supplemented by other levels of classification (subphyla, superclass, infraclass, *etc.*). The superclass ***Tetrapoda,*** for example, includes all vertebrates with four limbs (birds, most mammals, many reptiles and amphibians).

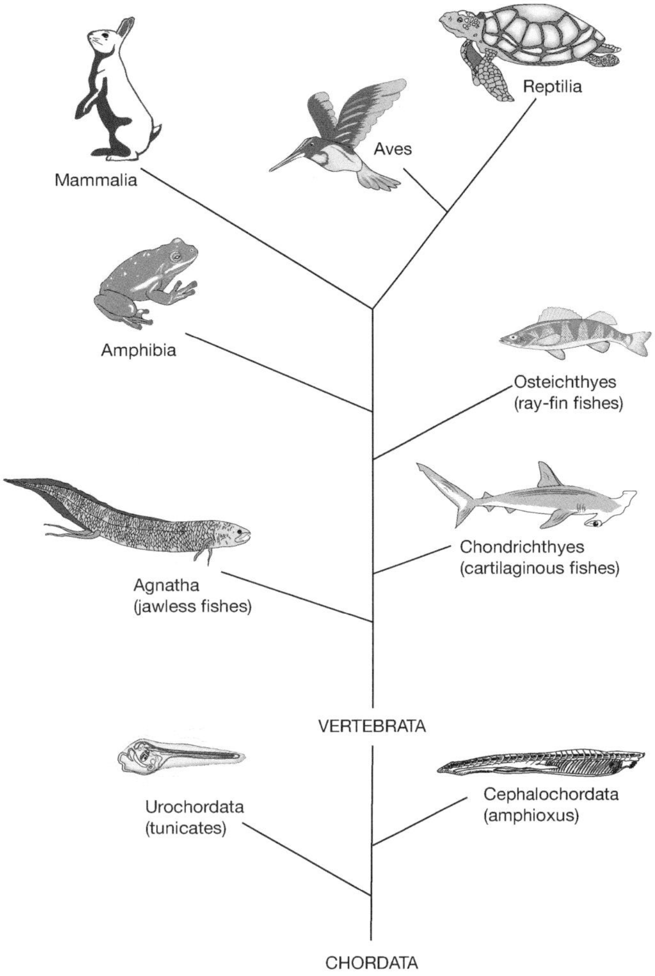

Figure 1–3

Major Subdivisions of the Phylum Chordata

There is no universally accepted taxonomic scheme. Some taxonomists group all fish together in a superclass (*Pisces*). Those who place significance on the development of jaws often separate *Agnatha* (jawless vertebrates) from the other six classes which are grouped together in the superclass *Gnathostomata* (jaw-mouthed vertebrates). Taxonomists who center their classification schemes around the development of extraembryonic membranes group the mammals, birds, and reptiles together as amniotes and the remaining four classes comprise the anamniotes.

Table 1-2 Taxonomy of Mankind

Kingdom	*Phylum*	*Class*	*Order*	*Family*	*Genus*	*Species*
Animalia	**Chordata**	**Mammalia**	**Primates**	**Hominidae**	**Homo**	**sapiens**

Objectives

5. Classify mankind taxonomically (phylum and subphylum, class, order, family, genus, species).

Human Anatomic Characteristics

There are several anatomical characteristics that set humans apart from most other animals:

1. **Brain size.** Humans have the largest brain mass/body mass ratio in the animal kingdom. Some animals have larger brains on an absolute scale but not when compared as a percentage of the overall size of the animal.
2. **Bipedal posture/locomotion.** With the exception of kangaroos and wallabies, mankind is the only mammal that is bipedal in its primary mode of locomotion. Most birds can function in the bipedal mode but are not known as great hikers. Even the monkeys and apes that can move bipedally use it sparingly and spend most of their time on all four limbs.
3. **Opposable thumbs.** The fact that the thumb can be folded across the palm of the hand greatly increases the grasping ability of the human hand. Some other animals (monkeys and apes) have this anatomic characteristic as well.
4. **Stereoscopic vision.** The ability to direct both eyes at the same object allows depth perception. Some other mammals and some birds also have stereoscopic vision.
5. **Vocal organ.** Although many animals can vocalize to a limited extent, none but man have evolved a complex, articulate form of speech. This involves intricate interactions of the larynx, tongue, oral cavity, teeth, and lips.
6. **Crooked teeth.** Very few human beings have perfect dentition (naturally). This is probably related to dietary changes over the last several thousand years which have resulted in shortening of the mandible and maxillae and crowding of the teeth.

In addition to these features, there are other characteristics that set mankind partially or totally apart from other animals. These include specific numbers of vertebrae, teeth, and the relative helplessness of neonates (newborn infants). The characteristics that distinguish one animal from another are called factors of morphological variation. These include species, sex, age, race, individual variations, and state of health.

Objectives

6. List at least five anatomical characteristics that are humanoid and indicate the one that is distinctly human.
7. List the anatomic features that distinguish each human being individually.

Levels of Organization

There are ten major levels of organization in the body ranging from subatomic particles and waves to organ systems. These are illustrated in Figure 1-4 along with some of the scientific disciplines which study them. Note that as one moves to the right on this chart, items at each higher level are composed of subunits from the level immediately to the left of it.

It is a well established fact that the smallest units of matter exist as **subatomic particles** and **waves**. The more familiar forms include **electrons**, **protons**, and **neutrons**, but nuclear physicists have identified many more including mesons, positrons, *etc.* In stable state matter, these particles and waves are organized into **atoms**. The number of protons in the nucleus of an atom determines what species (element) it is. Over one hundred **elements** have been identified, and certain ones predominate in the body. **Oxygen** (O), **carbon** (C), **hydrogen** (H), and **nitrogen** (N) are particularly abundant and form over ninety-five percent of the total body weight. Most of the remainder of the body mass is formed by **calcium** (Ca), **sulfur** (S), **phosphorus** (P), **potassium** (K), **sodium** (Na), **magnesium** (Mg), and **chlorine** (Cl), with trace amounts of many other elements. Although small amounts of some elements are present in their uncombined form in the body, most atoms are combined by chemical bonds to form **compounds**. The simplest of these are **inorganic compounds** such as water (H_2O), ammonia (NH_3), phosphoric acid (H_3PO_4), and carbon dioxide (CO_2). Within the body these exist mainly in ionic and/or hydrated forms (H_3O^+, NH_4^+, $H_2PO_4^-$, HCO_3^-).

Various inorganic compounds are combined with hydrocarbon chains to form **organic compounds** (building blocks). These are distinguished by their carbon content and more complex structure. The term *organic* refers to living organisms and the fact that these compounds are normally produced only by living things. The organic building blocks include **simple** (five and six carbon) **sugars**, **amino acids**, **fatty acids**, **glycerol**, and the **purine** and **pyrimidine bases** (adenine, thymine, uracil, guanine, cytosine). Organic molecules are combined by dehydration synthesis reactions to form **biological macromolecules**. The latter include **polysaccharides**, **proteins**, **lipids**, and **nucleic acids**.

Organelles are subparts of cells. Structurally they can be described as supramolecular assemblies of biological macromolecules. Organelles include ribosomes, lysosomes, mitochondria, golgi complex, endoplasmic reticulum (and several more). Even the nucleus and the cell membrane can be considered to be organelles. Organelles are suspended in cell fluid (cytoplasm) and surrounded by limiting membrane to form a cell. A **cell** may be defined as a unit of living matter delineated by a semipermeable membrane and capable of reproduction in an environment devoid of other life. All living things are composed of cells and cell products. There are many specific types of cells and each is specialized for different purposes. Some cells continually divide (reproduce), others do so only in certain situations, and others in the body have lost this ability completely.

Groups of cells and their products form **tissues**. There are only four **basic tissues** in the body: muscle (muscle tissue), epithelium (epithelial tissue), connective tissue, and nervous tissue. **Muscle tissue** is composed of cells which are specialized for contraction (shortening). There are three specific types of muscle tissue: cardiac muscle, skeletal muscle, and smooth muscle. **Cardiac muscle** is a major component of the heart and some of the large vessels near the heart. **Skeletal muscle** forms the contractile parts of the named skeletal muscles of the body. **Smooth muscle** is found within many of the organs of the body as well as at the bases of hair follicles.

Epithelial tissue covers the inner and outer surfaces of the body and forms the secretory portions of glands. Surface covering (membranous) epithelium protects the tissues adjacent to it and is classified into several subtypes based on its thickness (one cell thick = simple, two or more cells thick = stratified) and on the shape of the surface cells. Glandular epithelium is not further subdivided itself, but the glands of which it is a part are classified in many different ways. The most significant taxonomical criterion divides them into two groups depending on whether they secrete directly into the bloodstream (**endocrine glands**) or empty their secretion onto a free body surface (**exocrine glands**).

Connective tissue is distinguished from the other body tissues by the presence of large amounts of intercellular material. This material (called **matrix**) consists of fibers and an amorphous glue termed **ground substance**. Connective tissue has the widest range of functions and the greatest number of specific cell types of the four basic tissues. It is subdivided into several categories including **connective tissue proper**, **bone**, **cartilage**, **blood**, **adipose tissue** (fat), and some others (bone marrow, lymphatic tissue, and reticular connective tissue).

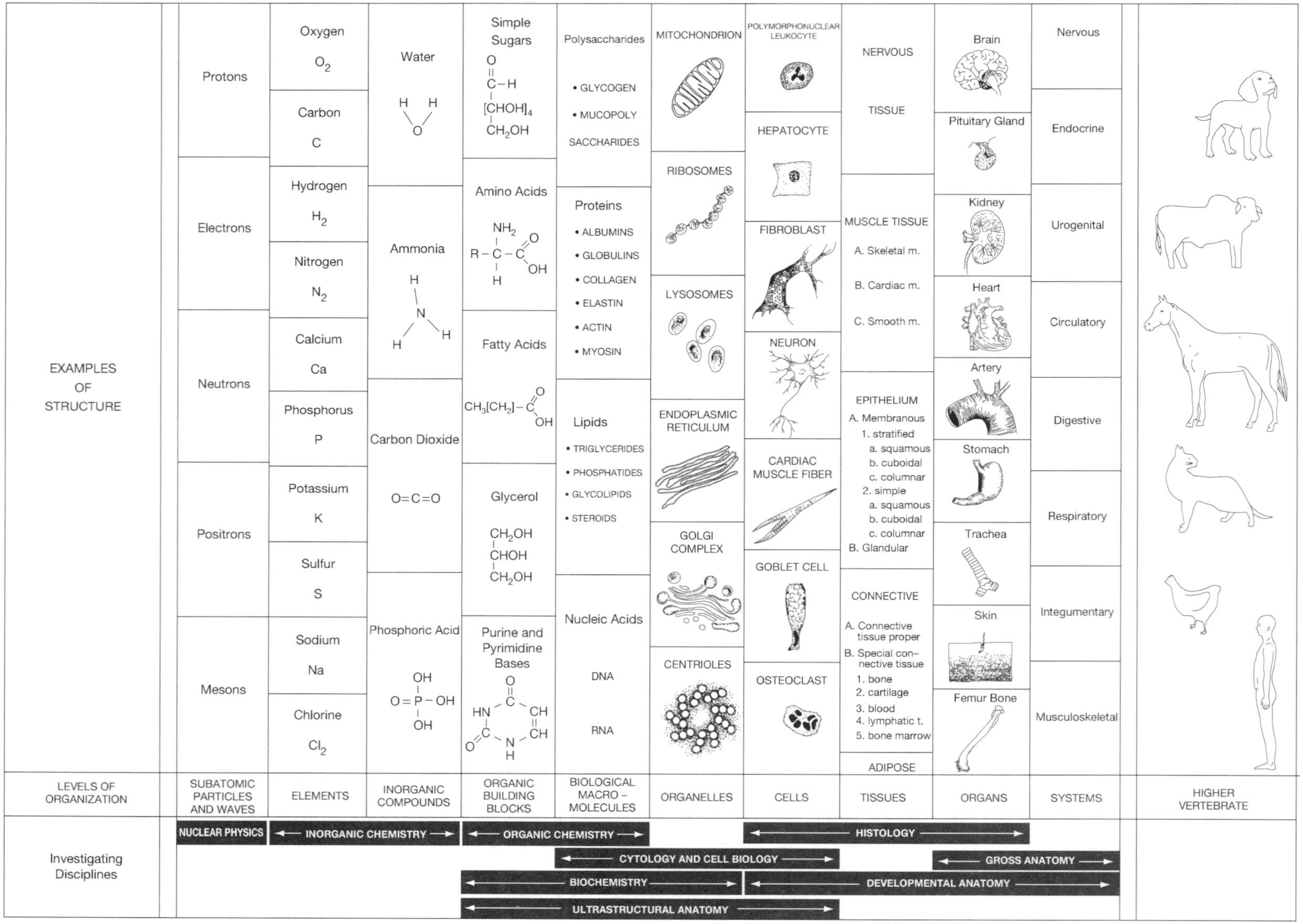

Figure 1–4

Ten Levels of Organization in Man and Other Vertebrates

(Note that this diagram demonstrates the "reduced" number of body systems (see text and Table 1-3).

Nervous tissue consists of cells called **neurons** that are specialized for the conduction of electrical impulses, and several kinds of supporting cells called **neuroglia**. **Sensory neurons** carry impulses which are interpreted and correlated by other neurons in the brain. **Motor neurons** send impulses that control the activity of muscle tissue and glandular epithelium.

An **organ** is a structure composed of two or more tissues. Organs include a broad range of entities, from structures as complex as the brain to entities as simple as capillaries. Many organs have a **lumen** (central hollow space) that may always or occasionally contain something else (air, ingesta, blood, urine, *etc.*). The main functional components of an organ collectively comprise its **parenchyma** and the structural framework is called the **stroma**. Most organs are composed of all four of the basic tissue types, although one or two may predominate. The femur bone, for example is an organ that consists predominately of bone tissue (one of the connective tissues) but it has cartilage on its ends, adipose tissue and bone marrow tissue within its medullary cavity, smooth muscle tissue, blood, and epithelium within its vascular network, a connective tissue proper encasement (periosteum) and lining (endosteum), and nervous tissue components within part of its structure.

Body systems are groups of organs with common functional goals. For example, the esophagus, stomach, intestine, and liver all belong to the digestive system (Figure 1-5). Mammals have a dozen organ systems (Table 1-3). The first five systems listed in Table 1-3 are called **visceral** body systems and the last seven are **somatic** systems. The visceral body systems possess three common characteristics which distinguish them from the somatic systems: a **tubular design**, **one or more openings at the body surface**, and a **mucous membrane** (**mucosa**) lining. The latter has three identifiable layers: a lining of membranous epithelium (next to the lumen), some connective tissue proper called lamina propria, and some muscle tissue (furthest from the lumen) called muscularis mucosae. Organs belonging to the visceral body systems are termed **viscera** (singular = viscus) or **visceral organs**. Note that none of the somatic systems are lined by a mucous membrane (an argument could be raised for the nervous system in regard to parts of the eye and ear) and none open (*per se*) at the body surface,

Table 1-3 Body Systems

System	*Major Components*
Digestive System	oral cavity, gullet, pharynx, esophagus, stomach, intestine, salivary glands, liver and gallbladder, pancreas
Respiratory System	nose, nasal cavity, larynx, trachea, bronchi, lungs
Urinary System	kidneys, ureters, urinary bladder, urethra
Male Reproductive System	testes, epididymides, ductula deferentia, penis, prostate, seminal vesicles, bulbourethral glands
Female Reproductive System	ovaries, uterine tubes, uterus, vagina, vulva
Integumentary System	skin, hair, nails
Skeletal System	bones, joints, ligaments
Muscular System	skeletal muscles
Endocrine System	endocrine organs: pineal body, pituitary gland, thyroid gland, parathyroid glands, adrenal glands
Cardiovascular System	heart, arteries, veins, capillaries, blood
Lymphatic System	lymphatic vessels, lymph nodes, tonsils, thymus, spleen
Nervous System	brain, spinal cord, nerves, ganglia, sensory receptors

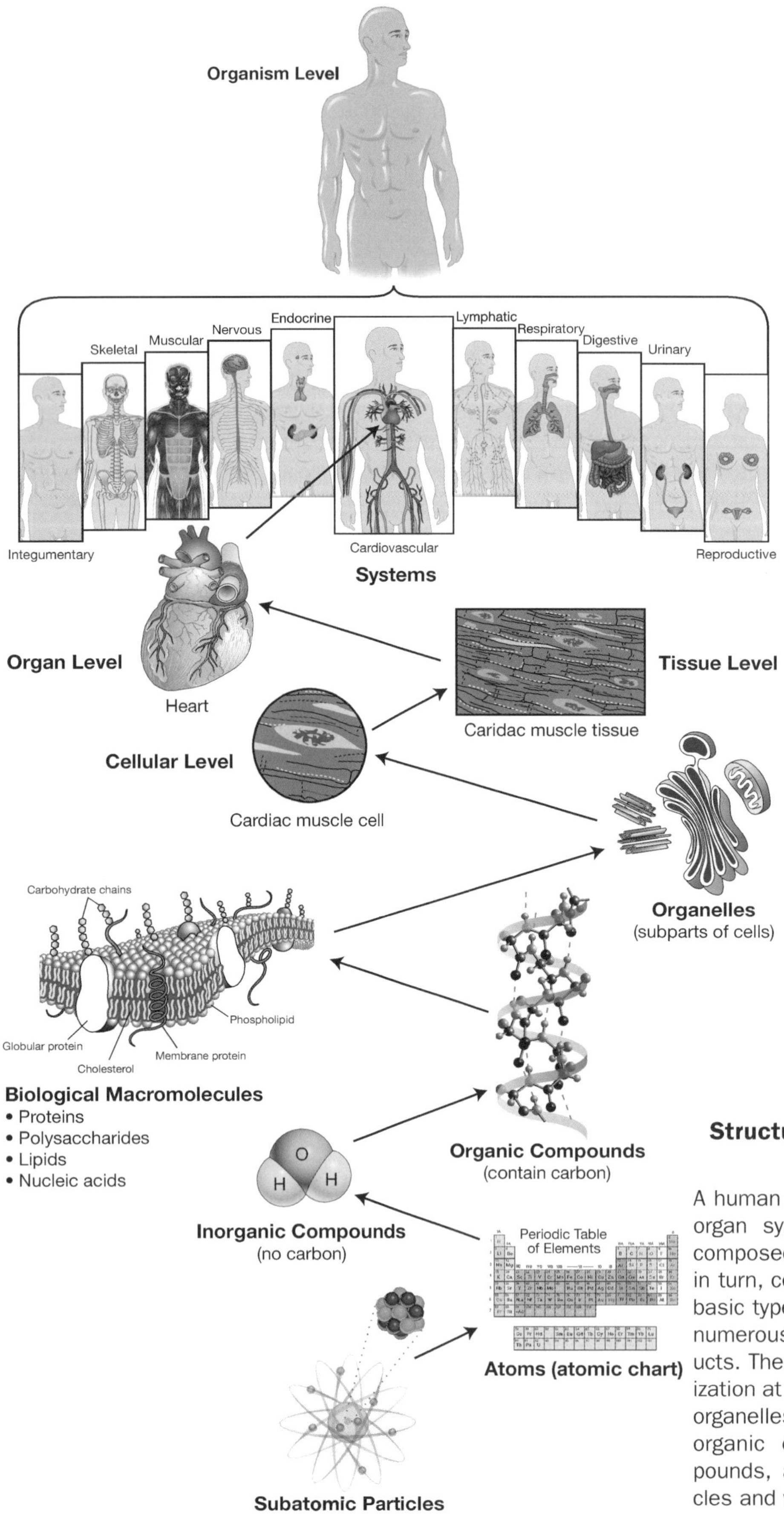

Figure 1-5

Structural Interrelationships in the Body

A human being is composed of eleven organ systems and each system is composed of several organs which are, in turn, composed of tissues. The four basic types of tissue are composed of numerous types of cells and their products. There are several levels of organization at the subcellular level including organelles, biological macromolecules, organic compounds, inorganic compounds, atoms, and subatomic particles and waves.

Table 1-4 Major Parts of the Body

I. **Head [caput]**—the superior extension of the body supported by the neck.
   A. **Cranium [cranium]**—the part of the head that houses the brain.
   B. **Face [facies]**—the anterior aspect of the head.
II. **Neck [collum]**—the portion of the body joining the head to the trunk.
III. **Trunk [truncus]**—the segment of the body to which the neck and limbs attach.
   A. **Back [dorsum]**—the posterior aspect of the trunk.
   B. **Thorax/chest [thorax/pectus]**—the anterosuperior part of the trunk (behind the thorax, abdomen and pelvis).
   C. **Abdomen [abdomen]**—the part of the trunk between the thorax and pelvis. It is commonly divided into four quadrants (left superior, right inferior, etc.) by the median plane and a transverse plane through the umbilicus.
   D. **Pelvis [pelvis]**—the anteroinferior portion of the trunk.
IV. **Superior Limbs [membra superioris]**—the paired limbs which attach to the lateral aspect of the thorax.
   A. **Deltoid (Shoulder) Region [regio deltoideus]**—the junction of the superior limb with the trunk.
   B. **Arm [brachium]**—the "upper" arm between the shoulder and elbow.
   C. **Elbow [cubitus]**—the junction of the brachium and antebrachium.
   D. **Forearm [antebrachium]**—the portion of the limb between the elbow and hand.
   E. **Hand [manus]**—the distal portion of the superior limb.
      1. **Wrist [carpus]**—the proximal part of the hand.
      2. **Metacarpus [metacarpus]**—the part of the hand to which the fingers attach.
      3. **Digits of the Hand [digiti manus I-V]**—the thumb and fingers.
V. **Inferior Limbs [membra inferioris]**—the paired limbs which attach to the pelvis.
   A. **Hip [coxa]**—the junction of the inferior limb with the trunk.
   B. **Thigh [femur]**—the part of the inferior limb between the hip and knee.
   C. **Knee [genu]**—the junction of the thigh and leg.
   D. **Leg [crus]**—the part of the inferior limb between the knee and foot.
   E. **Foot [pes]**—the distal portion of the inferior limb.
      1. **Ankle [tarsus]**—the proximal part of the foot.
      2. **Metatarsus [metatarsus]**—the part of the foot to which the toes attach.
      3. **Digits of the Foot [digiti pes I-V]**—the toes.

although the integumentary system is located there. However, parts of the cardiovascular, lymphatic, and nervous systems are tubular in general design.

Some authors reduce the number of body systems by combining closely related ones. For example, the muscular and skeletal systems are often considered together as the musculoskeletal system. The urinary and reproductive systems are often combined to form the urogenital system. The lymphatic system is often considered to be a subdivision of the cardiovascular system. The immune (body defense)system was not listed because it exists as a functional entity more than a physical structure and includes parts of several anatomic systems. **Splanchnology** includes the study of the visceral organs as well as those of the endocrine system (sometimes the heart, spleen, and great vessels are included, too).

Objectives

8. List and define the 10 levels of organization in higher organisms. Give some examples of body structures in each.
9. Name the 12 organ systems, identify the five that are considered to be visceral body systems, and list three characteristics which distinguish the visceral systems from the somatic systems.
10. Name the four basic ("primary") tissues.

Major Parts of the Body

In addition to a systemic organization, the body also has obvious regional subdivisions. There are five major regional body parts: head, neck, trunk, superior limbs, and inferior limbs. Each of these has numerous subdivisions as shown in Table 1-4 and each subdivision is composed of numerous anatomical parts.

Objectives

11. State the English and Latin names for each of the major subdivisions of the body.

Basic Principles of Morphology

There are five structural principles around which the body is organized: tubulation, stratification, zygomorphism, metamerism, and cavitation (Figure 1-6). **Tubulation** refers to the fact that many body parts are hollow or tubular in design (blood vessels, alimentary canal, urinary bladder, air passageways, *etc.*). The hollowness of the organs within a system continues from organ to organ. **Stratification** describes the distinct layering in many parts of the body (skin, intestinal wall, cornea of the eye, *etc.*). The principle of **zygomorphism** reflects the bilateral symmetry present in the body (*left* structures are identical to but mirror images of *right* structures). Examples include eyes, ears, limbs, ribs, *etc.* **Metamerism** is the longitudinal (linear) series of structures demonstrated by some parts of the body (vertebrae, ribs, intercostal muscles, superior and inferior limbs, *etc.*).

Cavitation refers to the fact that the head and trunk of the body are not solid structural masses. Instead, they have an outer wall surrounding and separated from internal organs. The space within the head houses the brain and is called the **cranial cavity**. The space within the thorax containing the heart, lungs, esophagus, and several other organs is termed the **thoracic cavity**. Similarly, the space within the abdomen (containing the liver, kidneys, stomach, intestines, *etc.*) is the **abdominal cavity**. The thoracic cavity is separated from the abdominal cavity below it by a partition of skeletal muscle termed the **diaphragm**. These two major body cavities within the trunk should not be confused with the four serous body cavities which they contain: left and right pleural cavities, pericardial cavity, and peritoneal cavity. The serous cavities are potential spaces lined by serous membranes that surround the lungs (**pleural cavities**), heart (**pericardial cavity**), and abdominal organs (**peritoneal cavity**). The serous cavities actually contain nothing except a tiny amount of serous fluid. Their relationships to organs with which they are associated is similar to that of a fist shoved into the side of a soft (half-inflated) balloon. The fist is not inside of the balloon but it is essentially surrounded by the balloon. The **serous membrane** (**serosa**) itself is a paper thin structure with two layers: an epithelial lining and a delicate outer layer of connective tissue proper (fibrous connective tissue) that binds the epithelium to the adjacent structures. Serous membranes (two layers) should be differentiated from mucous membranes (three layers). See the discussion covering visceral body systems in *Levels of Organization* in this chapter.

Objectives

12. Define five principles of morphology and give examples of each.

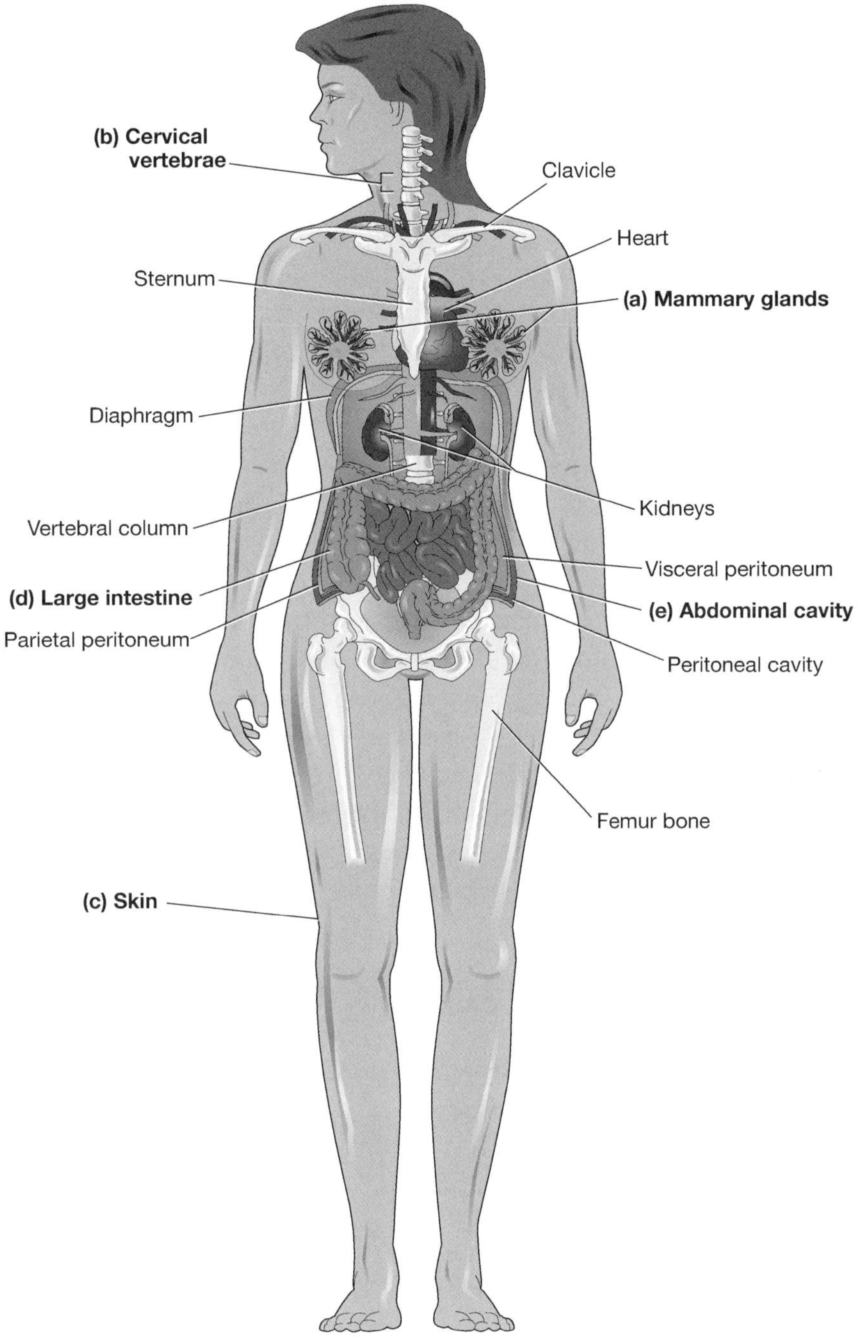

Figure 1-6

Examples of the Morphological Principles

Zygomorphism or bilateral symmetry (a) is exhibited by structures that occur in left–right pairs (eyes, ears, lungs, kidneys, limbs, many bones). Metamerism or linear sequencing of similar structures (b) is exhibited by the vertebrae, ribs, and the phalanges within the digits. Stratification or layering (c) is demonstrated by skin and most hollow organs. Tubulation, a hollowness that continues from organ to organ (d), is present in most organs of the digestive, respiratory, urinary, reproductive, and cardiovascular systems. Cavitation, the space inside the body walls (e), is demonstrated by the abdominal, thoracic, and cranial cavities (as well as the serous cavities within them).

Anatomic Planes

A **plane** is a flat surface, real or imaginary, along which any two points can be connected by a straight line. Planes in three major orientations, each perpendicular to the other two, are used to describe structural relationships in the body (Figure 1-7).

The **median** (**midsagittal**) **plane** is a vertically oriented plane which passes through the anterior (front) and posterior (back) midline of the body and divides the head, neck, and trunk into equal (left and right) halves. There is only one median plane and it can intercept only those structures located in the middle of the body (*i.e.,* between the anterior and posterior midlines). Planes parallel to the median plane (but off the midline of the body to one side or the other) are termed **sagittal planes**. The body can be intercepted (cut, sliced) by an infinite number of sagittal planes.

Frontal (**coronal**) **planes** are vertically oriented planes perpendicular to the median plane. They divide the body into anterior and posterior portions. There is an infinite number of frontal planes. Those through the tip of the nose will miss all other body parts except the feet. Frontal planes intercept the body as a whole longitudinally (lengthwise). However, they slice through the anterior aspects of the feet transversely.

Transverse planes are horizontally oriented planes that divide the head, neck, trunk, or limbs into superior (upper) and inferior (lower) portions. An infinite number of transverse planes exist at different horizontal levels and they are perpendicular to sagittal and frontal planes. Transverse planes intercept most body parts transversely (perpendicular to their long axes). However, structures with horizontally oriented long axes (feet, clavicles) are sliced longitudinally (lengthwise) by transverse planes. Note that transverse and frontal planes intercept the feet in conceptually opposite ways compared to other body parts. For example, frontal planes intercept the feet *transversely* and transverse planes intercept the feet *longitudinally*. This occurs because the feet turn ninety degrees forward at the ankles.

Objectives

13. Define in words and develop a working concept of the three main types of anatomic planes.
14. Explain how the abdomen can be divided into four quadrants around the umbilicus by two particular planes.

Directional Terms

A number of anatomic directional terms are used to describe positional interrelationships (Table 1-5). Some directional terms which are used in anatomic descriptions require no clarification. These include **right**, **left**, **central**, **peripheral**, **vertical**, **horizontal**, and other words commonly used in everyday communications. Note that most of them are paired with each member of a pair having a meaning opposite to that of its counterpart. It should be intuitively obvious that directional terms can be combined to indicate **oblique** (angled) orientations such as *proximomedially, anterolateral, etc.* All directional terms refer to the body in the **normal anatomical position** (see Figure 1-7). In this position, the body is standing erect with the head and feet directed forward, the arms hanging loosely at the sides, the fingers straightened and directed downward, and the palms directed forward. All structural interrelationships are described as though the body were in this position.

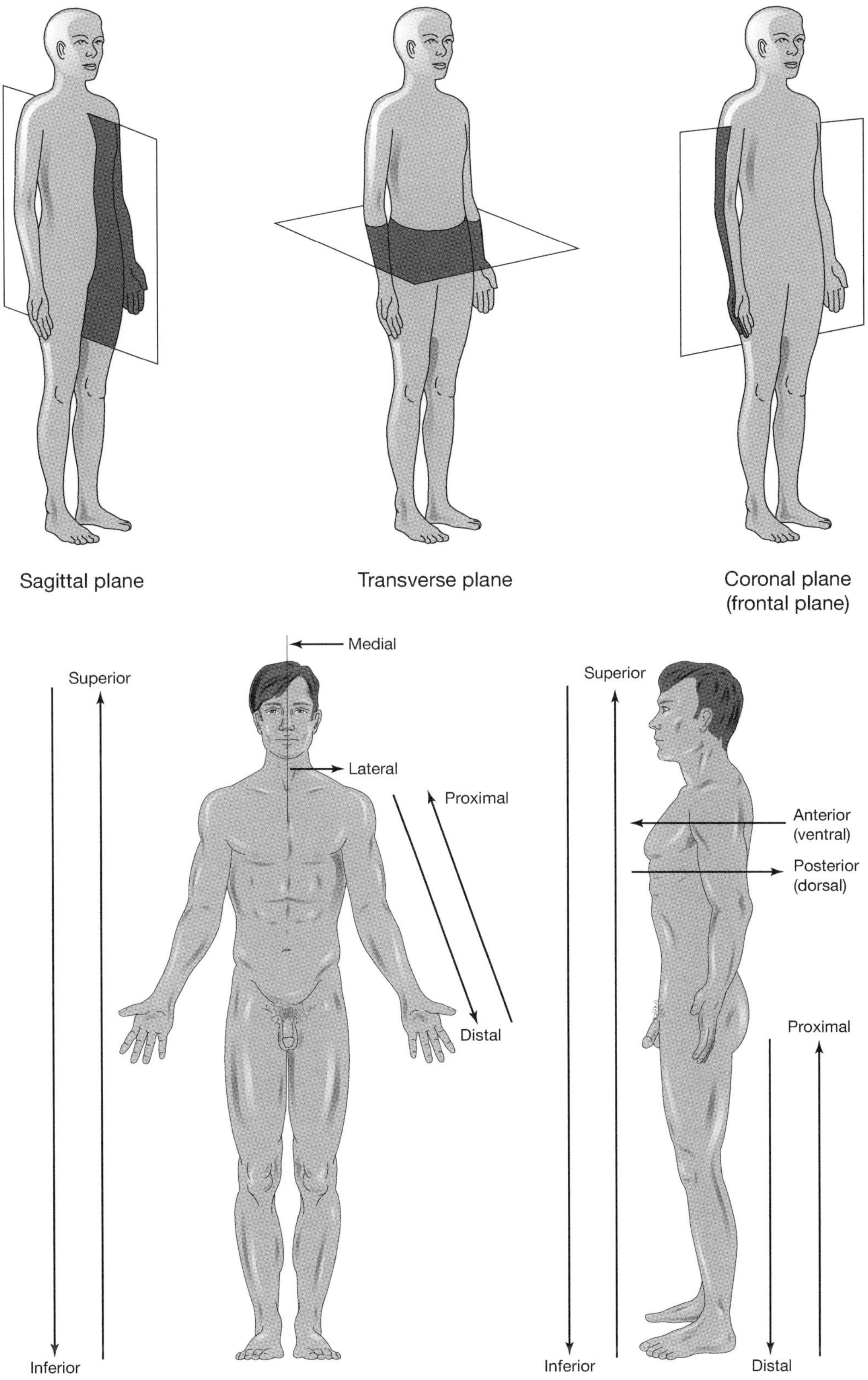

Figure 1-7

The Normal Anatomic Position

Anatomic planes have been superimposed on this figure and several directional terms are demonstrated. A sagittal plane through the midline is called the median (midsagittal) plane.

Table 1-5 Anatomic Directional Terms

Term	*Definition*
Anterior [anterior]	Toward or relatively closer to the front side of the body.
Posterior [posterior]	Toward or relatively closer to the back side of the body.
Medial [medialis]	Toward or relatively closer to the median plane.
Lateral [lateralis]	Away from or relatively further from the median plane.
Superior [superior]	Toward or relatively closer to the top of the head.
Inferior [inferior]	Away from or relatively further from the top of the head.
Proximal [proximalis]	Toward or relatively closer to the trunk (main body mass). This term is nearly always applied to the limbs where it has same conceptual meaning as *superior* (except in the foot).
Distal [distalis]	Away from or relatively further from the trunk. This term is nearly always applied to the limbs where it has the same general conceptual meaning as *inferior*.
Superficial/external [superficialis/externus]	Near or relatively closer to the outer aspect (surface) of the body or part.
Deep/internal [profundus/internus]	Near or relatively closer to the central aspect of the body or part.
Dorsal [dorsalis]	Literally implies toward or relatively closer to the "back." In practice it is most commonly applied to the posterior surface of the head, neck, trunk, or hand; or to the "superior" aspect of the foot.
Ventral [ventralis]	Literally implies toward or relatively closer to the "belly." In practice it is commonly used to refer to the lower aspect or underside of an organ or part.
Middle [medius]	A position between superior/inferior, anterior/posterior, proximal/distal, or superficial/deep.
Intermediate [intermedius]	A *side-to-side* position between medial and lateral structures.
Palmar [palmaris]	Toward or relatively closer to the anterior aspect of the hand (*i.e.,* the side where the *palm* is located).
Plantar [plantaris]	Toward or relatively closer to the sole (underside) of the foot where it is synonymous with inferior.
Radial [radialis]	Implies toward or relatively closer to the *lateral* aspect of the superior limb.
Ulnar [ulnaris]	Implies toward or relatively closer to the *medial* aspect of the superior limb.
Tibial [tibialis]	Implies toward or relatively closer to the *medial* aspect of the inferior limb.
Fibular [fibularis]	Implies toward or relatively closer to the *lateral* aspect of the inferior limb.
Longitudinal [longitudinalis]	Parallel to the long axis of the body or body part (lengthwise).
Transverse [transversalis]	Perpendicular to the long axis of the body or body part (across).
Ipsilateral [ipsilateralis]	On the *same* side of the body.
Contralateral [contralateralis]	On the *opposite* side of the body.

Objectives

15. Define and be able to use the anatomic directional terms.
16. Describe and assume the normal anatomical position.

Clinical Considerations

A complete **physical exam** by a physician evaluates all of the systems and many specific organs of the body. The integumentary system can be directly observed since its organs are located at the body surface. The skin is examined for color, smoothness, and resiliency. The presence of abnormalities may indicate developing tumors, localized hypersensitive reactions, or superficial infections. A number of specific diseases cause characteristic changes in the skin locally or symmetrically. Hair is examined noting its symmetrical distribution, texture, and sheen. Nails should exhibit symmetrical growth and a lack of splitting and delamination. They should have shiny, smooth surfaces, and no pain should be elicited by pressure along their lateral margins.

The skeletal system is evaluated by noting body symmetry, absence of pain when pressure is applied to bones, and normal gait and other body movements (especially those involving the limbs). More information can be gained using **radiography** to evaluate specific abnormalities.

The muscular system is examined subjectively by noting the symmetry and relative sizes of the major muscle masses. It is also routinely evaluated by eliciting a number of neuromuscular **reflexes** (such as the classic knee-jerk reflex). These reflexes evaluate peripheral nerves and the spinal cord as well as the skeletal muscles involved. The functions of specific muscles may be evaluated by electrically stimulating them (electromyography) and they may also be evaluated by biopsy (removal of a small sample of tissue and examining microscopic sections of it).

Some portions of the upper respiratory system can be directly examined including the nasal passageways and pharynx. The trachea, lungs, and bronchial tree are evaluated most commonly by **auscultation**. The sound of air moving through normal respiratory passageways is distinguishable from that moving through collapsed or partially blocked ones. Most organs of the respiratory system can be imaged radiographically, and direct examination of the lumina of the larynx, trachea, and bronchial tree can be performed with fiberoptic instruments (flexible, elongated, illuminating and viewing tubes).

Techniques used to evaluate the digestive organs include direct observation of structures in the oral cavity and **fiberoptic examination** of the esophagus, stomach, and intestine if warranted. Conventional radiography is often used to image digestive organs (especially teeth) and positive contrast radiography (regular radiography after a patient has swallowed a radiodense material such as barium sulfate) is sometimes used.

Most physical evaluation of the cardiovascular system centers around auscultation of the heart to detect normal versus abnormal sounds and measurement of **blood pressure** using a sphygmomanometer (blood pressure cuff). **Capillary refilling time** is noted by applying fingertip pressure to various parts of the body to blanch them and then noting the return of normal skin color after pressure is removed. Blood samples are routinely drawn in physical examinations for several specific analyses including the concentration of red blood cells, concentration and relative numbers of the various types of white blood cells, clotting time, and several other parameters.

The nervous system is evaluated by observing coordinated body movements, assessing speech, checking areas of skin for normal tactile sensation, and evaluating neuromuscular reflexes. The eye and external ear are also directly observed and are evaluated using instruments (ophthalmoscope, otoscope). Vision is tested using eye charts and color blindness illustrations. Hearing is assessed by conversation as well as by tuning forks, and more sophisticated instruments if defects are detected.

The lymphatic system is evaluated by palpating lymph nodes and observing the palatine tonsils. If warranted, a specialized radiographic technique called lymphangiography can be used in which radio-dense (iodine based) compounds are injected into lymphatic vessels to make them visible radiographically.

Except for the thyroid gland, which can be palpated, the endocrine system cannot be examined by regular physical means. Specific biochemical tests are used to check levels of some hormones. Abnormalities may be initially deduced by characteristic metabolic alterations or physical changes associated with abnormal levels of certain hormones.

The routine technique used to evaluate the urinary system is **urinalysis** (analysis of a urine sample). If warranted, this can be supplemented by radiographic and fiberoptic examinations. Kidney function can also be evaluated by monitoring plasma clearance of certain injected compounds.

The male reproductive system is evaluated by observation of the penis; palpation of the testes, epididymides, spermatic cord, and prostate; and by analysis of semen samples. The latter is not routinely performed unless infertility is suspected based on a wife's inability to conceive.

The female reproductive system is evaluated by a pelvic examination of the external genitalia, vagina, and cervix of the uterus. Cell samples from the cervical area are routinely collected (pap smear) and evaluated for changes associated with cervical cancer.

Clinical Case Studies

Case 1—A new mother was shocked to find that the fourth and fifth digits on the hands of her newborn baby daughter were fused together. The attending pediatrician suggested surgical correction (sometime in the future) and reassured the woman that the condition did not result from improper diet or care during her gestation period. What would cause this condition?

Case 2—In the early 1960's, a large number of infants were born with missing or grossly deformed limbs. These defects were soon related to a tranquilizer called thalidomide which the mothers took during gestation. One chemical form of the drug functioned well for its intended use, but a closely related form caused the defects. The early prescriptions for thalidomide contained a mixture of both forms. How can a chemical cause a failure of limb development?

Case 3—As a race, the Japanese people are shorter in stature than people of many other ethnic backgrounds. However, in recent decades the average mature height for these people has dramatically increased. Offer an explanation.

Points to Ponder

Although there are about 10,000 named gross parts of the human body, many of them are small subdivisions of larger structures. A superficial anatomic knowledge requires familiarity with about one thousand of the major structures. Medical students learn over three times that many in their first anatomy course. Body parts are the same from individual to individual except for slight differences related to race, age, individual variation, and of course, sexual dimorphism.

Gross anatomy can be studied systematically or regionally. In the systemic approach, the major components of each system are studied individually and as a group. This is the technique which seems to be most useful in introductory treatises. The regional approach involves study of all structures located in a particular gross part (*i.e.*, study of the abdomen, head, or superior limb). Regardless of approach, the study of anatomy involves three major facets of each structure encountered: name, location, and function.

Virtual (computer screen) anatomy certainly has its place—especially for review, self testing, and study at home or office where cadavers, specimens, and models are not available. However, by lacking the third dimension and not allowing students to heft, palpate, and gain a true feel of texture, firmness, and physical interrelationships, computer assisted learning programs have reinforced their own concept. They will likely remain to be computer *assisted* learning modes in the better anatomy programs throughout the world.

Students of comparative anatomy are often quite amazed at how similar human anatomy is to that of other mammals. The bodies of man and dog, for example have the same basic parts, and many organs and systems are quite similar to (in some cases almost indistinguishable from) each other. Consequently, anatomists who study quadrupedal mammals learn essentially the same structures and use the same nomenclature with the exception of emphasizing different directional terms (cranial/caudal *vs.* anterior/posterior and dorsal/ventral *vs.* superior/inferior).

The phylum Chordata to which mankind belongs is one of about 20 such major categories of animals distinguished from each other by various anatomic features. One phylum (Priapulida) contains only four species of little known worms. At the other end of the spectrum, the phylum Arthropoda contains nearly a million different species. Although the main taxons of classification are phylum, class, order, family, genus, and species, numerous other subdivisions have been added when necessary to allow subgroupings where very large numbers of species occur. Some of these lesser known taxons include "subs" of all of the major taxons (subkingdom, subphylum, subclass, *etc.*) as well as supra- and infraorders, and tribes (between subfamily and genus).

During physical exams, medical practitioners examine many structures of the body by observation, palpation, percussion, and auscultation. They first attempt to determine what is normal *vs.* abnormal. For abnormal findings an attempt is made to determine (possible/probable) causes and form tentative diagnoses. Additional information is often sought during this process in the form of laboratory tests (blood counts, urinalysis, glucose, tolerance tests, *etc.*) and/or diagnostic imaging techniques. The latter include standard and specialized forms of radiology, ultrasonography, magnetic resonance imaging (MRI), and radionuclide imaging.

Slang and Obsolete Nomenclature

UNOFFICIAL TERM	OFFICIAL DESIGNATION
paramedian plane	sagittal plane *[planum sagittalis]*
arm (whole limb)	superior limb *[membrum superioris]*
upper arm	arm *[brachium]*
leg (whole limb)	inferior limb *[membrum inferioris]*
upper leg	thigh *[femur]*
lower leg	leg *[crus]*
forefinger	index finger, second digit of hand *[index, digitus secundus (II)]*
pinkie	fifth digit/little finger *[digitus quintus/minimus]*
forefoot	metatarsus *[metatarsus]*
stomach (anterior, lower trunk)	abdomen *[abdomen]*

Review Questions

1. Which of the following definitions is incorrect?
   A. Human anatomy is the study of the body and its parts.
   B. Radiography is the science of using x-rays to produce photograph-like images.
   C. The *Nomina Anatomica* is the official world standard of anatomic nomenclature.
   D. A taxon is a name given to a particular level or grouping of organisms in a systematic classification scheme.
   E. Cells are components of tissues and tissues are components of organelles.

2. Which of the following does not demonstrate the morphological principle with which it is matched?
   A. head—cavitation
   B. ribs—metamerism
   C. stomach—zygomorphism
   D. skin—stratification
   E. artery—tubulation

3. The taxonomic order to which mankind belongs is ________________________.
   A. Primates
   B. *sapiens*
   C. Hominidae
   D. *Homo*
   E. Chordata

4. Which of the following anatomical directional terms is mismatched with its reference point?
   A. distal—top of head
   B. radial—lateral aspect of superior limb
   C. external—outer aspect of the body or part thereof
   D. lateral—median plane
   E. inferior—top of head

5. Which of the following is not one of the four basic tissues in the human body?
   A. epithelial tissue
   B. muscle tissue
   C. adipose tissue
   D. connective tissue
   E. nervous tissue

6. Which plane intercepts (cuts, intersects) the antebrachium longitudinally?
   A. sagittal plane
   B. midsagittal plane
   C. transverse plane
   D. median plane
   E. If more than one of the above intersect the antebrachium longitudinally, choose this response.

7. Which of the following characteristics is least helpful in setting humans apart from other animals?
   A. opposable thumbs
   B. bipedal locomotion
   C. brain mass/body mass ratio
   D. stereoscopic vision
   E. ability to produce sound

8. Which item is false?
   A. Serous membranes have two layers: epithelial tissue and connective tissue proper.
   B. Mucous membranes have three layers: epithelial tissue, smooth muscle, and connective tissue proper.
   C. The trunk is composed of two major body cavities: thoracic cavity and abdominal cavity.
   D. Splanchnology includes the study of visceral body organs as well as endocrine organs.
   E. The following are visceral organs: lung, liver, testis, uterus, and urethra.
   F. Choose this response if all the above (A-E) are true statements.
   G. Choose this response if two or more of the above (A-E) are lies.

9. Which one of the following has mismatched items?
   A. urinary system—ureter—visceral
   B. integumentary system—nails—somatic
   C. cardiovascular system—heart—visceral
   D. muscular system—diaphragm—somatic
   E. respiratory system—trachea—visceral
   F. nervous system—spinal cord—somatic

10. Which of the following is mismatched.
    A. Mammalia—three pairs of auditory ossicles—Class
    B. Hominidae—mankind is the only living member—Family
    C. Animalia—heterotrophs—Kingdom
    D. Chordata—notochord—Phylum
    E. Choose this response if all the above (A-D) are correctly matched.

Thought Questions

1. Do transverse planes cut (section, intercept) all parts of the body transversely? Name some structures of the body that would be longitudinally sectioned by a transverse plane.

2. All of the visceral body systems have (at least some) tubular organs. Give examples of tubular structures found in somatic systems.

3. By conceptually combining the reproductive and urinary systems into a single urogenital system, the muscular and skeletal systems (to form a musculoskeletal system), and by considering the lymphatic system to be part of the cardiovascular system, the total number of body systems would be ______________________. (Note that this was done in Figure 1-4).

4. What do radiography, MRI, and ultrasonography have in common? What feature of radiography is not found in MRI or ultrasonography?

5. Why isn't the "defense system" listed as one of the organ systems of the body?

6. Some obsolete names for body parts were based on the names of individuals who discovered these parts or did something significant in regard to them. Examples include the eustachian tube, fallopian tube, malpighian corpuscle, *etc.* Why were these kinds of names discarded when the official names for structures were selected?

7. Why does auscultation yield such a small volume of anatomical information?

8. *Homo sapiens* is the genus/species designation of all human beings. What factors make each individual unique?

9. If one conceptually combines the structural levels of inorganic compounds, organic compounds and biological macromolecules into one level (molecules) the total number of levels of organization in the body would be reduced from ____ to ____.

10. The visceral body systems have one or more openings at the surface of the body. Name two somatic systems which have organs located at the body surface.

11. Can every structure in the body be sectioned by a sagittal plane? By a coronal (frontal) plane? By a transverse plane?

12. Name a body landmark that can not be intercepted by any sagittal plane except the midsagittal (median) plane.

13. Name the smallest group of animals to which horses and humans both belong (taxonomically). Repeat the question for humans and snakes.

14. Which basic tissues...
    A. are in contact with air?
    B. are present in most organs?
    C. are present in *every* organ?

15. Why is having a standardizing (official) nomenclature so important in a science like anatomy?

16. Developmentally, all chordates possess a notochord. What does it become in the human body?

17. Which six anatomical directional terms should be included in a "bare bones" list. In other words, which six will allow the positions of all body structures to be related to each other?

18. Which two body systems are most difficult to examine by routine physical exam techniques? Which body systems have components located in the limbs?

19. Which subdivision of the trunk runs the full length of the trunk?

20. The abdominal organs are within the abdominal cavity but they are not inside of the peritoneal cavity. They are said to be invaginated into (but not inside of) the peritoneal cavity. Explain this physical relationship.

21. Is carbon dioxide an organic or inorganic compound?

Answers to Clinical Case Studies

Case 1—This condition is called *syndactyly* or *syndactylism* and is a heritable genetic trait. The degree of fusion is variable. Some cases involve soft tissue only while others have various degrees of skeletal fusion. Those without skeletal fusion are more easily correctable by surgical means.

Case 2—In early development, during the first trimester of gestation, the groups of cells and tissues that form various parts of the body segregate and differentiate by subtle chemical differences. Developmental biologists (embryologists) have shown that everything that occurs developmentally has a chemical basis.

Case 3—Until the last half of the twentieth century, Japan was largely an isolated nation with a diet based primarily on rice and fish. When Japan opened its doors to outside influences, the overall nutritional base of its people improved, as well. As a result, the last few generations of Japanese have been taller.

Answers to Review Questions

1. E. The first part of the statement is accurate but tissues are components of organs.

2. C. The stomach is not a bilateral organ.

3. A. The species is *sapiens*; Hominidae is the family; *Homo* is the genus; Chordata is the phylum.

4. A. *Distal* has various reference points but never the top of the head.

5. C. Adipose tissue is one of several subtypes of connective tissue.

6. A. Midsagittal (B) and median (D) planes miss the antebrachium completely. Transverse planes (C) can intercept the antebrachium, but they cut it horizontally (transversely).

7. E. Most higher animals can produce sound.

8. C. The trunk is *composed* of the chest, abdomen, back, and pelvis. It *contains* two major cavities: thoracic and abdominal.

9. C. The heart belongs to the cardiovascular system but the latter is a *somatic* system.

10. E.

Answers to Thought Questions

1. No. Transverse planes are horizontally oriented planes. They section many parts of the body transversely. However, elongated structures like the clavicle (collarbone) and metatarsus, whose long axes are horizontally oriented, will be longitudinally sectioned by them.

2. The brain and spinal cord (nervous system) are tubular, as are blood and lymphatic vessels (cardiovascular and lymphatic systems).

3. Eight.

4. All three diagnostic imaging techniques are non-invasive. Radiography uses ionizing radiation which is carcinogenic. Neither the magnetic field of MRI nor the sound waves of ultrasonography have been found to be deleterious to human health.

5. The "defense system" is not an anatomic system but rather it is a functional concept. Essentially all body systems have defensive roles, but the lymphatic and cardiovascular systems have major defensive functions.

6. Official names are selected which have instructive and descriptive value. Nomenclature based on names of individuals (eponyms) lacks descriptive and instructional values.

7. Most parts of the body do not make noise and those that do, don't necessarily describe themselves!

8. Sex, age, race, individual variation, state of health (the factors of morphological variation).

9. Ten – Eight.

10. Integumentary system (skin, hair, nails) and nervous system (eyes, ears).

11. Any structure in the body can be intercepted by at least one sagittal, one coronal, and one transverse plane.

12. Anterior and posterior midlines.

13. Mammals—vertebrates (a subgroup of the chordates).

14. A—epithelium (only)
    B—all four basic tissues
    C—connective tissue and epithelium (even the simplest organ like capillaries and serous membranes contain these two).

15. It reduces confusion and increases the efficiency of communication. The objective is to create a 1:1 relationship between names and structures.

16. Bodies of the vertebrae and intervertebral discs. It does not form the spinal cord.

17. Anterior, posterior, medial, lateral, inferior, superior.

18. The endocrine and lymphatic systems are most difficult to evaluate in a routine physical exam. The integumentary, nervous, cardiovascular, lymphatic, skeletal, and muscular systems. No components of the endocrine, digestive, respiratory, urinary or reproductive systems are found there.

19. The back [dorsum].

20. They have the same relationship to the peritoneal cavity that a hand shoved into the side of a large, soft balloon has to the inside of the balloon (where the air is trapped). The hand is shoved into (invaginated into) the side of the balloon but is not *inside* of the balloon.

21. Carbon dioxide does contain carbon, so it is technically an organic compound. However, it is such a simple compound that it is often grouped with the inorganic substances.

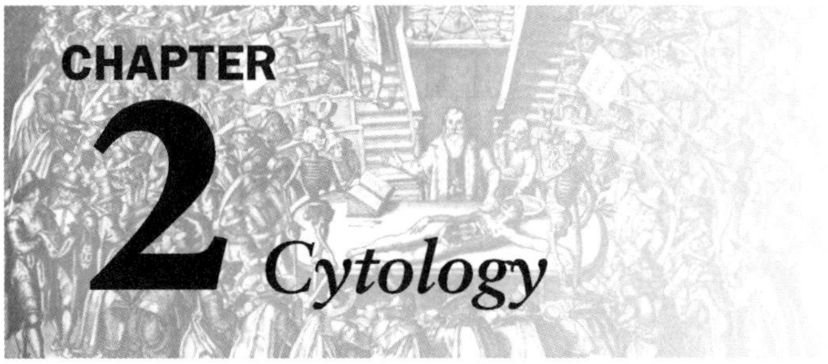

CHAPTER 2 Cytology

Chapter Outline and Key Concepts

INTRODUCTION

Cytology is the study of cells.

All living things are composed of cells and cell products, and (barring creation) cells are derived only from pre-existing cells; these are the tenets of the *Cell Theory.*

GENERAL CONCEPTS

All body cells develop from a single fertilized ovum (zygote).

Even though all cells in one human body have the same genome (DNA), several dozen cell types exist.

CYTOCHEMISTRY

Four elements form over 95% of the body mass: oxygen, carbon, hydrogen, and nitrogen.

Water (H_2O) constitutes about two-thirds of the body mass.

Basic (alkaline) chemicals are those that form aqueous solutions with a pH above seven and acidic ones form solutions with a pH below seven.

The normal pH of blood is 7.35-7.45.

The four major groups of biological macromolecules are proteins, polysaccharides, lipids, and nucleic acids.

Proteins are polymers of amino acids and form enzymes, antibodies, hormones, contractile elements, and structural components of cells.

Polysaccharides are polymers of monosaccharides and are important sources of cellular energy.

Lipids include glycerides, steroids, prostaglandins, and phospholipids.

DNA is formed by replication, all three kinds of RNA are formed by transcription, and proteins are assembled by translation.

CELL STRUCTURE

The three major parts of a cell are the nucleus, cytoplasm, and the cell membrane.

Simple diffusion, facilitated diffusion, osmosis, and active transport are membrane transport mechanisms at the ionic and molecular level.

Cell membrane modifications include microvilli, cilia, flagella, and several types of microstructures used to join cells to each other.

Cytoplasm is the cellular fluid (cytosol) plus the cellular organelles which are suspended in it.

Organelles are cellular subparts, suspended in the cytosol, that have specific functional roles.

The largest cellular organelle and the one that contains (most of) the DNA is the nucleus.

CELL CYCLE

Cellular life is divided into four major phases: G1, S, G2, and mitosis.

Mitosis (regular nuclear division) is divided into prophase, metaphase, anaphase, and telophase.

Formation of gametes (sperm and ova) involves reductive cell division - a two step process called meiosis in which the normal chromosome number (46) is reduced by half (to 23).

CLINICAL CONSIDERATIONS

Changes in cell size and number include atrophy, hypertrophy, and hyperplasia.

Metaplasia is the process of one cell type changing to another cell type.

Metaplasia resulting in more specialized cell types is called differentiation.

Mutations in the DNA of cells may result in inborn errors of metabolism (genetic defects).

Abnormalities in chromosome number include monosomies and trisomies.

Cancer (neoplasia) results from uncontrolled cell division.

Life threatening neoplasia is classified as malignant and less noxious forms are termed benign.

Selected Definitions

Active transport—a membrane transport mechanism requiring energy whereby chemical entities can be moved against the concentration gradient. Active transport requires carrier molecules and is powered by ATP.

Carbohydrate—an organic compound composed of carbon, hydrogen, and oxygen, often in a 1:2:1 ratio. Simple carbohydrates are joined by dehydration synthesis to form long chains called polysaccharides.

Cytokinesis—the cell divisional event wherein the cell membrane invaginates around two newly formed nuclei to form two separate cells. Cytokinesis begins during telophase of mitosis or meiosis.

Cytoplasm—a collective term for the fluid and organelles located between the cell membrane and nucleus. The fluid alone is termed *cytosol.*

Dehydration synthesis—the process wherein simple organic compounds are chemically combined to form biological macromolecules. A hydrogen atom (H^+) removed from one compound combines with a hydroxyl group (OH^-) removed from the second compound to form a molecule of water.

Differentiation—progression from less specialized cell types to more specialized ones. Primitive, undifferentiated cells are often termed stem cells and these may give rise to various forms of specialized definitive cells via differentiation.

Diffusion—random movement of chemical entities from higher to lower areas of concentration. If membranes are crossed, the term *simple* diffusion implies that no carrier molecules are involved and *facilitated* diffusion implies that carriers are required.

Diploid—the full chromosomal complement of regular body cells as opposed to the halved chromosomal number of sex cells. Since human body cells have 46 chromosomes (23 pair) the diploid (2N) number for human cells is 46 and the haploid number (N) is 23.

Endocytosis—cellular engulfment of particulate matter (phagocytosis) or a liquid droplet (pinocytosis) by surrounding the material with cell membrane. Similar movement of material out of a cell is called exocytosis.

Endoplasmic reticulum (ER)—an organelle consisting of double cytoplasmic membranes continuous with the nuclear membrane and golgi apparatus. Those areas on which ribosomes are currently attached (rough endoplasmic reticulum = RER) manufacture proteins for export and those without ribosomes (smooth endoplasmic reticulum = SER) synthesize lipids and carry out (perform) detoxification reactions.

Hypertrophy—increase in the size of a structure. Cellular hypertrophy can cause hypertrophy of an organ but the latter can also result from hyperplasia (increase in cell number).

Lipid—an organic compound composed of carbon, hydrogen, and oxygen that is insoluble in water. Lipids can be divided into four major categories: glycerides, steroids, prostaglandins, and phospholipids.

Meiosis—the nuclear events associated with gametogenesis (formation of sperm and ova). Meiosis is a "two" divisional process wherein the chromosome number is halved in the first division and sister chromatids are separated in the second one.

Mitosis—the nuclear part of regular cell division. Mitosis has four named stages (prophase, metaphase, anaphase, and telophase) based on the dissolution/reformation of the nuclear membrane and on chromosomal events.

Nucleic acid—a biological macromolecule composed of nucleotide subunits. The five carbon sugar component of each nucleotide subunit is either ribose (resulting in RNA) or deoxyribose (resulting in DNA).

Protein—a biological macromolecule composed of one hundred or more amino acids linked by peptide bonds. Proteins fulfill many intracellular and extracellular roles in the body including structural components, enzymes, receptors, contractile elements, hormones, and defensive chemicals.

pH—a quantitation of the hydrogen ion content of a fluid. A hydrogen ion concentration of 1×10^{-7} moles/liter (pH=7) is considered neutral. Higher concentrations of hydrogen ions (lower pH numbers) are acidic; lower concentrations (higher pH numbers) are basic.

Ribosome—the organelle formed of protein and ribosomal RNA which serves as the site of protein synthesis. Proteins that remain within the cell are synthesized on free ribosomes and those that are exported (secreted) are manufactured on membrane-bound ribosomes (attached to endoplasmic reticulum).
Replication—nucleic acid synthesis wherein DNA is used as a pattern to form more DNA. Replication precedes cell division so that each resulting (daughter) cell will have a complete genome.
Transcription—nucleic acid synthesis wherein one strand of a DNA molecule is used as a pattern (via complementary base pairing) for the formation of RNA. Three major kinds of RNA are formed: transfer RNA (tRNA), messenger RNA (mRNA), and ribosomal RNA (rRNA).
Translation—protein synthesis = peptide bond formation = using all types of RNA to manufacture protein. Translation is a constant occurrence in most body cells.

Etymology ***De nihilo nihil*—"Nothing comes from nothing."**

acidus (L), *sour*—acidosis
lipo (G), *fat*—lipid
ana (L), *up, throughout*—anaphase
lysis (G), *divide, destroy*—hydrolysis
basis (L), *a pedestal*—basic
meta (L), *middle, among*—metaphase
centrum (L), *center*—centromere
mito (G), *thread*—mitochondrion
chrom (G), *color*—chromosome
neo (G), *new*—neoplasia
diffusus (L), *to lead away*—diffusion
oides (G), *form, shape*—diploid
diplo (G), *double, two*—diploid
organum (L), *tool, instrument*—organelle
dyo (G), *two*—disaccharide
phago (G), *to eat*—phagocytosis
ellae (L), *little one resembling*—organelle
phasis (L), *to appear*—metaphase
gen (G), *to produce*—gene
pinein (G), *to drink*—pinocytosis
haplo (G), *single, simple*—haploid
pro (L), *before*—prophase
hydro (G), *water*—dehydration
sakcharon (G), *sugar*—monosaccharide
hyper (G), *over, above*—hyperplasia
soma (G), *body*—lysosome
inter (L), *between, among*—interphase
syn (G), *together*—synthesis
kinesis (G), *motion*—cytokinesis
telo (G), *end, completeness*—telophase
cyt (G), *cell*—cytology

Introduction

The study of cells is termed **cytology**. In the 1830's, two German scientists named Schleiden and Schwann hypothesized that all living things are composed of cells (and cell products). In 1858 Virchow completed this **Cell Theory** by advocating that cells are derived only from pre-existing cells. All scientific studies to date have upheld these basic premises, and today, cells are recognized as the universal building blocks of life as we know it.

General Concepts

A cell is a unit of life, surrounded by a semi-permeable membrane, that is capable of reproduction in an environment devoid of other living matter. The human body develops from a single cell which divides to form two cells, then four, then eight, *etc.*, until a mass of approximately one quadrillion cells is formed (that is a one followed by fifteen zeros). Each of these cells contains the same genetic material, but there are dozens of different cell types with different functional roles in the body.

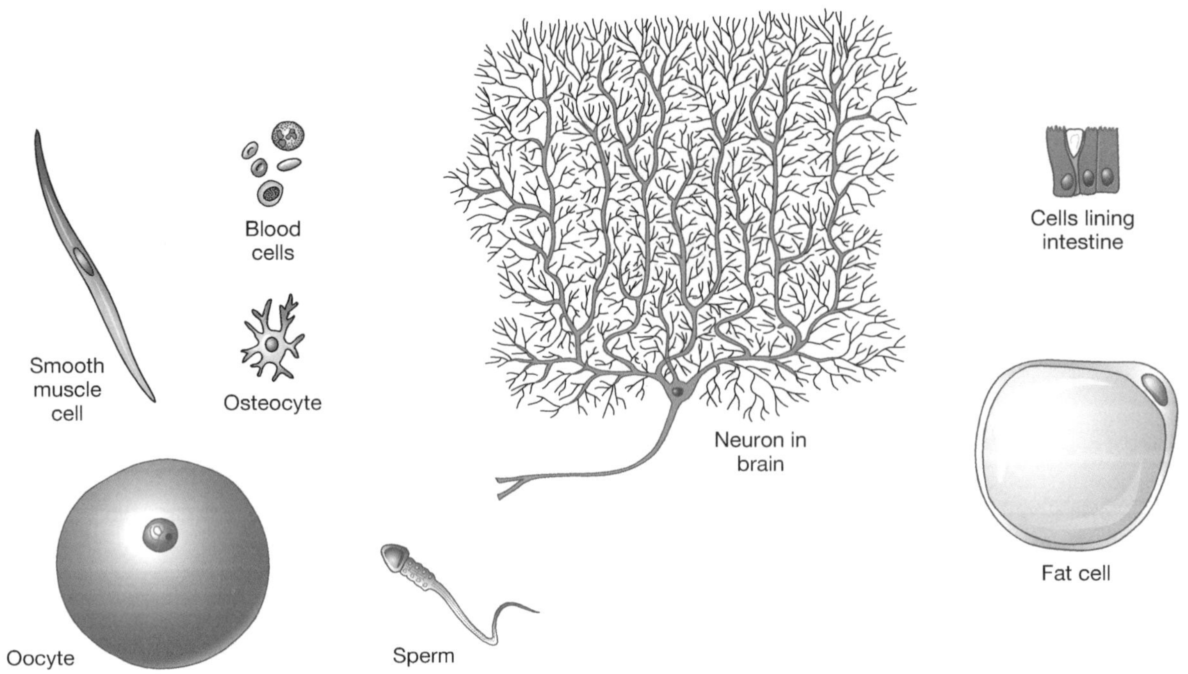

Figure 2-1

Examples of Various Body Cells (500X)

There are dozens of specific types of cells in the body. The sizes and shapes of different types of cells are related to different functions.

The largest cells (female egg cells or ova) are barely visible to the human eye and measure about 140 microns in diameter (one micron = 1/1,000,000 meter). Red blood corpuscles by comparison are among the smallest cellular units with a diameter of about seven microns and a volume several thousand times less than ova. Different cell types have a myriad of shapes from spherical to flattened and stellate (star-shaped) to cylindrical (Figure 2-1). Some cells (nerve cells in particular) are so markedly elongated that they are more than one meter in length.

Objectives

1. Define cell, cytology, and cell theory.
2. Discuss the diversity of human body cells.

Cytochemistry

As mentioned in the last chapter, four elements form over 95% of the body mass. By weight these are oxygen (65%), carbon (18%), hydrogen (10%), and nitrogen (3%). Most of the rest is formed by calcium, potassium, sodium, phosphorus, magnesium, chlorine, and sulfur with trace amounts of many others. Nearly all of these are chemically bonded to form inorganic and organic compounds.

Table 2–1 Functional Role of Proteins

Type	*Examples*
Structural proteins	Collagen, elastin, reticulin, keratin
Antibodies	Gamma globulins
Enzymes	Pepsin, trypsin, amylase
Hormones	Insulin, luteinizing hormone
Blood proteins	Hemoglobin, albumins, globulins, fibrinogen
Muscle proteins	Myoglobin, actin, myosin

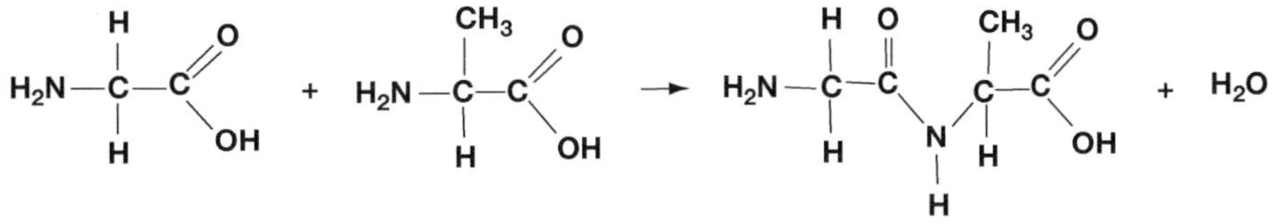

Figure 2-2

Formation of a Dipeptide

Combination of two amino acids (glycine and alanine) by dehydration synthesis to form a dipeptide. Note that a molecule of water is formed each time a dehydration synthesis reaction occurs. When the opposite reaction occurs (hydrolysis) water molecules are added back to form the original monomeric subunits (in this case, amino acids).

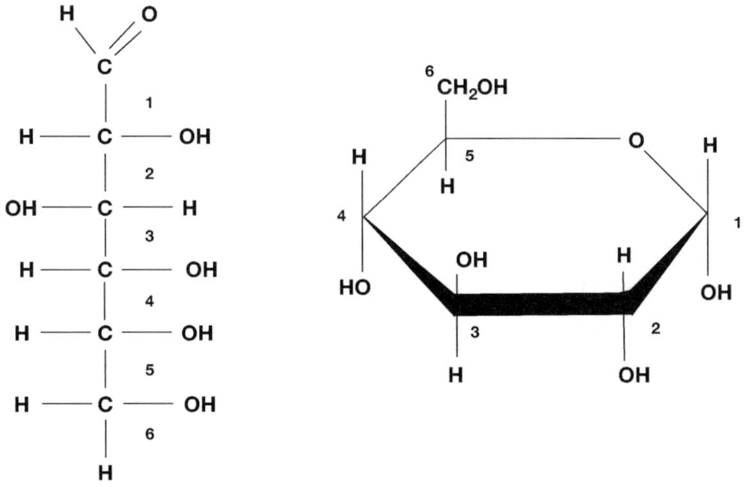

Figure 2-3

Linear and Ring Forms of a Six Carbon Sugar (Glucose)

Glucose ($C_6H_{12}O_6$) is a six carbon sugar that demonstrates the 1:2:1 ratio of carbon: hydrogen: oxygen that is present in many carbohydrates. Galactose and fructose are other six carbon sugars that have the same chemical formula ($C_6H_{12}O_6$) but have different structural formulae (physical arrangement of the hydrogen and oxygen atoms on the carbon chain).

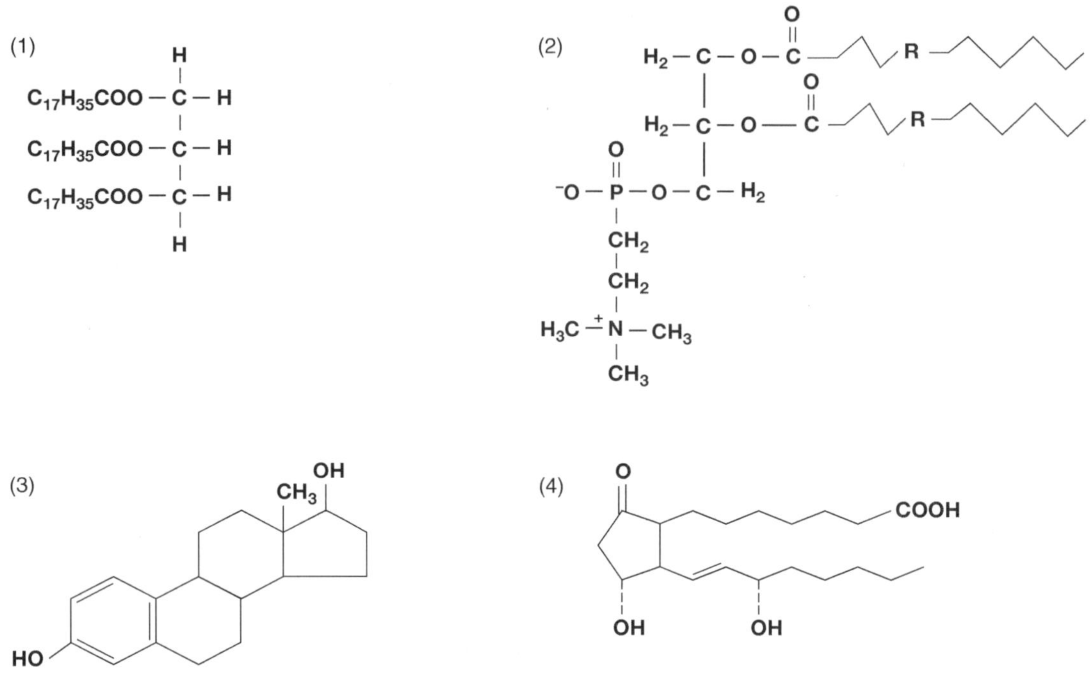

Figure 2-4

The Four Major Types of Lipids

Glycerides (1) are classified as mono-, di-, or triglycerides depending on the number (1, 2, or 3) of fatty acids that are joined to the three-carbon, glycerol core. Phospholipids (2) are any lipids that contain phosphorus. All steroids (3) have a characteristic ring structure and differ in the side groups that are attached to the ring portion. Prostaglandins (4) are long chain fatty acids with a five member cyclic group within their structure.

The most common compound in the body is water and it constitutes about two-thirds of the body mass. Water is an excellent solvent and also helps to maintain a constant body temperature because it absorbs and releases heat relatively slowly. Water is also a reactant in many cellular reactions. In fact, most of the larger organic compounds in cells (biological macromolecules) are formed by removing water as the subunits are bonded together. This process is called **dehydration synthesis**. When these compounds are subsequently broken down, water is replaced by a process called **hydrolysis** to separate the subunits.

Electrolytes are inorganic compounds that form **ions** (charged molecules) when dissolved in water. There are three major classes of electrolytes: acids, bases, and salts. **Acids** release excess hydrogen ions (H^+) which lower the body pH. Examples include hydrochloric acid (HCl), carbonic acid (H_2CO_3), and phosphoric acid (H_3PO_4). **Bases** release excess hydroxyl ions (OH^-) which raise the body pH. Examples include sodium hydroxide (NaOH), calcium hydroxide ($Ca[OH]_2$), and potassium hydroxide (KOH). When acids and bases react they form salts and water.

The pH scale (1-14) is a means of representing the acidity ("acidness") or alkalinity ("basicness") of an aqueous solution. Solutions that are neutral have a pH of seven. Those with pH's above seven are considered to be alkaline (basic) and those with a pH below seven are acidic. A change of one

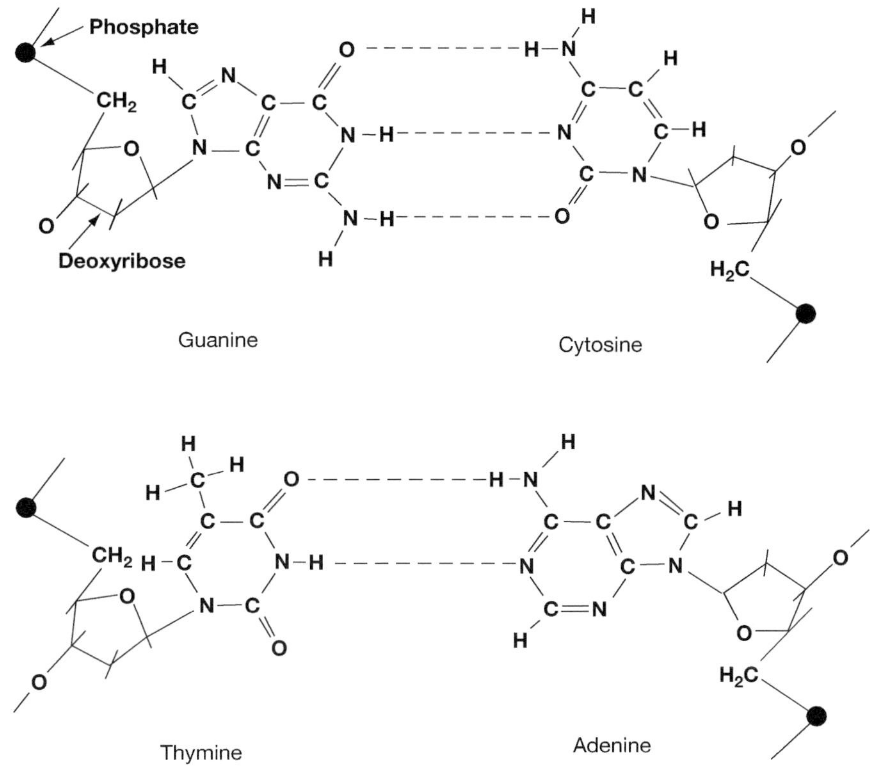

Figure 2-5

The Four Nitrogenous Bases Found in DNA

Hydrogen bonds between guanine and cytosine and between adenine and thymine (shown as dotted lines) hold the left and right polynucleotide strands of DNA together. RNA has three of these same four nucleotides in its structure but has a base called uracil instead of thymine.

whole pH number represents a 10-fold change in hydrogen ion concentration. A relatively narrow pH range must be maintained in the body (normal range for blood is 7.35 to 7.45). In fact, if the body pH extends beyond these limits, a coma or convulsions may occur and death is imminent unless the situation is corrected. For this reason, controlled reactions between acids and bases to form salts is a critical issue. Substances which are significantly involved in maintaining body pH within its critical boundaries are called **buffers** and include hemoglobin, bicarbonate ions (HCO_3^-), and a number of other compounds. Buffers act by "absorbing" (removing) excess hydrogen or hydroxyl ions from solution.

The organic compounds found within the body are those that contain carbon. The simpler organic compounds form the subunits of much larger biological macromolecules. These compounds, naturally found only in living organisms, are divided into four main groups: proteins, polysaccharides, lipids, and nucleic acids. **Proteins** are biological macromolecules composed of **amino acids**. There are about 20 different amino acids and they are combined by dehydration synthesis (removal of water) to form linear chains called **peptides** (Figure 2-2). A chain two amino acids long is called a **dipeptide**, and one formed from three amino acids is a **tripeptide**, *etc.* Chains of amino acids too long to easily count are called **polypeptides** and polypeptides of one hundred or more amino acids are called **proteins**. Proteins and polypeptides serve many roles in cellular (and extracellular) structure. Some of them act as buffers or hormones and others serve as carrier molecules that are involved in some kinds of membrane transport. Proteins are the receptor molecules for antibodies and hormones. The enzymes (chemical catalysts) which control chemical reactions within cells and within the lumens of the digestive organs are proteins as are the defense chemicals (antibodies). Some specific examples of protein in the body include myosin and actin (contractile proteins in muscle tissue); collagen, elastin, and reticulin (extracellular structural proteins which form fibers); hemoglobin, albumins, and globulins (in blood); and insulin (Table 2-1).

Carbohydrates are organic compounds which contain carbon, hydrogen, and oxygen in a ratio of 1:2:1. The more common biological ones include five carbon sugars (ribose and deoxyribose) and six carbon sugars (glucose, galactose, and fructose)(Figure 2-3). Five and six carbon sugars are called simple sugars (monosaccharides). These can be combined by dehydration synthesis to form **disaccharides** containing two monosaccharide subunits (such as sucrose, maltose, and lactose) or **polysaccharides** containing many monosaccharides (such as starch and cellulose). Carbohydrates form structural components in cells and are the preferred fuel (energy source) for cellular activity.

Lipids are organic compounds that have the same three major elemental components as carbohydrates (carbon, hydrogen, and oxygen) but with a smaller percentage of oxygen. The feature that distinguishes lipids from other chemical entities in cells is that they are insoluble in water. There are four major groups of lipids in the body: glycerides, phospholipids, steroids, and prostaglandins (Figure 2-4). **Glycerides** are compounds composed of glycerol (a three carbon alcohol) and long chain fatty acids. Compounds with only one fatty acid combined with glycerol are called **monoglycerides**, those with two are called **diglycerides**, and those with fatty acids bonded to all three alcohol groups of glycerol are called **triglycerides**. Triglycerides are the major chemical components in the fats and oils of the body. They are also an important alternate energy source. **Phospholipids**, as their name implies, contain phosphorus. Most of them are diglycerides with a phosphorus-containing group bonded to the third position on the glycerol. Phospholipids are important structural components of cellular membranes. **Steroids** are lipids that have a basic structural backbone of three, six-carbon rings and a five-carbon ring. Steroids vary from one another in the chemical groups (R-groups) that are joined to these rings. Some steroids, like cholesterol, are important structural components of cells. Others form hormones (like testosterone, estrogen, the cortisones, *etc.*). The last group of lipids, **prostaglandins**, are long-chain, cyclical fatty acids. They serve in several hormone-like capacities in the body.

Nucleic acids (DNA and RNA) are polymers of nucleotides. A **nucleotide** consists of a purine or pyrimidine nitrogenous base combined with a five-carbon sugar (ribose or deoxyribose) and with phosphoric acid (Figure 2-5). **Deoxyribonucleic acid** (**DNA**) is a double-stranded polymer of nucleotides that have deoxyribose as the sugar component and adenine, guanine, cytosine, and thymine as the nitrogenous bases. DNA forms the genetic material within each cell. It is combined with protein to form **chromatin**. When cells divide, the chromatin condenses to form chromosomes. Chromatin is duplicated before each regular cell division by a process called **replication** so that each new (daughter) cell has a complete and identical copy (set). **Ribonucleic acid** (**RNA**) is similar to DNA except that it is single stranded, has ribose instead of deoxyribose, and has uracil in place of thymine. RNA is manufactured from the DNA by a process called **transcription**. Three types of RNA exist. One type called **ribosomal RNA** (**rRNA**) forms part of the cellular organelles called ribosomes which serve as the site of protein synthesis. The other two types, called **transfer RNA** (**tRNA**) and **messenger RNA** (**mRNA**), are directly involved in the synthesis of proteins (a process called **translation**).

Objectives

3. Name (a) the four most common elements in the body, (b) the seven elements that form most of the rest of the body, and (c) the most common chemical compound in the body (and its percentage of the body weight).
4. State the normal pH range of blood.
5. Name the four main groups of biological macromolecules and define: amino acid, polypeptide, protein, mono- (di-, poly-) saccharide, glyceride, prostaglandin, steroid, phospholipid, and nucleotide.
6. State the differences between RNA and DNA and define replication, transcription, and translation.

Cell Structure

Although the cells of the body have a variety of specific features and functions, most of them have the same basic structural components: cell membrane, cytosol and organelles, and a nucleus (technically an organelle but usually considered separately). The **cell membrane** is a fluid mosaic of protein, phospholipids, and carbohydrates. It serves as the limiting membrane which contains all other cellular structures, controls what enters and exits the cell, and contains certain receptors and identifiers that have hormonal and antigenic significance. The cell membrane is semi-permeable (allows some kinds of molecules through, but not others). Factors that affect permeability include molecule size, ionic charge, lipid solubility, specific structure, and the presence of carrier molecules. There are several different mechanisms by which substances can enter or leave cells. Some of these are summarized in Table 2-2.

Table 2-2 A Comparison of Chemical Transport Across Cell Membranes

Mechanism	*Driving Force*	*Carrier Required*	*Energy Required*	*Can Move Against a Concentration Barrier*
Simple diffusion	Concentration gradient	No	No	No
Facilitated diffusion	Concentration gradient	Yes	No	No
Osmosis	Concentration gradient	No	No	No
Active transport	High energy compounds	Yes	Yes	Yes

1. **Simple diffusion:** the passive movement of a substance from an area of higher concentration of that substance to an area of lower concentration. Example: movement of oxygen and carbon dioxide across the air-blood barrier in the pulmonary alveoli.
2. **Facilitated diffusion:** a passive movement similar to simple diffusion except that a specific carrier molecule is required. Example: movement of glucose into a cell.
3. **Osmosis**: the passive movement of a solvent through a **semipermeable membrane** from an area of higher concentration of solvent to an area of lower concentration. This is similar to simple diffusion except that a semipermeable membrane is required and the substance diffusing is a solvent (Figure 2-6). In biological systems this solvent is always water and so biologists often define osmosis as *movement of water through a semipermeable membrane from a higher concen-*

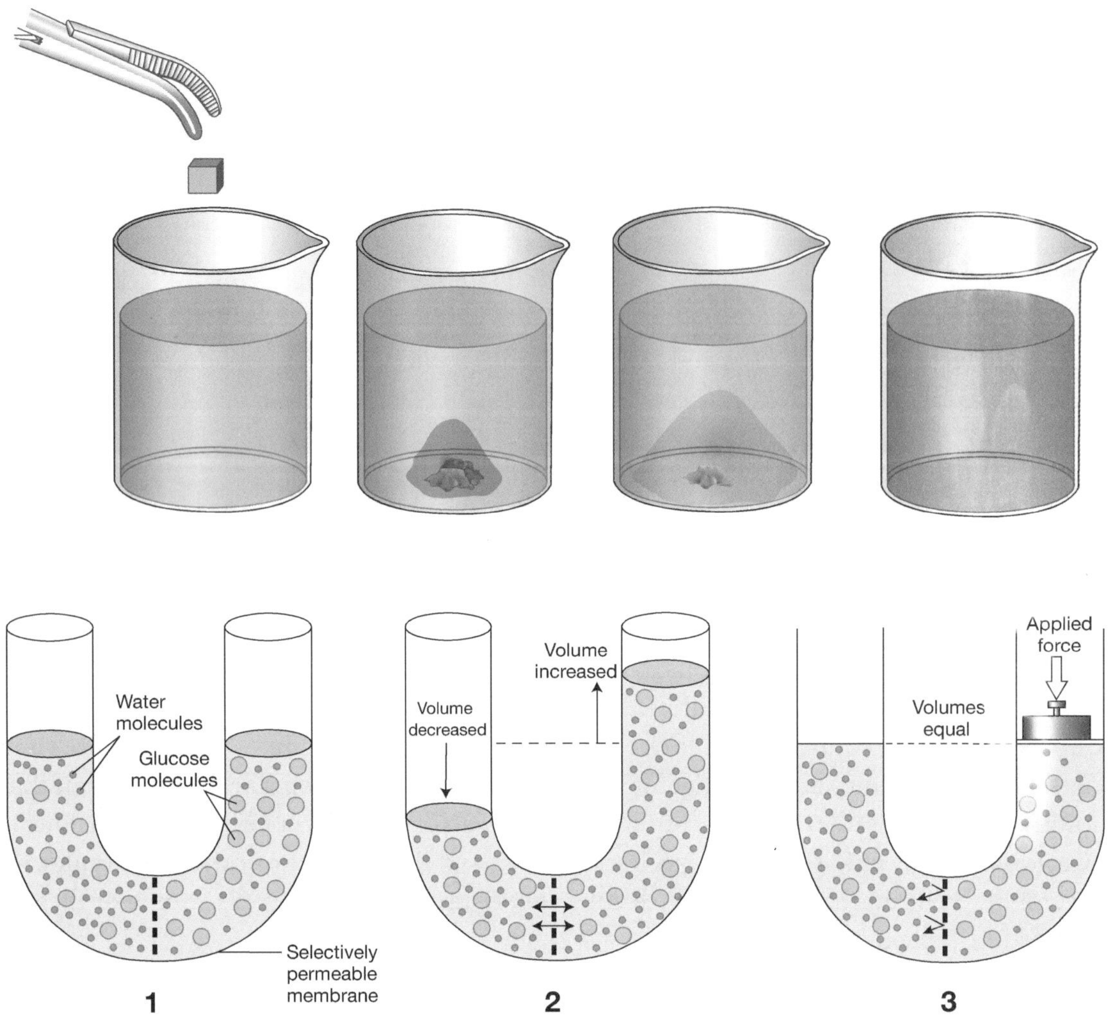

Figure 2-6

Simple Diffusion (above) and Osmosis (below)

Simple diffusion is the passive movement of a substance from an area of higher concentration to an area of lower concentration. It can occur within gases, liquids, or (as shown here) across different states of matter. Osmosis is the simple diffusion of a solvent through a semi-permeable membrane. In the body, the solvent is usually water and the membrane crossed typically belongs to the cell and/or its organelles. In this illustration, water molecules (small dots) can cross the membrane but glucose molecules (larger dots) cannot. The starting concentrations are shown in 1. At equilibrium (2), the concentration of solute (glucose) is the same on both sides of the membrane. The physical pressure required to prevent solvent movement (3) is called the osmotic pressure.

tration of water to a lower one. Example: movement of water molecules from filtrate (within renal tubules of the kidney) back into the medullary tissue and thence back into the bloodstream. This concentrates the urine and conserves body water.

4. **Active transport**: the active transport of molecules against a concentration gradient. Both a carrier and an energy source are required. Example: the sodium-potassium pump that moves three

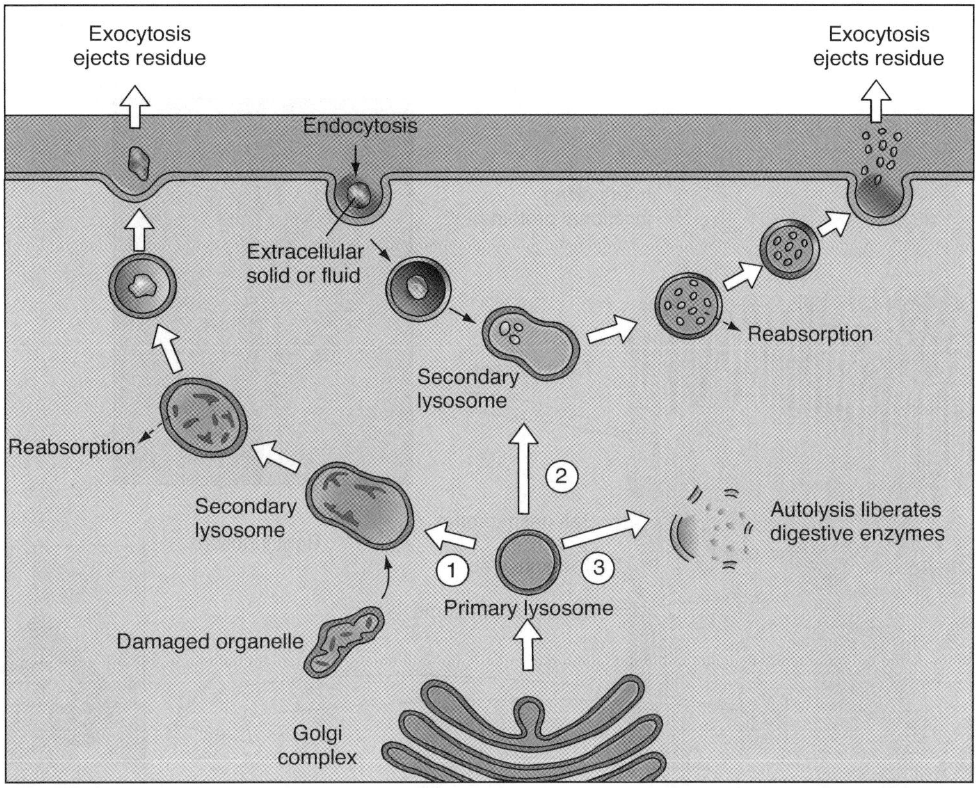

Figure 2-7

Cell Membrane Dynamics

When endocytosis occurs via pinocytosis or phagocytosis, a small amount of cell membrane is lost as it envelopes the newly engulfed material. Membrane is replaced as exocytosed vacuoles fuse to the cell membrane. Materials which leave the cell include the end results of lysosomal digestion (shown here) as well as other secretory products packaged by the golgi complex ("apparatus").

molecules of sodium out of the cell and two molecules of potassium into a cell for each high energy molecule (ATP) expended. This helps maintain the relatively low sodium/high potassium intracellular environment necessary for several aspects of metabolism.

5. **Pinocytosis**: the engulfment of *liquid* droplets into the cell by invagination of the cell membrane and pinching off of vacuoles.
6. **Phagocytosis**: the engulfment of *solid* particles by cell membrane manipulations similar to those of pinocytosis.

The cell membrane is modified in specific kinds of cells in several ways. Microvilli are tiny finger-like projections of the cell membrane that increase the surface area of the absorptive cells in the small intestine. Cilia are much larger membrane projections that the cell can actively move. Flagella are similar to cilia except that normally only one is present per cell (sperm cells are the only flagellated cells in the human body). Some specialized sensory cells in the internal ear have fine hair-like projections from the cell membrane that stimulate the cell when they are moved.

The cell membrane is a dynamic structure that is constantly being used and replaced (Figure 2-7). When vacuoles form by endocytosis (pinocytosis or phagocytosis), small amounts of cell mem-

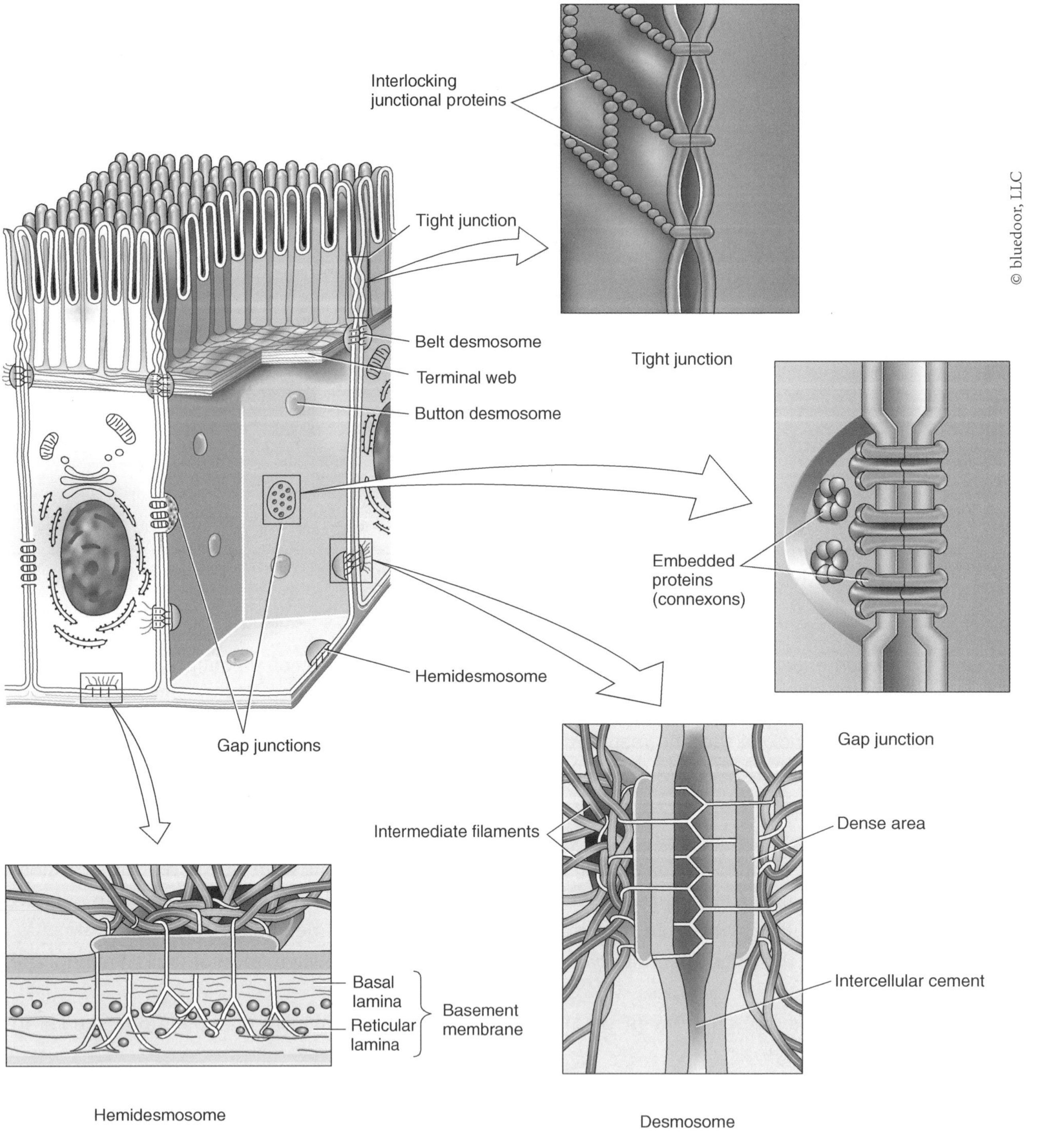

Figure 2-8

Attachments of Epithelial Cells

Most cells of the body are attached to adjacent cells and other cellular structures by various modifications of the cell membrane and by biological "glues" (see text).

brane are lost as the engulfed particles are "packaged" for cytoplasmic entry. Conversely, cells which are actively secreting (exocytosing) constantly add membrane to the cell via the packaging membranes manufactured by the golgi complex.

Most cells in the body are firmly attached to adjacent cells by various modifications to the cell membrane called gap junctions, tight junctions, intermediate junctions, and desmosomes (Figure 2-8). **Gap junctions** are formed by interlocking proteins that form tiny connecting channels between the cytoplasm of adjacent cells. These allow ions and small molecules to pass between the cells and are especially common in cardiac muscle tissue and smooth muscle tissue. **Tight junctions** are formed by the partial fusion of lipid portions of adjacent cell membranes. These are especially strong connections and are found between adjacent cells near exposed surfaces where they form a relatively impenetrable barrier against bacteria, acids, wastes, *etc.* **Intermediate junctions** are formed when adjacent cell membranes are "cemented" together by protein/polysaccharide complexes called *proteoglycans.* **Desmosomes** are cell membrane connections formed by very thin layers of proteoglycans reinforced by cytoplasmic fibrils. They are very common between adjacent cells at the surface of the skin.

The cytosol and organelles include everything inside the cell membrane except the cell nucleus (which technically *is* an organelle but is usually considered separately). The **cytosol** is the fluid in which the cellular organelles are suspended. It is about eighty-five percent water and the remainder is ions and molecules. This fluid and the organelles that are suspended within it are collectively called the **cytoplasm**. The cellular **organelles** are the formed structures within the cytoplasm (Table 2-3). The term organelle literally means *little organ* and there are several different types with each having its own peculiar structure and function in cellular metabolism.

Ribosomes are structures composed of ribosomal RNA and proteins. They serve as the site of protein synthesis (peptide bond formation). Some float freely in the cytoplasm and others are temporarily bound to endoplasmic reticulum (see below). Proteins that remain within the cell are manufactured on free ribosomes. Membrane-bound ribosomes produce the proteins that are exported from (secreted by) the cell.

Endoplasmic reticulum (**ER**) is a complex system of double membranes that extends through the cytoplasm from the nuclear membrane to the cell membrane. There are two categories of endoplasmic reticulum (rough and smooth). **Rough endoplasmic reticulum** (**RER**) is called *rough* because it is currently studded with ribosomes (Figure 2-9). These ribosomes produce proteins primarily for secretion from the cell. When attached ribosomes complete the protein strand dictated by the mRNA that they are translating, they detach from the ER and re-enter the cytosol. **Smooth endoplasmic reticulum** (**SER**) is *smooth* because it lacks attached ribosomes. It functions primarily in production of lipid materials and in certain types of detoxification reactions. For example, smooth ER in the liver cells of alcoholics is especially well-developed because of its role in alcohol metabolism. The **golgi complex** consists of a series of membranous sacs and vesicles near the nucleus that are interconnected to the endoplasmic reticulum. It manufactures carbohydrates and glycoproteins, and modifies and packages material for secretion from the cell. When these secreted materials leave the cell by exocytosis, their surrounding membranes fuse to and become part of the cell membrane. A cell that is actively in-taking and secreting materials may undergo a complete turnover of cell membrane in this manner in less than one hour.

Mitochondria are double-membrane-bound organelles that serve as the site of oxidative phosphorylation and electron transport reactions. These are the reactions that produce high energy compounds such as **adenosine triphosphate** (**ATP**) that are used in energy consuming (anabolic) reactions within the cell. Because of this role, mitochondria are often called the cellular *powerhouses.*

Table 2-3 Summary of Organelles and Other Cellular Components

Item	*Function(s)*
Cell membrane: fluid mosaic of lipid, protein, and carbohydrate components.	Physically surrounds cytoplasm and organelles, and controls substances entering/leaving the cell.
Cytosol: fluid (mostly water) in which organelles are suspended.	Serves as a medium in which chemical reactions occur.
Nucleus: double-membrane-bound area (usually centrally located) which contains most of cellular DNA.	Replicates prior to cell division (so that each daughter cell has a set of DNA) and serves as a template for the manufacture of RNA (transcription).
Nucleolus: one or more dark staining areas within the nucleus.	Contains the DNA used to manufacture ribosomal RNA.
Chromatin: the combination of DNA and protein that forms the structure of chromosomes.	Replicates before a cell divides and condenses to form chromosomes (heterochromatin). More commonly involved in the manufacture of RNA in a less organized form called euchromatin.
Mitochondria: double membrane bound organelles with highly folded inner membranes.	Contain enzymes and coenzymes involved in oxidative phosphorylation/electron transport reactions (*i.e.,* they produce ATP).
Ribosomes: structures composed of protein and ribosomal RNA.	Serve as the site of protein synthesis by "reading" the codes (three base sequences) on messenger RNA.
Golgi Complex: series of double membrane sacs and vesicles near the nucleus and connected to the endoplasmic reticulum.	Produces carbohydrates and glycoproteins and modifies and packages materials for cellular secretion.
Endoplasmic reticulum: double membranes extending throughout the cytosol from the nucleus to the cell membrane.	When ribosomes bind to it (rough endoplasmic reticulum = RER), it channels the proteins produced by the ribosomes to the golgi complex to be packaged for exocytosis. Without ribosomes (smooth endoplasmic reticulum = SER), ER is involved in lipid synthesis and detoxification reactions.
Lysosome: single-membrane-bound cytoplasmic sacs containing hydrolytic enzymes.	Fuse to other cytoplasmic structures in order to digest phagocytized material or hydrolyze worn out cell parts.
Vacuoles (vesicles): single-membrane-bound cytoplasmic sacs that may contain a variety of materials.	Often consists of recently endocytosed material awaiting lysosomic degradation or material to be exocytosed. Any (single) membrane-bound structure that cannot be specifically identified is termed a vacuole.
Peroxisomes: single-membrane-bound cytoplasmic sacs containing enzymes capable of producing hydrogen peroxide (H_2O_2).	Produce hydrogen peroxide and use it in oxidation reactions.
Centrioles: a pair of microtubular structures located in an area near the nucleus called the centrosome.	Organize the cellular microtubular structures and attach via them to the chromosomes during cellular division.
Cilia: hair-like projections of the cell membrane of some cells.	Can "beat" or "wave" in a coordinated fashion to move material along the cell's surface.
Flagellum: a single, elongated cilium-like projection forming the tail of a sperm.	Propels sperm forward in a "swimming-like" manner.
Microvilli: cell membrane projections similar in appearance to cilia but much smaller and immobile.	Increase the cell surface area to increase the efficiency of absorption.
Microfilaments: tiny, non-tubular filaments formed of protein.	Involved in cellular "contractions" and amoeboid movements.
Microtubules: tubular structures that extend throughout the cytosol.	Form the central parts of cilia, flagella, and the spindle apparatus involved in chromosomal organization during cell division.

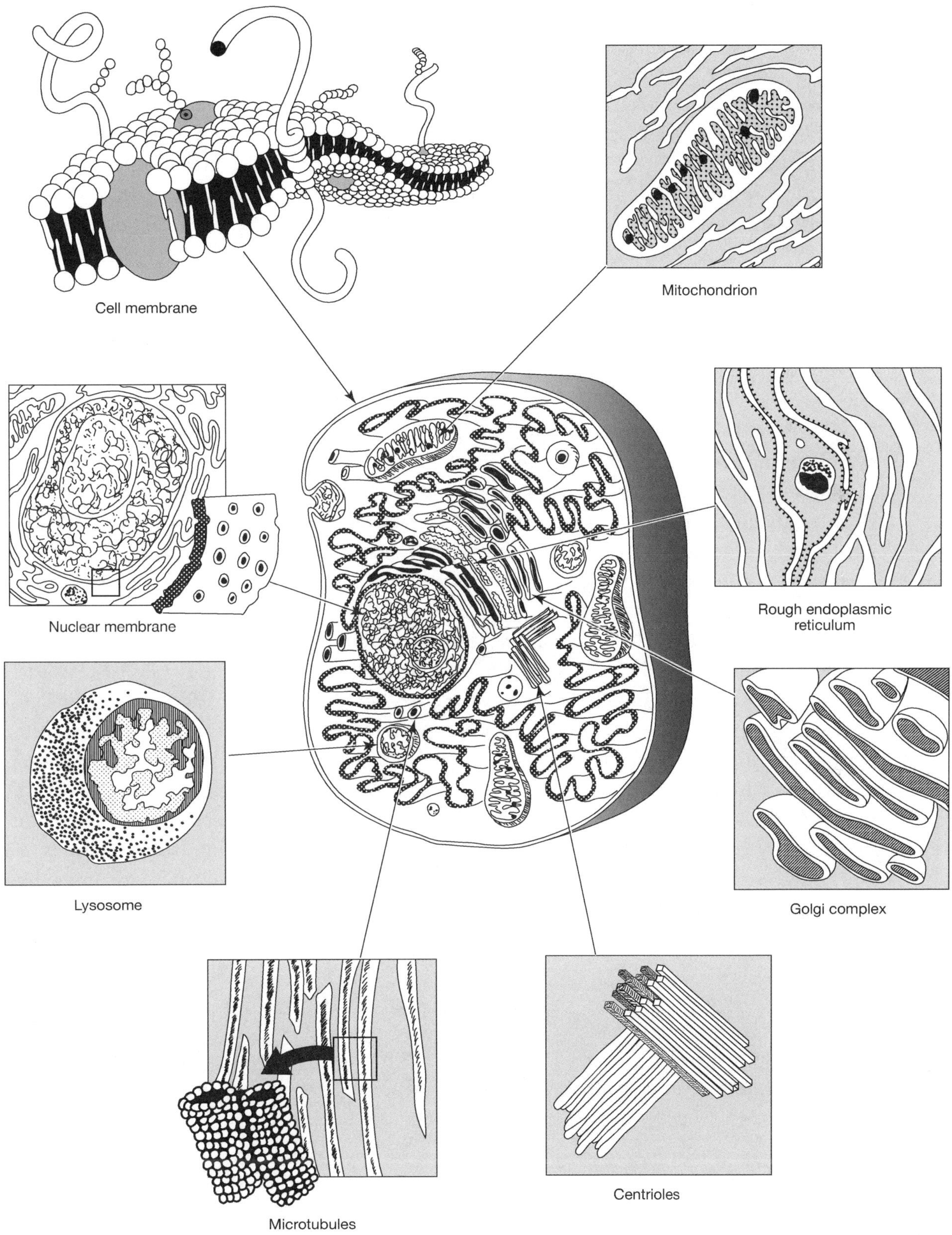

Figure 2-9

Typical Animal Cell and its Organelles

The cytoplasm contains several types of single-membrane-bound, free floating, structures including lysosomes, peroxisomes, and vacuoles. **Lysosomes** are membrane-bound sacs of digestive enzymes manufactured by the golgi complex. They digest foreign particles as well as worn-out cellular components. Newly formed lysosomes are called *primary lysosomes.* Those that are actively involved in digestive processes are called *secondary lysosomes.* Worn-out (non-functional) lysosomes are termed *residual bodies.* The decrease in uterine size after parturition (the birth of a baby) occurs by lysosomal digestion. Similarly, the regression of mammary tissue after weaning an infant is due to lysosomes. Lysosomal dysfunction is a factor in some diseases (like certain types of arthritis).

Peroxisomes are membranous sacs that are similar to lysosomes. They contain certain types of enzymes including some that produce hydrogen peroxide (H_2O_2). The latter is an important compound in the metabolism of certain types of phagocytes. **Vacuoles** are membranous sacs that temporarily store cellular compounds. They are often formed by pinocytosis or phagocytosis.

Centrioles are rod-like structures composed of microtubules that function during cell division to organize and properly distribute the chromosomes into the daughter cells. They are found only in cells that can divide. Non-dividing cells such as mature muscle cells and nerve cells lack centrioles.

Fibrils and **microtubules** are cytoplasmic components that impart structure and rigidity to the cytoplasm and also function in the movement of materials through it. Microtubules also extend out into the finger-like projections of the cell membrane termed **cilia**. They cause the cilia to move in a controlled rhythmic manner to propel matter along the cell surface. For example, the cells lining the trachea are ciliated to help move mucus up and out of the respiratory passageways. **Flagella** are structurally similar to cilia except that they are longer and each cell has fewer. The only human cells that are flagellated are spermatozoa. Flagella are used to move the cells.

The **nucleus** is typically located near the center of the cell. It is the largest single structure within the cell membrane and contains the genetic material (DNA). A few body cells (osteoclasts, skeletal muscle cells) are multinucleated and mature red blood corpuscles (RBC's) lack a nucleus. The nucleus is separated from the cytoplasm by a **nuclear membrane** that is continuous with the endoplasmic reticulum. The nuclear membrane is perforated by a number of **nuclear pores** that allow small materials into and out of the nucleus. The **nucleolus** is an area inside the nucleus where ribosomal RNA is actively manufactured. **Chromatin** is the name of the nuclear substance that is composed of DNA and protein. At cell division it undergoes organization into **chromosomes**. Human body cells contain 46 (23 pairs of) chromosomes. A portion of a chromosome containing the genetic code related to the synthesis of a single protein is called a **gene**. Each chromosome has thousands of genes within its structure.

Objectives

7. Name the three major parts of a cell (cytosol + organelles = one part).
8. State the functions of the cell membrane and list, define, and compare six ways that substances cross the membrane.
9. Match each organelle with its major role in cellular structure or function.

Cell Cycle

The sequence of events involved in a cell's existence from its formation through its division to form two new cells is called the **cell cycle** (Figure 2–10). Some cells divide every few hours, many divide less frequently, and some do not divide (in adults). The cell cycle consists of a non-dividing period

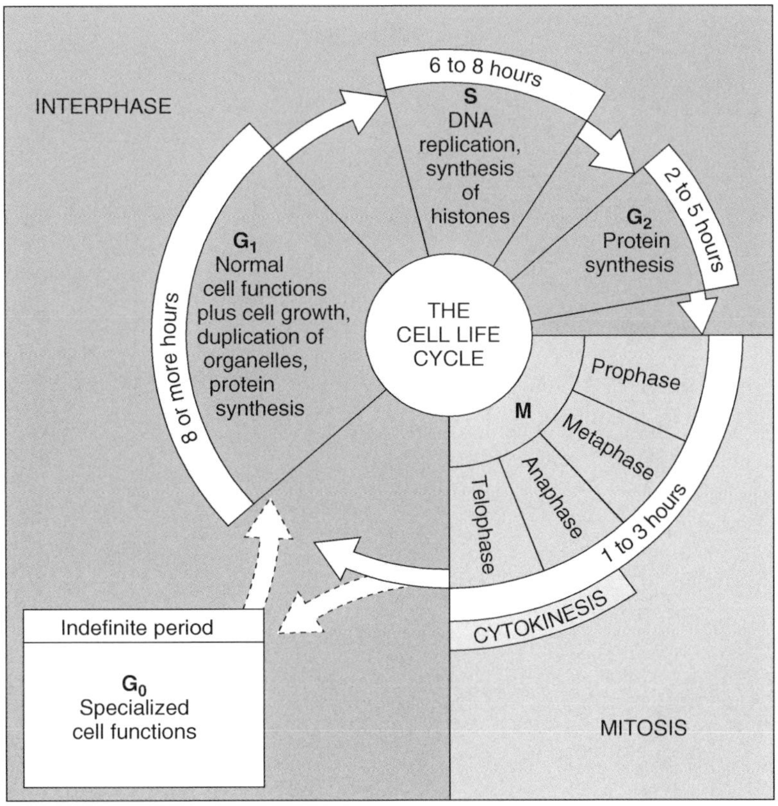

Figure 2–10

The Major Stages in the Cell Cycle

Note that the times given may vary considerably for different types of cells.

commonly called interphase and a dividing period called mitosis. During **interphase**, cellular growth and synthesis of compounds and organelles occur. Interphase is commonly divided into three phases: G1, S, and G2. The **G1** (first growth) **phase** is a period of rapid growth and metabolism terminating in the replication of the centrioles. During the **S** (synthesis) **phase**, the DNA replicates to form two identical sets so that both new cells formed at cell division will receive a complete set of genetic information. The **G2** (second growth) **phase** is used for synthesis of the enzymes and other compounds needed for cell division.

Mitosis is the nuclear division that occurs after the G2 phase (Figure 2-11). It is commonly divided into prophase, metaphase, anaphase, and telophase. During **prophase**, the chromatin condenses to form visible chromosomes. These were duplicated during the S phase of interphase and the duplicate members are joined to each other at a specific locus called the **centromere**. The nuclear membrane begins to disappear during prophase and the centrioles move to opposite poles of the cell. **Spindle fibers**, which attach to the chromosomes, become visible. During **metaphase**, the chromosomes are arranged along the equatorial plate with spindle fibers attached to the centromeres of each one. **Anaphase** is the period where the centromeres split and the sister chromatids of each pair are pulled toward opposite poles of the cell. During **telophase** the two new nuclear membranes appear and the chromosomes become unorganized chromatin. This is followed by division of the intervening cytoplasm (**cytokinesis**) to form two new cells identical to the original cell.

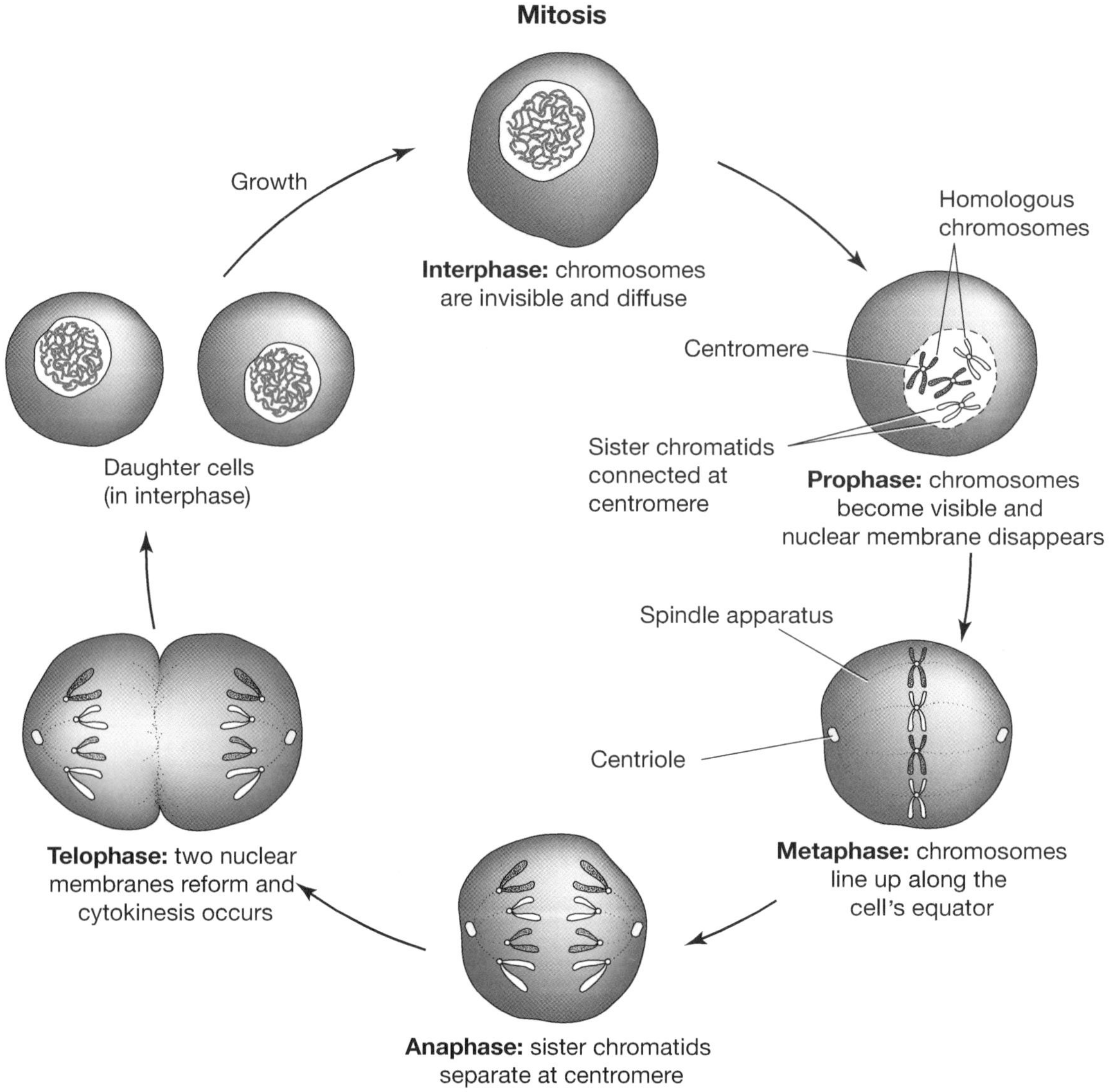

Figure 2-11
The Stages of Mitosis

Mitosis is the nuclear events that occur when regular body cells divide. The chromosome number is not reduced because when the centromeres split (which doubles the chromosome number) one sister chromatid migrates to each end (pole) of the dividing cell and becomes a chromosome in the resulting daughter cell. When this separation is complete at the end of anaphase, the cytoplasm and organelles are separated by cytokinesis and two daughter cells result. Although humans have 46 chromosomes (23 pairs) only four were shown here for clarity.

Meiosis is the special type of cell division that occurs during the formation of sex cells (spermatozoa and ova). It consists of two modified nuclear divisions during which the chromosome number is reduced from the **diploid** (**2N**) **number** (46) to the **haploid** (**N**) **number** (23). This process will be discussed more fully with the reproductive systems.

Objectives

10. Define the cell cycle in terms of its four major phases and the subdivisions of mitosis.
11. Differentiate mitosis and meiosis.

Clinical Considerations

Cells are remarkably adaptable as long as their basic nutritional and environmental needs are met. They can be injured in a number of ways including heat, cold, chemicals, radiation, and by bacteria and viruses. Cells react to these noxious and other stimuli in a variety of ways depending on the magnitude of the stimulus and the specific cell type. Changes in cell size and number are variously termed atrophy, hypertrophy, or hyperplasia. Cellular **atrophy** is a decrease in cell size, which in turn, causes a decrease in the size of the parent organ. Atrophy can occur due to disease, disuse, or senility. Cellular **hypertrophy** is an increase in cell size which results in enlargement of the parent organ. Hypertrophy occurs due to hormonal influences or due to increased metabolic demands which cause increased numbers of organelles and cytoplasmic volume. **Hyperplasia** is an increased number of cells. **Metaplasia** refers to a change in cell type such that one type of cell is transformed into another. Metaplasia which is accompanied by a change from more primitive cells to more specialized cell types is called **differentiation**. Considerable differentiation occurs during normal development since all of the types of cells found in the adult are formed from one original cell (zygote). Cells that are highly specialized are less likely to undergo metaplasia than other, more primitive cells. Some cells are so highly differentiated and specialized that they have lost all ability to divide. Consequently, injury to them can be quite serious because the body cannot manufacture replacements (*see Chapter 3*).

Mutations are changes that occur in the genetic material (DNA) of a cell. These can be induced by drugs, radiation, or they can occur naturally. Some mutations result in **inborn errors of metabolism** (genetic defects). These include several diseases caused by abnormal (non-functional) enzymes. Disease syndromes related to abnormal metabolism include albinism, phenylketonuria (PKU), Tay-Sachs disease, and several others. Some genetic problems are related to too few or too many chromosomes. A missing chromosome is called **monosomy**. A common form of monosomy is Turner's syndrome in which a phenotypically female individual has only one *X* chromosome. **Trisomy** is a condition in which an extra chromosome is present. The best known trisomy is trisomy 21 which is also called Down syndrome (formerly known as mongolism).

Cancer (**neoplasia**) is a disease state related to uncontrolled cellular division. Cancers are commonly classified as **benign** if the offending tissues grow slowly and are bound by a membrane that does not allow them to spread, or **malignant** if they grow more quickly and tend to spread (**metastasize**). Cancer causing agents are called **carcinogens** and include radiation, chemicals, and certain types of viruses. Interestingly, cancer itself is not life threatening. Deaths attributed to cancer occur when uncontrolled tissue growth sufficiently impedes some vital function(s).

Clinical Case Studies

Case 1—A lymph node biopsy (sample) was examined microscopically to assess prognosis in a cancer patient. Instead of the usual types of cells the histopathologist reported that the sample contained a large number of highly undifferentiated cells. What is the significance of this finding?

Case 2—A young housewife with no children complained of chronic fatigue in spite of efforts to eat a balanced diet and get sufficient rest. Analysis of her blood revealed a significant reduction in her red blood cell count and the presence of significant numbers of nucleated RBC's. Explain how her symptoms and test results are related.

Case 3—Before leaving the hospital with her newborn infant, a young mother was informed that her baby tested positive for PKU (phenylketonuria). Her pediatrician immediately placed the infant on an artificial diet that was low in the amino acid phenylalanine. Why?

Objectives

12. Define atrophy, hyperplasia, hypertrophy, metaplasia, and cellular differentiation.
13. Differentiate benign *vs.* malignant neoplasia.

Points to Ponder

Cells contain subparts called organelles which are composed of biological macromolecules formed from smaller organic subunits . . . and so it goes—down the various levels of organization. Going up, the levels of organization are tissues, organs, and systems which are discussed in other chapters. Cytology is the manna of cytologists and molecular biologists who still labor to unwind the cellular mysteries including the details of how and what these cellular organelles do. Nearly all of them are membranous, at least in part.

Cells multiply by dividing—a tricky mathematical maneuver that seems to be specifically challenging to that group of snakes known as "adders."

It is remarkable that all of the genetic information necessary to develop a full-size adult is contained in the single-celled zygote. This fact becomes even more difficult to comprehend when one realizes that the DNA simply determines the types of proteins that the cells of the developing embryo manufacture. There is no genetic code which determines the quantities of these proteins. Nothing in the genetic code directly determines how many eyes, ears, or limbs we have or where they are located on our bodies. The microenvironmental factors that control these kinds of constants remain largely unknown. It could be debated which is more amazing—that we develop the way we do embryologically—or that so relatively few times developmental processes fail to follow their normal patterns.

Most of the breeds of domestic animals have been developed in the past few hundred years by selective breeding. In recent decades, the concept of selective breeding has reached new heights. Today, a high-producing dairy cow can be pharmaceutically induced to superovulate (produce many more ova than normal). Excess ova can be collected, fertilized in vitro, and transferred into the uteri of grade cows who then gestate and surrogate the offspring. In this manner, exceptional genetic pools can be rapidly expanded and can quickly increase the efficiency of milk and meat production.

It has been shown that if the two cells resulting from mitotic division of the zygote are physically separated, each one can, with subsequent division, produce a complete individual. In other words, identical twins can be produced in this manner. The cloning of higher mammals has also been accomplished by removing cells from adults and developing complete and genetically identical individuals. The moral and ethical implications of these types of biological manipulations are complex and subject to heated debate.

When mankind manipulates reproduction, evolution (change) can be exponentially increased. Witness the development of dozens of different breeds of dogs in the last few hundred years. Some of them are so physically unsuited for life processes that they require iatric intervention to persist. For example, the heads of Boston Terrier fetuses at term are often larger than the bony limits of the birth canals of their mothers. Without veterinarians to assist at parturition, Boston Terriers would become extinct in a few decades by natural selection.

Selective breeding to increase productivity in food animals (and plants) is inherently logical. But is there justification for manipulating breeding to produce sideshow curiosities that have no purpose other than satisfying the visual whims of a public determined to create something else cute and unusual?

Slang and Obsolete Nomenclature

UNOFFICIAL TERM	OFFICIAL DESIGNATION
Golgi apparatus	golgi complex *[complexus golgiensis]*
sarcolemma	cell membrane *[membrana cellularis]* of a muscle cell
sarcoplasmic reticulum	endoplasmic reticulum *[reticulum endoplasmicum]* of a muscle cell

Review Questions

1. Which of the following statements is incorrect?
   A. Mitosis is the portion of the cell cycle in which the chromosomes are duplicated.
   B. Acids release hydrogen ions (H^+) which lower the body pH.
   C. Metaplasia is a change in cell type.
   D. Cytology is the study of cells.
   E. Hydrolysis is a process whereby biological macromolecules are broken down into their subunits.

2. Which form of cellular entry requires a carrier and energy?
   A. facilitated diffusion
   B. phagocytosis
   C. active transport
   D. osmosis
   E. simple diffusion

3. Which statement is false?
   A. Nucleotides are monomers of nucleic acids.
   B. Lipids are inorganic compounds with the same three major elemental components as carbohydrates but with a smaller percentage of oxygen.
   C. Carbohydrates are organic compounds which often contain carbon, hydrogen, and oxygen in a ratio of 1:2:1.
   D. Proteins are polymers of amino acids.
   E. Ribosomal RNA (rRNA) forms part of the cellular organelles called ribosomes which serve as the site of protein synthesis.

4. A decrease in cell size is called ________________.
   A. metaplasia
   B. malignancy
   C. hypertrophy
   D. hyperplasia
   E. atrophy

5. Which item is false?
   A. The nucleolus is an area inside the nucleus where ribosomal RNA is actively manufactured.
   B. Translation of DNA results in the formation of protein.
   C. The three basic components of a cell are the cell membrane, cytosol and organelles, and a nucleus.
   D. One of the functions of mitochondria is to produce ATP.
   E. The longest cells in the body are neurons.

6. Find the mismatch.
   A. protein—amino acid
   B. nucleic acid—nucleotide
   C. lipid—fatty acid
   D. amino acid—polypeptide
   E. carbohydrate—monosaccharide

7. Which of the following is not a membranous structure?
   A. mitochondria
   B. golgi complex
   C. SER
   D. nucleolus
   E. lysosome

8. Which statement is false?
   A. Fibrils impart structure and rigidity to the cytosol of cells.
   B. There are 1x 10^{15} cells in a human being.
   C. Cilia move materials along the cellular surface and flagella can move cells.
   D. Centrosomes attach to spindle fibers.
   E. Carcinogens are cancer-causing agents.

9. Which of the following is mismatched?
   A. prophase—condensation of chromatin
   B. anaphase—centromeres split
   C. telophase—two new nuclear membranes appear
   D. metaphase—chromosomes are arranged at the equatorial plate
   E. S phase—division of cytoplasm and organelles

10. Find the mismatch.
    A. centrioles—function in cellular division
    B. RER—protein production for exportation

C. vacuoles—storage of cellular compounds
D. ribosomes—site of peptide bond formation
E. mitochondria—site of oxidative phosphorylation
F. Choose this response if all of the above (A-E) are correctly matched.

Thought Questions

1. Since (essentially) all of the cells in a human body have the same genome (identical DNA) explain how different types of cells can exist.

2. Since red blood corpuscles (RBC's) lack nuclei, how are they reproduced?

3. Since the process for endocytosis reduces the total amount of cell membrane, how is it replenished?

4. (Biological) osmosis can be defined as the simple diffusion of water through a semipermeable membrane *or* as the diffusion of water through a semipermeable membrane from an area of higher water concentration to an area of lower water concentration. Which is the better definition?

5. Which cellular organelles are membranous?

6. Why are some cancers fatal while others are not life threatening?

7. What is the purpose of meiosis?

8. What are the three major differences between DNA and RNA?

9. Why is thymine involved in replication and transcription but not in translation?

10. Of the four major groups of biological macromolecules in the body, which ones are typically formed from monomers by dehydration synthesis?

11. What can cells do that viruses cannot?

12. What is the difference between polypeptides and proteins?

13. Which cell membrane modification aids absorption? Cell movement? Movement of other substances along a cell's membrane?

14. In most body cells, chromosomes cannot be observed (microscopically) most of the time. Why?

15. Which chemical transport mechanism can occur without the presence of a membrane?

16. What do free ribosomes do? Membrane bound ribosomes?

17. What do plant cells typically have that animal cells do not?

18. Some cells like skeletal muscle cells and osteoclasts are multinucleated. In theory, how can this occur?

19. Why does cellular hyperplasia typically result in hypertrophy of the parent organ? Can hyperplasia occur without hypertrophy?

20. Why cannot some body cells (like neurons in an adult) divide?

21. Which atom type (element) is present in the greatest number in a human body?

Answers to Clinical Case Studies

Case 1—Undifferentiated cells are more primitive cell types that are characteristic of many kinds of neoplasia. This suggests a malignant cancer and a grave prognosis for the patient.

Case 2—The significant reduction of red blood corpuscles constitutes anemia. This is manifested by reduced oxygen carrying capacity of the blood and would explain the patient's fatigue. The presence of nucleated RBC's indicates that the anemia has been present for some time and is the body's attempt to reverse the anemia by forcing RBC's into circulation before they have completed their maturation by losing their nuclei. The cause of the anemia in this patient must be determined so that appropriate corrective steps can be taken.

Case 3—Phenyl ketones in the urine indicate that one or more enzymes involved in phenylalanine metabolism is lacking or dysfunctional. Unfortunately, the phenyl ketones which accumulate as a result can interfere with brain development and function. By placing the infant on a diet low in the amino acid phenylalanine, these effects can be averted.

Answers to Review Questions

1. A. Chromosomes are replicated during S phase (not M phase).

2. C. Facilitated diffusion (A) requires a carrier but no energy. Phagocytosis (B) requires energy but no carrier. Osmosis (D) and simple diffusion do not require either one.

3. B. Lipids are *organic* compounds.

4. E. Metaplasia (A) is a change in cell type. Malignancy (B) implies a lethal cancer. Hypertrophy (C) is an increase in size. Hyperplasia (D) is an increase in cell number.

5. B. RNA is translated.

6. D. A-C and E demonstrate "polymer–monomer" relationships, D is a "monomer–polymer" relationship.

7. D. The nucleus has a membrane but the nucleolus does not.

8. D. The centrosome is an area near the nucleus of an interphase cell in which the centrioles are located.

9. E. Division of the cytoplasm and organelles occurs during cytokinesis *just after* mitosis.

10. F.

Answers to Thought Questions

1. Not all of the DNA is used (transcribed) in a given type of cell. In fact, large amounts of it are not used. For illustration purposes, assume that a library contained all human knowledge. Those individuals desiring to be physicians would need (use) primarily the information in the medical science area (only).

2. They (themselves) cannot reproduce because of the lack of a nucleus. RBC's are derived from bone marrow cells called hemocytoblasts that do have nuclei and *can* reproduce.

3. Endocytosis depletes the cell membrane but exocytosis replenishes it.

4. These definitions say the same thing and are equally accurate.

5. Nuclei, endoplasmic reticula (both types), mitochondria, lysosomes, golgi complexes, peroxisomes, and vacuoles.

6. Uncontrolled cell division (cancer) is not inherently life threatening. Only when the increased cell populations interfere with vital processes does a cancer threaten life. Some cancers (benign) grow so slowly that life is never threatened.

7. Meiosis reduces the regular cellular chromosome number (diploid, 2N=46) to the haploid (N=23) number. It consists of two divisions. In the first meiotic division, the chromosome number is halved (46 to 23), and in the second meiotic division, sister chromatids are separated at their connecting centromeres. Thus, at the end of the first meiotic division, a daughter cell has only 23 chromosomes—but each consists of two copies of that portion of the DNA. After the second meiotic division, each daughter cell has 23 chromosomes, each of which has a single copy of that part of the DNA. Thus, when a sperm (23 chromosomes) fertilizes an ovum (23 chromosomes) the diploid (2N) number is restored. This explains why some traits are inherited from one's father and others are derived from one's mother.

8. RNA typically is single stranded, contains a 5-carbon sugar (ribose), and contains the nitrogenous bases adenine, cytosine, guanine and uracil. DNA is double stranded, contains the 5-carbon sugar (deoxyribose), and contains the nitrogenous bases adenine, cytosine, guanine, and thymine (in place of uracil).

9. Thymine is found in DNA but not in RNA. Replication and transcription both involve DNA. Translation involves RNA only, and RNA contains no thymine.

10. All of them except some subtypes of lipids.

11. A cell can multiply (by dividing) in an environment that contains no other cells. Viruses are obligate intracellular parasites.

12. Size. By definition, a protein is a polypeptide of 100 or more amino acids.

13. Microvilli—flagella—cilia.

14. Chromosomes become visible just before cells divide. Most body cells are not dividing most of the time.

15. Simple diffusion.

16. Free ribosomes serve as the site of synthesis for polypeptides and proteins that remain in the cell. Membrane-bound ribosomes are the site of synthesis for polypeptides and proteins that are exported from the cells as part of a secretory product.

17. Cell walls formed of polysaccharides and chloroplasts. The plant cell membrane is within this cell wall.

18. Multinucleated cells can occur by fusion of single cells which pool their nuclei into a common cell membrane or by nuclear division without concurrent cytoplasmic division.

19. An increase in cell number in most cases necessitates an increase in organ size. Hyperplasia can occur, however, without an increase in overall size if the dividing cells get smaller. This happens during the first several cell divisions of the fertilized ovum. The cell number increases but the total mass of the conceptus remains unchanged.

20. They have become so differentiated (specialized) that they have lost the microtubules, *etc.*, involved in mitosis. RBC's cannot divide because they do not have a nucleus.

21. Hydrogen. Although hydrogen is only about 10% of the total body mass (*vs.* 65% for oxygen and 18% for carbon), hydrogen atoms are only 1/16 as heavy as oxygen atoms and only 1/12 as heavy as carbon atoms. Hydrogen's smaller percentage of the total body mass is more than offset by the small size of the hydrogen atoms.

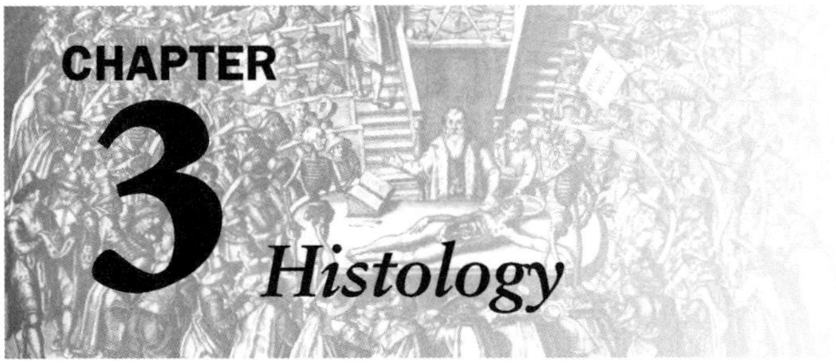

CHAPTER 3 Histology

Chapter Outline and Key Concepts

INTRODUCTION

Histology is synonymous with microscopic anatomy.

Tissues are groups of cells and the extracellular matrix in which they are embedded.

The four basic tissues (epithelial, muscle, nervous, and connective tissue) are derived developmentally from the three primary germ layers (ectoderm, mesoderm, endoderm).

MUSCLE TISSUE

Myocytes (muscle cells, myofibers) contain specialized cytoplasmic organelles called myofibrils that are directly involved in the contractile process.

Three kinds of muscle tissue are present in the body (skeletal, cardiac, and smooth).

Skeletal muscle cells are voluntary, striated, cylindrical, multinucleated, and the nuclei are peripherally located within the cells.

Cardiac muscle cells are involuntary, striated, branched, and usually have a single nucleus near the center of the cell.

Smooth muscle cells are involuntary, not striated, fusiform, and have a single nucleus near the center of the cell.

Skeletal muscle tissue is found primarily in skeletal muscles, cardiac muscle tissue is located primarily in the heart, and smooth muscle tissue is found in many loci—especially in the walls of vessels and visceral organs.

EPITHELIUM (EPITHELIAL TISSUE)

Epithelium is divided into two main subtypes: membranous and glandular.

Membranous epithelium is avascular and aneural, covers the outer surface of the body, and lines all luminal organs.

Membranous epithelium is classified as simple or stratified based on its thickness (single cell/multiple cells) and as cuboidal, columnar, or squamous based on the shape of the surface cells.

Two types of membranous epithelium do not fit the standard classification scheme: transitional epithelium and pseudostratified columnar epithelium.

Glandular epithelium has a blood and nerve supply and forms the secretory portion of glands.

Glands are classified as unicellular/multicellular based on the number of secretory cells and as endocrine/exocrine based on whether the secretory product is released into the bloodstream or onto a free body surface.

Exocrine glands are further classified based on the pattern of the duct system (simple/compound), the overall shape of the groups of secretory cells (tubular, acinar, tubuloacinar), and by the mode of secretion (eccrine, apocrine, and holocrine).

CONNECTIVE TISSUE

All types of connective tissue consist of cells suspended in an extracellular matrix of fibers and ground substance.

Connective tissue proper (fibrous connective tissue) is the major component of tendons, ligaments, fascia, and the ensheathments called epimysium, epineurium, and periosteum.

Connective tissue proper is classified by criteria related to its extracellular fibers as loose or dense, regular or irregular, and elastic, reticular, or collagenous.

Bone tissue has three major cell types and a mineralized matrix.

Cartilage is divided into three major types (elastic, hyaline, and fibrocartilage) based on the predominant fibers in the extracellular matrix.

Blood is the only liquid tissue.

Adipose tissue resembles connective tissue proper with a significant adipose (fat) cell content.

Other connective tissues include bone marrow tissue, reticular connective tissue, and primitive connective tissue (mesenchyme).

NERVOUS TISSUE

Nervous tissue is not divided into subtypes but has two major cell types (neurons and glial cells).

Neurons (nerve cells) conduct nervous impulses and are classified structurally as pseudounipolar, multipolar, or bipolar and functionally as sensory or motor and visceral or somatic.

Glial cells (neuroglia) include several types of cells that support neurons.

CLINICAL CONSIDERATIONS

The seriousness of an injury is partially determined by the regenerative capacity of the damaged tissues.

Surgical transplantations present two major challenges: the mechanics of the operation and possible immunological rejection of the transplant by the recipient.

Histopathology involves microscopic examinations of tissue removed during surgical or biopsy procedures.

Selected Definitions

Adipose tissue—a connective tissue characterized by the presence of large numbers of adipocytes (fat cells). It occurs subcutaneously, in the medullary cavities of bones, and elsewhere, serving as a stored source of body energy.

Apocrine secretion—a secretory mode of glandular epithelium in which part of the cell physically breaks away to form the secretory product. Apocrine secretion contrasts with merocrine (eccrine) secretion where no (visible) part of the cell enters the secretory product, and with holocrine secretion where the cells die and slough to become the secretion.

Basic tissue—any one of the four main categories of body tissue: epithelium, muscle tissue, connective tissue, and nervous tissue. Except for nervous tissue which has no subtypes, *per se*, the basic tissues are subdivided into specific tissues.

Biopsy—removal of cells or tissue from a living organism, typically for laboratory analysis. A common form of biopsy is removal of a blood sample, but many other tissue types can be biopsied, as well.

Blood—a liquid connective tissue. It is the only body liquid with a cell concentration high enough to deserve the label "tissue."

Bone marrow tissue—the major material occupying the medullary cavities of bones. It is a subtype of connective tissue and is called red bone marrow when actively hemopoietic; yellow bone marrow when it contains a high population of adipocytes, and gelatinous bone marrow when it involutes with senility.

Bone tissue—a mineralized subtype of connective tissue. It is the only body material routinely mineralized except for the enamel, dentin, and cementum of teeth, and it forms a major structural component of (the organs called) bones.

Cartilage—a connective tissue with a firm but typically unmineralized extracellular matrix. It is divided into three subtypes based primarily on the major type of proteinaceous fibers found in the matrix: elastic cartilage (containing elastic fibers), fibrocartilage (containing collagenous fibers), and hyaline cartilage (containing reticular fibers).

Connective tissue proper (fibrous connective tissue)—one of several subtypes of connective tissue. Connective tissue proper is the most widely distributed connective tissue and forms part of every organ.

Extracellular matrix—the material outside of and between cells. In many tissues it includes various types of proteinaceous fibers as well as amorphous protein/polysaccharide material called ground substance.

Fiber—a term used in various contexts to mean a muscle cell, a neuronal process, or a protein component of the extracellular matrix. Proteinaceous extracellular fibers include those composed of elastin, collagen, and reticulin.

Glandular epithelium—epithelium that is specialized for secretion. Although glandular epithelial cells are scattered within the surface epithelium of mucous membranes, most glandular epithelium is concentrated in the secretory organs called glands.

Ground substance—the protein/ polysaccharide component ("glue") of the extracellular matrix. The polysaccharide portion is often formed by polymers of chondroitin sulfate, keratin sulfate, and hyaluronic acid.

Histology—literally, "the study of tissue." In usage, histology is equivalent to microscopic anatomy which is the science of the minute structure of the body (organelles, cells, tissues, and organs).

Membranous (surface) epithelium—the tissue that forms all outer surfaces of the body and lines all of its lumina and cavities. Membranous epithelium is classified according to the shape of the surface cells (squamous, cuboidal, columnar) and whether it is one cell thick (simple) or more than one cell thick (stratified).

Mesenchyme—primitive connective tissue containing a large population of undifferentiated (stem) cells. Mesenchyme is concentrated in intervertebral discs and small amounts are present in the loose connective tissue around vessels.

Muscle tissue—the basic tissue functionally specialized for contraction. Three subtypes exist, skeletal muscle tissue (voluntary and striated), smooth muscle tissue (involuntary, not striated) and cardiac muscle tissue (involuntary and striated).

Neuroglial (glial) cell—a collective term encompassing the support cells of the nervous system. Neuroglia do not transmit impulses, but they support neurons physically and metabolically.

Neuron (nerve cell)—a cell specialized for impulse transmission. Each neuron has a single process termed the axon and one or more processes called dendrites.

Primary germ layer—any of the three defined strata that are formed during embryonic gastrulation: ectoderm, mesoderm, and endoderm. These germ layers differentiate to form the various tissues.

Regenerative capacity—the ability of a given type of cell or tissue to replace itself if lost, injured, or diseased. Epithelium and connective tissue have high regenerative capacity, but nervous tissue and muscle tissue have low regenerative capabilities.

Etymology *Modus vivendi*—**"A way of getting along together"**

adipo (L), *fat*—adipose
bio (G), *life*—biopsy
blasto (G), *formative*—blastocyst
chondro (G), *cartilage*—chondroclast
dendr (G), *tree*—dendrite
derma (G), *skin*—hypodermis
ekto (G), *outside*—ectoderm
endon (G), *within*—endoderm
epi (G), *upon, besides*—epithelium
erythro (G), *red*—erythrocyte
fibra (L), *small fiber*—myofibril
glia (G), *glue*—neuroglia
histo (G), *web, tissue*—histology
hormon (G), *to stimulate*—hormone
hyalin (G), *glassy*—hyaline
kerato (G), *horn*—keratin
klast (G), *to break*—osteoclast
kolla (G), *glue*—collagen
krinein (G), *to separate*—merocrine
leuko (G), *white*—leucocyte
matrix (L), *the womb, origin*—matrix
meso (G), *middle*—mesoderm
mikro (G), *small*—microvilli
myo (G), *muscle*—myomere
neuron (G), *nerve*—neuron
para (G), *beside*—paralysis
patho (G), *suffering, disease*—pathology
pseudo (G), *false*—pseudostratified
reticulatus (L), *netlike*—reticulum
squamo (L), *scales*—squamosal
thele (G), *nipple, teat*—epithelium

Introduction

The study of tissues is termed **histology** and is essentially synonymous with microscopic anatomy. **Tissues** are groups of similar cells and the **extracellular** matrix (products) in which they are embedded. The **matrix** is typically produced (secreted) by the cells and may be liquid (as it is in blood), semisolid, firm (as it is in cartilage), or quite hard (as it is in bone). Matrix consists of **extracellular fibers** (usually composed of protein) and an amorphous **ground substance** which is composed of carbohydrate/protein complexes called glycoproteins or mucopolysaccharides.

There are four basic types of tissue: muscle tissue, epithelial tissue (epithelium), connective tissue, and nervous tissue. These four basic types are further subdivided into specific types according to a number of structural criteria (Table 3-1). The whole body develops from one original cell at fertilization and thus all cells in the body have the same genetic material. Different types of cells (and thus tissues) occur because different cell types "read" (use) different parts of their genetic complement. About two weeks after fertilization, the cells of a developing embryo form three **primary germ layers**: ectoderm (outer layer), mesoderm (middle layer), and endoderm (inner layer). **Ectoderm** forms the outer epithelium and all of the nervous tissue of the body. **Mesoderm** forms all of the connective tissue, all of the muscle tissue, and the epithelium lining the vessels and serous body cavities. **Endoderm** forms the lining epithelium of most parts of the visceral body systems. The four basic tissues differ structurally in the amount and type of intercellular material and in the capacity of the cells to proliferate (regenerate) after injury.

Table 3–1 General Features of the Four Basic Tissues

	Epithelial Tissue	*Muscle Tissue*	*Connective Tissue*	*Nervous Tissue*
Nature and quantity of intercellular material	essentially none	a small amount of connective tissue proper	abundant fibers and ground substance	essentially none
Regenerative capacity	high	low	high	low
Major types	membranous and glandular epithelium	smooth, cardiac, and skeletal muscle tissue	c.t. proper, bone, blood, cartilage, adipose tissue, and several others	not subdivided into types (per se) but has two major cell types
Origin	endoderm, mesoderm, and ectoderm	mesoderm	mesoderm	ectoderm
Function	secretes and covers surfaces	contracts	joins (connects) other structures	conducts impulses

Objectives

1. Define: histology, extracellular matrix, ground substance, and extracellular fibers.
2. Compare the four basic tissues in regard to regenerative capacity, major subtypes, germ layer origin, type and quantity of intercellular material, and major function(s).

Muscle Tissue

Muscle tissue is the basic tissue functionally specialized for contraction. Muscle cells are called **myofibers** (**muscle fibers**) or **myocytes** and they contain elongated contractile organelles in their cytoplasm called myofibrils. **Myofibrils** are composed of alternating stacks of proteins (actin, myosin, and

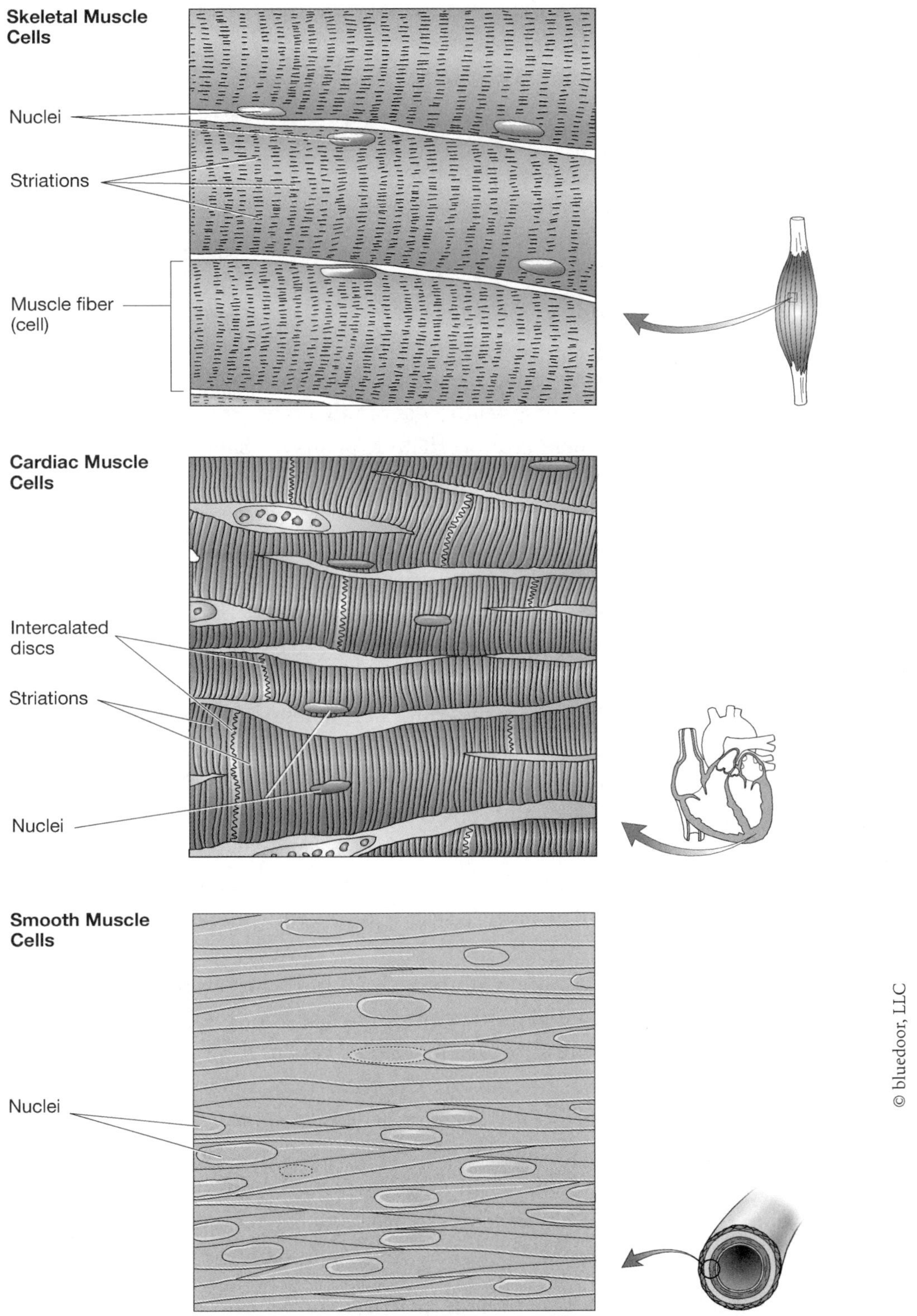

Figure 3-1

The Three Types of Muscle Tissue

Striations are more obvious in skeletal muscle cells than in cardiac muscle cells and note that smooth muscle cells are not striated. Skeletal muscle cells are multinucleated and so large that at this level of magnification, parts of only a few cells are illustrated. The different shapes of the three kinds of muscle cells (cylindrical, branched, spindle) are obvious.

others). The latter are called **myofilaments** and they cause physical shortening (contraction) of the cells by sliding together (interdigitating) in a manner similar to the physical way that the tines of two forks can be pushed together. Contraction of muscle cells causes movement of materials through the body as well as movement of the body as a whole. This process will be discussed in further detail in Chapter 8. There are three types of muscle tissue: skeletal muscle, cardiac muscle, and smooth muscle. These all have the common property of contraction but differ from each other in several structural and physiological ways (Table 3-2). Muscle cells produce very little intercellular matrix but each cell is invested with a delicate connective tissue sheath (*see Chapter 8*). Two types (skeletal and cardiac) have essentially no regenerative capacity.

Skeletal muscle tissue forms the contractile parts of the named muscles that move various parts of the body resulting in grossly observable body motion. Skeletal muscle is under the direct (voluntary) control of the nervous system. In fact, skeletal muscle cells have no inherent rhythmicity (innate contractile ability). Consequently, loss of innervation results in loss of contraction of skeletal muscle tissue and subsequent atrophy. This explains the small diameter of the limbs in individuals that suffer some kinds of paralysis. Skeletal muscle cells are large, cylindrically-shaped cells which may be several centimeters long (Figure 3-1). Each skeletal muscle cell has several nuclei located near the peripheral aspects of the cytoplasm. The multinucleated characteristic results from failure of complete cytoplasmic division during mitosis. The nuclei are displaced to the periphery of the cell because the cytoplasm is so tightly packed with myofibrils. The alternating stacks of the myofilaments (actin and myosin) in the myofibrils causes a differential cross-hatched or striated appearance in routine histological preparations.

Cardiac muscle tissue makes up the contractile parts of the heart and extends out into the walls of the large vessels near the heart (ascending aorta and pulmonary trunk). Contraction of cardiac muscle provides the propelling force that pumps blood through the cardiovascular system. Cardiac muscle has inherent rhythmicity and thus is involuntary, but the periodicity of its contractions can be increased or decreased by the autonomic nervous system. Cardiac muscle cells are branched (*Y*-shaped), striated, and considerably smaller than skeletal muscle cells. Each cardiac muscle cell has a centrally located nucleus and adjacent cells are joined end-to-end by specialized structures termed **intercalated discs**.

Smooth muscle tissue is found within the walls of blood vessels, in the walls of visceral organs, at the base of hair follicles, and within the iris and ciliary body of the eye. In blood vessels, smooth muscle helps control blood pressure. In the visceral organs it provides the force that helps to move materials through the lumina (peristalsis). Contraction of smooth muscle at the base of hair follicles causes the piloerection associated with gooseflesh (*cutis anserina*). Smooth muscle in the iris of the eye controls the pupillary diameter and thus the amount of light that strikes the retina. The smooth muscle in the ciliary body of the eye influences the thickness of the lens to allow images of near/far objects to be properly focused on the retina. Like cardiac muscle tissue, smooth muscle tis-

Table 3–2 A Comparison of Three Types of Muscle Tissue

Type	*Nervous Control*	*Appearance*	*Cell Shape*	*Cell Size*	*Number and Position of Nuclei*
Skeletal m.	voluntary	striated	cylindrical	50 μ x 20,000 μ	many/peripheral
Cardiac m.	involuntary	striated	"Y"-shaped	15 μ x 75 μ	one/central
Smooth m.	involuntary	non-striated	fusiform	5 μ x 125 μ	one/central

sue is involuntary and has inherent rhythmicity, and is under the influence of the autonomic nervous system. Smooth muscle cells are fusiform in shape with single, centrally located nuclei. They have a lower degree of organization of the myofibrils than cardiac and skeletal muscle cells. Consequently the contractile proteins in adjacent myofibrils are not in register (lined up). For this reason, smooth muscle lacks the histological striations found in skeletal and cardiac muscle tissue.

Objectives

3. Differentiate the three types of muscle tissue in regard to: voluntary/involuntary, presence/absence of striations, cell shape, number and position of nuclei, and location in body.

Table 3–3 Classification and Location of Membranous Epithelia

Type	*Location/Example*
Simple epithelia (one cell layer thick):	
simple squamous epithelium	lining vessels (endothelium), serous body cavities (mesothelium), pulmonary alveoli
simple cuboidal epithelium	lining renal tubules, thyroid follicles, and some ducts
simple columnar epithelium	lining intestinal lumen (not ciliated) and lining uterine tube (ciliated)
pseudostratified columnar epithelium	lining respiratory passageways (ciliated in most locations)
transitional epithelium	lining urinary bladder, ureters, and urethra
Stratified epithelia (two or more cell layers thick):	
stratified squamous epithelium	outer part of skin (keratinized) and lining of oral cavity, vagina, and anal canal (non-keratinized)
stratified cuboidal epithelium	larger ducts of sweat glands, salivary glands, and pancreas
stratified columnar epithelium	exists only where other types join (blend together)

Epithelial Tissue (Epithelium)

Epithelial tissue covers the inner and outer surfaces of the body (membranous epithelium) and forms the secretory portions of glands (glandular epithelium). Membranous epithelium forms protective boundaries between the environment and more deeply located structures. Glandular epithelium manufactures a myriad of secretory products including sweat, milk, cerumen (ear wax), sebum (skin oil), hydrochloric acid, bile, pancreatic juice, mucus, saliva, sperm, ova, and several others. Epithelium has a relatively small amount of intercellular matrix. In fact, epithelial tissue consists almost exclusively of tightly packed epithelial cells. They have a remarkably high ability to regenerate. Some epithelial tissues, like those lining the stomach, regenerate completely every 48 hours.

Simple Membranous Epithelia

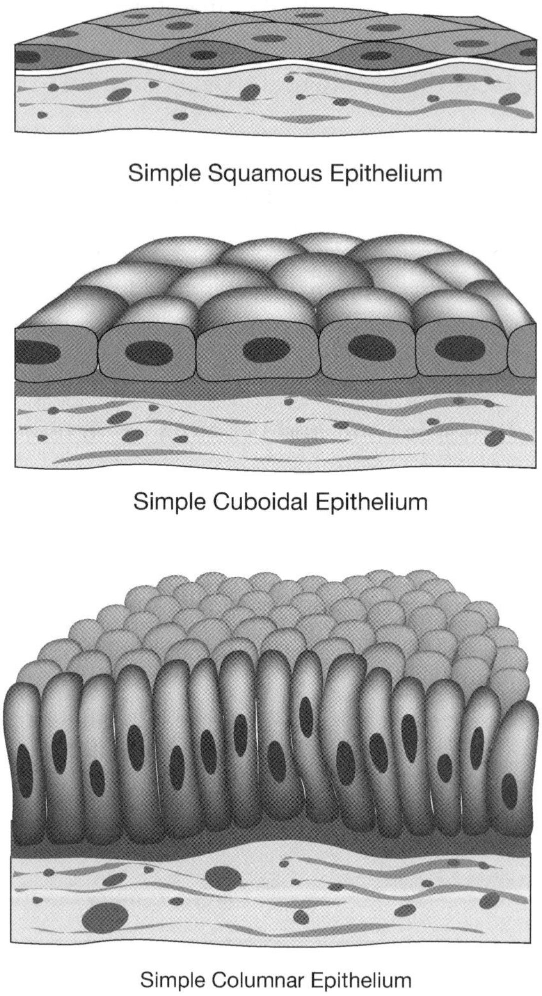

Figure 3-2
Simple Membranous Epithelia

Simple epithelia are only one cell thick and the cells may be squamous, cuboidal, or columnar in shape.

Membranous epithelium is sometimes called *surface epithelium* because it covers outer surfaces and lines the inner surfaces of the body. It is avascular, aneural, and varies in thickness from one cell to several dozen cells thick (Figures 3-2 and 3-3). The cells are separated from the underlying tissues by a thin structure termed the **basement membrane**. This consists of extracellular glycoprotein material that is manufactured by the epithelial cells themselves. Since membranous epithelium lacks blood vessels, it exchanges nutrients and wastes with adjacent tissues solely by diffusion. It is classified into several categories by two basic criteria: thickness (number of cells) and shape of the surface cells. Epithelial tissue that is only one cell thick (one cell between the basement membrane and the surface or lumen) is termed a **simple epithelium**. Epithelium with two or more cell layers is termed **stratified epithelium**. Epithelial cells may be **squamous** (flattened), **cuboidal** (globular), or **columnar** (elongated) in shape. Those near the basement membrane may be shaped differently

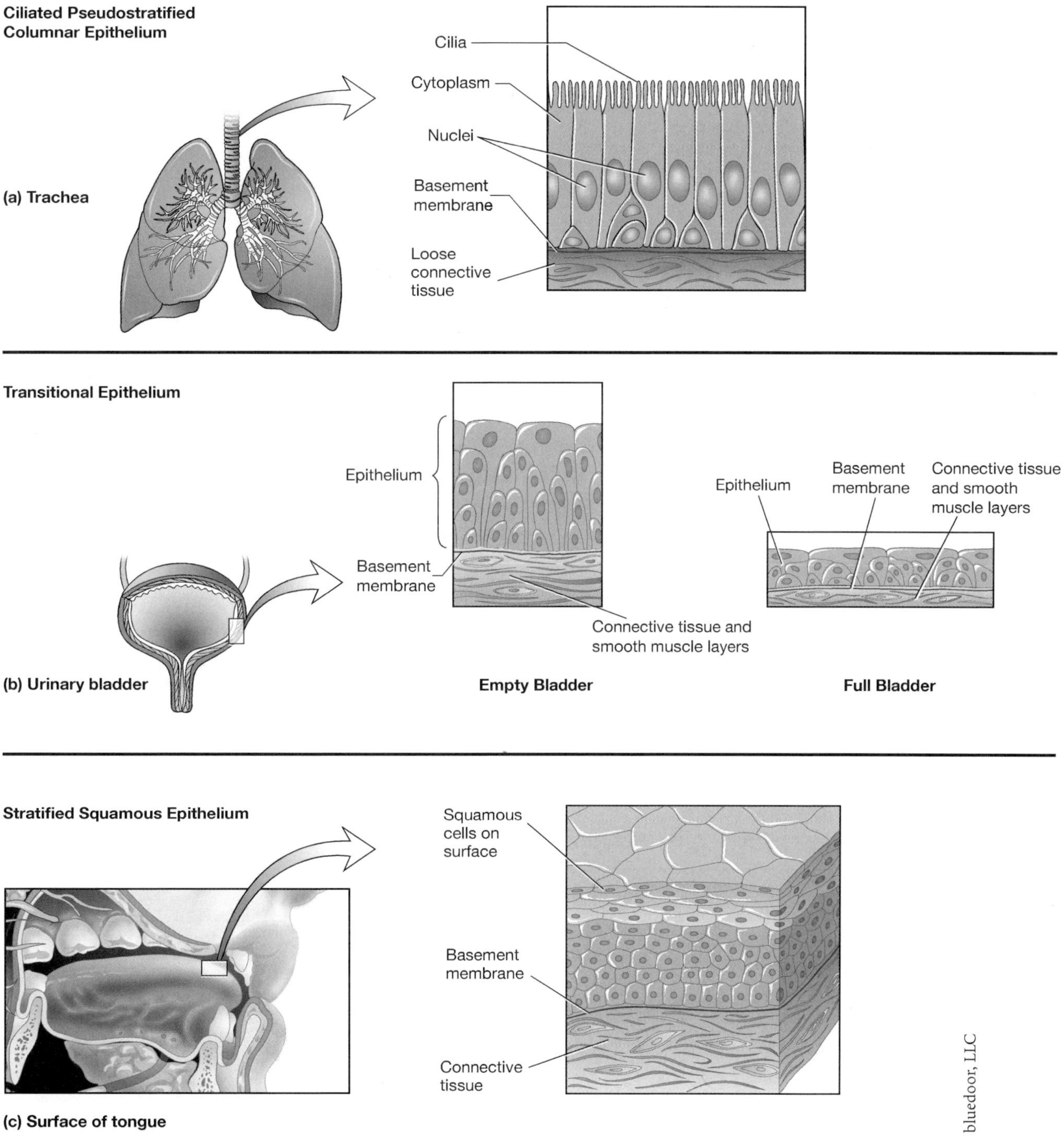

Figure 3-3

Other Membranous Epithelia

Stratified epithelia are two or more cells thick. Note that pseudostratified epithelium (a) and transitional epithelium (b) are usually considered to be simple epithelia because all cells make contact with the basement membrane. Note that "unstretched" transitional epithelium looks like stratified cuboidal epithelium. The latter, however, is never more than two cells thick.

Table 3–4 Modes of Secretion of Glandular Epithelium

Mode	*Description*	*Examples*
Eccrine (Merocrine)	watery secretion, no structural parts of the secretory cells become part of the secretion	some sweat glands, salivary glands, liver, pancreas
Apocrine	parts of secretory cells are lost into (become part of) the secretion	mammary glands and some sweat glands
Holocrine	entire cells of the gland are lost into (become part of) the secretion	sebaceous glands of skin, ceruminous glands of external acoustic meatus

than those at the surface. Only the shape of the cells at the surface is used when classifying epithelia. These two criteria (number of cells thick and shape of the surface cells) allow a classification of membranous epithelial tissue into several categories (Table 3-3).

At this point, the principles of classification of membranous epithelium should be understood, but it is not necessary to commit to memory the example location of each type. Two types require additional explanation: pseudostratified columnar epithelium and transitional epithelium. **Pseudostratified columnar epithelium** appears to be more than one cell thick because some cells are quite short and do not reach the surface. However, since all cells are in contact with the basement membrane, it is technically only one cell layer thick. The name pseudostratified (*false stratified*) is descriptive. This type of epithelium lines the air conducting passageways of the respiratory system and is sometimes called "respiratory epithelium". **Transitional epithelium** lines the urinary bladder, ureters, and part of the urethra. It appears to be composed of several layers of cuboidal cells, but like those of pseudostratified columnar epithelium, all cells make contact with the basement membrane. When the urinary bladder fills with urine and expands, these cells become more flattened in appearance (*i.e.,* they undergo a *transition* in shape). Because the cells get stretched "side-

Table 3–5 Selected Exocrine Glands and Products

Gland	*Product*	*Function*
Salivary glands	saliva	lubrication of ingesta
Pancreas	pancreatic juice	hydrolysis of ingesta
Liver	bile	emulsification of lipids
Sudoriferous glands	sweat	thermoregulation
Sebaceous glands	sebum	pliability of skin
Testis	sperm	reproduction
Ovary	ova	reproduction
Ceruminous glands	cerumen (earwax)	maintenance of tympanum
Mammary glands	milk	nutrition of neonate
Kidney	urine	homeostasis
Gastric glands	HCl and pepsinogen	hydrolysis of proteins
Prostate	prostatic secretions	buffering of vaginal secretions

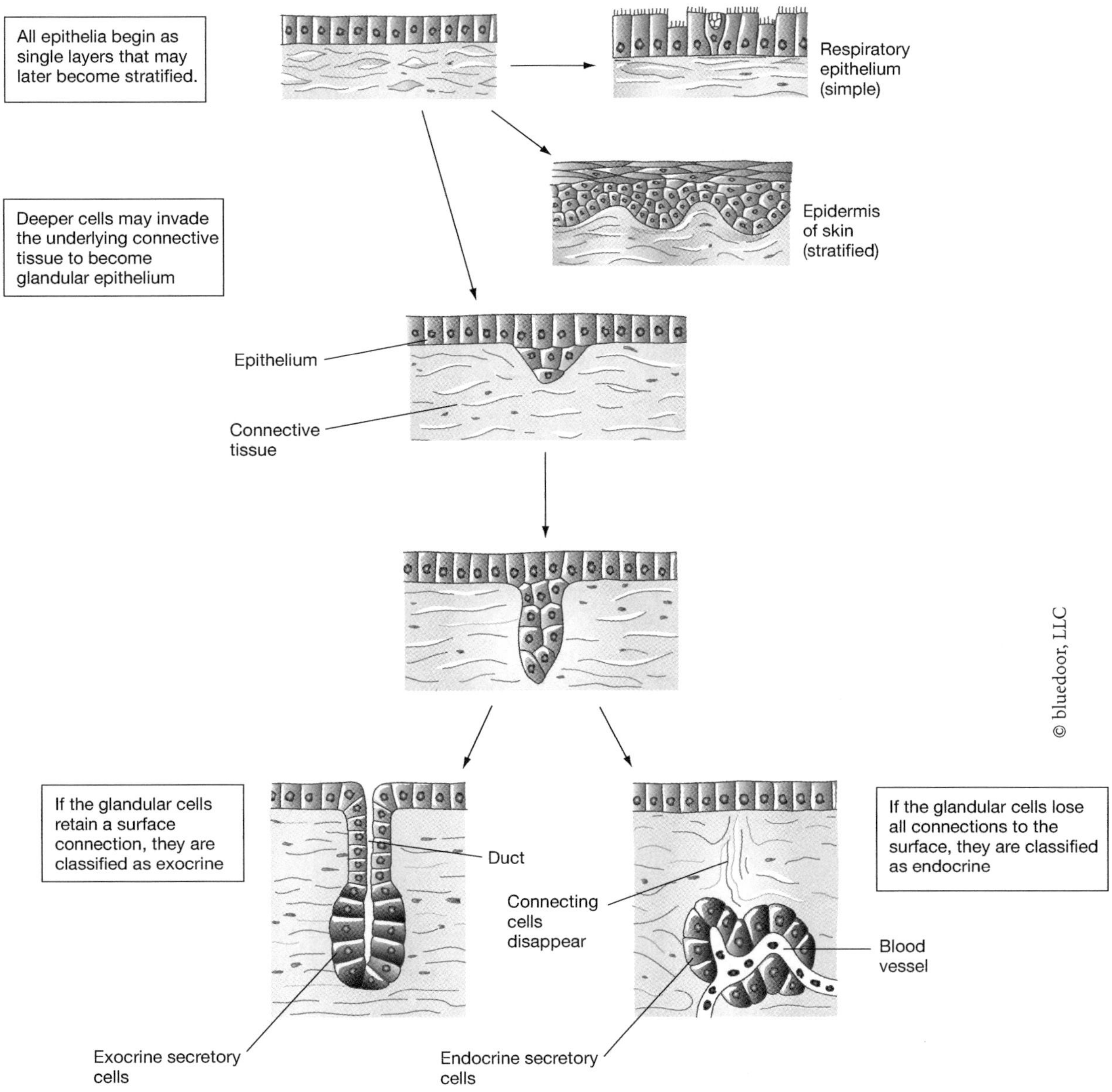

Figure 3-4

Development of Glandular Epithelium from Membranous Epithelium

All glandular epithelium develops from surface (membranous) epithelium. Membranous epithelium that becomes glandular (secretory) may remain on the surface, may maintain a surface contact in the form of a duct, or may lose surface contact altogether. In the first two instances, the glandular epithelium secretes exocrine products onto a free body surface and if all surface contact is lost, the epithelium secretes endocrine products (hormones) into the bloodstream.

ways" and flatten as the urinary bladder fills with urine, a distended urinary bladder wall appears to have fewer layers of epithelial cells in its lining than the wall of a non-distended bladder.

There are several modifications that the surface cells in membranous epithelia may possess. Some have **cilia** which are relatively long projections that the cells use to propel materials along the surface. When cilia are present, the word *ciliated* is added to the name (ciliated pseudostratified columnar epithelium). Some cells specialized for absorption (like those lining the intestine or parts

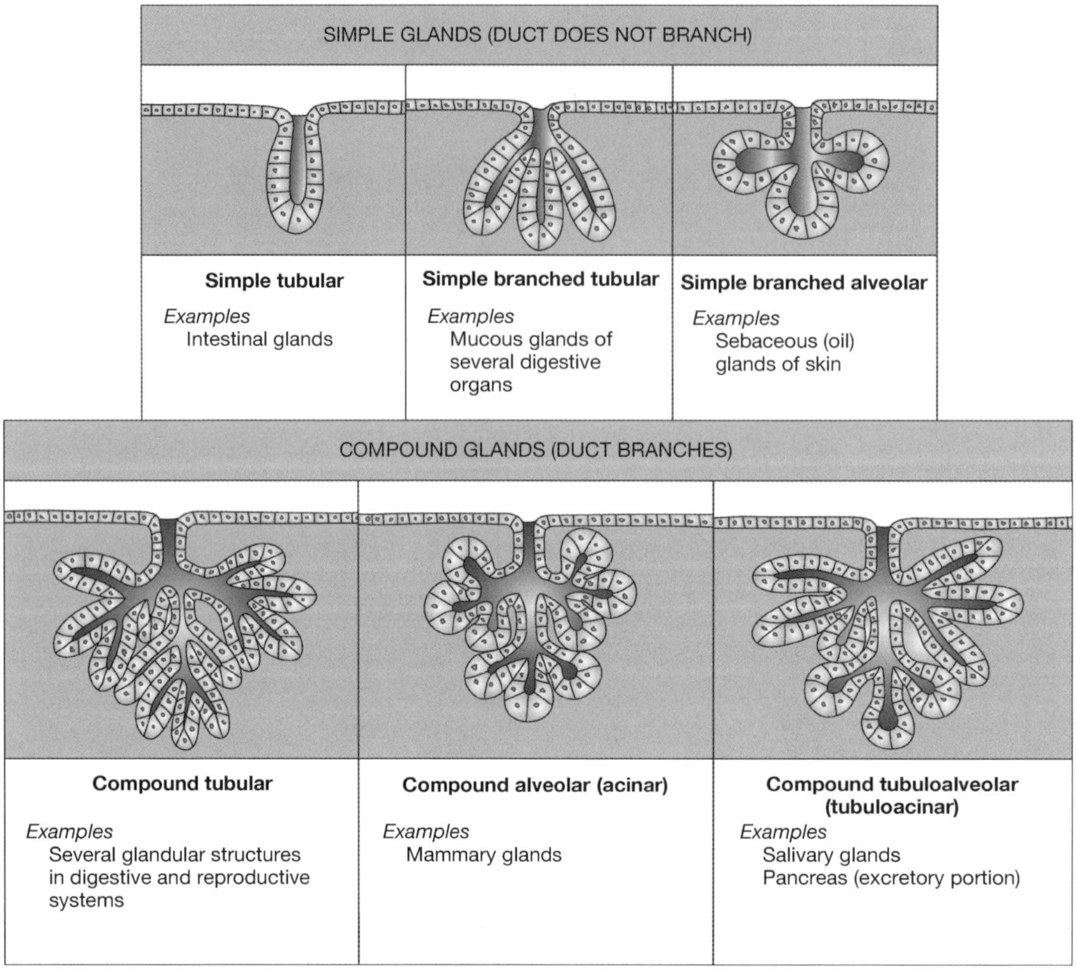

Figure 3-5

Classification of Multicellular Exocrine Glands

Simple and *compound* are used to indicate whether the duct is single or multiple. *Tubular, acinar* (alveolar), *tubuloacinar* (tubuloalveolar) are used to describe the overall shape of the mass of secretory cells.

of the renal tubules) have numerous projections similar to cilia but much smaller. These are called **microvilli** (singular = *microvillus*). Microvilli cannot be moved by the cell. Their apparent function is to increase the surface area in order to facilitate absorption. A third modification of the surface cells is keratinization. **Keratin** is a dense protein that is manufactured by the stratified squamous epithelium of the skin. It remains within the cells but imparts physical strength and resistance to desiccation (drying).

Glandular epithelium forms the secretory portion (parenchyma) of glands. The latter are organs that contain a significant structural framework (stroma) of connective tissue proper as well as several other kinds of tissue. Glandular epithelium differs structurally from membranous epithelium in three significant ways: it is highly vascularized, innervated, and lacks a basement membrane. Developmentally, all glandular epithelium is derived from membranous epithelium (Figure 3-4). Glandular epithelium that maintains a surface or lumen connection by being physically located at the surface (goblet cells) or by having a duct that reaches a body surface (or lumen) forms the secretory

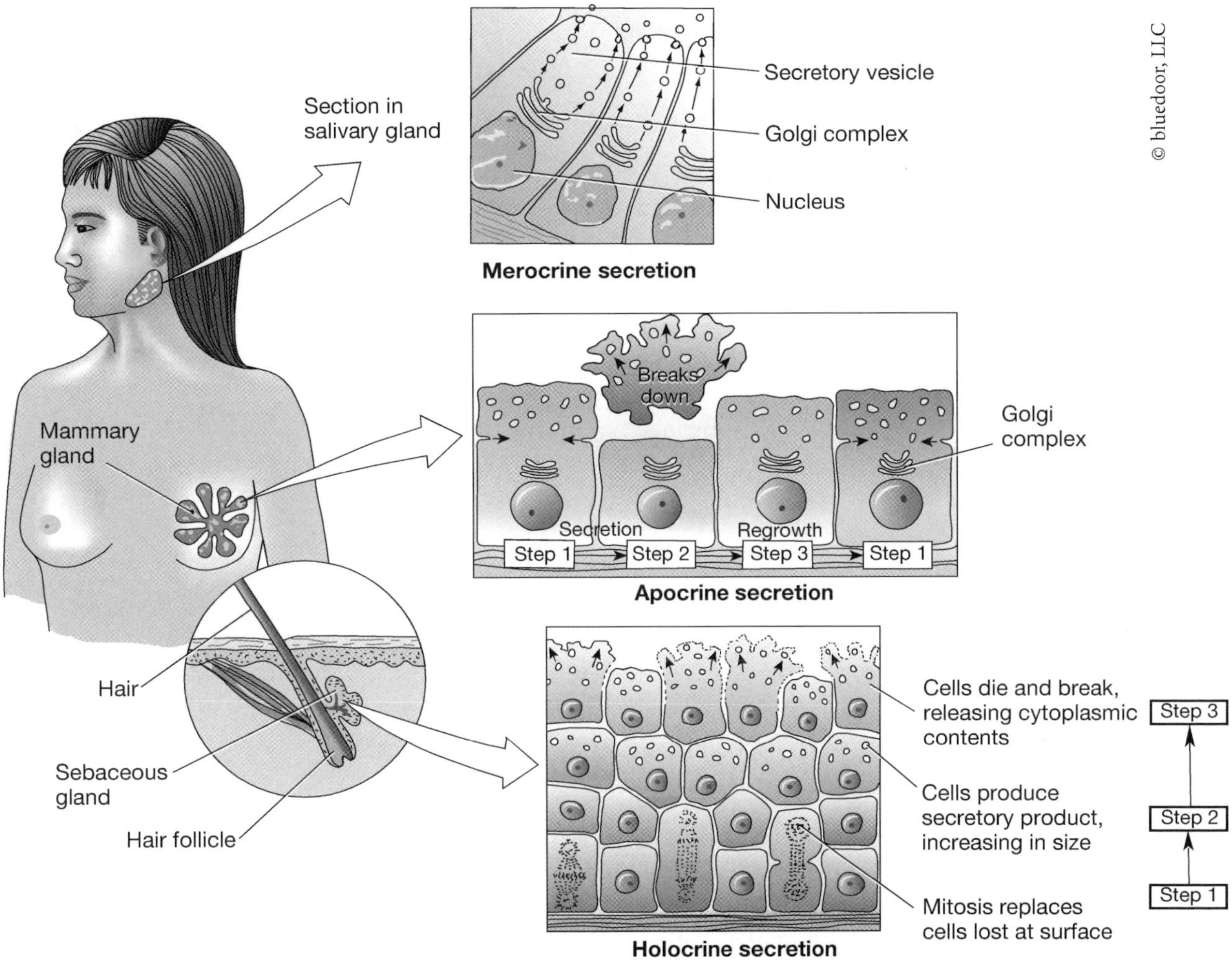

Figure 3-6

Modes of Secretion of Glandular Epithelial Cells

Glandular epithelium classified as merocrine (eccrine) secretes with no loss of microscopically visible portions of the cell structure. In apocrine secretion, a portion of the cell breaks away to form the secretory product. Holocrine secretion involves loss of whole cells into the secretory product.

portions of **exocrine glands**. These produce a variety of secretions as noted previously. Glands that lose all connections to the surface and secrete their products directly into the bloodstream are often called "endocrine glands" and their secretory products are called **hormones**. Officially (*Nomina Anatomica, 1989*), the term **endocrine gland** is reserved for the five glands that have no known function *except* hormone production (*see Chapter 14*). The term *ductless* is also used for endocrine glands by some authors but it is descriptively incorrect since it literally includes any gland lacking a duct. Therefore, it also includes goblet cells—the mucus producing unicellular exocrine glands within pseudostratified columnar epithelium in the respiratory passages and within the simple columnar epithelium of the intestinal lining. Some glands secrete both exocrine and endocrine products and are referred to as mixed glands (examples include the pancreas, intestine, testes, ovaries, *etc.*).

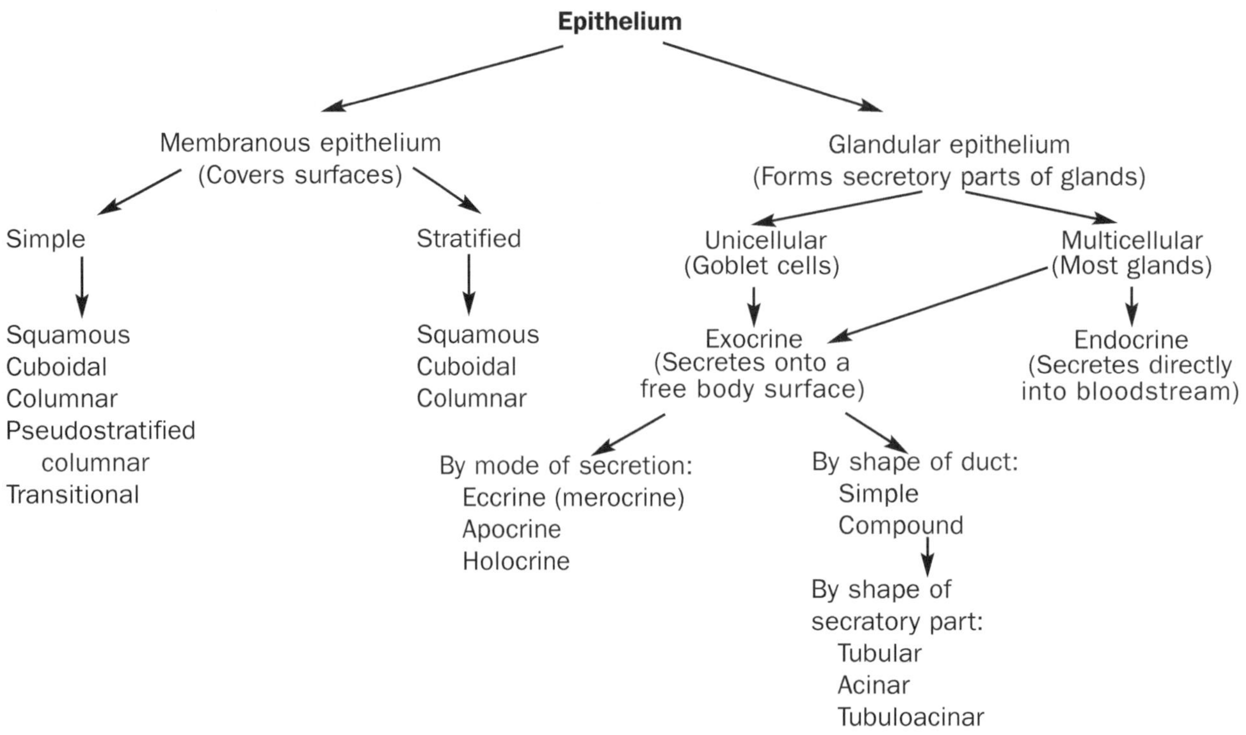

Figure 3-7

Classification of Epithelial Tissues

Endocrine glands are not further subdivided but exocrine glands are classified according to their mode of secretion as eccrine (merocrine), apocrine, or holocrine glands (Table 3-4 and Figure 3-6). They are also classified by the shape of their secretory units as *acinar* (spherical), *tubular*, *tubuloacinar*, and by the branching (*compound*) or non-branching (*simple*) of their ducts (Figure 3-5). Selected exocrine glands and their products are listed in Table 3-5. A flow chart of the taxonomy of epithelium is shown in Figure 3-7.

Objectives

4. Differentiate the two major categories of epithelium on the basis of blood supply, presence of basement membrane, and general location in body.
5. Classify membranous epithelium into six categories on the basis of its thickness (one cell/more than one cell) and the shape of the surface cells (squamous, cuboidal, columnar).
6. Name and state the location of two types of membranous epithelium that do not fit the usual classification scheme. Indicate what is meant by "respiratory" epithelium.
7. Discuss the kinds and functions of modifications found in the surface cells of membranous epithelium.
8. Define the following terms used to classify glandular epithelium and glands: endocrine/exocrine; simple/compound; acinar, tubular, tubuloacinar; eccrine (merocrine), apocrine, and holocrine.
9. Differentiate the development of endocrine *vs.* exocrine glands.

Connective Tissue

Connective tissue binds various parts of the body together, forms the structural framework of many body parts, and is also involved in the transport and exchange of nutrients and wastes. It consists of several types of **cells**, and an abundant **extracellular matrix** (usually) secreted by the cells. The latter includes **fibers** and **ground substance**. Because it retains a number of primitive (undifferentiated) cell types, connective tissue has a high regenerative capacity. In fact, traumatic injuries to muscle and nervous tissue (which have low regenerative capabilities) are repaired by the formation of a connective tissue scar. There are many different types of connective tissue (Table 3-6). These are differentiable on the basis of the types of cells, fibers, and ground substance present.

Connective tissue proper (**c.t. proper**) is also called **fibrous connective tissue** (Figure 3-8). It forms many structural parts of the body and is present to some degree in essentially all organs. There are several different kinds of cells in connective tissue proper, but the major one is called a fibroblast. **Fibroblasts** (called **fibrocytes** when they become older and relatively inactive) secrete three kinds of extracellular fibers as well as the ground substance of the matrix. The extracellular fibers include **collagenous fibers** (composed of a protein called **collagen**), **elastic fibers** (composed of a protein called **elastin**), and **reticular fibers** (made of a protein called **reticulin**). Collagenous fibers are relatively inelastic but are quite strong. Elastic fibers have a rubber-band-like ability to stretch and return to their original shape. Reticular fibers are structurally similar to very thin collagenous fibers. The ground substance present in connective tissue proper is an amorphous, jelly-like material chemically composed of protein/polysaccharide complexes. *Connective tissue proper* is classified by three simple criteria involving the fibers: **fiber density** (loose/dense), **fiber arrangement** (regular/irregular), and the major (predominant) **fiber type** present (Table 3-7). The loose/dense criterion is a subjective one referring to whether the fibers are tightly packed (dense) or have considerable space around them (loose). The regular/irregular criterion indicates whether the fibers are oriented in a relatively parallel manner (regular) or are not parallel to each other (irregular). The fiber type criterion simply indicates which fiber type predominates (all three types are present to some degree in most fibrous connective tissues). Using these criteria, a connective tissue proper that is classified as *dense, regular, collagenous connective tissue proper* has tightly packed fibers of collagen that are parallel to each other. *Loose, irregular connective tissue proper* (also known as areolar connective tissue) has loosely packed fibers that are not parallel to each other. The lack of a fiber type designation indicates that it is either unknown or not germane to the point being made. *Loose* connective tissues are always *irregular* (*i.e.*, loose regular c.t. proper does not exist in the body). Table 3-8 lists a number of structures that are composed primarily of c.t. proper.

Bone tissue is the main (but not only) structural component of the named bones of the body (Figure 3-9). It has three cell types: **osteoblasts** (which secrete the fibers and ground substance), **osteocytes** (old osteoblasts which become entrapped in little cavities within the matrix called **lacunae**), and **osteoclasts** (multinucleated giant cells that reabsorb bone tissue). The major fiber type secreted by osteoblasts is collagenous fibers. The feature that makes bone so hard is its mineral content. The mineral is modified forms of calcium phosphate and precipitates onto the collagenous fibers. Bone tissue is in a constant state of flux because there is slow but continuous formation and resorption. This will be discussed in greater detail in Chapters 5 and 6.

Cartilage has three cell types analogous to those of bone tissue: chondroblasts, chondrocytes, and chondroclasts. The matrix usually remains un-mineralized but is quite firm. This firm nature keeps the matrix from collapsing and forms lacunae around the **chondrocytes** and **chrondroblasts**. **Chondroblasts** (immature chondrocytes) arise from mesenchyme and form the extracellular matrix

Table 3-6 A Comparison of Different Types of Connective Tissue*

Type	*Major cells present*	*Fibers*	*Major subtypes*	*Locations in body*	*Peculiar features*
Connective tissue proper (Fibrous c.t.)	fibroblasts, fibrocytes, (and several others)	collagenous, elastic, reticular	loose/dense, regular/irregular, and fiber type taxonomy (collagenous, elastic, reticular)	tendons, ligaments, fascia, periosteum, endosteum, epimysium, plus a framework for most organs	present to some degree in all organs
Bone tissue	osteoblasts, osteocytes, osteoclasts	collagenous	compact, spongy	within the named bones of the body	has hard matrix because of mineral deposits, has cells in lacunae
Cartilage	chondroblasts, chondrocytes, chondroclasts	collagenous, elastic, "reticular"**	fibrocartilage, elastic cartilage, hyaline cartilage	articular surfaces of bones, costal cartilages, intervertebral discs, pinna of ear, tracheal cartilages	has firm matrix, has cells in lacunae
Blood	RBC's, WBC's	potential fibers (fibrinogen)		within organs of cardiovascular system	the only "liquid" tissue
Adipose tissue	adipose cells	collagenous		within subcutaneous tissue, medullary cavities of bones, peritoneum, pericardium	consists of many adipocytes within connective tissue proper
Reticular connective tissue	reticular cells	reticular		lymph nodes, spleen, thymus, medullary cavities of bones	requires special stains to demonstrate
Bone marrow tissue	hemocytoblasts and all of their derivatives	reticular		within medullary cavities of many bones	consists of reticular connective tissue plus differentiating blood cells
Primitive connective tissue (mesenchyme)	mesenchymal cells	very few present		nucleus pulposus of intervertebral discs, around vessels	can undergo rapid metaplasia for repair of damage

*The mineralized connective tissues associated with teeth (enamel, dentin, cementum) are mentioned in Chapter 17.

**These are very delicate collagenous fibers that resemble classical reticular fibers but vary slightly in structure. They are called reticular fibers by some authors.

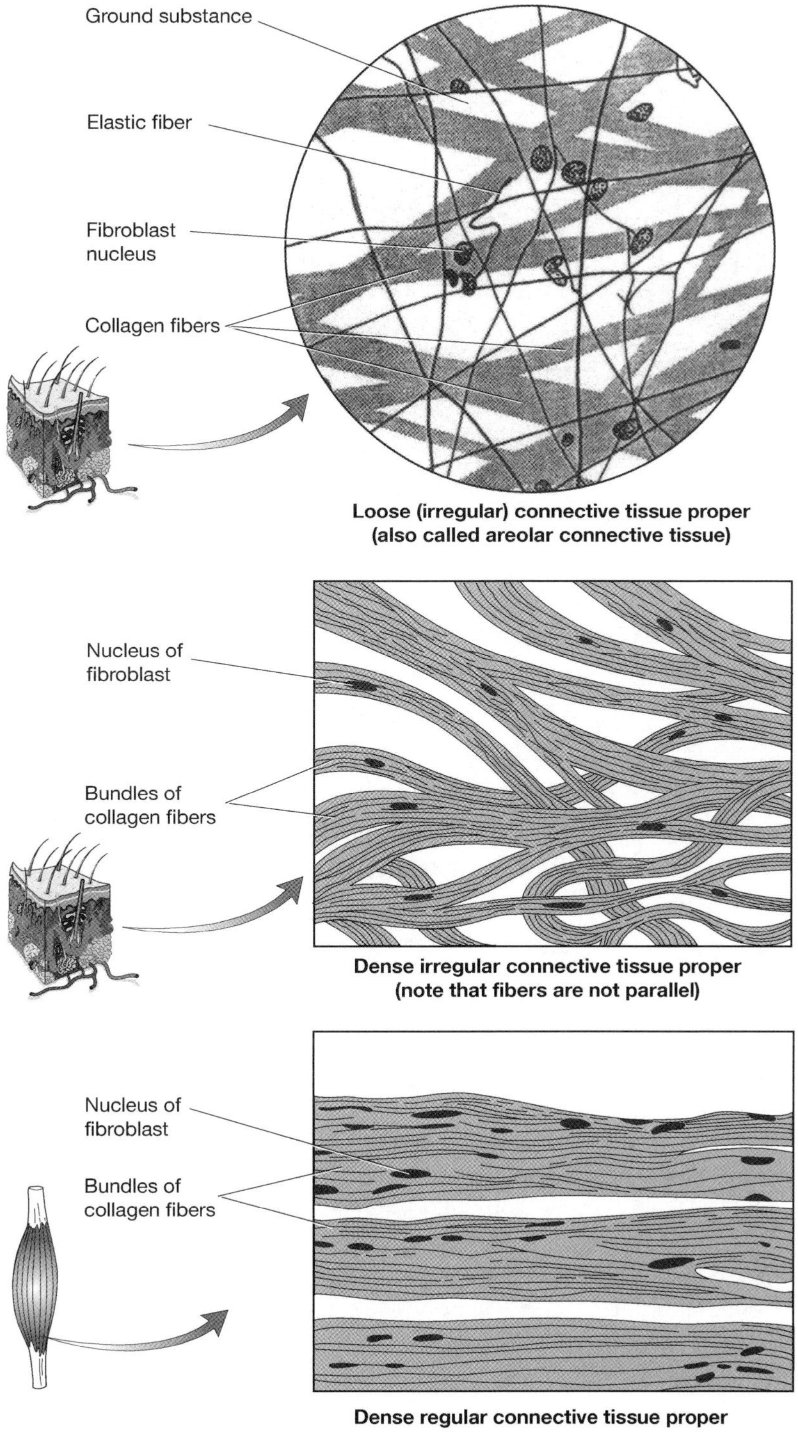

Figure 3-8

Examples of Connective Tissue Proper

Also known as fibrous connective tissue, connective tissue proper is classified on the basis of the density (dense/loose), and arrangement (regular/irregular), of its extracellular fibers. If the predominant type of protein in the fibers is known (collagenous, elastic, reticular), that, too, may be added to the name. Areolar connective tissue is abundant in the superficial fascia (hypodermis) that binds the skin to the underlying structures. Dense irregular connective tissue occurs in the dermis of the skin and in numerous other loci. Dense regular connective tissue occurs in tendons, ligaments, and retinaculae. Note that the cytoplasm/cell membrane of the fibroblasts are not clearly represented.

by secreting the fibers and ground substance. A **chondroclast** is a giant cell that absorbs cartilage. Like membranous epithelium, mature cartilage is avascular and receives all of its nutrition through diffusion. There are three types of cartilage based on the predominant fiber type present: fibrocartilage, elastic cartilage, and hyaline cartilage. In **fibrocartilage**, the dense collagenous fibers in the matrix impart strength and resistance to tearing and compression (Figure 3-10). Fibrocartilage forms the outer parts of the intervertebral discs (between the vertebrae) and forms menisci within some of the joints (*see Chapter 7*). There is also fibrocartilage present in the pubic symphysis which joins the two halves of the bony pelvis. **Elastic cartilage** has significant numbers of elastic fibers in the matrix which impart flexibility (Figure 3-10). It is found in the external ear and in parts of the larynx. **Hyaline cartilage** has delicate collagenous ("reticular") fibers within its matrix (Figure 3-10). The matrix itself has a clear (glassy) appearance when viewed microscopically (hyaline = *glassy*). Hyaline cartilage is found on the articular surfaces of bones where it is often called *articular cartilage*. This type of cartilage also forms the costal cartilages of the ribs, the cartilages within the trachea and bronchi, and some of those in the larynx. In addition, most of the bones are formed first of hyaline cartilage and later become osseous (*see Chapter 6*). Unlike bone tissue, once cartilage is formed, it is relatively static and has a very low turnover rate. Chondroclasts (cartilage resorbing cells) are present only in mineralized cartilage that is being removed as part of the endochondral ossification process (*see Chapter 6*). Selected cartilaginous structures are listed and defined in Table 3-9.

Blood is the only liquid tissue (Figure 3-11). It has all of the regular connective tissue components (cells, fibers, ground substance), but the ground substance is fluid because of its high water content and because its fibers (fibrinogen) remain soluble unless the clotting mechanism is activated (*fibrinogen* is converted to insoluble *fibrin*). The cells of blood include **red blood corpuscles** (**erythrocytes**) and several kinds of **white blood cells** (**leucocytes**). Blood transports nutrients, wastes, and hormones, and plays important roles in thermoregulation, acid/base balance, and body defense. It will be discussed in more detail in Chapter 15.

Table 3-7 Types of C.T. Proper Based on Fiber Density and Arrangement

Types	*Location/Comment*
Loose (irregular)* c.t. proper	Forms superficial fascia (hypodermis) which binds skin to underlying structures. This type is also called areolar connective tissue.
Dense irregular c.t. proper	Widely distributed structural component of many organs. It forms periosteum, endosteum, epi-, peri-, and endomysium, as well as epi- and perineurium.
Dense regular c.t. proper	The principle component of tendons, ligaments, and retinacula.

* Loose regular c.t. proper does not exist in the body.

Adipose tissue is a connective tissue that contains a large number of **adipose** (fat) **cells** (Figure 3-12). It occurs within subcutaneous tissues, within the medullary cavities of many bones, and is also deposited within the connective tissue layer of peritoneum and pericardium. Adipose tissue serves as a mobilizable stored energy source (some folks have more stored energy than others). In an average individual, over 10% of the total body weight is fat and this represents about a 40 day reserve of energy. Fat is the most efficient form of stored energy because it weighs less and occupies less volume than a calorie equivalent of carbohydrate or protein. Since man and other higher animals feed intermit-

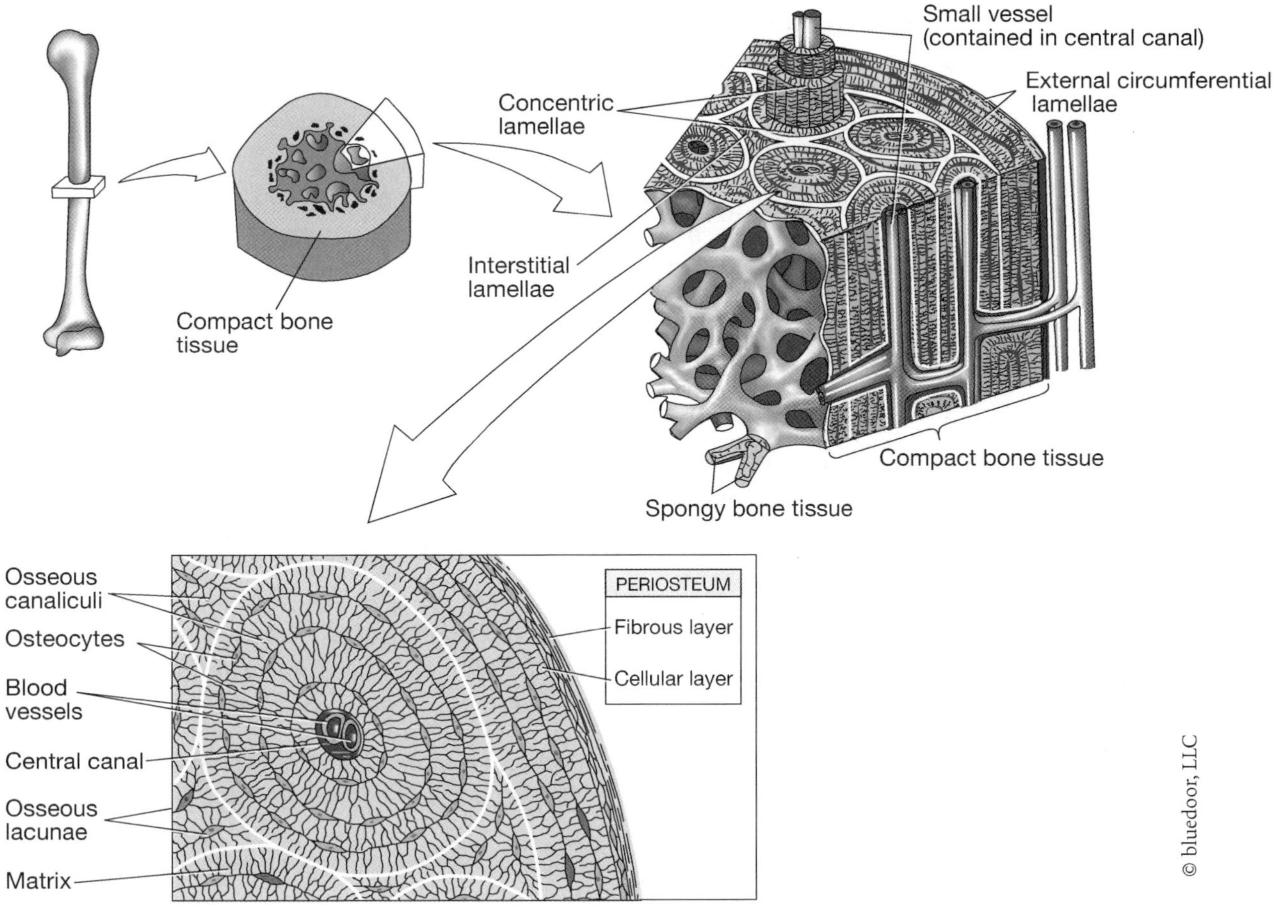

Figure 3-9

Bone Tissue

The cells found in the lacunae of bone tissue are called osteocytes. Before they became entrapped in the layers of extracellular matrix (lamellae) they were osteoblasts. The multinucleated bone tissue reabsorbing cells (osteoclasts) are not illustrated here. The periosteum on the outside of a bone is dense, irregular, collagenous connective tissue proper.

tently but consume energy continuously, adipose tissue plays a dynamic role in the body's energy cycle. Fat accumulates in periods of excess food intake, and is hydrolyzed, releasing fatty acids for energy during periods of fasting.

There are several other types of connective tissue including reticular connective tissue, bone marrow tissue, and primitive connective tissue. **Reticular connective tissue** consists of modified fibroblasts called **reticulocytes** that secrete reticular fibers. This specialized type of connective tissue is present in lymph nodes, spleen, thymus, and within the medullary cavities of the bones. **Bone marrow tissue** occurs in the medullary cavities of many bones. It consists of a myriad of blood cell precursor cells (hemocytoblast derivatives) interspersed in a framework of reticular connective tissue. **Primitive** (undifferentiated) **connective tissue** (also called **mesenchyme**) is found around blood vessels and within the intervertebral discs. It can undergo rapid metaplasia and differentiation when needed.

Table 3-8 Structures Composed Primarily of Connective Tissue Proper

Tendon	A dense regular collagenous c.t. proper band (cord) that attaches a muscle belly to its site of origin or insertion. Most muscles have at least two tendons. A broad, flat, sheet-like tendon is called an aponeurosis.
Ligament	A dense regular collagenous (usually) c.t. proper band that stabilizes skeletal structures at a joint. (Note: there are other ligaments that are associated with soft tissue structures and some of them are formed by serous membranes).
Fascia	The loose or dense irregular collagenous (usually) c.t. proper that binds the skin to underlying structures, vessels and nerves into neurovascular bundles, and muscle bellies into groups. Fascia is classified by location as superficial (= hypodermis = subcutaneous tissue) or deep.
Periosteum, endosteum	The dense irregular collagenous c.t. proper that encases a bone (periosteum) and lines its medullary cavity (endosteum).
Joint capsule	The dense irregular collagenous c.t. proper that surrounds/encloses the joint cavity of a synovial joint. It is lined by a synovial membrane.
Epi-, peri-, and endomysium	The dense irregular collagenous c.t. proper that encases a whole muscle belly (epimysium), a bundle of muscle cells within a muscle belly (perimysium), or an individual muscle cell (endomysium).
Epi-, peri, and endoneurium	The dense irregular collagenous c.t. proper that encases a whole nerve (epineurium), a bundle of fibers within a nerve (perineurium), or an individual nerve fiber (endoneurium).
Retinaculum	A dense regular collagenous c.t. proper band that binds tendons together and holds them in certain locations.
Periodontium	The dense irregular collagenous c.t. proper (sometimes called "periodontal membrane") that "glues" the roots of teeth into the dental alveoli to form gomphoses (dento-alveolar joints).
Dental pulp	The loose irregular connective tissue proper within the pulp cavities of teeth including the nerves and vessels therein.
Lamina propria	The loose or dense irregular c.t. proper that forms the middle (second) of the three layers of a mucous membrane (mucosa).
Submucosa	The loose or dense irregular c.t. proper that is found external to (superficial to) the mucosa that lines many of the visceral organs.
Meninx	Any of the three dense irregular collagenous c.t. proper encasements of the brain and spinal cord. They are named (from without inward): dura mater, arachnoid mater, and pia mater.
Adventitia	The loose or dense irregular collagenous c.t. proper that encases blood vessels and covers viscera in locations where serous membranes are not present.
Sclera	The dense irregular collagenous c.t. proper that forms much of the fibrous tunic of the eyeball. It is commonly called the "white" of the eye.
Dermis	The dense irregular collagenous c.t. proper that forms the deeper of the two main layers of the skin. It blends into the superficial fascia (hypodermis) which lies deep to it.
Hypodermis	The loose irregular connective tissue proper that binds the skin to underlying structures. (Hypodermis = subcutaneous tissue = superficial fascia.)

Table 3-9 Selected Cartilaginous Structures

Articular cartilage	The hyaline cartilage that forms bearing surfaces in synovial joints.
Articular disc	The fibrocartilaginous structure which separates the articulating surfaces in the radiocarpal*, acromioclavicular, sternoclavicular, and temporomandibular joints.
Articular meniscus	One of the two fibrocartilaginous structures found within each knee joint. These stabilize the joint and help distribute synovial fluid over the articular surfaces.
Auricular cartilage	The elastic cartilage that stiffens the external ear.
Cartilage of the auditory tube	The hyaline cartilage that supports the wall of the cartilaginous portion of the auditory ("eustachian") tube.
Cartilaginous external acoustic meatus	The hyaline cartilage portion of the external acoustic meatus. It lies lateral to the bony channel.
Costal cartilage	The hyaline cartilage extension of the bony part of a rib.
Epiphyseal cartilage ("growth plate," "epiphyseal plate")	The hyaline cartilage that separates the ossified portions of growing bones.
Glenoid labrum, acetabular labrum	The fibrocartilaginous rims around the glenoid cavity of the scapula and the acetabulum of the os coxae, respectively. These deepen the "sockets" formed.
Interpubic disc	The fibrocartilaginous pad that connects the pubic bones to form the pubic symphysis.
Intervertebral disc	The fibrocartilaginous connection between the bodies of adjacent vertebrae.
Laryngeal cartilage	Any of the nine hyaline and elastic cartilages that stiffen the larynx (thyroid, cricoid, epiglottic, and paired arytenoid, cuneiform and corniculate cartilages).
Nasal cartilage	Any of the hyaline or elastic cartilages that lend stiffness but flexibility to the antero-inferior aspect of the nose and the nasal septum. These include lateral nasal, greater and lesser alar, nasal septal, vomeronasal, and accessory nasal cartilages.
Tracheal cartilage	Any of the C-shaped hyaline cartilages that add rigidity to the tracheal wall. Smaller pieces of hyaline cartilage stiffen the bronchial walls.
Xiphoid process	The inferior portion of the sternum. It has an osseous and a hyaline cartilage component. The latter tends to ossify with age.

In addition to these structures, there are tiny cartilages within the cricothyroid ligament, within the edges of the eyelids, and sometimes (inconsistently) in the vocal ligaments and lateral head of the gastrocnemius muscle. The hyaline cartilages forming the cranial synchondroses have no other anatomical designations. Mineralization of these structures as well as others listed above may occur with time.

*Some references indicate that this cartilage is associated with the distal radio-ulnar joint. Positionally, however, it completes the articulation between the antebrachial skeleton and the proximal row of carpal bones. Therefore, associating it with the radiocarpal joint seems more appropriate.

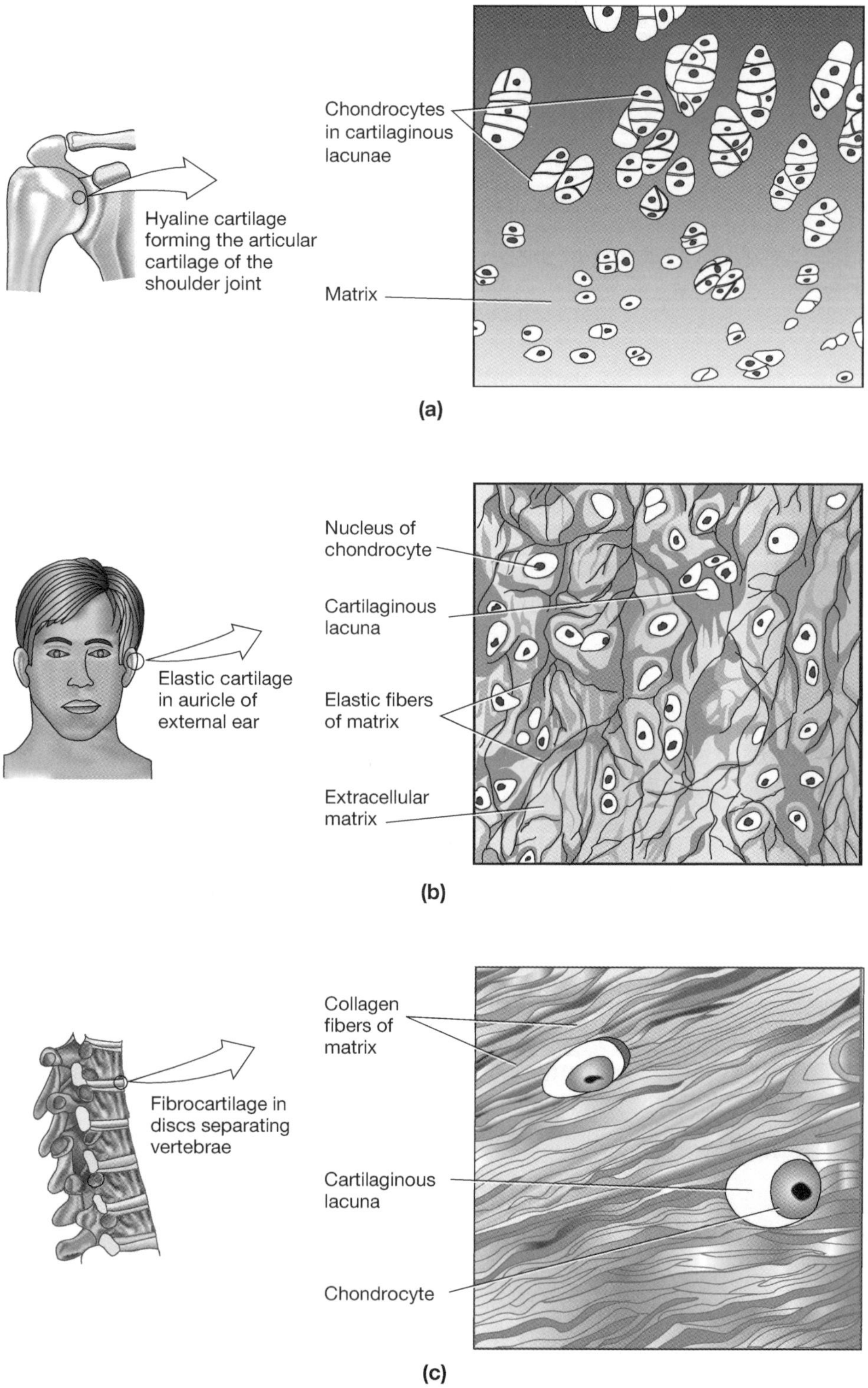

Figure 3-10

The Three Types of Cartilage

The three types of cartilage have different kinds of extracellular fibers. In hyaline cartilage (a) the fibers are delicate and made of reticulin-like protein. They have the same refractive index as the ground substance and therefore cannot be distinguished histologically. In sections of elastic cartilage (b) and fibrocartilage (c) the fibers (elastin and collagen, respectively) are easily seen.

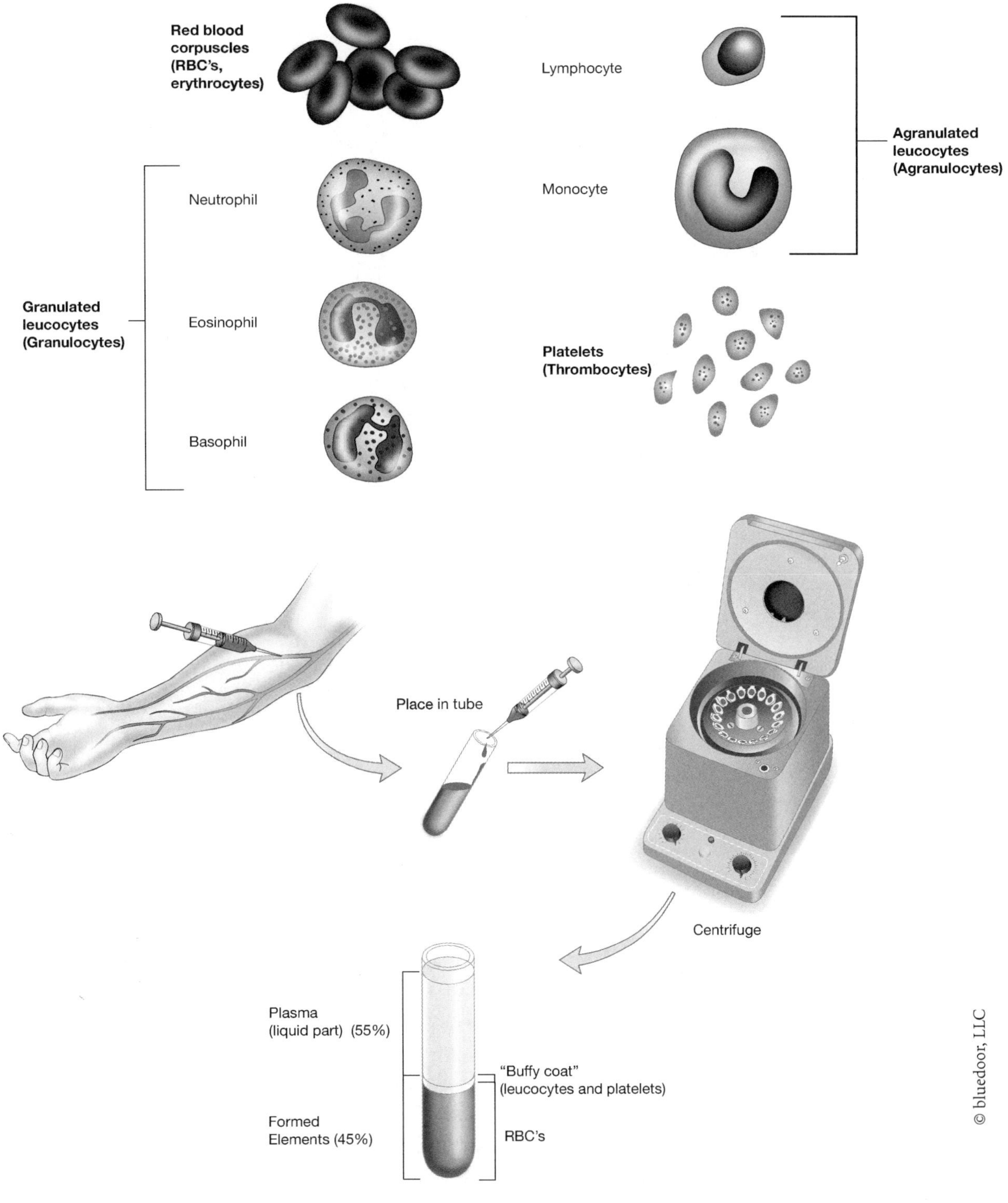

Figure 3-11

The Components of Blood

Blood is the only liquid tissue. (The cellular content of lymph is so low that it is usually not considered to be a tissue.) The ground substance of blood is mostly water and the "fibers" occur in the form of a water-soluble protein called fibrinogen. Only when the clotting mechanism is activated does fibrinogen become insoluble to form true extracellular fibers called fibrin.

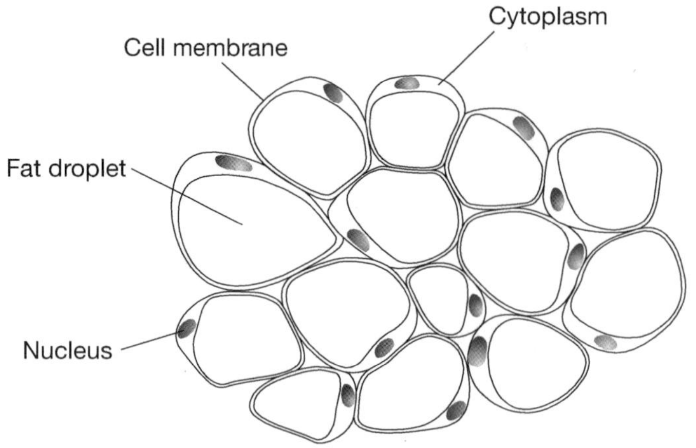

Figure 3-12
Adipose Tissue

Adipose tissue consists of large groups of fat cells (adipocytes) within connective tissue proper. The fat cells have huge fat deposits (droplets) within their cytoplasm.

Objectives

10. List three components found in all connective tissues, list the major types of connective tissue, and state where they are located in the body.
11. Classify connective tissue proper (fibrous connective tissue) on the basis of density, arrangement, and fiber composition.
12. Name the subtypes of cartilage and state the predominant fiber type present in each.

Nervous Tissue

Nervous tissue is specialized for the conduction of electrical impulses. Like epithelium, nervous tissue contains very little intercellular material (except for some connective tissue proper encasements of peripheral nerve cell processes). It consists of neurons (nerve cells) and several types of supporting cells termed neuroglia. **Neurons** are so specialized that they cannot divide. Thus, nervous tissue has a low regenerative capacity and injuries to it are serious and often permanent. A neuron consists of a central portion called the **cell body** and two or more processes which conduct impulses (Figure 3-13). Processes that conduct impulses toward the cell bodies are termed **dendrites**. Some neurons have only one dendrite and others have several. Neuronal processes that carry impulses away from the cell bodies are called **axons**. Most neurons have only one axon but it may branch. Based on the number and arrangement of their processes, neurons are classified morphologically as multipolar, bipolar, or pseudounipolar (*see Chapter 9*). The impulses carried by some neurons transmit sensory (incoming) information into the spinal cord and brain. Other neurons transmit motor (outgoing) information that is ultimately distributed to muscle and gland cells. The axonic and dendritic processes of neurons which carry these impulses are often collectively called **nerve fibers**.

Neuroglia (**neuroglial cells**) include several (six) types of supporting cells found in nervous tissue. They do not conduct nervous impulses but perform a number of other functions. Neuroglia and neurons will be more fully discussed in Chapter 9.

Objectives

13. Differentiate the two groups of cells found in nervous tissue.
14. Define axon and dendrite.

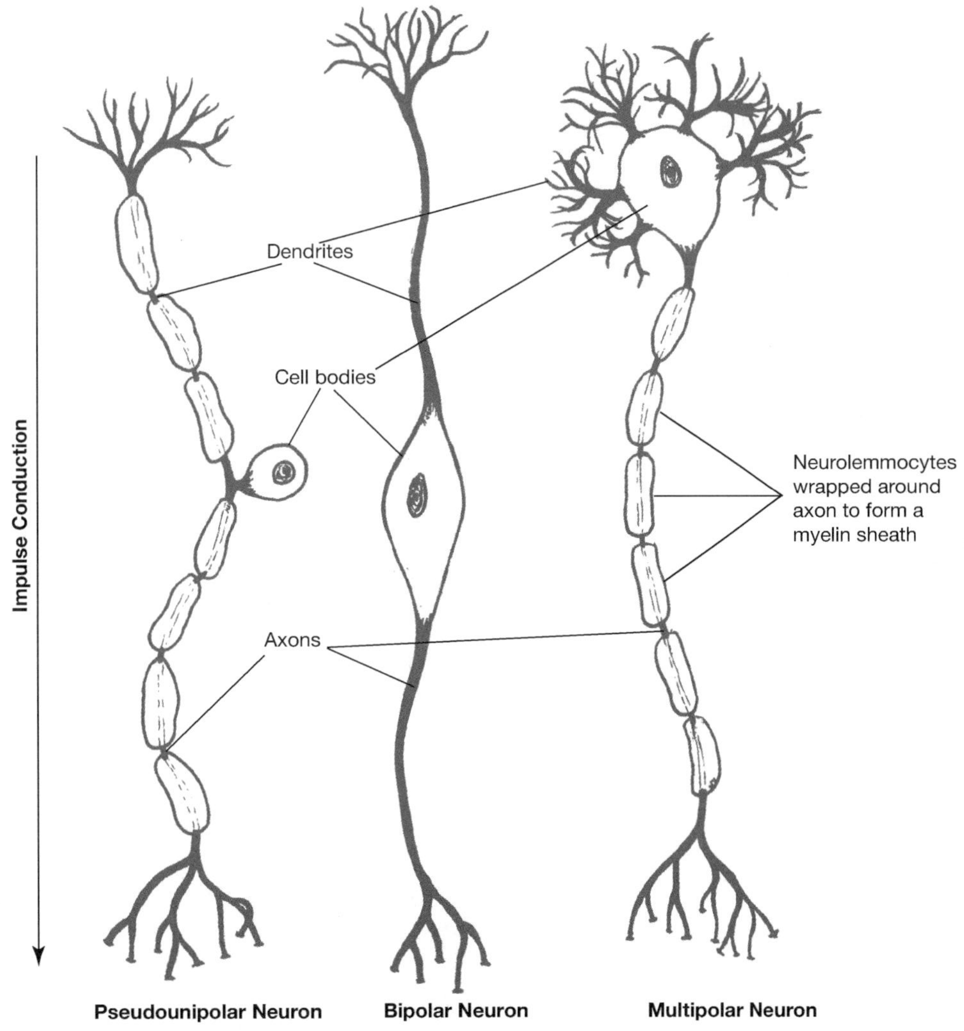

Figure 3-13

Anatomic Types of Neurons

Neurons are specialized for the conduction of nervous impulses. Their processes are classified on the basis of the direction of impulse conduction as dendrites (toward cell body) or axons (away from cell body). Some neurons are myelinated, which speeds up the conduction of impulses.

Clinical Considerations

The **regenerative capacity** of the various tissues (low in muscle and nervous tissue, high in epithelium and connective tissue) is significant in predicting the long term outcome of various types of injuries. Organs composed primarily of epithelium and connective tissue (skin, liver) can recover from serious and/or continuous insults to a much greater degree than structures containing larger portions of muscle and/or nervous tissue. Neurons and skeletal muscle cells in adults totally lack the ability to divide. Consequently, each of these cells that is lost due to an injury cannot be replaced.

Skeletal muscle tissue has a close physiological relationship with its nerve supply. Lacking inherent contractility, skeletal muscle tissue is totally dependent on its motor nerve supply. A relatively small wound that severs a peripheral nerve will **paralyze** all skeletal muscles supplied by that nerve (distal to the point of injury). However, since nerves are composed of only the processes of neurons, the motor neuron cell bodies may survive the injury and regenerate their axonal processes. Unfortunately, in many cases scar tissue (c.t. proper) may preclude the re-establishment of any connection between the axons and the skeletal muscle cells that they originally supplied. In these cases, the loss of contractile ability remains permanent and the skeletal muscles involved undergo rapid atrophy.

Scarring in the skin (and in many other structures) results from the proliferation of connective tissue proper after an injury. Skin scars can be minimized by close apposition of the wound edges and careful attention to asepsis. Connective tissue proper also "heals" ruptured skeletal muscles by physiologically "gluing" the severed ends back together. In some cases, proliferation of c.t. proper has deleterious effects. For example, individuals who consume large volumes of alcohol injure their liver cells (glandular epithelium). The latter readily divide and regenerate. However, the scarring that also occurs due to connective tissue ingrowth crowds out the liver cells. The resulting loss of the liver's ability to perform its functions in the body (detoxification, intermediary metabolism, *etc.*) can eventually result in death.

One of the relatively recent developments in medicine is **transplant technology** wherein major organs (heart, lungs, kidneys) can be removed from one individual (donor) and implanted in another one (recipient). These are remarkable achievements given the number of intricate connections which must be re-established and the delicate nature of the structures involved. An additional obstacle which must be minimized is rejection of the foreign tissues by the recipient. Like blood, many other tissues of the body have "types" that may elicit an immune response in the recipient that ultimately causes transplantation failure (rejection). For that reason, close blood relatives (and ideally identical twins) typically make good transplant donors. In some cases, rejection can be averted with chemotherapy.

Histopathology is the branch of medicine involved in the microscopic examination and evaluation of body tissues. Samples may be collected from tissues removed during surgery or by a special procedure (**biopsy**) where a small sample is harvested especially for histopathological examinations. Some pure tissue samples such as blood, mature cartilage, and some membranous epithelia can be taken without being contaminated by other types of tissues. Tissue samples may undergo complex chemical preparation to form permanent sections for microscopic viewing, or they may be subjected to a quicker but less permanent procedure called frozen sectioning.

Clinical Case Studies

Case 1—During a surgical approach to the hip joint, an orthopedic surgeon needed to reflect a skeletal muscle from the surgical field. Rather than transect (cut) the muscle and then retract (pull) the severed ends out of the way, he chose to cut the bony prominence where the tendon of the muscle inserted and reflect the whole muscle including the freed piece of bone. At the conclusion of the surgery, integrity of the muscle was restored by replacing the avulsed piece of bone and stabilizing it with a stainless steel bone screw. Why did the surgeon elect to cut bone tissue rather than muscle or its tendon?

Case 2—A 35-year-old college professor had noticeably unstable knees and shoulders. He had to undergo surgery to stabilize recurring dislocations of his left shoulder. All of his problems occurred in spite of the fact that he had never participated in high risk activities. Analysis of collagen from a biopsy of one of his tendons indicated an abnormal amino acid sequence. How could this fact relate to his clinical problems?

Case 3—A 40-year-old truck driver sought medical advice regarding a very hard, dime-sized knot that formed on his leg after healing of a wound suspected of being a brown recluse ("fiddleback") spider bite. Histopathologic exam of a biopsy from the lesion indicated the presence of heavy calcification and no living cells were present in the center of the mass. What conclusion did the pathologist draw?

Points to Ponder

The tissues forming the organs of the human body demonstrate a remarkable degree of stratification. Outer surfaces and luminal linings are always formed of membranous epithelium (which itself is typically layered). Adjacent to the epithelium is connective tissue proper, and the next tissue is usually muscle. Taking the intestinal wall as an example and beginning on its luminal surface, the tissues encountered are epithelium, connective tissue proper, muscle tissue, connective tissue proper, and then muscle, connective tissue proper, and finally epithelium on the outside. Each of these layers has specific functional roles including absorption, peristalsis, serving as an avenue of penetration for vessels and nerves, *etc.*

Developmentally, tissues differentiate primarily due to the types of proteins that their component cells manufacture. For example, cells that become muscle cells manufacture large amounts of actin and myosin—two of the contractile proteins characteristic of muscle cells. The types of proteins manufactured depend primarily on which parts of a cell's DNA are transcribed. The exact mechanisms that determine the parts of the DNA utilized remain largely unknown. However, considerable active research is ongoing in this area.

During surgical procedures, physicians are cognizant of the organs and tissues that they must, of necessity, damage. A surgeon forced to transect a muscle, for example, will attempt to do so near the junction of the contractile portion and its tendinous attachment(s). This minimizes the damage to the nerve and blood supply (which usually enters the belly of the muscle). In addition, the fibrous connective tissue scar which forms to heal the transection will have less effect on the contractile ability of the muscle after healing occurs if it is located at the periphery of the muscle belly.

Diseases often significantly affect the structure of the tissues within one or more organs. Consequently, microscopic examinations of surgical or biopsy specimens can often lead to a diagnosis or prognosis. To view organs microscopically, extremely thin sections are cut on specialized machines called microtomes and subjected to staining procedures to color the tissues.

Just as human blood has "types", there are tissue types that may lead to immunological incompatibilities and possible postsurgical rejection after organ transplants. This problem and the mechanics of the surgery itself are the two greatest challenges in organ transplantation procedures. The most successful types of transplants involve movement of structures within the same individual—such as translocating some normal skin to a severely burned area on the same individual. These types of autotransplants avoid immunological incompatibilities altogether. In homotransplants (same species, different individuals) or heterotransplants (different species) rejection of the transplant by the recipient is quite common. Transplant surgeons try to minimize rejection as much as possible via matching recipient and donor tissue. Immuno-suppressive drugs also are used post-surgically to increase chances of success.

Although technology exists to successfully transplant most organs, brains and spinal cords remain beyond abilities of medical science at the present time. The connections that would have to be made are too numerous and too intricate. If this is accomplished in the future, one cannot help but wonder to whom one might be speaking—the donor or the recipient!

Slang and Obsolete Nomenclature

UNOFFICIAL TERM	OFFICIAL DESIGNATION
respiratory epithelium	ciliated pseudostratified columnar epithelium *[epithelium pseudostratificatum columnare ciliatum]*
bone (the tissue)	bone tissue *[textus osseus]*
Wharton's jelly	mesenchyme *[mesenchyma]*
bone marrow	bone marrow tissue *[textus myeloideus]*
smooth muscle (the tissue)	smooth muscle tissue *[textus muscularis nonstriatus]*
skeletal muscle (the tissue)	skeletal muscle tissue *[textus muscularis skeletalis]*
cardiac muscle (the tissue)	cardiac muscle tissue *[textus muscularis cardiacus]*
basic germ layer	(primary) germ layer *[stratificatio germinalis]*
primary tissue	basic tissue

Review Questions

1. Find the false statement.
   A. The cells of nervous tissue that conduct impulses are called neurons.
   B. Reticular connective tissue is a major component of many lymphatic organs.
   C. Adipose tissue resembles connective tissue proper that contains a lot of fat cells.
   D. Cells, fibers, and ground substance are the three major components of any connective tissue.
   E. Cartilage is a connective tissue that has a mineralized matrix.

2. Which item is false?
   A. Membranous epithelium is called "simple" if it is one cell thick and "stratified" if it is two or more cells thick.
   B. Smooth muscle tissue is striated.
   C. Muscle tissue and connective tissue have more than two major subtypes each.
   D. Skeletal muscle tissue has cells a few centimeters long and is voluntary.
   E. Epithelial tissue and nervous tissue have very little intercellular material.

3. Which of the following is not a subtype of connective tissue?
   A. blood
   B. bone tissue
   C. bone marrow tissue
   D. cartilage
   E. fibroblast

4. Which of the following is not one of the named cell shapes found in membranous epithelia?
   A. cuboidal
   B. spherical
   C. squamous
   D. columnar
   E. Choose this response if all of the above are names of cell shapes found in membranous epithelia.

5. Find the mismatch.
   A. epithelial tissue—endoderm—high regenerative capacity
   B. connective tissue—mesoderm—low regenerative capacity
   C. muscle tissue—mesoderm—low regenerative capacity
   D. nervous tissue—ectoderm—low regenerative capacity
   E. Choose this response if all the above (A-D) are correctly matched.

6. Find the incorrect statement.
   A. Glandular epithelium is derived from membranous epithelium.
   B. Merocrine glands secrete watery secretions containing parts of the secretory cells.
   C. Eccrine glands secrete watery secretions.
   D. Ear wax is secreted by a holocrine gland.
   E. Only surface epithelia have basement membranes.

7. Which of the following is mismatched.
   A. skeletal muscle tissue—biceps brachii muscle—involuntary
   B. cardiac muscle tissue—aorta—involuntary
   C. smooth muscle tissue—most arteries—nonstriated
   D. cardiac muscle tissue—heart—striated
   E. smooth muscle tissue—mucous membrane—fusiform

8. Find the false statement.
   A. Scarring results from the proliferation of c.t. proper after an injury.
   B. Neurons are composed of dendrites, axons, and cell bodies.
   C. There are several (six) different types of neuroglial cells.
   D. Fibrous connective tissue can be found to some degree in all body organs.
   E. Primitive connective tissue can undergo rapid hyperplasia when needed.

9. Find the mismatch within the following associations.
   A. adipose tissue: collagenous fibers—adipose cells—subcutaneous tissue
   B. blood: potential fibers—RBC's—veins
   C. bone tissue: elastic fibers—osteoblasts—clavicle
   D. bone marrow tissue: reticular fibers—hemocytoblasts—medullary cavity of a bone
   E. cartilage: elastic fibers — chondrocytes—pinna of ear

10. Find the false statement.
   A. Smooth muscle tissue and skeletal muscle tissue have inherent rhythmicity.
   B. Blood is the only liquid tissue.
   C. Both bone and cartilaginous tissues have lacunae.
   D. Most exocrine glands have ducts.
   E. Keratin is a dense proteinaceous material that imparts strength and resistance to desiccation in the skin.

Thought Questions

1. What is the difference between...
   A. Bone tissue and a bone?
   B. Skeletal muscle tissue and a skeletal muscle?
   C. Glandular epithelium and a gland?

2. Do all exocrine glands have ducts? Explain.

3. Outline which of the four basic tissues develop from which of the three primary germ layers.

4. Although only four basic tissues are recognized, some cells in the body blur the taxonomical boundaries between them. Which *two* basic tissues do each of the following seem to emulate?
   A. The specialized cardiac muscle cells of the heart (called purkinje fibers) that are involved in transmitting the impulses that initiate cardiac muscle contraction.
   B. Neurons in the supraoptic and paraventricular nuclei of the hypothalamus that secrete oxytocin and antidiuretic hormone.
   C. Myoepithelial cells in the mammary gland that are involved in milk ejection.

5. Any structure that has a blood supply contains blood vessels which include connective tissue (blood in the lumen and c.t. proper in the vessel walls), muscle tissue (smooth muscle in the blood vessel wall), and epithelium (lining the lumina). What structures in the body are avascular?

6. A structure is said to be apocrine. What else does this word imply about the item?

7. What is the fiber density and fiber arrangement of areolar connective tissue?

8. Collagen fibers may be much larger than the cells (fibroblasts) that secrete them. How is this possible?

9. Why are injuries to epithelium and connective tissue less debilitating (in general) than injuries to muscle tissue and nervous tissue?

10. One cannot reach muscle tissue without first passing through which two other basic tissues?

11. Loss of nerve supply to skeletal muscles paralyzes them but loss of innervation to smooth muscle tissue does not prevent contraction. Explain this difference.

12. Blood is the only liquid tissue but not the only liquid found in the body. Why are the other liquids not considered to be tissues?

13. Name the two basic tissues present in all organs.

14. What cell manufactures the components of the extracellular matrix in fibrous connective tissue?

15. Which two types of membranous epithelium do not exemplify the standard membranous epithelium classification criteria? Where are each of these found in the body?

16. Why are alternative names for some specific types of tissue developed (*i.e.*, areolar tissue for loose connective tissue proper and *respiratory epithelium* for ciliated pseudostratified columnar epithelium)?

17. How can the rhythmic "beating" (movements) of cilia move materials along a cell's surface? (When the cilia go back to their original position for another "stroke", why doesn't that motion move the material back to its original position?

18. Since muscle cells don't regenerate, how does a transected muscle heal?

19. What are the three major differences between bone tissue and cartilage?

20. List the differences between membranous and glandular epithelium.

21. Which organs contain only three of the four basic tissues?

Answers to Clinical Case Studies

Case 1—Surgeons avoid transecting the bellies of skeletal muscles whenever possible because disruption of the blood and nerve supply, coupled with the fact that skeletal muscle tissue does not regenerate, will reduce the postsurgical contractile ability. Tendons are sometimes transected, but they are not easily reconstructed. Bone tissue, on the other hand, readily regenerates, is readily replaced by the body, and heals with no loss of function.

Case 2—The abnormal amino acid sequence in collagen could likely explain the relative weakness in this individual's joints. Collagen is the principle fiber type in several connective tissue proper structures of the body including tendons and ligaments. Since this patient suffered multiple problems which all appeared to be related to weak, stabilizing connective tissue structures, it would be logical to assume that he had a genetic (DNA) defect resulting in an inborn error of metabolism which produced the weakened collagen.

Case 3—Abnormal presence of mineralization in soft tissues sometimes occurs but the exact cause remains unclear. This lesion, dubbed "metaplastic calcification" by the pathologist who examined the biopsy, caused the patient no particular problems but was analyzed to rule out the possibility of cancer. Over a several year period, the lesion did not enlarge and did not change in character.

Answers to Review Questions

1. E. Cartilage can mineralize, but most cartilage contains very little mineral.

2. B. Lack of histological striations is why it is called *smooth* muscle tissue.

3. E. Fibroblasts are cells.

4. B. Some cuboidal cells may be almost spherical, however.

5. B. Connective tissue is derived from mesoderm but it has high regenerative capacity.

6. B. The description given is true for apocrine glands.

7. A. Skeletal muscle tissue is voluntary. Cardiac muscle tissue is striated, involuntary and is found in the heart and in some large vessels near the heart.

8. E. Primitive connective tissue can undergo rapid metaplasia when needed.

9. C. Mature bone tissue does not contain elastic fibers.

10. A. Skeletal muscle tissue (and even some smooth muscle tissue) lacks inherent rhythmicity.

Answers to Thought Questions

1. The first item listed in all three instances is a specific kind of *tissue*. The second item is an *organ* that contains several kinds of tissue.

2. Most exocrine glands have ducts but not all of them do. The unicellular glands called goblet cells are located on a surface so no duct is needed to transport the secretory product.

3. Nervous tissue is derived from ectoderm, muscle tissue and connective tissue proper are derived from mesoderm. Epithelium is derived from all three primary germ layers (ectoderm, mesoderm, and endoderm).

4. A. Muscle tissue and nervous tissue.
   B. Nervous tissue and epithelium.
   C. Muscle tissue and epithelium.

5. Membranous epithelium and its derivatives (nails, hair), serous membranes, mature cartilage.

6. Apocrine also implies *exocrine* and *glandular epithelium.*

7. Areolar connective tissue is loose and irregular in regard to its fiber density and arrangement.

8. Fibroblasts manufacture subunits (tropocollagen) that are assembled as they leave the cell into (onto) growing collagen fibers.

9. Epithelium and connective tissue have high regenerative capacity. Thus, when damaged, they are capable of healing the injury by proliferating the same tissue. Nervous tissue and muscle tissue have much lower regenerative capacity.

10. Epithelium (membranous) which covers/lines all surfaces of the body and connective tissue (proper) which lies deep to all membranous epithelia.

11. Skeletal muscle tissue lacks inherent rhythmicity. Consequently it must have a nerve supply to contract. Smooth muscle tissue (and cardiac muscle tissue) do have inherent rhythmicity and therefore do not need a nerve supply to contract. They are innervated, however, and the nerve supply affects the *frequency* of contraction.

12. Their cell content is too low to qualify them as tissues.

13. Epithelium and connective tissue. The simplest organs include capillaries and serous membranes.

14. Fibroblasts typically manufacture both components of the extracellular matrix (fibers and ground substance).

15. Transitional epithelium (lining the ureters, urinary bladder, and initial part of the urethra) and (ciliated) pseudostratified columnar epithelium (lining the conducting passageways of the respiratory system).

16. Some of the official descriptive names are unwieldy and cumbersome.

17. Cilia use the same general principle involved in the wing beats of a bird or the swimming strokes of a freestyler—the *power* stroke and the *recovery (re-cock)* stroke are *not* the exact same motions in reverse.

18. Connective tissue proper proliferates to form a scar that fuses the severed ends together.

19. Different types of cells are present in each, different ground substances, and bone tissue has a significant mineral content while cartilage does not.

20. Membranous epithelium is aneural, avascular, and the cells occur in three general shape categories (cuboidal, columnar, and squamous). Glandular epithelium has a nerve and blood supply and the cells are typically cuboidal (only).

21. We can't think of any—but some organs have only two (see Item 13 above).

CHAPTER

4 Integumentary System

Chapter Outline and Key Concepts

INTRODUCTION

The integumentary system has only three major components: skin, hair, and nails.

All of the external body surfaces (except the openings of the visceral body systems and the eyeballs) are covered by integumentary organs.

FUNCTIONS OF THE INTEGUMENTARY SYSTEM

The major functions of the integumentary system relate to homeostasis and protection.

Specific functions include thermoregulation, hydroregulation, physical and chemical protection, sensory reception, vitamin D synthesis, and communication.

SKIN

Skin is the largest body organ and accounts for over ten percent of the body weight.

The skin consists of two major layers (epidermis and dermis) and is bound to underlying structures by connective tissue proper called hypodermis (superficial fascia).

The epidermis is stratified squamous epithelium (several dozen cells thick) that is divided into four or five named layers depending on location.

The dead cells of the outer-most layer of the epidermis (stratum corneum) contain a protein (keratin) that imparts abrasion resistance.

The dermis is connective tissue proper and is divided into a papillary layer (superficial) and a reticular layer (deep).

Skin color is imparted by melanin, carotene, and hemoglobin.

GLANDS OF THE SKIN

Glands associated with the skin include sweat, sebaceous, ceruminous, and mammary glands.

Eccrine sweat glands are found in the skin covering most areas of the body.

Apocrine sweat glands are found primarily in the axillary and perineal regions.

Sebaceous glands secrete sebum and their ducts, like those of apocrine sweat glands, open into hair follicles.

Ceruminous glands secrete cerumen (earwax) to keep the tympanic membranes soft and pliable.

Mammary glands are modified sweat glands that produce milk.

HAIR

Hair is found on all external aspects of the body except the palms of the hand, soles of the feet, lips, nipples, nails, and some parts of the genitalia.

There are nine types of body hair identified including lanugo, capilli, supercilia, cilia, barba, tragi, vibrissae, pubes, and hirci.

A hair consists of an apex, shaft, root, and bulb (all composed of dead or dying cells).

Hair texture is related to the cross-sectional shape of the hair shaft and hair color depends on the presence of melanin (black, brown, blond), trichosiderin (red), or the absence of pigment (white/gray).

Hair growth results from mitosis of hair follicle cells—some of which die and become part of the hair bulb and root.

NAILS

A nail consists of a body (epithelium) and an underlying nail bed (dermis).

The hardness of nails is due to an especially well-developed stratum corneum of the epidermis.

The edges of a nail consist of two lateral borders, a blind (proximal) border, and a free (distal) border.

The thin skin overlying the blind border is the eponychium and the thickened skin under the free border is the hyponychium.

SURFACE ANATOMY

Many of the body's superficial landmarks are produced by structures which underlie the skin.

Surface features are important orientational markers for medical practitioners.

CLINICAL CONSIDERATIONS

Inflammation of the skin (dermatitis) has many causes.

Skin cancer is a common disorder related to exposure to sunlight.

Traumatic skin injuries include lacerations, abrasions, avulsions, and puncture wounds.

Scarring in wound healing results from proliferation of connective tissue proper in the dermis.

Selected Definitions

Dermis—the deeper of the two major layers of skin. The dermis is composed of connective tissue proper and is divided into a superficial papillary layer and a deeper reticular layer.

Epidermis—the outer one of the two major layers of skin. The epidermis is composed of keratinized stratified squamous epithelium, several dozen cells thick, and is divided into four or five named strata (depending on locus).

Eponychium—the cuticle located near the proximal border of a nail. It is a narrow band of epidermis that extends onto the nail surface.

Hair (pilus)—a nonviable epidermal derivative scattered over the body surface except for the palms of the hands, the soles of feet, nipples, lips, and parts of the external genitalia. Specific names are given to hair in different loci including capilli, supercilia, cilia, barba, tragi, vibrissae, hirci, and pubes.

Hair follicle—the group of living cells around the bulb and root of a hair. These cells, continually dividing in scalp hair and facial hair in men, die and are cemented together to form the hair itself.

Hypodermis—the connective tissue proper, continuous with and deep to the reticular layer of the dermis, that loosely binds the skin to deeper structures. The hypodermis is also known as superficial fascia and subcutaneous tissue.

Keratin—a tough, abrasion resistant protein present in the outer layer (stratum corneum) of the epidermis. Keratin begins its development as the cells degenerate and die in the stratum granulosum.

Laceration—a torn, ragged wound through the skin. Lacerations are distinguished from abrasions (scrapes), avulsions (tissue torn completely away), punctures, and contusions (bruising).

Mammary gland—a modified sweat gland that produces milk in lactating females. Each breast contains several mammary glands and their ducts open on the mammary papilla (nipple).

Melanin—a black pigment which contributes to skin and hair color. Melanin is produced by melanocytes and a genetic defect prevents its production in albinos.

Nail (unguis)—the smooth epidermal derivative which covers the distal, dorsal aspect of each finger and toe. Nails are composed of dead stratum corneum cells containing significant amounts of keratin.

Nail bed (matrix)—the dermis which underlies a nail. It is well vascularized and innervated in contrast to the nail itself which is avascular and aneural.

Sebaceous gland—a cutaneous gland that produces sebum (oil). Sebaceous glands typically open into hair follicles (which the oil follows to the skin surface) and their secretions waterproof the skin and increase its pliability.

Skin (cutis)—the organ which covers the external surface of the body. The skin is the largest body organ by weight and has two principal named layers: epidermis and dermis.

Stratum basale—the layer of cells adjacent to the basement membrane in stratified squamous epithelium. These cells are actively mitotic, and together with the cells of the stratum spinosum, constitute the stratum germinativum.

Stratum corneum—the outer most layer of stratified squamous epithelium. These cells are flattened and dead, and in some loci (epidermis), they are keratinized (cornified).

Stratum granulosum—the layer of epidermis, several cells thick, just superficial to the stratum spinosum. The grainy histological appearance of these dying cells is caused by the clumping of their degenerating organelles.

Stratum lucidum—a clear layer, several cells thick, of epidermis. It is found only in the thick skin of the palms of the hands and soles of the feet.

Stratum spinosum ("prickle cell layer")—the layer of stratified squamous epithelium, several cells thick, just superficial to the stratum basale. Its name is derived from its peculiar histological appearance.

Sudoriferous gland—a cutaneous gland that secretes sweat. Two kinds exist: eccrine sudoriferous glands scattered over the skin surface (primarily thermoregulatory) and apocrine sudoriferous glands located in the axillary and groin areas that become functional at puberty and produce pheromones.

Trichosiderin—an iron containing pigment which contributes a red color to hair. The hair of redheads also contains a variable amount of melanin.

Etymology *Res age, tute eris*—**"Wash that man right out of your hair."**

albus (L), *white*—albino
apo (G), *away from*—apocrine gland
avulsio (L), *to tear off*—avulsion
basale (L), *situated at the base*—stratum basale
cera (L), *wax*—ceruminous gland
corneus (L), *horny*—stratum corneum
cutis (L), *skin*—cutaneous
ec (L), *out of, outside of*—eccrine gland
holos (G), *complete, entire*—holocrine gland
integumentum (L), *to cover*—integument
karotin (G), *carrot*—carotene
krinein (G), *to separate*—eccrine gland
lanugo (L), *down*—lanugo
lucidus (L), *clear*—stratum lucidum
lunula (L), *crescent-shaped ornament*—lunula
melano (G), *black, dark*—melanocyte
meros (G), *part*—merocrine gland
onych (L), *nail of digit*—eponychium
onyx (L), *nail of digit*—perionyx
pilus (L), *hair*—arrector pili muscle
sebum (L), *tallow, grease*—sebaceous gland
stratum (L), *spread, bed, layer*—stratum corneum
sudor (L), *sweat*—sudoriferus gland
therme (G), *heat*—thermodynamic

Introduction

Based on the number of its component organs, the **integumentary system** is the simplest of the body systems because it has only three major organs: skin (and its associated glands), hair, and nails. These organs are collectively called the **common integument**. They cover all aspects of the outer surface of the body and are interrupted only by the penetrating orifices of the visceral body systems and the outer surfaces of the eyeballs.

Objectives

1. Name the three major components of the integumentary system.

Functions of the Integumentary System

The organs of the integumentary system serve several roles related to homeostasis and protection. Specific functions include:

1. **Thermoregulation**. Increasing or decreasing the blood flow to the deep layer of the skin when the core temperature of the body increases or decreases helps to prevent major changes in body temperature. Sweat produced by the sudoriferous glands of the skin helps to prevent overheating.
2. **Hydroregulation**. The organs of the integumentary system prevent desiccation of the body by forming a waterproof barrier at the surface.
3. **Physical and chemical protection.** Not only do the organs of the integumentary system protect the rest of the body from temperature extremes and desiccation, they also form a physical barrier to microbial invaders, prevent direct trauma to deeper organs, and the nails can even serve as formidable weapons in certain situations. Secretions produced by glands associated with the skin have antibacterial activity. Hair protects (to some degree) the skin from the potentially harmful effects of overexposure to the ultraviolet rays of the sun. The skin does not prevent passage of certain organic toxins.
4. **Sensory reception.** The integumentary organs are invested with numerous sensory receptors. These include exteroceptors that respond to heat, cold, touch, pressure, pain, and movement.
5. **Vitamin D production.** Ultraviolet light interacts with lipids in the skin to produce vitamin D. Overexposure to UV light can cause skin cancer.
6. **Nonverbal communication.** The skin itself is not a major organ of communication. Although changes in its color may reflect embarrassment or shock, most communication ascribed to the skin is, in reality, associated with changes in facial expression.

Objectives

2. State the functions of the integumentary system.

Skin

The **skin** is the largest body organ and accounts for over ten percent of the body weight. It consists of two distinct layers: epidermis and dermis. The **epidermis** is stratified squamous epithelium and the underlying **dermis** is connective tissue proper (Figure 4-1). The dermis is connected to the deeper structures of the body by a layer of areolar connective tissue called the **hypodermis** (Figure 4-2). This tissue is also called **subcutaneous tissue** or **superficial fascia**.

The **epidermis** is 0.07 to 0.12 mm thick over most regions of the body but it may be 1.00 to 1.50 mm thick on the palms and soles. It consists of several dozen layers of cells. The surface cells are continually sloughed off and replaced by cells that arise in the basal layers below. New cells that are formed there are displaced toward the surface by the continuing generation of cells underneath them. As they near the surface, the cells form **keratin** which is the dense protein responsible for their abrasion resistance. There are five named layers in the epidermis: stratum basale, stratum spinosum, stratum granulosum, stratum lucidum, and stratum corneum. The **stratum basale** is a single layer of cells which sits on the basement membrane. The basal cells continually divide and some of the daughter cells are forced toward the surface. The **stratum spinosum** is composed of several layers of cells. Its name is derived from the fact that tight intercellular connections cause the formation of spine-like cellular processes in histological sections of skin. There is some mitotic activity in this layer. Consequently, the stratum basale and stratum spinosum are sometimes collectively termed the "stra-

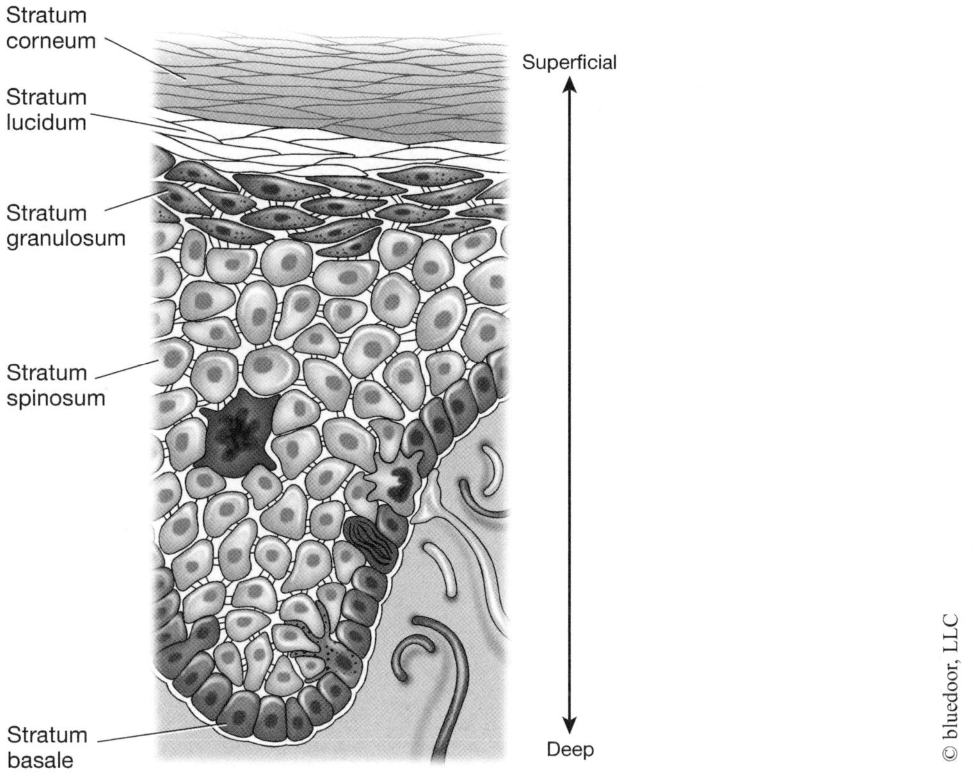

Figure 4-1

Layers of the Epidermis

The cells of the stratum basale and stratum spinosum continually divide to form new cells. Over a period of weeks, these new cells are forced toward the surface by the dividing cells deep to them and finally are sloughed at the external surface of the stratum corneum. The stratum lucidum is present only in the skin on the palms of the hands and the soles of the feet. Stratum germinativum is a name applied collectively to the stratum basale and stratum spinosum.

tum germinativum." The **stratum granulosum** is so-named because of the granular appearance of the cytoplasm of its cells. These cells are flattened and are degenerating because they are so far removed from the blood supply in the dermis (recall that membranous epithelium is avascular). The process of keratinization (cytoplasmic keratin formation) begins in this layer. The **stratum lucidum** is a layer present only in the skin of the palms of the hands and soles of the feet. The cytoplasmic organelles are so degenerated in this layer that they are no longer visible. The **stratum corneum** is the outer layer formed by two or three dozen layers of dead squamous cells. These have significant quantities of keratin in their cytoplasm (*see Chapter 3*). Because of this keratin, the epithelium of the skin is often called **cornified** or **keratinized stratified squamous epithelium**. In contrast, the stratified squamous epithelium lining the oral cavity and esophagus is non-keratinized. The surface of the epidermis is not smooth but has natural ridges and grooves. The ridges are especially well-developed on the palms of the hands and the soles of the feet. These are individual-specific and are the basis for identification by finger-printing. Lines and creases (caused by repeatedly moving body joints in the same manner) are present in several loci, especially on the hands and feet.

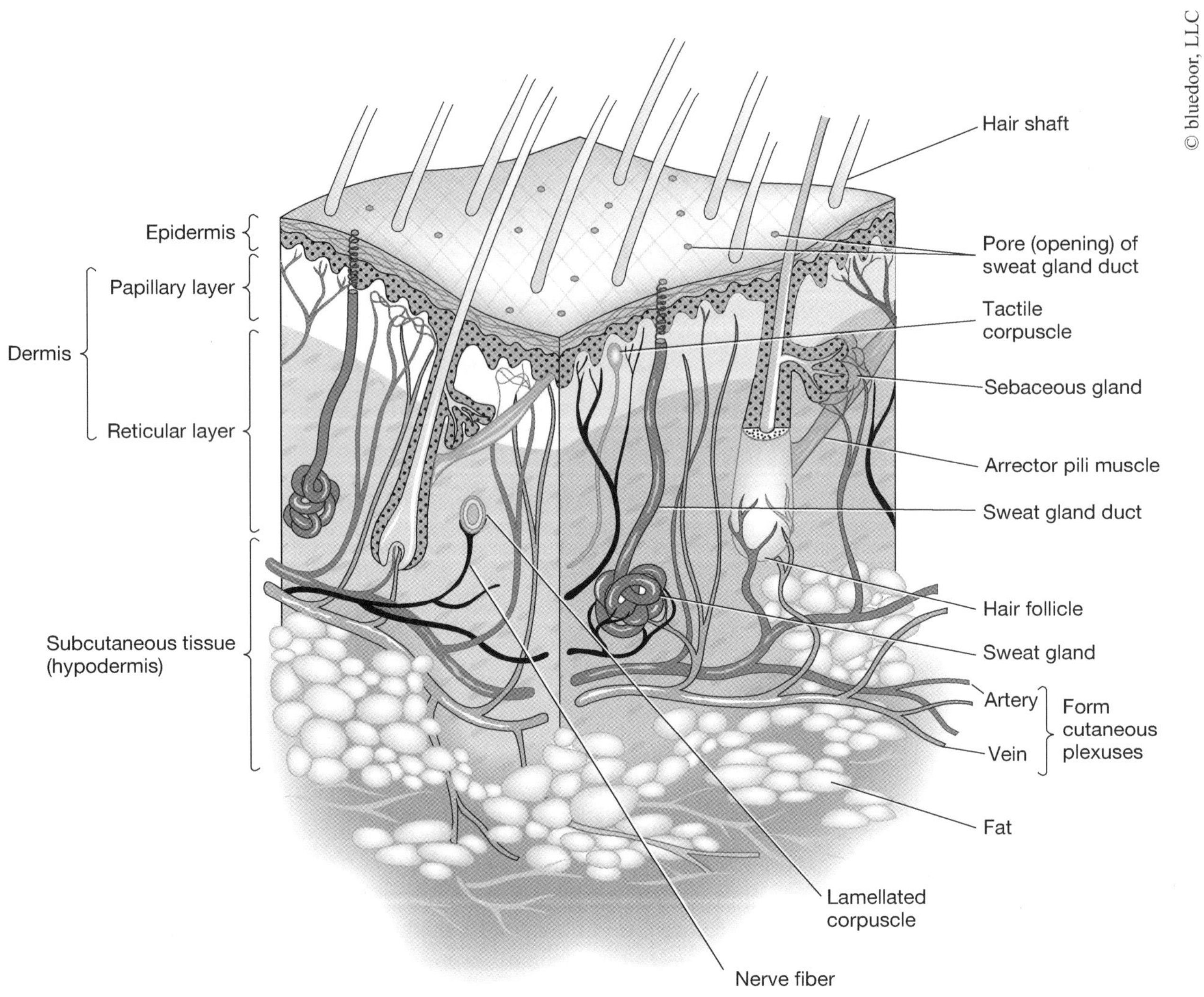

Figure 4-2

Anatomy of the Skin (Epidermis and Dermis) and Hypodermis

Note that the hair follicles and glandular structures are located in the dermis and penetrate through the epidermis to reach the surface.

The **dermis** is the deep layer of the skin, composed of connective tissue proper and is divided into two layers: papillary and reticular. The **papillary layer** is the thinner superficial portion which lies directly under the epidermis. It has numerous projections and ridges which support the surface patterns that cause fingerprints. The **reticular layer** lies deep to the papillary layer and is continuous with the underlying subcutaneous tissue. Both layers of the dermis are highly vascularized and contain significant numbers of elastic and collagenous fibers. Tearing of some of these fibers with subsequent scarring results in the so-called "**stretch marks**" often called "**lineae albicans**" visible on the abdomen, shoulders, thighs, and breasts of some individuals.

Skin coloration (tone) results from a summation of several different pigments. **Melanin** is a dark (almost black) pigment that is produced by **melanocytes**. These cells are located within the stratum basale and stratum spinosum and are interspersed among the basal and spinous cells. Individuals of all skin colors have about the same number of melanocytes. The amount of pigment they produce and the degree that it is dispersed within their cytoplasm determine whether an individual is black, brown, or white-skinned. Exposure to ultraviolet light causes increased melanin production which accounts for the so-called "suntan." Individuals whose melanocytes cannot produce melanin are termed **albinos**. Due to a genetic defect, their melanocytes lack an enzyme necessary for melanin production. In addition to melanin, **hemoglobin** (the red pigment in red blood corpuscles) and **carotene** (a pigment found in many dark green, leafy, and yellow vegetables) contribute to skin color. Carotene exists in four isomeric forms (α, β, γ, δ) and in colors ranging from violet to orange and yellow. β carotene is the main precurser of vitamin A and the photopigment called retinal.

Objectives

3. Name the two major layers of the skin, classify them histologically, name their sublayers, and differentiate them from hypodermis.
4. List the pigments that contribute to skin color.

Glands of the Skin

The skin has several types of exocrine glands associated with it including sweat glands, sebaceous glands, ceruminous glands, and mammary glands (Table 4-1). **Sweat (sudoriferous) glands** produce a watery secretion that has a thermoregulatory function. Two types are present: eccrine and apocrine. **Eccrine (merocrine) sudoriferous glands** are located over the whole skin surface except for the margins of the lips, the glans penis, and the areas covered by nails. They are simple, coiled tubular glands with the secretory portion deep within the dermis. The openings of their ducts at the surface are called **sudoriferous pores. Apocrine sudoriferous glands** resemble their eccrine counterparts structurally but open into hair follicles. They are located primarily in the axillae and perineal regions. Their secretory portions are more deeply located (within the hypodermis) and they begin to function at puberty. Their secretion is more viscous and odoriferous than that of the eccrine sweat glands because it contains sloughed portions of the secretory cells.

Sebaceous glands are holocrine, oil-producing glands. Their secretion is called **sebum** and it helps to make the skin more pliable and waterproof. Most sebaceous glands secrete into hair follicles but some open freely on the skin surface (Figure 4-3). When their ducts become blocked and infection occurs, **acne** results.

Ceruminous glands are specialized glands found only in the skin of the external acoustic meatus. They secrete the **cerumen** (earwax) which is responsible for keeping the tympanic membrane pliable.

Mammary glands are modified sweat glands that produce milk (Figure 4-4). They are found within the **breasts** which overlie the pectoralis major muscle on each side. The several **lactiferous ducts** from the mammary glands open at the **nipple**. The pigmented skin surrounding the nipple is termed the **areola**. Small projections within the areola are formed by areolar glands which secrete a substance thought to prevent chapping during lactation. Sensory cells within the areola contribute to the milk let-down process.

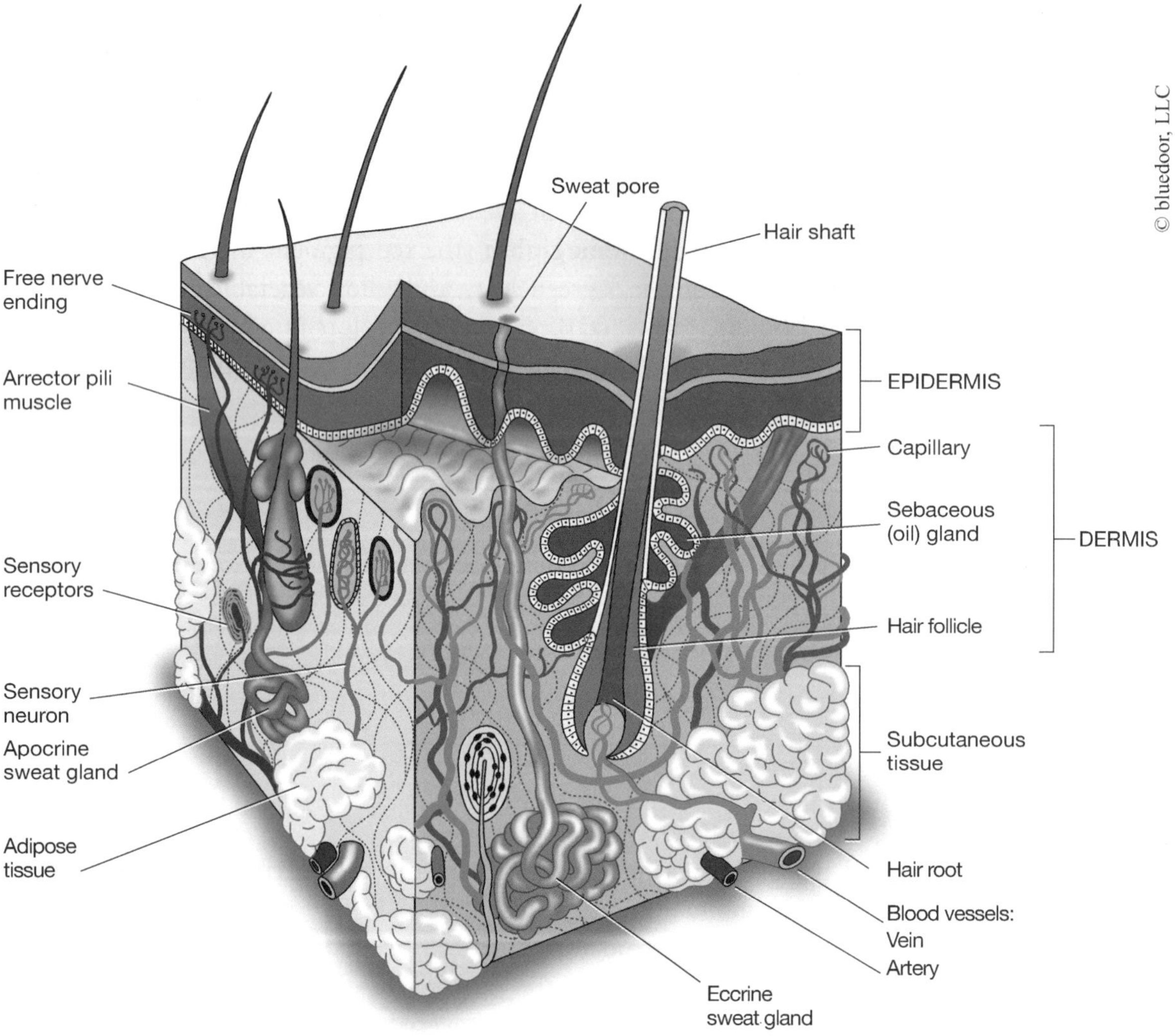

Figure 4-3

Sweat and Sebaceous Glands

The ducts of sebaceous glands and apocrine sweat glands typically open into hair follicles. Ducts of eccrine (merocrine) sweat glands open freely at the epidermal surface.

Table 4–1 Glands of the Skin

Types of Gland	*Mode of Secretion*	*Secretory Product*	*Function*
Eccrine sudoriferous	eccrine/merocrine	sweat	thermoregulation
Apocrine sudoriferous	apocrine	sweat	pheromone
Sebaceous	holocrine	oil	lubricate skin
Ceruminous	holocrine	wax	lubricate eardrum
Mammary	apocrine	milk	nutrition

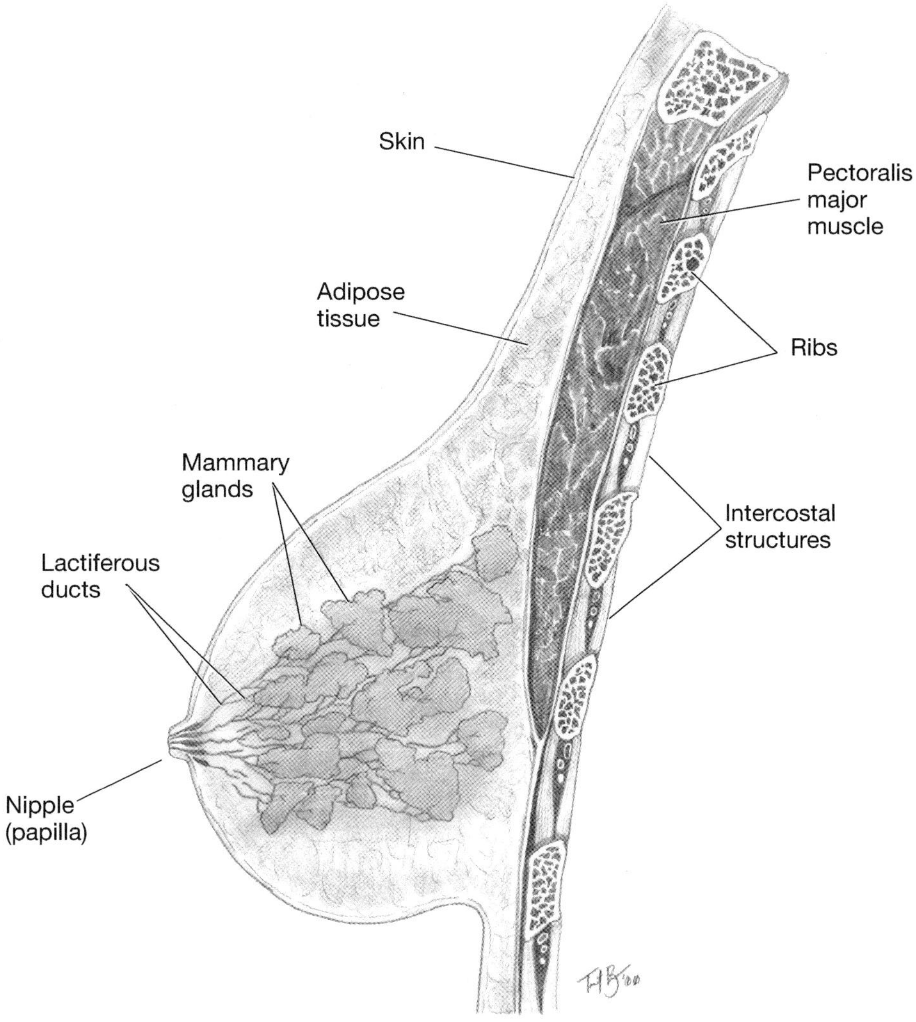

Figure 4-4 Breast of a Female

The mammary glands secrete through lactiferous ducts which open separately at the nipple.

Objectives

5. Differentiate the glands associated with the skin in regard to location, type of secretion, mode of secretion, and function.

Hair

Compared to most other mammals, the human body is only sparsely covered with **hair**. Hair is not present on the nails, palms of the hands, soles of the feet, lips, nipples, and some parts of the genitalia. It is especially dense on the cephalic, pubic, perineal, and axillary regions. Males and females have about the same amount of body hair, but the individual hairs are often coarser and more darkly pigmented in men due to the influence of testosterone.

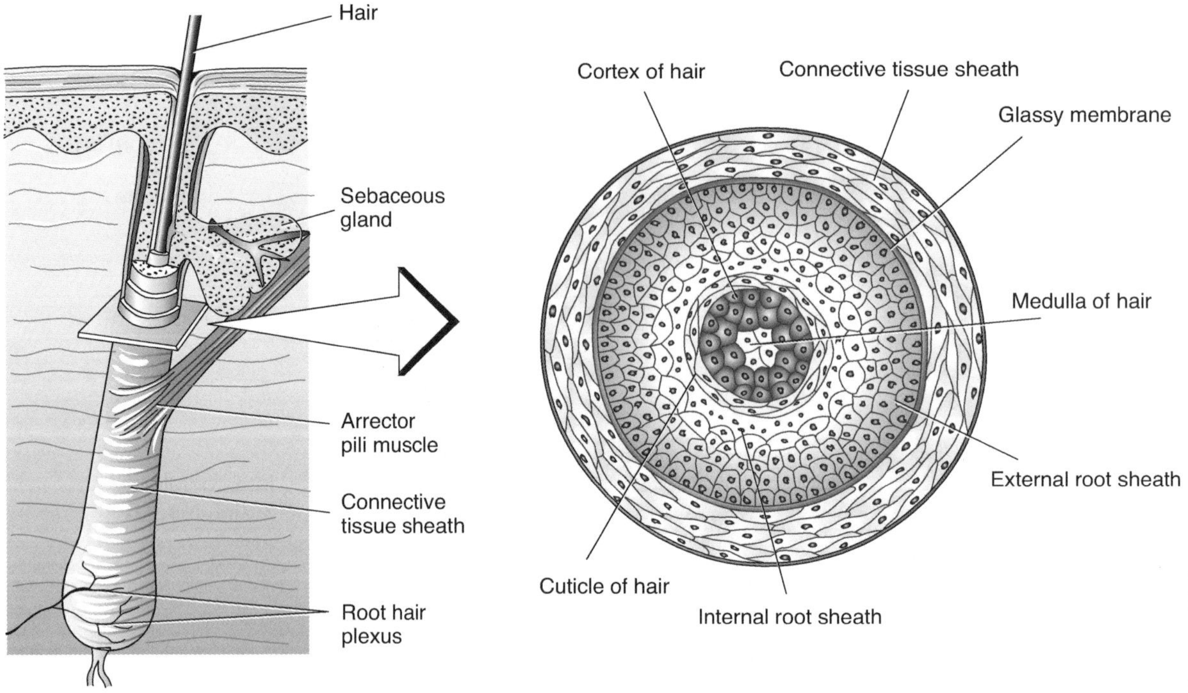

Figure 4-5 Anatomy of a Hair and Hair Follicle

The hair itself consists of dead cells cemented together and is divided into a bulb (at the bottom), root, shaft and apex. The latter two parts project above the skin surface.

Several different types of body hair develop in humans (Table 4-2). The fine hair that is present on developing fetuses is called **lanugo hair**. It is shed and replaced by coarser hair. Most body hair elongates to a certain length and then ceases growing. This includes all body hair except scalp hair in both sexes and the facial hair in males. Hairs remain in place for a few months (eyelashes) to a few years (scalp hairs). Those lost are replaced by new ones growing from the base of the follicles. Scalp hairs elongate at a rate of about 1.0 cm/month. Several dozen scalp hairs are shed each day.

An individual hair consists of an apex, shaft, root, and bulb. The **apex** (tip) and **shaft** are exposed above the skin surface and the **root** and **bulb** project down into the dermis (Figure 4-5). The bulb is the deepest portion and is larger in diameter than the rest of the hair. It is embedded in an epidermal encasement called the **hair follicle**. The cells of the follicle surrounding the bulb divide to cause hair growth, but they die as they are forced closer to the surface and further from the nutrient supply. Therefore, the exposed portion of a hair is a non-living structure. In transverse section, a hair shaft has three layers: an inner medulla, surrounded by a cortex which is, in turn, covered by a cuticle. The **medulla** consists of loosely packed cells and air pockets. The **cortex** and **cuticle** are formed by hardened, more tightly packed cells. A smooth muscle fasciculus called **arrector pili muscle** attaches to the hair follicle. When stimulated by the sympathetic part of the autonomic nervous system this fasciculus erects the hair shaft and causes gooseflesh (cutis anserina), also called goose bumps.

Hair color is due mainly to the type and amount of pigment imparted to the cells when they are formed at the base of the hair follicle. Increasing amounts of **melanin** are responsible for blonde, brown, and black hair. Red hair contains an iron-based pigment termed **trichosiderin**. Gray and white hair are caused by the lack of pigment and the presence of increasing amounts of air in the medullary portions of the hair shafts. Hair texture is due to the diameter and shape of the hair shafts with round shafts resulting in straight hair, and oval and flattened shafts causing wavy and kinky (tight-curly) hair, respectively.

Table 4–2 Different Types of Hair

Lanugo—embryonic hair	***Supercilia***—eyebrows	***Vibrissae***—nose hair
Capilli—scalp hair	***Barba***—facial hair	***Pubes***—pubic hair
Cilia—eyelashes	***Tragi***—ear hair	***Hirci***—axillary hair

Objectives

6. Differentiate a hair from a hair follicle and explain the phenomenon of "goose bumps".
7. State the specific names for hair located in different regions of the body and discuss the substances that contribute to hair color.
8. Explain the relationship between the texture of hair and cross-sectional shapes of hair shafts.

Nails

Nails are present on each digit where they function in a protective capacity. Their hardness is due to an especially well-developed stratum corneum layer (Figure 4-6). A nail consists of a body and a matrix. The **body** is the epithelial portion and the **matrix** (**nail-bed**) is the dermis to which the body is attached. The nail is overlapped along its **blind** (**proximal**) **border** and two **lateral borders** by a fold of skin termed the **wall of the nail**. The thin layer of skin adherent to the nail over its proximal border is the **eponychium**. Its remnant which separates away is the **perionyx** (commonly called the **cuticle**). The **hyponychium** is the thickened layer of epidermis under the **free** (**distal**) **border** of the nail. The half-moon shaped, pale area along the proximal border of some nails is called the **lunula**.

Objectives

9. Sketch a nail and label its parts including its four borders and the lunula.
10. Define cuticle, eponychium, hyponychium, and matrix as they apply to nail structure.

Surface Anatomy

There are many areas of the body surface that are given specific identifying names. Some of these simply refer to the name of the major segment of the body involved (brachial region, crural region, [*see Table 1-4*]). Other names refer to more specific landmarks. A few of the latter are outlined in Table 4-3 and Figure 4-7. Many superficial landmarks are produced by structures which underlie the skin. These surface features have clinical significance as surgical and diagnostic orientational mark-

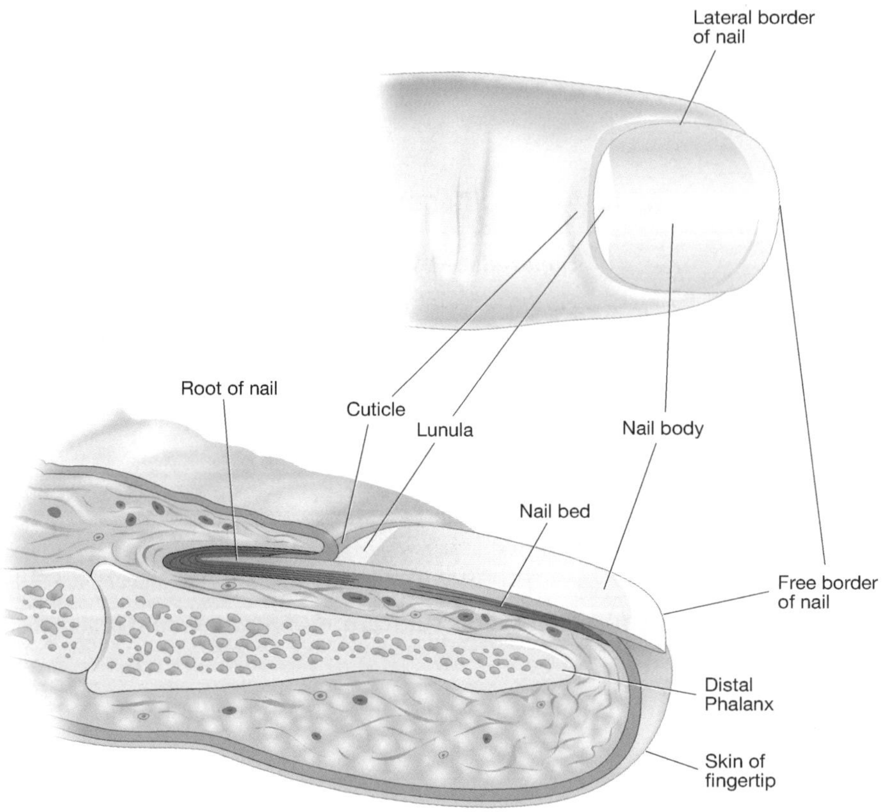

Figure 4-6 Architecture of a Nail

The main part of a nail is formed by a thick layer of epidermal stratum corneum. The germinal epithelium which produces the epidermis is buried within the surrounding dermis at the blind (proximal) border.

ers. For example, digital pressure in the carotid triangle, a subdivision of the anterior cervical triangle (Table 4-3, Figure 4-7), can be used to monitor the pulse. An emergency tracheostomy (incision directly into the trachea to bypass a blocked airway) is made on the anterior midline between the inferior aspects of the left and right muscular triangles (Table 4-3, Figure 4-7). Digital pressure in the femoral triangle (Table 4-3) can be used to control severe hemorrhage from the distal part of the inferior limb.

Objectives

11. Define the boundaries of the anterior cervical triangle and the posterior cervical triangle.
12. Find the landmarks listed in Table 4-3 on your body.

Clinical Considerations

Inflammation of the skin is termed **dermatitis** and has numerous causes (Table 4-4). Some of these are infectious agents and others damage the skin by physical means. **Burns** are thermal injuries whose seriousness depends on their size and severity. They are classified as first, second, or third degree based on whether the skin is reddened, blistered, or charred. The latter often require skin grafts if they cover large areas. Not only do severe burns destroy the body's natural barrier to invading microbial agents, but they destroy the ability to control surface fluid loss. Consequently, keeping burn victims properly hydrated and in electrolyte balance is a major challenge.

Skin cancer is a very common disease and appears to be directly related to exposure to ultraviolet light from the sun. Most forms of skin cancers (basal cell and spinous cell carcinomas) respond favorably to surgical excision if it is performed early enough in the course of the disease. Malignant melanoma is a form of skin cancer which is especially dangerous. Any mole which enlarges or undergoes changes in color or shape should be considered suspect and examined by a physician.

Traumatic injuries involving the skin include lacerations, abrasions, avulsions, and puncture wounds. **Lacerations** are tears as opposed to cuts, which are more like surgical incisions. Both may

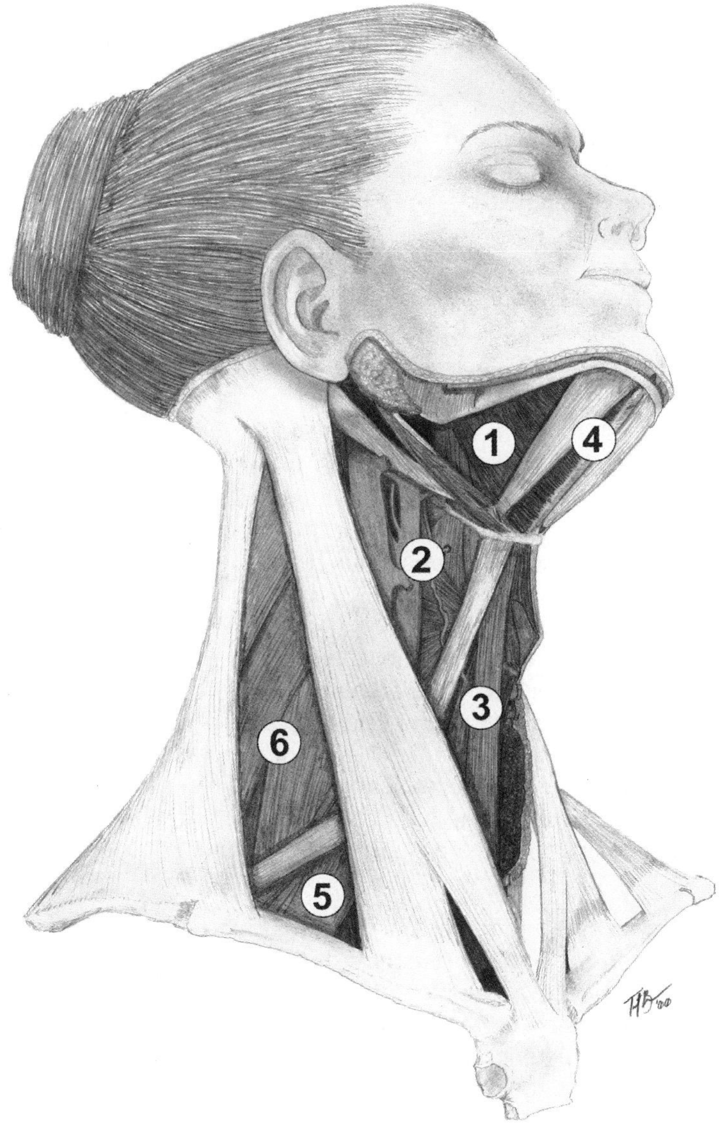

Figure 4-7 The Triangles of the Neck

The anterior cervical triangle is subdivided into the (1) submandibular, (2) carotid, (3) muscular, and (4) submental triangles. The posterior cervical triangle is subdivided into the (5) omoclavicular and (6) occipital triangles.

Table 4–3 Major Surface Features

Head and Neck

"Scalp"*—the skin covering the cranium.
Eyebrow—the small patch of hair above each eye.
Vertex—the top of the head.
Occiput—the back of the head.
Forehead (brow)—the area between the scalp and eyes.
Mentolabial groove—the transverse groove between the lower lip and chin.
Anterior cervical triangle (region)—a paired (left/right) area bounded by the anterior midline, body of the mandible, and sternocleidomastoideus muscle. It is subdivided into four other triangles:
- **Submandibular triangle**—the area bounded by the body of the mandible and the two bellies of the digastricus muscle.
- **Carotid triangle**—the area bounded by the omohyoid m., sternocleidomastoideus m., and posterior belly of the digastricus muscle.
- **Muscular (omotracheal) triangle**—the area bounded by the anterior midline, superior belly of the omohyoid muscle, and the sternocleidomastoideus muscle.
- **Submental ("suprahyoid") triangle**—the area bounded by the anterior midline, anterior belly of the digastricus m., and the hyoid bone.

Posterior cervical triangle (region) (lateral cervical region)—the area bounded by the superior border of the clavicle, trapezius muscle, and posterior border of the sternocleidomastoideus muscle. It is subdivided into two other triangles:
- **Omoclavicular ("subclavian") triangle**—the area bounded by the clavicle, omohyoideus muscle, and sternocleidomastoideus muscle.
- **Major supraclavicular fossa** = "Occipital triangle"—the area bounded by the omohyoideus m., trapezius m., and sternocleidomastoideus muscle.

Sternocleidomastoid region—the lateral cervical region occupied by the sternocleidomastoideus muscle.
Lesser supraclavicular fossa ("Zang's space")—the triangular area bordered by the clavicle and the two inferior heads of the sternocleidomastoideus muscle.

Trunk

Clavipectoral ("deltopectoral", "infraclavicular") triangle—a depression bounded by the clavicle and adjacent borders of the deltoideus and pectoralis major muscles.
Axilla (armpit)—the depression under the shoulder joint. It is bounded by anterior and posterior axillary folds which overlie the major pectoral and latissimus dorsi muscles.
Umbilicus—the navel.
Regions of the abdomen:
- **Umbilical region**—the area surrounding the umbilicus.
- **Right and left lateral abdominal regions**—the areas to the right and left of the umbilical region.
- **Hypogastric region**—the area between the umbilical region and pubis.
- **Right and left inguinal regions**—the area on each side of the hypogastric region.
- **Epigastric region**—the area between the umbilical region and thorax.
- **Right and left hypochondriac regions**—the area on each side of the epigastric region.

Perineal region—the area comprising the inferior aspect of the trunk between the thighs.

Superior Limb

Medial and lateral bicipital grooves—the depression on either side of the biceps brachii muscle.
Cubital fossa—the depression on the anterior aspect of the elbow.
Palm of the hand—the anterior surface of the hand excluding the wrist and digits.
"Anatomical snuffbox"—the depression on the posterolateral aspect of the carpus when the thumb is abducted and its joints are fully extended.
Hypothenar eminence—the elongated, bulb-like swelling extending proximally from the palmar aspect of the base of the little finger.
Thenar eminence—the large bulb-like swelling at the base of the thumb on the lateral aspect of the palm.
"Flexion creases"—on the anterior aspect of the hand; the distinct lines in the skin where it folds during flexion of the carpal and digital joints.
"Interdigital webs"—the skin and underlying soft tissues which extend between the bases of adjacent digits.

* Items with quotes are unofficial names.

Table 4–3 Major Surface Features (continued)

Inferior Limb

Crena ani (natal cleft)—the groove between the buttocks.
Gluteal groove—the furrow between the inferior aspect of the buttock and the posterosuperior aspect of the thigh.
Femoral triangle—the triangular area at the anteromedial aspect of the proximal thigh bounded by the sartorius m., adductor longus m., and inguinal ligament.
Popliteal fossa—the area on the posterior aspect of the knee.
Sole of foot—the inferior aspect of the foot.
Ball of foot—the round, padded portion of the sole of the foot.

involve only the skin or they may damage deeper organs. Lacerations and cuts heal very quickly if the wound edges are apposed and infection does not occur. **Abrasions** are scrapes. Depending on how much epidermis is lost, these may require a much longer recovery time than lacerations. **Avulsions** are injuries in which structures are torn away and lost. These require extended recovery times and often result in severe scarring. **Puncture wounds** are often not serious injuries themselves, but bacteria introduced by the puncturing object often cause bothersome subcutaneous infections. Of particular concern is the fact that the body tissues often lack sufficient oxygen levels to inhibit the growth of *Clostridium tetani* (the bacterium which causes "lockjaw") and a fatal tetanus syndrome may ensue. This is the reason that puncture wounds cause such great concern.

Scarring occurs when wounds or other morbid processes heal by the proliferation of excessive connective tissue proper. If wound edges are properly apposed (pulled together) and infection is controlled, scarring is often minimal.

Skin grafts are often employed to aid the recovery of burn victims and those who have lost large areas of skin from other causes. Healthy skin from other parts of the body is physically transferred to denuded and properly prepared recipient areas.

Table 4–4 Types of Dermatitis

Cause	*Examples*
Trauma	Abrasions, avulsions, lacerations
Overexposure to UV light	Sunburn, actinic dermatitis
Heat	Burns
Cold	Frostbite
Exposure to irritants	Poison ivy affliction
Mycotic infection	Ringworm, blastomycetic dermatitis
Bacterial infection	Boils, acne
Arthropod infection	Scabies, acarine dermatosis
Immunologic reactions	Hives, wheals

Objectives

13. Define/differentiate the common types of skin injuries including lacerations, abrasions, punctures, and avulsions.
14. Explain what causes scarring.

Clinical Case Studies

Case 1—A 30-year-old attorney noticed a yellow and white discoloration near the distal margin (free border) of the nail of his right big toe. Over the next several months the discolored area progressively enlarged. When he trimmed the nail, it appeared thickened and brittle in the involved region, and the nail seemed to be elevated somewhat from the underlying nail bed by a light colored "powdery" material that caused the nail discoloration. What caused the changes in the character of the nail?

Case 2—A 45-year-old executive noticed moderate enlargement in a small mole located on his left shoulder. Eight months later he died from cancer diagnosed as malignant melanoma. Was his cancer related to the mole?

Case 3—A forensic pathologist was asked to testify by the defense in a homicide case where the defendant was linked to the crime by several pieces of circumstantial evidence including blond hair found at the crime scene. After comparing hair samples from the defendant with those found at the crime scene, the pathologist presented convincing arguments that cleared the defendant. Upon what could the pathologist have based his argument for innocence?

Points to Ponder

"Beauty is only skin deep..." emphasizes the importance of this largest of all organs to the physical aspect of interpersonal relationships—and as noted herein, beauty is a thin disguise, at best. Not satisfied with nature's endowments, Revlon,® Maybelline,® Mary Kay,® and Avon® offer embellishments and camouflage to hide imperfections, emphasize assets, and increase allure in general. To bolster their edge in the highly competitive "look at me" market, individuals spend considerable time and money on the other two components of the integumentary system: hair and nails. Natural, artificial, every color and shape imaginable is tried and retried. Some, dissatisfied or perhaps pleased with the results, continue the artificial adornment scheme with an array of metallic objects inserted through unnatural openings. No part of the skin surface is immune to the more adventuresome of these skewers.

Enter the tattoo. Once a symbol of some sailors, bikers, and "tuff"guys, tattoos in recent decades have been appearing with a greater degree of frequency. The big drawback, a permanence well beyond that of body piercing adornments, is sometimes overcome by laser-assisted tattooectomy techniques.

One of the cruelest pranks physiology plays on the human race is the acneic dermatitis that afflicts a large portion of junior high and high school age young people. This typically hormonal induced tragedy occurs at that delicate adolescent time when self-esteem is already quite fragile and can have very long term or even permanent affects on psychological development.

The many roles that skin plays in body defense, protection, and homeostasis are largely taken for granted until one loses a significant patch of skin to a severe burn or unscheduled close association with an abrasive object (motorcycles and pavement are bad about this). Lacerations (even quite long ones) usually heal quite rapidly ("side-to-side" and not "end-to-end" as every surgical student knows). However, when large areas of skin are completely lost, healing can require a significant amount of time and considerable medical help in the form of nursing care and even surgical transplantation.

Ironic, isn't it, that the golden brown, naturally tanned body has a very high chance of developing skin cancer due to exposure to ultraviolet light—and that loss of the ozone layer appears to be increasing the risk at an alarming rate! Gustav Eckstein in *The Body Has a Head* (Harper and Row, 1970) put it so eloquently: "Skin is a defense against many assaults of many kinds, cold winter, hot summer. The way it tans defends, the dark pigment rising from the deeper layers of the skin blocking further absorption of the ultraviolet of the sunlight, defending thus the depths from further exposure to that assailant. How permanently damaging that exposure may be has come to be known only in later years." He continues that the skin "...furthermore is greased. A thin sheet of fat lies on it, fabricated by sebaceous glands, and each time a hair moves, it squeezes out a bit of fat, and somewhere a hair is always moving. A polite fat—does not get rancid. An aggressive fat—its fatty-acids and soaps kill bacteria. A friendly fat—prevents us from drying, moisturizes us, keeps us pliable, causes one human being not to be averse from touching another . . ."

Slang and Obsolete Nomenclature

UNOFFICIAL TERM	OFFICIAL DESIGNATION
suprahyoid triangle	submental triangle *[trigonum submentale]*
subclavian triangle	omoclavicular triangle *[trigonum omoclaviculare]*
occipital triangle	greater supraclavicular fossa *[fossa supraclavicularis major]*
Zang's space	lesser supraclavicular fossa *[fossa supraclavicularis minor]*
deltopectoral triangle	clavipectoral triangle *[trigonum clavipectorale]*
infraclavicular triangle	clavipectoral triangle *[trigonum clavipectorale]*
anatomic snuffbox	(none exists)
belly button	navel *[umbilicus]*

Review Questions

1. Find the truth.
   A. Secretions by glands associated with the skin have antibacterial activity.
   B. The integumentary system assists in desiccation of the body.
   C. The integumentary system is the most complex of the 12 body systems because it has only three organs.
   D. The skin is composed of epidermis, dermis, and hypodermis.
   E. Vitamin K production is one of the functions of the integumentary system.

2. Which of the following layers of the epidermis is directly superficial to the stratum granulosum on the sole of the foot?
   A. dermis
   B. stratum basale
   C. stratum corneum
   D. stratum lucidum
   E. stratum spinosum

3. Skin tone (color) results from a summation of different pigments. Which of the following is responsible for a "pinkish/reddish" skin tone?
   A. carotene
   B. hemoglobin
   C. keratin
   D. melanin
   E. melatonin

4. Which of the following structures associated with hair is furthest removed from a blood supply?
   A. arrector pili muscle
   B. hair bulb
   C. hair follicle
   D. hair root
   E. hair shaft

5. Which of the following is the Latin term for hair located in the armpit?
   A. barba
   B. capilli
   C. hirci
   D. tragi
   E. vibrissae

6. Which of the following forms the lateral (anterior) border of the femoral triangle?
   A. adductor longus muscle
   B. crena ani
   C. gluteal groove
   D. inguinal ligament
   E. sartorius muscle

7. Which of the following is not a function of the integumentary system?
   A. thermoregulation
   B. vitamin D production
   C. sensory reception
   D. hydroregulation
   E. protection
   F. Choose this response if all of the above (A-E) are functions of the integumentary system.

8. Find the glandular mismatch.
   A. apocrine sudoriferous: sweat—pheromone—apocrine
   B. ceruminous: wax—lubricant—holocrine
   C. sebaceous: oil—lubricant—holocrine
   D. eccrine sudoriferous: sweat—thermoregulation—merocrine
   E. mammary: milk—nutrition—holocrine

9. Which of the following is not a boundary of either the anterior or posterior cervical triangles?
   A. body of mandible
   B. sternocleidomastoid muscle
   C. latissimus dorsi muscle
   D. clavicle
   E. anterior midline

10. Which of the following organs would not be found in the left superior quadrant of the abdomen?
   A. spleen
   B. pancreas

C. splenic vein
D. stomach
E. transverse colon
F. Choose this response if all of the above (A-E) can be found in the named region.

Thought Questions

1. What are the unique features of the integumentary system (compared to the other body systems)?

2. Which of the eight types of body hair in an adult continually elongate? Does cutting hair cause it to grow faster?

3. Why do teenagers (and adults) have more body odor than second graders?

4. Why is there no pain associated with haircuts and manicures (except in the pocket book)?

5. Why will a hair usually regrow even if it is pulled out "by the root?"

6. Which hair color is due to a particular (unique) pigment?

7. Why does lacerated skin heal so quickly and readily?

8. Why is a severely bruised finger/toe nail so painful?

9. Which two of the four major types of skin wounds should heal the fastest? What slows the rate of healing in the other two?

10. Which superficial landmark would be of most value to...
    A. A surgeon making an anterior midline abdominal incision?
    B. A phlebotomist drawing a routine blood sample?
    C. An anatomy student looking for his own pisiform bone?
    D. An EMT trying to apply pressure to slow severe hemorrhage from an injured foot?

11. Why is sweat from eccrine (merocrine) sweat glands less odiferous than sweat from apocrine sweat glands or sebum from sebaceous glands?

12. What causes cellular death in the superficial layers of the epidermis?

13. What function does the integumentary system share with the ______________ system?
    A. urinary
    B. cardiovascular
    C. skeletal

14. Most of the "communication" ascribed to skin should really be attributed to the __________ system.

15. Why are chemical toxins dissolved in water less noxious (as a group) when applied to skin than toxins dissolved in organic solvents?

16. Why are the stratum basale and stratum spinosum layers of the skin collectively grouped as stratum germinativum?

17. In general, how long does it take for a cell to "move" from the basement membrane to the free surface in the epidermis of the skin?

18. Assuming that contraction of an arrector pili muscle causes the bottom end of a hair follicle to swing *toward* the muscle and the hair shaft to swing (angle) in the opposite direction, on which side of a hair shaft should a "goose bump" occur? (*i.e.*, on the arrector pili muscle side or on the opposite side?

19. Gray (white) hair is less dense (mass/volume) than hair of other colors because....

20. In overweight individuals, muscle definition cannot be observed as easily as in thinner individuals because of the increased adipose tissue depositions... (where)?

21. What is a keloid?

Answers to Clinical Case Studies

Case 1—This condition is caused by a fungal infection of the nail. It is a very slowly progressing disease that some individuals seem much more susceptible to than others. There are medications that can "cure" the disease but they must be administered orally, are relatively expensive, and require an extended period of therapy to be effective. Topical medicaments do not have any effect. The incidence of recurrence after successful treatment is quite high. The fungus invades the stratum corneum of the nail and disrupts its normal architecture.

Case 2—Perhaps, but not necessarily. Any change in size or character of an existing mole should be brought to the immediate attention of a medical practitioner because of the high correlation of such incidents with cancer.

Case 3—The diameters of the hair shafts and their cross-sectional shapes could have been compared to those from the defendant as well as chemical analyses for certain trace minerals.

Answers to Review Questions

1. A. (B) "Helps prevent dessication", (C) "least" not most, (D) no hypodermis in skin, (E) vitamin "D" not K.

2. D.

3. B. Found in hemoglobin, (E) is a hormone.

4. E.

5. C. (A, B, D, and E are facial, scalp, ear and nose hairs, respectively).

6. E. (A) Is the medial border, (D) is the superior border.

7. F.

8. E. Mammary glands are apocrine.

9. C.

10. F.

Answers to Thought Questions

1. The integumentary system contains the largest body organ (skin), the fewest organs, and it is the only system located totally on the external surface of the body.

2. Capilli (scalp hairs) in both sexes and barba (facial hair) in men. Cutting hair has no effect on its growth rate.

3. Apocrine sweat glands become functional at puberty (*see Question 11*).

4. Hair and nails are composed of dead cells and there are no sensory nerve endings within them.

5. The living cells responsible for hair growth are in the hair follicle, many of which remain intact and in place when a hair is pulled out.

6. Red hair is due to the presence of an iron containing pigment called trichosiderin. Most other colors (black, brown, blond) are due to the relative amount of melanin present. White/gray hair occurs when pigment is replaced by air.

7. Its two major tissue components (stratified squamous epithelium and connective tissue proper) both have high regenerative capacity.

8. The extravasated blood collects deep to the body of the nail and forcefully separates it from the underlying matrix. The latter is well endowed with sensory nerve endings.

9. Lacerations and puncture wounds should heal quite quickly since there is no tissue "lost" in the injury. Abrasions and avulsions require more time to heal because the tissue lost must be replaced.

10. A. Umbilicus B. Cubital fossa C. Hypothenar eminence D. Femoral triangle

11. Eccrine (merocrine) secretory products contain no dead/dying (*i.e.*, degenerating) cells or cell parts.

12. Membranous epithelium is avascular. The deepest layers of cells receive adequate nutrition via diffusion but the more superficial layers of cells die and degenerate because their nutrition is inadequate.

13. A. hydroregulation B. defense and thermoregulation C. protection

14. Muscular system (it is responsible for facial expressions).

15. Organic solvents penetrate the skin more readily than water (and carry the toxins with them).

16. Mitosis occurs in both layers and "germinativum" implies this.

17. Several weeks.

18. On the opposite side.

19. It has air within the hair shaft.

20. Within the hypodermis (subcutaneous tissue).

21. A progressively enlarging scar due to the formation of excessive connective tissue proper. It is often disfiguring and seems to be a sequel to wound healing in certain individuals but not in the population at large.

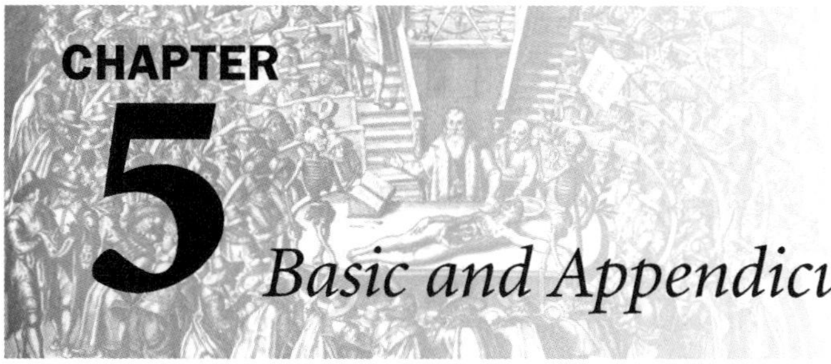

CHAPTER 5 Basic and Appendicular Osteology

Chapter Outline and Key Concepts

INTRODUCTION

Osteology is the study of bone tissue and the study of bones (the organs).

STRUCTURE OF BONE TISSUE

Bone tissue is composed of three kinds of cells (osteoblasts, osteocytes, and osteoclasts), extracellular collagenous fibers, ground substance, and mineral.

Bone mineral (primarily hydroxyapatite) imparts the hardness to bone tissue and accounts for about two-thirds of the dry weight.

As bone forming cells (osteoblasts) secrete the organic part of bone tissue, some of them become entrapped in their own secretory products and become osteocytes.

Layers of osteocytes and extracellular matrix called lamellae are classified by their specific arrangement and position as concentric, interstitial, or circumferential.

Throughout life, bone tissue is continually being formed by osteoblasts and reabsorbed by osteoclasts.

Bone tissue exists in two forms: compact and spongy.

Bone tissue is one of the types of connective tissue, but named bones are organs.

Bones are organs containing bone tissue as well as several other types of tissue.

FUNCTIONS OF BONES (AND BONE TISSUE)

Physical functions of bones include body shape, protection, and locomotion.

Metabolic functions include hemopoiesis, serving as a fat depository, and calcium/phosphorus storage.

CLASSIFICATION OF BONES BY POSITION

The appendicular skeleton includes all bones associated with the limbs.

The axial skeleton includes bones of the head, vertebral column, ribs, and sternum.

Those axial and appendicular bones that support the free parts of the limbs are collectively called the pectoral and pelvic girdles.

CLASSIFICATION OF BONES BY SHAPE

There are five categories of bones by shape: long, short, flat, irregular, and sesamoid bones.

The appendicular skeleton contains long, short, flat, and sesamoid bones.

The axial skeleton is composed of flat and irregular bones (only).

GENERAL ANATOMIC FEATURES OF BONES

Most of the outer surface of a bone is covered by a connective tissue proper encasement called periosteum.

Periosteum does not occur where tendons, ligaments, and joint capsules attach, and at articular surfaces (which are covered by articular cartilage).

The central, hollow part of a bone, called the medullary cavity, contains bone marrow tissue.

The solid bone tissue making up most of a bone's structure is called compact bone.

Thin spicules of bone invaginating the medullary cavity comprise spongy bone.

Nerves and vessels enter and penetrate a bone through nutrient foramina/nutrient canals.

In long bones, the ends are called epiphyses and the central part (shaft) is the diaphysis.

Specific features and landmarks, unique to each bone, are given specific names.

BONES OF THE SUPERIOR LIMB

The 34 bones within a superior limb include two flat bones, 22 long bones, eight short bones, and two sesamoid bones.

The pectoral girdle forms the bony support for the free parts of the superior limbs and is composed of four appendicular bones (scapulae and clavicles) and one axial bone (sternum).

The clavicle ("collarbone") is a flat bone that has the appearance of a long bone.
Features of the scapula ("shoulder blade") include three borders, three angles, and two surfaces.
The humerus is the largest bone in the superior limb and forms the skeleton within the brachium.
The radius and ulna form the skeletal support for the antebrachium.
The eight carpal bones are arranged in two rows and constitute the only short bones in the superior limb.
The five metacarpal bones are numbered 1-5 from lateral to medial.
Phalanges (singular=phalanx) are the long bones within the digits.

BONES OF THE INFERIOR LIMB

The 33 bones within each inferior limb include one flat bone, 22 long bones, seven short bones, and three sesamoid bones.
The os coxae (hip bone) is formed by the fusion of an ilium, ischium, and pubis.
The pelvic girdle forms the bony support for the free parts of the inferior limbs and includes the two os coxae and the bony sacrum.
The femur bone forms the skeleton within the thigh and is the longest bone in the body.
The patella ("kneecap") is the largest sesamoid bone in the body.
The tibia and fibula form the skeleton within the crus.
The seven tarsal bones form two irregular rows and constitute the only short bones in the inferior limb.
The five metatarsal bones are numbered 1-5 from medial to lateral.
The phalanges within the toes resemble their counterparts in the digits of the hands.

CLINICAL CONSIDERATIONS

The clinical conditions involving bones include entities from every major disease category: degenerative conditions, anomalies, metabolic diseases, neoplasia, infections, and trauma.

Selected Definitions

Appendicular skeleton—that portion of the skeleton associated with the limbs. It includes the clavicles, scapulae, ossa coxae, and all of the bones in the free parts of the limbs.

Articular cartilage—the hyaline cartilage that covers those load bearing surfaces of bones that are involved in synovial joints. Some hyaline cartilage is not involved in joints (costal cartilage), some is not involved in synovial joints (epiphyseal cartilage), and cartilaginous structures found in some synovial joints are not composed of hyaline cartilage (*e.g.*, articular discs and menisci).

Axial skeleton—the sternum and ribs, and the bones of the vertebral column and head. These bones are all flat or irregular in shape.

Compact (cortical) bone tissue—bone tissue that is "solid" (*i.e.*, not in the form of small spicules separated by bone marrow tissue). Compact bone tissue is also called "dense" bone tissue.

Epiphysis—either end of a long bone. Specific landmark names are applied to epiphyses depending on the anatomic features located there (head of the humerus, base of a metacarpal bone, tuberosity of a distal phalanx, *etc.*).

Flat bones—those bones that are obviously flattened in one dimension (sternum, ribs, scapulae, clavicles, ossa coxae, and many bones in the skull).

Hydroxyapatite—the principal inorganic component of bone tissue. Hydroxyapatite is a complex calcium phosphate salt that has the chemical formula $Ca_{10}(PO_4)_6(OH)_2$ and it is also the primary mineral in the enamel, cementum, and dentin of teeth.

Irregular bones—the vertebrae and several bones of the head which have jutting processes. Exact numbers of irregular bones and flat bones are typically not stated because some bones have parts that are flat and other portions that are irregular (temporal and occipital bones).

Long bones—those bones designated as such by convention. The 88 long bones are found in the free parts of each superior limb (humerus, radius, ulna, five metacarpal bones, and 14 phalanges) and each inferior limb (femur bone, tibia, fibula, five metatarsal bones, and 14 phalanges).

Medullary cavity—the space within a bone that contains bone marrow tissue, adipose tissue, and blood. The connective tissue proper that lines the medullary cavity (thinner but similar to periosteum) is called endosteum.

Osseous lacunae—the tiny spaces within bone tissue that contain osteocytes. Osteocytes in neighboring lacunae communicate physically and metabolically by extending cytoplasmic processes through tiny passageways called osseous canaliculi.

Osseous lamella—a layer of mineralized osteoid. Those parallel and adjacent to the periosteum and endosteum are called external and internal circumferential lamellae. Those in the intervening compact bone are called concentric (osteonal) and interstitial lamellae.

Osteoblast—a bone tissue forming cell. Osteoblasts secrete the organic part of the extracellular matrix of bone tissue and become osteocytes when they become trapped therein.

Osteoclast—a multinuclear bone cell involved in bone tissue absorption. Osteoclasts dissolve the mineral with acidic secretions and hydrolyze the osteoid enzymatically.

Osteoid—the non-cellular organic portion of bone tissue. It is manufactured by osteoblasts and consists of collagenous fibers embedded in a protein/polysaccharide ground substance.

Osteology—the study of bone tissue and of bones. Bones are organs that contain all of the various connective tissues as well as smooth muscle tissue, nervous tissue, and simple squamous epithelium.

Periosteum—the dense, irregular connective tissue proper that forms the outer encasement of bones. Periosteum covers all of the external surfaces except for articular surfaces, attachments of tendons, ligaments, retinacula, joint capsules, and ports of entry for nerves and vessels.

Sesamoid bones—"seed-like" bones that are embedded in a few tendons and serve as bearing surfaces for them. The patellae (kneecaps) are the largest sesamoid bones, and two smaller ones are typically found at the base of each thumb and big toe.

Short bones—the carpal and tarsal bones. There are 30 short bones total (eight in each wrist and seven in each ankle). Some short bones are physically longer than some of the long bones.

Spongy (trabecular) bone tissue—bone tissue formed of small spicules between intervening regions of bone marrow tissue. This form of bone tissue is often found within the ends of long bones and is also called "cancellous" bone tissue.

Etymology ***Malus ad osteum*—"Bad to the bone."**

acetabulum (L), *a cup*—acetabular fossa
calcaneum (L), *the heel*—calcaneus
clavis (L), *a key or lock*—clavicle
cuneus (L), *a wedge*—medial cuneiform bone
cortex (L), *bark of a tree*—cortex
diaphysis (G), *a growing through*—diaphysis
glene (G), *a socket*—glenohumeral joint
hamulus (L), *a hook*—hamulus of hamate bone
hamatus (L), *furnished with a hook*—hamate bone
hem (G), *blood*—hemopoiesis
humerus (L), *upper part of arm*—humeral condyle
ischion (G), *hip*—ischial spine
korone (G), *a crow*—coronoid process
lacuna (L), *lake, cavity*—lacuna
lamella (L), *a thin plate*—interstitial lamellae
luna (L), *moon*—lunate bone
malleolus (L), *small hammer*—malleolar groove
navis (L), *a ship*—navicular bone
obturare (L), *to stop up*—obturator foramen
olene (G), *elbow*—olecranon
osteon (G), *a bone*—osteoporosis
phalanx (L), *line of battle*—distal phalanx
physis (G), *nature*—metaphyseal growth
pisium (L), *pea*—joint of pisiform bone
poiesis (G), *a making*—leucopoiesis
popliteus (L), *ham*—popliteal fossa
pub (L), *of the groin*—pubic crest
ramus (L), *branch of a tree*—inferior ramus of pubis
scaph (L), *light boat, skiff*—scaphoid bone
scapula (L), *shoulder blade*—spine of scapula
sesame (G), *sesame seed-like*—sesamoid bone
skeleton (G), *a mummy or dried body*—axial skeleton
trabs (L), *a beam*—trabecula
triquetra (L), *three-cornered*—triquetral bone
troch (L), *pulleys*—trochlear notch
ulna (L), *elbow*—ulnar notch

Introduction

Osteology is the study of bone tissue as well as the study of the individual bones of the skeleton. Bone tissue is one of the subtypes of connective tissue and is a major (but not the only) tissue component of the named bones of the body (humerus, radius, femur bone, *etc.*). Named bones are organs because they are composed of several tissues.

Structure of Bone Tissue

Bone tissue is the third hardest substance in the body (enamel and dentin of the teeth are harder). The hardness comes from its high mineral content which comprises about two-thirds of its dry weight. The organic portion of bone (one-third of the dry weight) consists of the same three general components as the other connective tissues: cells, fibers, and ground substance. There are three types of bone cells: osteoblasts, osteocytes, and osteoclasts. **Osteoblasts** are single-nucleated, metabolically active cells that are found on the surface of bone tissue. They secrete the fibers and the organic part of the ground substance. The fibers of bone are collagenous in nature and the ground substance is a protein-polysaccharide. Taken together, these form the organic part of the matrix which, in bone, is called **osteoid**. **Osteocytes** are relatively sedentary cells which are entrapped within the extracellular matrix. They are, in effect, *former osteoblasts* which become imprisoned in the products of their own secretion. **Osteoclasts** are large, multinucleated cells which are active in bone reabsorption. The mineral portion of bone is composed of complex forms of calcium phosphate. The most common form is **hydroxyapatite** which has the chemical formula: $Ca_{10}(PO_4)_6(OH)_2$. In addition to calcium and phosphate ions, there are a number of other minerals present in trace amounts in bone tissue. Bone minerals are deposited on (actually, they precipitate on) the collagenous fibers after the osteoblasts manufacture and extrude them.

When osteoblasts are actively secreting the collagenous fibers and ground substance of bone tissue, they are located on a surface. As they extrude their secretory products, some of them become imprisoned by the intercellular matrix (extracellular matrix) that they produce. Thereafter, they occupy small cavities called **lacunae** and are known as osteocytes. Mitotic divisions of the osteoblasts at the surface prevent their numbers from decreasing. The alternating layers of entrapped osteocytes and matrix are called **lamellae** and there are four types: concentric, interstitial, and external and internal circumferential lamellae (Figure 5-1). Lamellae that surround neurovascular channels within the cortex of bone are termed **osteonal** or **concentric lamellae**. A set of concentric (osteonal) lamellae and the neurovascular structures which they surround is termed an **osteon**. In long bones, most osteons are longitudinally oriented and their neurovascular passageways are called **central canals**. Neurovascular passageways that pass through bone perpendicular to the long axis often lack surrounding lamellae and are known as **nutrient canals (perforating canals)**. Tiny channels through the lamellae called **canaliculi** (*little canals*) contain cytoplasmic processes of the osteocytes and allow those located close to the vessels to exchange nutrients and wastes with those located farther from the vessels.

Osteons are the functional subunits of bone. New osteons are formed after osteoclasts "cut" channels through the bone by reabsorbing it. This process, termed bone remodeling, is a continuous one that helps maintain the proper blood calcium levels. First, an osteoclast creates a channel in bone tissue by dissolving the mineral with localized pH changes and enzymatically degrading the collagen fibers and ground substance. Primitive cells associated with the vessels that follow the osteoclasts differentiate into osteoblasts. These osteoblasts then begin depositing matrix and forming new lamellae on the surface of the wall of the newly created channel beginning with the outermost layer and continuing inward (layer by layer). Since osteoclasts do not stay within osteonal boundaries when they reabsorb bone, they leave partial remnants of existing lamellae next to the channels that they form. These incomplete remnants of concentric and external circumferential lamellae are termed **interstitial lamellae**. The several layers of lamellae that surround (encase) a whole bone are termed **external circumferential lamellae**. Corresponding ones that line the medullary cavities of mature bones are termed **internal circumferential lamellae**.

Bone tissue exists in two physical forms: compact and spongy. **Compact (cortical) bone** is also known as "dense" bone. This form is relatively solid and forms the majority of the substance of most bones. **Spongy (trabecular) bone** is also called "cancellous" bone. It consists of slender spicules and reinforcing struts which lend strength without excessive bulk. Spongy bone is found between the inner and outer layers of compact bone of the braincase, and also within the ends of long bones where it provides reinforcement for the overlying articular surfaces.

Objectives

1. Discuss bone tissue including its organic and inorganic components, its three kinds of cells, four kinds of lamellae, and histological architecture.
2. Explain why interstitial lamellae are always "older" than adjacent concentric lamellae.

Bone is a Tissue; Named Bones are Organs

A clear distinction should be made between the substance (tissue) bone (Figure 5-2) and named bones such as the scapula, tibia, *etc.*, which are organs. Although bone tissue is a major component of the named bones of the body, one should note that the latter are organs because they contain numerous other tissues *in addition* to bone. For example, bones are covered and lined by connective

Table 5-1 Tissues Present in a Bone

Tissue	*Location*
Bone tissue	Throughout most of structure
Connective tissue proper	Periosteum and endosteum
Cartilage*	Covering articular surfaces
Adipose tissue	Within medullary cavity
Bone marrow tissue	Within medullary cavity
Smooth muscle tissue	Within vascular network
Simple squamous epithelium	Within vascular network
Nervous tissue	Throughout most of structure
Blood	Within vascular network

*A few bones lack cartilage

tissue proper and usually have cartilage covered ends. They contain bone marrow tissue and adipose tissue within their medullary cavities and even some smooth muscle and epithelium within the walls of their vascular network and blood within their vascular lumina. Finally, as anyone who has suffered a fracture can attest, bones are invested with nervous tissue (Table 5-1). The context in which the term *bone* is used often clarifies the intended meaning as bone the *tissue* versus bone the *organ*.

Objectives

3. Differentiate bone tissue from named bones by listing the tissues found in any named bone in addition to bone tissue.

Functions of Bone(s)

Bones have many functional roles. They lend physical support to the body and give it a permanent shape. They also form joints with each other to allow body movement. Bones surround many vital organs and form protective enclosures. The brain, for example, is completely encased by skeletal components and the heart and lungs are protected by the thoracic cage formed by the sternum, vertebrae, and ribs. In addition to these physical functions, bones have a number of important metabolic roles. They house the bone marrow tissue which produces most of the blood cells. The medullary cavities of bones also serve as a depository for excess adipose tissue (unfortunately, there is a limit to how much fat can be stored there!!). The minerals in bone tissue serve as a readily mobilizable storehouse of calcium and phosphorus which helps the body maintain the critical blood levels of these minerals compatible with life. The various functions of bone are summarized in Table 5-2.

Table 5-2 Functions of Bones and Bone Tissue

Physical Functions	*Metabolic Functions*
Body shape—allows permanent shape and upright posture	**Hemopoiesis**—formation of RBC's and many types of WBC's
Protection—encasement of brain, thoracic, and pelvic organs	**Fat depository**—a normal metaplastic change with age
Locomotion—interaction with skeletal muscles to produce body movement	**Calcium/phosphorus storage**—within the hydroxyapatite

Objectives

4. State the functions of bones and bone tissue and divide them into two large categories: physical and metabolic.

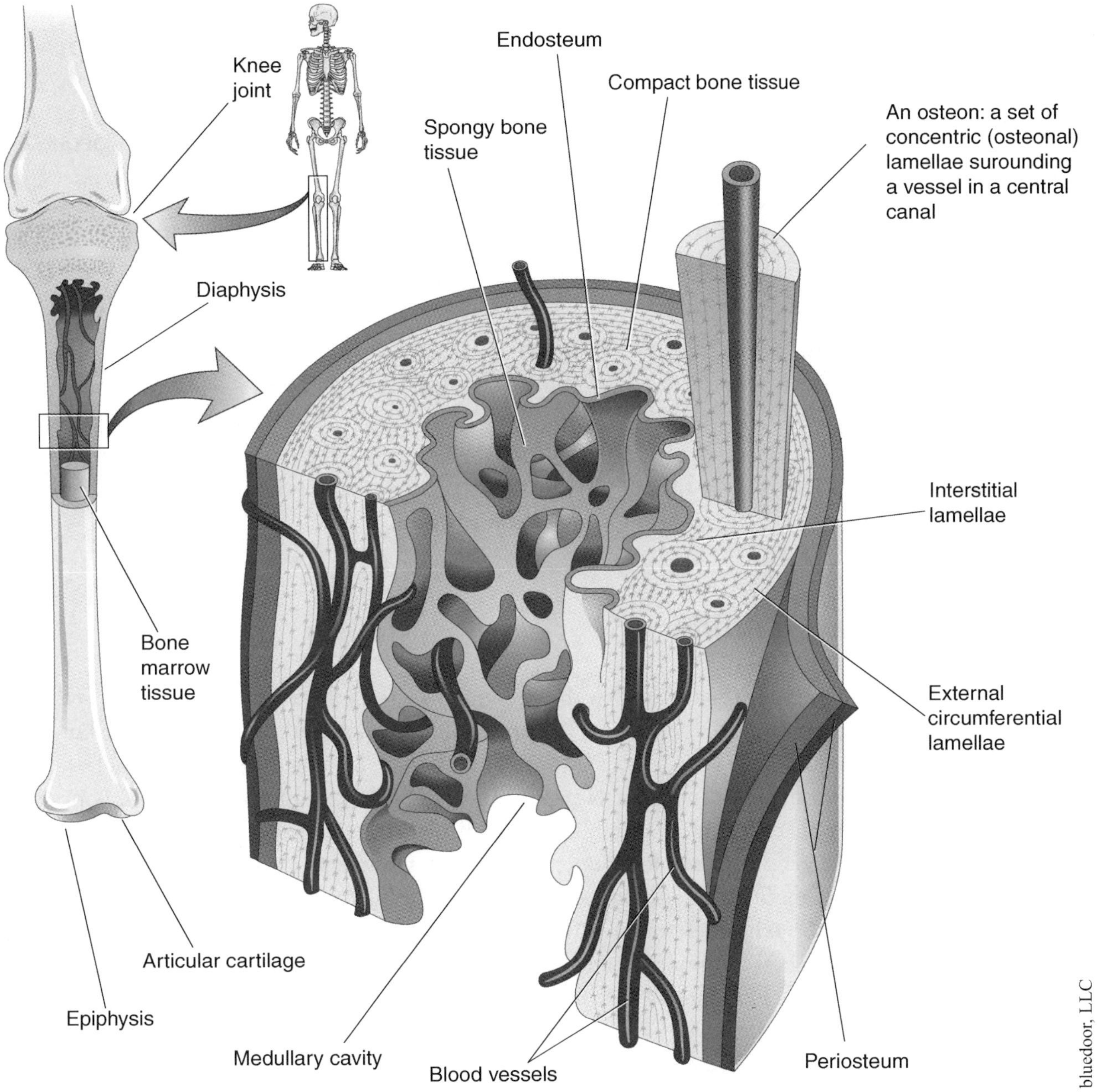

Figure 5-1

Structure of Bone Tissue

A cortical segment of a long bone has been removed and enlarged to show architectural detail. The basic structural unit is a set of concentric lamellae surrounding a central canal and is called an osteon. Interstitial lamellae are remnants of "old" concentric or external circumferential lamellae that remain after osteoclasts have excavated channels and new osteons have filled them in. Internal circumferential lamellae (not well illustrated) lie adjacent to the endosteum in mature bones.

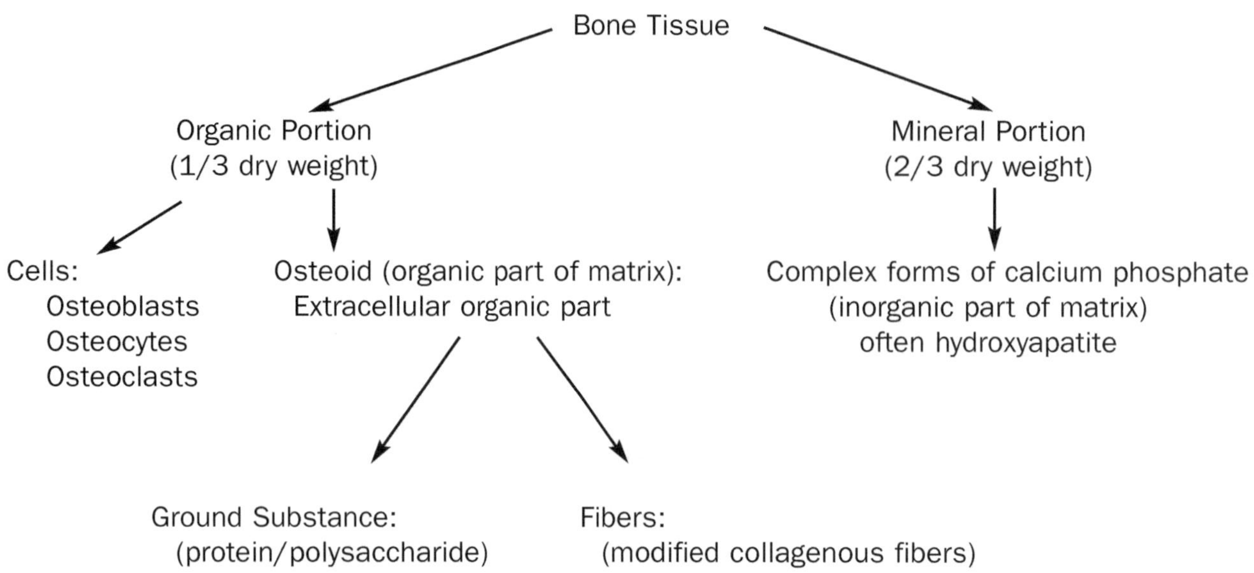

Figure 5-2
The Composition of Bone

Classification of Bones by Position

The 214 bones of the body (Figure 5-3) are divided into two groups based on their position in the body: appendicular skeleton and axial skeleton. The **appendicular skeleton** includes all of the bones associated with the limbs (Table 5-3). For each superior limb these include the clavicle, scapula, humerus, radius, ulna, eight carpal bones, five metacarpal bones, 14 phalanges and two sesamoid bones (at the base of the thumb). For the inferior limb the appendicular skeleton is composed of the os coxae (hip bone), femur bone, patella (a sesamoid bone), tibia, fibula, seven tarsal bones, five metatarsal bones, 14 phalanges, and two more sesamoid bones (at the base of the big toe).

The bones of the **axial skeleton** are divided into several groups consisting of those found within the head, the vertebral column, ribs, and sternum (Table 5-3). The bones of the head include eight that form the cranial cavity and 14 that form the skeleton of the face. In addition, there are three pairs of auditory ossicles (malleus, incus, stapes) in the head and a single hyoid bone. The vertebral column is typically composed of 26 components that represent 33 originally separate vertebrae. The sacral vertebrae fuse to form the bony sacrum and the coccygeal vertebrae fuse to form the coccyx. There are 12 pairs of ribs and cartilaginous extensions from all but the inferior two pairs extend medially to make direct or indirect contact with the sternum.

At the junction of the appendicular and axial skeletons, some bones from each form the skeletal support for the free parts of the limbs. These supporting bones comprise the pectoral girdle and the pelvic girdle. The **pectoral girdle** supports the free parts of the superior limbs which begin at the shoulders and extend distally. It includes the sternum (a flat bone of the axial skeleton), and the two clavicles and two scapulae (flat bones belonging to the appendicular skeleton). The **pelvic girdle** supports the free parts of the inferior limbs which begin at the hip joint and extend distally. It includes the bony sacrum (an irregular bone from the axial skeleton) and the right and left os coxae (flat bones from the appendicular skeleton).

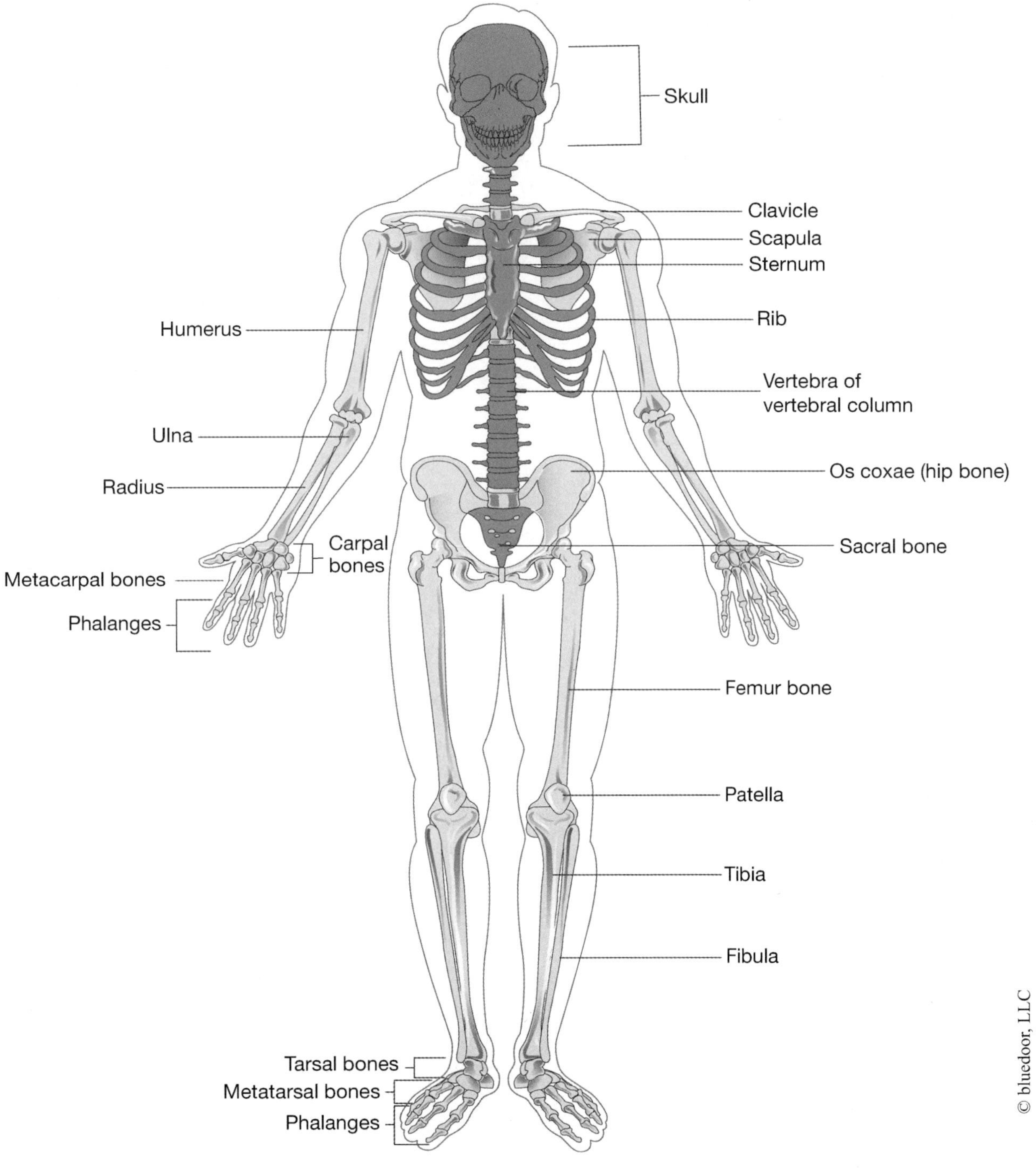

Figure 5-3

Anterior View of the Human Skeleton

The bones of the limbs (shown white above) comprise the appendicular skeleton and the others (those of skull, thoracic cage, and vertebral column shown in gray) comprise the axial skeleton.

Table 5-3 Classification of Bones by Position

There are typically 214* bones in the adult human body.

Axial Skeleton (80)			**Appendicular Skeleton (134)**	
Head (29)	Vertebral Column (26)	Thoracic cage (without vertebrae) (25)	Superior Limbs (68) (34 in each limb):	Inferior Limbs (66) (33 in each limb)
8 cranial bones	7 cervical vertebrae	24 ribs (12 pair)	within pectoral girdle	within pelvic girdle
14 facial bones	12 thoracic vertebrae	true ribs (1-7)	1 clavicle	1 os coxae
6 auditory ossicles	5 lumbar vertebrae	false ribs (8-12)	1 scapula	free part of limb
1 hyoid bone	within pelvic girdle	floating ribs (11-12)	free part of limb	1 femur bone
	1 bony sacrum	within pectoral girdle	1 humerus	1 patella
	1 coccyx	1 sternum	1 radius	1 tibia
			1 ulna	1 fibula
			8 carpal bones	7 tarsal bones
			5 metacarpal bones	5 metatarsal bones
			14 phalanges	14 phalanges
			2 sesamoid bones*	2 sesamoid bones*

Osseous Trivia

1. The longest bone is the femur bone.
2. The smallest bone is the stapes ("stirrup").
3. The most frequently fractured bone is the clavicle.
4. The patella is the largest sesamoid bone in the body.
5. The coccyx is formed by a fusion of (typically) four coccygeal vertebrae.
6. The bony sacrum is formed by a fusion of (typically) five sacral vertebrae.
7. Each os coxae is formed by fusion of an ilium (not ileum), ischium, and pubis.
8. The axial skeleton is composed of flat and irregular bones (no long, short or sesamoid bones).
9. There are 56 phalanges (20 proximal phalanges, 16 middle phalanges, and 20 distal phalanges).
10. Disregarding vertebrae, only the sternum, hyoid bone, mandible, and five bones of the skull are unpaired.
11. The shortest long bone (often the middle phalanx of the fifth toe) is much shorter than the longest short bone (calcaneus).
12. The free part of each limb contains only long bones, short bones, and sesamoid bones (no flat or irregular bones).
13.* The two sesamoid bones at the base of each thumb and the two at the base of each big toe are often ignored (when totaling the skeletal components). Some individuals have other, inconstantly present, sesamoid bones associated with the digits.
14. The pelvic girdle supports the free parts of the inferior limbs and includes three bones: both os coxae and the bony sacrum.
15. The pectoral girdle supports the free parts of the superior limbs and includes five bones: both clavicles, both scapulae, and the sternum.

Classification of Bones by Shape

Bones are classified into five categories on the basis of their general shape: long bones, short bones, flat bones, irregular bones, and sesamoid bones (Table 5-4). **Long bones** are those which are elongated in one dimension. They are found only in the limbs where they act as supporting columns and articulate with each other to form joints and levers for locomotion. There are 88 long bones in the body (44 pairs) and 56 of them are the phalanges within the fingers and toes. **Short bones** include the eight carpal bones within each wrist and seven tarsal bones within each ankle (thirty total). Most of them are somewhat cuboidal in shape. **Flat bones** are significantly reduced in one dimension. They include the clavicles, scapulae, ribs, sternum, ossa coxae (bones of the pelvis), and many bones of the head. **Irregular bones** are characterized by jutting processes. They include the vertebrae and several bones of the head. **Sesamoid bones** are small (seed-like) bones embedded in some tendons. They function as bearing surfaces and protect the tendons from frictional deterioration as they work back and forth over bony prominences. The largest sesamoid bones in the body are the patellae (kneecaps). Two smaller sesamoid bones are located at the base of each thumb and big toe, bringing the usual total number to ten (some individuals have fewer and others have more).

Table 5-4 Classification of Bones by Shape

Type	*Location/Comment*	
Long bones	*in each superior limb* (22): humerus radius ulna metacarpal bones (5) phalanges (14)	*in each inferior limb* (22): femur bone tibia fibula metatarsal bones (5) phalanges (14)
Short bones	*within each carpus* (8): scaphoid bone lunate bone triquetral bone pisiform bone trapezium bone trapezoid bone capitate bone hamate bone	*within each tarsus* (7) talus calcaneus navicular bone medial cuneiform bone intermediate cuneiform bone lateral cuneiform bone cuboid bone
Flat bones	scapulae (2), clavicles (2), sternum, ribs (24), os coxae (2), several bones in the skull	
Irregular bones	vertebrae (26), several bones in the skull	
Sesamoid bones	patellae (2), sesamoid bones at the base of each thumb (2), sesamoid bones at the base of each big toe (2); additional sesamoid bones may be present	

Note: the auditory ossicles and the hyoid bone are usually ignored by shape taxonomists.

Objectives

5. Classify the bones of the skeleton into two groups by position and five groups by shape.
6. State which bone shape types are found in the appendicular *vs.* axial skeleton.

Table 5-5 General Surface Features of Bones

Type	*Example and Definition*
Articulating surfaces	Condyle—a rounded articular surface Head—a rounded articular surface Trochlea—a smooth, pulley-like articular surface upon which another bone glides
Non-articulating surfaces	Border—the edge of a bone Face, surface—a designated part of the external surface Fossa—a shallow depression; some fossae articulate Epicondyle—non-articulating area adjacent to a condyle
Non-articular projections	Tubercle, tuberosity, tuber, trochanter—a roughened process that typically serves as a site for muscle attachment Process—a pointed projection that typically serves as a site for muscle attachment Crest—a ridge-like, elongated projection Spine—a name given to some ridges and some projections Ramus—a branch-like projection from a bone
Openings, cavities, and passageways	Foramen—a rounded opening Fissure—a narrow, crack-like opening Meatus, canal—a tubular channel through a bone Sinus—an empty (air-filled) space within a bone
Depressed areas and indentations	Groove, sulcus—an elongated depression Notch—an indentation in a bone Fovea—a small pit or depression; some are articular and some are not
Other landmarks	Neck—a portion of a bone that connects the head to the body of a bone Body—a specific name for the main portion of a bone Base—a term designating the proximal epiphysis of a metacarpal bone, metatarsal bone, or phalanx

General Anatomic Features of Bones

Although each bone of the body has its own peculiar landmarks and shape, there are a number of general structural features common to essentially all bones. The general terms **epiphysis** (end) and **diaphysis** (body) apply only to long bones. The epiphyses of a long bone are typically enlarged in comparison to the diaphysis in order to create larger weight-bearing surfaces for articulations (joints). All bones are encased in a connective tissue proper envelope called **periosteum.** The periosteum covers all of the outer aspects except for articular surfaces, attachments of tendons, ligaments, and joint capsules, and ports of entry of nerves and vessels (Figure 5-4). It is firmly anchored to the underlying bone tissue by microscopic **perforating fibers** composed of collagen. The inner portion of a bone is hollow and is termed the **medullary cavity**. It is lined by a thin sheet of connective tissue proper termed the **endosteum** and houses the bone marrow tissue. The latter is actively hemopoietic in young individuals and is called **red bone marrow**. In many bones it changes to **yellow** (fatty) **bone marrow** with age, and may even become **gelatinous bone marrow** with senility. The bone tissue between the endosteum and periosteum in most areas of most bones is compact bone and is called the **cortex**. It is penetrated by neurovascular structures in several locations. The periosteal openings of these passageways are called **nutrient foramina** (singular = foramen) and the passageways themselves are **nutrient canals**. The nerves and vessels they contain supply the medullary tissue and small branches from them form the neurovascular components within the central canals of the osteons. The external aspects of bones which contact other skeletal components are nearly always covered by cartilage. In the freely moving (synovial) joints of the body, this is a specialized type of hyaline cartilage termed **articular cartilage**. Some bones are joined solidly to each other by either hyaline cartilage or fibrocartilage (cartilaginous joints) and a few are united by fibrous connective tissue without cartilage present.

The landmarks and features of bones are given specific names (*styloid process of the ulna, greater tubercle of the humerus, medial condyle of the femur bone, etc.*). Although each one of these specific names refers to only one entity, there are some general definitions of osteological terms like process, tubercle, foramen, *etc.*, which should be studied and understood (Table 5-5). None of these terms represent specific anatomic structures by themselves, but they serve as parts of more complete names and have definitional significance therein.

Objectives

7. Sketch and label the features of a typical long bone and indicate which features are found in long bones only.

Bones of the Superior Limb

The 34 bones forming the skeleton of each superior limb include two flat bones (clavicle, scapula), 22 long bones, (humerus, radius, ulna, five metacarpal bones, 14 phalanges), eight short bones (carpal bones), and two sesamoid bones (at the base of the thumb). The only point of articulation between the bones of the superior limb and the axial skeleton is the sternoclavicular joint. The incomplete ring of skeletal components formed by the two scapulae, two clavicles, and the intervening manubrium of the sternum is called the **pectoral girdle**. As previously noted under *Classification of Bones by Shape*, this girdle supports the free parts of the superior limbs and provides extensive attachment for muscles which attach the limb to the trunk.

The **clavicle** is the most frequently fractured bone in the body. Even though classified as a flat bone, it is somewhat cylindrical throughout much of its length and resembles a long bone (Figure 5-5). The clavicle consists of a central **body**, a **sternal extremity** ("end") which articulates with the clavicular notch of the sternum, and a flattened **acromial extremity** ("end") that articulates with the acromion of the scapula. The **conoid tubercle** projects from the posterior border of the clavicle near the acromial extremity.

The **scapula** is a triangularly-shaped flat bone with three named borders (superior, medial, and lateral), three angles (superior, inferior, and lateral), and two surfaces (anterior and posterior). The **posterior surface** is divided by a prominent ridge termed the **spine** into a smaller **supraspinous fossa** and a larger **infraspinous fossa** (Figure 5-6). The spine ends laterally in a projection termed the **acromion**. The **medial** and **lateral borders** are fairly straight, but the **superior border** is indented by the **scapular notch**. The **superior** and **inferior angles** are unremarkable but the **lat-**

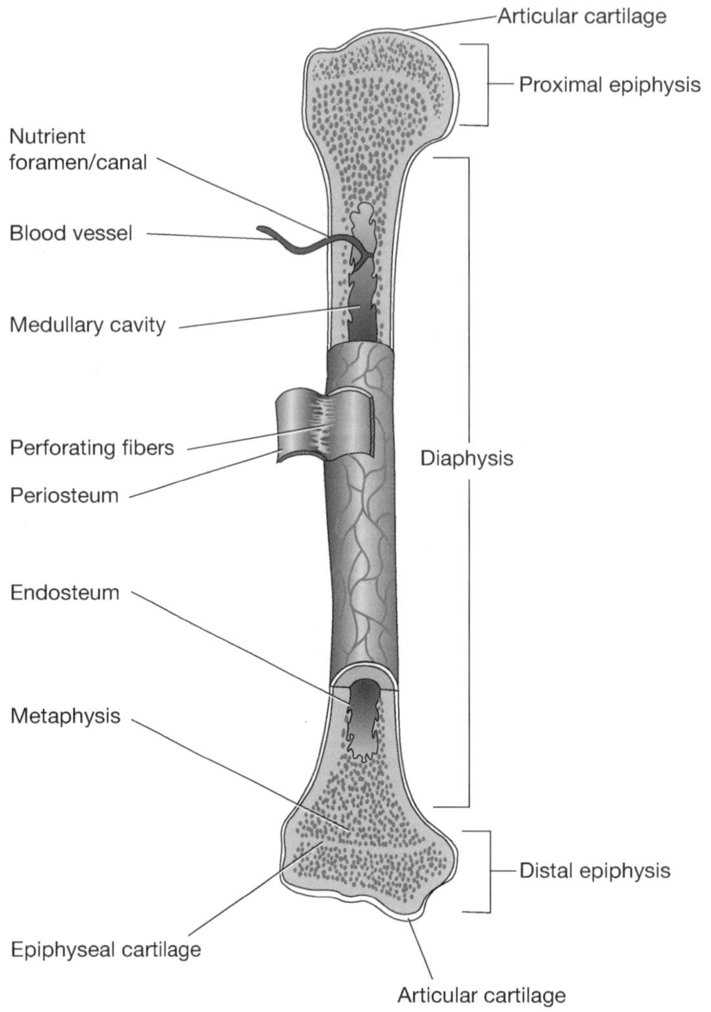

Figure 5-4

Features of a Typical Growing Long Bone

The epiphyseal cartilages ("growth plates") separate the epiphyses from the diaphysis. The metaphyses are portions of the diaphysis adjacent to the epiphyseal cartilages. The channels through which vessels penetrate the cortex are called nutrient canals, and their periosteal openings are called nutrient foramina.

eral (**glenoid**) **angle** is occupied by the **glenoid cavity**. The latter is a depressed area that articulates with the head of the humerus to form the shoulder joint. The constricted portion just medial to the glenoid cavity is the **neck of the scapula**. The prominent, laterally directed projection from the area near the scapular notch is the **coracoid process**. The **anterior** (**costal**) **surface** of the scapula is relatively flat, and most of it is occupied by the **subscapular fossa** which provides attachment for the subscapularis muscle.

The **humerus** is the largest bone in the superior limb and forms the skeleton within the brachium (Figure 5-7). The proximomedial end of the humerus is dominated by the rounded **humeral head** that articulates with the glenoid cavity of the scapula to form the shoulder joint. The two non-articular projections near the head are the **greater tubercle** (laterally) and the **lesser tubercle** (anteriorly). These are separated by the **intertubercular groove** which transmits the tendon of the long head of the biceps brachii muscle. The constricted region distal to the head and tubercles is the **surgical neck** of the humerus. This should be distinguished from the **anatomical neck** which lies immediately adjacent to the articular margin of the head. As is true of all long bones, the diaphysis of the humerus is named the **body**. Near its middle, a subtle roughened area called the **deltoid tuberosity** projects from the anterolateral aspect. The distal articular surface of the humerus is termed the **humeral condyle** and is divided by an unnamed ridge into the rounded **capitulum** (laterally) and the **trochlea** (medially). The non-articular **medial** and **lateral epicondyles** form the palpable bony prominences just proximal to the condyle. A prominent, palpable ridge termed the **lateral supracondylar crest** extends proximally from the lateral epicondyle. The **olecranon fossa** is the deep depression on the posterior side of the distal epiphysis that receives the olecranon of the ulna when the elbow joint is fully extended. A pair of shallower depressions on the anterior aspect called the **coronoid fossa** (medially) and **radial fossa** (laterally) receive the coronoid process of the ulna and the head of the radius when the elbow joint is markedly flexed.

The radius and ulna form the skeleton within the antebrachium (Figure 5-8). The **radius** is lateral to the ulna and its proximal epiphysis is termed the **head**. The radial head has a depressed **articular fovea** that articulates with the capitulum of the humeral condyle and a smooth **articular circumference** that articulates with the radial notch of the ulna to form the proximal radio-ulnar joint. The **neck** of the radius is a constricted area just distal to the head which joins the latter to the radial body. The **body** of the radius encompasses most of its length. The obvious projection at its proximal end is the **radial tuberosity** which serves as the site of insertion for the biceps brachii muscle. The roughened medial surface of the radial body is termed the **interosseous border** and serves as the attachment for the antebrachial interosseous membrane. This dense band of fibrous connective tissue joins the radius and ulna, side-to-side, throughout much of their length. The distal end of the radius is occupied by the **carpal articular surface** which articulates with the proximal row of carpal bones (primarily the scaphoid and lunate bones). The **styloid process** projects distally from the lateral aspect of the distal epiphysis. On the medial side of the distal epiphysis is a depression termed the **ulnar notch** that articulates with the ulna to form the distal radio-ulnar joint.

The **ulna** is positioned medial to the radius within the antebrachium and is longer than the radius. The proximal projection of the ulna that forms the point of the elbow is the **olecranon**. The olecranon serves as the point of insertion for the triceps brachii and anconeus muscles. The large depression distal to the olecranon is the **trochlear notch**. This notch articulates with the trochlea of the humeral condyle. At the distal extent of the trochlear notch is an anterior projection termed the **coronoid process**. The **radial notch** of the ulna is an indentation in the lateral aspect of the coronoid process that articulates with the articular circumference of the radius. The body of the ulna has an **interosseous border** on its lateral aspect which corresponds to and faces that of the radius. The **head** of the ulna forms the palpable "knob" on the posteromedial aspect of the distal antebrachium. The head includes the **articular circumference** which articulates with the ulnar notch of the radius and the pointed projection termed the **styloid process**. In contrast to the radius, the ulna does not articulate directly with carpal bones and the small gap is filled in by a triangularly-shaped articular disc.

The bones of the hand include eight carpal bones within the wrist, five metacarpal bones within the metacarpus, 14 phalanges within the digits, and two sesamoid bones near the base of the thumb (Figure 5-9). The **carpal bones** are arranged in two rows. The **scaphoid bone** is the lateral bone in the proximal row and is the most frequently fractured bone in the wrist. The rounded projection from its anterior aspect is the **tubercle** of the scaphoid bone. The **lunate bone** lies just medi-

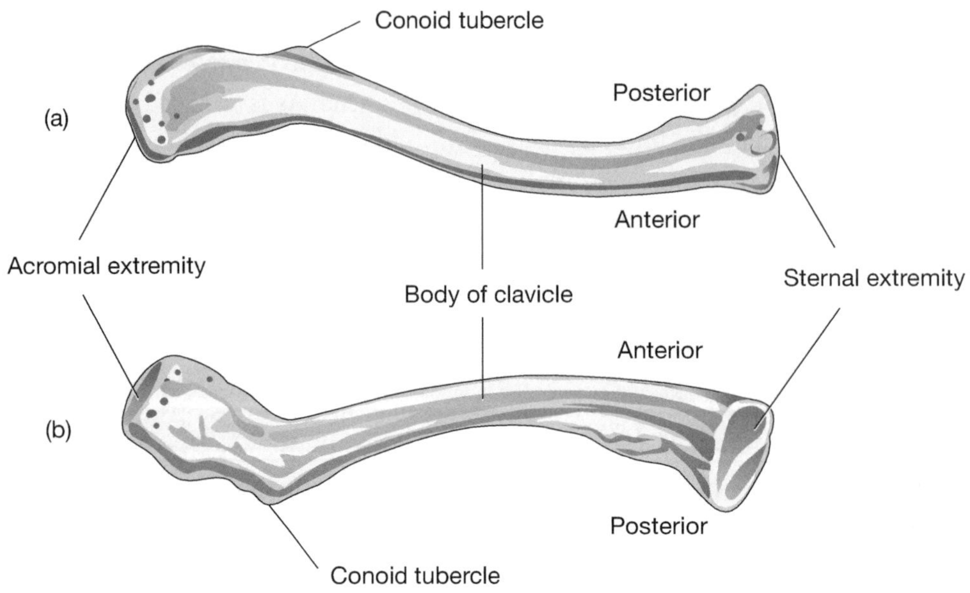

Figure 5-5
Superior (a) and Inferior (b) Views of the Right Clavicle

al to the scaphoid bone and the **triquetral bone** lies medial to the lunate bone. The **pisiform** (pea-shaped) **bone** is the smallest carpal bone. It is positioned anteromedial to the triquetral bone and forms the palpable, bony prominence at the proximal-most extent of the medial aspect of the palm of the hand. The distal four carpal bones are the **trapezium**, **trapezoid**, **capitate**, and **hamate bones** from lateral to medial, respectively. The capitate bone is the largest carpal bone and is positioned proximal to the third metacarpal bone. The trapezium bone has an anterior projection termed the **tubercle** and the hamate bone has an anterior projection termed the **hamulus** (hook). These serve as points of attachment for the flexor retinaculum which is a band of fibrous connective tissue that binds the flexor tendons and accompanying nerves and vessels into the anterior concavity (**carpal groove**) formed by the carpal bones.

The five **metacarpal bones** are numbered **1-5** from lateral to medial (Figure 5-9). Each one has a proximally located **base**, a **body**, and a distally oriented **head**. The heads of the metacarpal bones form the knuckles at the distal end of the metacarpus when a tight fist is formed. The third metacarpal bone has a posterolateral projection from its base termed the **styloid process**. The latter serves as a point of insertion for the extensor carpi radialis longus muscle.

The **phalanges** (**phalanx** is the singular form) are the bones within the digits (Figure 5-9). Each digit of the hand contains three phalanges (proximal, middle, distal) except for the thumb which lacks a middle phalanx and thus has only two. Each phalanx has a proximally located **base** and a central **body**. The distal epiphyses of the proximal and middle phalanges are termed **heads**. The distal epiphyses of the distal phalanges end in widened processes termed **tuberosities**.

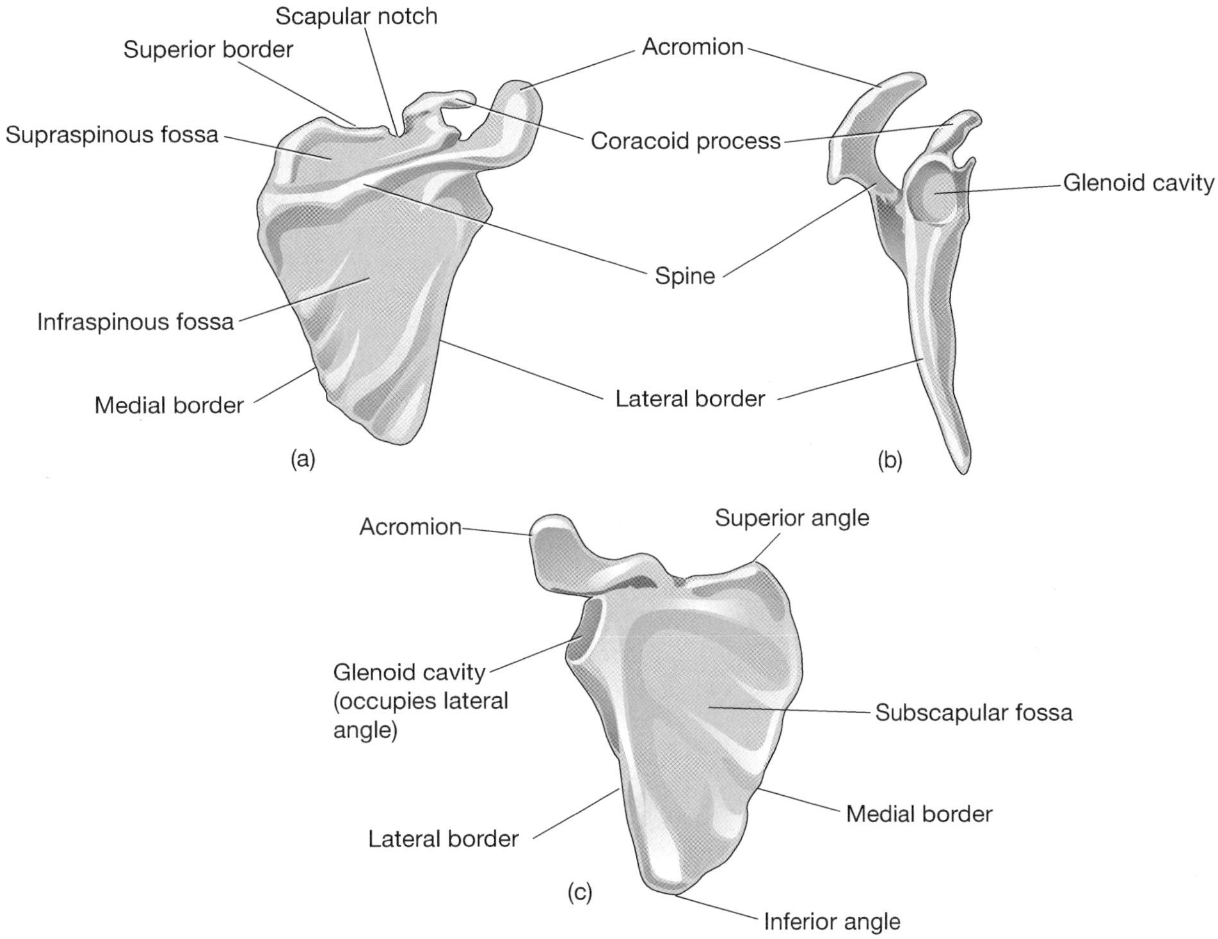

Figure 5-6

Posterior (a), Lateral (b), and Anterior (c) Views of the Right Scapula

Objectives

8. Name the bones of the superior limb and classify them by shape.
9. State the function of the pectoral girdle, list the bones that form it, and indicate which ones belong to the appendicular skeleton.
10. Define phalanx, phalanges, and digit. Explain why "three phalanges comprise a digit" is false but "most digits contain three phalanges" is true.

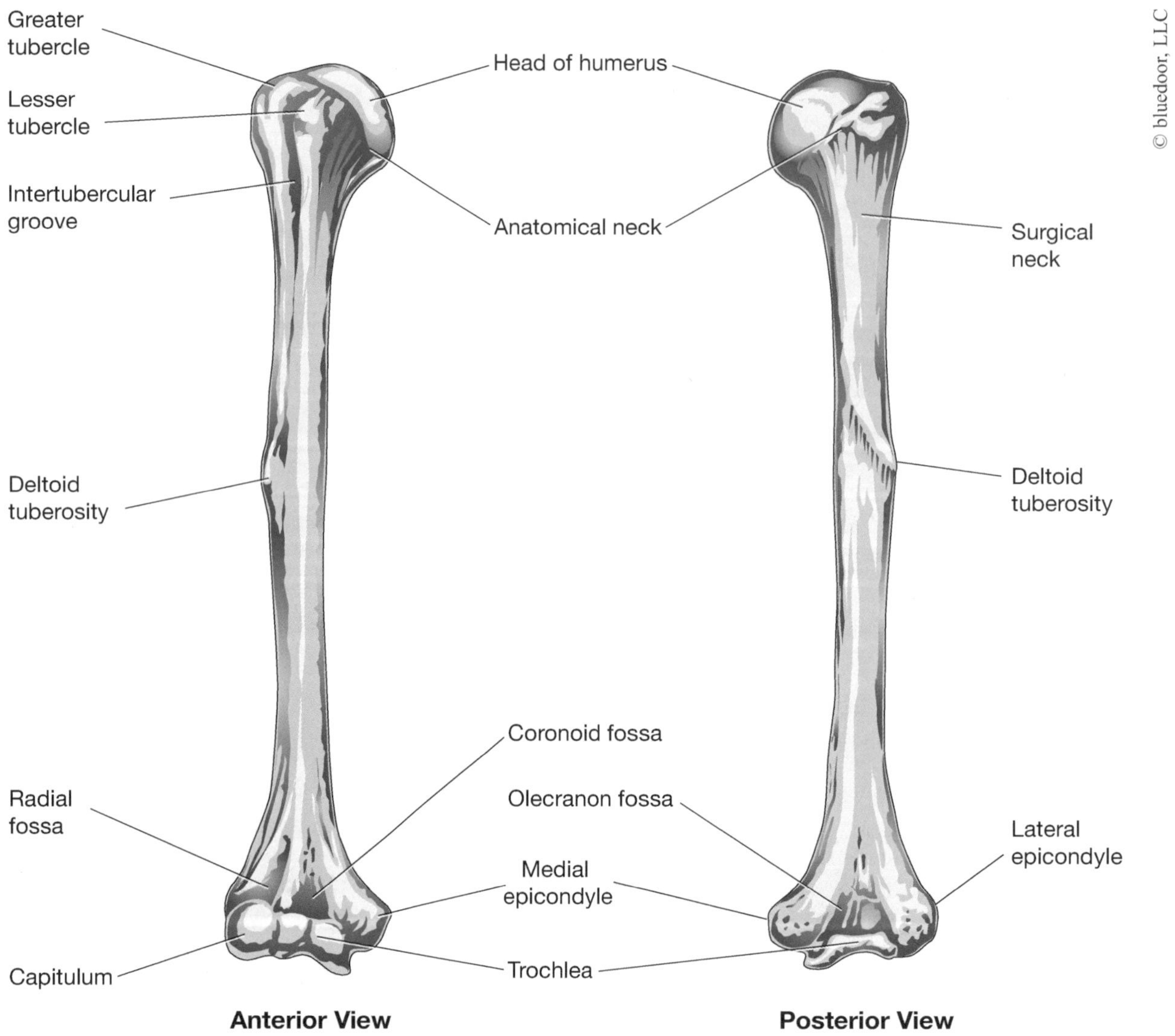

Figure 5-7

Anterior and Posterior Views of a Right Humerus

The whole articular surface at the distal end (including the capitulum and the trochlea) is called the humeral condyle.

Bones of the Inferior Limb

The 33 bones forming the skeleton of each inferior limb include one flat bone (os coxae), 22 long bones (femur bone, tibia, fibula, five metatarsal bones, 14 phalanges), seven short bones (tarsal bones), and three sesamoid bones (two at the base of the big toe and the patella). The left and right ossa coxae are joined anteriorly at the pubic symphysis to form the **bony pelvis**. They articulate with the axial skeleton at the sacroiliac joints. The complete ring of skeletal components formed by the two **ossa coxae** and the bony sacrum is called the **pelvic girdle** (Figure 5-10). It supports the free

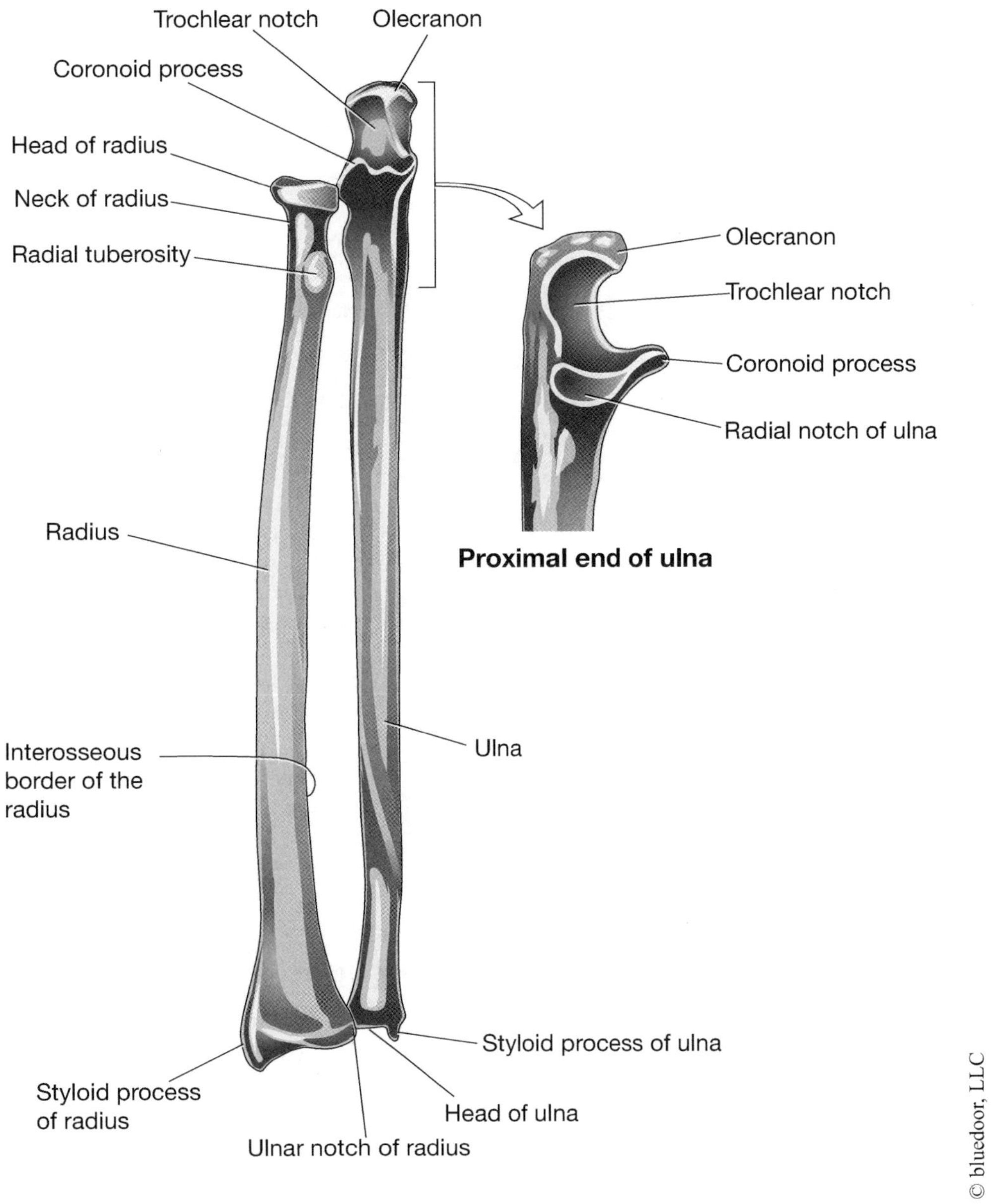

Figure 5-8
Right Radius and Ulna

parts of the inferior limbs and is a site of origin for muscles which act on the limb. The passageway through the pelvic girdle is commonly called the "pelvic canal". The superior end of this passageway is called the **superior pelvic opening** ("pelvic inlet") and the inferior end is the **inferior pelvic opening** ("pelvic outlet"). This narrow portion of the pelvic girdle is called the **minor** (lesser or "true") **pelvis** *vs.* the wider flair of the bone above it which constitutes the **major** (greater or "false") **pelvis.** Various diameters of the pelvic canal are assessed prior to parturition to insure that natural

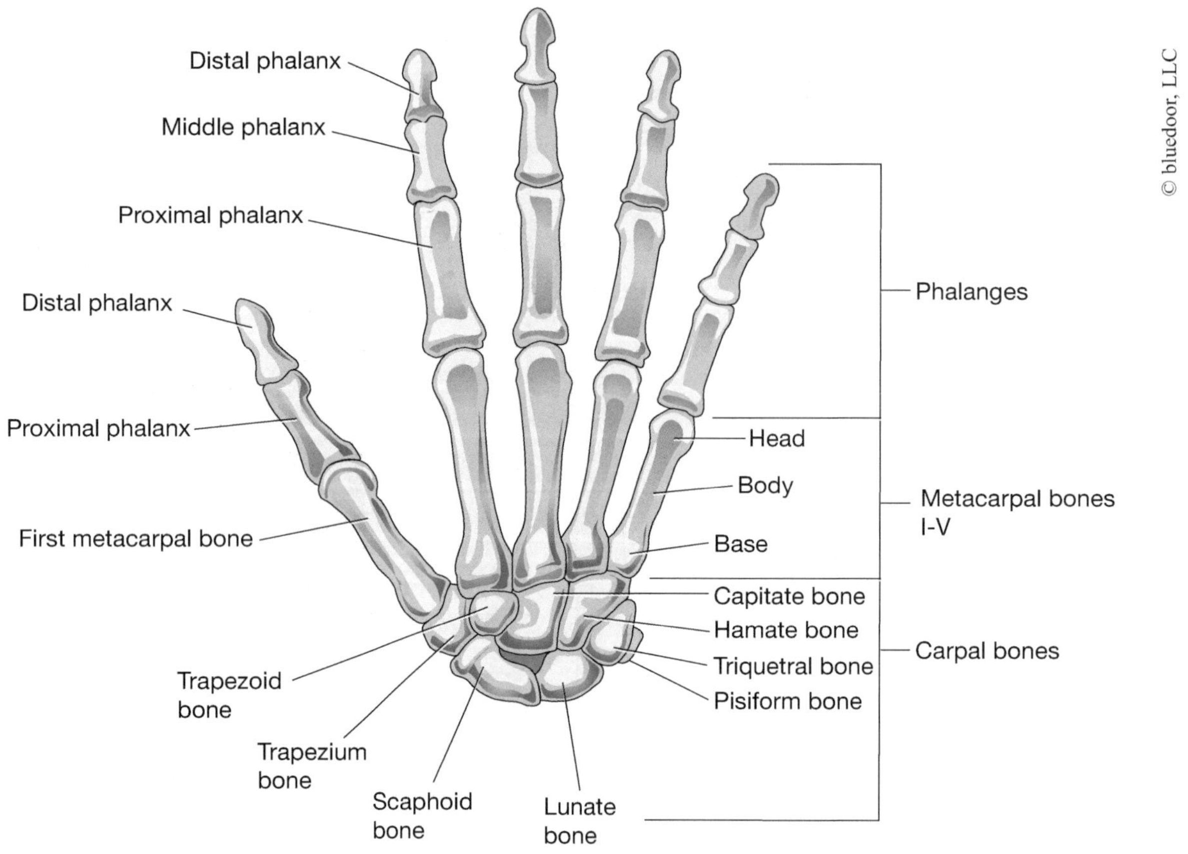

Figure 5-9

Posterior View of the Bones of the Right Hand

Each of the five metacarpal bones has a base, body, and head. The phalanges have similarly named landmarks except that the "heads" of the distal phalanges are flattened to form tuberosities. Note that the pair of sesamoid bones at the base of the thumb cannot be seen in this perspective.

delivery can occur (*see Clinical Considerations in Chapter 6*). There is subtle sexual dimorphism in the pelvic girdle structure. Males have more massive pelvises but relatively narrower pelvic canals than females. Males also tend to have oval *vs.* triangular obturator foramina and smaller subpubic angles (the angle of the pubic arch) than females (Figure 5-11).

The **os coxae** (hip bone) is formed by the fusion of three other bones: ilium, ischium, and pubis (Figure 5-12). Where these join each other, a laterally oriented depression called the **acetabulum** is formed which receives the head of the femur bone to form the hip joint. The articular portion of the acetabulum is somewhat "half-moon" in shape and is called the **lunate surface**. The non-articular portion of the acetabulum is called the **acetabular fossa**. It extends out to the inferior aspect of the acetabular margin (edge) where it causes a defect called the **acetabular notch**. Inferior and medial to the acetabulum is the large **obturator foramen** which transmits the obturator nerve.

The **ilium** is the fan-shaped, flat bone forming the superior two-thirds of the os coxae (Figure 5-12). Its inferior portion is called the **body** and forms the superior part of the acetabulum. The wider, superior part of the ilium is called the **ilial wing**. The superior border of the ilial wing is called the **iliac crest**. It forms the obvious bony prominence near the waist on the side of the trunk. Anteriorly, the iliac crest ends in an obvious prominence termed the **anterior superior iliac spine.** A few centimeters below it is the **anterior inferior iliac spine**. A similar pair of prominences is present at the posterior aspect of the ilial wing (**posterior superior iliac spine** and **posterior inferior iliac spine**). The marked indentation below the posterior inferior iliac spine is called the **greater sciatic notch**. The broad, flat posterolateral aspect of the ilial wing is called the **gluteal surface**. It is crossed by anterior, posterior, and inferior **gluteal lines**. These subtle ridges and the adjacent smooth areas serve as attachment sites for the gluteal muscles. The flattened, anteromedial aspect of the wing of the ilium is the **sacropelvic surface**. A small portion of the posterior part of the sacropelvic surface, called the **auricular surface**, articulates with the sacral bone to form the sacroiliac joint. Just above it is a roughened non-articular area termed the **iliac tuberosity**. The smooth, anterior part of the sacropelvic surface is called the **iliac fossa** which serves as an attachment site for the iliacus muscle.

The **ischium** is the flat bone forming the posteroinferior part of the os coxae (Figure 5-12). The thick vertical part which contributes to the formation of the acetabulum is the **body** of the ischium. The triangular, posteriorly-directed projection from the ischial body, just below the greater sciatic notch, is the **spine** of the ischium. The indentation below the ischial spine is the **lesser sciatic notch**. The inferior portion of the ischium is called the **ramus** of the ischium. It forms the posterolateral margin of the obturator foramen and projects anteriorly to join the inferior ramus of the pubis. Roughened projections from the posterior aspects of the left and right ischial bodies called the **ischiatic tubers** form the bony prominences on which we "sit."

The **pubis** is the flat bone comprising the anteroinferior portion of the os coxae (Figure 5-12). It forms the anteromedial margin of the obturator foramen and is divided into three major parts: body, superior ramus, and inferior ramus. The **body** of the pubis is the portion on which the **symphyseal surface** is located. This surface articulates with its contralateral counterpart to form a fibrocartilaginous joint termed the *pubic symphysis*. The anterior portion of the body is termed the **pubic crest**. It ends laterally in a subtle projection termed the **pubic tubercle**. The **superior ramus** of the pubis is the portion that projects superiorly to contribute to the acetabulum. The sharp ridge on the anterosuperior aspect of the ramus is the **pecten of the pubis**. The **inferior ramus** of the pubis projects posteriorly to join the ramus of the ischium. The curved rim of bone formed by the posterior borders of the left and right pubes is called the **pubic arch**. The measurable angle between the pubes as they join to form the pubic arch is called the **subpubic angle** (Figure 5-11). In males this angle tends to be smaller than in females.

The **femur bone** is the longest bone in the body and forms the skeleton within the thigh (Figure 5-13). The rounded **head** of the femur bone articulates with the acetabulum to form the coxal joint. In the central part of the articular surface of the femoral head is a non-articular depression called the **fovea** of the femoral head. It serves as an attachment for the ligament of the femoral head. The **neck** of the femur bone is the constricted area just distal to the femoral head. At its junction with the femoral body are two large prominences that serve as attachment sites for muscles: a larger **greater trochanter** (laterally) and a smaller **lesser trochanter** (medially). These are joined by two bony ridges: the **intertrochanteric crest** on the posterior side and the less obvious **intertrochanteric line** on the anterior side. The **body** of the femur bone comprises most of the length of the bone. The roughened elongated area on the posterior aspect of the body is the **linea aspera**. In the distal aspect of the bone the

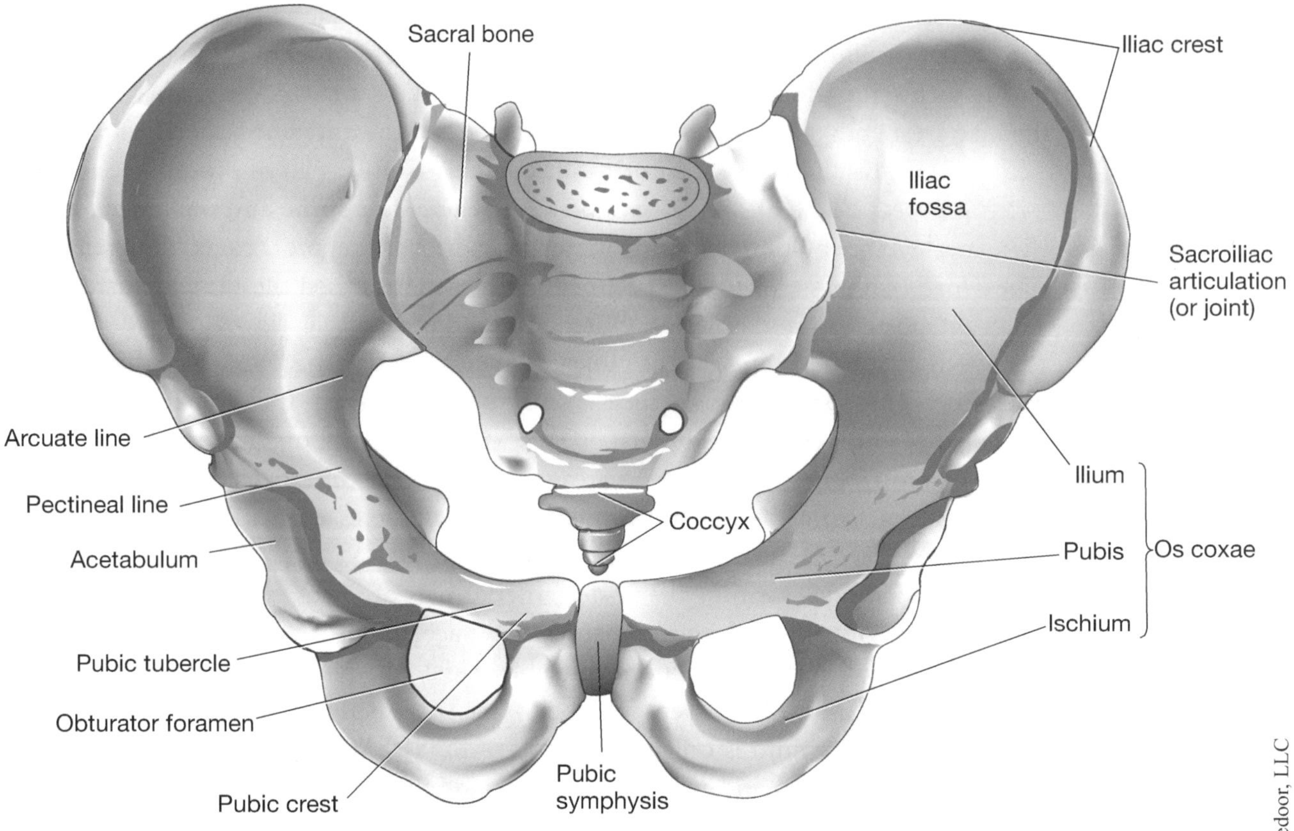

Figure 5-10

Anterior View of the Pelvic Girdle and Coccyx

The pelvic girdle supports the free parts of the inferior limbs and includes left os coxae, right os coxae, and sacral bone.

linea aspera fades and blends into the smooth **popliteal surface**. The distal end of the femur bone has two large, rounded articular surfaces termed **medial** and **lateral femoral condyles**. These join anteriorly to form the **patellar surface**. Posteriorly, the femoral condyles are separated by the **intercondylar fossa**. The non-articular areas just above the condyles on each side of the femur bone are the **medial** and **lateral epicondyles**. The medial epicondyle has a well-developed prominence termed the **adductor tubercle**.

The **patella** is the largest sesamoid bone in the body and is readily palpable (Figure 5-14). It has **anterior** and articular ("posterior") **surfaces**, a proximally located **base,** and a distally oriented projection called the **apex**. The patella is intercalated into the tendon of the quadriceps femoris muscle.

The **tibia** is the medial and larger of the two bones forming the skeleton within the crus (Figure 5-14). It and the distal phalanges within the digits are the only long bones which lack a landmark termed the *head*. Proximally, the tibia has **medial** and **lateral condyles** that articulate with those of the femur bone to form the femorotibial joint (part of the knee joint). The non-articular region

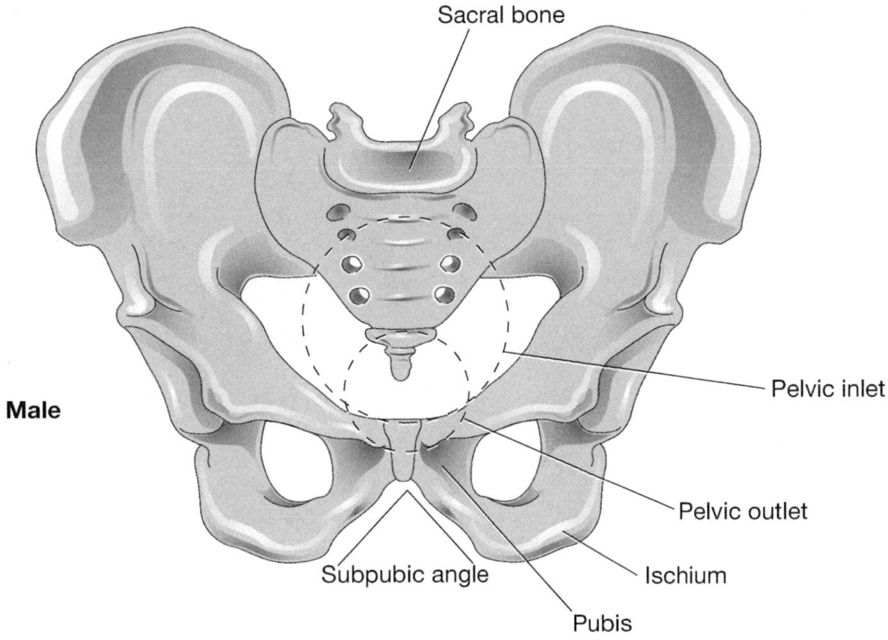

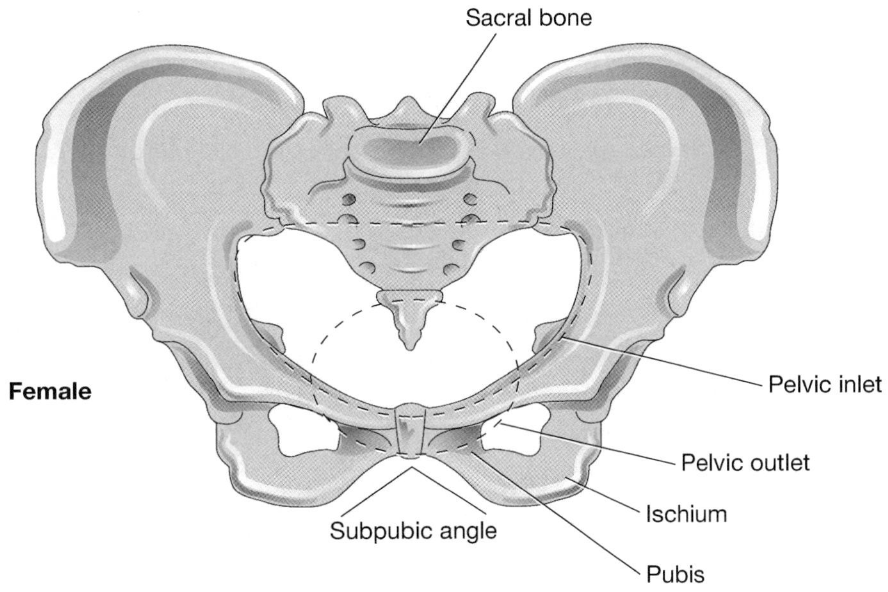

Figure 5-11

Sexual Dimorphism in the Human Pelvis

Males have a smaller subpubic angle (90° or less) and a narrower pelvic canal than females. In addition, the obturator foramina are more rounded in males and more oval-shaped in females.

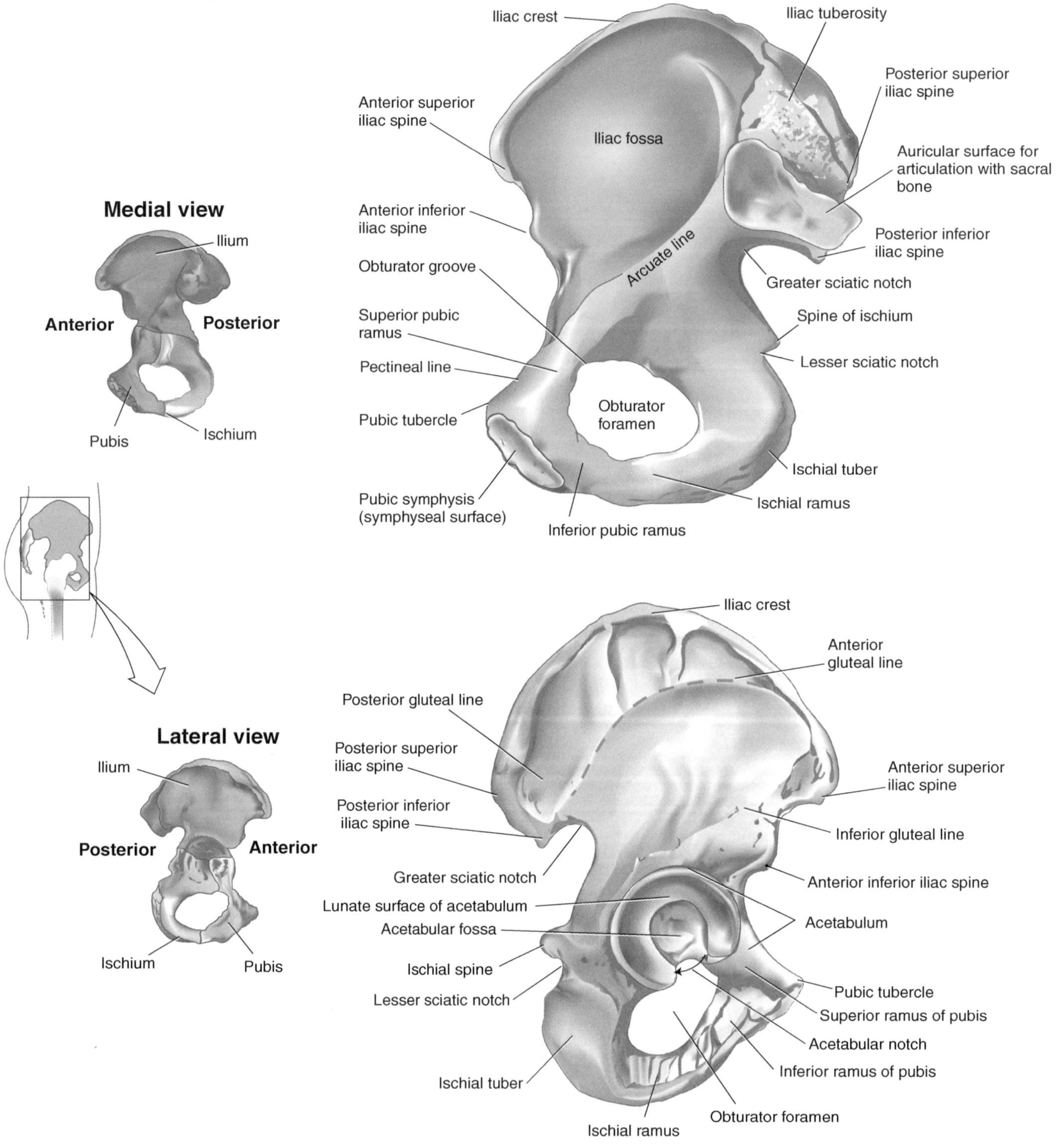

Figure 5-12

Medial and Lateral Views of the Os Coxae

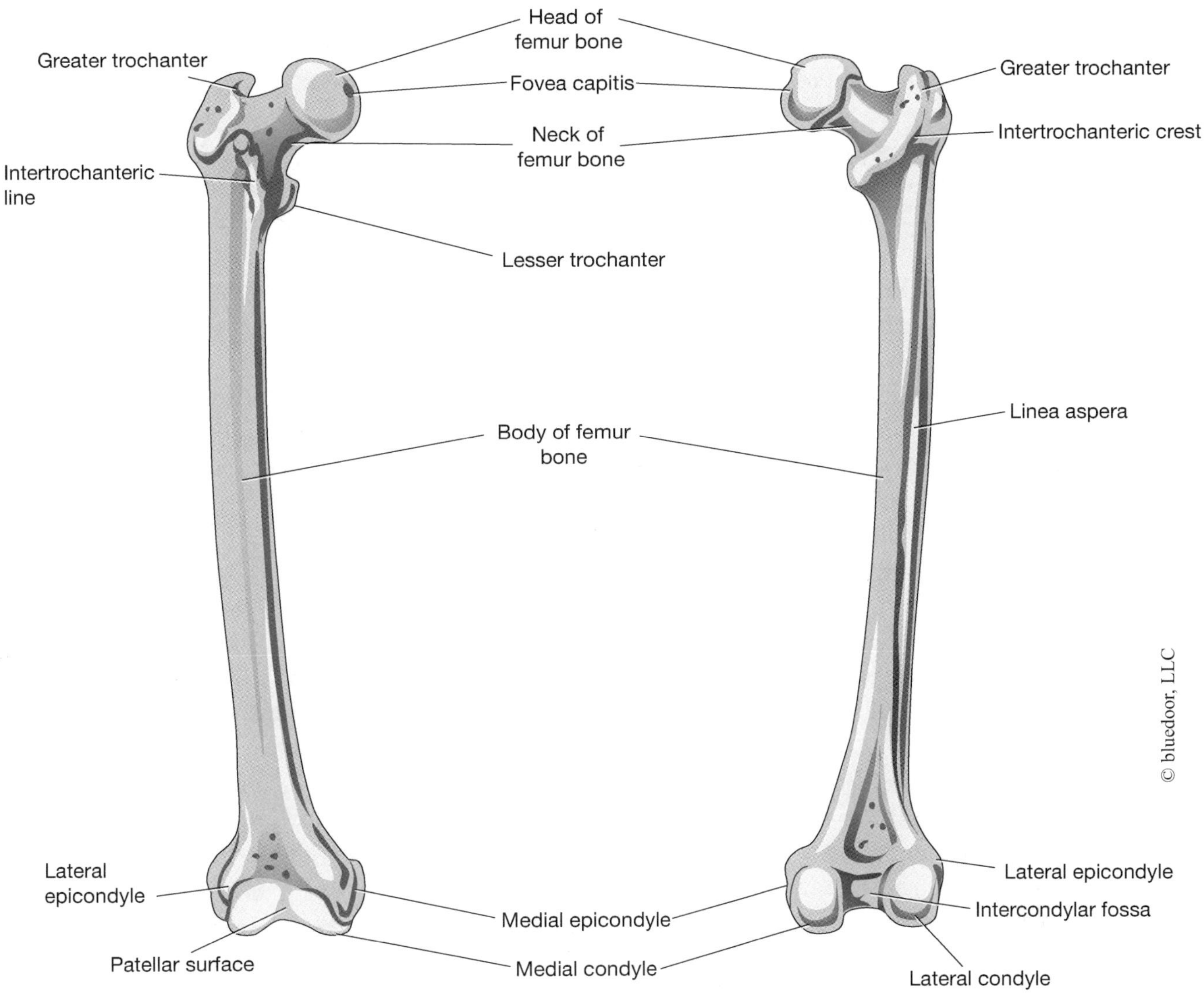

Figure 5-13

Anterior (left) and Posterior (right) Views of Right Femur Bone

Femur, used alone, is Latin for thigh. The os femoris (bone of the thigh) is Anglicized as femur bone or bone of the thigh.

between the tibial condyles is divided into the anterior and posterior **intercondylar areas** by an intercondylar eminence. The **intercondylar eminence** is formed by a pair of protrusions termed **medial** and **lateral intercondylar tubercles**. A **fibular articular surface** lies on the lateral aspect of the lateral condyle. The **body** of the tibia is triangular in transverse section with medial, lateral, and posterior surfaces, and anterior, medial, and interosseous borders. The anteriorly-directed, angular projection from the anterior border a few centimeters distal to the proximal end of the bone is the **tibial tuberosity**. This serves as the point of attachment for the patellar ligament. The obliquely oriented, linear, roughened area on the proximal aspect of the posterior tibial surface is called the **soleal**

line (line of attachment for the soleus muscle). The medial surface of the tibia is readily palpable but the lateral surface is covered by muscles. Distally the tibia has a large, medially directed, knob-like enlargement called the **medial malleolus**. This forms the obvious bony projection on the medial aspect of the crus just proximal to the ankle. On the distolateral aspect of the tibia is the **fibular notch** which forms a fibrous joint with the lateral malleolus of the fibula. The **inferior articular surface** of the tibia articulates with the talus.

The **fibula** is the slender bone forming the lateral component of the crural skeleton (Figure 5-14). It has four major parts: head, neck, body, and lateral malleolus. The fibular **head** is the proximal epiphysis. It ends superiorly in a pointed projection termed the **apex**, and medially it articulates with the tibia at the **articular surface of the fibular head**. The **neck** of the fibula is the indistinctly constricted region distal to the head that joins the fibular body. The **body**, like that of the tibia, is somewhat triangular in transverse section with lateral, medial, and posterior surfaces, and anterior, posterior, and interosseous borders. The distal epiphysis of the fibula is termed the **lateral malleolus**. It forms the large knob-like projection on the lateral aspect of the distal crus. Medially, the lateral malleolus has a **malleolar articular surface** that articulates with the talus. Just posterior to this surface is a depression (**fossa of the lateral malleolus**) and further posteriorly is an indentation called the **malleolar groove** which transmits some tendons.

The bones of the foot include seven tarsal bones within the ankle, five metatarsal bones within the metatarsus, 14 phalanges within the digits, and two sesamoid bones at the base of the big toe. The seven **tarsal bones** form the skeleton within the ankle and are arranged in two irregular rows (Figure 5-15). The **talus** is the medial bone in the proximal row and is the only one that articulates with the tibia and fibula. Its proximal rounded portion is called the **trochlea of the talus**. Distal to the trochlea is a constricted region comprising the **body** and **neck** of the talus. The **head of the talus** is the distal portion that articulates with the navicular bone. The talus has a number of named surfaces and other landmarks. One projection termed the posterior process of the talus sometimes remains separate from the main part of the bone and forms an eighth tarsal bone called the os trigonum (triangular bone).

The **calcaneus** is the longest tarsal bone and it projects posteriorly to form the **tuber calcanei**. The tuber calcanei serves as a point of attachment for the calcanean tendon and is subtly divided into **medial** and **lateral tubercles**. Like the talus, the calcaneus has a number of named landmarks and articular surfaces. Projecting from its medial aspect is a prominence termed the **sustentaculum tali** that extends behind and under the talus.

The **navicular bone** is positioned just distal to the head of the talus on the medial aspect of the tarsus. It has a prominent medial projection termed the **tuberosity of the navicular bone** that is palpable. Distal to the navicular bone are three wedge-shaped tarsal bones termed the **medial**, **intermediate**, and **lateral cuneiform bones**. Lateral to these and distal to the calcaneus is the **cuboid bone**.

The five **metatarsal bones** are numbered 1-5 from medial to lateral and form the skeleton within the metatarsus (Figure 5-15). Like their metacarpal counterparts, each metatarsal bone has a proximally located **base**, a **body**, and a distally located **head**. The first metatarsal bone supports the big toe and is slightly shorter but considerably stouter than the other four. The first and fifth metatarsal bones have **tuberosities** on the inferior aspect of their bases that serve as attachment sites for tendons.

Fourteen **phalanges** form the skeleton within the toes (Figure 5-15). These resemble their counterparts in the manus with each digit having three phalanges (**proximal**, **middle**, **distal**) except for the big toe which lacks a middle phalanx. As in the manus, each phalanx in the pes has a proximally located **base** and a **body**. Distally, the proximal and middle phalanges end in **heads** and the distal phalanges end in **tuberosities**.

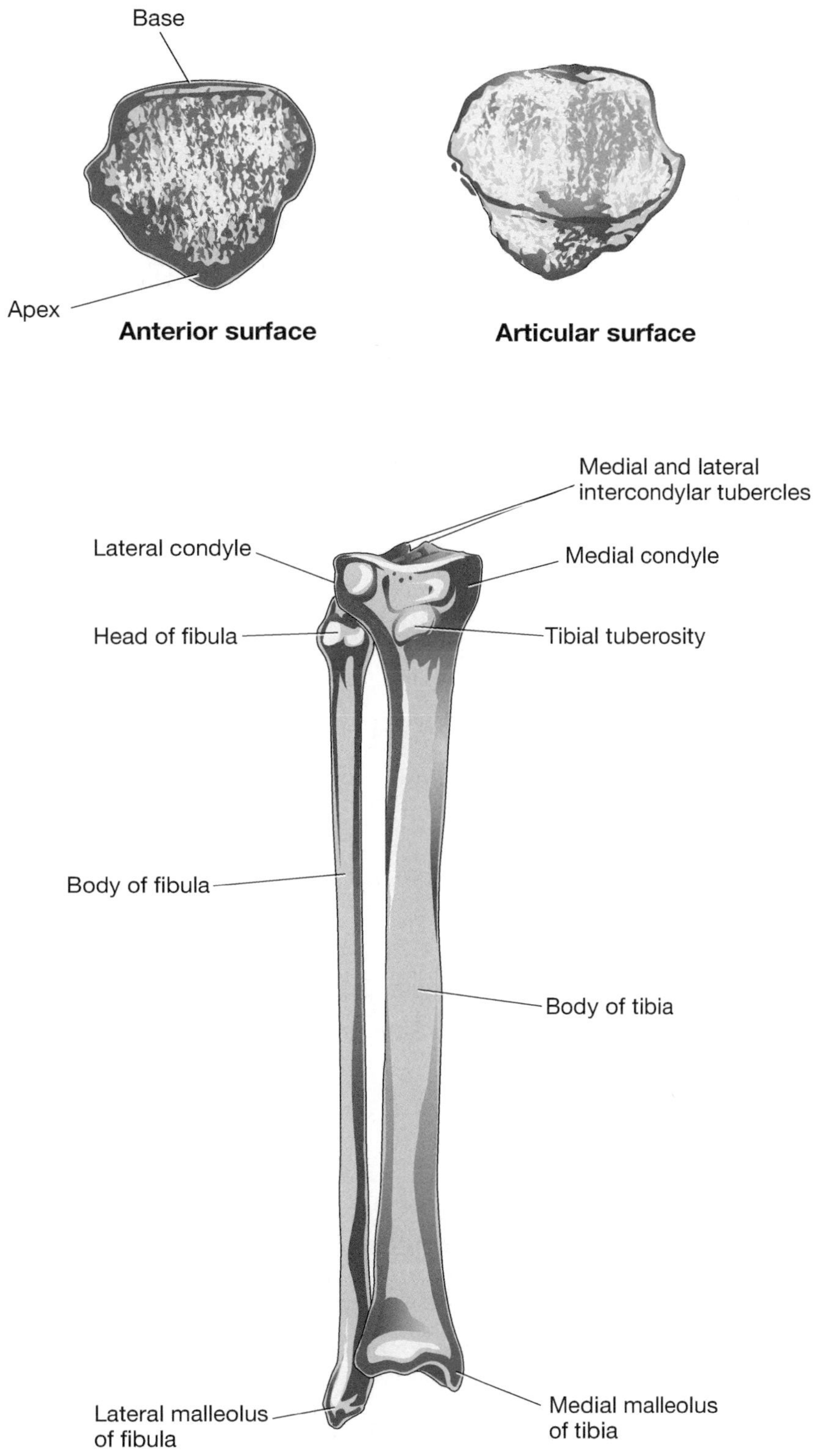

Figure 5-14

Patella (above) and Right Tibia and Fibula (below)

Not drawn to scale.

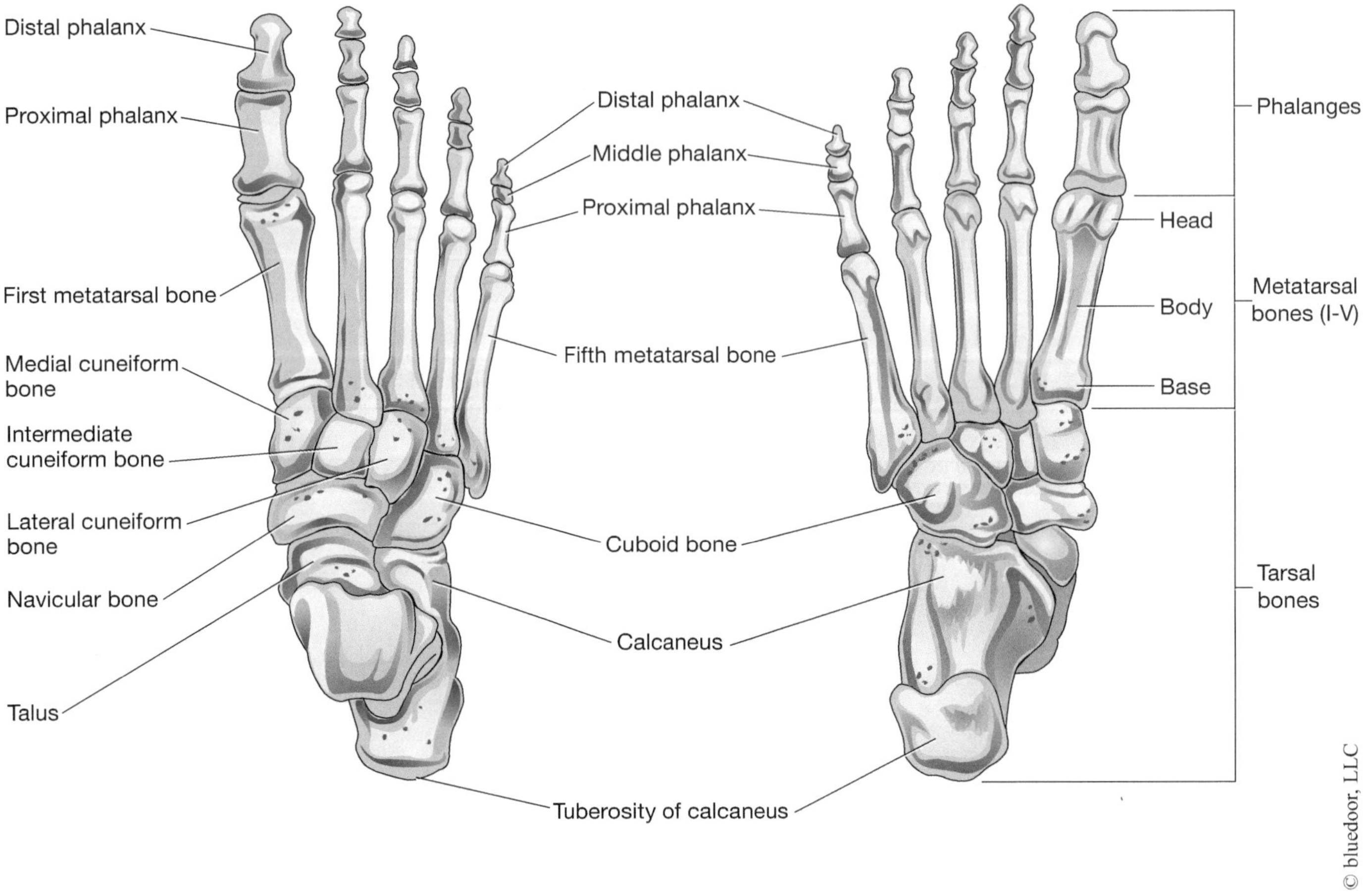

Figure 5-15

Bones of Right Foot, Superior and Inferior Views

Objectives

11. Name the bones of the inferior limb and classify them by shape.
12. State the function of the pelvic girdle, list the bones that form it, and indicate which ones belong to the appendicular skeleton.
13. Differentiate the major (greater, "false") pelvis from the minor (lessor, "true") pelvis.
14. List the bones that fuse to form the os coxae.
15. Compare the phalanges of the foot to those of the hand and identify any given phalanx by using proximal, middle, or distal (as appropriate) and stating the number or name of the digit of which it is a part.
16. Note which appendicular bones have "bone" in their name and which do not.

Clinical Considerations

Medical, veterinary, and dental students are sometimes taught to use the "**DAMN IT**" differential when diagnosing and analyzing disease syndromes. This mnemonic is an acronym for *degenerative, anomalous, metabolic, neoplastic, infectious*, and *traumatic*, which are the six major etiological categories of disease.

Degenerative problems involving the skeletal system include a number of arthritic conditions which are more prevalent in, but not limited to, elderly individuals (*see Chapter 7*). Older people lose skeletal mass due to mild demineralization associated with their reduced activity. This same phenomenon has been shown to temporarily occur in individuals subjected to the weightless environment of space. Excessive skeletal demineralization is a major problem among the elderly and is termed **osteoporosis**. Reduced hormone levels, especially estrogen, have been shown to play a role in this disease. Bones thus weakened by excessive demineralization are frequently subject to fracture (*see Chapter 6*).

Anomalies of the skeletal system include complete failure of certain bones to develop and abnormal sizes, positions, and shapes of skeletal components. In the late fifties and early sixties a large number of babies were born with shortened limbs (**micromelia**) or absent limbs (**amelia**). The cause was traced to a drug called thalidomide taken by the pregnant mothers to relieve morning sickness during early pregnancy. **Spina bifida** is a congenital defect of the vertebral column wherein the left and right laminae of the vertebral arch have failed to fuse and completely encase the spinal cord. **Cleft palate** occurs when the left and right maxillae and/or palatine bones fail to meet and fuse to complete the skeletal support of the bony palate. The resulting open communication between the nasal and oral cavities causes difficulties which require surgical intervention.

Metabolic disorders of the skeletal system include nutritional and hormonal disorders. Secretion of too little growth hormone by the pituitary gland of a child results in **dwarfism**. Secretion of too much growth hormone causes **giantism** if it occurs before the skeletal system matures. After skeletal maturity, excess growth hormone results in a condition called **acromegaly** in which limited and sometimes disfiguring enlargement occurs in the bones of the hands, feet, and face. The nutritional disease of most significance in the skeletal system is caused by vitamin D deficiency. This results in inadequate absorption of calcium from the intestine and improper incorporation of calcium and phosphorus into bone tissue. In growing children this causes **rickets** which is a deformation of some bones in the inferior limbs that are not strong enough to support the body weight. In adults, vitamin D deficiency causes a demineralization syndrome called **osteomalacia**. This disease is more prevalent in women on poor diets who have numerous children.

Tumors originating in bone are usually accompanied by pain. Malignant ones (**osteogenic sarcomas**) often metastasize (spread) through the bloodstream where the tumor cells may be trapped in the capillary beds of other organs, especially the lungs. Non-malignant bone tumors are called **osteomas**. Tumors of soft tissues may metastasize to bone.

Infectious diseases of bones often occur in association with open fractures and may severely hamper the healing process. These may be caused by bacteria or fungi. Traumatic injuries involving bone are discussed in Chapter 6.

Objectives

17. Explain the "DAMN IT" mnemonic as used to categorize the causes of disease.
18. Define osteomalacia and osteoporosis.

Clinical Case Studies

Case 1—A 33-year-old college professor suffered a severely fractured ankle when he rolled his foot sideways while making a sudden directional change on a racquetball court. The emergency room physician described the fracture over the phone to the orthopedist on duty as a "trimalleolar" fracture. What was broken?

Case 2—A second grade boy, falling from a playground monkey bar, fractured his right radius through its distal epiphyseal cartilage just proximal to the wrist. The ipsilateral ulna remained intact. The physician who stabilized the radial fracture with an external cast told the boy's parents that the fracture should heal uneventfully but he warned that the limb might require a corrective osteotomy of the radius within a few years to prevent foreshortening and curvature of the involved antebrachium. Why?

Case 3—When a youngster failed to crawl properly several months after his older siblings had developed that milestone ability, the parents had the child examined by their pediatrician. After physical and radiographic examination, the child was diagnosed as suffering developmental hip dysplasia and his inferior limbs were immobilized for several months in a "wide stance" position via a spacing rod joining both casted limbs. How could this positioning aid subsequent development of his shallow acetabula?

Points to Ponder

The three kinds of bone cells make an interesting study. Like the daydreaming floor painter who finds himself trapped in a corner, osteoblasts that are especially productive in the fiber and ground substance departments find themselves surrounded by and entrapped within their own secretory products. Known thenceforth as osteocytes and damned to a celibate and hermitic existence within cramped spaces called lacunae, their only contact with other similar misfortunates is via cellular processes that extend through tiny channels called canaliculi. Those fortunate enough to be near the central canal of an osteon get first dibs on nutrients and pass the excess (unwanted) material on to the others located in outer (Siberian) lamellae. The negative side of being located in an inner lamella is that waste products are passed centrally through the canaliculi from cell to cell such that the inner osteocytes have to handle everyone else's wastes as well as their own. (Outside every silver lining there is a cloud!)

Osteoclasts are among the few multinucleated cells in the body. It has been suggested that they arise when a group of nonconformist osteoblasts go on strike, join forces and pool their cytoplasmic, nuclear, and cell membrane resources into one large conglomerate. Multiple nuclei (as the saying goes) are better than one and their combined DNA seems to revive the lost art of acid production which osteoclasts use to advantage in dissolving the calcium phosphates in the mineralized matrix.

We cannot help but admire the paleontologist who, when presented with a single fossil bone, can often name the species and expound at length regarding the animal as a whole. Likewise, the forensic pathologist who can often surmise the likely scenario of an individual's demise from a single fragment of broken bone. These types of individuals are not psychic—their interpretations are based on a huge body of knowledge tempered by a significant measure of common sense.

Much of animal paleontology involves the skeletal system because the latter is readily preserved (fossilized) for future study millennia later. Organs of the other systems are, for the most part, lost and subject only to conjecture and speculation based on what is known from the preserved skeletal structures. Likewise, the tenacity of modern mankind's bones in warding off the degenerative aspects of decay leave a record of life and death and the trauma incurred in both. Skeletons and parts thereof have been resurrected years after their original owner has expired for evidence leading to guilt and innocence in numerous trials.

The shape, strength, and features of a bone are largely determined by the forces acting on it. This has been repeatedly demonstrated by the fracture healing process. With time, the excess bone tissue laid down during fracture healing is reabsorbed and the injured bone slowly reshapes itself toward its original form. The biomechanics of this process involves microelectrical charges produced when the mineral (crystalline) portion of bone tissue is subjected to mechanical forces. This phenomenon, known as the piezoelectric effect, has been used therapeutically to aid fracture healing in certain cases.

Bone tissue is in a dynamic equilibrium with some reabsorption and some synthesis continually occurring. This dynamic reabsorption/synthesis equilibrium is controlled by two hormones: parathyroid hormone and calcitonin. These chemical regulators help keep the blood calcium levels within the narrow range that is compatible with life. When bones are actively growing, the synthesis of bone tissue exceeds the rate of reabsorption. When bones lose mass in old age or in astronauts subject to a weightless environment (with fewer stresses) reabsorption exceeds synthesis. In a normal adult, the turnover of bone tissue is extremely slow.

Medical practitioners who specialize in the skeletal system include orthopods, osteopaths, and chiropractors. Orthopods specialize in surgery, osteopaths emphasize a naturalistic approach, and chiropractors utilize manipulative techniques to correct disorders.

Slang and Obsolete Nomenclature

UNOFFICIAL TERM	OFFICIAL DESIGNATION
collar bone	clavicle *[clavicula]*
shoulder blade	scapula *[scapula]*
spinous process of scapula	spine of scapula *[spina scapulae]*
acromion process of scapula	acromion *[acromion]* of scapula
bicipital groove of humerus	intertubercular groove *[sulcus intertubercularis]* of humerus
shaft of humerus, radius, *etc.*	body of humerus, radius, etc. *[corpus humeri, radii]*
olecranon process of ulna	olecranon *[olecranon]* of ulna
radial notch	radial notch *[incisura radialis]* of ulna
styloid process	styloid process *[processus styloideus]* of radius/ulna/ third metacarpal bone/temporal bone, *etc.*
radiale	scaphoid bone *[os scaphoideum]*
navicular bone (within wrist)	scaphoid bone *[os scaphoideum]*
ulnare	triquetral bone *[os triquetrum]*
greater multangular bone	trapezium bone *[os trapezium]*
lesser multangular bone	trapezoid bone *[os trapezoideum]*
triquetrum, scaphoid, *etc.*	triquetral bone, scaphoid bone, *etc.* (*see above*)
metacarpals	metacarpal bones *[ossa metacarpi/metacarpalia I-V]*

marrow cavity	medullary cavity *[cavitas medullaris]*
epiphyseal (growth) plate	epiphyseal cartilage *[cartilago epiphysialis]*
Sharpey's fibers	perforating fibers *[fibra perforans]*
Haversian system	osteon *[osteonum]*
Haversian canal	central canal *[canalis centralis]* of an osteon
cancellous bone	spongy/trabecular bone *[substantia spongiosa/trabecularis]*
dense bone	compact/cortical bone *[substantia compacta/corticalis]*
innominate bone	hip bone, os coxae *[os coxae]*
coxa (the bone)	hip bone, os coxae *[os coxae]*
ischial tuberosity	ischiatic tuber *[tuber ischiadicum]*
femur (the bone)	femur bone (bone of the thigh) *[os femoris]*
fibular tarsal bone	calcaneus *[calcaneus]*
tibial tarsal bone	talus *[talus]*
astragalus	talus *[talus]*
metatarsals	metatarsal bones *[ossa metatarsi/metatarsalia I-V]*
first/second/third cuneiform bones	medial/intermediate/lateral cuneiform bones *[os cuneiforme mediale, intermedium, laterale]*

Review Questions

1. Which of the following is mismatched?
   A. humerus—long bone—free part of superior limb
   B. clavicle—long bone– pectoral girdle
   C. navicular bone—short bone—free part of superior limb
   D. scapula—flat bone—pectoral girdle
   E. ulna—long bone—free part of superior limb
   F. Choose this response if more than one of the above (A-E) is mismatched.

2. Which of the following is mismatched?
   A. pectoral girdle: five flat bones—four appendicular bones—one axial bone
   B. pelvic girdle: two flat bones—one irregular bone—two appendicular bones
   C. pectoral girdle: five bones total—four flat appendicular bones—one flat axial bone
   D. pelvic girdle: three bones total—two flat appendicular bones—one flat axial bone
   E. pectoral girdle: supports free parts of superior limbs
   F. pelvic girdle: supports free parts of inferior limbs
   G. Choose this response if all the above (A-F) are correctly matched.

3. Find the truth.
   A. The longest bone in a superior limb is the femur bone.
   B. More than 25 percent of the bones in the body are phalanges.
   C. The most frequently fractured bone in the axial skeleton is the clavicle.
   D. There are six sesamoid bones in the two superior limbs.
   E. The shortest long bone (in a hand) is the proximal phalanx of the little finger.

4. Which of the following is incorrect?
   A. medullary cavity—hollow inner portion of most bones
   B. periosteum—outer-most bony layer of a bone
   C. sesamoid bone—seed-like bones located within tendons
   D. articular cartilage—specialized hyaline cartilage located between adjacent, articulating bone surfaces
   E. yellow bone marrow—what red bone marrow typically becomes with age

5. Find the correct definition.
   A. internal circumferential lamellae—lamellae located adjacent to the periosteum
   B. interstitial lamellae—incomplete remnants of a lacuna
   C. osteoblast—bone cell located within a lacuna
   D. trabecular bone—consists of slender spicules within inner and outer layers of spongy bone
   E. Choose this response if all of the above (A-D) are incorrect.

6. Which of the following parts of a bone is composed of osseous tissue?
   A. physis
   B. epiphyses
   C. endosteum
   D. medullary cavity
   E. bone marrow

7. Which of the following is not part of a digit of the hand?
   A. muscles
   B. phalanges
   C. blood vessels
   D. metacarpal bone
   E. skin
   F. nails

8. Find the false statement.
   A. There are 34 bones in the skeleton of each superior limb (just count them!).
   B. A typical bone is composed of more than seven different tissues.
   C. There are no long or short bones in the skeletal girdles.
   D. There are more short bones in the superior limb than in the inferior limb.
   E. Lacunae-bound osteocytes become osteoblasts when liberated by osteoclasts.

9. Find the mismatch.
   A. patella—sesamoid bone—free part of inferior limb
   B. bony sacrum—irregular bone—pelvic girdle
   C. fibula—long bone—crus
   D. intermediate cuneiform bone—long bone—pes
   E. talus—short bone—tarsus

10. Which of the following is mismatched?
    A. ilium—superior—os coxae
    B. head—distal—ulna
    C. trapezium bone—lateral—manus
    D. head—distal—talus
    E. tuberosity—posterior—first metatarsal bone
    F. head—proximal—tibia
    G. Choose this response if all the above (A-F) are correctly matched.

Thought Questions

1. The humeri and femur bones are the most proximal bones in the free parts of the limbs. What constitutes the free part of a limb?

2. The human radius and ulna are significantly less massive than the human tibia and fibula, but in quadrupeds the antebrachial skeleton is relatively larger. Suggest a logical reason.

3. Parathyroid hormone causes the blood calcium levels to rise. What effect would high levels of this hormone (as might occur due to neoplasia of the parathyroid gland) have on the mineral content of bone tissue?

4. Which of the functions of bones are related primarily to the organ level of body organization and which ones are related to the bone tissue level?

5. The components of osteoid are manufactured only by the osteoblasts on the surface. Explain, then, how osteoblastic activity can follow an osteoclast which is excavating a tiny cylindrical channel through solid (dense) bone tissue.

6. "Osteocytic osteolysis" refers to the fact that osteocytes may be involved in breaking down some of the extracellular matrix surrounding their lacunae when the blood levels of calcium ions need to be increased. What probably stimulates this "osteoclastic" type of activity?

7. Within a set of concentric lamellae, what can be assumed regarding their relative ages (*i.e.*, which one was formed first/last)?

8. Which categories of bone shapes are not found in the axial skeleton?

9. How are tubercles, tubers, tuberosities, and trochanters distinguished from each other?

10. How do osteoclasts break down the mineral components of bone tissue?

11. Which one of the two major categories of epithelium is not found in a bone? Which two categories of muscle tissue are not found in bones?

12. An obsolete name for the scaphoid bone is navicular bone. What confusion did this name cause?

13. Is bone tissue involved in blood cell formation? Explain.

14. Are the pectoral and pelvic girdles composed of axial or appendicular skeletal components?

15. Indicate where the appendicular skeletons of the superior and inferior limbs meet (join) the axial skeleton.

16. Which bones of the inferior limbs exhibit sexual dimorphism?

17. In an adult, the levels of osteoclastic and osteoblastic activity are about equal. What happens if osteoclastic activity exceeds osteoblastic activity?

18. Which areas on the outer surface of a bone lack periosteum?

19. Why do all of the carpal bones, and most of the tarsal bones have "bone" in their name, but the calcaneus and talus lack the word bone?

20. What effect does heavy exercise have on bone density?

21. What "advantage" does spongy bone tissue provide in comparison to compact bone tissue?

Answers to Clinical Case Studies

Case 1—The lateral and medial malleolus of the tibia and fibula were separated from their parent bones and the medial malleolus was broken into two major fragments. These three "malleolar" fragments account for the name of this relatively common fracture. It was stabilized with five pins and two pieces of wire and healed uneventfully. The patient continued to suffer some discomfort until the pins and wire were removed eight months later.

Case 2—The growing radius has two epiphyseal cartilages (one proximal, one distal) that contribute to its overall length increase between the elbow and carpus. The ulna has two epiphyseal cartilages, as well, but only one of them contributes to the increase in ulnar length between the elbow and carpus. During growth, the two in the radius must produce the same total bone length increase as the one in the ulna. Otherwise, disparate elbow-to-carpus lengths in the radius and ulna occur and result in curvatures of the antebrachium. Sometimes, when fractures occur through actively growing epiphyseal cartilages, growth is reduced or stopped altogether. If this occurred in this patient, the ulna would outgrow the radius and produce such a curvature. This can be corrected, by transecting the radius near the middle of its body and allowing the cut ends to separate (distract) as the ulna lengthens and then heal together when the desired (definitive) antebrachial length has been reached.

Case 3—Hip dysplasia is characterized by shallow acetabula and unstable hip joints. When it is detected in young children, the deformity can be largely corrected by stabilizing the inferior limbs in an abducted (splay-legged) position. This forces the femoral heads into the acetabula and encourages development of their normal, deep-socket configuration.

Answers to Review Questions

1. F. The clavicle is a *flat* bone (B) and the navicular bone is in the *inferior* limb (C).

2. D. The pelvic girdle includes two flat appendicular bones and one *irregular* axial bone.

3. B. A. should be in *inferior* limb, C. should be in the *appendicular* skeleton, D. should be in the inferior limb, and E. should be the *distal* phalanx.

4. B. Periosteum is not a bony layer but a *c.t. proper* layer.

5. E. A. should be adjacent to *endosteum*, B. should be a remnant of an *osteon*, C. should be an *osteocyte*. D. would be true of some bones of the skull if *spongy* were changed to *compact* bone.

6. B.

7. D. Metacarpal bones are part of the *metacarpus*, not digits.

8. E. Osteocytes do not become osteoblasts when liberated from lacunae (they are killed by the low pH of osteoclastic secretions).

9. D. The intermediate cuneiform bone is not a long bone but a *short* bone.

10. F. All long bones have heads except tibias and distal phalanges.

Answers to Thought Questions

1. The free parts of the limbs are those portions which extend away from the trunk and can be freely moved relative to the trunk.

2. In most quadrupeds, slightly more than half of the total body weight is supported by the front limbs. Consequently, the antebrachial skeleton is relatively larger.

3. Parathyroid hormone stimulates osteoclastic activity which causes demineralization of bone tissue. A parathyroid tumor can cause such extensive demineralization that bones may fracture quite easily.

4. All of the physical functions of bones and even fat storage occur at the organ level. Hemopoiesis is a function of bone marrow tissue but not of bone tissue. Only calcium/phosphorus storage is truly a bone *tissue* function.

5. Osteoblasts *are* only found on a surface but "surface" includes the walls of the microscopic tunnels left behind after osteoclastic activity.

6. Hormones—especially an increase in circulating parathyroid hormone, which is normally released from the parathyroid gland in response to lowered blood calcium levels.

7. The outermost lamella was formed first, followed, in order, by each one toward the central canal. The lamella around the central canal was the last one formed.

8. There are no long, short, or sesamoid bones in the axial skeleton. All bones of the axial skeleton are flat or irregular in shape.

9. They represent different names for the same general type of feature—a roughened process typically serving as a muscle attachment site. One cannot look at one of these and determine which term is used in its name.

10. They are believed to be able to secrete hydrogen ions which lower the pH at their microenvironmental locations enough to dissolve the mineral. This puts the mineral back into circulation and plays a role in the homeostasis of calcium and phosphorus. (The organic components of the osteoid are hydrolyzed by enzymes that the osteoclasts produce).

11. Glandular epithelium, cardiac muscle tissue, and skeletal muscle tissue are not found within bones.

12. There is a tarsal bone with this name.

13. No, not at the tissue level. However, bones (the organs) do house the bone *marrow* tissue which is hemopoietic in some bones at some ages.

14. Both girdles contain bones from the axial *and* appendicular skeletons.

15. In the superior limbs, at the junction of the clavicle and sternum (sternoclavicular joint). In the inferior limbs, at the junction of the ilium and sacral bone (sacroiliac joint).

16. The bony pelvis (left and right hip bones) of a male tends to have oval obturator foramina (versus more triangular ones in females). There are other subtle differences as well.

17. The bone weakens due to demineralization—a condition called osteomalacia/osteoporosis.

18. Those areas covered by cartilage, tendinous insertions, ligamentous attachments, and the attachments of joint capsules.

19. That's just the way it is (TJTWII)! There is no logic or rule of thumb.

20. Exercise increases bone density because the osteoblasts respond to the added stress by secreting osteoid. Conversely, lack of exercise leads to a decrease in bone density. This fact has been vividly demonstrated by astronauts who have spent extended time in space. Their bones demineralize because of the reduced stresses placed on them by the weightless environment.

21. Spongy bone tissue has a superior strength/weight ratio. Just as an airplane wing is hollow to allow a certain shape without the added weight that a "solid" design would include, spongy bone tissue occurs in places where a certain size/shape is required but the additional strength that compact bone tissue would provide is unwarranted.

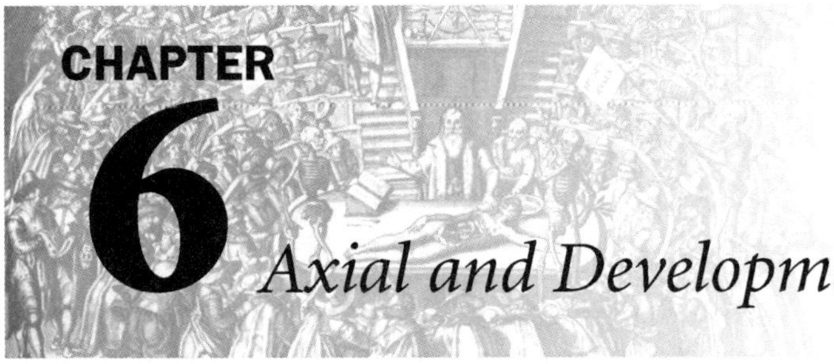

CHAPTER 6 Axial and Developmental Osteology

Chapter Outline and Key Concepts

INTRODUCTION

Most of the bones of the axial skeleton are positioned along the long axis of the body which is located between the vertex of the head and a point equidistant between the feet.

BONES OF THE HEAD

Bones in the head include eight which form the braincase, 14 which form the face, three pairs of auditory ossicles, and the single hyoid bone.

The 22 bones of the braincase and the face collectively comprise the skull.

Six of the skull bones are single entities and eight of them are paired.

The viscerocranium is composed of the inferior nasal conchae, mandible, vomer, maxillae, and the zygomatic, palatine, nasal, and lacrimal bones.

The neurocranium is composed of the frontal, parietal, occipital, temporal, sphenoid, and ethmoid bones.

VERTEBRAE

General vertebral features include a vertebral body, arch, foramen, and three kinds of processes: spinous(1), transverse(2), and articular(4).

Vertebrae are grouped regionally into five types represented by the vertebral formula $C_7T_{12}L_5S_5Cy_4$.

The seven cervical vertebrae are distinguished by the presence of transverse foramina, and the first two (atlas and axis) have some unique features.

The 12 thoracic vertebrae articulate with ribs and have long spinous processes and short bodies.

The five lumbar vertebrae have stout bodies and long transverse processes.

The five sacral vertebrae typically fuse to form the sacral bone ("sacrum") and the four coccygeal vertebrae fuse to form the coccyx.

In general, the vertebrae get larger in the lower part of the vertebral column.

The bodies of most vertebrae are separated from their adjacent counterparts by intervertebral discs.

STERNUM

The sternum is the unpaired "breastbone" formed by the fusion of the manubrium, body, and xiphoid process of the sternum.

RIBS

The ribs are 12 pairs of flat bones that articulate with the thoracic vertebrae.

The anterior, cartilaginous extensions of the ribs are called costal cartilages.

Ribs whose costal cartilages make direct contact with the sternum (first seven pairs) are called *true* ribs *vs.* the lower five pairs which are called *false* ribs.

The false ribs whose costal cartilages end freely in the body wall (last two pairs) are called *floating* ribs.

DEVELOPMENT OF BONES

Bones develop by two different mechanisms called endochondral (intracartilaginous) and intramembranous ossification.

Endochondral ossification is a four step process involving the formation, mineralization, and reabsorption of a hyaline cartilage model before bone tissue is formed.

Intramembranous ossification involves "direct" (no cartilage model) bone tissue formation within a connective tissue proper membrane.

Most bones are initially formed by endochondral ossification and long bones grow in length primarily by this mechanism.

Some bones (and parts of other bones) form initially by intramembranous ossification and most bones increase their diameters by this mechanism.

The first area of a bone to mineralize is called the primary center of ossification; later separate areas that mineralize are secondary centers of ossification.

Epiphyseal cartilages ("growth plates") are hyaline cartilage structures that separate ossified portions of bones and allow continued elongation as the skeleton enlarges.

CLINICAL CONSIDERATIONS

Fractures (broken bones) are a common traumatic disorder of the skeletal system.

The two most important principles in promoting fracture healing are stability and reduction.

Fractures that take an exceptionally long time to heal are called delayed unions.

Some delayed unions progress to pseudoarthroses (false joints).

Pelvic measurements constitute the science of pelvimetry and are of interest to gynecologists and anthropologists.

Selected Definitions

Chondrocranium—that part of the neurocranium forming the base of the skull. Parts of several bones are involved and endochondral ossification occurs.

Costal cartilages—the hyaline cartilage structures that attach to the anterior ends of the ribs. Those of the true ribs articulate directly with the sternum, those of ribs 8, 9, and 10 form the costal arch on each side, and those of ribs 11 and 12 end in the soft tissue of the body wall.

Endochondral (intracartilaginous) ossification—bone tissue formation that involves an initial hyaline cartilage model. Endochondral ossification is a multi-step process involving mineralization and then resorption of the cartilage before bone tissue is formed.

Epiphyseal cartilage—a hyaline cartilage "growth plate" in an immature bone. A developing long bone typically has an epiphyseal cartilage at each end of its diaphysis.

Epiphyseal line—radiographic evidence of recent mineralization of an epiphyseal cartilage. Epiphyseal lines become less distinct with time and ultimately disappear altogether.

Fontanel—a "soft spot" in the skull of a neonate occurring along sutures where adjacent flat bones are incompletely ossified. Six of these are typically present: unpaired anterior and posterior fontanels, and paired anterolateral and posterolateral fontanels.

False rib—a rib whose costal cartilage does not make direct contact with the sternum. The lower five ribs on each side are false ribs, and the last two pairs of false ribs whose costal cartilages end blindly in the soft tissues of the body wall are (also) called floating ribs.

Fracture—a crack or break in a bone typically caused by trauma. If properly "set" (reduced, stabilized) to prevent movement, and if the blood supply to the fragments (pieces) remains intact, fractures may heal in a few weeks or require several months.

Intercostal spaces—the spaces between adjacent ribs and costal cartilages. These spaces are occupied by intercostal muscles, vessels, and nerves.

Intervertebral foramina—the paired openings on the sides of the vertebral column that transmit the spinal nerves. These foramina are formed by the juxtaposition of the superior and inferior vertebral notches of the adjacent vertebral arches.

Intramembranous ossification—direct osteogenesis occurring within a thin sheet of connective tissue proper (a "membrane"). All bones utilize at least some intramembranous ossification on their outer surfaces as they grow in diameter, and some flat bones use this form of ossification exclusively.

Metaphysis—the portion of a developing diaphysis that lies next to an epiphyseal cartilage. This area has very high metabolic activity and is often the focus of neoplastic and infectious processes.

Neurocranium—the cranial vault that surrounds and protects the brain. It is formed by eight bones: the unpaired frontal, occipital, ethmoid, and sphenoid bones, and the paired parietal and temporal bones.

Osteon—a group of concentric (osteonal) osseous lamellae surrounding a central canal. Osteons are formed when an osteoclast "drills" a passageway through compact bone tissue and is followed by osteoblasts which secrete concentric layers of osteoid.

Paranasal sinus—an air-filled diverticulum in the frontal bone, maxillae, sphenoid bone, or ethmoid bone. Similar small diverticuli from the tympanic cavities invaginate the temporal bones (mastoid cells).

Primary center of ossification—the first locus in a developing bone that contains bone tissue. Subsequent separate areas that ossify in the same bone are called secondary centers of ossification.

Sutural ("wormian") bones—small "islands" of bone tissue that sporadically occur within the sutures that unite the flat bones of the skull (especially the lambdoid suture). These have no clinical significance and their nomen was coined when they were incidentally observed.

Thoracic ("rib") cage—the bony framework formed by the sternum, ribs, and thoracic vertebrae. It surrounds and protects deeper thoracic organs.

True rib—a rib whose costal cartilage makes direct contact with the sternum. The first seven ribs on each side are true ribs.

Vertebral column—the spine. It is formed by twenty-six bones: seven cervical, twelve thoracic, and five lumbar vertebrae, as well as the os sacrale and os coccyx.

Viscerocranium—the skeleton that supports and shapes the face. It is formed by fourteen bones: the unpaired vomer and mandible, and the paired maxillae, inferior nasal conchae, zygomatic, palatine, nasal and lacrimal bones.

Etymology *Alea iacta est*—**"The die is cast."**

costa (L), *a rib*—costal cartilage
cribratus (L), *a sieve*—cribriform foramina
crista (L), *comb of a cock*—crista galli
ethmos (G), *strainer*—ethmoidal sinus
fontanelle (Fr), *fountain*—anterolateral fontanel
gallina (L), *relating to poultry*—crista galli
incussus (L), *an anvil*—incudostapedial joint
kokkyx (G), *cuckoo's beak*—coccygeal vertebra
manubrium (L), *hilt, handle*—manubriosternal symphysis
mastos (G), *breast*—mastoid process
magnus (L), *great*—foramen magnum
malleus (L), *a hammer*—incudomalleolar joint
parietalis (L), *a wall*—parietal bone
petra (L), *a stone*—petrous portion of temporal bone
sella (L), *a seat*—dorsum sellae
sphen (G), *wedge*—sphenoid bone
stapes (L), *stirrup*—tympanostapedial syndesmosis
sternon (G), *the breast bone*—sternum
turcica (L), *Turkish*—sella turcica
viscus (L), *inner parts of body*—viscerocranium
xiphos (G), *a sword*—xiphoid process
zygon (G), *a yoke*—zygomatic arch

Introduction

The axial skeleton is composed of all of the bones that are not located in the limbs. Included are the bones of the head, vertebral column, ribs, and sternum. These are called axial bones because of their close relationship to the long axis of the body. The long axis is a virtual landmark beginning at the top of the head (vertex) and extending inferiorly to a point equidistant between the feet.

Bones of the Head

The bones of the head include eight which form the cranial vault around the brain (**neurocranium**) and fourteen which form the skeleton of the face (**viscerocranium**) (Table 6-1). In addition, there are six auditory ossicles (three in each middle ear) and the hyoid bone at the base of the tongue. The **auditory ossicles** are the tiny bones located within the air-filled cavity of the middle ear (Figure 6-1). Each

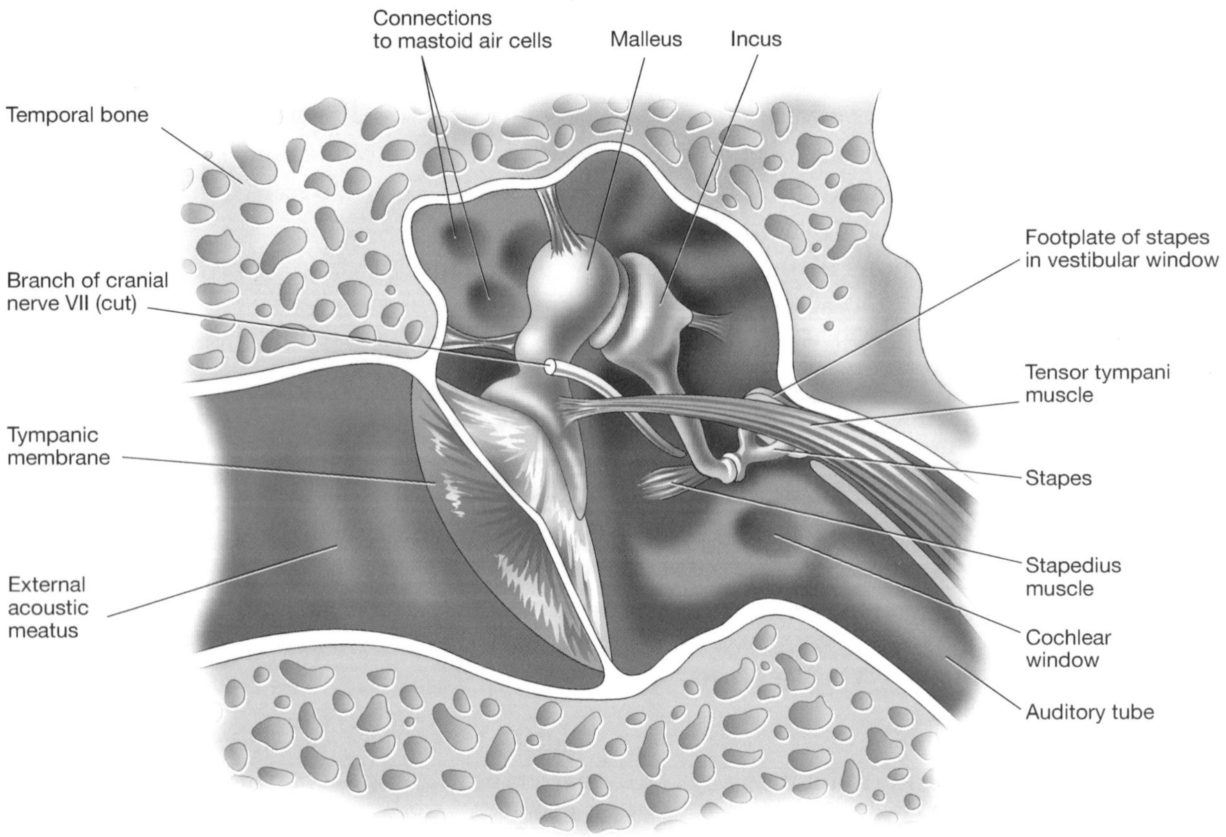

Figure 6-1

Frontal Section through the Right Ear Showing the Auditory Ossicles

The three auditory ossicles found in each tympanic cavity are the smallest bones in the body. They articulate with each other to form the incudomallear joint and the incudostapedial joint.

middle ear contains a **malleus** (attached to the tympanic membrane), an **incus**, and a **stapes** (*see Chapter 13*). These bones vibrate (when the tympanic membrane vibrates) and thereby conduct the vibrations to fluid associated with the internal (inner) ear. The **hyoid bone** is embedded in the muscles at the base of the tongue. It does not articulate with the rest of the skeleton (Figure 6-2).

Objectives

1. Divide the bones of the head into four groups and list and enumerate the bones in each group.

Skull

The 22 bones forming the neurocranium and viscerocranium are collectively and commonly called the **skull**. Six of these are single entities and eight of them are paired (Table 6-1). The anterior aspect of the skull is dominated by the two **orbits** which house the eyes, and by the **anterior nasal**

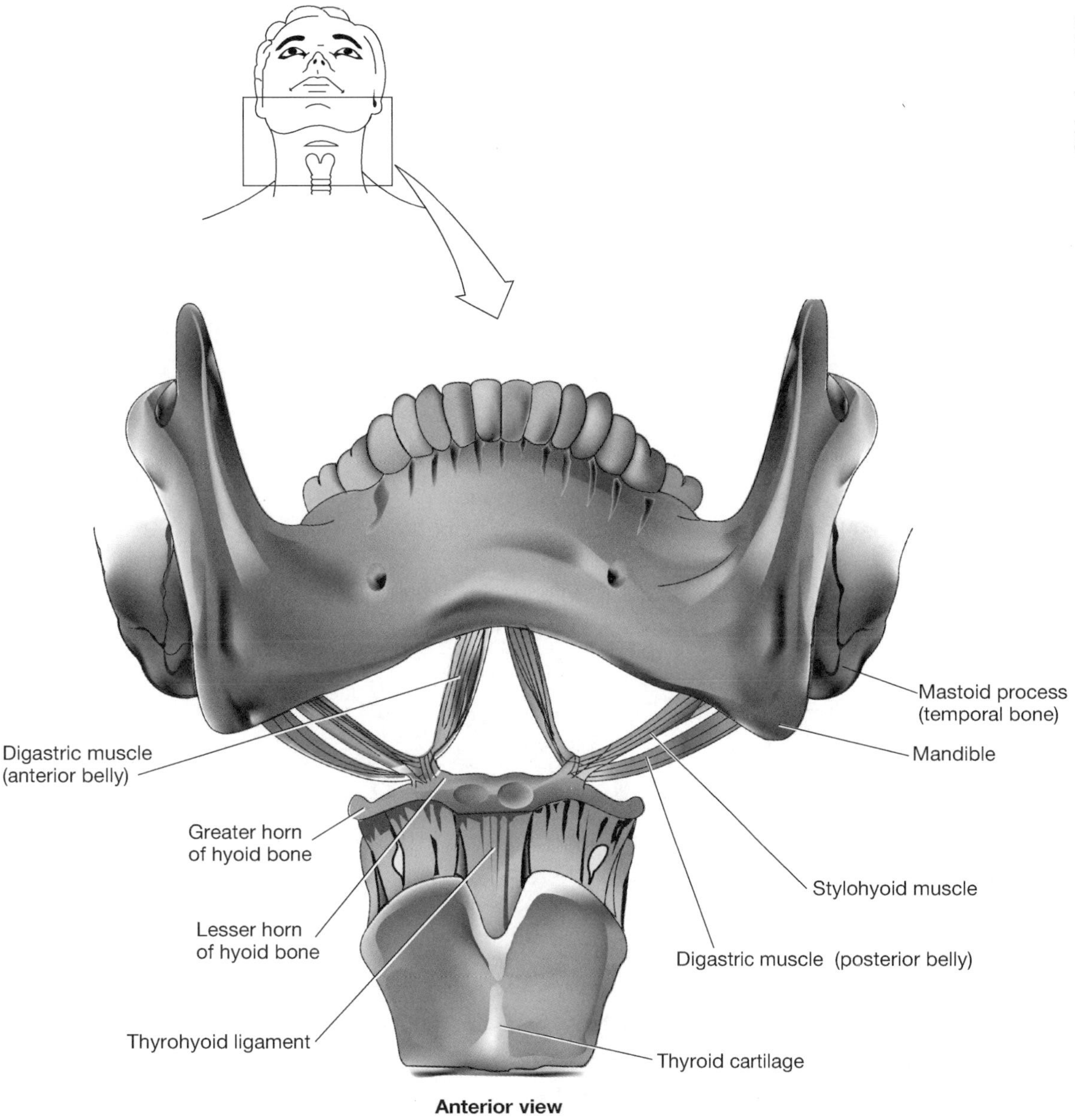

Figure 6-2
Anterior View of the Hyoid Bone

aperture which transmits the nasal passageways (Figure 6-3). Each orbit is formed by parts of seven bones and is penetrated posteriorly by three neurovascular passageways: optic canal, superior orbital fissure, and inferior orbital fissure (Table 6-2, Figure 6-4). The most obvious landmark on the side of the skull is the **zygomatic arch** which is formed by parts of the temporal and zygomatic bones (Figure 6-3). Inferiorly, the skull has numerous neurovascular passageways, but the most obvious feature is the large **foramen magnum** which transmits the spinal cord (Figure 6-5).

The superior aspect of the skull is called the **calvaria** and consists of parts of four bones: frontal bone, left and right parietal bones, and occipital bone (Figure 6-3, 6-6). Islands of bone within the

Table 6-1 Bones of the Head

Subgroup	*Name*		*Number*
Cranial bones	Frontal bone		1
	Parietal bone		2
	Occipital bone		1
	Temporal bone		2
	Sphenoid bone		1
	Ethmoid bone		1
		total	8
Facial bones	Zygomatic bone		2
	Maxilla		2
	Palatine bone		2
	Nasal bone		2
	Lacrimal bone		2
	Vomer		1
	Inferior nasal concha		2
	Mandible		1
		total	14
Auditory ossicles	Malleus		2
	Incus		2
	Stapes		2
		total	6
Hyoid bone	—		1

joints of the calvaria are called **sutural** (wormian) **bones**. The most common sutural bones are found in the lambdoid suture (the joint between the parietal and occipital bones). In newborn babies, the bones of the calvaria are not completely ossified and the connective tissue proper membranes between them and adjacent bones form the so-called "soft spots", officially named **fontanels (fontanelles)** (Figure 6-7). The most notable midline fontanels are the **anterior fontanel** at the junction of the two halves of the frontal bone and the two parietal bones, and the **posterior fontanel** at the junction of the two parietal bones and the occipital bone. The anterior-most of the two fontanels on each side of the skull is called the **anterolateral fontanel** (located at the junction of the frontal, parietal, temporal, and sphenoid bones) and the posterior-most is called the **posterolateral fontanel** (located where the occipital, parietal, and temporal bones meet). As infants mature, these areas complete their ossification.

Internally, the floor of the cranial cavity is divided by two pairs of ridges (Figure 6-5). The anterior pair is formed by the sphenoid bone and the posterior pair is formed by the petrous part of the temporal bone. These ridges separate the **anterior**, **middle**, and **posterior cranial fossae** which accommodate different parts of the brain. The posterior cranial fossa is the largest and deepest of the three. The foramen magnum is located within it.

Objectives

2. Define skull, calvaria, fontanel, foramen magnum, and zygomatic arch.

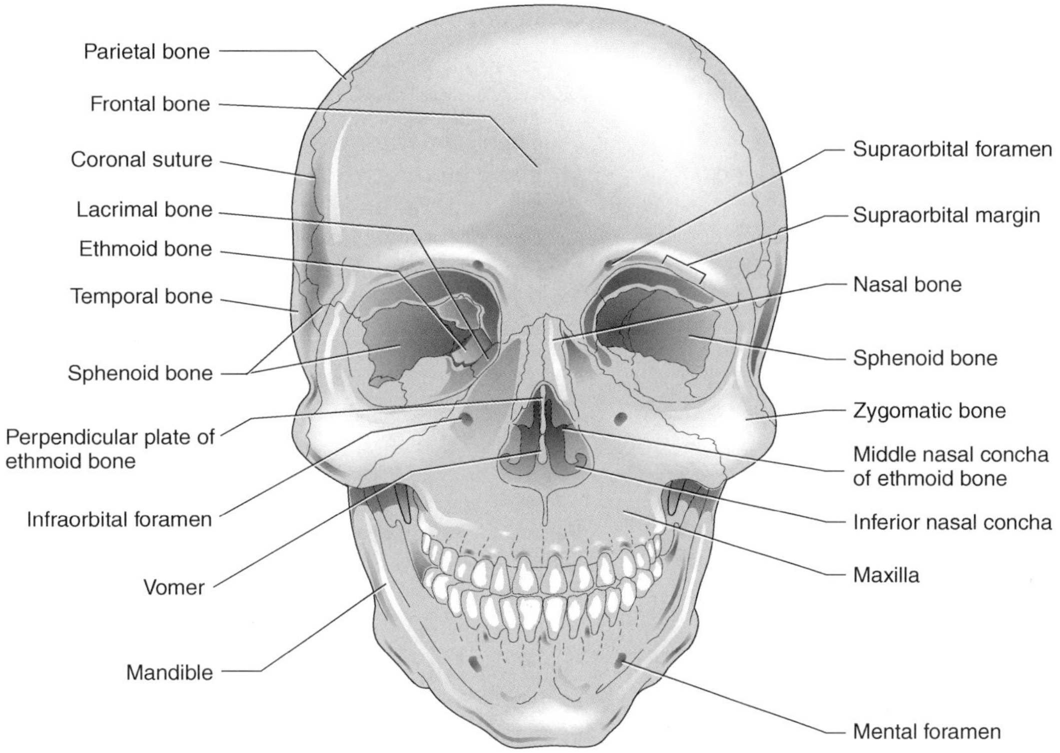

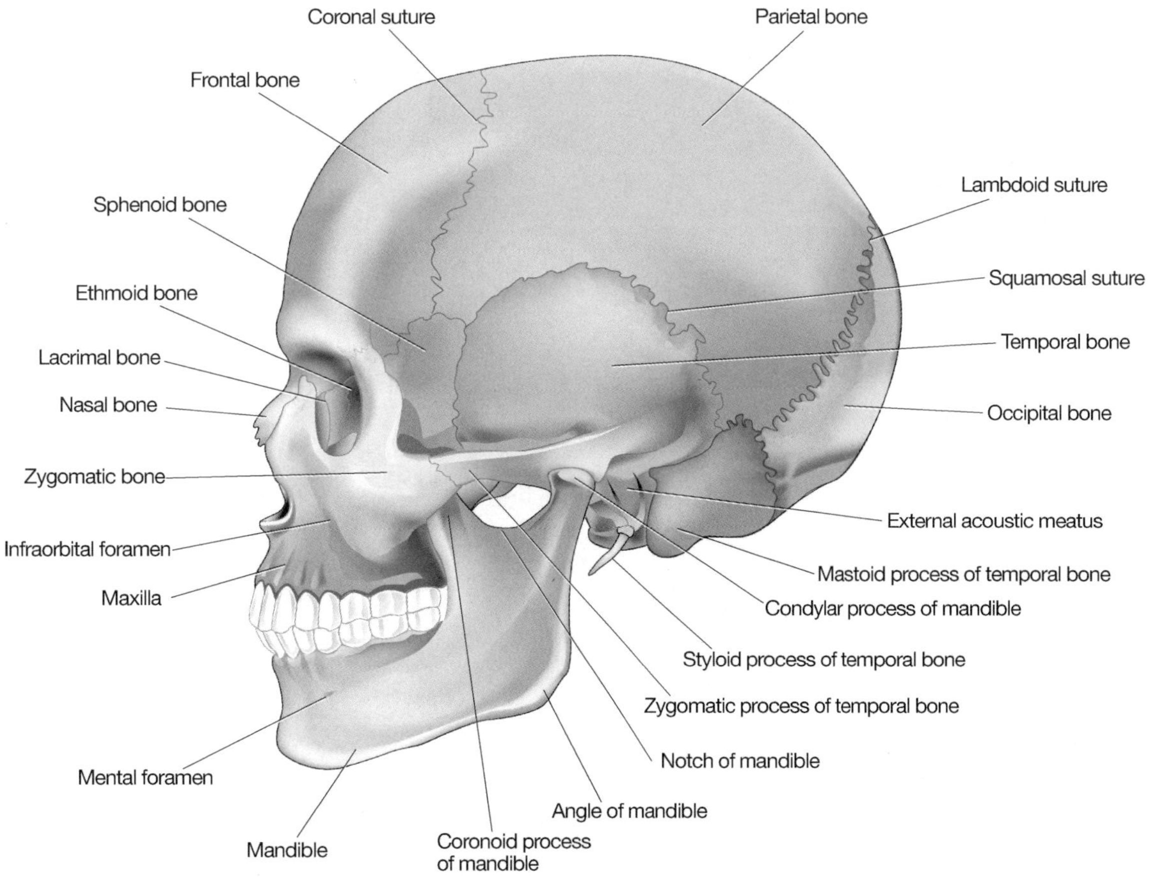

Figure 6-3

Anterior and Lateral Views of the Skull

Table 6-2 Osseous Components of the Orbit

Bone	*Portion of Orbit Formed*
Frontal Bone	Superior portion
Zygomatic Bone	Inferolateral aspect
Maxilla	Inferomedial aspect
Lacrimal Bone	Part of medial wall
Ethmoid Bone	Part of medial wall
Palatine Bone	Part of inferior aspect
Sphenoid Bone	Posterior wall

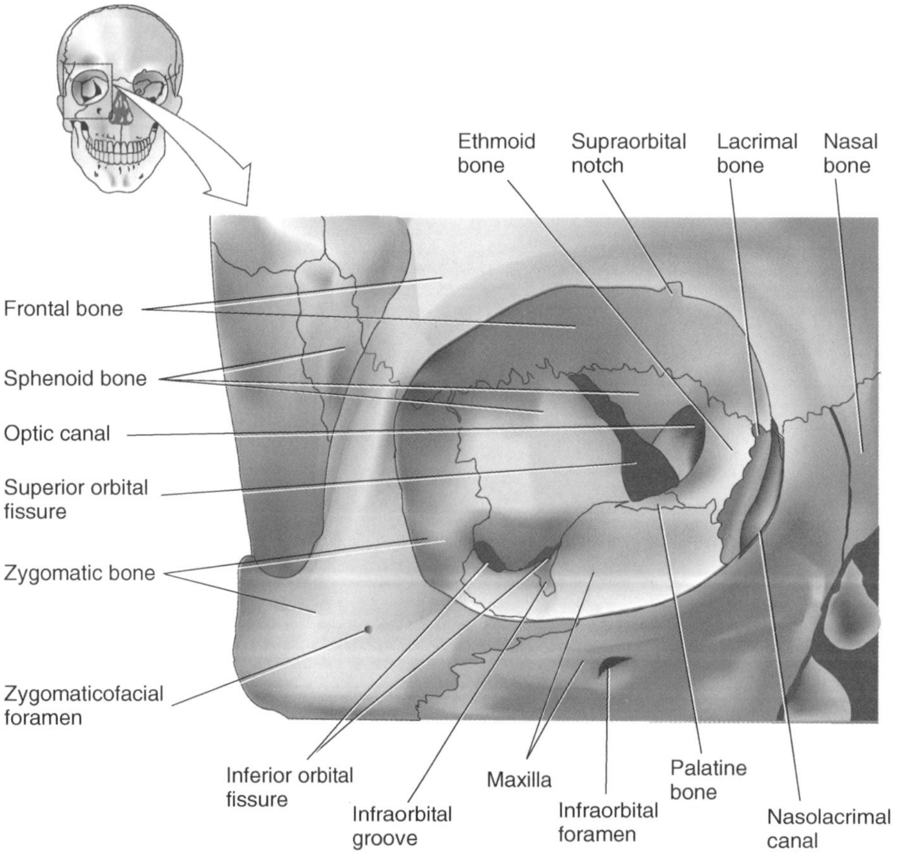

Figure 6-4

Bones of the Orbit

Seven bones contribute to the orbit: frontal, zygomatic, palatine, lacrimal, ethmoid, and sphenoid bones and the maxilla.

Neurocranium

The unpaired **frontal bone** (Figure 6-3) forms the anterosuperior aspect of the skull. It forms most of the brow (forehead), the roof of the nasal cavity, and the superior aspects of the orbits. The frontal bone actually develops from separate right and left halves. However, these usually fuse (ossify) at a young age so tightly and completely that the frontal bone of an adult is considered to be a

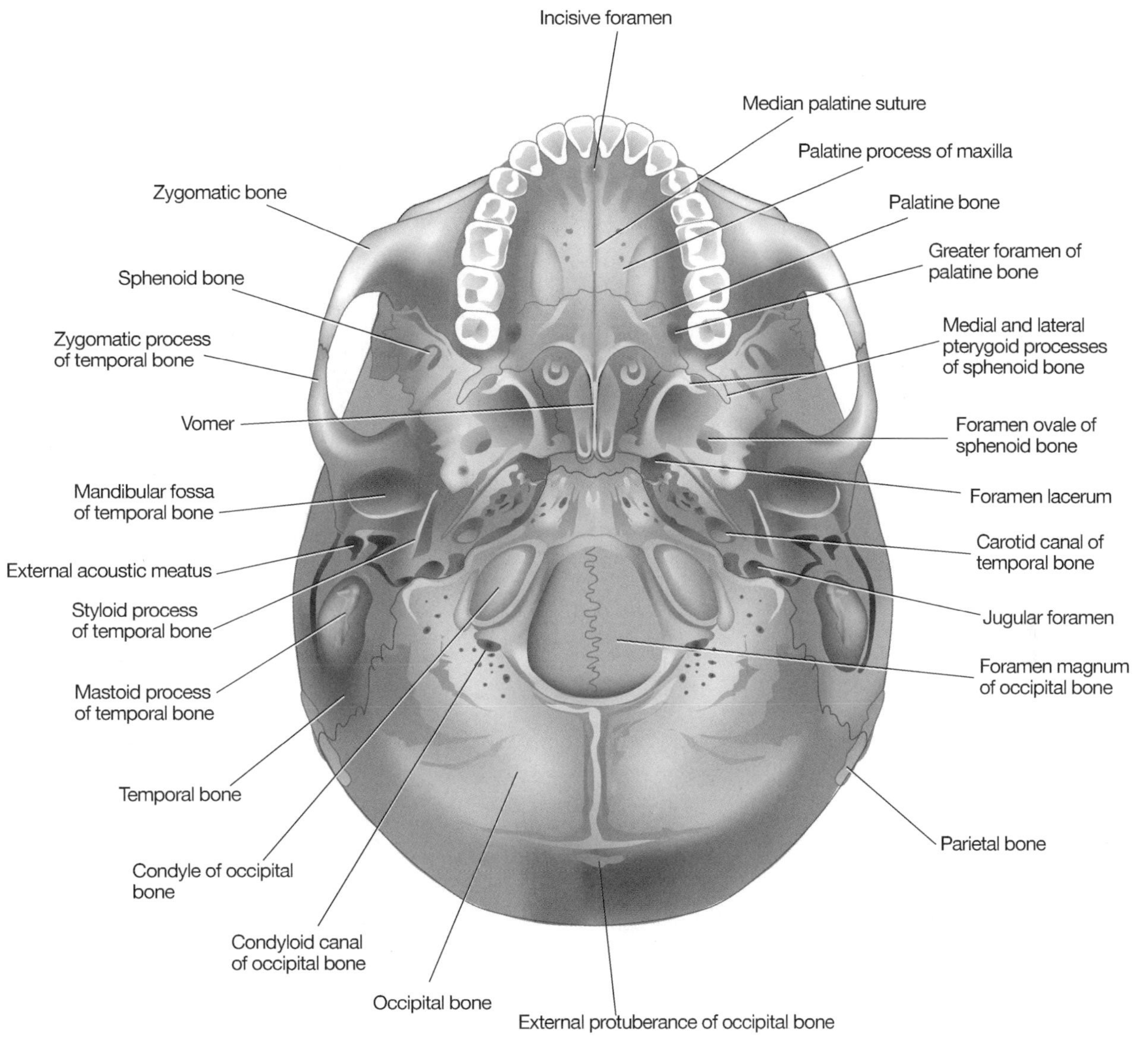

Figure 6-5A
Inferior View of the Skull

single (unpaired) structure. At a level of about one-third of the way toward the back of the calvaria, the frontal bone joins the left and right parietal bones to form the coronal suture. The largest portion of the frontal bone is called the **squama frontalis** and forms the brow and the anterior part of the temple. Much smaller **nasal** and **orbital parts** extend inferiorly from the squamous portion. Air-filled, mucous membrane lined cavities within the frontal bones called **frontal sinuses** communicate with the nasal cavity.

The left and right **parietal bones** form the middle half of the top of the cranial vault (Figures 6-3, 6-6). They meet along the median plane to form the jagged sagittal suture. Each parietal bone has **frontal**, **occipital**, **sphenoid**, and **mastoid angles** as well as occipital, squamous, sagittal, and frontal borders named according to the adjacent bone, bony landmark, or suture. Laterally each parietal bone articulates with the squamous part of the ipsilateral temporal bone at the squamous suture. Posteriorly, each parietal bone articulates with the occipital bone at the lambdoid suture.

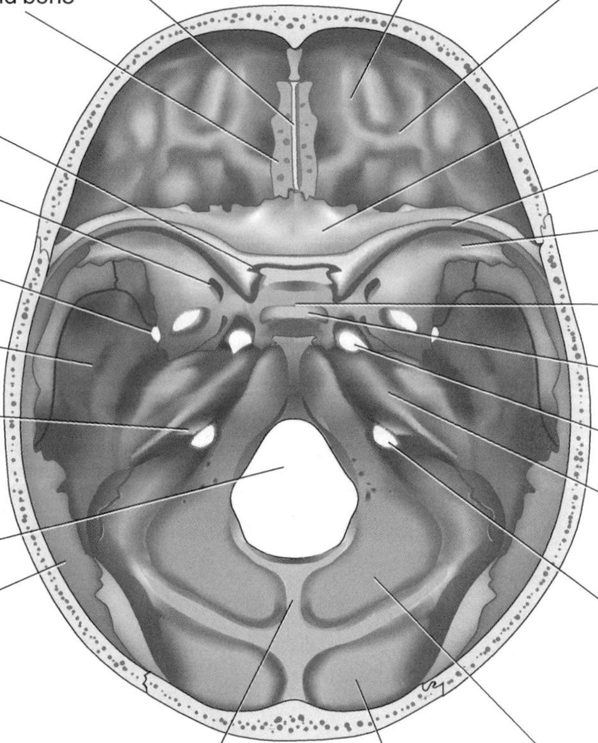

Figure 6-5B
Internal Base of the Skull

The unpaired **occipital bone** forms the posterior aspect of the skull as well as the posterior part of its inferior portion (Figure 6-5). Inferiorly, the occipital bone transmits the spinal cord through the foramen magnum. On each side of the foramen magnum are the right and left **occipital condyles** which articulate with the first cervical vertebra. The bony "knot" on the lower aspect of the posterior portion of the skull is the **external occipital protuberance**.

The paired **temporal bones** form the lateral parts of the skull around the ears as well as part of the central portion of the floor of the cranial cavity (Figure 6-8). Each temporal bone is divided into three major portions: squamous, tympanic, and petrous parts. The **squamous part** includes the flattened lateral portion above the ear as well as the **zygomatic process** which projects forward to meet the zygomatic bone and forms the zygomatic arch. Posterior to the zygomatic arch is the **mandibular fossa** which articulates with the head of the mandible to form the temporomandibular joint. The **tympanic part** of the temporal bone surrounds the **external acoustic meatus** through which atmospheric sound vibrations pass en route to the tympanic membrane. The **petrous part** of the temporal bone is the inferior portion which surrounds the structures of the middle and internal ears.

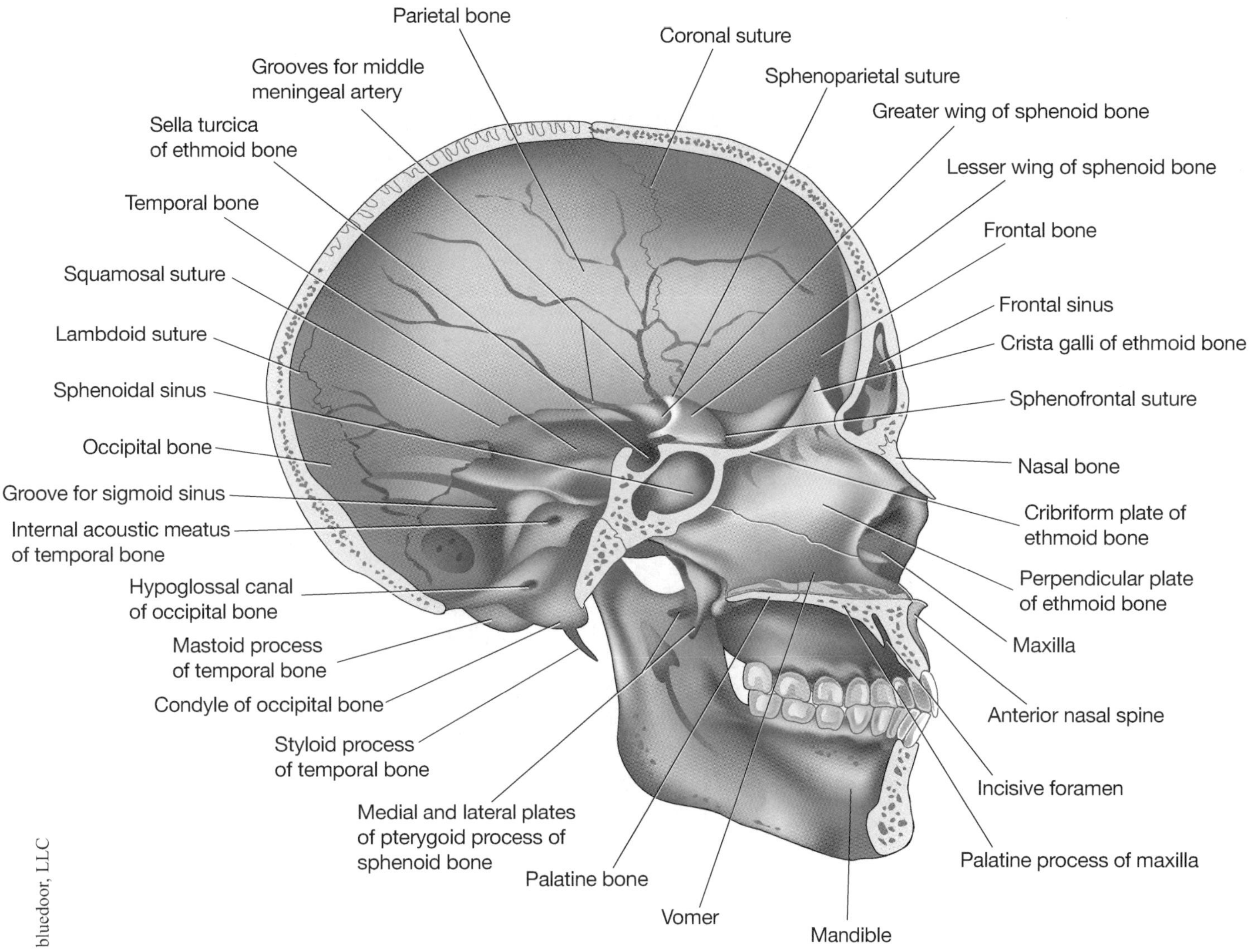

Figure 6-6A
Sagittal Section of the Skull

The rounded bony projection of the petrous part just posterior and inferior to the ear is the **mastoid process** of the temporal bone. Just anterior to the mastoid process is the pointed **styloid process** which projects inferiorly. The small **stylomastoid foramen** which transmits the seventh cranial (facial) nerve is located between the base of the styloid process and the mastoid process.

The unpaired **sphenoid bone** forms part of the anterior floor of the cranial cavity as well as a small portion of the lateral aspect of the skull (in the inferior part of the small temporal region) (Figures 6-5, 6-9). The sphenoid bone includes a central **body** with (paired) **greater** and **lesser wings**. The left and right **pterygoid processes** extend inferiorly from the greater wings. Each process is composed of a medial and lateral plate (lamina). Air-filled diverticuli of the nasal cavity within the body of the sphenoid bone constitute the **sphenoidal sinus**. Another major landmark of the body of the sphenoid bone is the median plane depression called the **sella turcica** in which the pituitary gland sits. The sphenoid bone transmits the optic nerves through the **optic canals** (anterolateral to the sella

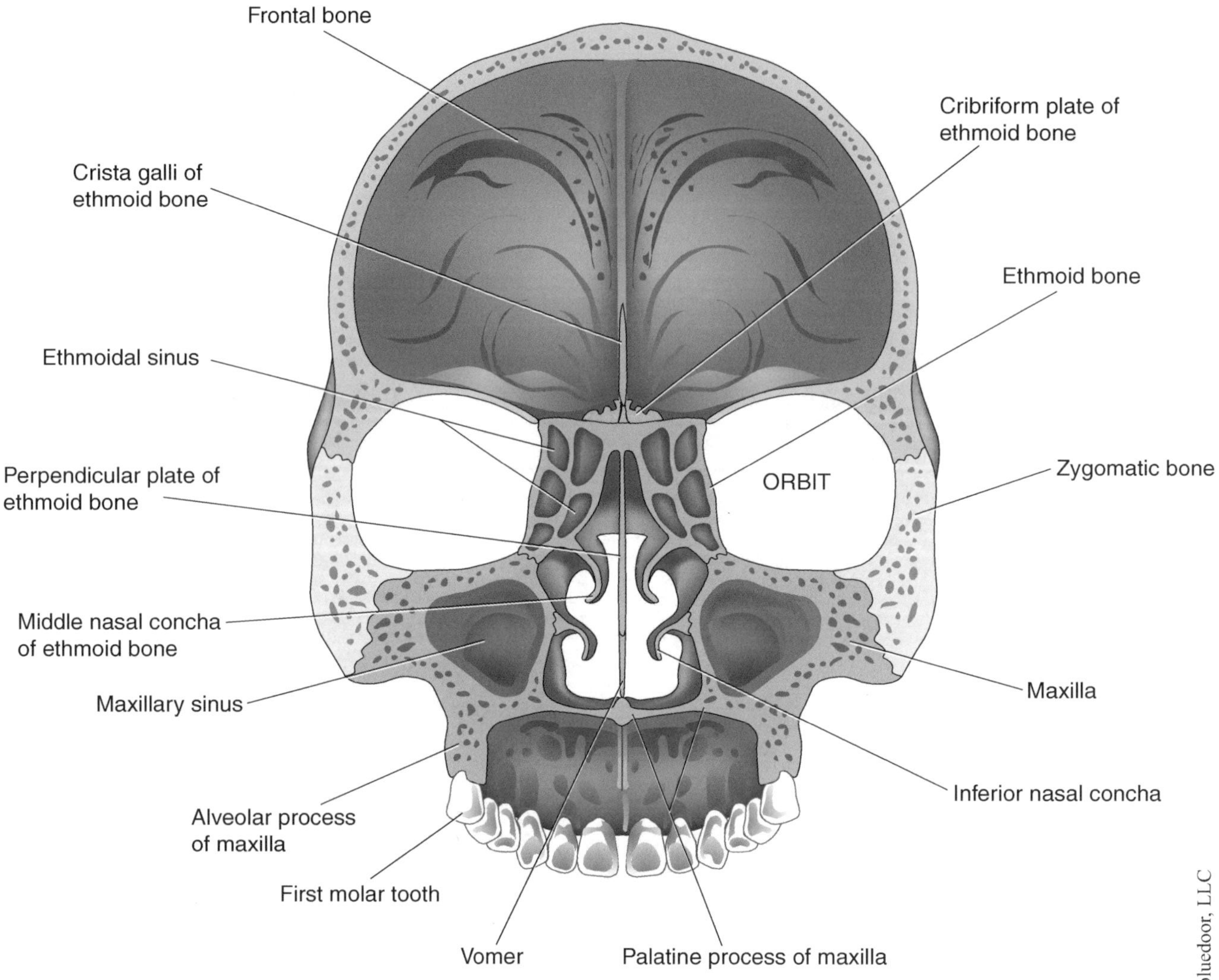

Figure 6-6B
Frontal Section of the Skull

turcica) and the **mandibular** and **maxillary nerves** through the oval and round foramina, respectively. These are located lateral to the sella turcica.

The unpaired **ethmoid bone** contributes to the formation of both orbits and forms part of the nasal septum that divides the nasal cavity (Figure 6-10). Air-filled diverticuli within the ethmoid bone are collectively termed the **ethmoidal sinus** and are individually termed ethmoidal cells. The superior portion of the ethmoid bone, called the **cribriform plate**, forms a small portion of the cranial vault on the midline. It has a median ridge called the **crista galli** and is penetrated by numerous **cribriform foramina** through which the fibers of the first cranial (olfactory) nerves pass. The portion of the ethmoid bone that contributes to the nasal septum is the **perpendicular plate**. Thin, scroll-like projections of bone called the **superior** and **middle nasal conchae** project into the nasal cavity from the ethmoid bone. The larger, inferior nasal concha is a separate bone.

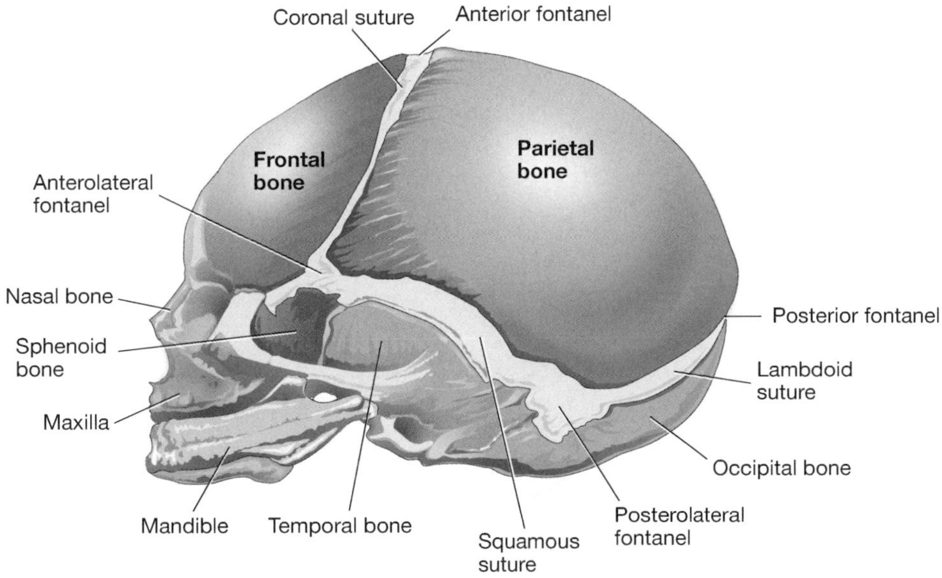

Figure 6-7

Lateral Aspect of Fetal Skull Illustrating the Fontanels

The six fontanels are "soft spots" formed by non-ossified fibrous connective tissue. The unpaired anterior and posterior fontanels are centered on the midline. The paired (left and right) anterolateral and posterolateral fontanels are located on the lateral aspects of the skull. The fontanels ossify and fuse as the skeleton matures.

Objectives

3. State which bones of the neurocranium and which ones of the viscerocranium contribute to the orbit (Table 6-2).

Viscerocranium

The fourteen facial bones include six which are paired and two which are single. The facial bones inferolateral to the orbits which form the so-called "cheek bones" are the **zygomatic bones** (Figure 6-3). Each zygomatic bone has a **frontal process** which extends superiorly to meet the frontal bone and complete the lateral encasement of the orbit (Table 6-2). The **temporal process** of the zygomatic bone projects posteriorly to join the zygomatic process of the temporal bone and complete the formation of the **zygomatic arch**.

The left and right **maxillae** form most of the anterior portion of the skull below the orbits (Figure 6-11). Each maxilla consists of frontal, zygomatic, palatine, and alveolar processes. The **body** is the large central portion that contributes to the orbit, forms part of the lateral wall of the nasal cavity, and surrounds the **maxillary sinus**. Just below the orbit, the body of the maxilla is penetrated by the **infraorbital foramen** which transmits the infraorbital nerve and vessels. The **frontal** and **zygomatic processes** of the maxilla are the portions that articulate with the frontal and zygomatic bones. The **palatine processes** of the left and right maxillae meet along the midline to form the skeletal support for the anterior portion of the **bony palate**. The **alveolar processes** support all of the superior teeth in sockets called **dental alveoli**.

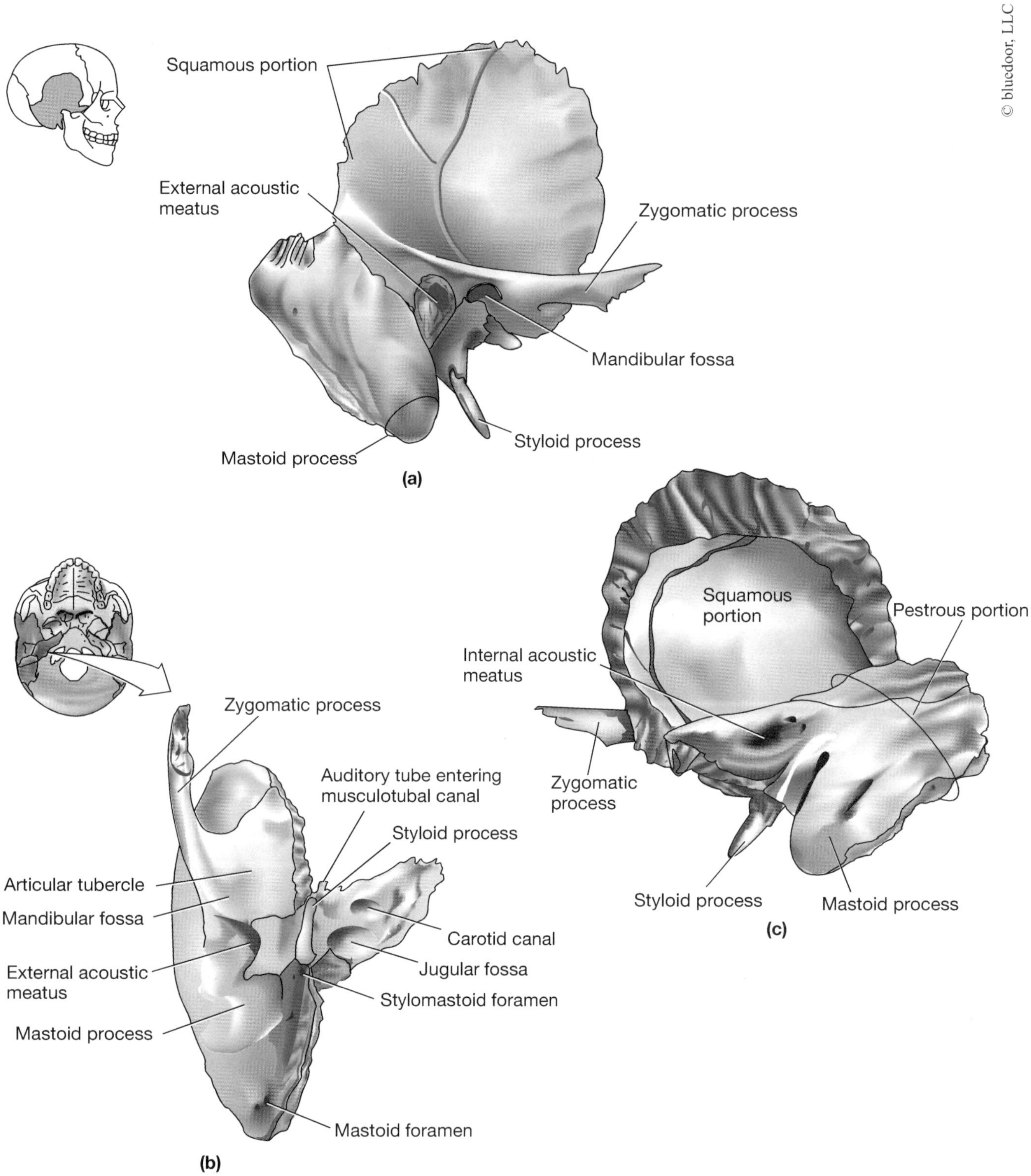

Figure 6-8

Lateral (a), Inferior (b), and Medial (c) Views of the Right Temporal Bone

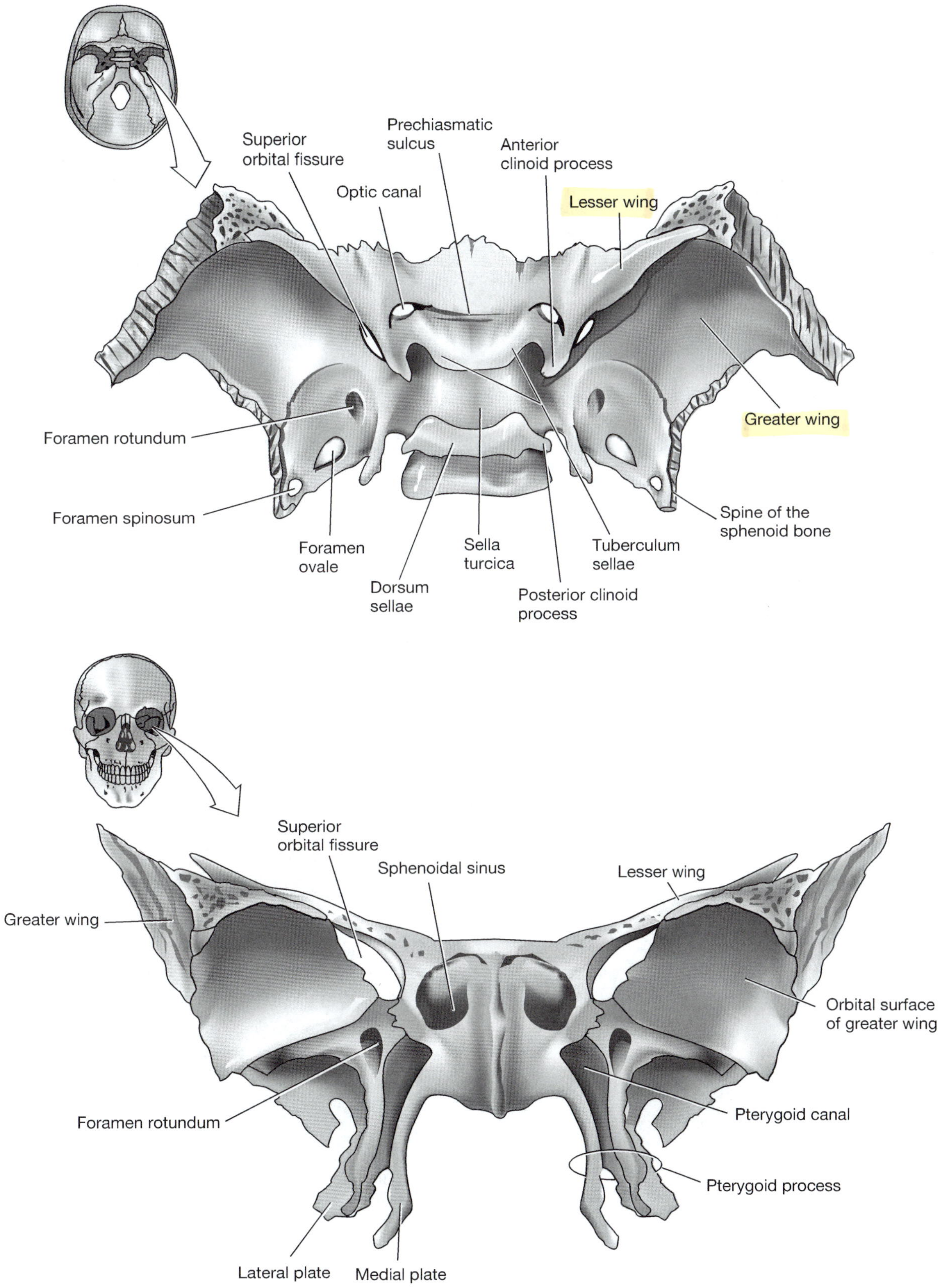

Figure 6-9

Superior and Anterior Views of the Sphenoid Bone

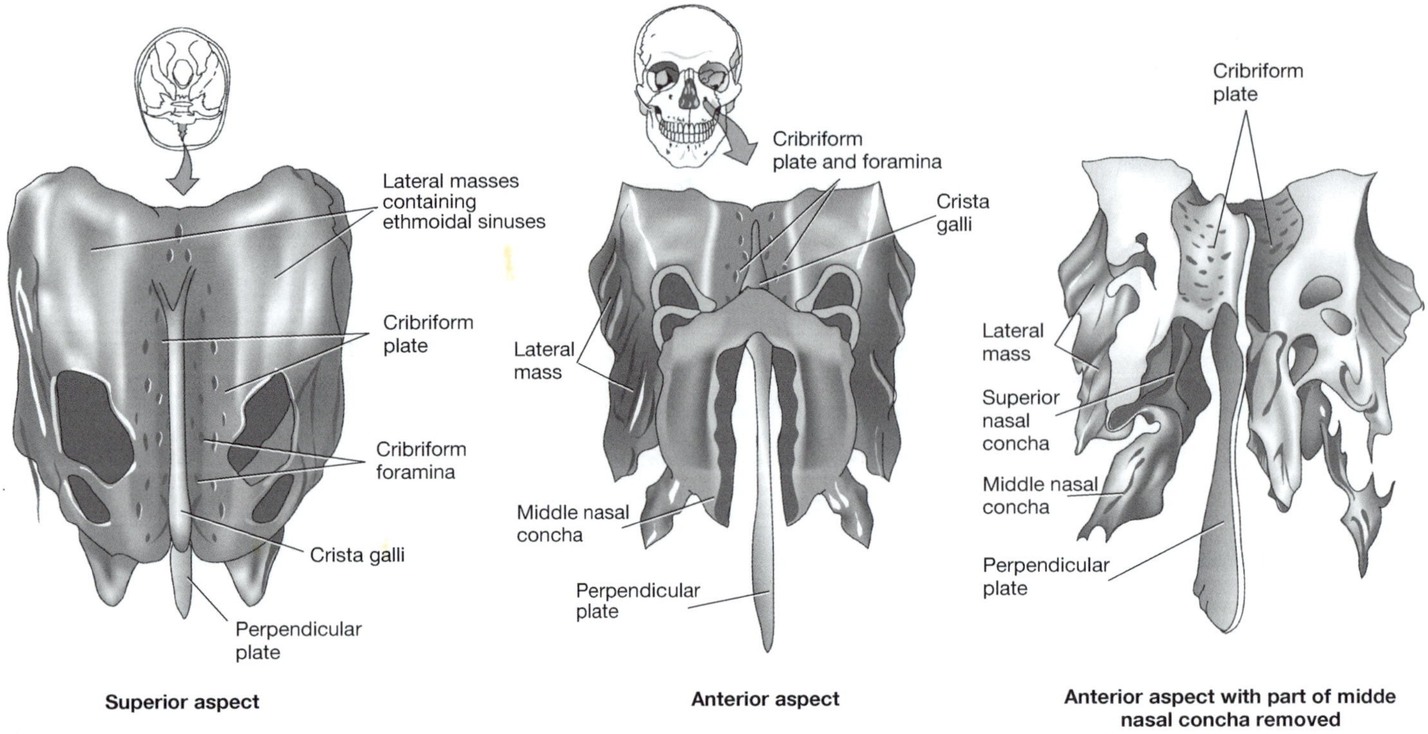

Figure 6-10

Three Views of the Ethmoid Bone

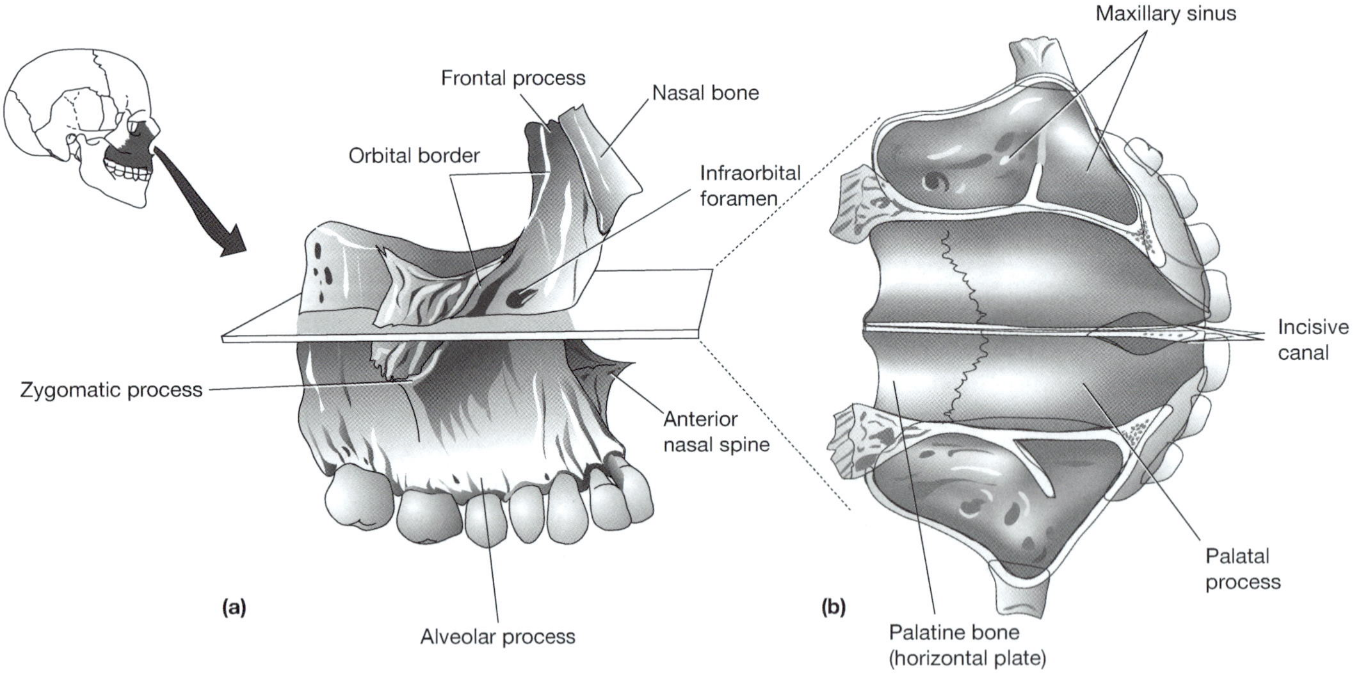

Figure 6-11

Maxilla

(a) Lateral view of right maxilla

(b) Transverse section through both maxillae

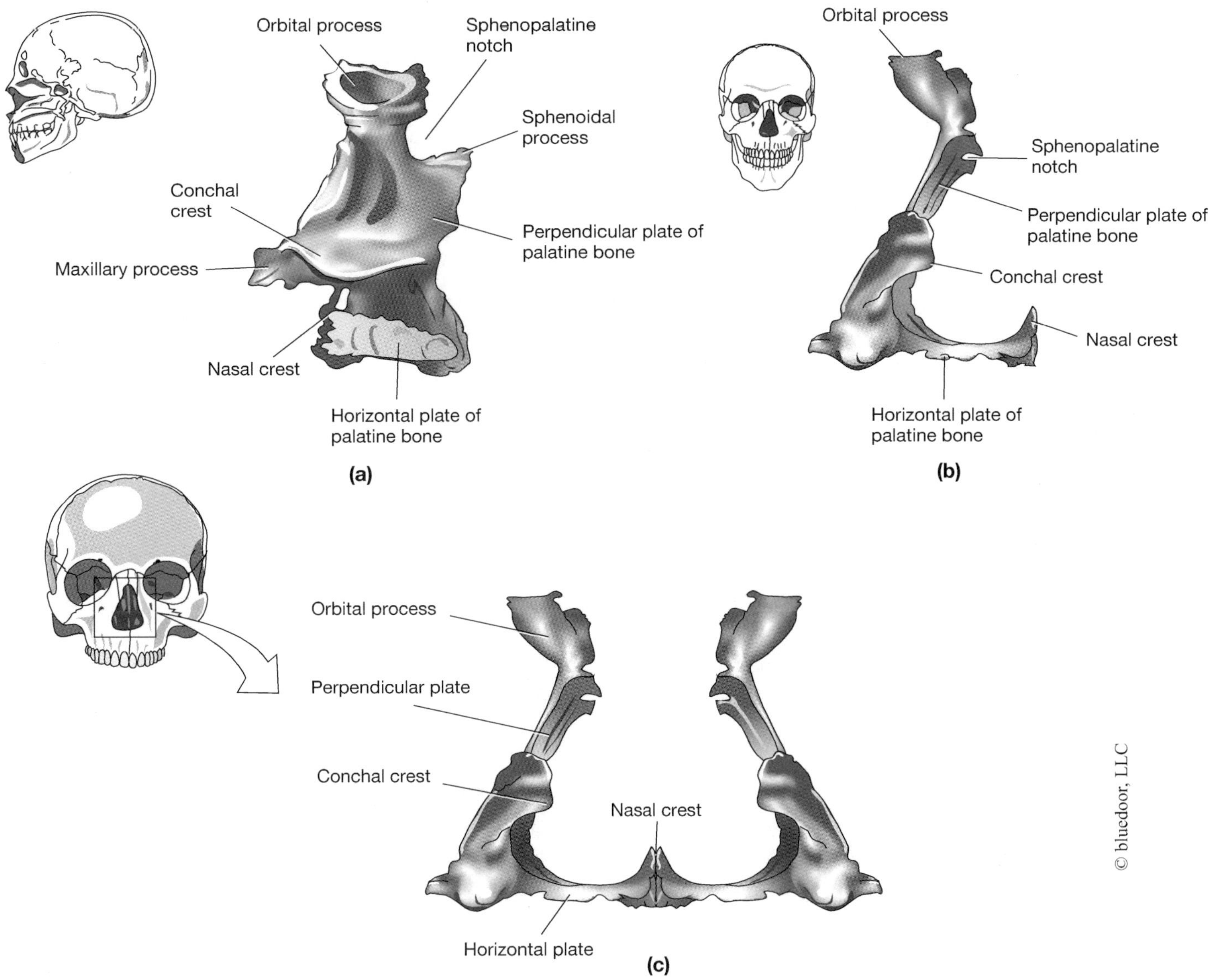

Figure 6-12
Palatine Bone
(a) Medial view of right palatine bone
(b) Anterior view of right palatine bone
(c) Anterior view of both palatine bones

The paired **palatine bones** are positioned just posterior to the maxillae (Figure 6-12). Each palatine bone has a horizontal plate and a vertically oriented perpendicular plate. The **horizontal plates** of the palatine bones form the skeletal support for the posterior portion of the hard palate. The **perpendicular plate** of each palatine bone projects superiorly to form part of the lateral wall of the nasal cavity and a tiny portion of the ipsilateral orbit.

The small, paired **nasal bones** form the skeletal support for the bridge (dorsum) of the nose (Figure 6-3). They articulate with the frontal bones superiorly, with the maxillae laterally, and with each other along the midline. The unpaired **vomer** forms a large part of the inferior portion of the

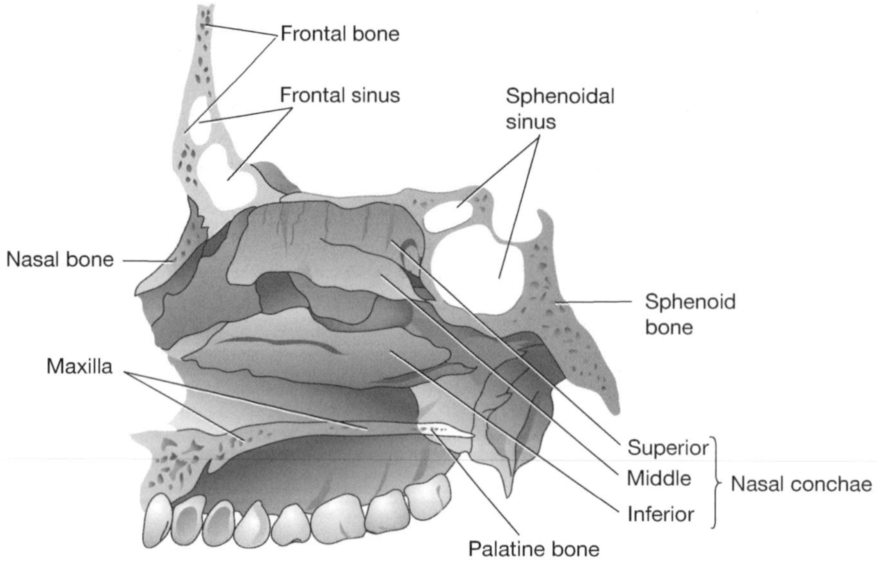

Figure 6-13

Bones of the Lateral Wall of the Nasal Cavity

The superior and middle nasal conchae are parts of the ethmoid bone (see Figure 6-10). The inferior nasal concha is a separate bone. Note that both left and right maxillae and both palatine bones contribute to the bony palate.

osseous part of the nasal septum. The left and right **lacrimal bones** form parts of the medial wall of each orbit (Figure 6-4). The paired **inferior nasal conchae** project medially from the maxillary portions of the lateral walls of the nasal cavity (Figure 6-13). Nasal mucosa covering these bones increases the total surface area of the wall of the nasal cavity which assists in cleaning and moisturizing inspired air as well as regulating its temperature.

The **mandible** is the unpaired bone in which all of the inferior teeth are embedded (Figure 6-14). It consists of a horizontally oriented body and two vertically oriented rami. The left and right halves of the **body** develop separately and fuse on the midline to form the **mandibular symphysis**. The superior portion of the mandibular body is called the **alveolar part** because of the **dental alveoli** which support the inferior teeth. Small openings along the anterolateral aspects of the body, called **mental foramina**, transport the mental nerves. The bony prominence along the posteroinferior aspect of the mandibular ramus is the **angle of the mandible**. The medial (internal) aspect of each mandibular ramus is penetrated by a **mandibular foramen** which transmits the inferior alveolar nerve (a branch of the mandibular nerve) and vessels. The superior aspect of each **mandibular ramus** consists of a **coronoid process** (anteriorly) and a **condyloid process** (posteriorly) separated by the **mandibular notch**. The condyloid process includes the rounded **head of the mandible** that articulates with the mandibular fossa of the temporal bone to form the temporomandibular joint.

Objectives

4. State how the inferior nasal conchae differ from the superior and middle nasal conchae.

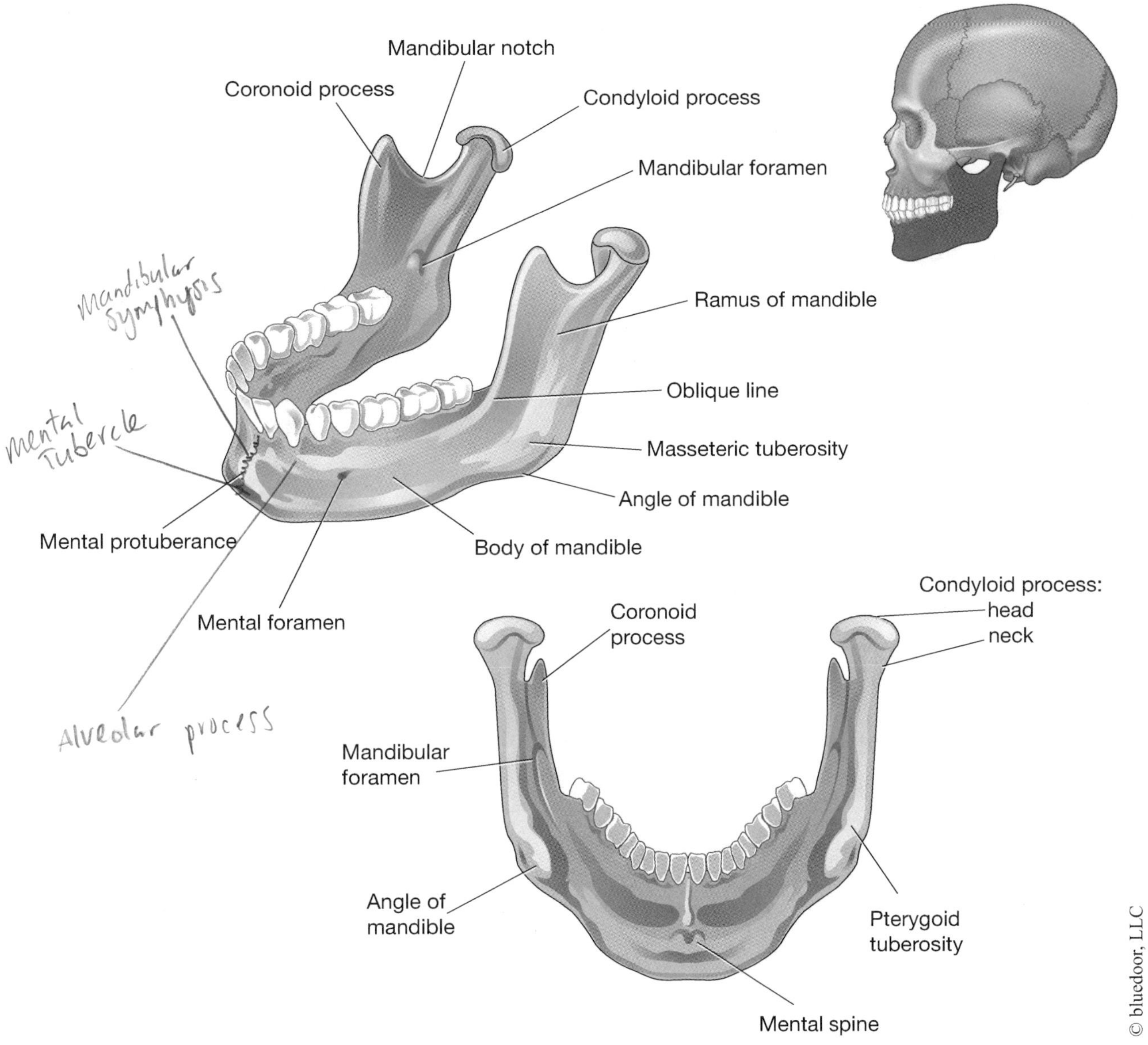

Figure 6-14

Mandible (Lateral and Inferior Aspects)

The two halves of the maxilla are joined synostotically along the median plane by the ossified mandibular (mental) symphysis (not labeled).

Vertebrae

Vertebrae have some general features which include a vertebral body, vertebral arch, and some processes. The **vertebral body** is the large solid portion which is located anteriorly. The bodies of adjacent vertebrae (except between C1 and C2) are separated by **intervertebral discs** (*see Chapter 7*). These join the bodies to each other, allow limited movement, and act as shock absorbers. The **vertebral arch** is the posterior portion of each vertebra that surrounds the spinal cord. Developmentally each arch is formed by left and right **pedicles** and by left and right **laminae** which fuse to each other and to the vertebral body to complete a bony encasement around the spinal cord

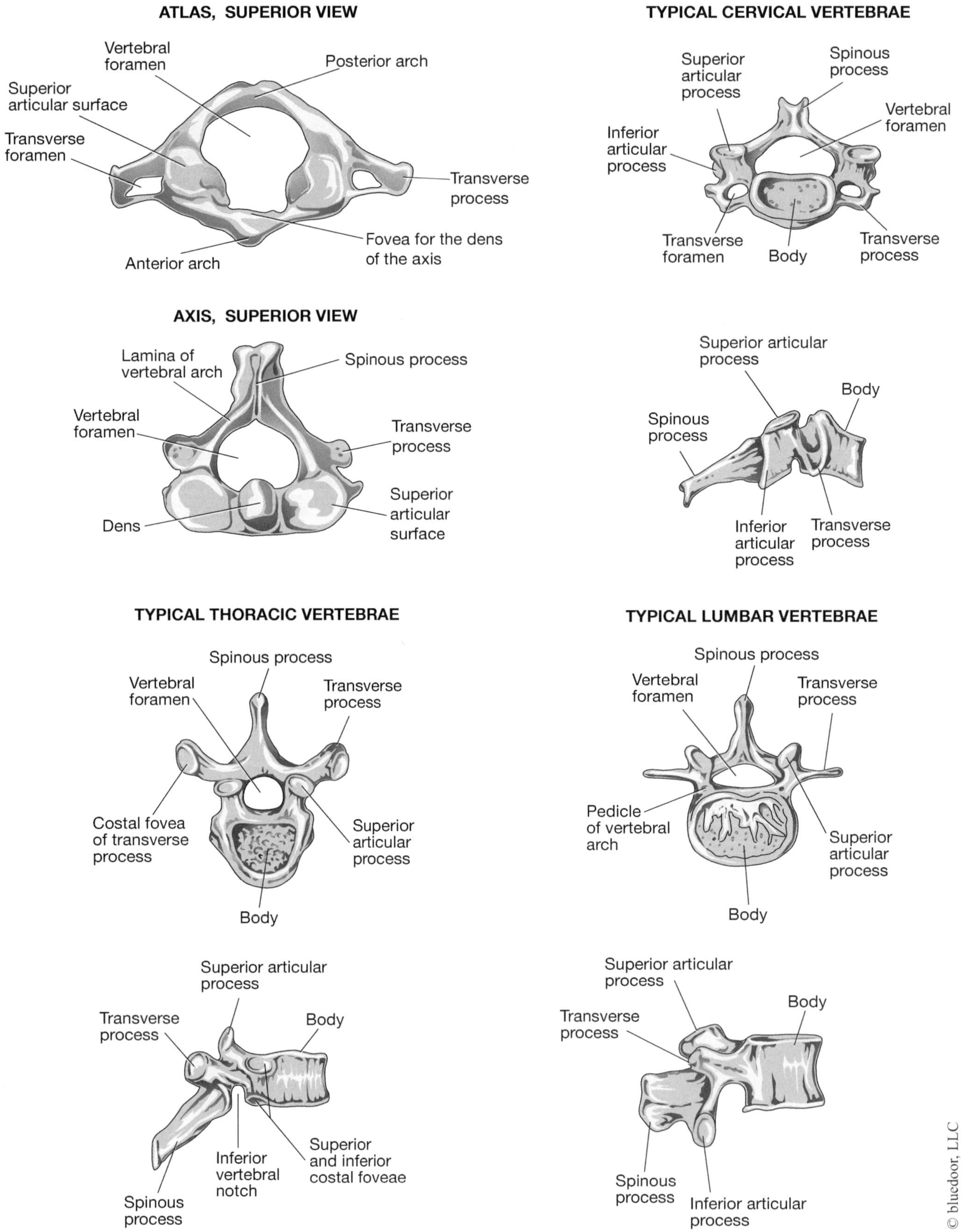

Figure 6-15
Cervical, Thoracic, and Lumbar Vertebrae

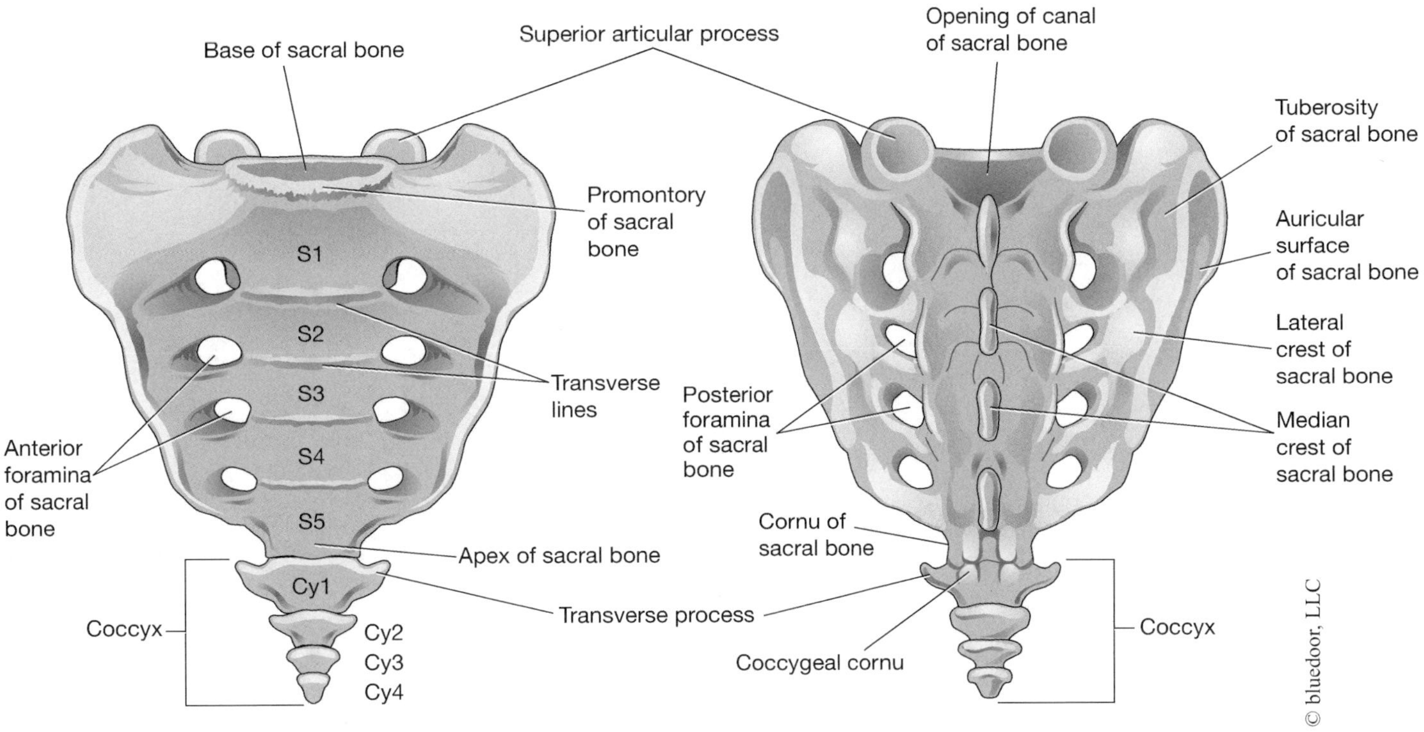

Figure 6-16
The Sacral Bone and Coccyx

(Figure 6-15). The large passageway thus formed is called the **vertebral foramen** and the collective vertebral foramina of adjacent vertebrae constitute the **vertebral canal**. Only parts of the arches of adjacent vertebrae touch each other. The lateral gaps that exist are called **intervertebral foramina** and transmit the spinal nerves (Figure 6-15). Each intervertebral foramen is formed by indentations in the arches of adjacent vertebrae called **inferior** and **superior vertebral notches**. The processes of a vertebra include a single (palpable) **spinous process** which projects posteriorly from the arch, a pair of **transverse processes** which extend laterally from the arch, and four small **articular processes** (left/right superior, left/right inferior) which also project from the arch and articulate with those of adjacent vertebrae (Figure 6-15).

Vertebrae are divided into five groups (cervical, thoracic, lumbar, sacral, and coccygeal) and are numbered superiorly to inferiorly within each group. The seven **cervical vertebrae** are found within the neck. The **first cervical vertebra**, also known as **C1** or **atlas**, is somewhat atypical because it has no spinous process and no body (Figure 6-15). It articulates with the occipital bone of the skull. The **second cervical vertebra** (**C2** or **axis**) has an especially broad spinous process, but its most obvious feature is a large superior projection from its body, called the **dens**, which represents the "lost" body of the atlas. The remaining cervical vertebrae are unremarkable (Figure 6-15). The vertebra at the base of the neck with the most palpable spinous process is called the **prominent vertebra**. It is usually C7 but may be the sixth cervical or first thoracic vertebra. The transverse processes of all cervical vertebrae are penetrated by **transverse foramina** which transmit the vertebral nerves and vessels.

The 12 **thoracic vertebrae** articulate with the 12 pairs of ribs (Figure 6-15). They have relatively long spinous processes, short bodies, and short transverse processes. The thoracic vertebrae have **costal foveae** on their bodies where the heads of the ribs articulate and most of them also have costal foveae

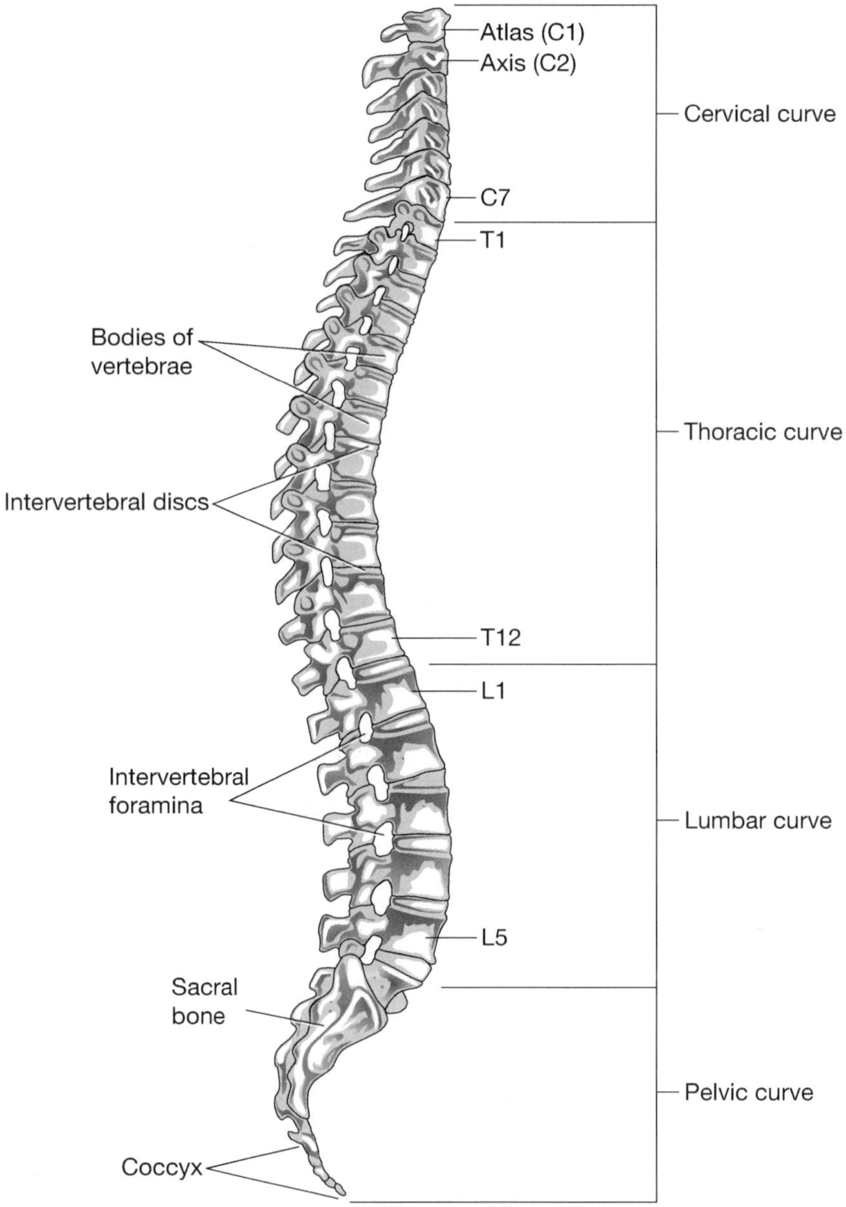

Figure 6-17
Lateral Aspect of the Vertebral Column

on their transverse processes for articulation with the tubercles of the ribs. The five **lumbar vertebrae** have stout bodies reflecting the larger percentage of the body weight that they support (Figure 6-15). They are located in the lower back and are characterized by well-developed transverse processes. The five (sometimes only four) **sacral vertebrae** fuse to form a solid bony mass called the **sacral bone** (*os sacrale*). This is usually shortened to "sacrum" (Figure 6-16). The bony sacrum articulates with the ilium of the os coxae to form a slightly movable but solid connection between the axial skeleton and the appendicular skeletons of the inferior limbs. The bony sacrum is much wider at its **base** (superior end) than at its **apex** (inferior end). Four pairs of **anterior sacral foramina** penetrate the pelvic surface (anterior aspect) of the bony sacrum. The dorsal surface (posterior aspect) is similarly penetrated by four pairs of **posterior sacral foramina**. The spinous processes of the fused sacral vertebrae form the

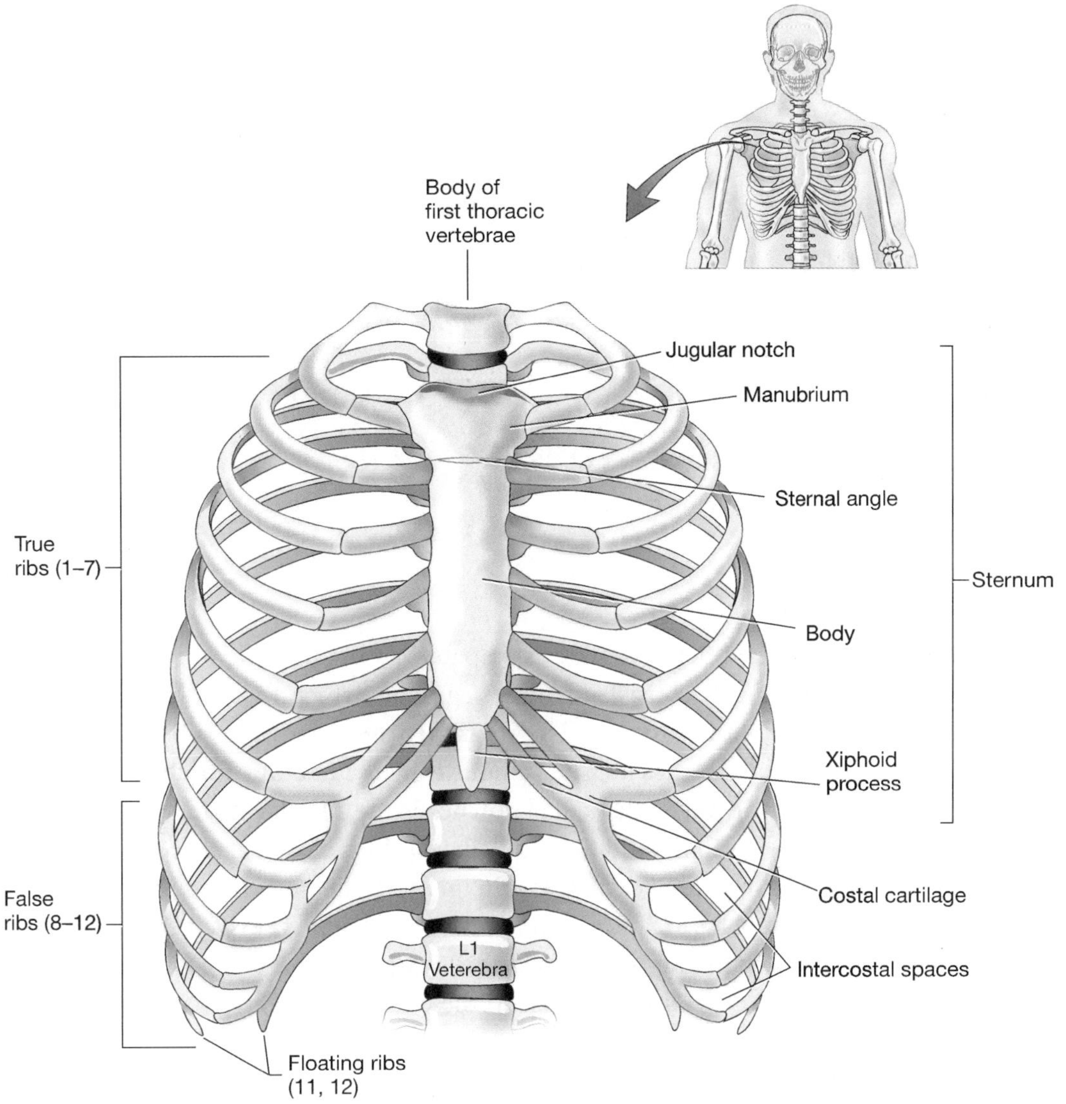

Figure 6-18

Anterior Aspect of the Sternum, Ribs, and Costal Cartilages

The first seven pairs of ribs are true ribs and the last five pairs are false ribs. The last two pairs of false ribs are also known as floating ribs. Three kinds of notches occur on the various parts of the sternum: the unpaired jugular notch (at the top), a pair of clavicular notches (where the left and right sternoclavicular joints occur) and seven pairs of costal notches (where the costal cartilages of the seven pairs of true ribs articulate).

median sacral crest. The four **coccygeal vertebrae** fuse to form a small bony mass known as the **coccyx**. It is wider superiorly and tapers inferiorly (Figure 6-16). Note that adults are still considered to have five sacral vertebrae and four coccygeal vertebrae even though these fuse to form only two bony masses (os sacrum and os coccyx) counted as one each when totalling the bones in the skeleton.

The vertebrae and intervening intervertebral discs collectively form the **vertebral column**. It should be straight as viewed from an anterior or posterior perspective but has four curvatures when viewed laterally (Figure 6-17). Two of these curvatures are convex anteriorly (cervical and lumbar curves) and two (thoracic and pelvic curves) are concave anteriorly. The vertebral formula, $\mathbf{C_7T_{12}L_5S_5Cy_4}$, is a shorthand method of describing the number of each type of vertebrae found in the column. Note: sometimes Co is used in place of Cy.

Objectives

5. Sketch and label a typical vertebra (superior view).
6. Write and be able to use the human vertebral formula.
7. Sketch a curved line representing the vertebral column in lateral perspective and label the cervical, thoracic, lumbar, and pelvic curvatures. Note which two are concave and which two are convex anteriorly (as viewed from the lateral aspect).

Sternum

The **sternum** is the unpaired flat bone that is palpable on the midline of the anterior aspect of the thoracic wall (Figure 6-18). It consists of three segments which fuse to form a single bony mass: manubrium, body, and xiphoid process. The **manubrium** is the wide superior portion. It articulates with the left and right clavicles at indentations called **clavicular notches**. The median indentation between and superior to the clavicular notches is the **jugular notch**. Along each side of the manubrium and body are seven indentations called **costal notches** where costal cartilages of the ribs join the sternum. The second costal cartilages join the sternum at the fused junction of the manubrium with the sternal **body**. This location is marked by a palpable transverse ridge in most individuals and is known as the **sternal angle**. The **xiphoid process** is directed inferiorly. It remains cartilaginous until the third year and does not fuse to the body of the sternum until later in life.

Objectives

8. List the three bones that fuse to form the sternum.

Ribs

There are 12 pairs of **ribs** in most individuals numbered **1-12** from superior to inferior (Figure 6-18). The first pair is quite short, the next six pairs get progressively longer, and the last five pairs are progressively shorter. Each rib has a head, neck, and body. The **head** is the rounded end which articulates with the costal foveae on the bodies of the thoracic vertebrae (Figure 6-19). The heads of most ribs articulate with two adjacent vertebrae, and have divided articular surfaces. Heads of ribs *1*, *10*, *11*, and *12* articulate only with the correspondingly numbered thoracic vertebra. The **neck** of a rib is the constricted portion immediately adjacent to the head. The **body** constitutes the largest portion of a rib. The bodies of most ribs have a small **tubercle** near the neck which articulates with the costal fovea of the transverse process of the similarly numbered thoracic vertebra. Tubercles are reduced or completely lacking on ribs *10*, *11*, and *12* because the costovertebral articulations of these

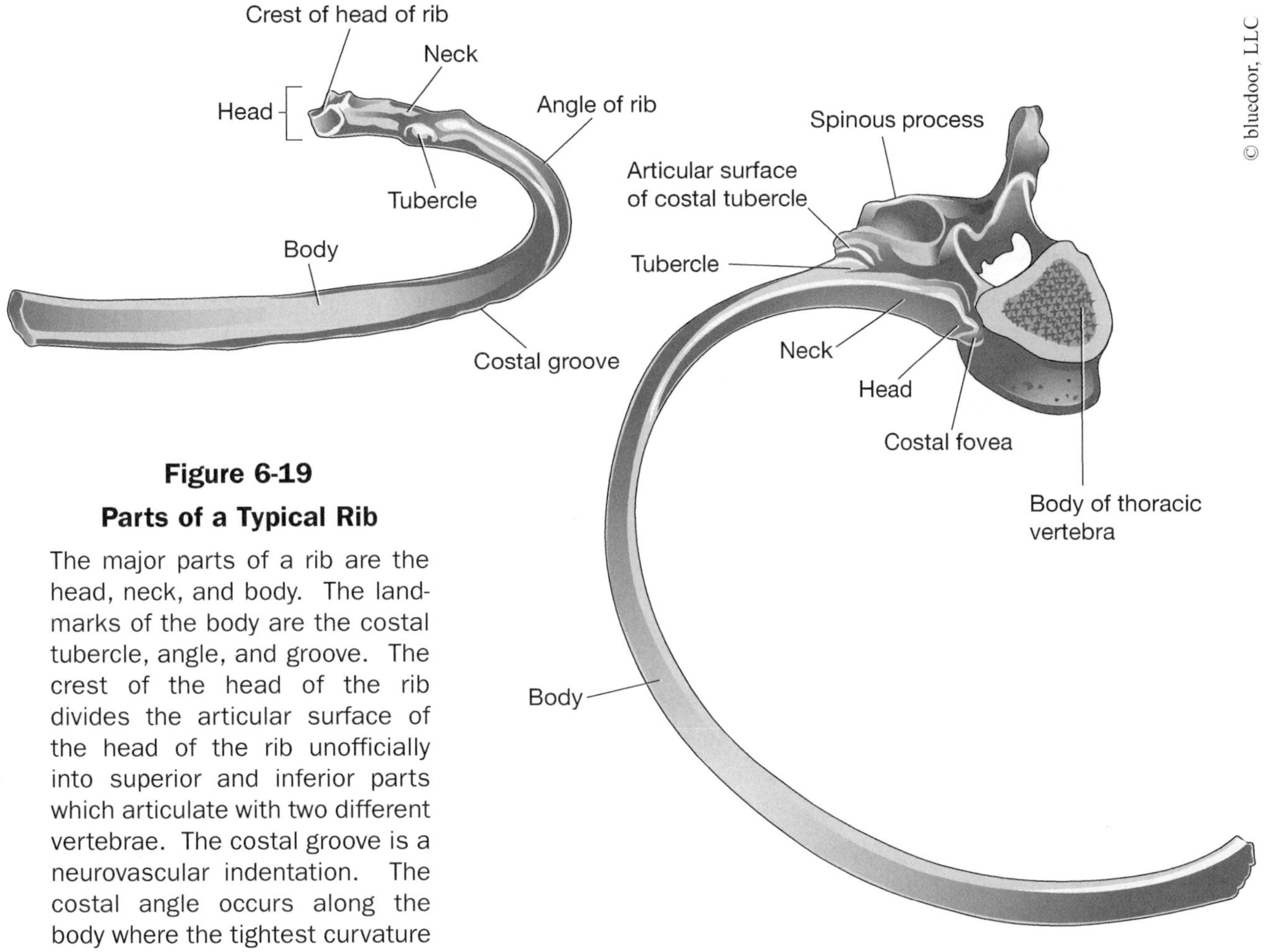

Figure 6-19
Parts of a Typical Rib

The major parts of a rib are the head, neck, and body. The landmarks of the body are the costal tubercle, angle, and groove. The crest of the head of the rib divides the articular surface of the head of the rib unofficially into superior and inferior parts which articulate with two different vertebrae. The costal groove is a neurovascular indentation. The costal angle occurs along the body where the tightest curvature is located.

ribs are located only between the costal heads and vertebral bodies. The portion of the body that makes the tightest bend is called the **costal angle**. It forms the most posterior aspect of most ribs. The linear depression along the internal surface of the inferior border of a rib is called the **costal groove**. It is occupied in life by intercostal vessels and nerves. The ossified bodies of the ribs attach to hyaline cartilages. Since the costal cartilages of the first seven pairs of ribs articulate directly with the sternum, these ribs are called **true ribs** (Figure 6-18). The remaining five pairs of ribs are called **false ribs** because their costal cartilages do not directly contact the sternum. Those of ribs 8, 9, and 10 on each side attach to each other and to that of rib 7 to form the **costal arch**. This forms the palpable inferior aspect of the rib cage. Because the costal cartilages of ribs 11 and 12 end freely within the abdominal wall, these ribs are often termed **floating ribs**. The 11 gaps between adjacent ribs and costal cartilages on each side are called **intercostal spaces**. In life these are occupied by intercostal muscles, blood vessels, and nerves.

Objectives

9. Draw and label the major parts of a typical rib (head, neck, body). Note that the tubercle, angle, and costal groove are landmarks on the body of a rib.

Development of Bones

Bones develop by two different mechanisms: endochondral ossification (also called intracartilaginous ossification) and intramembranous ossification. **Endochondral ossification** involves four distinct steps (Figure 6-20):

1. A hyaline cartilage model of the bone forms from tissues derived from the mesoderm. This model resembles the bone it is to become in shape (but it is smaller).
2. The cartilage mineralizes to become calcified cartilage. The latter is hard like bone tissue, but differs in several respects (the cells are chondrocytes versus osteocytes and the matrix has a different composition).
3. The mineralized cartilage is reabsorbed by chondroclasts.
4. As the cartilage is reabsorbed, cells differentiate into osteoblasts, secrete osteoid, and then bone salts (minerals) precipitate onto the collagenous fibers to complete the formation of definitive bone tissue.

The first area in a developing bone where these four steps are completed is typically near the center of the bone and is called the **primary center of ossification** (Figure 6-20). Days (or sometimes weeks) later, other areas in the same bone will complete the same four steps outlined above. These areas are called **secondary centers of ossification**. A typical long bone has a minimum of three separate centers of ossification: one primary center and at least one secondary center within each epiphysis. The ossification front proceeds slowly but steadily outward from the original sites and with time, very little of the original cartilage model of the bone remains. The thin plates of such cartilage that separate the expanded centers of ossification are called **epiphyseal cartilages** or **physes** ("growth plates"). These plates of hyaline cartilage do not completely disappear until skeletal maturity. In fact, chondroblasts therein actively divide and secrete matrix to form more cartilage. This new cartilage enters step two (of the four step endochondral ossification sequence) and then completes the ossification process to become bone tissue. This allows growing bones to increase in length. In long bones, the portions of the **diaphysis** (body) adjacent to the epiphyseal cartilages are called **metaphyses**. They are the most metabolically active areas in immature bones. When an individual ceases growing, the epiphyseal cartilages ossify, and then remain radiographically visible for a time as **epiphyseal lines**. Eventually the epiphyseal lines disappear as remodeling of the mature bone occurs. Endochondral ossification is the mechanism by which the majority of bones in the body initially develop. It is also (as noted above) the primary method by which most long bones increase in length.

Intramembranous ossification does not require a cartilaginous model or mineralization and resorption thereof. Instead, fibroblasts or undifferentiated stem cells within connective tissue proper membranes (hence the name intramembranous) simply undergo metaplasia and differentiate into osteoblasts. These osteoblasts then form osteoid to complete the process. Intramembranous ossification is involved in the original formation of some flat bones of the body and also is the major mechanism by which most bones grow diametrically. This form of ossification occurs on the deep side of the periosteum to form the external circumferential lamellae. The internal circumferential lamellae are formed by the same process adjacent to the endosteum. The latter lamellae are not formed until the osteoclastic activity responsible for the enlargement of the medullary cavity during growth is basically complete. Some bones, such as the scapula, have some portions that develop initially by endochondral ossification and other parts that are formed by intramembranous ossification.

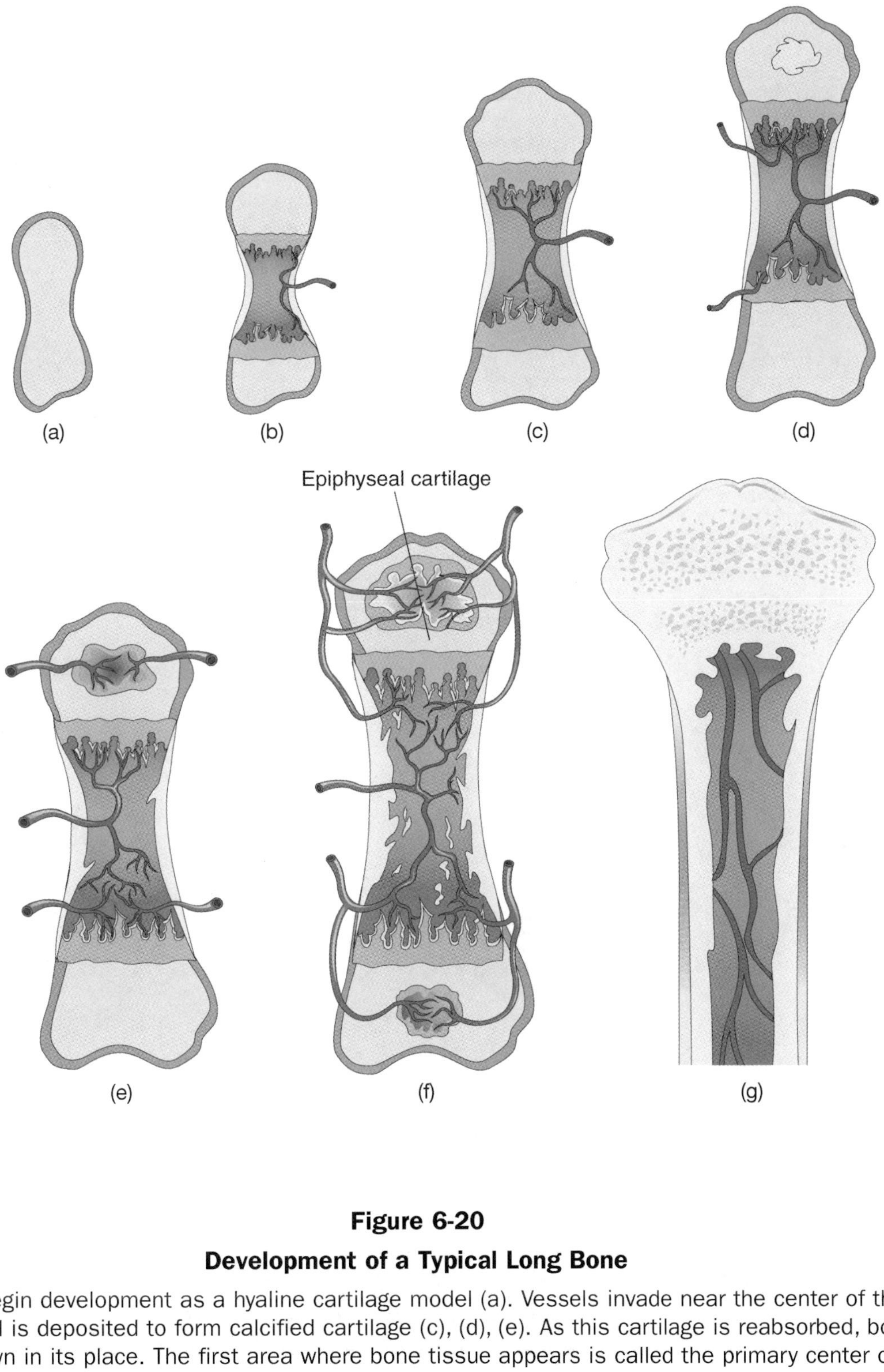

Figure 6-20

Development of a Typical Long Bone

Most bones begin development as a hyaline cartilage model (a). Vessels invade near the center of the bone (b) and mineral is deposited to form calcified cartilage (c), (d), (e). As this cartilage is reabsorbed, bone tissue is laid down in its place. The first area where bone tissue appears is called the primary center of ossification. Other (separate) areas which ossify later are called secondary centers of ossification. At least one secondary center occurs in each epiphysis (e), (f). The thin, unmineralized cartilage that remains as the bone continues to elongate (for several years) is called an epiphyseal cartilage (f). Eventually, at skeletal maturity, even the epiphyseal cartilage is ossified (g).

Objectives

10. Compare endochondral *vs.* intramembranous ossification in regard to what they each contribute to skeletal development and the specific steps involved.
11. Define and differentiate primary *vs.* secondary centers of ossification.
12. Explain how the medullary cavity gets larger in a growing long bone.

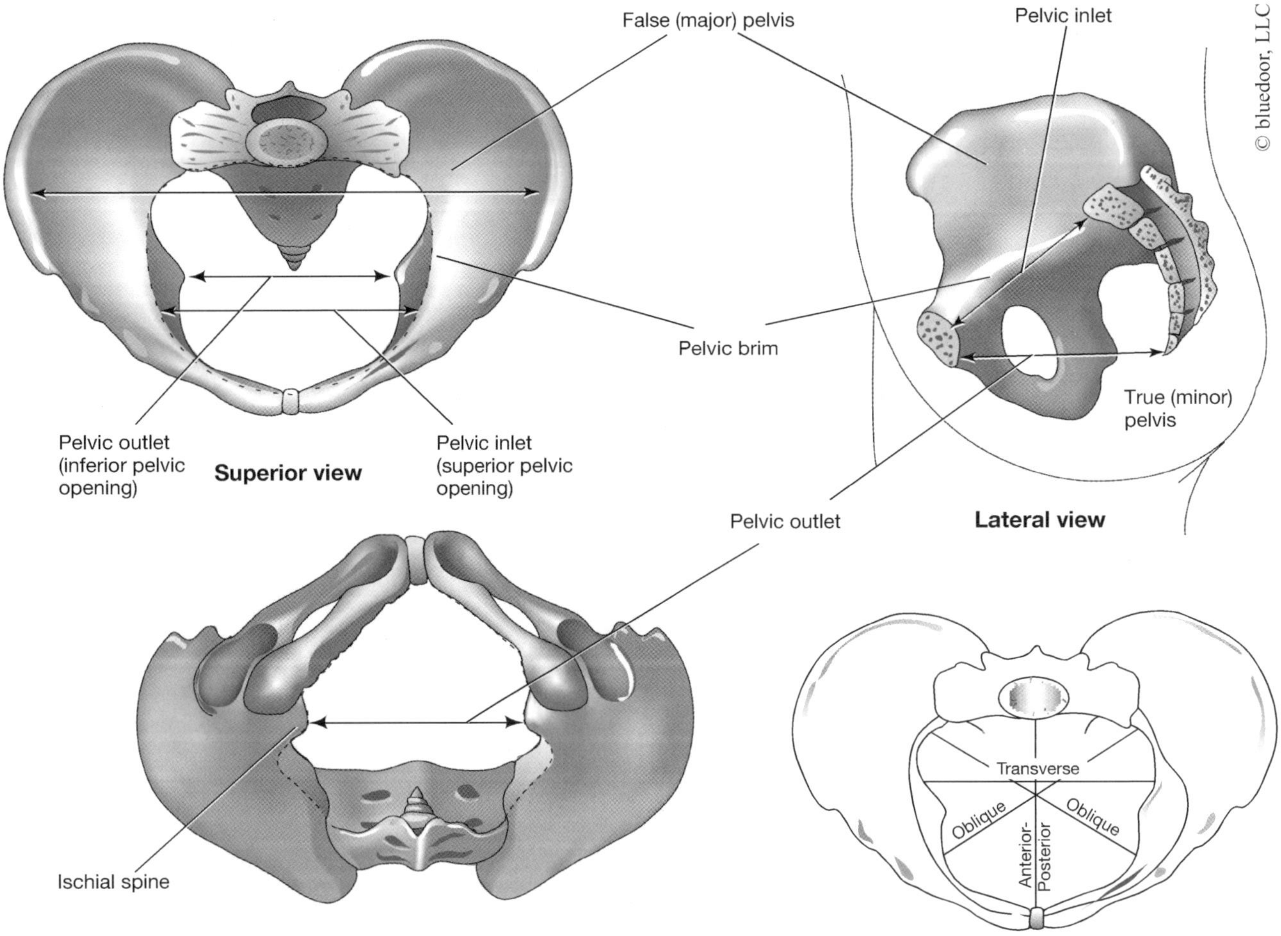

Figure 6-21
Pelvimetry

Clinical Considerations

The bone disorders most familiar to the general populace (often from personal experience) are fractures. **Fractures** involve the cracking or breaking of a bone and are classified clinically into several dozen descriptive types. A **comminuted** fracture is one in which the bone has been broken into a number of pieces. An **avulsion** fracture involves the traumatic tearing away of a bone fragment at the site of attachment of a tendon or ligament. Greenstick fractures often occur in long bones of children where incomplete separation of the fragments occurs as in breaking a green (living) stick. A few of the major terms used to describe fractures are presented in Table 6-3. Although fractures usually involve a traumatic incident, a number of other factors can weaken a bone and predispose it to a fracture which might not otherwise occur. These include disuse atrophy, demineralization related to menopause, senility, or to hypersecretion of parathyroid hormone.

Healing of fractures involves several steps similar to those of ossification and may require several weeks or even several months depending on the location and severity of the break. If the broken portions of the bone are not correctly positioned, physicians will *reduce* the fracture by placing the broken ends in proper alignment. The popular term for this process is "setting" the break and in some cases it requires surgery. Fixation of a fracture refers to the stabilization that is added to prevent movement during the healing process. This may include casts, pins, wires, plates, screws or various combinations thereof. Severely damaged bones may require bone grafts (bone transplants) to heal. **Delayed union** refers to a fracture that takes an exceptionally long time to heal. Some fractures never heal and false joints termed **pseudoarthroses** develop. Fractures in children that involve the growing areas of immature bones sometimes interfere with cell division in the epiphyseal cartilages. This may cause premature mineralization ("closure") of the physes and can cause a given bone to be relatively shorter than its counterparts. Depending on the degree of shortening, this may cause mild to severe disability. Most cases can be corrected or at least improved by surgical intervention. Measurements of the diameters of the pelvis are called **pelvimetry**. Those documented include the transverse diameter, conjugate (anterior-posterior) diameter, and oblique diameters. The conjugate diameter varies according to the plane in which it is measured and is the diameter of most significance in regard to adequate room for passage of a fetus at birth (Figure 6-21). These measurements may be made during pelvic examinations and/or they may be determined radiographically.

Table 6-3 Classification of Fractures

Criterion	*Comments and Descriptive Terms*
Skin penetration	fractured bone does (open, compound) or does not (closed, simple) penetrate the skin
Orientation of fracture line	may be described as *transverse*, *longitudinal*, or *oblique* relative to the long axis of the bone
Part of bone involved	described as *epiphyseal* or *diaphyseal*, (and in young bones perhaps as *metaphyseal* or even *physeal*)
Degree of break	*partial* (a crack), *complete*, *greenstick*
Position of fracture fragments relative to each other	*displaced*, *non-displaced*, *overriding* (the fractured ends have slipped past each other), *distracted* (ends are pulled apart)

Objectives

13. Indicate the meaning of each of the following terms in describing fractures: open, closed, transverse, longitudinal, oblique, epiphyseal, diaphyseal, metaphyseal, physeal, greenstick, displaced, overriding, comminuted.
14. Define delayed union, pseudoarthrosis, pelvimetry.

Clinical Case Studies

Case 1—A distance runner noticed a palpable mass in the lower left side of his back that was not present on the right. There was no pain or related symptoms, but he sought medical attention because of concern that the mass might indicate something serious. Radiography confirmed that he had only eleven ribs on the right side but had 12 on the left. The attending physician determined that the mass he felt was nothing more than the end of the costal cartilage on his left twelfth rib. What caused this situation?

Case 2—A ski acrobat suffered a broken neck when he landed on his head while attempting a new aerial trick. His practice partner, who happened to be a certified EMT, saw the accident and had the foresight not to allow the victim to be moved until trained emergency personnel arrived and stabilized the injured area. What was the EMT's concern?

Case 3—When breast-feeding her newborn son for the first time, a young mother noticed that milk dribbled from his nose and he frequently choked. When the infant was examined by her pediatrician, a tiny cleft in the palate was noticed that had been previously overlooked. How could this cleft be related to the infant's difficulty in feeding?

Points to Ponder

How does one repair a fracture? Put the broken pieces back into reasonably close proximity (known in the business as "reducing" the fracture and on the street as "setting" the break) and then stabilize the skeletal components to keep subsequent motion to a minimum. Osteoblastic activity will knit the broken ends back together providing movement is minimized during the healing process. The logic here is somewhat akin to the process of gluing parts of a model together—one does not move the parts while the glue dries lest it not hold once it has set. Stabilization can be variously accomplished with casts, pins, plates, screws, wire, *etc.* The exact regimen chosen for a given fracture depends on a number of factors including the location and severity of the break, amount of displacement of the fracture fragments, age of the individual, personal preference of the surgeon, *etc., etc.* Some fractures aren't even treated, *per se.* Included here are non-displaced fractures of a single metacarpal or metatarsal bone and some clavicular and phalangeal fractures. These may be bandaged to prevent further trauma and are usually painful enough that the owner gingerly protects them from physical abuse. Physicians who specialize in surgical procedures involving bones and joints are called orthopods (orthopedic surgeons).

One cannot observe orthopedic surgery without being impressed by how rough and physical some aspects of it can be. An orthopod's surgical packs contain saws, drills, hand chucks, hammers, chisels, reams, files, screwdrivers, screws, plates, and pins. Many of the instruments resemble those found in any mechanic's tool box, but they are manufactured to especially close tolerances, and are made of the very finest materials for the intended use. After a gentle approach to a bone or joint, taking care to preserve neurovascular structures, Dr. Jekyll, the soft tissue surgeon, becomes Mr. Hyde, the wood-working cabinet maker. Holes are drilled and tapped, and wedges of bone are removed as fractures are reduced and stabilized, angles are changed, and prosthetic devices are installed. Even biologically compatible glues are used in some instances to hold parts together or join prostheses to normal bone structures.

Like specialists in other branches of medicine and surgery, orthopods first complete medical school and then they train for 3-5 years under board certified orthopedic surgeons typically in a medical residency position. After this 10-15 years of formal training (counting pre-med) they must successfully complete board exams in orthopedic surgery which include both written and practical portions. Considering all of the expensive training which they must undergo, it should not be surprising that the services of board certified specialists are somewhat pricey to obtain!

After graduation from Purdue's veterinary college, I earned some extra money while attending graduate school by serving as a relief veterinarian for some of the local practitioners around Lafayette, Indiana. One day amidst the usual vaccinations, declaws, and teeth cleanings that monopolize most of a veterinarian's time, a small "moppet" mixed breed dog came in with a broken humerus compliments of the front tire of a Buick. Radiography showed it to be a simple fracture of the distal end of the bone that would likely do well if stabilized with an intramedullary pin and given a few weeks of time. Spurning my instincts which told me to refer the case to the nearby small animal clinic at Purdue, I anesthetized the dog and repaired the fracture using the techniques we'd been taught in surgery class. The dog healed nicely and the owner was pleased. Retrospectively, I realized that I'd been fortunate. I did not have the experience to tackle that type of case—it just happened to go well. As one of our instructors in vet school used to remind us—"Just don't do anything to hurt 'em, because most of them will get better on their own!" [Of course, this doesn't apply to most fracture cases.]

Slang and Obsolete Nomenclature

UNOFFICIAL TERM	**OFFICIAL DESIGNATION**
maxillary bone	maxilla *[maxilla]*
optic foramen of sphenoid bone	optic canal *[canalis opticus]* of sphenoid bone
external/internal acoustic canal	external/internal acoustic meatus *[meatus acousticus externus/internus]* of temporal bone
olfactory foramina	cribriform foramina *[foramina cribosa]*
inferior concha	inferior nasal concha *[concha nasalis inferior]*
wormian bone	sutural bone *[os suturalis]*
spinal column	vertebral column *[columna vertebralis]*
sacrum	bony sacrum (sacral bone) *[os sacrum/os sacrale]*
odontoid process of axis	dens of axis *[dens axis]*
demifacets for head of rib	inferior/superior costal fovea *[fovea costalis superior/inferior]* of vertebra
articular facets of vertebra	inferior/superior costal fovea *[fovea costalis superior/inferior]* of vertebra
demifacets of rib	articular surfaces of costal head *[facies articularis capitis costae]*
vertebrosternal ribs	true ribs *[costae verae I-VII]*
vertebrochondral ribs	false ribs *[costae spuriae VIII-XII]*
breastbone	sternum *[sternum]*
rib cage	thoracic cage *[compages thoracis]*
soft spots (of infant skull)	fontanels (fontanelles) *[fonticuli]*

Review Questions

1. Find the false statement.
   A. Most bones develop initially by endochondral ossification.
   B. Bones increase in diameter by intramembranous ossification.
   C. The medullary cavity enlarges due to osteoblastic activity.
   D. Endochondral ossification is responsible for the formation of the metaphysis.
   E. Most long bones have three or more centers of ossification.

2. Which of the following is the correct sequence of events during endochondral ossification?
   a. reabsorb mineralized cartilage
   b. cells differentiate into osteoblasts
   c. formation of a hyaline cartilaginous model
   d. formation of calcified cartilage
   e. bone salts precipitate onto fibers
   A. a—b—c—d—e
   B. e—c—d—a—b
   C. c—d—a—e—b
   D. d—c—a—b—e
   E. c—d—a—b—e

3. Which item is false?
   A. The youngest concentric lamellae within an osteon are located furthest from the central canal.
   B. The youngest internal circumferential lamellae are formed by intramembranous ossification adjacent to the endosteum.
   C. Radiologically, physes can be observed as black (dark) lines between the metaphyses and epiphyses of growing long bones.
   D. Pseudoarthroses may result from fractures that do not heal.
   E. A bone has only one primary center of ossification, but can have numerous secondary centers of ossifications.

4. Find the mismatch.
   A. cranial bones—eight pairs
   B. auditory ossicles—three pairs
   C. ribs—12 pairs
   D. articular processes of a vertebra—two pairs
   E. Choose this response if all the above (A-D) are correctly matched.

5. Which of the following statements is false?
   A. There are seven pairs of true ribs, five pairs of false ribs, and two pairs of floating ribs.
   B. There are seven cervical vertebrae, twelve thoracic vertebrae, five lumbar vertebrae, five sacral vertebrae, and usually four coccygeal vertebrae.
   C. There are 24 ribs in males.
   D. The osseous sacrum is a single bone resulting from the fusion of several sacral vertebrae.
   E. Choose this response if all the above (A-D) are true statements.

6. Which statement is incorrect?
   A. The bony sacrum is composed of five fused vertebrae.
   B. The sternum is composed of three fused parts.
   C. The calvaria is composed of four bones.
   D. There are 29 bones in the head (including the auditory ossicles).
   E. There are more intercostal spaces than there are vertebrae.

7. Which of the following is an incorrect anatomical term?
   A. hyoid bone
   B. palatine bone
   C. incus
   D. vomer bone
   E. mandible

8. Find the vertebral lie.
   A. transverse processes/typical vertebra—2
   B. spinous processes/typical vertebra—1
   C. vertebral foramina/typical vertebra—1
   D. pedicles (of the vertebral arch)/typical vertebra—2
   E. intervertebral discs (superior to bony sacrum)—24

9. Find the incorrect statement.
   A. The viscerocranium consists of 14 bones.
   B. There are only seven osseous components of the orbit.
   C. All ribs have a head, neck, body, angle, groove, and tubercle.
   D. The sternum is composed of a manubrium, body and xiphoid process.
   E. Choose this response if all the above (A-D) are true.

10. Which item is false?
   A. The cranium surrounds the brain.
   B. The osseous components of the antebrachium lie parallel to each other.
   C. The ribs have bony attachments to vertebrae and to the sternum.
   D. The orbit protects the eye.
   E. There is only one weight bearing bone between the acetabulum of the os coxae and the weight bearing bone of the crus.

Thought Questions

1. Name the structures found in growing long bones that are not present at skeletal maturity.

2. Explain why a growing bone has numerous external circumferential lamellae but often no identifiable internal circumferential lamellae.

3. Assume two tiny stainless steel marker screws were inserted into the body of the humerus of an eight year old child: one near the longitudinal center of the bone and the second one 2 cm further distally. How far apart would the two screws be when the individual turned twenty years of age?

4. What is the difference between bone tissue and mineralized cartilage?

5. Which is more important in fracture healing: good reduction (putting the broken ends back into proper alignment) or good stabilization (prevention of movement during the healing process)?

6. A fracture of the femur bone was described as closed, oblique, and over-riding. What does each term indicate?

7. "Bones of the head" and "bones of the skull" are not quite synonymous. Explain the difference.

8. When evaluating fractures by radiography, at least two exposures are usually made at right angles to each other. Why?

9. The radius has two physes between the elbow joint and radiocarpal joint, but the ulna has only one. Since the two bones acquire the same overall length increase as they grow, what can be said about the relative rate of elongation at the three involved physes?

10. Which bones of the skull can be palpated?

11. What is the difference between an epiphyseal cartilage and a cartilaginous epiphysis?

12. Differentiate the following passageways associated with the vertebral column: vertebral foramen, vertebral canal, intervertebral foramen, and transverse foramen.

13. Which bones form the thoracic ("rib") cage?

14. How many bones of the total (214) in a human body have a landmark termed the head of that bone?

15. Name several definitive bones that form by the fusion (synostosis) of other named bones.

16. What determines the shape of a bone?

17. Why are the vertebra in the lumbar region of the vertebral column much larger and more massive than those in the cervical region?

18. In the skull of a young, growing individual, which named bone borders all of the fontanels?

19. Explain how the total number of ribs (24) includes 14 true ribs, 10 false ribs, and four floating ribs.

20. Although most bones of the head are paired (left and right), some are not. Name the unpaired bones of the head.

21. How many bones are intercepted by a median (midsagittal) plane? (Don't count any bones of the skull).

Answers to Clinical Case Studies

Case 1—Different numbers of ribs on the right and left sides of the body occasionally occur with no clinical consequence. The cause remains unknown.

Case 2—When vertebrae are fractured, the resulting instability puts the spinal cord at considerable risk. Injury to the spinal cord at any level is serious but greater disability occurs with injuries at higher levels. In fact, if the spinal cord is disrupted above the origins of the phrenic nerves which supply the diaphragm, death can result from asphyxiation.

Case 3—The palate separates the nasal cavity (above) from the oral cavity (below). Its osseous portion is formed from left and right primordia that must grow toward each other, meet on the midline, and fuse. Failure of its complete development results in the defect called cleft palate. When this deformity is present, it interferes with suckling by making it difficult/impossible for the infant to form the vacuum necessary to suck on the nipple and it interferes with normal swallowing because the tongue forces milk up into the nasal cavity through the cleft.

Answers to Review Questions

1. C. Should be *osteoclastic* activity.

2. E.

3. A. The ones furthest from the central canal were formed first.

4. A. There are only two pair of cranial bones and numerous single bones (but there are eight paired bones of the skull).

5. E.

6. E. There are 22 intercostal spaces (11 on each side) and 26 vertebrae in an adult (the sacral bone and coccyx are considered to be single bones in an adult.

7. D. *Vomer* stands alone!

8. E. There are 23 i.v. discs superior to the bony sacrum (there is no i.v. disc immediately above or below the atlas).

9. C. Not all ribs have tubercles (ribs 11 and 12 and sometimes 10).

10. C. There is no bony connection between ribs and the sternum.

Answers to Thought Questions

1. Physes (epiphyseal cartilages) and metaphyses.

2. Bones grow in diameter by the deposition of external circumferential lamellae via intramembranous ossification on the deep aspect of the periosteum. During growth, the endosteal surface is under continual osteoclastic degradation as the medullary cavity is enlarged. Consequently, internal circumferential lamellae are not formed in growing bones.

3. The screws would remain the same distance apart. Length increases in long bones occur at the physes (epiphyseal cartilages) which are located near the ends of the bones.

4. They contain different cells, different ground substance, and different fibers. Even the mineral content is different. The only things they have in common are lacunae and the fact that mineral is present.

5. Both are important, but stabilization is much more important. If the bone fragments are well stabilized, healing will occur even if the reduction is suboptimal.

6. *Closed* means the skin was not broken by the fracture. *Oblique* indicates the plane of the fracture line was angled relative to the long axis of the bone. *Over-riding* means the broken ends had slipped past each other (due to muscle contraction or to the force of the traumatic incident).

7. The skull does not include the auditory ossicles nor the hyoid bone.

8. A radiograph is a two-dimensional representation of three dimensions. Unless two views are obtained at right angles, the spatial relationships of structures cannot be evaluated.

9. The ulnar elongation at the single physis must equal the total elongation at both radial physes. If this does not occur, deviation (curvature) of the antebrachium occurs.

10. All of them. The ethmoid bone and inferior nasal concha are hard to reach.

11. An epiphyseal cartilage is a "growth plate" ("epiphyseal plate"). The term cartilaginous epiphysis was coined to describe the epiphysis of a (very) young growing bone which is entirely cartilaginous.

12. The vertebral foramen is the vertically oriented passageway through the arch of any one vertebra which transmits the spinal cord. Collectively, the vertebral foramina form the vertebral canal around the spinal cord. Notches on the sides of the vertebral arches form the intervertebral foramina in the articulated vertebral column. Spinal nerves emerge through these passageways. The transverse foramina, located only in the transverse processes of the cervical vertebrae, transmit the vertebral artery, vein, and nerve.

13. Ribs, thoracic vertebrae, sternum.

14. All proximal and middle phalanges (36), all ribs (24), humeri (2), radii (2), ulnae (2) all metacarpal and metatarsal bones (20), femur bones (2), fibulae (2), tali (2), mandible (1), and malleus (2). Total 95. Note that the mandible (one bone) actually has two heads.

15. Os coxae, bony sacrum, sternum, coccyx.

16. The forces which act on a bone in some way influence osteoblastic and osteoclastic activity. It has been shown that the crystalline structure of hydroxyapatite (bone mineral) demonstrates a piezoelectric effect (differential charging) when subjected to physical forces. These charges may influence the activity of the bone cells.

17. Lumbar vertebrae carry much more weight than cervical vertebrae (which only have to support the head). Consequently, they are subjected to more compressive forces, *etc.*

18. Parietal bone(s).

19. The 14 true ribs attach directly to the sternum and the other 10 are called false ribs. The four floating ribs (the last two pairs) are four of the 10 false ribs. In other words, floating ribs are also false ribs.

20. Frontal bone, mandible, sphenoid bone, occipital bone, vomer, ethmoid bone, hyoid bone.

21. Twenty-eight. All of the vertebrae (seven cervical, twelve thoracic, five lumbar, one bony sacrum, and one coccyx) plus the hyoid bone (not included in the skull) and the sternum.

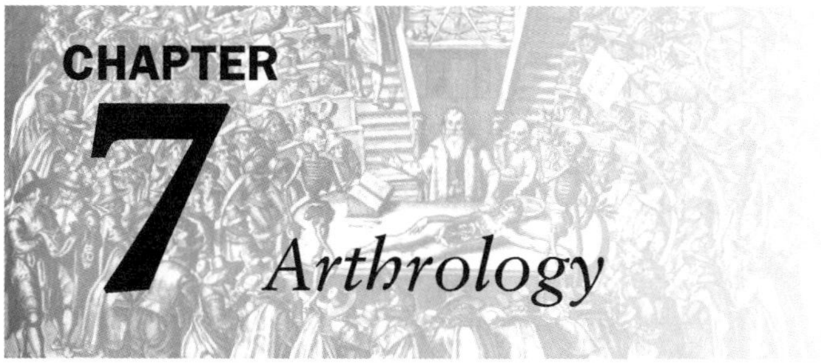

CHAPTER 7 Arthrology

Chapter Outline and Key Concepts

INTRODUCTION

Joints are the structures formed when two or more bones or cartilages are united to each other or to teeth by some type of connective tissue.

Simple joints involve two skeletal structures and composite joints involve three or more.

TAXONOMY OF JOINTS

There are three major categories of joints: fibrous joints (synarthroses), cartilaginous joints, and synovial joints (diarthroses).

Fibrous joints include sutures, syndesmoses, and gomphoses (dentoalveolar joints).

Cartilaginous joints include symphyses (fibrocartilaginous joints) and synchondroses (hyaline cartilage joints).

Synovial joints are divided into seven categories based on the type of movement that the shapes of their articular surfaces allow.

Joints vary significantly in the amount of motion that they allow.

PARTS OF A SYNOVIAL JOINT

Synovial joints have a joint cavity filled with synovial fluid.

The joint cavity is created by a joint capsule which has (outer) fibrous and (inner) synovial membrane layers.

Specialized cells in the synovial membrane secrete synovial fluid which has lubricating and nourishing roles.

The articular surfaces of synovial joints are covered with hyaline cartilage called articular cartilage.

Ligaments are connective tissue proper bands (cords) that stabilize the skeletal components of joints.

The ligaments associated with synovial joints are classified as intracapsular, extracapsular, or capsular based on their location relative to the joint capsule.

Menisci and articular discs are fibrocartilaginous structures found between the articulating bones in some synovial joints.

JOINTS OF THE AXIAL SKELETON

Joints of the head include a number of sutures, a few synchondroses, the dentoalveolar joints (gomphoses), temporomandibular joints, atlanto-occipital joint, and joints of the auditory ossicles.

Joints of the vertebral column include the atlanto-axial joint, the intervertebral symphyses, and the zygapophyseal joints (between articular processes of vertebrae).

Joints of the thoracic cage include the joints joining the heads and tubercles of the ribs to the vertebrae, the junctions of the ribs and costal cartilages, joints between costal cartilages and between these cartilages and the sternum, and the two joints between the three parts of the sternum.

JOINTS OF THE SUPERIOR LIMB

All joints involving the skeleton of the superior limb are synovial except for the radio-ulnar syndesmosis.

The joints of the pectoral girdle are those at both ends of the clavicles.

The major joints in the free parts of the superior limbs include the shoulder, elbow, carpal, and "digital" joints.

The shoulder joint is the simple joint between the humeral head and the glenoid cavity of the scapula.

The elbow joint is the composite articulation with three named subparts: humeroradial, humero-ulnar, and proximal radio-ulnar joints.

The carpal joint includes the radiocarpal, intercarpal, and carpometacarpal articulations.

The "digital" joints of the hand include the metacarpophalangeal and interphalangeal joints.

JOINTS OF THE INFERIOR LIMB

All joints of the inferior limb are synovial except for the pubic symphysis and the tibiofibular syndesmosis.
The hip joint is a classic ball and socket (spheroidal) joint with a well-developed intracapsular ligament.
The knee joint contains two menisci and two strong intracapsular ligaments.
The tarsal (ankle) joint, like its counterpart in the superior limb, includes numerous articulations.
The "digital" joints of the foot resemble those of the hand.

BASIC JOINT MOTIONS

Flexion and *extension* involve angular changes within sagittal planes.
Flexion is a decrease in the size of a joint's designated flexor angle.
Adduction (to, toward) and *abduction* (away from) involve motions within coronal (frontal) planes.
Rotation (pronation, supination, inversion, eversion) involves movement of a body part around its long axis.

LEVER SYSTEMS IN LOCOMOTION

Bones, muscles, and joints form lever systems that effect locomotion and posture.
A lever system requires a rigid bar (lever arm), a force, a point of rotation (fulcrum) and a resistance.
Lever systems are divided into three classes (first, second, third) depending on the relative positions of the force, fulcrum, and resistance on the lever arm.
Most lever systems in the body are third class.
All simple levers at equilibrium can be quantified by the moment arm equation ($F \times D_F = R \times D_R$) where F and R are the force and resistance and D_F and D_R are the distances of the force and resistance from the fulcrum.

CLINICAL CONSIDERATIONS

Arthritis (inflammation of a joint) has numerous causes.
Dislocations of joints are termed luxations (if complete) or subluxations (if partial).
Bony union of a joint is termed a synostosis and may be normal or pathological.
Surgical invasion of a joint is termed arthrotomy (or arthroscopy, if fiberoptic procedures occur).
Intervertebral disc disease occurs when bulging or ruptured intervertebral discs put pressure on nerves or the spinal cord.
Abnormal curvatures of the vertebral column are termed kyphosis, lordosis, or scoliosis depending on their orientation.

Selected Definitions

Adduction—movement of a body part within a frontal plane. Limbs, digits, and hands can be adducted/abducted, and reference is made to the joint at which motion occurred.

Articular disc—a fibrocartilaginous structure that occurs within a few synovial joints. The two "articular discs" in each knee joint are called *articular menisci.*

Cartilaginous joint—a joint in which cartilage unites the skeletal structures. In some cartilaginous joints (synchondroses), hyaline cartilage serves as the uniting material and in others the uniting material is fibrocartilage (symphyses).

Composite joints—a joint with three or more skeletal components. Composite joints include the carpal, tarsal, and cubital joints.

Flexion—movement of joint components such that the flexor angle decreases in size (or the extensor angle increases in size). The flexor/extensor surfaces of all joints are defined.

Gomphosis (dentoalveolar joint)—a fibrous joint between the root(s) of a tooth and the dental alveolus in which it is embedded. The fibrous connective tissue connecting the bone and tooth is called periodontium or periodontal ligament ("periodontal membrane").

Intervertebral discs—the fibrocartilaginous structures located at the intervertebral symphyses. The gelatinous center of an i.v. disc (nucleus pulposus) is sometimes forced through the outer part (anulus fibrosus) resulting in pressure on the spinal cord or roots of a spinal nerve.

Joint (articular) capsule—the connective tissue capsule that surrounds a synovial joint cavity. It has a fibrous connective tissue outer layer and a synovial membrane lining.

Joint (articular) cavity—the space inside an articular capsule of a synovial joint. In some composite joints, this space is common to several or all compartments of that joint.

Joint (articulation)—the structure formed by the junction of two or more bones, cartilages, or teeth. Joints are classified as simple or composite (based on the number of participating components) and as fibrous, cartilaginous, or synovial (based on the type of uniting tissue and the presence of a fluid-filled cavity).

Ligament—a band (cord) of c.t. proper that stabilizes the skeletal structures in synovial joints. A ligament can be extracapsular, capsular, or intracapsular and a given joint can have more than one type.

Luxation (dislocation)—a malalignment of the skeletal components at a joint. Usually traumatic in origin, luxations typically involve significant ligamentous and joint capsule damage.

Simple joint—a joint with only two skeletal components (bone to bone, bone to cartilage, cartilage to cartilage, bone to tooth). Simple joints include the shoulder joint, hip joint, and all interphalangeal joints.

Suture—a fibrous joint between flat bones of the skull. Thirty-three sutures are named and most of them are zygomorphic.

Symphysis—a fibrocartilage joint. In the intervertebral symphyses, the bones are united by fibrocartilaginous structures called intervertebral discs, and the pubic symphysis is stabilized by the interpubic disc.

Synarthrosis—a joint stabilized by fibrous connective tissue and lacking a cavity (*i.e.,* a fibrous joint). The three subtypes of synarthroses are sutures, syndesmoses, and gomphoses.

Synchondrosis—a hyaline cartilage joint. Synchondroses include the costochondral joints, some of the joints in the base of the neurocranium and the joints formed by the epiphyseal cartilages in growing bones.

Syndesmosis—a fibrous joint between the radius and ulna, tibia and fibula, or stapes and temporal bone. The connective tissue joining the bones in the radio-ulnar syndesmosis is called the antebrachial interosseous membrane, and that in the tibiofibular syndesmosis is called the crural interosseous membrane.

Synostosis—a bony union. Synostoses occur with normal maturation in many loci, can be iatrogenically induced, and in some cases are pathological.

Synovial fluid—the lubricating and nourishing fluid secreted by the synoviocytes located in synovial membranes. Injury to a joint often induces hypersecretion of synovial fluid ("water on the knee.")

Synovial joint—any joint which has, as one of its features, a joint (articular) cavity containing synovial fluid. Synovial joints include most of those found in the limbs and many of the joints in the axial skeleton.

Etymology *Satis verborum*—**"Let's have some action."**

chondr (G), *cartilage*—chondrocyte
ginglymos (G), *hinge*—ginglymus
gomphosis (G), *a bolting together*—gomphosis
kyphosis (G), *humpback, bent*—kyphosis
lordosis (G), *bent backward*—lordosis
luxatus (L), *dislocated*—luxation
meniskos (G), *small moon*—meniscus
sella (L), *saddle*—sellar joint
skoliosis (G), *crookedness*—scoliosis
sub (L), *below, partial*—subluxation
sutura (L), *seam*—suture
symphysis (L), *state of growing together*—symphysis
syn (G), *together with*—synchondrosis
syndesmos (G), *to bind together*—syndesmosis
zygon (G), *a yoke*—zygapophyseal joint

Introduction

Arthrology is the study of joints. The **joints (articulations)** of the body allow various degrees of movement. They are formed when two or more bones or cartilages are united to each other or to teeth by connective tissue proper or cartilage. A joint with only two skeletal components is termed a **simple joint** and one with three or more skeletal components is a **composite joint.** Joints are further classified into three major categories depending on the type and configuration of the intervening connective tissue: fibrous, cartilaginous, and synovial joints (Table 7-1).

Objectives

1. Define joint and classify joints into two categories based on the number of articulating skeletal components and three categories based on the type of uniting connective tissue and presence of a joint cavity.

Taxonomy of Joints

In **fibrous joints**, also known as **synarthroses** (singular = synarthrosis), the skeletal components are united by fibrous connective tissue (connective tissue proper). These joints have little or no movement and are divided into three subtypes: syndesmoses, sutures, and gomphoses (Figure 7-1). **Syndesmoses** (singular = *syndesmosis)* are fibrous joints with a relatively large amount of fibrous connective tissue between the skeletal components. There are few of these in the body and they include the side-to-side joints between the radius and ulna in each superior limb and those between the tibia and fibula in each inferior limb. **Sutures** are the fibrous joints between flat bones of the skull. These bones fit together so tightly that only a small amount of connective tissue proper is present. The *Nomina Anatomica* lists 33 sutures (Table 7-2) and the positions of most of them can be derived from their names. Sutures are subdivided into four categories based on the manner in which the edges of the bones meet: serrated suture, squamous suture, planar suture, and schindylesis. In **serrated sutures,** the bones are united by interlocking processes resembling the teeth of a saw (*serra* = saw) or in some cases the tabs of the pieces in a jigsaw puzzle (as in the sagittal suture). In **squamous sutures**, the bones meet in beveled overlapping edges (as in the articulation between the parietal bone and the squamous portion of the temporal bone on each side of the skull). In **planar sutures** there is simple apposition of the articulating bones with no overlapping and no interlocking (as in the lacrimomaxillary suture). A **schindylesis** is a variant type of suture in which a thin

Table 7-1 Classification of Joints

Category	*Uniting Connective Tissue*	*Movement*
Fibrous Joints (Synarthroses):		
Syndesmosis	Connective tissue proper	
Suture	Connective tissue proper	Essentially none
Gomphosis	Connective tissue proper	
Cartilaginous Joints:		
Synchondrosis	Hyaline cartilage	Little or none
Symphysis	Fibrocartilage	
Synovial Joints (Diarthroses):		
(Seven subtypes based on the shape of the articular surfaces)	Connective tissue proper (have an articular cavity)	"Freely" movable

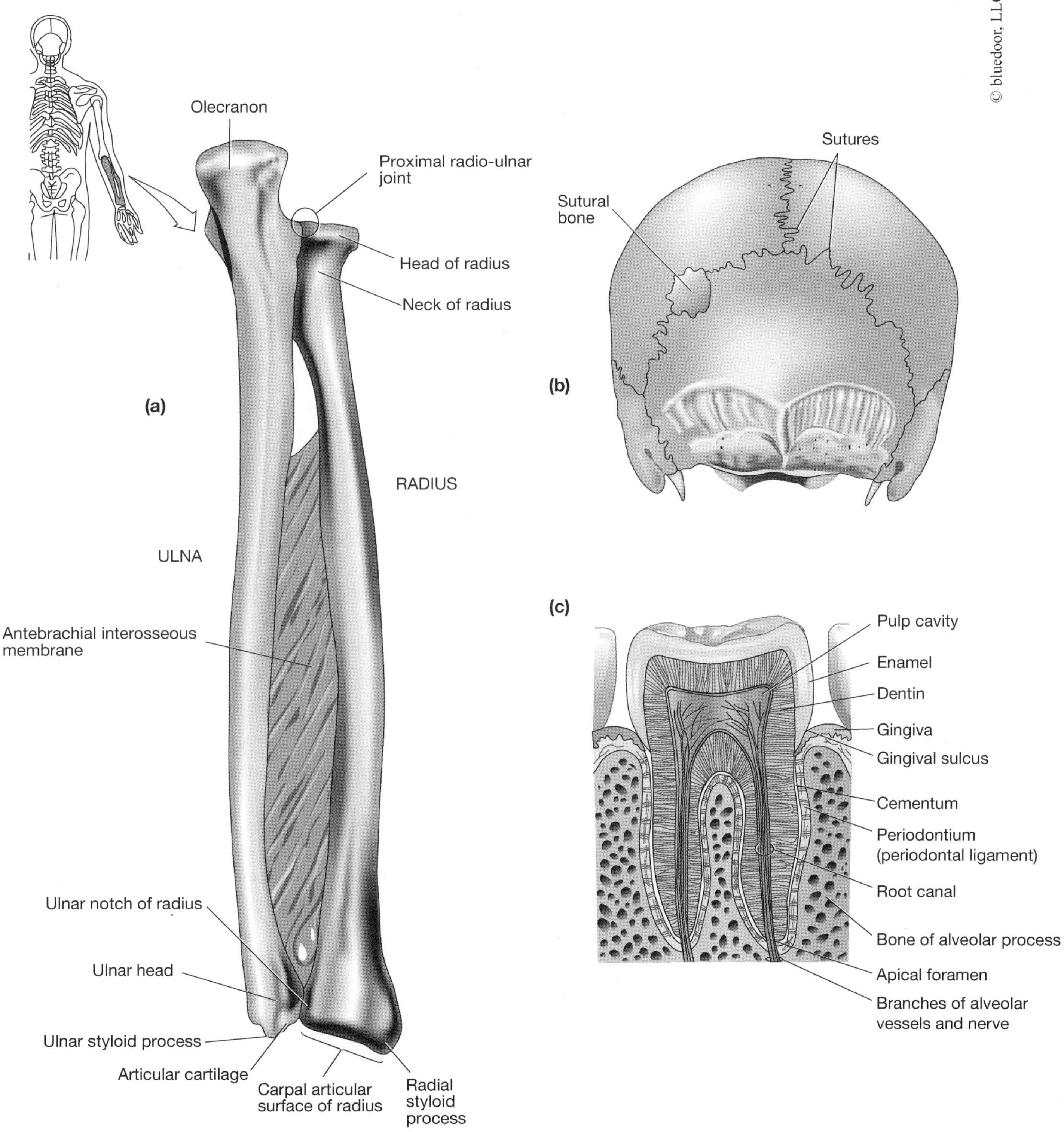

Figure 7-1

Examples of the Three Subtypes of Fibrous Joints

(a) Syndesmosis (radio-ulnar syndesmosis) (b) Suture (between flat bones of the skull) (c) Gomphosis (dentoalveolar joint)

Table 7-2 Sutures of the Head (Name-Location)

Coronal s.—frontal bone (anteriorly)/ parietal bones (posteriorly)
Sagittal s.—between the left and right parietal bones
Lambdoid s.—parietal bones (anteriorly)/occipital bone (posteriorly)
Occipitomastoid s.—occipital bone (medially)/mastoid processes of temporal bones (laterally)
Sphenofrontal s.—greater wings of sphenoid bone (inferolaterally)/frontal bone (superiorly)
Spheno-ethmoidal s.—body of sphenoid bone/orbital lamina of ethmoid bone
Sphenosquamous s.—greater wing of sphenoid bone (anteriorly)/squamous portion of temporal bone
Sphenoparietal s.—greater wings of sphenoid bone (anterolaterally)/parietal bones (posterosuperiorly)
Squamous s.—squamous portion of temporal bones (laterally)/parietal bone (superiorly)
Frontal s.*—between frontal bones (usually it fuses during childhood)
Parietomastoid s.—parietal bone (superoposteriorly)/mastoid process of temporal bones (inferoposterior)
Squamomastoid s.—squamous portion/mastoid process of temporal bone (usually ossifies early in life)
Frontonasal s.—frontal bone (superiorly)/nasal bone (inferiorly)
Fronto-ethmoidal s.—frontal bone (in anterior cranial fossa)/cribriform plate of ethmoid bone
Frontomaxillary s.—frontal bone/frontal processes of maxilla
Frontolacrimal s.—orbital part of frontal bone (superiorly)/lacrimal bone
Frontozygomatic s.—zygomatic process of frontal bone/zygomatic bone
Zygomaticomaxillary s.—zygomatic bone/zygomatic process of maxilla
Ethmoidomaxillary s.—orbital part of ethmoid bone/orbital surface of maxilla
Ethmoidolacrimal s.—orbital part of ethmoid bone (posteriorly)/lacrimal bone (superiorly)
Sphenovomerine s.—medial pterygoid process of sphenoid bone/wing of vomer
Sphenozygomatic s.—greater wing of sphenoid bone (posteriorly)/zygomatic bone (anterolaterally)
Sphenomaxillary s.—pterygoid process of sphenoid bone (posteroinferiorly)/maxilla
Temporozygomatic s.—zygomatic process of temporal bone/temporal process of zygomatic bone
Internasal s.—between the nasal bones (medially)
Nasomaxillary s.—nasal bone (medially)/maxilla (laterally)
Lacrimomaxillary s.—lacrimal bone (superiorly)/orbital part of the maxilla
Lacrimoconchal s.—lacrimal bone (superiorly)/inferior nasal concha (inferiorly)
Intermaxillary s.—between the maxillae just below the anterior nasal spine
Palatomaxillary s.—orbital part of palatine bone/orbital part of the maxilla
Palato-ethmoidal s.—orbital part of palatine bone/orbital part of ethmoid bone
Median palatine s.—between the horizontal part of the palatine bones and between the maxillae (medially)
Transverse palatine s.—horizontal part of palatine bone (posteriorly)/palatine process of maxilla (anteriorly)

*If the frontal suture persists beyond its normal fusion time, about six years of age, it is called a *metopic suture.*

plate of one bone articulates in a cleft of another one, as in the articulation of the vomer with the ethmoid bone. Occasionally, small islands of bone tissue occur within the course of sutures. These are called **sutural bones** (or "wormian" bones). **Gomphoses** (singular = gomphosis) are the fibrous joints between teeth and the bony sockets in which they are embedded (dental alveoli). They are also known as **dentoalveolar joints** and have been called "peg joints" because of their configuration. The thin layer of connective tissue proper which "glues" the root(s) of a tooth into the alveolus is termed **periodontium (periodontal membrane)**.

The skeletal components of **cartilaginous joints** are united by cartilage. They allow little or no movement and two subtypes are recognized based on the type of cartilage present: hyaline cartilage joints and fibrocartilage joints (Figure 7-2). **Hyaline cartilage joints**, also known as **synchondroses**, are so named because the uniting connective tissue is hyaline cartilage. Examples include costo-

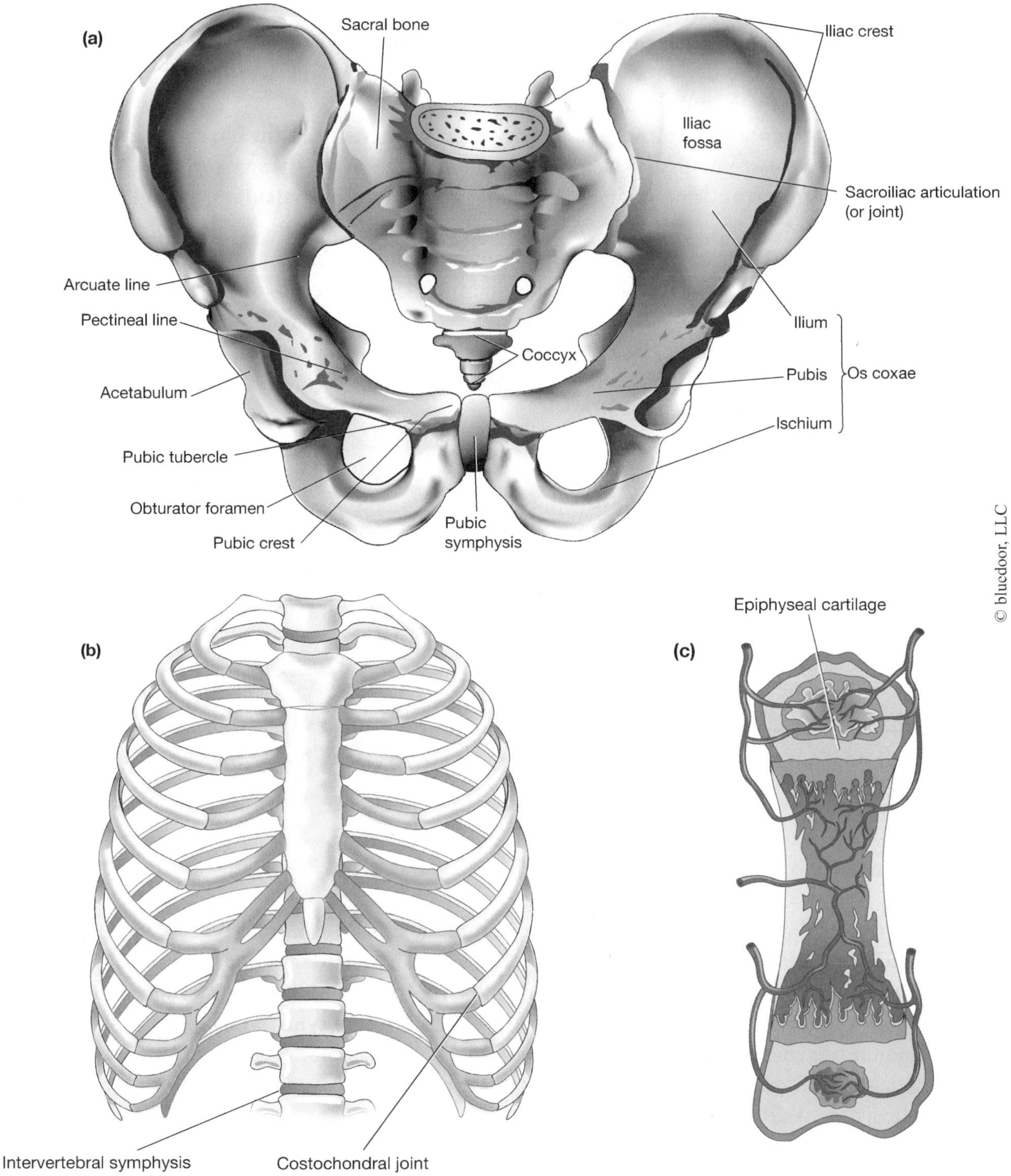

Figure 7-2

Examples of the Two Subtypes of Cartilaginous Joints

The pubic symphysis (a) where the interpubic disc is located and intervertebral symphyses (b) where intervertebral discs are located are fibrocartilaginous joints. Hyaline cartilage joints (synchondroses) include costochondral joints (b) and the articulations stabilized by epiphyseal cartilages in growing long bones (c). The joints between the three components of the sternum (manubriosternal symphysis and xiphisternal synchondrosis) are also cartilaginous joints. Synchondroses are also found between some bones at the base of the skull.

chondral joints, epiphyseal cartilages (physes) in growing bones, and several joints uniting bones of the skull. In **fibrocartilage joints**, also known as **symphyses** (singular = symphysis), the skeletal structures are united by fibrocartilage. Examples include the intervertebral symphyses, the pubic symphysis, and the manubriosternal symphysis.

Synovial joints are also known as **diarthroses**. In these joints, the bones or cartilages are united by fibrous connective tissue (as in fibrous joints) but they *also* have an articular ("synovial") cavity between the articulating surfaces. The latter are covered by **articular cartilage** which is a specialized type of hyaline cartilage. Synovial joints are usually freely moveable in one or more planes, and are usually stabilized by ligaments. They include most of the familiar joints within the limbs as well as the joints associated with the heads and tubercles of the ribs, the articular processes of the vertebrae, and the atlanto-occipital, atlanto-axial, and temporomandibular joints. There are seven subtypes of synovial joints based on the shapes of the articulating surfaces and (subsequently) on the type of movement which they allow (Table 7-3, Figure 7-3). Some are embellished by the presence of articular discs or articular menisci.

A **synostosis** is a bony union (fusion) created when skeletal components are united by osseous tissue (*i.e., bone*). Any joint (regardless of original classification) becomes a synostosis if bone replaces the fibrous connective tissue or cartilage originally present. This occurs naturally at epiphyseal plates and some sutures. It may also occur pathologically and is sometimes intentionally induced surgically (ankylosis of a joint).

Objectives

2. Divide the three major categories of joints into their various subtypes and indicate what distinguishes each subtype (syndesmosis, suture, gomphosis, synchondrosis, symphysis, *etc.*).

Parts of a Synovial Joint

The feature that distinguishes synovial joints from the other major joint types is the presence of an **articular (joint) cavity** surrounded and enclosed by an **articular (joint) capsule**. The joint capsule has a fibrous layer externally, composed of dense, irregular, collagenous connective tissue proper and a synovial membrane lining (Figure 7-4). Cells of the **synovial membrane** secrete a small amount of **synovial fluid (joint fluid, synovium)** into the joint cavity. This fluid lubricates and nourishes the relatively thin, avascular **articular cartilage** (1-2 mm thick) on the surfaces of the articulating skeletal components.

Synovial joints are reinforced by **ligaments** which are fibrous connective tissue bands and cords extending from one skeletal component to another. Ligaments that consist of regional thickening in the fibrous layer of the joint capsule are called **capsular ligaments** (Table 7-4). Those that are well developed, physically distinct bands of connective tissue located outside of the fibrous layer of the articular capsule are called **extracapsular ligaments**. Extracapsular ligaments that are located on each side of the major plane of motion in a joint are often termed **collateral ligaments** and are present in most joints of the limbs. Some joints have ligaments internal to the fibrous part of the joint capsule. These are called **intracapsular ligaments** and are present in the coxal, genual, tarsal, and carpal joints.

Table 7-3 Subtypes of Synovial Joints

Subtype	*Movement*	*Example*
Spheroidal (ball and socket)	Free movement in all planes	Shoulder and hip joints
Ellipsoid (condylar)	Movement in two planes (but not rotation)	Radiocarpal joint
Bicondylar (two rounded surfaces, two depressions)	Mostly in one plane	Genual (knee) joint
Ginglymus (hinge)	Movement in one plane	Interphalangeal joints
Trochoid (pivot)	Rotation only	Proximal radio-ulnar joint
Sellar (saddle)	Movement in two planes	Carpometacarpal joint of the thumb
Planar (gliding)	Gliding movement in any direction	Zygapophyseal joints and some parts of the carpal and tarsal joints

The congruence of the articular surfaces in some synovial joints is improved by the presence of fibrocartilaginous structures between the articular surfaces of the skeletal components. Their purpose is to "fill in the gaps" and to help spread synovial fluid over the articular surfaces for lubrication and for nourishment of the chondrocytes. When these structures completely separate the articular cartilages and thereby subdivide the articular cavity they are called **articular discs** and are found associated with the radiocarpal joints, acromioclavicular joints, sternoclavicular joints, and the temporomandibular joints. Two incomplete articular discs called **articular menisci** are found in the genual joint. They are "C" or "half-moon" -shaped fibrocartilages that do not completely separate the femoral condyles from the tibial condyles. The articular menisci of the knee joint are commonly called "cartilages" of the knee and are often torn during traumatic injuries (especially the medial one).

Objectives

3. Schematically draw and label a typical synovial joint.
4. State the functional roles of synovial fluid.
5. Define ligament as used in reference to joints and differentiate three types based on their positional relationship to the fibrous part of the joint capsule.
6. List the joints of the body that have intracapsular ligaments and the ones that contain menisci or articular discs.
7. Explain why joints that contain menisci or articular discs are not considered to be fibrocartilaginous joints (since that is the material composing the menisci/discs).

Joints of the Axial Skeleton

The joints of the axial skeleton include the joints of the head, vertebral column, and thorax (Table 7-5, Figure 7-5). The joints of the head include sutures, synchondroses, all of the dentoalveolar joints (gomphoses), the temporomandibular joints, atlanto-occipital joint, and the joints associated with the auditory ossicles (discussed with the ear in a later chapter). The left and right **temporo-**

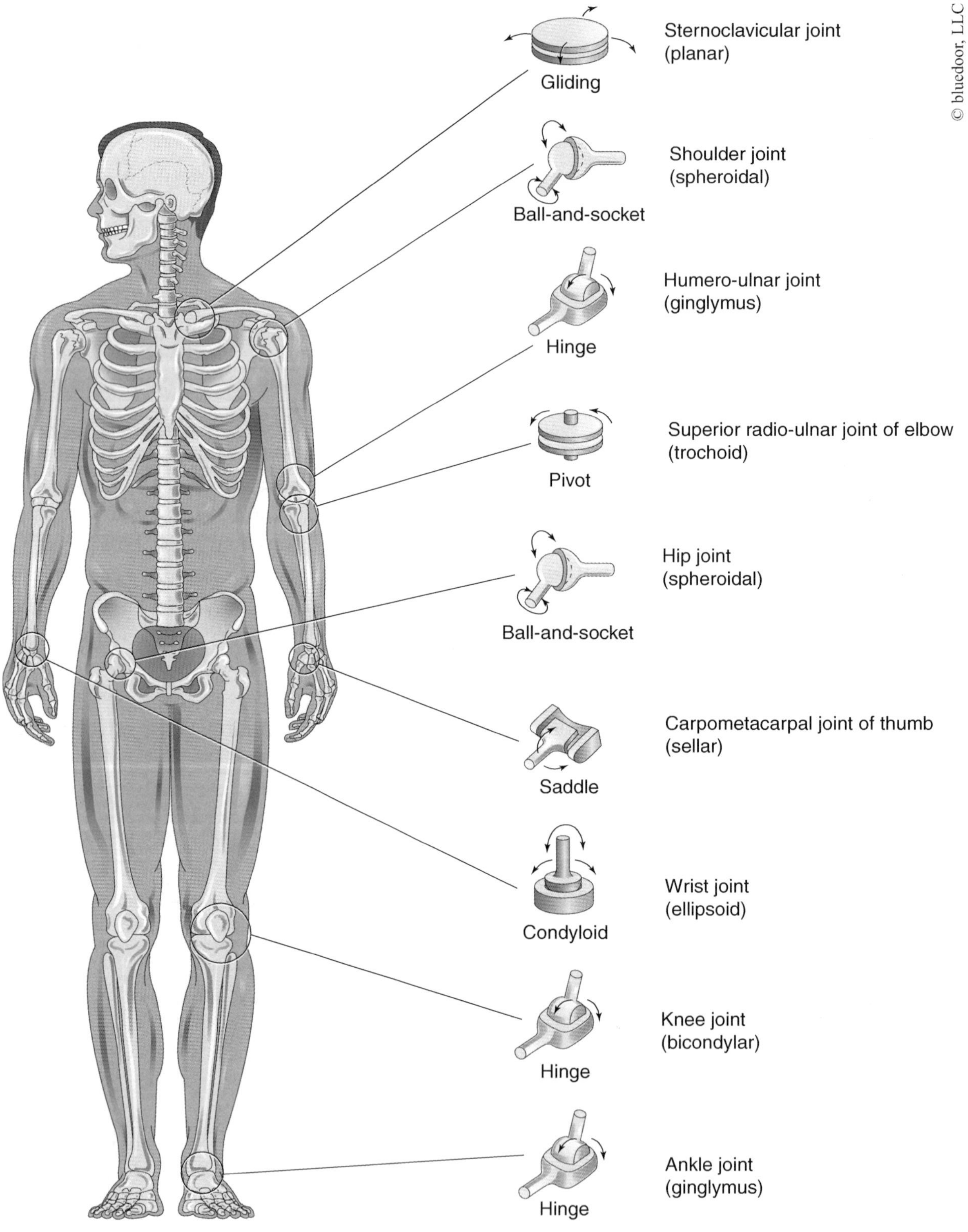

Figure 7-3

Subtypes of Synovial Joints

Synovial joints can be subdivided into seven subtypes based on the shapes of their articular surfaces (*see Table 7-3*). The reason that these subtypes are sometimes de-emphasized in anatomy courses is that they are based solely on the shapes of the articulating surfaces.

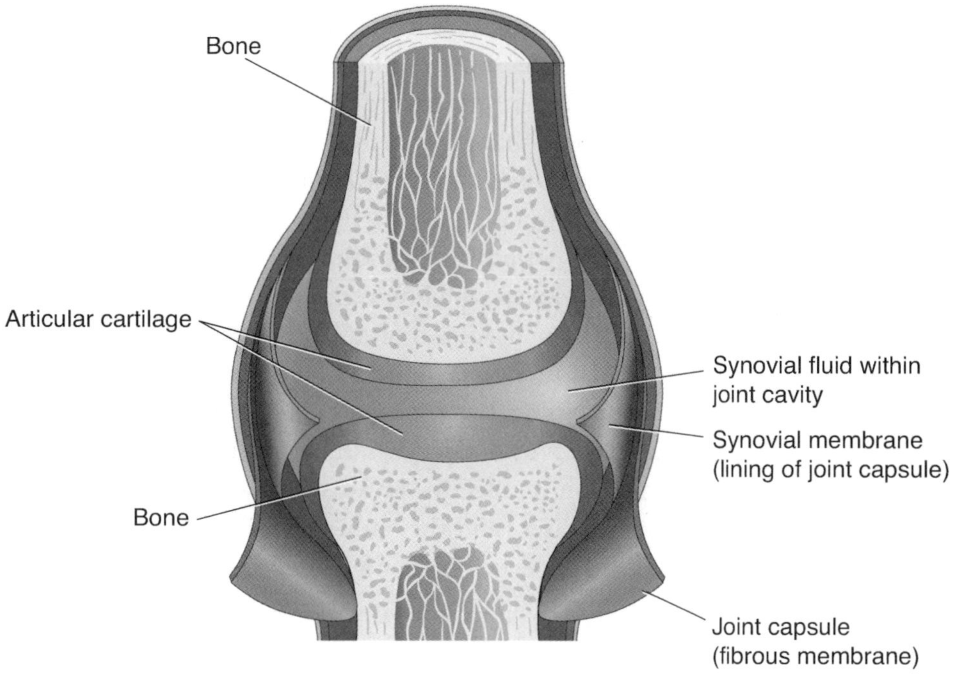

Figure 7-4
Parts of a Typical Synovial Joint

At least two articular cartilage covered skeletal structures and a synovium-secreting joint capsule must be present. In addition, synovial joints have stabilizing ligaments and a few of them contain fibrocartilaginous structures (articular discs/menisci) that add stability and help distribute synovial fluid over the articular surfaces.

Table 7-4 Ligaments Associated with Synovial Joints

Type	*Example*	*Location*
Capsular ligaments	Glenohumeral ligament	Shoulder joint
	Ischiofemoral ligament	Hip joint
	Pubofemoral ligament	Hip joint
	Iliofemoral ligament	Hip joint
Extracapsular ligaments	Tibial collateral ligament	Knee joint
	Fibular collateral ligament	Knee joint
	Collateral ligaments of the digital joints	Metacarpophalangeal and interphalangeal joints
Intracapsular ligaments	Radiate ligament of the heads of the ribs	Joints of the heads of the ribs
	Ligament of femoral head	Hip joint
	Anterior and posterior cruciate ligaments	Knee joint
	Intercarpal ligaments	Carpal joints
	Intertarsal ligaments	Tarsal joints

mandibular joints are ellipsoid synovial joints positioned between the temporal bones and the heads of the mandible. Each one has an intervening articular disc and allows the mouth to be opened and closed, as well as side-to-side and front-to-back motions. The **atlanto-occipital joint** is a paired condylar synovial articulation between the superior articular surfaces of the atlas and the occipital condyles. This is the main joint flexed and extended when miming "yes". Developmentally, the left and right halves of the mandible are joined anteriorly by a fibrocartilaginous joint termed the mandibular symphysis. This becomes synostotic but the name mandibular symphysis is retained.

The joints of the vertebral column include the atlanto-axial joint, the zygapophyseal joints, and the intervertebral symphyses. The **atlanto-axial joint** is a synovial articulation between the atlas and axis. It is the joint primarily moved when miming "no". The **zygapophyseal joints** are the planar synovial joints between articular processes of adjacent vertebrae. Most vertebrae have four of these since they have four articular processes (left/right, superior/inferior). The **intervertebral symphyses** are the fibrocartilaginous joints between the bodies of adjacent vertebrae. The intervening fibrocartilage is called an **intervertebral disc** (not to be confused with a synovial "articular disc"). Its outer fibrocartilaginous portion is called the **anulus fibrosus** and its gelatinous core is the **nucleus pulposus**. The intervertebral discs (and the bodies of the vertebrae) are derived from the notochord of the embryo. The discs absorb shock and allow limited movement at each intervertebral joint. They are the major stabilizers that keep the vertebrae in proper alignment. Because the nucleus pulposus slowly compresses during periods of sitting or standing, humans are measurably taller after lying down for a period of time (sleeping).

The joints of the thorax include those associated with the ribs and sternum. The **joints of the heads of the ribs** are synovial joints between the rib heads and the bodies of the thoracic vertebrae. The heads of most ribs articulate with the bodies of two adjacent vertebrae. Those of the last three rib pairs, however, usually articulate only with one thoracic vertebra. The tubercle of each rib articulates with a fovea on the ipsilateral transverse process of the thoracic vertebra of the same number. These synovial joints are called **costotransverse joints**. At the other end of each rib is a **costochondral joint** where the rib joins its costal cartilage. These are hyaline cartilage joints. The **sternocostal joints** are the articulations (mostly synovial) between the costal cartilages of the first seven pairs of ribs and the costal notches of the sternum. The synovial unions between the costal cartilages of ribs 7-10 on each side form the **interchondral joints**. The three segments of the sternum (manubrium, body, xiphoid process) are joined by the **manubriosternal symphysis** (a fibrocartilaginous joint) and the **xiphisternal synchondrosis** (a hyaline cartilage joint).

Objectives

8. Divide the joints of the axial skeleton into three categories (joints of the head, vertebrae, and thoracic cage) and name the joints in each area.
9. Explain why people are measurably shorter after sitting or standing for several hours (and in senility).

Joints of the Superior Limb

The joints of the superior limb include those within the pectoral girdle and those within the free part of the limb (*i.e.*, from the shoulder distally). All of these are synovial joints except for the radio-ulnar syndesmosis (Table 7-6, Figure 7-6). The superior limb articulates directly with the axial skeleton

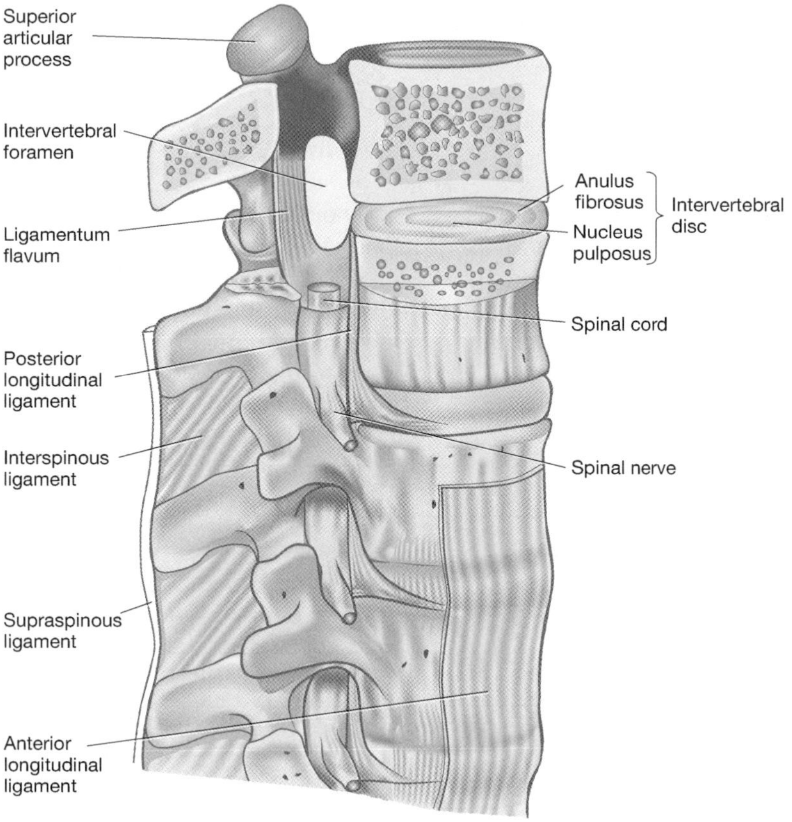

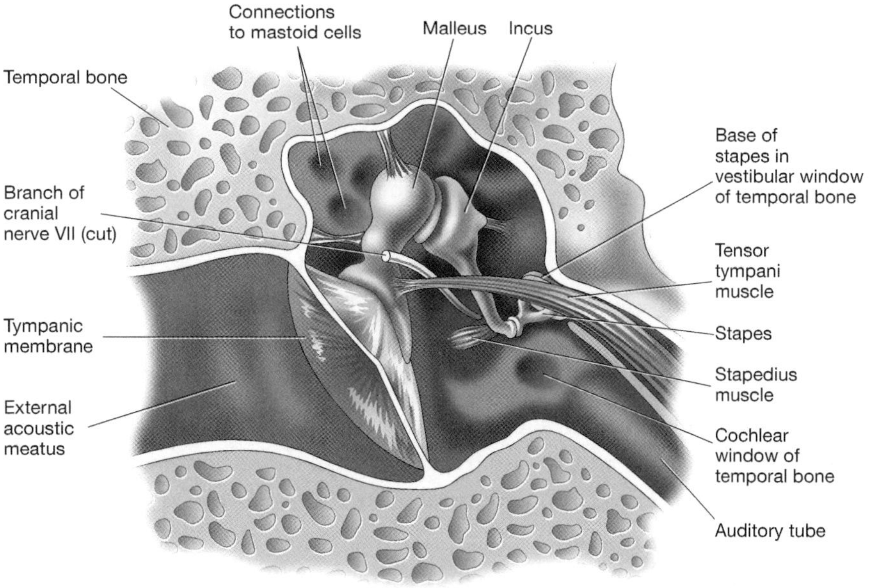

Figure 7-5

Selected Joints of the Axial Skeleton

Within the middle ear, the joints between the malleus and the incus and between the incus and stapes are synovial. However, the base ("footplate") of the stapes joins the temporal bone via a syndesmosis. The vertebral column has fibrocartilaginous joints between the bodies of adjacent vertebrae and synovial joints between the articular processes of the vertebrae.

Table 7-5 Joints of the Axial Skeleton*

Joints of the Head	*Type*	*Location*
Cranial sutures	Suture	*(see Table 7-2)*
Cranial synchondroses:		
Spheno-occipital syn.	Synchondrosis	Sphenoid/occipital bones
Sphenopetrosal syn.	Synchondrosis	Sphenoid/temporal bones
Petro-occipital syn.	Synchondrosis	Temporal/occipital bones
Intra-occipital syn.	Synchondrosis	Between occipital bones
Spheno-ethmoidal syn.	Synchondrosis	Sphenoid/ethmoid bones
Dentoalveolar joints	Gomphosis	Between teeth and dental alveoli
Temporomandibular joint	Synovial	Head of mandible/mandibular fossa of temporal bone
Atlanto-occipital joint	Synovial	Atlas/occipital condyles
Joints of the Vertebrae	*Type*	*Location*
Atlanto-axial joint	Synovial	Atlas/axis
Zygapophyseal joints	Synovial	Articular processes of adjacent vertebrae
Intervertebral symphyses	Symphysis	Between bodies of adjacent vertebrae
Joints of the Thoracic Cage	*Type*	*Location*
Joints of heads of ribs	Synovial	Heads of the ribs/bodies of the thoracic vertebrae
Costotransverse joints	Synovial	Tubercles of ribs/transverse processes of thoracic vertebrae
Costochondral joints	Synchondrosis	Bony part of ribs/costal cartilages
Sternocostal joints	Synovial	Costal cartilages of the ribs/costal notches of the sternum
Interchondral joints	Synovial	Costal arch
Manubriosternal symphysis	Symphysis	Manubrium/body of sternum
Xiphisternal synchondrosis	Synchondrosis	Body of sternum/xiphoid process

* See Chapter 13 for the joints associated with the auditory ossicles.

only at the **sternoclavicular joint**. This is a planar synovial joint between the sternal extremity of the clavicle and the clavicular notch of the sternum. The lateral end (acromial extremity) of the clavicle articulates with the acromion of the scapula at the **acromioclavicular joint**. The **shoulder (humeral) joint** is a spheroidal joint between the glenoid cavity of the scapula and the head of the humerus. It allows a wide range of motion in several planes.

The **cubital (elbow) joint** is a composite articulation involving the humeral condyle, the trochlear notch of the ulna, and the radial head. It has three named subdivisions: **humero-ulnar joint, humero-radial joint**, and the **proximal radio-ulnar joint**. It allows both flexion/extension and rotation (supination/pronation). The proximal radio-ulnar joint at the elbow is one of three side-to-side joints involving the antebrachial skeleton. The other two are the **radio-ulnar syndesmosis** (which extends most of the lengths of the bones) and the **distal radio-ulnar joint**. The radio-ulnar syndesmosis is the only fibrous joint in the superior limb. It is stabilized by a dense sheet of fibrous connective tissue called the **antebrachial interosseous membrane** that joins the bodies of the radius and ulna together side-by-side.

The joints of the manus include the carpal joint(s), the intermetacarpal joints, the metacarpophalangeal joints, and the interphalangeal joints. The **carpal joints** are those involving the carpal bones. Several of these have individual names. The **radiocarpal joint** is the articulation between the distal end of the radius and the scaphoid and lunate bones. It is the site of the major part of wrist

Table 7-6 Joints of the Superior Limb*

Joints of the pectoral girdle:
- **Sternoclavicular jt.**—clavicular notch of sternum/sternal extremity of clavicle
- **Acromioclavicular jt.**—acromial extremity of clavicle/acromion of scapula

Joints of the free part of the superior limb:
- **Shoulder (humeral) jt.**—glenoid cavity of scapula/head of the humerus
- **Elbow (cubital) jt.**—humeral condyle/trochlear notch of ulna and head of radius
  - **Humero-ulnar jt.**—trochlea of humeral condyle/trochlear notch of ulna
  - **Humeroradial jt.**—capitulum of humerus/articular fovea of the radial head
  - **Proximal radio-ulnar jt.**—articular circumference of the radial head/radial notch of the ulna
- **Radio-ulnar syndesmoses**—interosseous border of radius/interosseous border of ulna
- **Distal radio-ulnar jt.**—ulnar notch of the radius/articular circumference of the ulnar head
- **Carpal jts.**—any articulation involving carpal bones
  - **Radiocarpal jt.**—carpal articular surface of the radius/proximal row of carpal bones (excluding the pisiform bone)
  - **Intercarpal jts.**—between adjacent carpal bones
    - **Joint of the pisiform bone**—pisiform bone/triquetral bone
    - **Middle carpal jt.**—proximal row of carpal bones/distal row of carpal bones
  - **Carpometacarpal jts. (1-5)**—distal row of carpal bones/bases of metacarpal bones
- **Intermetacarpal jts.** (three total)—between the bases of metacarpal bones 2, 3, 4, 5
- **Metacarpophalangeal jts.****—heads of metacarpal bones/bases of proximal phalanges
- **Interphalangeal jts.****—between adjacent phalanges
  - **Proximal interphalangeal jts.**—heads of proximal phalanges of digits 2-5/bases of middle phalanges of digits 2-5
  - **Distal interphalangeal jts.**—heads of middle phalanges of digits 2-5/bases of distal phalanges of digits 2-5
  - **Interphalangeal joint of the thumb**—head of the proximal phalanx/base of the distal phalanx of the pollex

*All of these joints are synovial except for the radio-ulnar syndesmosis.
**These are often grouped as the "digital joints of the hand" for purposes of discussion.

motion. (Most of the rest occurs at the middle carpal joint, see below). The **intercarpal joints** are the joints between carpal bones (side-to-side as well as end-to-end). The collective intercarpal joints between the proximal row of carpal bones and the distal row comprise the **middle carpal joint**. The **carpometacarpal joints** occur between the distal carpal bones and the bases of the metacarpal bones. These are numbered 1-5 in reference to the involved metacarpal bones.

The **intermetacarpal joints** are the three side-to-side articulations between the bases of the metacarpal bones 2-5. There is no intermetacarpal joint between the first and second metacarpal bones because they do not touch. **Metacarpophalangeal joints** occur between the heads of the metacarpal bones and the bases of the proximal phalanges. These are numbered 1-5 in reference to the involved metacarpal bones. **Interphalangeal joints** occur between the phalanges. There is only one interphalangeal joint in the thumb because there are only two phalanges. Digits 2-5 have two interphalangeal joints each: **proximal interphalangeal joint** (between proximal and middle phalanges) and **distal interphalangeal joint** (between middle and distal phalanges).

Objectives

10. Name the joints of the superior limb including the subdivisions of the elbow and carpal joints. Note the only one which is not synovial.

(a)

(b)

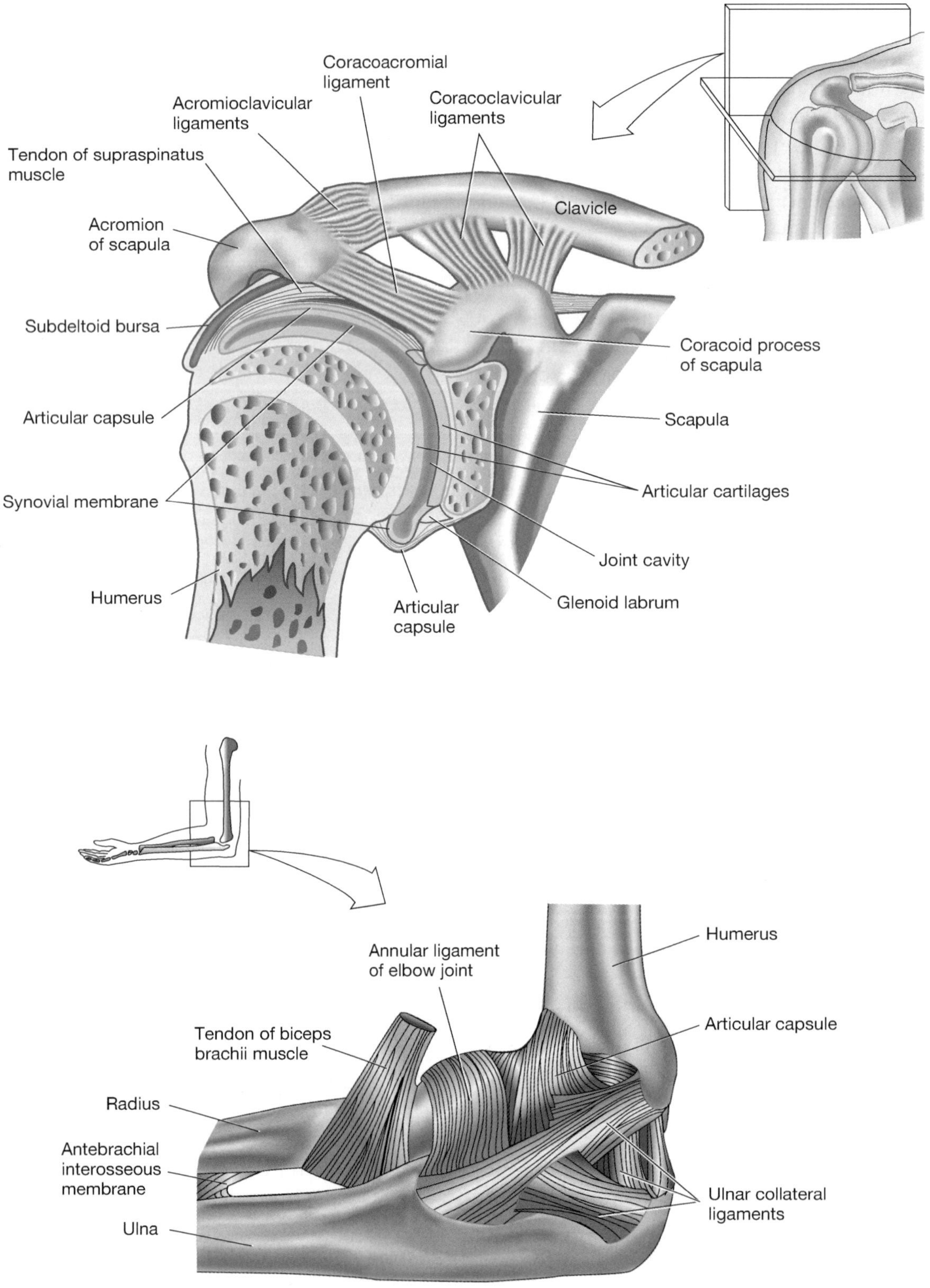

Figure 7-6 Selected Joints of the Superior Limb

(a) Humeral (shoulder) joint, (b) Cubital (elbow) joint.

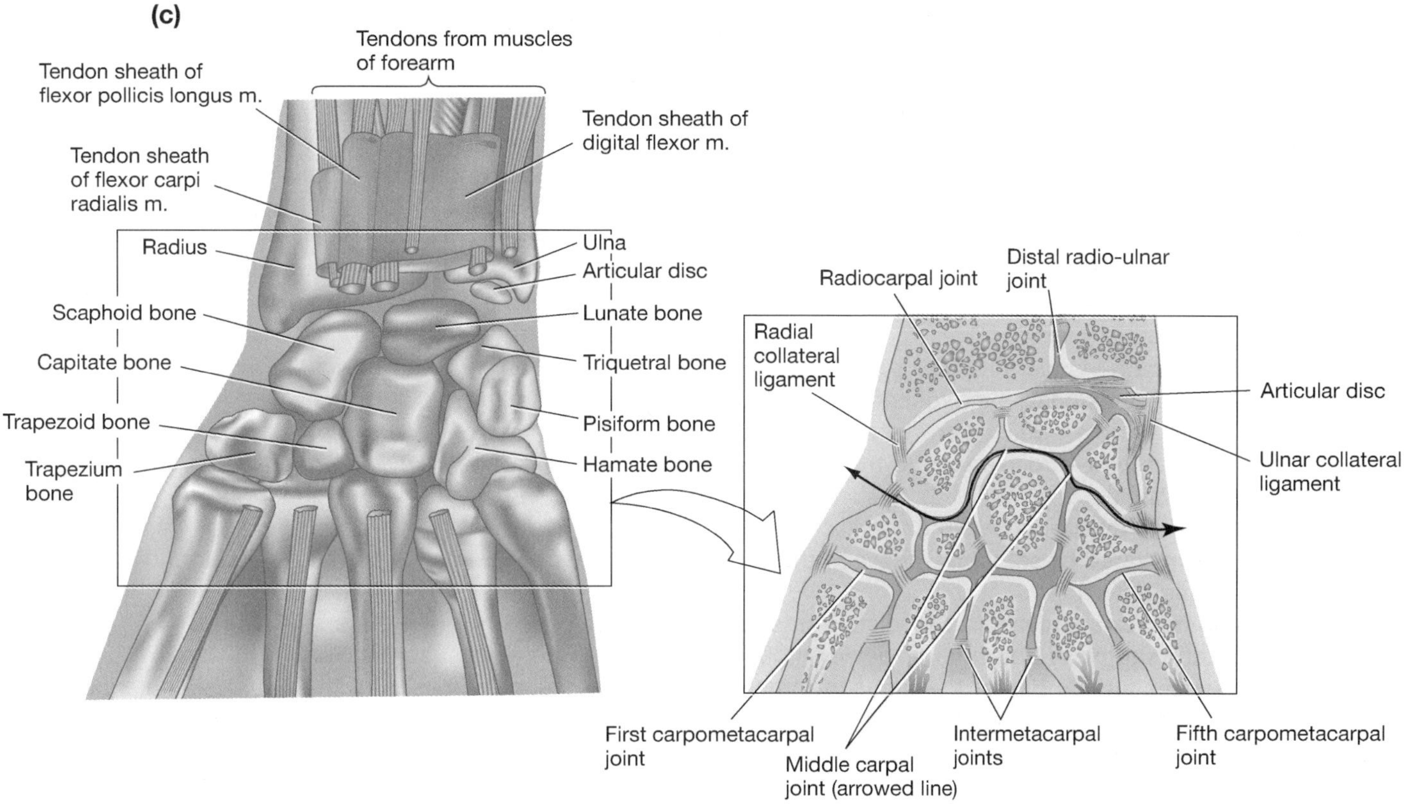

Figure 7-6 (continued)

(c) Joints of the carpal region.

Joints of the Inferior Limb

The joints of the inferior limb include those within the pelvic girdle and those within the free part of the inferior limb (Figure 7-7). All of the joints of the inferior limb are synovial with the exception of the tibiofibular syndesmosis and the pubic symphysis (Table 7-7). The inferior limb is joined to the axial skeleton at the **sacroiliac joint**. This planar synovial joint can develop fibrous or fibrocartilaginous adhesions later in life between the auricular surfaces of the sacral bone and ilium. The bodies of the pubic bones are joined together at the **pubic symphysis**. The fibrocartilaginous pad between the symphyseal surfaces of the pubic bones that stabilizes this joint is called the **interpubic disc**.

The proximal-most joint of the free part of the inferior limb is the **coxal** (**hip**) **joint**. This joint is a spheroidal synovial joint formed by the junction of the acetabulum of the os coxae with the femoral head. Capsular ligaments from all three bones of the os coxae attach to the femur bone to help stabilize the hip joint. A well-developed intracapsular ligament called the ligament of the femoral head extends from the fovea of the femoral head to the acetabular fossa. The fibrocartilaginous acetabular labrum (lip) helps to deepen the acetabulum. The hip joint has a wide range of motion and the numerous muscles of the hip mobilize and stabilize it.

The **genual** (**knee**) **joint** is a modified hinge joint at the junction of the thigh and crus (leg). For descriptive purposes it can be (unofficially) divided into the femoropatellar joint and the femorotib-

Table 7-7 Joints of the Inferior Limb*

Joints of the pelvic girdle:

- **Pubic symphysis**—between the symphyseal surfaces of the pubic bones
- **Sacroiliac joint**—auricular surfaces of the sacral bone and auricular surfaces of the ilia

Joints of the free part of the inferior limb:

- **Coxal (hip) joint**—acetabulum of the os coxae and the femoral head
- **Genual (knee) joint**—medial and lateral condyles of the femur bone with the medial and lateral condyles of the tibia ("femorotibial joint"), and the patellar surface of the femur bone and articular surface of the patella ("femoropatellar joint")
- **Tibiofibular joint**—fibular articular surface of the tibia and articular surface of the fibular head
- **Tibiofibular syndesmosis**—interosseous borders of the tibia and fibula
- **Tarsal joints**—joints involving any tarsal bones
  - **Talocrural joint**—trochlea of the talus, inferior articular surface of the tibia, and the malleolar articular surface of the fibula
  - **Intertarsal joints**—between any adjacent tarsal bones
    - **Transverse tarsal joint**—between the talus and calcaneus proximally and the navicular and cuboid bones distal to them
  - **Tarsometatarsal joints (1-5)**—distal tarsal bones and the bases of the metatarsal bones
- **Intermetatarsal joints** (four total)—between bases of adjacent metatarsal bones
- **Metatarsophalangeal joints****—heads of the metatarsal bones and the bases of the proximal phalanges
- **Interphalangeal joints****—between phalanges within each digit of the foot
  - **Proximal interphalangeal joints**—heads of the proximal phalanges and bases of the middle phalanges of digits 2-5
  - **Distal interphalangeal joints**—heads of the middle phalanges and the bases of the distal phalanges of digits 2-5
  - **Interphalangeal joint of the hallux**—head of the proximal phalanx and base of the distal phalanx of the big toe

*All of these are synovial joints except for the pubic symphysis and tibiofibular syndesmosis.
**These are often grouped as the "digital joints of the foot" for purposes of discussion.

ial joint. The stability of the latter is compromised by the rounded femoral condyles which articulate with the flattened tibial condyles. This incongruity is partially filled in by the **medial** and **lateral menisci**. These fibrocartilaginous "C"-shaped structures fill in the gaps between the bones and thus provide stability. Within the capsule are two ligaments that are positioned anterior/posterior near the center of the joint. The **anterior cruciate ligament** attaches to the anterior intercondylar area of the tibia and to the posterior part of the intercondylar fossa of the femur bone. The **posterior cruciate ligament** attaches to the posterior intercondylar area of the tibia and to the anterior part of the intercondylar fossa of the femur bone. Outside of the capsule, the **tibial** and **fibular collateral ligaments** connect the medial and lateral epicondyles of the femur bone to the tibia and the fibula, respectively. Anteriorly, the **patellar ligament** extends from the patella to the tibial tuberosity. The "terrible triad" is a common athletic injury of the genual joint. It includes a damaged medial meniscus, tibial collateral ligament, and anterior cruciate ligament.

The **tibiofibular joint** is the planar joint between the fibular articular surface of the tibia and the articular surface of the fibular head. Some anatomists mistakenly call this the "proximal" tibiofibular joint. The side-to-side fibrous joint between the interosseous borders of the fibula and tibia is the **tibiofibular syndesmosis**. The fibrous membrane which connects the bones is called the **crural interosseous membrane** and extends to their distal extremities. Some anatomists refer to the distal end of the tibiofibular syndesmosis as the "distal" tibiofibular joint even though there is no synovial joint present. The remaining joints within the inferior limb are grouped as the joints of the foot. They include the tarsal, intermetatarsal, metatarsophalangeal, and interphalangeal joints.

Tarsal joints include any joints involving the seven tarsal bones. The **talocrural joint** is the ginglymus between the trochlea of the talus, the inferior articular surface of the tibia, and malleolar articular surface of the fibula. The joint is shaped like a schindylesis with the trochlea of the talus fitting into a "slot" formed by the medial malleolus of the tibia, inferior articular surface of the tibia, and the lateral malleolus of the fibula. This joint provides most of the flexion/extension movement of the tarsal joint. **Intertarsal joints** are synovial joints between adjacent tarsal bones. Several of these joints have specific names based on the articulating bones (cuneonavicular joint, talocalcaneonavicular joint, *etc.*). The **transverse tarsal joint** is a composite proximal-to-distal joint between the proximal two tarsal bones (talus and calcaneus) and the two bones distal to them (navicular and cuboid bones). The middle carpal joint in the hand is homologous to this joint. The articulations between the distal tarsal bones (cuneiform bones and cuboid bone) and the bases of the metatarsal bones are referred to as the **tarsometatarsal joints**. They are numbered 1-5 according to the corresponding number of the involved metatarsal bone.

The four side-to-side synovial joints between the bases of the metatarsal bones are called the **intermetatarsal joints**. These are homologous to the three intermetacarpal joints. The remaining joints of the foot (**metatarsophalangeal** and **interphalangeal joints**) resemble their counterparts in the superior limb and are named in the same manner.

Objectives

11. Name the joints of the inferior limb including the subdivisions of the tarsal joint. Note the two which are not synovial.
12. Explain why the inferior limb has no "distal tibiofibular joint" in contrast to the superior limb (in which a distal radio-ulnar joint is present).

Basic Joint Motions

All joints allow some movement between the skeletal components. In fibrous and cartilaginous joints this is often negligible or minimal. Synovial joints are said to be "freely moveable" in one or more planes but some of them allow only a very limited range of motion. Joint movements may be produced by contraction of skeletal muscles, by gravitational pull, or by the "rebound" of elastic components of the body that have been stretched. There are several types of general and special joint movements (Figure 7-8).

Flexion and extension are joint motions that involve angular changes within sagittal planes. **Flexion** implies a *decrease* in size of the flexor angle of a joint in an anterior/posterior plane. **Extension** is an *increase* in size of the flexor angle. The **flexor angle** of each joint is specifically identified by convention. In the free part of the superior limb, the flexor angle is located on the anterior aspect of all joints. In the free part of the inferior limb, the flexor angle is anterior in the coxal and tarsal joints but it is posterior or plantar in all others. The angle opposite the flexor angle (*i.e.*, on the other side of the joint) is the **extensor angle**. Thus, flexion of a joint decreases the size of the flexor angle, and simultaneously, it increases the size of the extensor angle. Extension of a joint

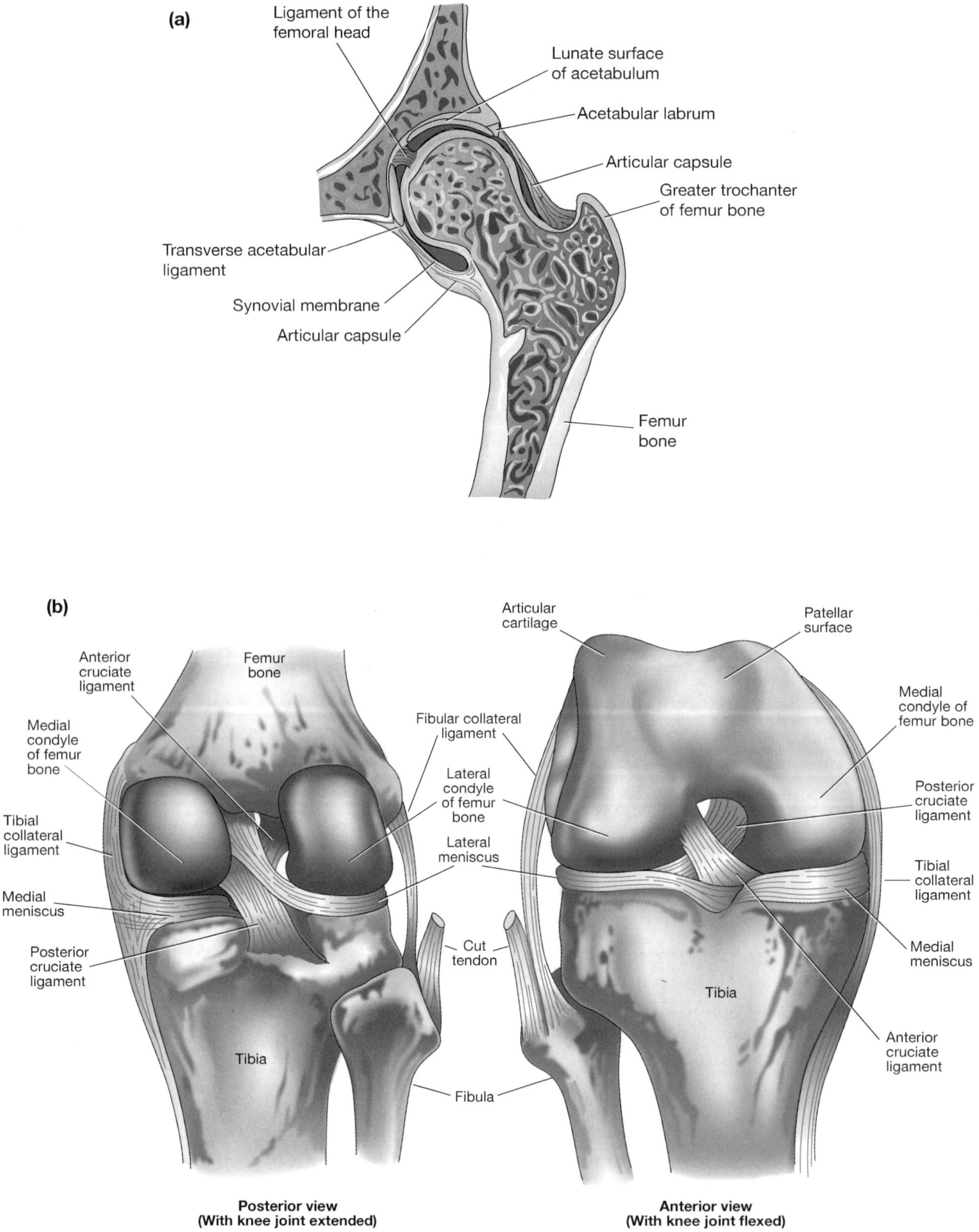

Figure 7-7 Selected Joints of the Inferior Limb

(a) Coxal (hip) joint (b) Genual (knee) joint

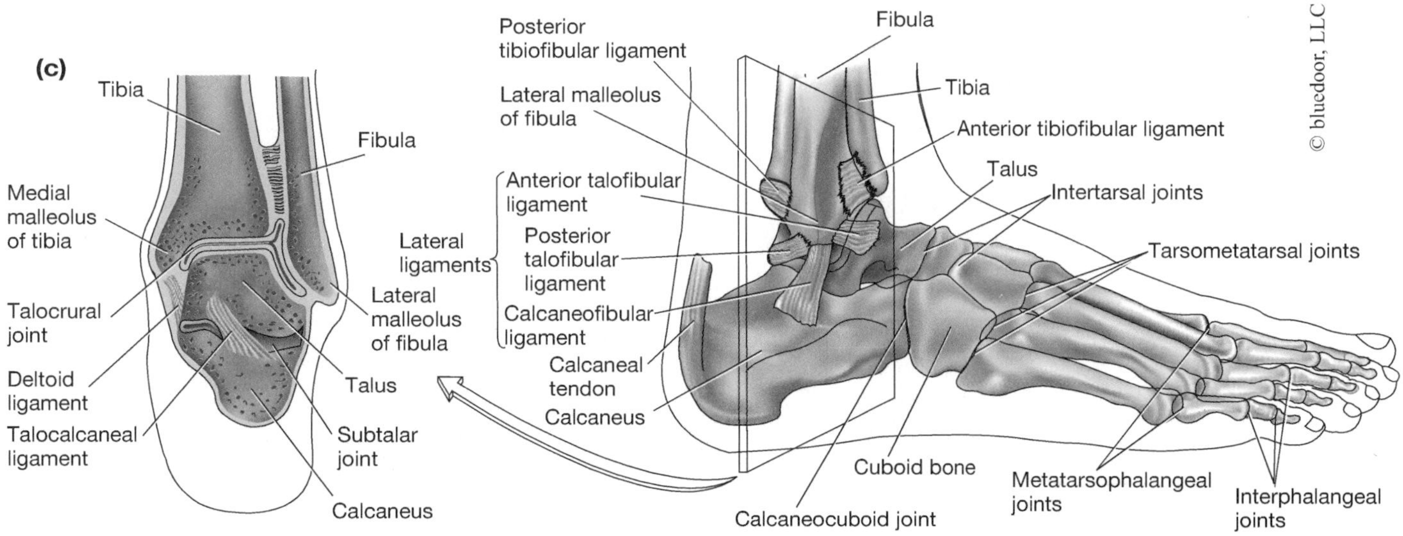

Figure 7-7 (continued)

(c) Joints of the foot.

increases the size of the flexor angle and decreases the size of the extensor angle. In the joints of the vertebral column, the flexor angle is on the anterior aspect. Thus, bending one's head down or rolling one's body up into a ball *flexes the joints of the vertebral column,* and arching one's back by protruding the chest (or tilting the head up) extends these joints. Joints that are markedly extended or flexed are often said to be **hyperextended** (or **hyperflexed**). Some authors reserve the use of hyperextension/hyperflexion for those situations where the joint components have been angled beyond 180° (others do not follow this convention). Some individuals, for example, can extend (hyperextend) their digital joints beyond 180° —thus partially curling their fingers in the "wrong" direction. The misnomer "double-jointed" is sometimes used for this situation. Physicians use hyperextension in a different way (see *Clinical Considerations*). At the tarsal joint, flexion is often termed **dorsiflexion** (as when easing off the accelerator pedal) and extension (rising up on one's toes) is termed **plantar flexion**. When using *flexion/extension* to describe joint movements, one should always name the *joint* (or *joints*) that is flexed or extended—never an unbendable part of the body. For example, one can flex or extend the cubital *joint* but not the brachium, antebrachium, limb as a whole, or a muscle (muscles are *contracted*).

Movement of a whole limb, hand, or digit in a lateral/medial orientation is termed *ab*duction or *ad*duction. **Abduction** is movement *away from* a point of reference and **adduction** is movement *toward* that reference. For the major parts of the limbs, the point of reference is the median plane. The body part moved and the joint at which the movement occurs should be identified. Thus, swinging an arm laterally (up to 90°) from the normal anatomic position is *abduction of the superior limb at the shoulder joint.* Returning the limb to the anatomical position is *adduction of the superior limb at the shoulder joint.* Swinging it on vertically from the 90°, fully abducted position or moving it toward the median plane in front of or behind the rest of the body is also considered to be *adduction* by some anatomists. Others consider the vertical continuation from a fully abducted 90° position to be further *abduction* because they combine the median plane reference with proximity to the normal anatomic position. Movement at the carpal joint which angles the hand medial to the axis of the limb is *adduction of the manus at the carpal joint.* The opposite motion is *abduction of the manus at the carpal joint.* In the inferior limb, adduction/abduction can occur only at the hip and metatarsopha-

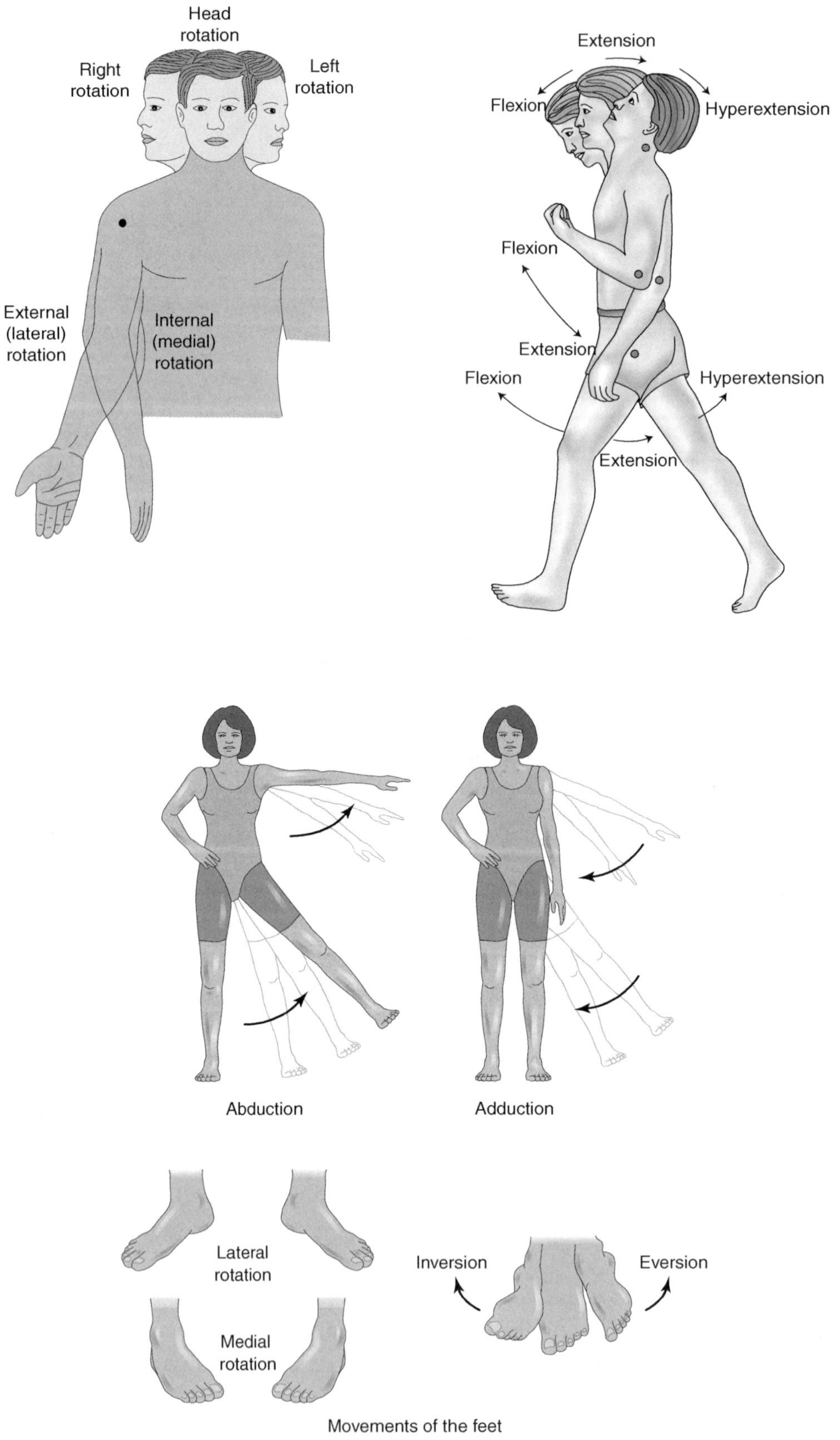

Figure 7-8
Examples of Joint Motion

langeal joints. The reference for abduction/adduction of the digits is the longitudinal axis of the limb. This axis passes through the middle finger of the hand and second toe of the foot. Thus, spreading one's fingers or toes is *abduction of the digits (at the metacarpophalangeal or metatarsophalangeal joints)*. The opposite motion is *adduction of the digits.*

Rotation is movement of a body part around its long axis. Rotation in the superior limb can occur at the shoulder joint and at the radioulnar joints. Internal (medial) rotation that turns the palmar aspect of the manus medially and then posteriorly is called **pronation**. External (lateral) rotation which turns a pronated manus back toward the normal anatomical position is called **supination**. In the inferior limb, rotation can occur at the coxal joints and to a lesser degree at the genual joint. External rotation of the limb which directs the toes further laterally is often termed *abduction of the forefoot* by those in sports medicine. Similarly, internal rotation of the inferior limb which turns the toes toward the median plane is often termed *adduction of the forefoot.* The intervertebral joints of the neck can be rotated left and right as in miming "no". Similar composite movements of the intervertebral joints in the thoracic and lumbar regions can produce left or right rotation (twisting) of the trunk.

In addition to *flexion/extension, abduction/adduction*, and *rotation*, there are several other terms used to describe particular movements including *inversion/eversion, protraction/retraction*, and *circumduction.* Elevation of the medial border of the foot such that the plantar surface is directed slightly medially is termed **inversion** of the foot. The opposite motion (elevation of the lateral border such that the plantar surface is directed somewhat laterally) is **eversion**. Movement of the mandible or of a whole limb anteriorly is termed **protraction**. This involves motion at only the temporomandibular joints in the case of the mandible, but in the limbs, protraction may involve simultaneous movement at several joints. Posterior movement of these same body parts is **retraction**. **Circumduction** is circular motion involving a finger, hand, foot, or whole limb such that a cone shape is described (formed, outlined) in space. Careful examination of circumduction will reveal that it is composed of extension, flexion, abduction, and adduction, *etc.* Notice that the movement involving circumduction of a finger occurs at a metacarpophalangeal joint. Circumduction involving a hand results from motion at the radiocarpal joint. Circumduction of the free part of a superior limb involves motion primarily at the shoulder joint.

Objectives

13. Define and properly use extension , flexion, dorsiflexion, plantar flexion, adduction, abduction, rotation, supination, pronation, inversion, eversion, protraction, retraction, and circumduction.
14. Note the position of the flexor angle (surface) of each appendicular joint.

Lever Systems in Locomotion

Bones, muscles, and joints interact as **lever systems** to effect locomotion and posture. Four components are needed for a functional lever system: a rigid bar to serve as a **lever arm**, a point of rotation along the bar called the **fulcrum**, an applied **force**, and a **resistance**. In vertebrates, the lever arms are formed by skeletal components, the applied force is usually supplied by muscle contraction or gravity, and the resistance is provided by gravitational pull (weight), by the inertia of body parts,

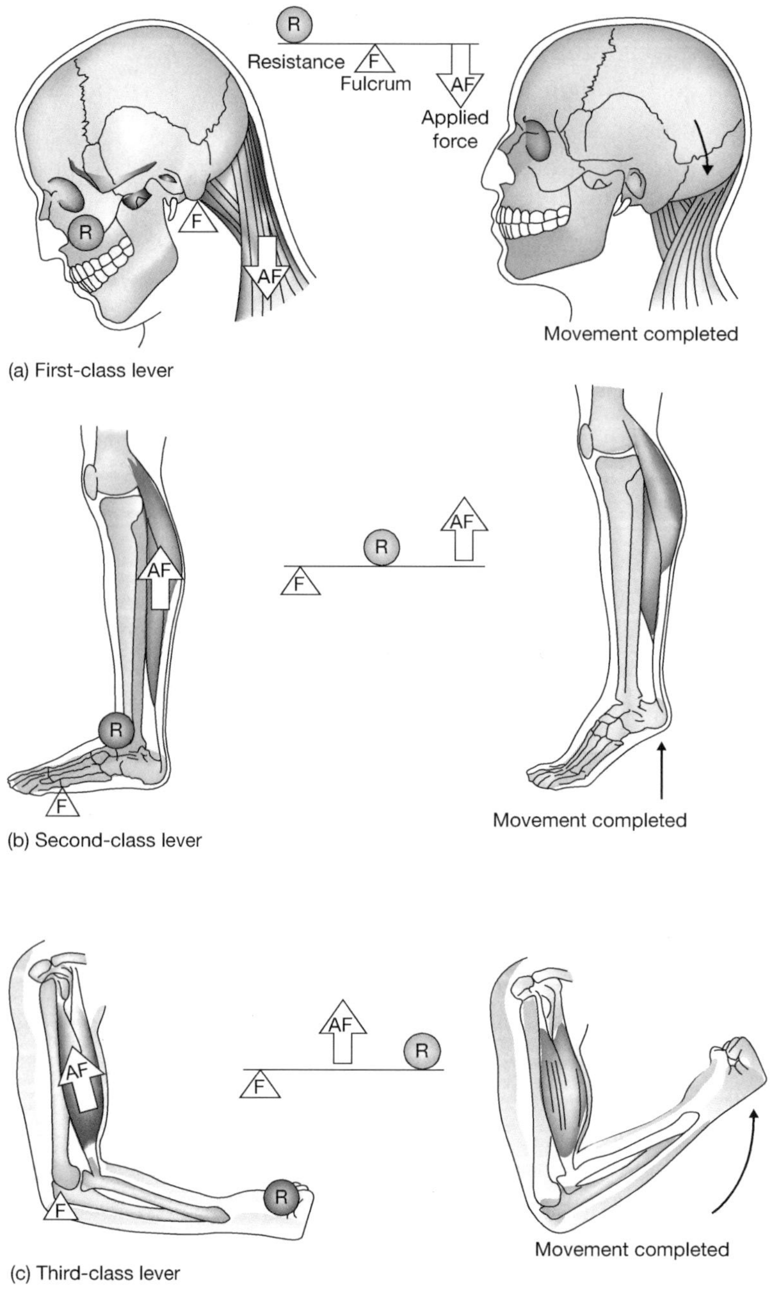

Figure 7-9

The Three Classes of Levers

The fulcrum, applied force, and resistance can be positioned in three relative ways along the lever arm. The moment arm equation applies equally to all three classes. In the body, third class levers are more common than first or second class levers.

or by the placement of body parts against objects. The fulcrum occurs at the point of least movement along the lever arm and is located either at a joint or where a limb contacts a surface (the ground, a table, *etc.*).

Lever systems are designated as first, second, or third class depending on the relative positions of the fulcrum, resistance, and applied force along the lever arm (Figure 7-9). In **first class levers** the

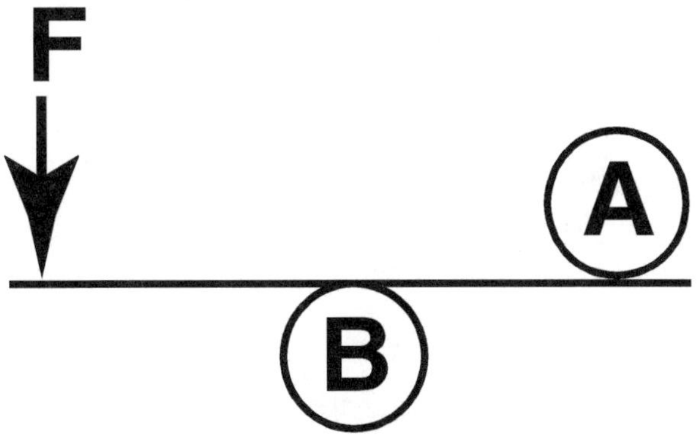

Figure 7-10

Interconvertibility of Some First and Second Class Levers

Assume that a lever arm is positioned between two structures (A and B) and a force (F) is applied as shown. If A is more easily moved than B, then A is the resistance, B becomes the fulcrum, and the lever system is first class. However, if B is more easily moved than A, B becomes the resistance, A is the fulcrum and the lever is second class.

fulcrum is positioned between the force and resistance. In **second class levers** the resistance occupies the middle position, and in **third class levers** the applied force is central. A lever system is said to be in equilibrium if the applied force produces a resultant force just large enough to balance the resistance. When lever systems are in equilibrium, all three types obey the same simple mathematical relationship: $\mathbf{F} \times \mathbf{D_F} = \mathbf{R} \times \mathbf{D_R}$ where **F** = force, **R** = resistance, $\mathbf{D_F}$ = distance from the force to the fulcrum, and $\mathbf{D_R}$ = distance from the resistance to the fulcrum. This formula is sometimes called the **moment arm equation**. Force and resistance must be in the same units (pounds, ounces, kilograms, *etc.*) and the two distances must be measured in the same units (inches, feet, centimeters, *etc.*).

At equilibrium, the applied force (F) may be larger, equal, or smaller in magnitude than the resistance (R). If the force is smaller than the resistance, the lever system *gains* **mechanical advantage** (*i.e.*, a smaller force can move a larger resistance). If F is larger than the resistance, the lever system *loses* mechanical advantage. If F = R, mechanical advantage is neither gained nor lost. Second class levers always gain mechanical advantage and third class levers always lose mechanical advantage. First class levers gain mechanical advantage if the fulcrum is closer to the resistance than to the force and they lose advantage if the fulcrum is closer to the force. When mechanical advantage is lost, a lever system has more speed and magnitude of movement of the lever arm at the resistance (R) than at the force (and vice versa). This is generally advantageous because the relatively small linear contraction of a muscle belly can move a given body part through a much greater distance.

In the body, there are more third class levers than first or second class. An example of a third class lever system is flexion of the cubital joint by the biceps brachii muscle. In this case, the fulcrum occurs at the elbow joint, and the applied force is produced by the biceps brachii muscle where it pulls proximally on the radial tuberosity. The resistance is the weight of the antebrachium and manus (plus anything picked up by the hand). An example of a second class lever system in the body is contraction of the gastrocnemius muscle causing one to rise up on one's toes. In this case, the fulcrum is located at the ball of the foot and the bones of the tarsus and metatarsus form the lever arm. The force is located at the posterior end of the tuber calcanei (where the gastrocnemius muscle attaches) and is directed superiorly. The resistance is the weight of the body resting on the talus. Notice that as long as one is on a firm surface, this lever system is second class because the anterior metatarsal region doesn't move (*i.e.*, it is on the ground) and is by definition the fulcrum. However, this same muscle-lever arm-joint system acts as a first class lever when one pushes down on the accelerator pedal of a car. In this case the resistance (R) is located under the ball of the foot, the applied force is in the same location (tuber calcanei), and the fulcrum is located at the talocrural joint. Many first and second class lever systems can be interconverted in this manner (Figure 7-10).

Objectives

15. Explain how bones, muscles, and joints interact to form lever systems for locomotion.
16. Compare the three kinds of levers in regard to relative positions of the applied force, fulcrum, and resistance on the lever arm, mechanical advantage, and relative motion (or speed) at the applied force vs the resistance.
17. Understand and be able to use the moment arm equation for lever systems in equilibrium ($F \times D_F = R \times D_R$).

Clinical Considerations

The most common clinical condition involving joints is **arthritis** (joint inflammation). Over two dozen subtypes have been described including traumatic, degenerative, infectious, rheumatoid and gouty arthritis. These differ from one another in pathoetiology (cause) and in some of their clinical manifestations. **Traumatic arthritis** is caused by physical damage to joint components. In synovial joints, the synovial membrane often reacts by producing excessive synovial fluid causing distension of the joint capsule and severe pain. Drainage of the fluid by **arthrocentesis** (joint puncture) may cause immediate relief, but pain often returns as the capsule is re-distended. Some degree of **degenerative arthritis** occurs as an age-related phenomenon in most individuals. **Infectious arthritis** occurs when a joint is invaded by infectious organisms (usually, but not always, by bacteria). **Rheumatoid arthritis** is a chronic proliferative type of synovial joint arthritis that involves defects in connective tissue metabolism. It is progressive, is more common in women than in men, and is characterized by erosion of the articular cartilage and thickening of the synovial membrane. **Gouty arthritis** is synovial joint inflammation resulting from deposit of urate crystals within the joint cavity. Men are affected to a greater degree than women. Conformational defects of the skeleton often result in subsequent arthritic changes.

Dislocations (luxations) of joints can occur with or without fractures of the involved bones. If the skeletal components are only partially out of alignment such that parts of the articular surfaces remain in contact, the dislocation is termed a **subluxation** (partial dislocation). Luxations always involve injury to the soft tissues that stabilize the joint including the joint capsule and ligaments and they most commonly occur in the joints of the limbs. They are described using directional terms that refer to the relative position of the distal joint component in relation to the proximal joint component. For example, a medial luxation of the elbow joint is one in which the proximal epiphyses of the radius and ulna (*distal* components of the joint) are *medial* to the humeral condyle (the *proximal* skeletal component of the joint).

Bony fusion of a joint is termed **synostosis** or sometimes **ankylosis**. This may occur after severe injury and it is sometimes a complicating consequence of some of the degenerative changes that occur in some forms of arthritis. Iatric (physician induced) ankylosis is sometimes performed in cases of severely damaged or degenerative joints. Once fusion occurs, pain associated with the diseased joint typically subsides.

Surgical invasion of a joint is termed **arthrotomy**. If fiber optic instrumentation is used, the incision can be kept quite small and the procedure is called **arthroscopy**. In the last decade, several specialized instruments have been developed that allow many joint surgeries to be performed with arthroscopes. Arthroscopy allows very small incisions, and results in less tissue damage and faster post-operative recovery.

Intervertebral disc disease occurs when the nucleus pulposus of an intervertebral disc puts pressure on adjacent spinal nerves or directly on the spinal cord itself by bulging or protruding completely through the anulus fibrosus. This causes a pain/paralysis syndrome depending on severity and is commonly (but erroneously) called a "slipped" disc. Medical and/or surgical intervention may be required to expedite recovery.

Abnormal curvatures of the vertebral column are classified as kyphosis, lordosis, or scoliosis depending on the direction of the deviation. **Kyphosis** is a "hunch-backed" posture characterized by exaggeration of the thoracic curvature. **Lordosis** is exaggeration of the lumbar curvature which results in anterior protuberance of the chest. This posture is sometimes called "saddle back" or "hollow back." **Scoliosis** is a lateral curvature of the vertebral column. These abnormal curvatures may involve simple or compound deviations. They may be fixed (unmovable) as a result of muscle or bone deformity or mobile as a result of unequal muscle contraction.

Clinical hyperextension of the joint occurs when a joint is forced to extend further than its normal physiological limits. This may damage the articular capsule and supporting ligaments to various degrees.

Objectives

18. Define arthritis and differentiate its common subtypes.
19. Define luxation and subluxation and explain the use of directional terms that are often used to describe these conditions.
20. Explain why pain or even paralysis can result from intervertebral disc disease.
21. Differentiate kyphosis, lordosis, and scoliosis.
22. For any named joint, indicate the specific skeletal components that articulate.

Clinical Case Studies

Case 1—A 23-year-old college co-ed severely traumatized her right knee in a fall while downhill skiing. Although she could bear weight on the joint after the injury, and radiographs were negative, the knee remained swollen, painful, and unstable. A clinical exam revealed that the proximal crus of the affected limb could be shifted anterior/posterior about 1 cm relative to the distal thigh. What anatomic structure does this instability implicate?

Case 2—A 35-year-old attorney suffered pain in the general area of his left shoulder that got progressively worse in the following few months. He also noted a weakness in his left grip and he occasionally had tingling sensations in his left arm. Radiography of his cervical vertebrae revealed intervertebral disc spaces that were narrower (thinner) than normal. How does this relate to the patient's clinical signs?

Case 3—A 42-year-old longshoreman suffered a crushing injury of his right ankle when a crane operator accidently swung a long crate against him and trapped his limb against a piling. Among the bones with multiple fractures were the distal tibia and fibula, talus, calcaneus, and navicular bone. After the initial swelling subsided, the attending orthopod put the ankle in a plaster cast and immobilized it for five months. What was the physician's objective?

Points to Ponder

In a synovial joint the articular surfaces of the skeletal components are either disparate in size or only partially in contact with each other. Otherwise, joint motion would, of necessity, cause at least subluxation. Synovial joints vary considerably in the freedom of motion afforded their skeletal components and the degree to which they can be subluxed without serious damage to their ligaments and joint capsules.

Does popping one's knuckles (fingers, toes, *etc.*) cause joint enlargement? No—but we lie about it to our children to keep them quieter in church! The actual "pop" is caused by the break in vacuum related to the sudden parting of the synovial (articular) surfaces—something similar to the noise produced when one pulls a suction cup off a pane of glass. The reason that one cannot "re-pop" the same joint immediately is apparently related to the fact that there is some gasification of the synovial fluid in a recently popped joint that must be reabsorbed before the phenomenon can be repeated.

How many synovial joints are in the body? Depends, of course, on how they are counted. Are you counting "1" for elbow joint or "2" (since they are paired)? Are you counting "3" for each elbow joint since there are three named subdivisions? If you think that's a headache, try to enumerate the intercarpal joints! Some questions are best left unasked because the answers are just plain messy.

Artificial (prosthetic) joints have been developed to replace severely arthritic or traumatized ones in certain locations. Prosthetic hips and knees were developed first and tested on dogs and monkeys. Artificial joints for several other areas soon followed. Made of high quality stainless steel, titanium, and wear resistant plastics, they are relatively expensive and fraught with numerous post-surgical complications including infection, rejection, loosening, and fatigue/failure. Nonetheless, they have been very beneficial to many recipients—tremendously increasing the quality of their lives. The surgical procedures involved in their installation are complex and frequently performed by teams of orthopedic specialists who may do only one or a few specific types of joint replacement. Recipients of prosthetic joints are in accord with their proclamation that to be able to move again with little or no pain is worth the surgery—even if the device must be replaced.

One of the areas in which the *Nomina Anatomica* has some serious deficits is in the nomenclature of joints. The mandibular symphysis and manubriosternal symphysis normally become synostotic and the xiphisternal synchondrosis sometimes does, as well. The costochondral joints are really synchondroses and the sacro-iliac joint has a symphytic portion. The classification of joints is even more seriously bobbled in many intermediate level anatomy/physiology texts by authors determined to use a functional taxonomy based on the movement allowed by a given articulation. They throw "amphiarthrosis"—a term that not even the most respected medical dictionaries can agree on—into the mix for "slightly moveable" joints and confuse the whole taxonomic scheme. Some try to redeem themselves by presenting an anatomical classification as well as a functional classification. This esoteric approach has nothing to recommend it and is undermined by the fact that some fibrous joints have more motion than some synovial joints. Taxonomy should serve science—not confuse it—and flawed taxonomy deserves the delete key!

Slang and Obsolete Nomenclature

UNOFFICIAL TERM	OFFICIAL DESIGNATION
proximal tibiofibular joint	tibiofibular joint *[articulatio tibiofibularis]*
distal tibiofibular joint	distal part of tibiofibular syndesmosis *[syndesmosis tibiofibularis]*
medial collateral ligament (knee jt.)	tibial collateral ligament *[ligamentum collaterale tibiale]* of knee joint
lateral collateral ligament	fibular collateral ligament *[ligamentum collaterale fibulare]* of knee joint
patellar tendon	patellar ligament *[ligamentum patellae]*
round ligament of the femoral head	ligament of the femoral head *[ligamentum capitis femoris]*
compound joint	composite joint *[articulatio composita/complexa]*
peg joint	gomphosis *[gomphosis]*
"yes" joint	atlanto-occipital joint *[articulatio atlanto-occipitalis]*
"no" joint	atlanto-axial joint *[articulatio atlanto-axialis]*
ACL	anterior cruciate ligament *[ligamentum cruciatum anterius]* of knee joint
PCL	posterior cruciate ligament *[ligamentum cruciatum posterius]* of knee joint
MCL	tibial collateral ligament *[ligamentum collaterale tibiale]* of knee joint
LCL	fibular collateral ligament *[ligamentum collaterale fibulare]* of knee joint
tibiotalar joint	talocrural joint *[articulatio talocruralis]*
TM joint (TMJ)	temporomandibular joint *[articulatio temporomandibularis]*

Review Questions

1. In a lateral subluxation of the cubital joint...
   A. the proximal end of the humerus is located lateral to the proximal ends of the radius and ulna.
   B. the distal ends of the radius and ulna are located medial to the humerus.
   C. the joint is medial to its normal position.
   D. the joint is lateral to its normal position.
   E. the proximal ends of the radius and ulna are lateral to the distal end of the humerus.

2. A typical thoracic vertebra articulates with the bodies of _______ other vertebra, with the tubercles of _________ ribs, and with the heads of _________ ribs.
   A. 2—4—2
   B. 1—2—4
   C. 2—2—4
   D. 1—4—2
   E. 3—2—4

3. Which of the following is part of every synovial joint?
   A. articular cartilage
   B. intracapsular ligament(s)
   C. articular menisci
   D. three or more bones
   E. bursae
   F. articular disc

4. Which of the following statements is incorrect?
   A. Articular menisci and articular discs are fibrocartilaginous structures that fill the incongruencies of some synovial joints.
   B. Elevation of the medial border of the foot (with the lateral border still on the floor) results in a motion called inversion.
   C. The applied force in most lever systems of the human body is supplied by muscle contraction or by gravity.
   D. In second class lever systems, the resistance is always located between the applied force and the fulcrum and this system always gains mechanical advantage.
   E. Choose this response if all of the above (A-D) are correct.

5. Using the moment arm equation, determine the resistance in a lever system at equilibrium if the applied force is 50 pounds, D_R is 5 inches, and D_F is 15 inches.
   A. 16.7 pounds
   B. 15 pounds
   C. 25 pounds
   D. 167 pounds
   E. 150 pounds
   F. 70 pounds

6. Which item is false?
   A. There are three types of cartilage in the body but only two types (subtypes) of cartilaginous joints.
   B. Synovial joints always allow more motion than synarthroses.
   C. Articular cartilage is lubricated and nourished by synovial fluid.
   D. Synostosis is a bony union created when skeletal components are united by osseous tissue.
   E. The skeletal components of fibrous and synovial joints are united (joined) by connective tissue proper.

7. Find the mismatch (joint—type of uniting tissue—shape category of the skeletal components).
   A. costotransverse joint—c.t. proper—flat and irregular
   B. intervertebral symphysis—fibrocartilage—irregular and irregular
   C. radiocarpal joint—fibrous connective tissue—long and short
   D. tibiofibular syndesmosis—c.t. proper—long and long
   E. pubic symphysis—fibrocartilage—irregular and irregular
   F. squamous suture—connective tissue proper—flat and flat

8. Find the correct match.
   A. lordosis—posture characterized by exaggeration of the thoracic curvature of the vertebral column
   B. arthritis—inflammation of a joint
   C. synostosis—fibrous fusion of a joint
   D. arthrotomy—joint luxation
   E. moment arm equation—velocity of superior limb motion divided by the length of its osseous components

9. Find the false statement.
   A. Flexion of the elbow occurs when the flexor angle at the cubital joint decreases.
   B. Rotation of the vertebral column occurs when left or right movement (around the long axis of the body) occurs primarily at the zygapophyseal joints.
   C. Adduction of the inferior limb at the hip joint occurs when the free part of the inferior limb is moved (at the hip joint) toward the median plane.
   D. Retraction of the mandible occurs when the mandible is moved posteriorly at the temporomandibular joint.
   E. Eversion of the foot occurs when the lateral border of the foot is elevated.

10. Find the incorrect statement.
   A. Syndesmoses, gomphoses, and sutures are all synarthroses.
   B. If the posterior cruciate ligament of the knee joint is ruptured, the femoral condyles can be moved (displaced) a few millimeters posteriorly relative to the tibial condyles.
   C. Plantar flexion of a tarsal joint implies the same motion as extension of a tarsal joint.
   D. A joint is being extended if its flexor angle is getting larger.
   E. We are usually shorter in the evening due to compression of the intervertebral discs while sitting or standing during the day.

Thought Questions

1. There is hyaline cartilage in synovial joints and hyaline cartilage in synchondroses. How are the two different?

2. Which sutures of the head have names that cannot be directly related to the names of the involved bones?

3. Why are *mandibular symphysis* and *costochondral joint* misnomers?

4. Which collateral ligament is most likely to be torn by the buckling motion caused by a heavy, medially directed blow to the lateral side of the knee?

5. Which specific type (not general category) of joint is least common in the body?

6. What is the difference between an intervertebral disc and an intervertebral symphysis?

7. What is the difference between the antebrachial interosseous membrane and the radio-ulnar syndesmosis?

8. The amount of direct, articular cartilage-to-articular cartilage contact between the femoral and tibial condyles is not significantly altered by surgical removal of a meniscus. Why?

9. Synovial joints subjected to traumatic incidents often become painfully swollen. This is due to hypersecretion of synovial fluid by the synovial membrane. Since articular cartilage is avascular and aneural, what causes the pain?

10. Why do injuries to tendons and ligaments often take longer to heal than fractured bones?

11. Can joints be "broken" (like bones)?

12. Why are surgeries involving prosthetic joint components so expensive?

13. What color (black, white, gray) do the images of cartilaginous structures typically appear on a developed radiograph?

14. Why is only a small amount of fibrous connective tissue found in sutures?

15. Which joints can normally be hyperextended (in most people)? What is meant clinically by *hyperextension?*

16. Name the six bones with which a typical thoracic vertebra forms synovial joints.

17. The sternocostal joints involving the costal cartilages of which pair of ribs typically occur at the level of the sternal angle (manubriosternal joint)?

18. Why are there only three intermetacarpal joints but four intermetatarsal joints?

19. How many intervertebral discs should be present in a vertebral column if none are found above/below the atlas and none occur within or inferior to the sacrum?

20. Explain why, in a *lateral subluxation of the elbow joint,* the distal humerus is somewhat *medial* to its proper position on the radius and ulna.

21. What does an epiphyseal cartilage have in common with an intervertebral disc and the antebrachial interosseous membrane?

Answers to Clinical Case Studies

Case 1—This anterior/posterior instability, called the drawer sign, is diagnostic for rupture of the anterior cruciate ligament (ACL). This intracapsular ligament angles anteriorly from its origin in the intercondylar fossa of the femur bone to its insertion in the anterior intercondylar area of the tibia. Its disruption allows the tibia to be shifted anteriorly about 1.0 cm relative to the distal femur bone. Other structures that are commonly injured whenever the ACL is ruptured include the tibial ("medial") collateral ligament and the medial meniscus of the genual joint.

Case 2—Narrowed disc spaces occur when the nucleus pulposus bulges or ruptures out of the anulus fibrosus. Either of these conditions can put pressure on the spinal nerves as they leave the spinal cord. This pressure could explain the patient's weakness and tingling sensations.

Case 3—Immobilization of a joint for several months will result in ankylosis (bony fusion/synostosis). In this case, the orthopod noted the multiple fractures of bones at the ankle region and elected to allow the ankle to fuse rather than try to repair numerous fractures that would probably result in an arthritic joint. Given the options of producing a stiff, painless joint or a painful one that could be moved, the choice was easily made.

Answers to Review Questions

1. E. "Lateral" refers to the relative position of the distal skeletal component (radius and ulna) to the proximal component (humerus).

2. C.

3. A. B. through F. occur in *some* (but not all) synovial joints.

4. E.

5. E.

6. B. Compare the radio-ulnar syndesmosis (some motion) to the interchondral joints (very little motion).

7. E. The pubis is a flat bone.

8. B.

9. B. The motion (rotation) occurs primarily at the intervertebral symphyses.

10. B. The tibia can be displaced posteriorly, so the femur bone "moves" anteriorly.

Answers to Thought Questions

1. Synchondroses (hyaline cartilage joints) are so named because the hyaline cartilage physically unites the skeletal components. In synovial joints the skeletal components are physically united by fibrous connective tissue and the hyaline cartilage that is present (articular cartilage) forms smooth bearing surfaces for the articulation.

2. Sagittal, lambdoid, squamous, and coronal sutures. The names of the other 29 cranial sutures can be related to the names of the involved bones. (See Table 7-2).

3. The mandibular symphysis is synostotic and the costochondral joint is a synchondrosis.

4. Tibial ("medial") collateral ligament.

5. Syndesmosis—only three pairs of these occur. They are located between the radius and ulna, tibia and fibula, and between the stapes and temporal bone.

6. Intervertebral symphysis is the name of the fibrocartilaginous joint between the bodies of two adjacent vertebrae. The structure that occurs there to physically unite the bones is the intervertebral disc.

7. The antebrachial interosseous membrane is the specific name for the heavy sheet of fibrous connective tissue that unites the radius and ulna (side-to-side) to form the radio-ulnar syndesmosis.

8. The menisci fill in the "gaps" between the edges of the articular surfaces but they are not physically interposed between the bearing surfaces.

9. Stretch receptors in the joint capsule are responsible for pain sensations. Often, when a swollen joint is drained by removing excess synovial fluid, the pain subsides (at least temporarily, until the joint swells again).

10. Bones have a greater blood supply.

11. No. Joints are typically said to be luxated or subluxated but not "broken." Physicians do speak of fractures through epiphyseal cartilages.

12. The devices themselves, fashioned of very high quality stainless steel, are very expensive to manufacture. Their research and development budgets and clinical trials in dogs or other animals often cost millions of dollars. Installation may require a team of surgical specialists.

13. Black. Cartilage is not mineralized and so it is relatively radiolucent (meaning that it does not stop the x-ray beam).

14. The contours of the edges of the articulating bones fit together so well that little connective tissue is needed to bind the bones together.

15. Carpal joints (radiocarpal joint), metacarpophalangeal joints, tarsal joints, metatarsophalangeal joints, joints of the vertebral column. Clinical hyperextension implies traumatic injury associated with forcing a joint into a (hyper) extended position.

16. The vertebrae above and below (zygapophyseal joints) and four ribs (heads of all four and tubercles of two of them).

17. Those of the second ribs.

18. The first metacarpal bone is positioned far enough from the second one that no intermetacarpal joint occurs between them.

19. 23.

20. Directional terms applied to the description of a luxation/subluxation indicate the relative position of the *distal* skeletal component(s) at the dislocation. In this case, the distal skeletal components (radius and ulna) have been displaced *laterally* and so the distal humerus must be *medial* to its proper position relative to them. The term *subluxation* implies a partial (incomplete) dislocation.

21. All three structures stabilize the skeletal components in the joints where they are found. An epiphyseal cartilage "glues" an epiphysis to a diaphysis to form a sychondrosis in a growing bone. An intervertebral disc "glues" the bodies of two adjacent vertebrae together to form an intervertebral symphysis. The antebrachial interosseous membrane stabilizes the adjacent bodies of the radius and ulna to form the radio-ulnar syndesmosis. Other structures that fulfill a homologous role include the crural interosseous membrane and the interpubic disc. On the other hand, articular discs and menisci do not physically join (unite) the skeletal components in their parent joints and, thus, do not fulfill this same role.

CHAPTER 8 Skeletal Myology/Muscular Systems

Chapter Outline and Key Concepts

INTRODUCTION

Skeletal muscles are organs, but skeletal muscle tissue is one of the three types of muscle tissue.
About half of the body mass is composed of skeletal muscles.

FUNCTIONS OF SKELETAL MUSCLES

When they contract, various skeletal muscles are involved in locomotion, posturing, respiration, prehension, mastication, deglutition, orifice closure (and opening), the abdominal press, vocalization, eye movement, and venous return.
Heat production is a by-product of muscle contraction rather than a primary function.

GROSS STRUCTURE OF SKELETAL MUSCLES

The two major parts of a skeletal muscle are the belly and tendinous attachments.
Tendons occur in two forms: bands of c.t. proper ("regular" tendons) and flat sheets of c.t. proper (aponeuroses).
Origin refers to the attachment at the less moveable end of the muscle belly and insertion is the attachment at the more moveable end.
Connective tissue proper encasements called epimysium, perimysium, and endomysium surround whole muscle bellies, groups of muscle cells (fascicles), and individual muscle cells, respectively.

ACCESSORY STRUCTURES ASSOCIATED WITH SKELETAL MUSCLES

Deep fascia binds groups of muscle bellies together.
Retinacula hold (bind) tendons into certain loci.
Bursae (partially) and tendon sheaths (totally) surround tendons and protect them from frictional degradation.
Sesamoid bones act as bearing surfaces for the tendons of a few muscles.

MUSCLE MICROSTRUCTURE AND CONTRACTION

Muscle cells (myocytes, myofibers) shorten (contract) when contractile proteins slide together (interdigitate) lengthwise.
The cytoplasmic organelles of contraction are called myofibrils and they contain the contractile proteins (thin and thick myofilaments).
The myofilaments are arranged (stacked) in the myofibrils in a very organized fashion in skeletal and cardiac muscle cells which produce histological cross striping termed striations (bands).
The dark (A) bands are produced by the stacks of thick myofilaments (myosin).
The lighter stained spaces between the A bands are called I bands.
Several other histological landmarks are present (Z line, H band, M line).
A functional subunit of a myofibril extending from one Z line to the next one is called a myomere ("sarcomere").

MUSCLE ACTIONS AND INTERACTIONS

The action of a muscle is the potential movement that may occur when the muscle contracts.
Some muscles have only one stated action, others have two or more.
When a muscle contracts, there may be no movement, the stated action, or the opposite (antagonistic) action.
Muscles with the same stated actions are synergists and those with opposite actions are antagonists.
A fixator muscle is one that is antagonistic to one or more actions of a multi-actioned muscle.

CONTROL OF MUSCLE ACTIVITY

Skeletal muscles are under direct voluntary control of the CNS.
A motor unit is one motor neuron and all of the

skeletal muscle cells that it supplies.

Motor units vary in size from a few muscle cells (precise control muscles) to hundreds of muscle cells (muscles with less precise control).

MUSCLE NOMENCLATURE

Terms used to name muscles are descriptive and are reflective of the muscle's shape, size, fiber orientation, action, location in the body, number of subdivisions, attachments and/or the part of the body acted upon.

MAJOR GROUPS OF SKELETAL MUSCLES

There are about 600 skeletal muscles in the human body (most are paired).

The seven major groups of muscles are muscles of the head, neck, back, thorax, abdomen, superior limbs, and inferior limbs.

MUSCLES OF THE HEAD

The muscles of the head are divided into six groups: muscles of the face, eye, auditory ossicles, mastication, tongue, and palate/fauces.

MUSCLES OF THE NECK

Muscles of the neck are divided into six groups: suboccipital, suprahyoid, infrahyoid, pharyngeal, and laryngeal muscles plus an unnamed group.

MUSCLES OF THE THORAX

The 11 muscles of the thorax are not subdivided into groups.

MUSCLES OF THE ABDOMEN

The muscles of the abdomen include those that form the anterior, lateral, and posterior abdominal walls as well as those forming the pelvic and urogenital diaphragms.

MUSCLES OF THE BACK

These muscles act primarily to bend the vertebral column and can be divided into an epaxial group (behind the transverse processes of the vertebrae) and a hypaxial group (in front of the latter).

MUSCLES OF THE SUPERIOR LIMB

The muscles of the superior limb can be divided into six groups: those of the shoulder/scapula, anterior brachium, posterior brachium, anterior antebrachium, posterior antebrachium, and manus (three subgroups).

MUSCLES OF THE INFERIOR LIMB

The muscles of the inferior limb can be divided into nine groups: three groups of hip muscles (anterior, posterior, medial), three groups of thigh muscles (anterior, posterior, medial), anterolateral muscles of the crus, posterior muscles of the crus, and muscles of the foot (three subgroups).

DEVELOPMENT OF SKELETAL MUSCLES

Skeletal muscles develop from various portions of the mesoderm.

The central part of the mesoderm divides to form over 40 block-like segments called somites.

Muscle cell precursors called myoblasts develop in parts of the somites called myotomes.

CLINICAL CONSIDERATIONS

Paralysis of muscles results from loss of innervation.

Muscles undergo hypertrophy when exercised and atrophy when they are not utilized.

Muscle cramps are involuntary painful contractions related to electrolyte imbalances.

Selected Definitions

A bands (anisotropic bands)—the darker of the microscopically observable, alternating dark and light striations across myofibrils. The A bands represent those areas where thick myofilaments are located.

Action—the potential motion(s) associated with the muscle contraction. When a muscle contracts, this motion may or may not occur (depending on opposing forces).

Antagonist—a muscle that has an opposing action to another muscle. When a given body motion occurs, the opposite can be effected by antagonists, gravity, or elastic recoil.

Belly of a muscle—the contractile part of a skeletal muscle. It is attached to other structures by tendons at each end and is sometimes divided into named subparts.

Epimysium—the outer connective tissue proper encasement of a skeletal muscle. At the ends of a muscle belly, epimysium condenses with the ensheathments formed by perimysium (around muscle fascicles) and endomysium (around individual muscle cells) to form the tendons of the muscle.

Fascicle—a small bundle of muscle, nerve, or tendon fibers. *Dorland's Medical Dictionary* has over 80 entries under *fasciculus* and the majority of them are named fiber tracts in the CNS.

Fixator—a muscle whose action is antagonistic to one or more actions of a multi-actioned muscle. Fixators are contracted to "limit" or "select" certain actions of multi-actioned muscles by negating (neutralizing) one or more of their unwanted actions.

I bands (isotropic bands)—the lighter of the microscopically observable, alternating dark and light striations across a myofibril. I bands occur between the A bands in those loci where the central parts of thin myofilaments are not overlapped by thick myofilaments.

Innervation—the nerve supply of a muscle or another body structure. Knowledge of the nerve supply of body structures has numerous clinical applications.

Insertion (termination) of a skeletal muscle—the site of attachment of the more moveable end of a skeletal muscle. In the limbs, the insertion is typically at the distal site of attachment.

Locomotion—body movement. Most locomotion is effected by contraction of skeletal muscles, but gravity and elastic recoil also play a role.

Motor unit—a motor neuron plus the group of skeletal muscle cells that are innervated by it. Skeletal muscles contain many motor units which vary in size from small ones (involving a few muscle cells) to large ones (involving a few hundred muscle cells).

Myofiber—a muscle cell (myocyte, muscle fiber). The contraction of an individual muscle fiber is "all or none".

Myofibril—a contractile organelle found in the cytoplasm of a muscle cell. The strength of contraction of a given muscle cell is related to the number of myofibrils that it contains.

Myofilament—a proteinaceous contractile element found within a myofibril. Two major myofilaments are recognized: thick myofilaments composed primarily of myosin, and thin myofilaments composed mainly of actin (along with significant amounts of troponin and tropomyosin).

Origin of a muscle—the site of attachment of the less moveable end of a skeletal muscle. In the limbs, the origin is always the proximal site of attachment.

Retinaculum—a band of connective tissue that courses transversely across one or more tendons to hold (bind) them in a certain location. Retinacula, ligaments, and tendons are similar structurally and they vary mainly in locus and function.

Synergist—a muscle that has the same action as another muscle. To effect a given motion, several synergists typically contract simultaneously.

Synovial bursa—a fluid-filled structure, similar to a synovial joint capsule, located between a bony prominence and the tendon or belly of a muscle. Functionally, a synovial bursa reduces frictional degradation as the muscle moves reciprocally over the prominence.

Synovial tendon sheath—a synovial "bursa" that completely envelopes a tendon. It has the same function as a bursa.

Tendon—the fibrous connective tissue structure found at each end of a skeletal muscle belly. It is the non-contractile part of a muscle which attaches the belly to other structures (bone, cartilage, or another muscle).

Etymology ***Quod erat faciendum*—"We have done the work we were required to do."**

agonista (L), *combatant*—agonist
ancon (L), *elbow*—anconeus muscle
aponeurosis (G), *to pass into a tendon*—epicranial aponeurosis
corrugatus (L), *to wrinkle*—corrugator supercilii muscle
hallux (L), *big toe*—m. adductor hallucis
hypo (L), *under, beneath*—hypothenar eminence
masticatus (L), *to gnash the teeth*—mastication
opponeus (L), *to oppose*—opponens pollicis muscle
platysma (G), *flat piece, plate*—platysma
deglutitus (L), *to swallow down*—deglutition muscle

pollex (L), *thumb*—m. opponens pollicis
thenar (L), *palm of hand*—thenar muscles
gemellus (L), *twin*—m. gemellus superior

Table 8-1 Tissues Found in a Skeletal Muscle

Type	*Location*
Skeletal muscle tissue	belly of the muscle
Connective tissue proper	tendons and ensheathments
Smooth muscle tissue	within the walls of blood vessels
Epithelium	lining the lumina of blood vessels
Nervous tissue	nerve fibers supplying the muscle
Blood	within the blood vessels of muscles

Introduction

Skeletal myology is the study of skeletal muscle tissue as well as the study of the voluntary (skeletal) muscles of the body. These are the muscles that are involved in body support and movement. As a group, the skeletal muscles comprise the muscular system which is one of the seven somatic body systems. The **muscular system** is the largest body system and forms nearly half of the body weight. Skeletal muscle is one of the three types of muscle tissue and, like smooth and cardiac muscle, it develops from the middle embryonic germ layer (mesoderm). The named skeletal muscles of the body are organs because they are composed of several tissues in addition to skeletal muscle (Table 8-1). In fact, the relationship between skeletal muscle tissue and named skeletal muscles (like the biceps brachii muscle) is the same as that between bone tissue and a named bone such as the humerus.

Objectives

1. Differentiate skeletal muscle tissue from skeletal muscles (which are organs) by listing the tissues present in any skeletal muscle.

Functions of Skeletal Muscles

The most obvious functions of skeletal muscles involve locomotion and posturing. **Locomotion** encompasses all aspects of body movements, but in its more limited sense it can be considered to be the grossly observable motions of the head, neck, trunk and/or limbs. **Posturing** involves the maintenance of body position in spite of gravitational or other extrinsic forces. In addition to these roles, skeletal muscles function in respiration, digestion, orifice opening and closure, the abdominal press, vocalization, eye movements, venous return, and heat production. In **respiration**, the increase in size of the thoracic cavity caused by contraction of the diaphragm (a skeletal muscle) and some of the other thoracic muscles produces a partial vacuum in the pleural cavities that results in inspiration. Relaxed expiration is largely a passive process, but forced expiration involves an abdominal press. Skeletal muscles have several minor roles in digestion including the locomotor aspects of **prehension** (getting food and drink into the oral cavity), **mastication** (chewing it) and **deglutition**

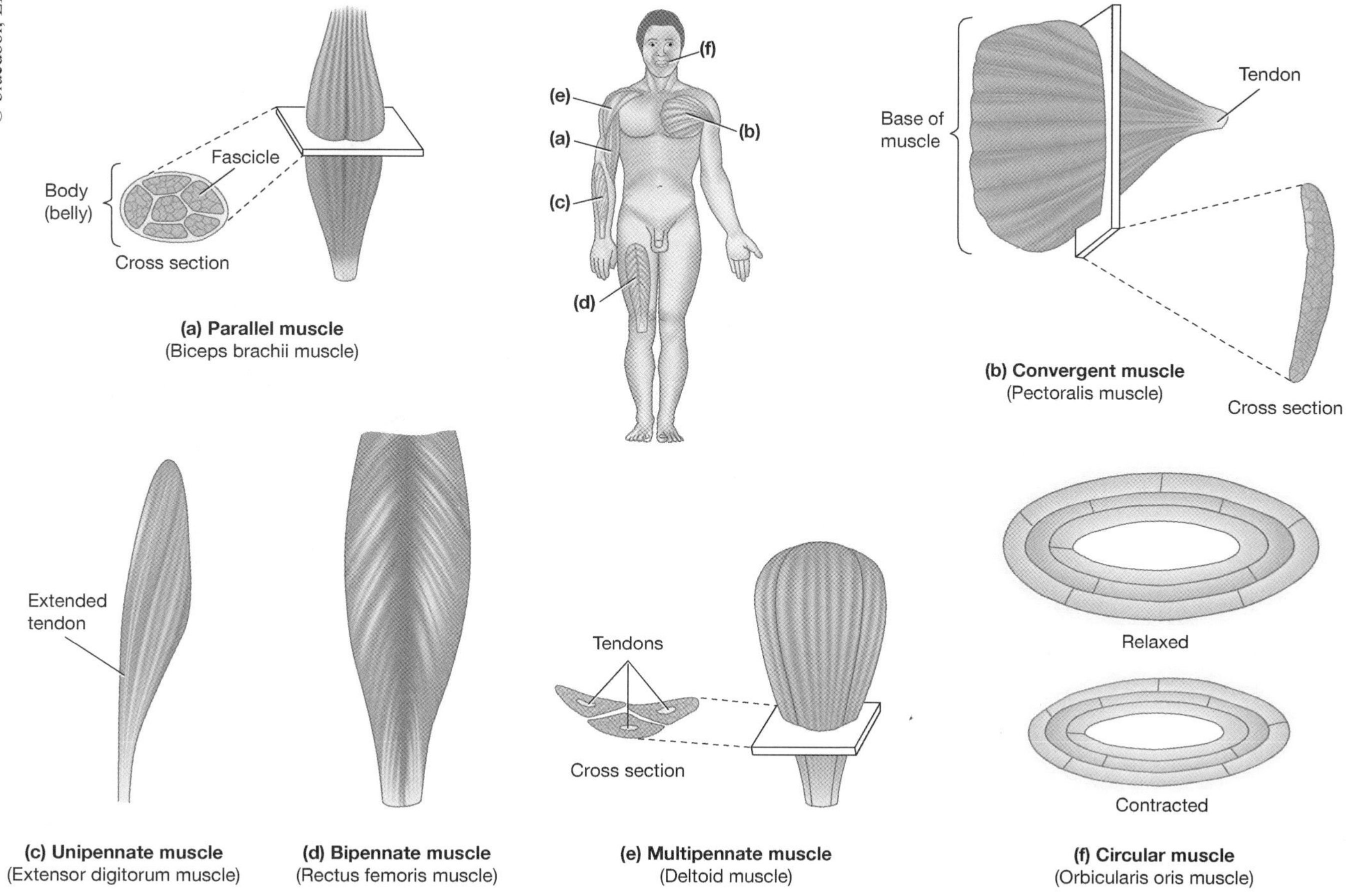

Figure 8-1

Various Configurations of Skeletal Muscle Cells Within Muscle Bellies

Contraction of muscles pulls the attachments closer to each other except for sphincter (circular) muscles where it decreases the diameter of the openings that the muscles surround.

(swallowing). At the other end of the alimentary canal, fecal excretion is partially controlled by the external anal sphincter muscle. This function (**orifice closure**) is also exhibited by skeletal muscles surrounding the mouth and each eye. The **abdominal press** involves contraction of the diaphragm and the muscles forming the abdominal wall to increase the pressure within the abdominal and thoracic cavities. This is useful in vomition, defecation, parturition, urination (hurried), as well as in coughing, sneezing, and forceful expiration. **Vocalization** involves contraction of several small skeletal muscles associated with the larynx to vary the tension on the vocal folds as well as their position relative to each other and to the airstream that passes between them. Vocalization also requires at least some contraction of the diaphragm (the verbal encouragement required to get children to clean up their rooms may need to be delivered with full blown abdominal presses!). **Eye movements** are controlled by several small skeletal muscles that anchor each eyeball into its orbit. These are capable of highly controlled, coordinated contractions that allow the visual axes to be precisely directed. The role of skeletal muscles in **venous return** is a passive one and does not play a major role in cardiovascular physiology. Contraction of muscles in the limbs assists movement of blood through the appendicular veins simply by squeezing on them in those loci where the veins are sandwiched

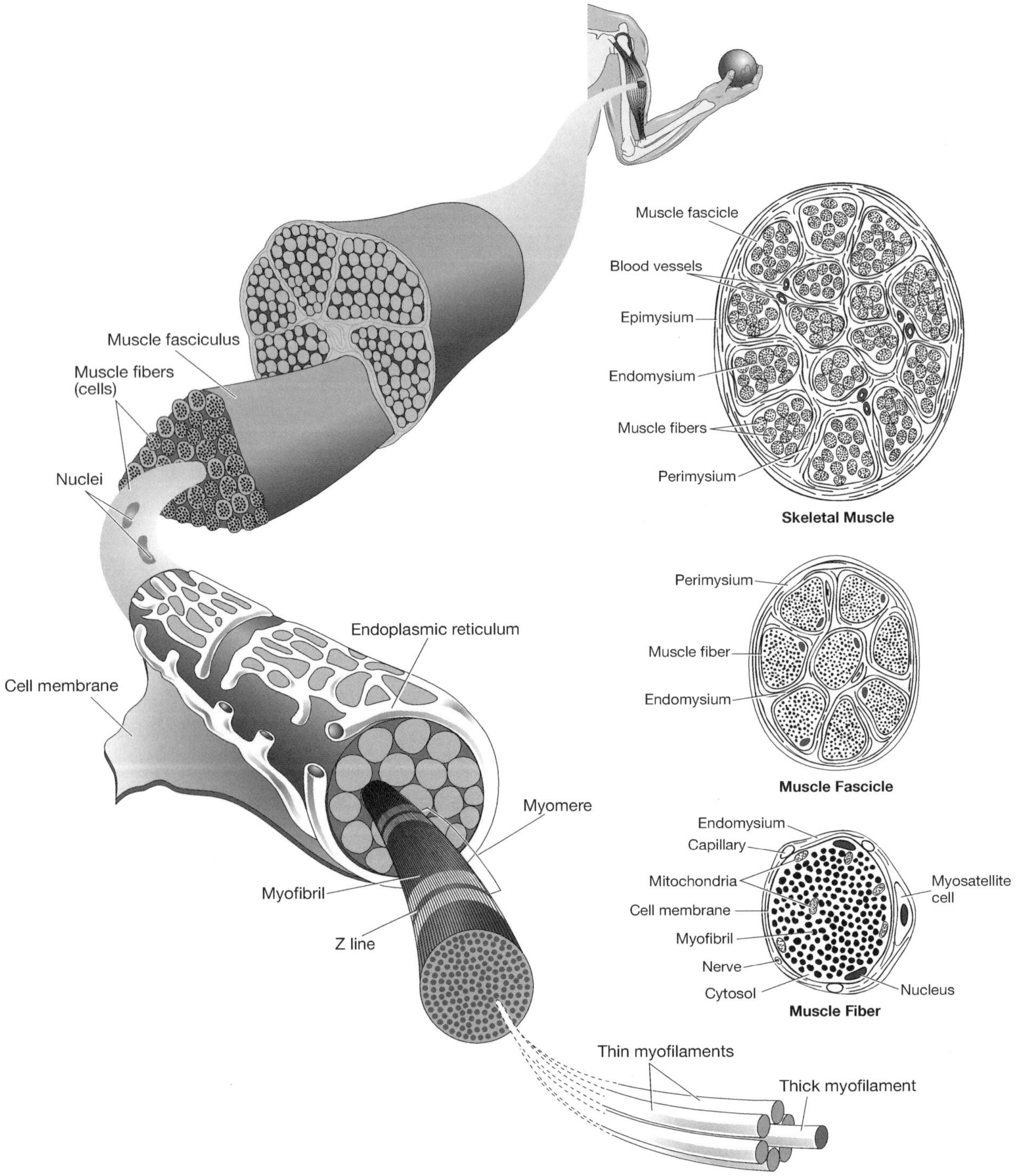

Figure 8-2

Skeletal Muscle Structure

Individual skeletal muscle cells are called muscle fibers or myocytes. They contain specialized cytoplasmic organelles called myofibrils and the latter contain myofilaments made of myosin and actin (and other proteins). Myosatellite cells are fibrocyte-like cells that form the endomysium around individual muscle cells.

between muscle bellies. Because these veins have valves that prevent backflow, this pressure forces blood to flow in one direction (back toward the heart). The role of skeletal muscles in **heat production** is sometimes overemphasized. Most assuredly, skeletal muscles produce heat when they contract. Whether this should be considered as a function, *per se*, of skeletal muscles is philosophically debatable. Quadriplegics are able to maintain their body temperature without the use of a significant portion of their skeletal muscle mass. On the other hand, shivering (uncontrolled contraction/relaxation of skeletal muscles) is a physiologic mechanism used by the body in its attempts to prevent or reverse hypothermia.

Objectives

2. List the various functions which skeletal muscles perform in the body.

Gross Structure of Skeletal Muscles

A typical skeletal muscle consists of a contractile portion called the **belly** and fibrous connective tissue attachments called **tendons**. The bellies of skeletal muscles have a variety of shapes including fusiform (spindle-shaped), triangular, and quadrate (four-sided). Muscles described as sphincter muscles (*external anal sphincter m.*) or orbicular muscles (*orbicularis oris m.*) encircle openings. Muscles having bellies in which the muscle cells angle into their tendons and resemble the feathers of birds are described as pennate muscles and include unipennate (half of a feather), bipennate (a whole feather) and multipennate (several feathers) (Figure 8-1).

Most tendons occur in the form of rope-like bands (cords) of connective tissue proper. In some cases, tendons are so short that the muscle belly appears to be directly anchored to bone via a so-called "direct" or "fleshy" attachment. Some bellies attach by broad, sheet-like tendons termed **aponeuroses**.

A few skeletal muscles do not attach to skeletal components, or do so only indirectly (*orbicularis oris, external anal sphincter, etc.*). Regardless of specific conformation (tendon, aponeurosis), the attachment of a muscle belly to the more fixed part of the skeleton (*i.e.,* the less moveable end of a muscle belly) is termed the **origin**. Conversely, the **insertion** is the attachment at the moveable end of a muscle belly. Skeletal muscles with more than one origin are said to have multiple **heads**. These may blend into a common belly or may remain separate throughout most or all of their length. When it remains unclear which end of a muscle moves more or less than the other, the terms *origin* and *insertion* are often ignored and the more generalized term (**attachments**) may be used.

Skeletal muscle bellies are ensheathed in a fibrous connective tissue covering termed **epimysium**. Thin partitions termed **perimysium** extend inward from the epimysium and segment the muscle cells into groups termed **fasciculi** or **fascicles** (Figure 8-2). In transverse sections of muscles, several gradations of perimysium can be seen ranging from those which are relatively thick and surround large groups of fibers to much thinner ones which envelope smaller fascicles. Delicate, fibrous connective tissue septae, continuous with the perimysium, envelope each individual muscle cell and are termed **endomysium**. All three of these ensheathments (epimysium, perimysium, endomysium) serve as avenues of penetration for nerves and vessels. They are continuous with each other and merge near the ends of the belly to form the tendons and aponeuroses by which bellies are attached.

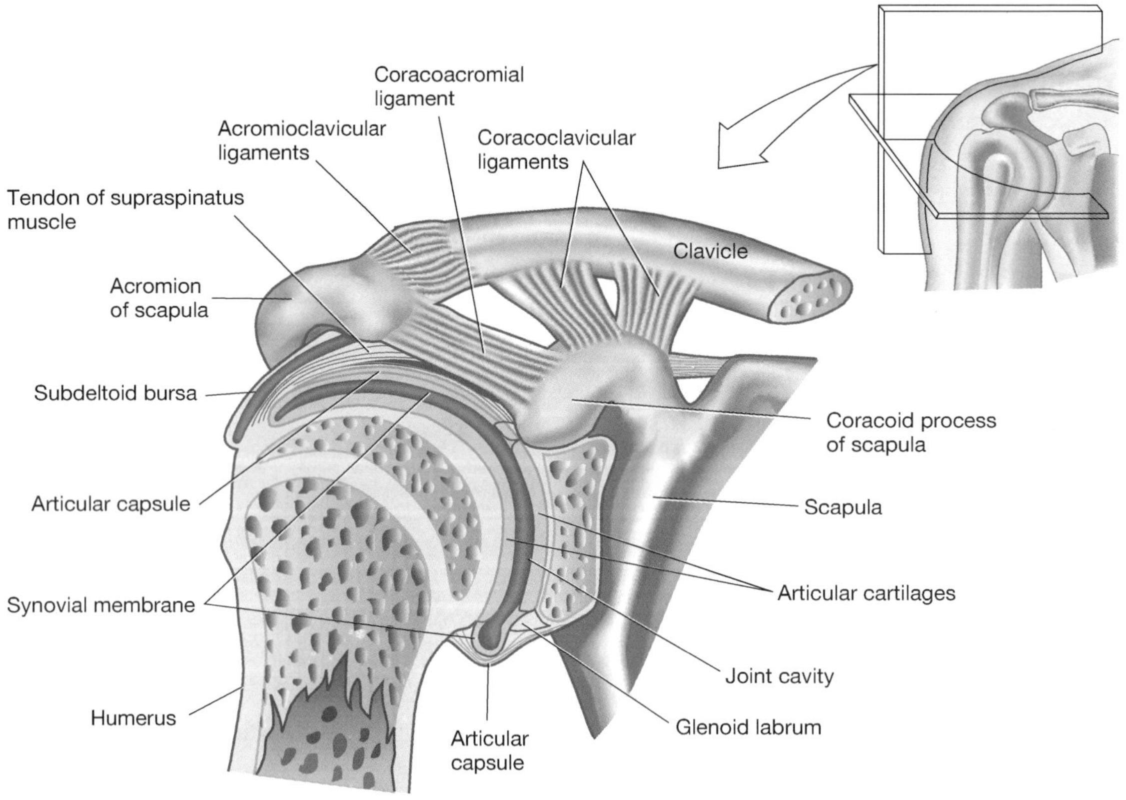

Figure 8-3

Structure of Tendon Sheaths and Bursae

A bursa is a synovial fluid-filled sac that protects a tendon from an adjacent bony prominence (see upper part of diagram). A tendon sheath is structurally and functionally similar to a bursa except that it completely encapsulates a tendon.

Objectives

3. Define the following as they relate to skeletal muscle structure: belly, tendon, aponeurosis, origin, insertion, epimysium, perimysium, endomysium, and fascicle.

Accessory Structures Associated with Skeletal Muscles

There are a number of structures that are closely associated with skeletal muscles but are not parts of them. These include fascia, retinacula, bursae, and tendon sheaths. **Fascia** is the irregular collagenous connective tissue proper that bonds the skin to the underlying musculature, binds muscles into groups, and serves as an avenue of penetration for vessels and nerves. That which is directly under the skin is called **superficial fascia** (**hypodermis**, **subcutaneous tissue**). Its fibers are usually loosely packed. The **deep fascia** which surrounds groups of muscles has densely packed, irregular fibers and is continuous with the epimysium of each muscle.

Retinacula are bands of dense regular collagenous connective tissue that bind tendons into groups and hold them in certain locations. Structurally, they are similar to ligaments, both in composition and in their "bone-to-bone" attachments. The **carpal flexor retinaculum**, for example, encloses the carpal groove formed by the carpal bones to form the **carpal canal** through which the tendons of the digital flexor muscles pass at the wrist.

Bursae are synovial fluid-filled sacs that are structurally similar to joint capsules (they have a fibrous outer layer and a synovial membrane lining). Bursae occur between tendons and adjacent bony prominences where they cushion (protect) the tendons and reduce sliding friction. Some bursae are continuous with joint capsules and others have no connection to them. Bursae that completely surround tendons and form closed, fluid-filled encapsulations are called **tendon sheaths** (Figure 8-3). Many of the tendons near the wrists and ankles are encased in tendon sheaths.

Even **sesamoid bones** can be considered to be accessory structures of skeletal muscles since they serve as bearing surfaces and protect tendons from frictional degeneration. The patellae are the largest sesamoid bones and are embedded in the tendons of the quadriceps femoris muscles. The pair of sesamoid bones at the base of each thumb are embedded in the tendons of the flexor pollicis brevis muscles. The pair at the base of each big toe is located in the tendons of the flexor hallucis brevis muscles.

Objectives

4. Explain how each of the following relate to or interact with skeletal muscles: fasciae, retinacula, bursae, tendon sheaths, and sesamoid bones. Name the three muscles whose tendons usually contain sesamoid bones.

Muscle Microstructure and Contraction

Muscle contraction involves the sliding together (interdigitation) of linear filaments composed of the contractile proteins actin and myosin. This process is called the **sliding filament mechanism** and is essentially identical in all three types of muscle tissue. To comprehend how contraction occurs, the microstructure of the contractile components of muscle cells must be understood.

Individual **myocytes** (muscle cells) are also called **myofibers** (muscle fibers)(Figure 8-4A, B). This usage of the term *fibers* (meaning muscle *cells*) should be differentiated from nerve fibers (referring to nerve cell *processes*) and from collagenous, elastic, and reticular fibers (which refer to extracellular proteinaceous strands). The cell membrane of a myocyte is called myolemma (formerly "sarcolemma"). The cytoplasm contains numerous specialized organelles called **myofibrils**. Each myofibril is an elongated cylinder that contains the rod-like contractile structures called **myofilaments**. These consist of thinner proteinaceous filaments composed primarily of **actin, troponin,** and **tropomyosin** and thicker proteinaceous filaments composed primarily of **myosin**. The filaments are arranged in partially overlapping alternating "stacks" throughout the length of each myofibril. This alternating arrangement imparts the striated (striped) appearance to skeletal and cardiac muscle cells because the thicker (myosin) filaments stain more darkly than the thinner (actin) filaments. Smooth muscle cells do not appear striated because the myofibrils in their cytoplasm are less neatly arranged. Consequently, the stacks of thick and thin filaments in adjacent myofibrils are staggered (*i.e.*, they are not in register).

Electron microscopy has been used to demonstrate the details of the striations. The dark cross bands produced by the thick myofilaments polarize visible light and are designated as **A (anisotropic) bands**. The light cross bands extend from the edge of one stack of thick filaments (myosin) to the edge of the next stack of myosin. They are called **I (isotropic) bands** because they do not polarize visible light. Some individuals use the memory aid: A (d<u>a</u>rk) and I (l<u>i</u>ght). The I bands contain only the thinner (actin) myofilaments but it should be noted that the thin filaments extend (overlap) partially into A band regions. These areas of overlap occur at each end of the A bands and cause the ends of each A band to stain somewhat more darkly than its central region. The lighter central region of each A band consists of thick filaments only and is designated as the **H band**. In its very center is a darker transverse line called the **M line**. This is caused by cross linking proteins that bind the thick filaments together and keep them in proper alignment. The center of each I band is crossed by a similar dark band called the **Z line** formed by cross linking proteins that bind the thin myofilaments together. The basic unit of skeletal muscle microstructure from Z line to Z line is called a **myomere**.

When contraction occurs, a nervous impulse causes electrochemical changes in the actin and myosin which make them electrostatically attractive to each other and they slide together (interdigitate) in the same manner that the tines of forks can be interdigitated. This occurs throughout the length of each myofibril and results in the overall shortening of the muscle cell. It should be obvious from a study of Figures 8-4A, 8-4B that the A band does not get shorter as a muscle cell contracts but the I band, H band, and the distances between adjacent Z lines and M lines do get narrower. A given muscle cell is either contracted or relaxed at any given moment. Differences in the strength of contraction of a whole muscle result from different numbers of muscle cells contracting.

Objectives

5. Differentiate myofiber, myofibril, myofilament, and myomere.
6. Schematically represent the arrangement of the thick and thin myofilaments in a myofibril and indicate what causes the A band, I band, H band, M line, and Z line.
7. State which ultrastructural features get shorter during contraction.

Muscle Actions and Interactions

The stated **action** of a skeletal muscle is the *potential movement* that contraction of that muscle evokes. Some muscles can cause only one particular movement while others have two or more stated actions. Each action can be logically deduced from the position of muscle attachments. The *biceps brachii muscle*, for example, has three actions: flexion of the elbow joint, supination of the antebrachium, and flexion of the shoulder joint. Flexion of the elbow joint is easily understood because the muscle crosses the anterior aspect of the elbow joint. Supination can be explained by careful examination of the position of its insertion on the radial tuberosity. Because the radial tuberosity projects somewhat medially from the radial body, the tension produced by the biceps brachii muscle pulls (rotates) it anteriorly resulting in lateral rotation (supination) of the antebrachium. Flexion of the shoulder joint is possible because the biceps brachii crosses the anterior aspect of the shoulder joint to attach to the scapula. Since it bridges (crosses) the anterior aspect of the shoulder joint, it can cause the humerus to rotate anteriorly about the shoulder joint (flexion of the shoulder joint). It should be understood that when a muscle contracts, three possibilities exist

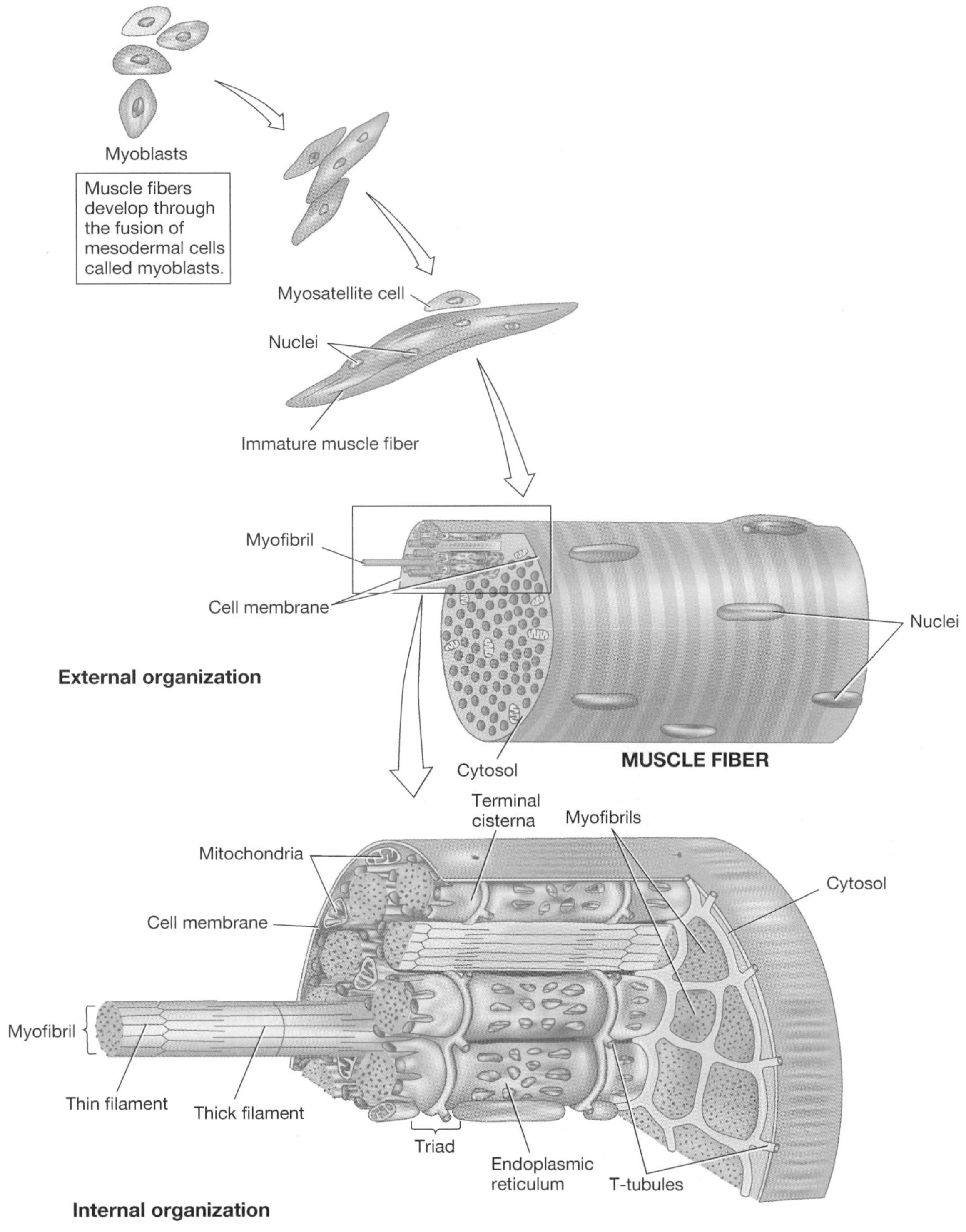

Figure 8-4A

Microstructure of Skeletal Muscle Tissue

Each skeletal muscle cell (= myocyte = myofiber) is multinucleated and contains contractile organelles called myofibrils in its cytoplasm ("sarcoplasm"). The myofibrils contain thick and thin contractile proteins collectively called myofilaments (*see Figure 8-4B*).

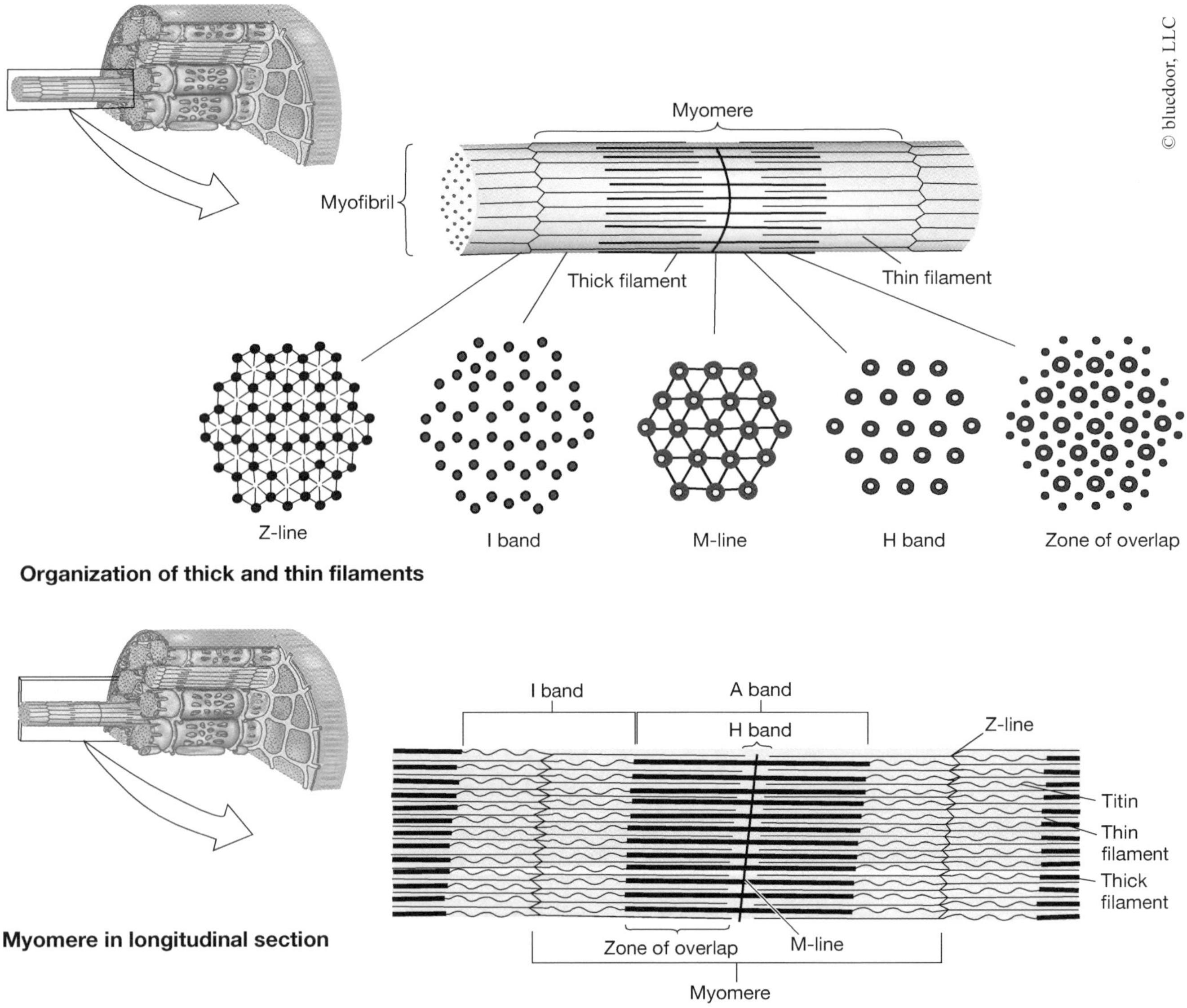

Figure 8-4B

Ultrastructure of a Skeletal Muscle Myofibril

Part of one myofibril is shown with the thick myofilaments (myosin) represented in the transverse section below as the bigger dots and the thin myofilaments shown as the smaller dots. The dark (A) bands occur where the thick myofilaments are located and they are separated by intervening light (I) bands (where no thick myofilaments are present). Cross linking proteins cause the Z line in the center of each I band and the M line in the center of each A band to stain more darkly than the adjacent areas. The H band is a somewhat lighter staining area in the central section of each A band where no overlapping thin myofilaments occur.

in regard to its stated action: (1) no movement, (2) the movement described by its stated action, (3) the *opposite* movement from its stated action. No movement occurs if contraction produces insufficient force to overcome the resistance. In fact, the opposite (antagonistic) motion can occur if the resistance is larger than the applied force. Theoretically, if a muscle spans (crosses) a joint, it can act on that joint. However, in some cases the action is so minimal that it is inconsequential.

Table 8-2 Categories of Terms Used in Skeletal Muscle Nomenclature

Category	Terms			
Configuration	trapezius rhomboideus teres splenius	pyramidalis serratus pterygoideus platysma	gracilis triangularis semitendinosus semimembranosus	longissimus scalenus piriformis quadratus
Size	maximus minimus	magnus vastus	major minor	longus brevis
Fiber Orientation	transversus rectus	obliquus orbicularis	longitudinalis verticalis	sphincter angularis
Action	flexor extensor adductor abductor	supinator pronator rotator levator	depressor opponens constrictor tensor	corrugator masseter compressor erector
Position	superficialis profundus medialis lateralis	superior inferior anterior posterior	externus internus dorsales palmares	plantares medius latae frontalis
Number of Parts	biceps triceps	quadriceps digastricus	gemelli multifidi	tertius unipennatus
Location	subcostalis abdominis thoracis cervicis temporalis pectoralis	anconeus peroneus articularis lumborum subclavius latissimus	interossei pharyngeus radialis tibialis laryngeus epicranius	articularis intercostalis popliteus mentalis interspinalis ulnaris
Attachments	deltoideus hyoideus puborectalis supraspinatus	infraspinatus subscapularis iliocostalis thyrohyoideus	iliococcygeus sternothyroideus sternohyoideus zygomaticus	geniohyoideus omohyoideus coracobrachialis tympani
Part of Body Acted Upon	digiti pollicis hallucis capitis carpi	labii auricularis oculi oris palatini	buccinator ani glossus spinalis nasalis	femoris brachii colli stapedius urethrae

Note: Many of the names in this table could be placed in another category with equal logic. This is especially true of the position, location, and attachment groups.

Muscles rarely act individually to effect a given body movement. Instead, whole groups of muscles contract simultaneously. Muscles which have the same action (as each other) are said to be **synergists** and those with opposing actions are called **antagonists**. These are relative terms and depend on the particular point of reference (agonist). An **agonist** can be any muscle that is contracting. Muscles with the same action as the agonist are then designated as synergists and those with opposing actions are antagonists. When muscles contract, they attempt to pull their points of attachment closer together. **Multi-actioned muscles** (those with more than one stated action) cannot intrinsically single out one or another of their actions. For example, when the *biceps brachii muscle* contracts, it "attempts" to pull its attachments (radial tuberosity and the scapula) closer together. This may result in the movement related to one, two, or all three of the possible actions of the biceps brachii. The reason that all three of the actions may not occur is that the force of contraction may be insufficient to cause movement, or contraction of other muscles may oppose (neutralize) one or two actions. Other muscles which can contract to reduce or prevent one or more actions of a given muscle (while allowing other actions of the muscle to occur) are said to be fixators. **Fixators** can be defined as antagonists to one or more actions of multi-actioned muscles. Their net effect is to reduce or limit selected actions of multi-action muscles in certain situations. For example when the *biceps brachii* is contracted to flex the elbow joint, simultaneous contraction of antebrachial pronators is needed to prevent supination of the antebrachium. The pronators would be acting as fixators in that instance. A given muscle may act as an agonist in one situation and function as a synergist, antagonist, or fixator in other situations. It should be noted that not all body movement is produced by muscular contraction. Gravity and elastic recoil of certain body components (that have been stretched) can also produce body movement.

Objectives

8. Define the action of a skeletal muscle and state three things that can happen when a muscle contracts.
9. Define and properly use the terms agonist, synergist, antagonist, and fixator.
10. Explain why single-actioned muscles can be fixators but cannot have fixators.
11. State two things that can produce body movement besides muscle contraction.
12. Explain why some muscles can have only one stated action whereas others can have two or even more actions.

Control of Muscle Activity

Skeletal muscles are under the direct voluntary control of the central nervous system. Since they have no inherent contractility, skeletal muscles must be stimulated by nervous impulses each time that contraction is initiated. If the nerve supply to a given skeletal muscle is disrupted, flaccid paralysis and subsequent muscular atrophy occur. Each skeletal muscle cell receives motor innervation from the nervous system. A single motor neuron and the group of myofibers that it controls collectively comprise a **motor unit**. Motor units vary in size from relatively small ones (with only a few skeletal muscle cells) to large ones containing several hundred muscle cells. Smaller motor units are found in those muscles capable of very precise movements (eye muscles), and larger motor units are found in muscles which lack such precise control. The named nerve whose branches supply each skeletal muscle (*i.e.*, the innervation of each muscle) is relatively consistent from one individual to another. This fact is useful clinically in the diagnosis of locomotor deficits.

Objectives

13. Define motor unit and explain why muscles over which we have precise control are composed of small motor units.

Muscle Nomenclature

Like other anatomic nomenclature, the names of muscles have descriptive significance (Table 8-2). There is, however, considerable difference from one muscle to the next in regard to how much and what kind of information that the name imparts. Some muscles have short names that convey only a limited quantity of data. The name of the *zygomaticus* muscles, for example, alludes only to their origin (zygomatic bone). The name of the *sternocleidomastoideus muscle* indicates all of its attachments (sternum, clavicle, mastoid process of the temporal bone). Longer names like *extensor carpi radialis longus muscle* catalogue much more information including action (*extension*), joint acted on (*carpal joint*), location (*adjacent to the radius*), and size (*long*).

Objectives

14. Glean as much information as possible from the name of any skeletal muscle.

Major Groups of Skeletal Muscles

There are approximately 230 named skeletal muscles in the body. Since most of them are paired, and several have named subdivisions, the total number of muscles is about 600. These are divided regionally into seven groups: *muscles of the head, neck, back, thorax, abdomen, superior limb and inferior limb.* The major subgroups within each group will be discussed but it is beyond the intended scope of this text to consider each muscle individually except as presented in Appendix I. In addition to the data presented there (name, origin, insertion, action) a complete description of a skeletal muscle includes innervation, blood supply, shape, and relationships with other structures.

Objectives

15. List the seven major groups of skeletal muscles.

Muscles of the Head

The muscles of the head are divided into six groups: muscles of the face, eye, ear, and tongue, muscles of mastication, and those associated with the palate and gullet (Table 8-3). Relatively few of them can be specifically identified by inspection or palpation. The **muscles of facial expression** include those that are superficially located on the scalp and face (Figure 8-5). Most of them originate from the bones of the skull and insert into subcutaneous tissue of the head. They allow a wide range of non-verbal communications and have protective functions related to the eyes (closing them and squinting). The muscles of facial expression are all supplied by the left and right seventh cranial nerves (facial nerves). Loss of this innervation on one side causes ipsilateral flaccid paralysis (Bell's palsy) which often progresses to a point where the mouth and lips are drawn toward the opposite side by the normal tone and contraction of the contralateral musculature.

The **muscles of the eye** include four rectus muscles (superior, inferior, medial, and lateral), two oblique muscles (superior and inferior), and the *levator palpebrae superioris muscle.* The rectus and

Table 8-3 Muscles of the Head

Muscles of the Face (22)	
m. epicranius	m. depressor anguli oris
m. procerus	m. transversus menti
m. nasalis	m. risorius
m. depressor septi nasi	m. zygomaticus major
m. orbicularis oculi	m. zygomaticus minor
m. corrugator supercilii	m. buccinator
m. depressor supercilii	m. mentalis
m. auricularis anterior	m. levator anguli oris
m. auricularis superior	m. levator labii superioris
m. auricularis posterior	m. depressor labii inferioris
m. orbicularis oris	m. levator labii superioris alaeque nasi
Muscles of the Eye	
m. rectus superior	m. obliquus superior
m. rectus inferior	m. obliquus inferior
m. rectus medialis	m. levator palpebrae superioris
m. rectus lateralis	
Muscles of the Ear	
m. tensor tympani	m. stapedius
Muscles of Mastication	
m. masseter	m. pterygoideus lateralis
m. temporalis	m. pterygoideus medialis
Muscles of Palate and Fauces	
m. levator veli palatini	m. palatoglossus
m. tensor veli palatini	m. palatopharyngeus
m. uvulae	
Extrinsic Muscles of the Tongue	
m. genioglossus	m. chondroglossus
m. hyoglossus	m. styloglossus

oblique muscles direct the visual axis by rotating the eyeball to the left and right and tilting it up and down. The *levator palpebrae superioris muscle* opens the eye by raising (elevating) the superior eyelid. These muscles are supplied by the oculomotor, trochlear, and abducens nerves (cranial nerves 3, 4 and 6). They will be discussed in more detail in Chapter 12.

The muscles associated with the ear include the **muscles of the auditory ossicles** as well as several vestigial intrinsic muscles extending from one part of the ear to the other. These latter muscles are extremely small vestiges which have essentially no real actions, and are not listed in Appendix I. The muscles of the auditory ossicles include only the tiny *tensor tympani muscle* that inserts on the malleus and the diminutive *stapedius muscle* that inserts on the stapes. These muscles reduce the amplitude of vibrations caused by very loud noises (*see Chapter 13*).

The **muscles of mastication** include the *masseter, temporalis, medial pterygoid* and *lateral pterygoid muscles* which are all innervated by branches of the mandibular nerve (a branch of cranial nerve 5) (Figure 8-6). Most of them elevate the mandible, but the lateral pterygoid muscle protracts it. The medial pterygoid muscle moves the mandible laterally in addition to elevating it. The two strongest muscles of mastication are the masseter and temporalis muscles. The *masseter muscle* is easily palpat-

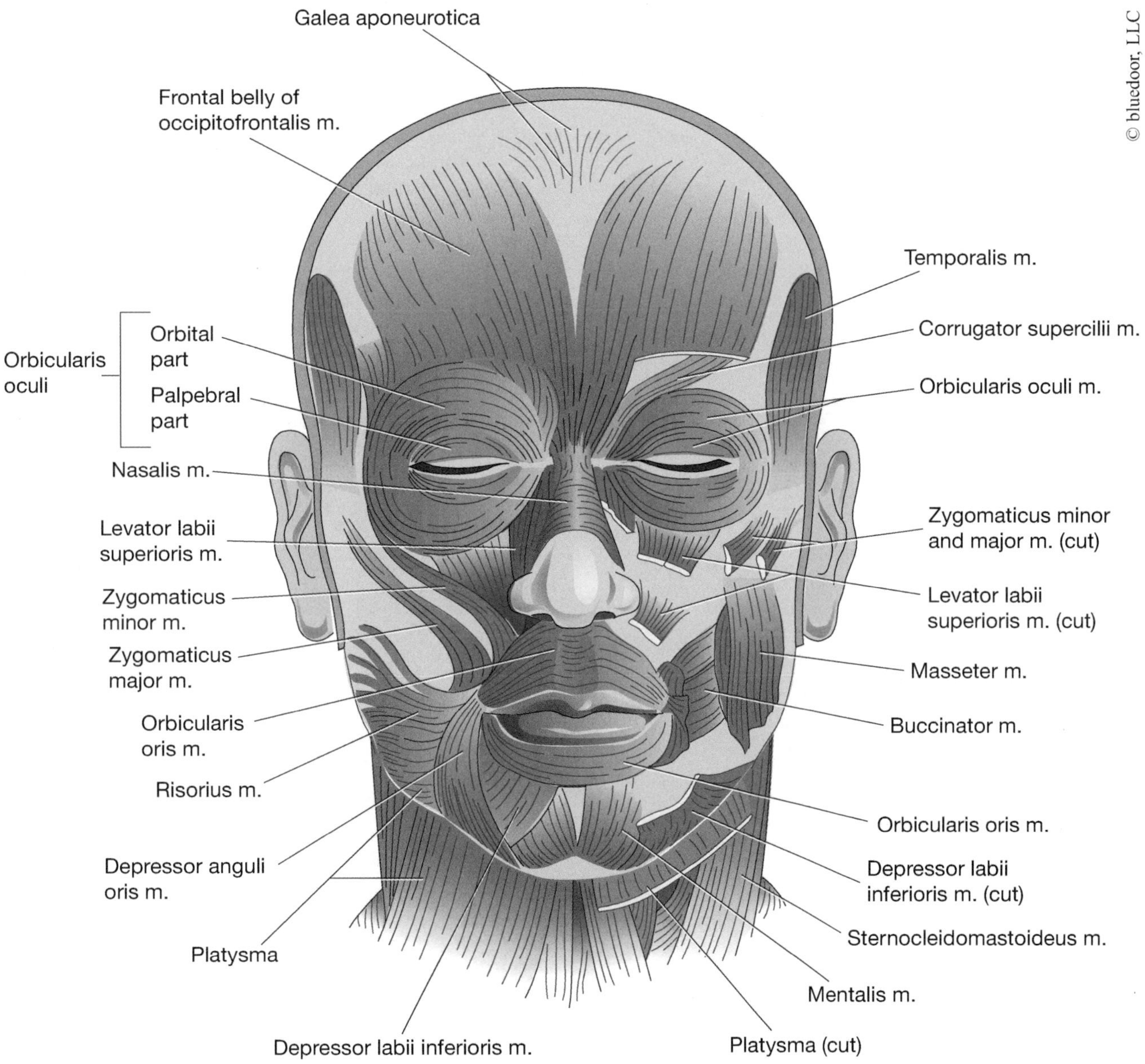

Figure 8-5A
Anterior View of Superficial Muscles of the Head

ed subcutaneously on the lateral side of the mandible near its angle. The *temporalis muscle* occupies the temporal fossa of the skull and can be palpably identified by feeling it tense when the teeth are clenched. The muscles of mastication are the first muscles to become tetanic in the disease caused by the bacterium *Clostridium tetani*. This disease is commonly called "lockjaw" or *tetanus*.

There are eight **muscles of the tongue**. Four of them are intrinsic muscles that are located totally within the tongue. These include *superior* and *inferior longitudinal muscles* as well as *transverse* and *vertical lingual muscles*. The more familiar extrinsic muscles originate on structures outside the tongue and are named accordingly (Appendix I, Part A and Figure 8-7). All of the lingual muscles are supplied by the hypoglossal nerve (cranial nerve 12). Individuals vary considerably in their ability to configure the tongue into specific shapes.

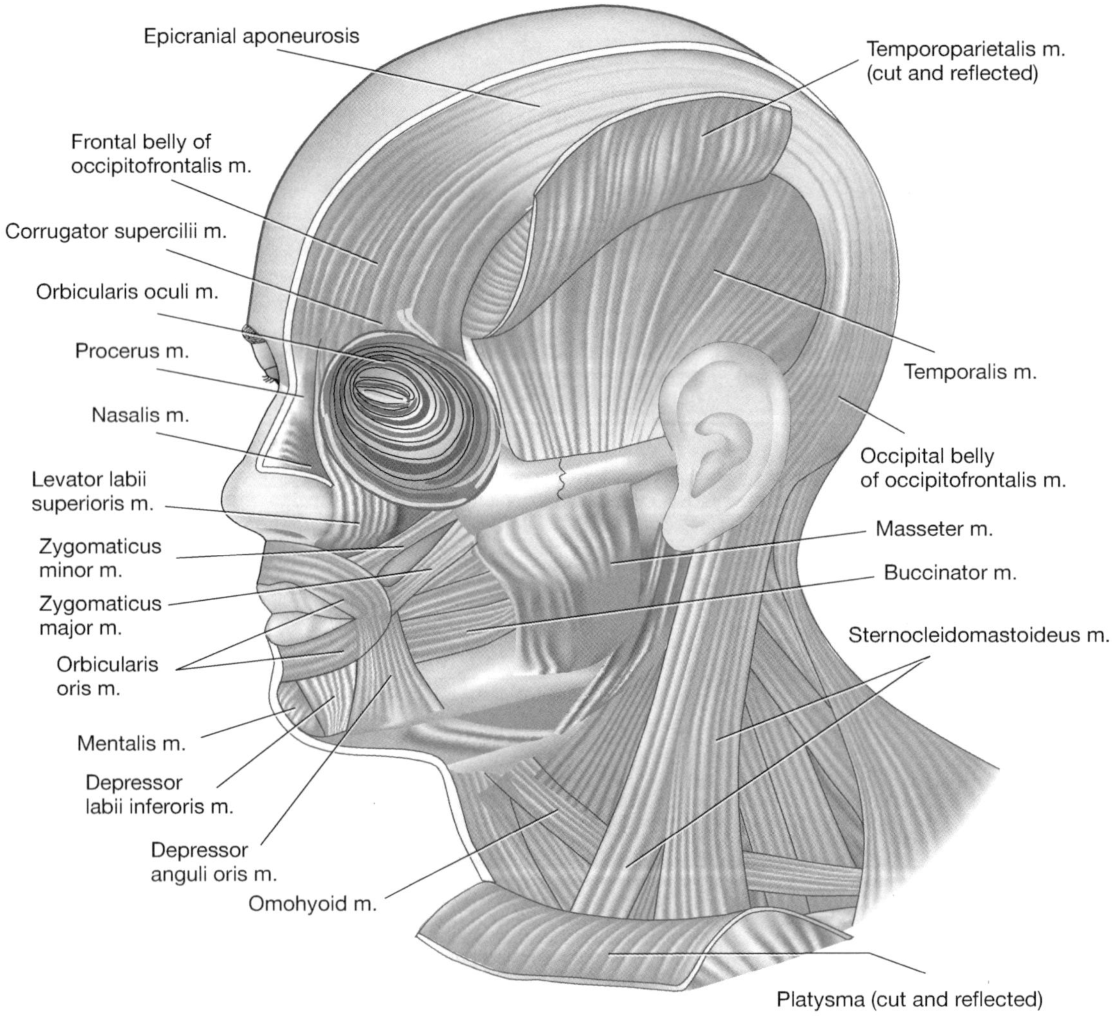

Figure 8-5B

Lateral View of Superficial Muscles of the Head

There are five **muscles of the palate and fauces** (**gullet**). They constrict the isthmus of the fauces during deglutition. Four of them are innervated by branches of the pharyngeal plexus (a network of nerve fibers from cranial nerves 9, 10, and 11) and one (*tensor veli palatini muscle*) is innervated by the trigeminal nerve (cranial nerve 5) (Figure 8-8).

Objectives

16. Divide the muscles of the head into six groups.

Muscles of the Neck

The muscles of the neck can be divided into six groups: suboccipital, suprahyoid, infrahyoid, pharyngeal and laryngeal muscles, as well as an unnamed group that includes the three scalenus muscles, the longus capitis and longus colli, the platysma, and the sternocleidomastoideus muscles (Table 8-4). The **suboccipital muscles** include four *rectus capitis muscles* and two *obliquus capitis muscles.* They are located on the back of the neck below the occipital bone and move the joints of the cervical part of the vertebral column (extension and rotation).

The four **suprahyoid muscles** are positioned above the hyoid bone. All of them can move the hyoid bone (and thus the base of the tongue). The digastricus muscle can also open the mouth by depressing the mandible. The four **infrahyoid muscles** are located below the hyoid bone. They depress the hyoid bone, elevate the larynx, or approximate the hyoid bone to the larynx.

The five **pharyngeal muscles** all have "pharyngeus" in their names. They narrow the pharynx and elevate it as part of the physical process of deglutition. The seven **laryngeal muscles** either move or change the tension on the vocal folds. During vocalization, the folds must be moved toward the median plane (adducted) and during regular respiration they are abducted. When the vocal folds are under greater tension, a higher pitched sound is produced.

The seven remaining muscles of the neck do not have a subgroup designation. They include three *scalenus muscles* (that elevate the ribs), the *longus capitis* and *longus colli* muscles (that rotate and flex the joints of the cervical region), the *platysma*, and the *sternocleidomastoideus muscle* (Figure 8-9). The *platysma* depresses the lower lip (and wrinkles the skin on the anterior cervical region in the process). It is a broad flat muscle whose action on the skin of the neck can be easily demon-

Table 8-4 Muscles of the Neck

Suprahyoid Muscles	
m. digastricus	m. mylohyoideus
m. stylohyoideus	m. geniohyoideus
Infrahyoid Muscles	
m. sternohyoideus	m. sternothyroideus
m. omohyoideus	m. thyrohyoideus
Suboccipital Muscles	
m. rectus capitis anterior	m. rectus capitis lateralis
m. rectus capitis posterior major	m. obliquus capitis superior
m. rectus capitis posterior minor	m. obliquus capitis inferior
Pharyngeal Muscles	
m. constrictor pharyngeus superior	m. stylopharyngeus
m. constrictor pharyngeus medius	m. salpingopharyngeus
m. constrictor pharyngeus inferior	
Laryngeal Muscles	
m. cricothyroideus	m. thyro-arytenoideus
m. crico-arytenoideus posterior	m. arytenoideus obliquus
m. crico-arytenoideus lateralis	m. arytenoideus transversus
m. vocalis	
Other Muscles of the Neck	
platysma	m. scalenus medius
m. longus colli	m. scalenus posterior
m. longus capitis	m. sternocleidomastoideus
m. scalenus anterior	

strated by the facial expression required for a loud scream. The *sternocleidomastoideus muscle* courses obliquely down the side of the neck in an anteromedial direction to attach to the superior aspect of the sternum near the midline. Contraction of the muscle turns the head toward the opposite side. If the left and right muscles contract simultaneously, they cause the head to bow forward (*i.e.*, they flex the joints of the cervical part of the vertebral column). The *sternocleidomastoideus muscle* can be demonstrated by turning the head sharply to one side. This will cause it to stand out from the neck, especially near its sternal attachment.

Objectives

17. Divide the muscles of the neck into six groups.

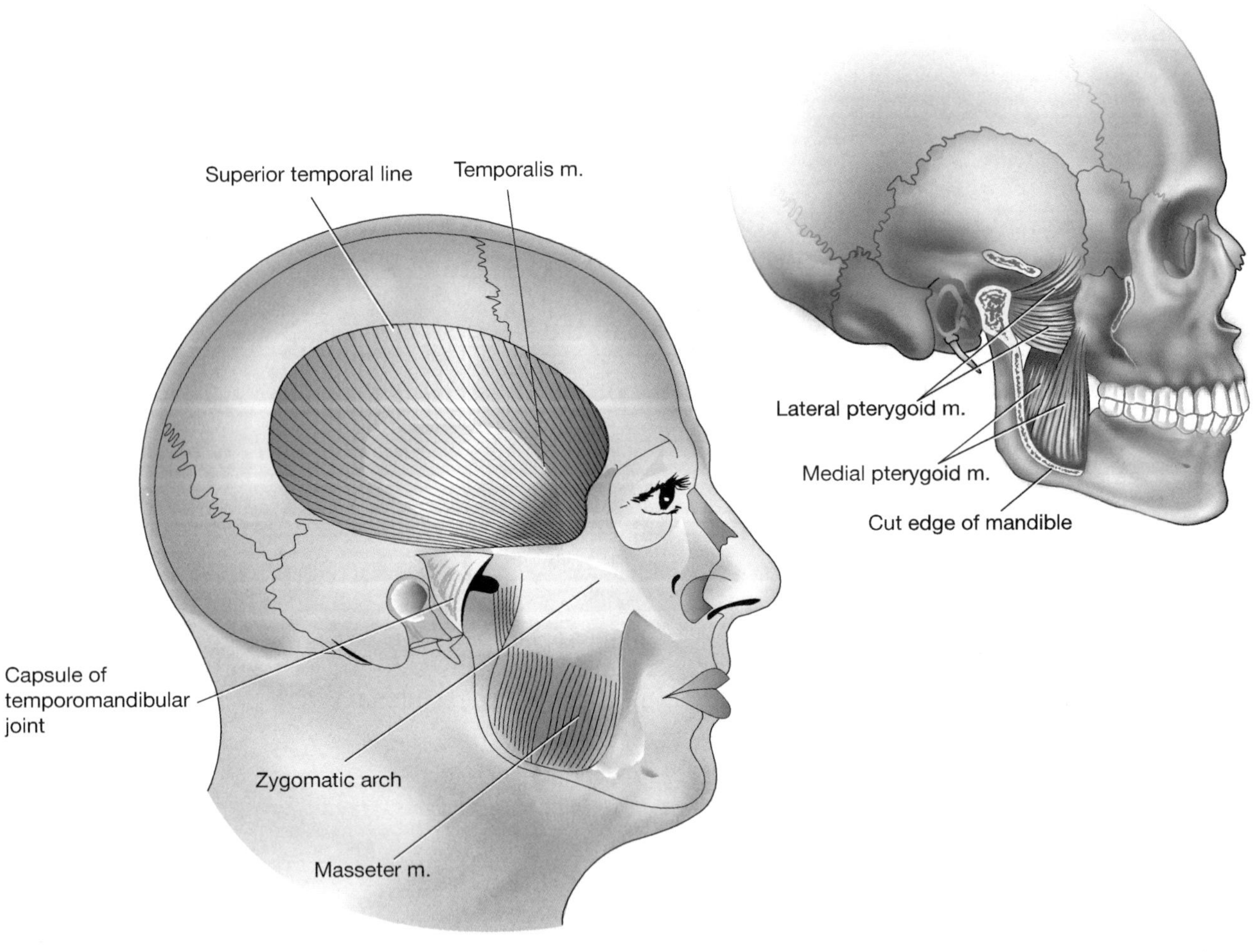

Figure 8-6

Muscles of Mastication (Lateral View)

The deeper (pterygoid) muscles can be observed only after the temporalis and masseter muscles have been removed.

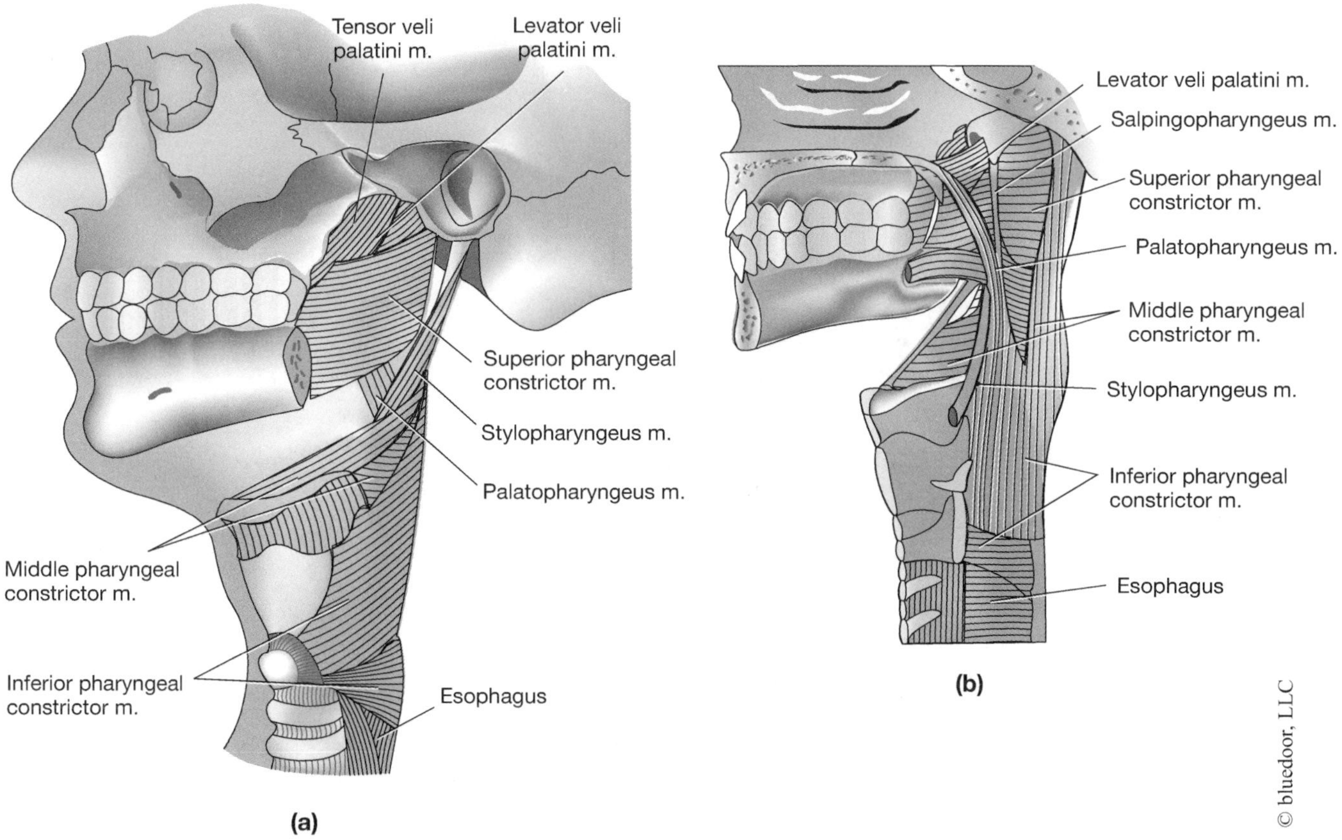

Figure 8-7

Suprahyoid, Infrahyoid, and Pharyngeal Muscles (a) Lateral View (b) Midsagittal Sectional View

Muscles of the Thorax

The 11 muscles of the thorax are not anatomically subdivided into smaller groups (Appendix I, Part C). The largest muscle of the thorax is the *major pectoral muscle* which forms a bulge lateral to the sternum on the anterior aspect of the thorax (Figure 8-10). The major pectoral muscle has three subparts (clavicular, sternocostal, and abdominal parts) named according to their origins. Functionally, it is the most powerful flexor of the shoulder joint. The smaller *minor pectoral muscle* is completely covered by the major one. The *serratus anterior muscle* joins the scapula to the ribs. Its name was derived from the "saw-tooth" appearance of the shape of its costal attachments. The location of the small *subclavius muscle* can be derived from its name. There is a series of *levatores costarum longi muscles* and *levatores costarum breves muscles* which extend inferolaterally from the vertebrae to the ribs. Their action, as implied by their name, is to elevate (raise) the ribs. The *intercostal muscles* are located between adjacent ribs (Figure 8-10). They include external, internal, and intimate groups. These three groups of intercostal muscles draw the ribs closer together. The external intercostals are slanted down and forward as they course from one rib to the next. The internal and intimate intercostal muscles (located deep to the externals) slant down and back from one rib to the next. The *subcostales muscles* are inconstantly present muscle fascicles that resemble the internal intercostals but pass deep to one or more ribs (*i.e.,* they "skip" ribs). The *transversus thoracis muscle* extends from the sternum

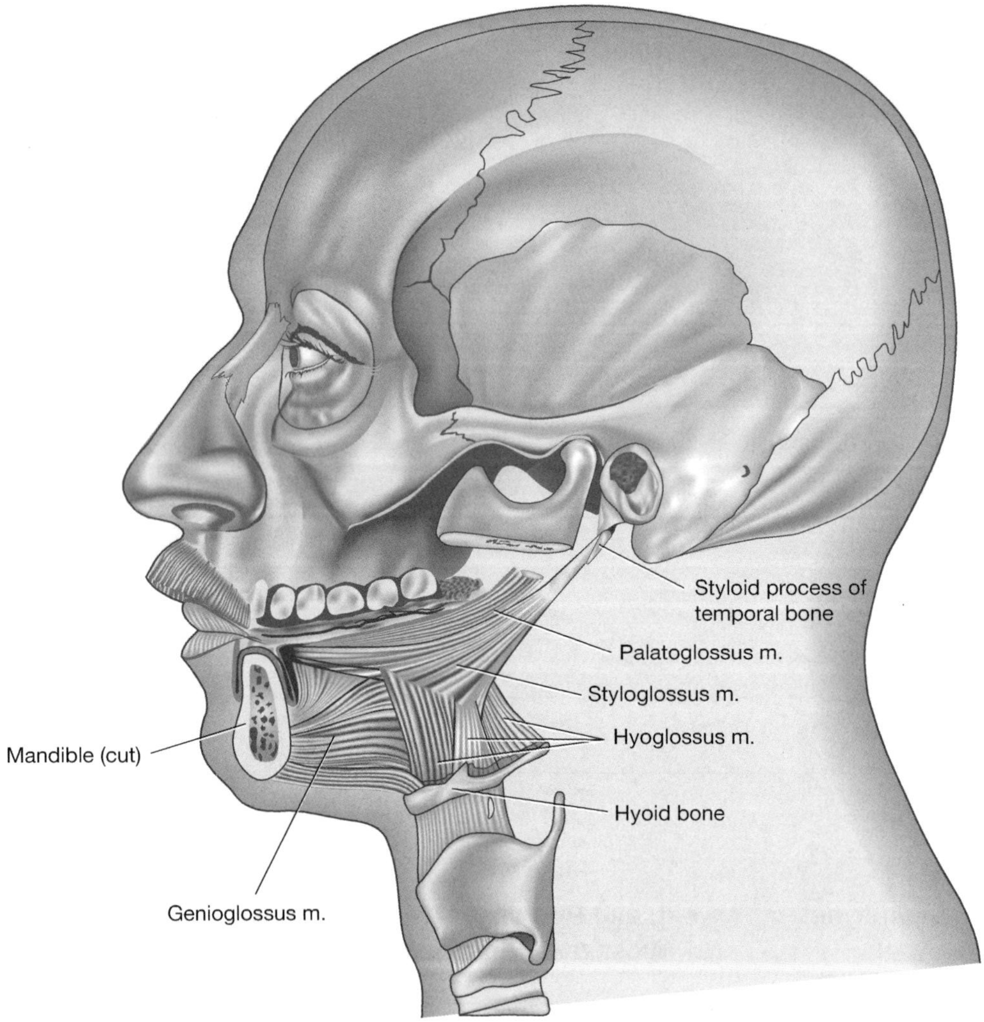

Figure 8-8

Extrinsic Muscles of the Tongue

The tongue contains four intrinsic muscles in addition to these four extrinsic muscles.

to the second through sixth costal cartilages. Its action is to narrow the thorax (*i.e.,* it assists forced expiration). The *diaphragm* is the major muscle of inspiration. It separates the thoracic and abdominal cavities. The diaphragm will be discussed in more detail in chapter 18.

Muscles of the Abdomen

The muscles of the abdomen include the ones that form the anterior, lateral and posterior abdominal wall as well as those which form the *pelvic diaphragm* (*i.e.,* the posterior floor of the pelvic cavity) and the *urogenital diaphragm* (the anterior floor of the pelvic cavity) (Appendix I, part D). The most anterior muscles of the abdominal wall are the strap-like, left and right *rectus abdominis muscles* which extend from the sternum to the pubic bones (Figure 8-11). Their bellies are crossed transversely by *tendinous intersections* which impart a rippled appearance to the anterior abdominal wall

(a)

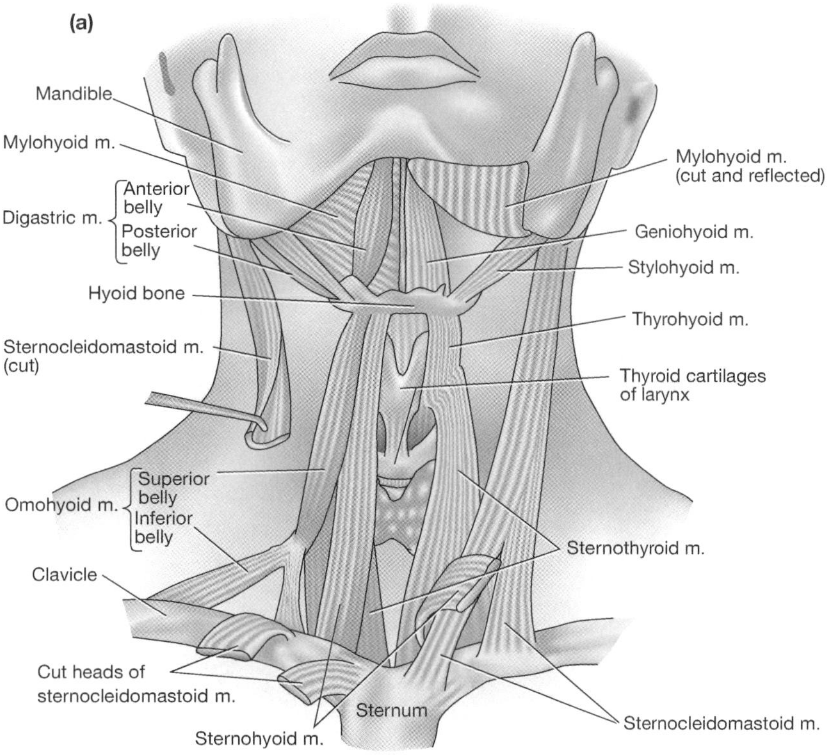

(b)

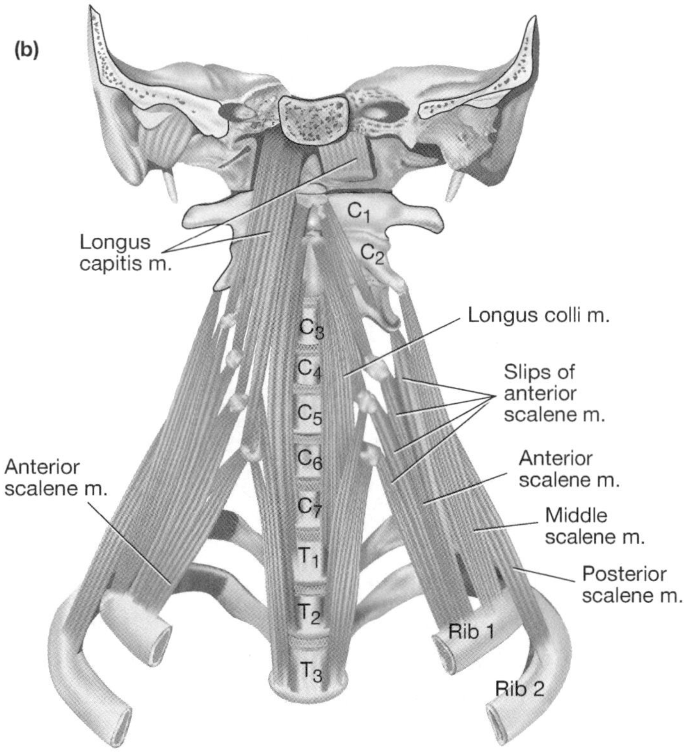

Figure 8-9

Muscles of the Anterior Cervical Region
(a) Superficial Muscles (b) Deep Muscles

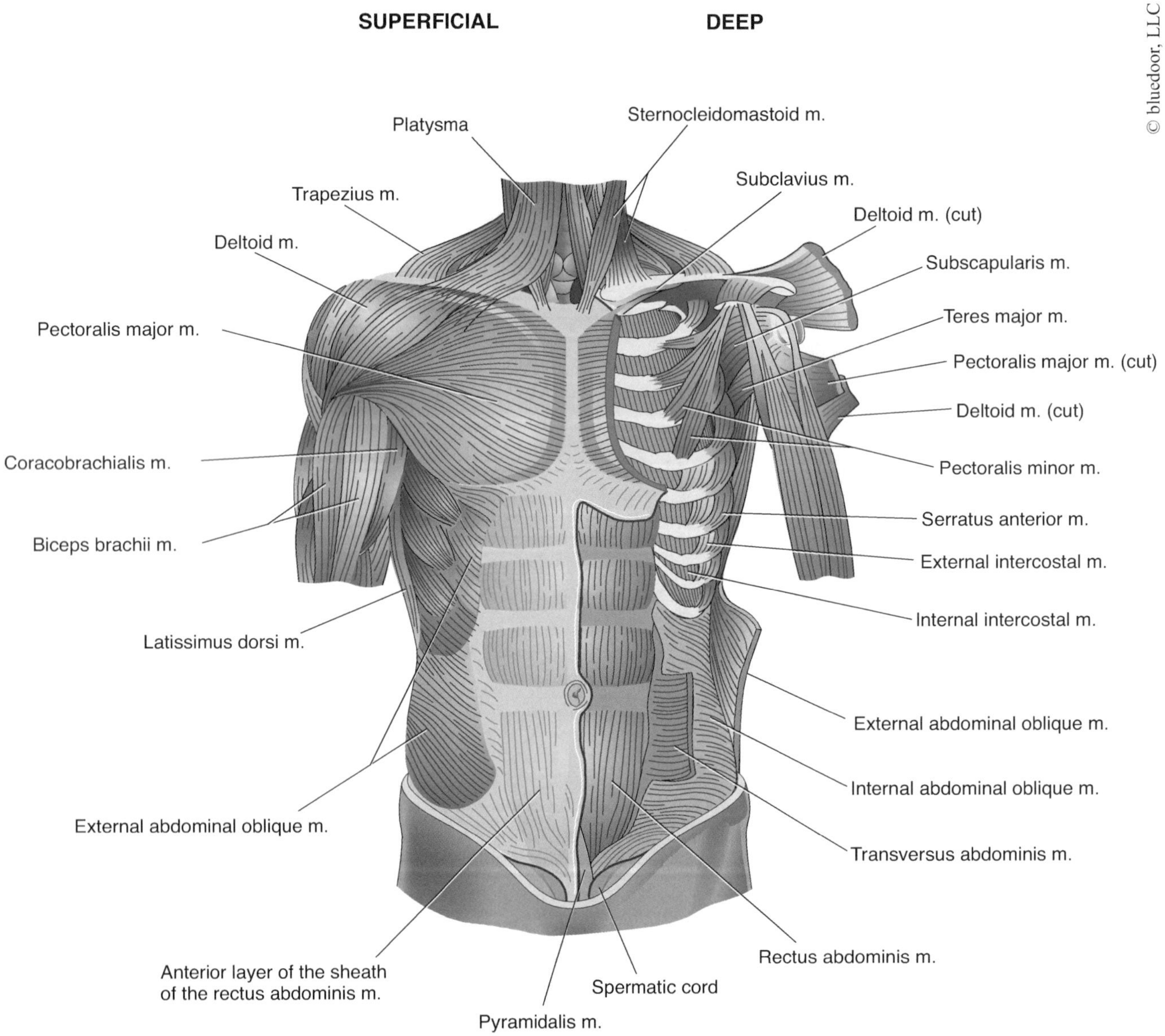

Figure 8-10
Muscles of the Anterior Trunk

in a well-developed individual. Near the pubis, the rectus abdominis is partially covered by the triangularly-shaped *pyramidalis muscle*. The *quadratus lumborum muscle* is a muscle of the posterior abdominal wall. It is a hypaxial muscle closely applied to the vertebral column.

The lateral aspects of the abdominal wall are formed by a tri-layer: *external abdominal oblique* (externally), *internal abdominal oblique*, and *transversus abdominis muscles*. The bellies of these muscles do not reach the anterior midline but are continued to it by aponeuroses. These aponeuroses pass on each side of the rectus abdominis muscle and form an encasement called the *sheath of the rectus abdominis*. The aponeurosis from the external abdominal oblique muscle courses anterior to the ipsilateral rectus abdominus muscle to form the main portion of the anterior lamina of this sheath. The aponeurosis of the transversus abdominus muscle courses posterior to the rectus

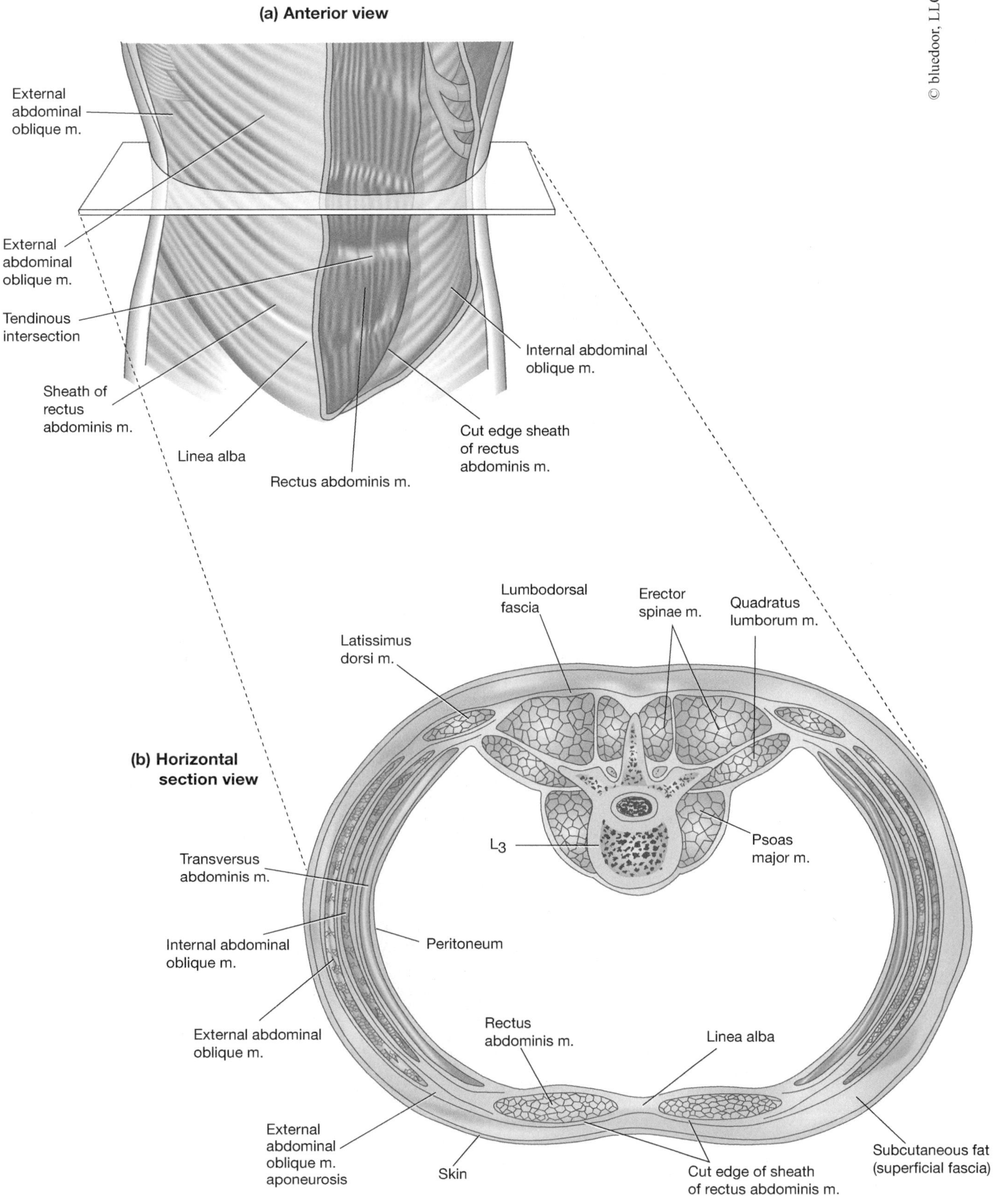

Figure 8-11

Transverse Section of the Anterior Abdominal Wall

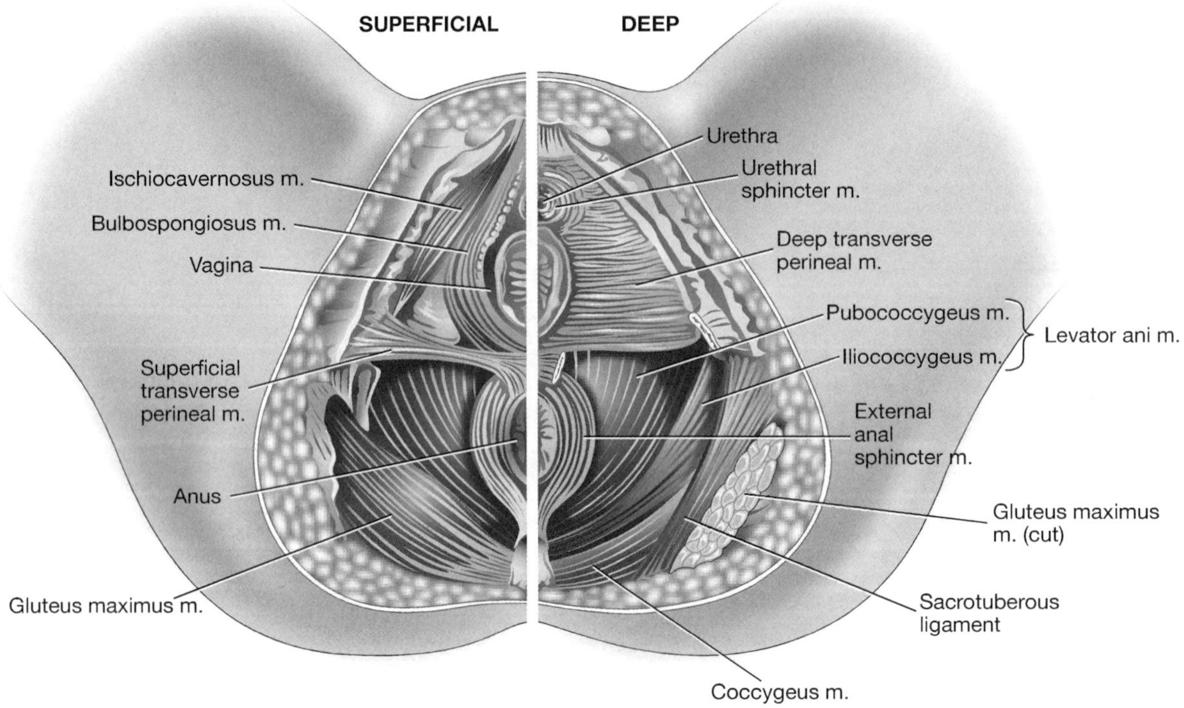

Figure 8-12
Muscles of the Perineal Region (Female)

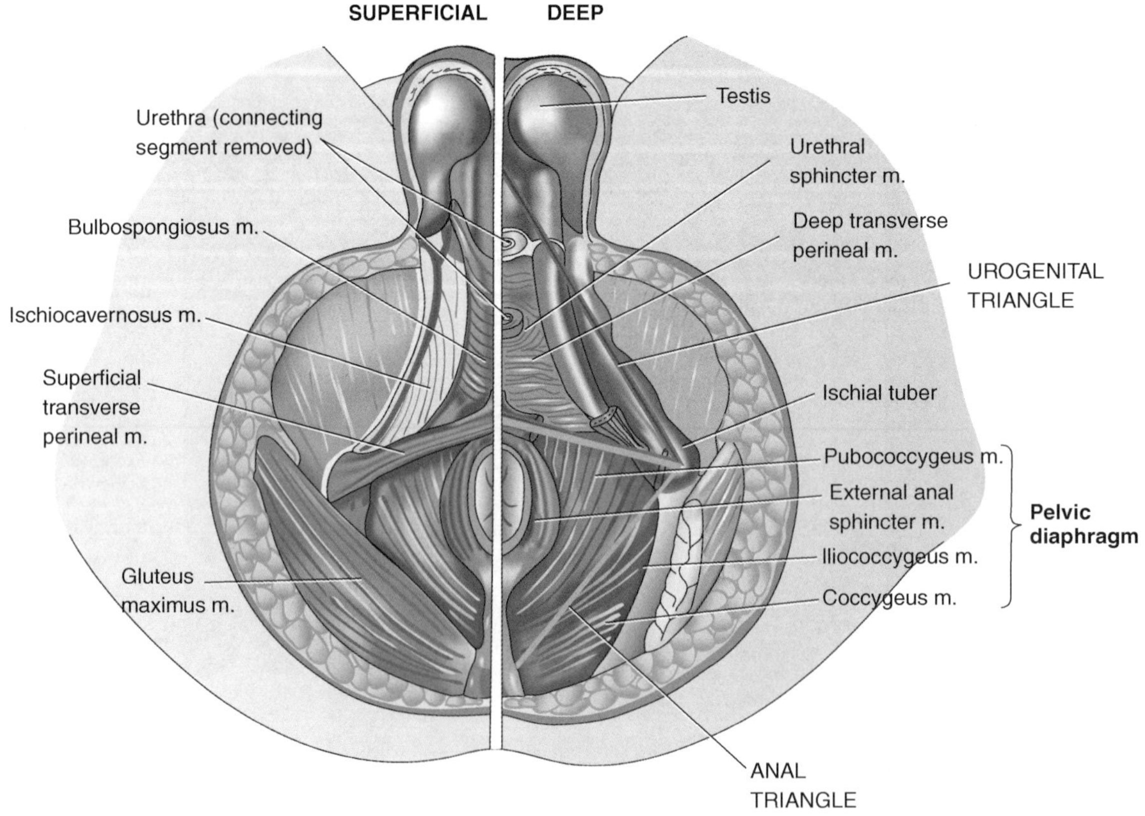

Figure 8-13
Muscles of the Perineal Region (Male)

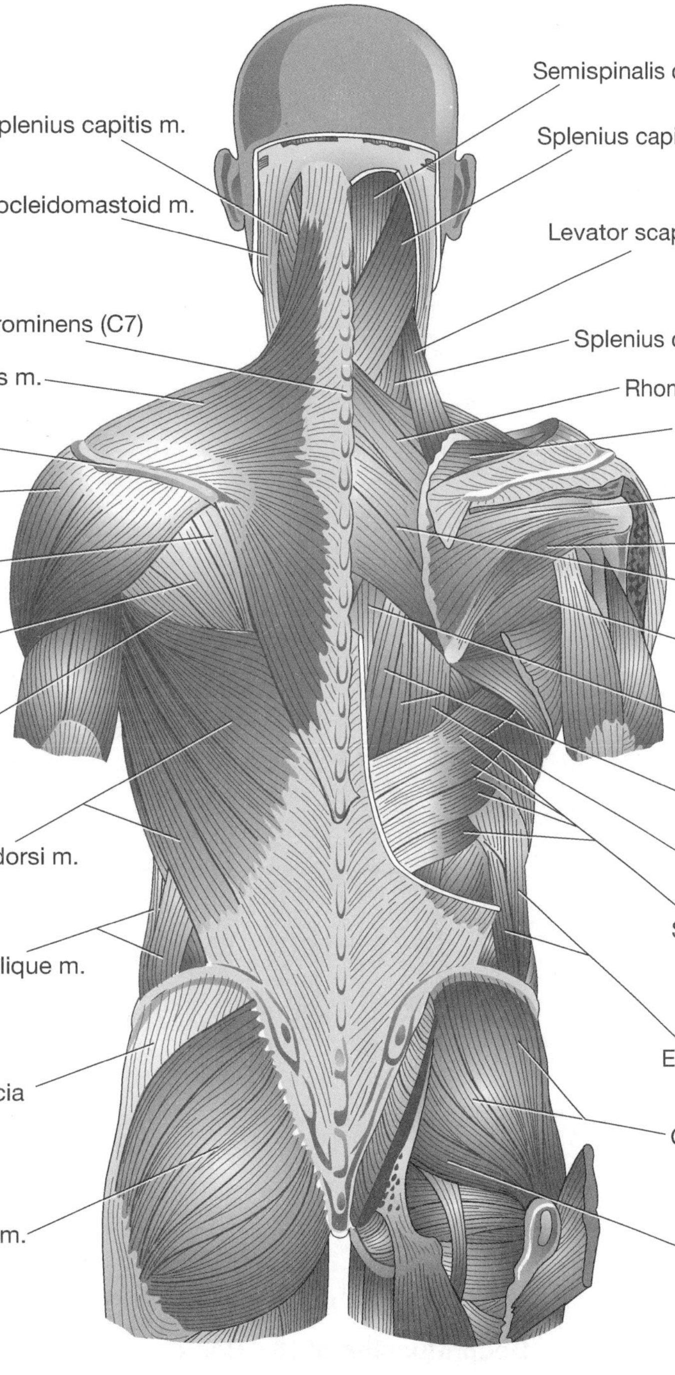

Figure 8-14
Superficial Muscles of the Back

abdominus muscle to form the main portion of the posterior lamina of the sheath. The aponeurosis of the internal abdominal oblique muscle splits with part of it contributing to the anterior lamina and part contributing to the posterior lamina. The left and right sheaths meet on the midline to form a connecting raphe (median junction) known as the **linea alba** (Figure 8-11). Surgical incisions into the abdominal cavity can be made through the linea alba without disrupting any muscle fibers. Surgeons can also avoid transecting muscle bellies when making non-midline abdominal incisions by using a "grid" technique in which the muscle cells in each muscle layer are divided par-

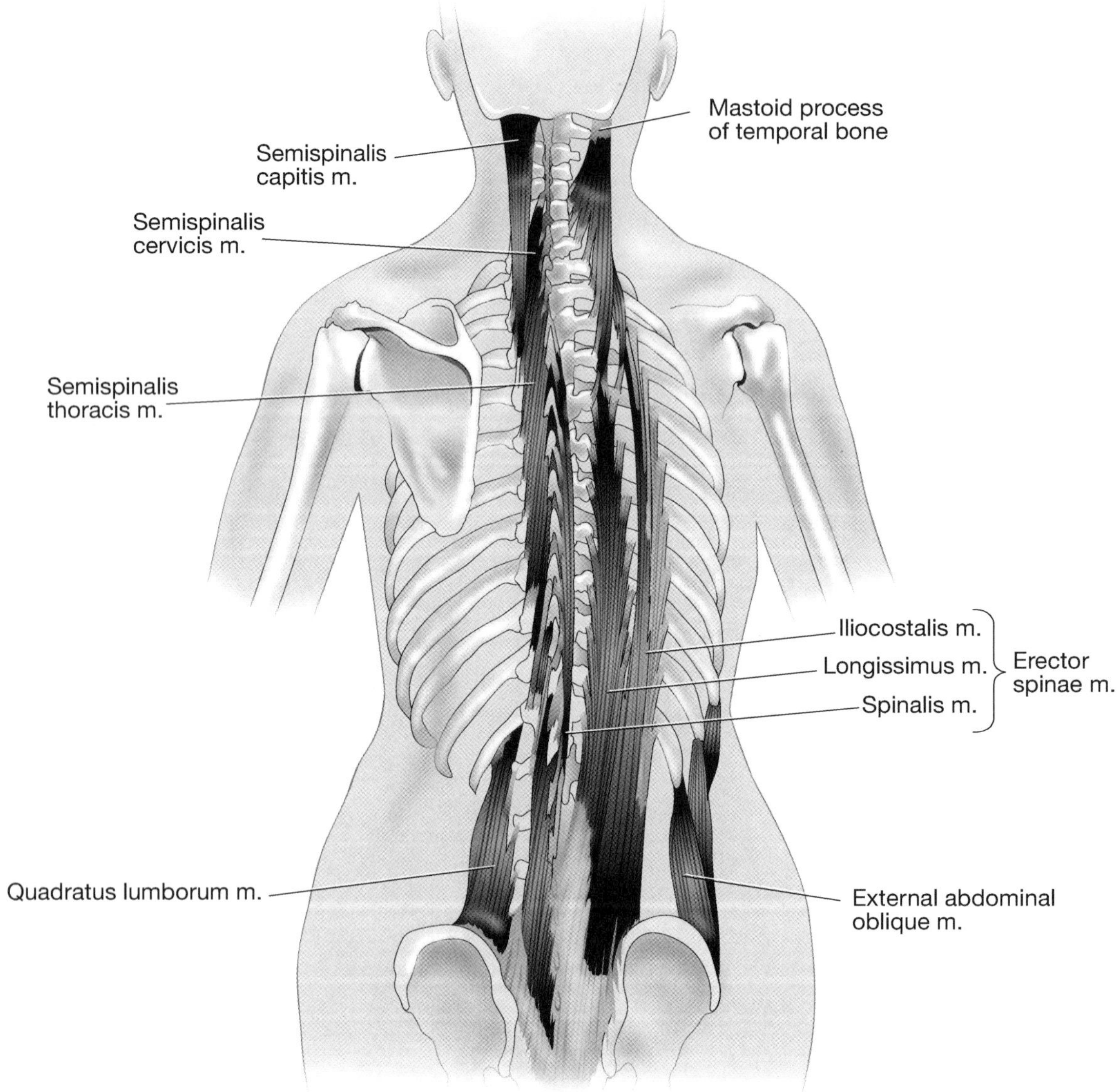

Figure 8-15
Deep Muscles of the Back

allel to their orientation. Contraction of the muscles of the abdominal wall causes an abdominal press and flexes the joints of the vertebral column.

The muscles of the pelvic diaphragm include the *levator ani* (which has four subparts), *coccygeus*, and *external anal sphincter muscles* (Figure 8-12). These muscles occupy the area between the pubis, ischium, and rectum. The muscles of the urogenital diaphragm include a superficial group (*ischiocavernosus, bulbospongiosus*, and *transversus perinei superficiales muscles*) as well as a deep group (*urethral sphincter, urethral compressor, urethrovaginal* and *transversus perinei profundus muscles*) (Figure 8-13). They are positioned between the rectum and the pubis in the perineal region.

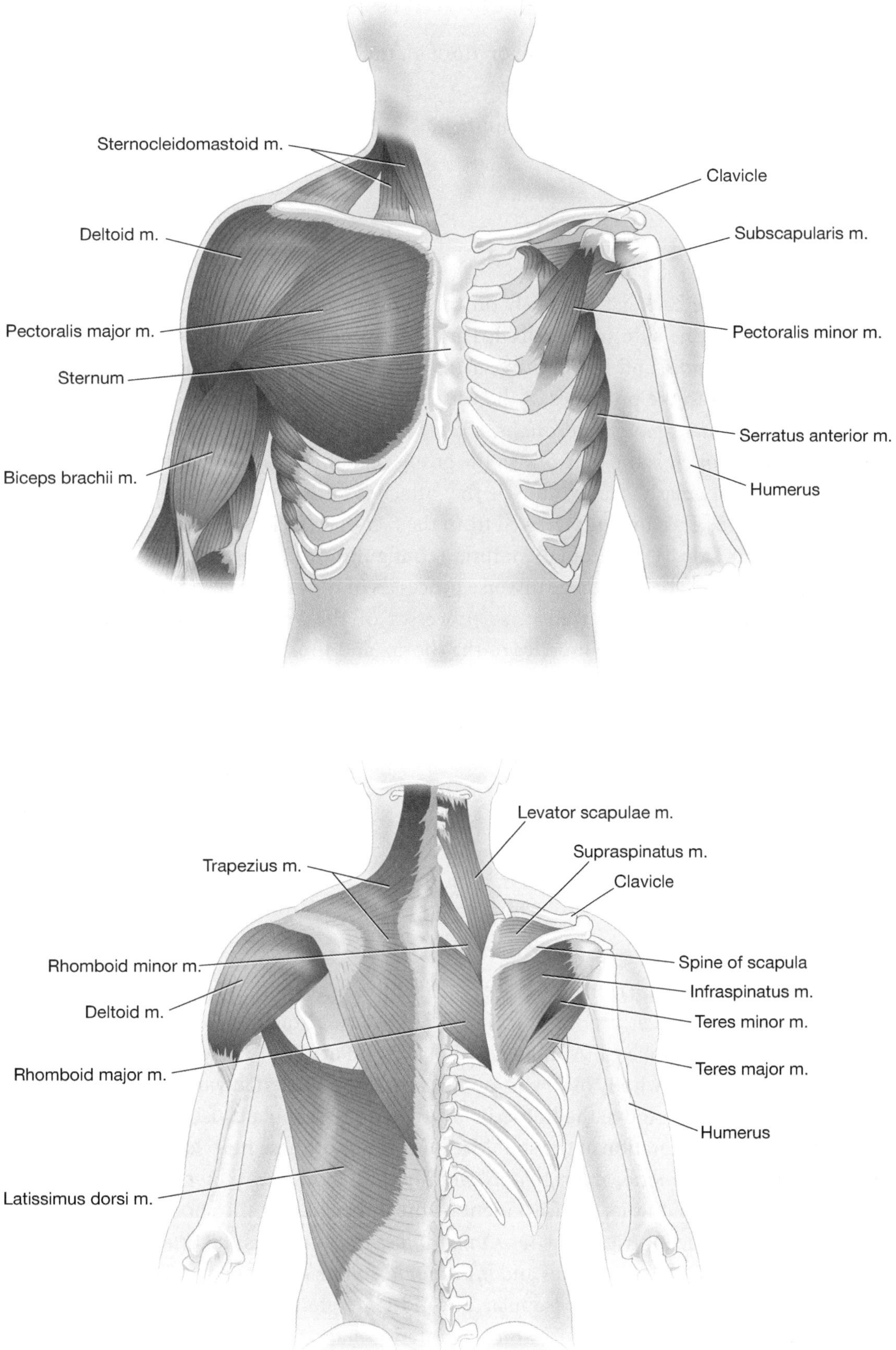

Figure 8-16
Muscles of the Shoulder and Upper Trunk

Objectives

18. Schematically represent a transverse section through the anterior abdominal wall and label the bellies and aponeuroses of the muscles involved.
19. Differentiate the pelvic and urogenital diaphragms.

Muscles of the Back

The muscles of the back act primarily on the joints of the vertebral column, extending them and bending them to one side (Appendix I, Part E). Some of them, like the *erector spinae, transversospinalis, interspinalis*, and *intertransversarius muscles* extend along much of the length of vertebral column attaching to the processes of the vertebrae (Figure 8-14). Four of these muscles act on the scapula (*rhomboideus major* and *minor, levator scapulae*, and *trapezius muscles* (Figure 8-15). The *latissimus dorsi muscle* is the only one in the group that attaches to the humerus. The *trapezius muscle* is a large triangularly-shaped muscle that attaches to the spine of the scapula in addition to the vertebral column. Its name was derived from the fact that the left and right trapezius (taken together) have a four-sided (trapezoidal) outline (configuration). The muscles of the posterior trunk which are positioned behind the transverse processes of the vertebrae are often termed **epaxial** muscles. Those anterior to the transverse processes of the vertebrae are called **hypaxial** muscles. Hypaxial muscles include the muscles of the thorax and those of the abdomen.

Objectives

20. Define hypaxial and epaxial muscles.

Muscles of the Superior Limb

The muscles of each superior limb are divided into six groups. These include muscles of the (1) shoulder and scapula; (2) anterior brachium; (3) posterior brachium; (4) anterior antebrachium; (5) posterior antebrachium; and (6) manus (Appendix I, Part F). The seven **muscles of the shoulder and scapula** originate wholly or in part on the scapula and insert at various loci on the proximal half of the humerus. They move the humerus relative to the scapula causing flexion, extension, adduction, abduction, and rotation at the shoulder joint. Four of these muscles contribute to the infamous **rotator cuff**: *supraspinatus, infraspinatus, subscapularis*, and *teres minor muscles* (Figure 8-16). This term refers to the tendinous reinforcement of the upper half of the shoulder joint capsule which is often torn in athletic injuries. The *teres major muscle* also rotates the brachium but it is not part of the rotator cuff. The *supraspinatus* and *infraspinatus muscles* form part of the palpable muscle mass above and below the spine of the scapula. The most lateral muscle in this group is the *deltoideus (deltoid)* which forms the muscle mass on the anterior, lateral, and posterior aspects of the shoulder region. The *coracobrachialis muscle*, as its name implies, extends from the coracoid process of the scapula into the brachium where it inserts on the humerus.

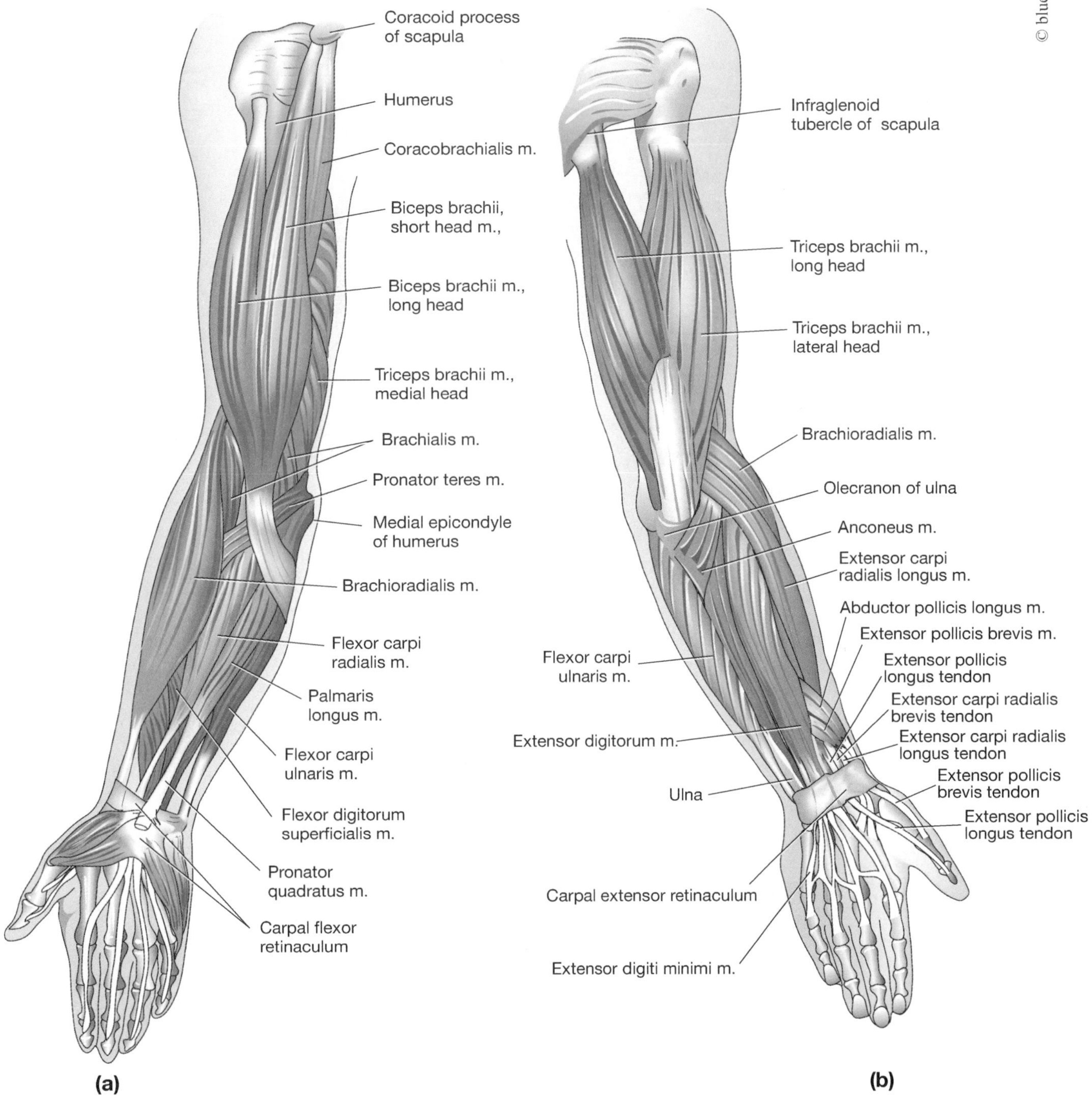

Figure 8-17

Muscles of the Brachium and Antebrachium
(a) Supinated View (b) Pronated View

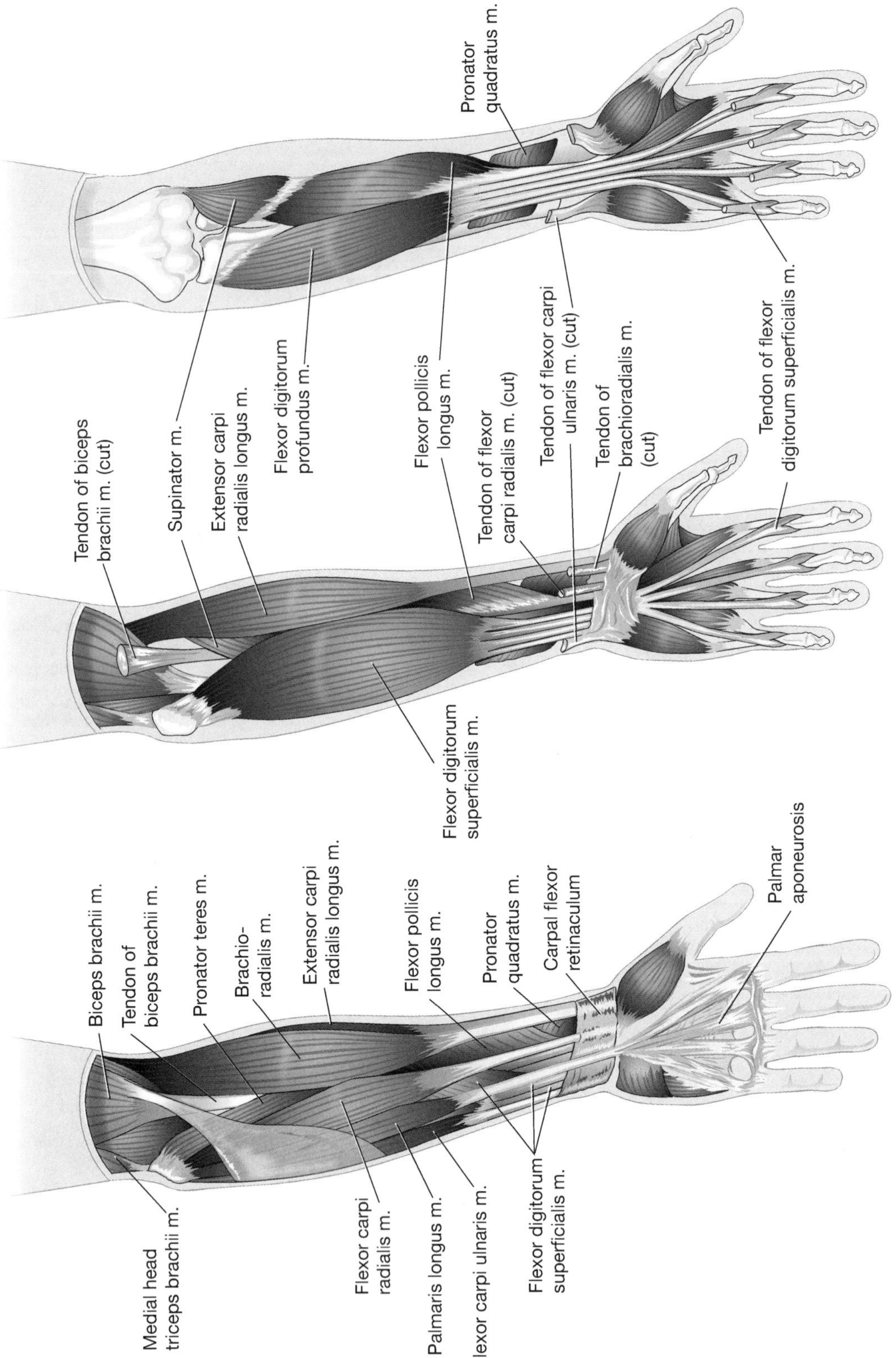

Figure 8-18A
Anterior Antebrachial Muscles

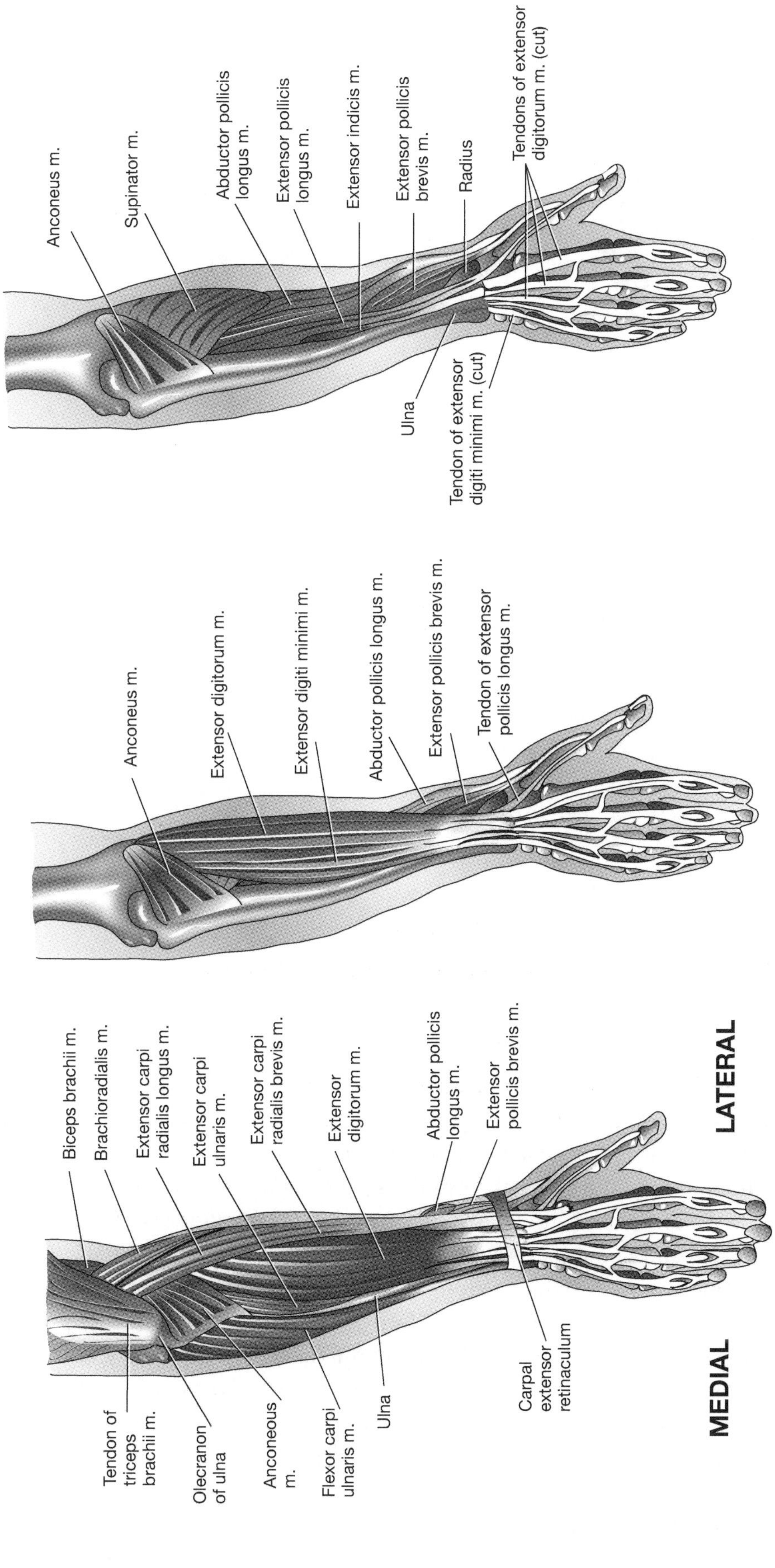

Figure 8-18B
Posterior Antebrachial Muscles

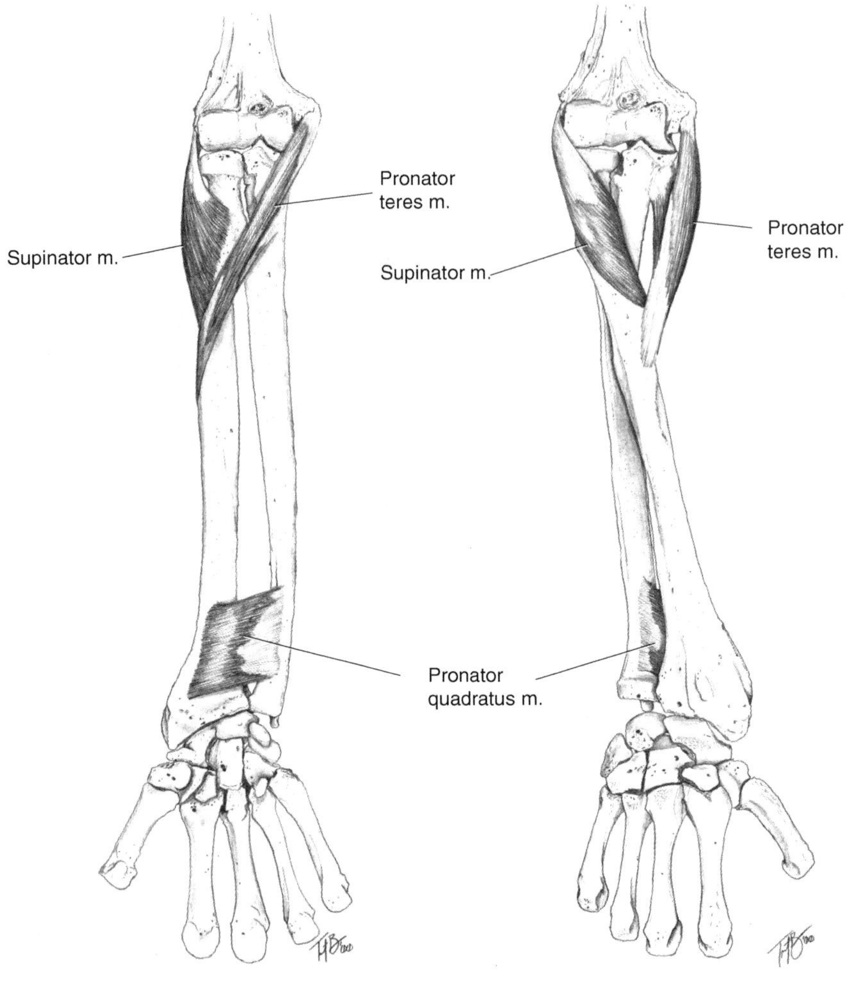

Figure 8-19
The Rotator Muscles of the Antebrachium

The three **anterior muscles of the brachium** all have *brachi* in their names: biceps brachii, brachialis, and brachioradialis muscles (Figure 8-17). The *biceps brachii muscle* is the largest and most anterior of these. It is the strongest flexor of the elbow joint and also is the strongest antebrachial supinator. Because it originates from the scapula and courses across the anterior aspect of the shoulder, it can also flex the shoulder joint. The *brachialis muscle* is sandwiched between the biceps brachii muscle and humerus. It has only one action (flex the elbow joint). A significant portion of the *brachioradialis muscle* courses along the lateral aspect of the antebrachium. It rotates the antebrachium, pronating a markedly supinated limb and supinating a markedly pronated one.

The two **posterior muscles of the brachium** are the (large) triceps brachii muscle and the much smaller anconeus muscle (Figure 8-17). The *triceps brachii muscle* is so named because it has three heads (medial, lateral, long). The long head originates on the scapula, inserts on the olecranon and therefore has two main actions: extension of the elbow and shoulder joints. The medial and lateral heads originate on the humerus and merge distally with the tendon of the long head. They do not cross the shoulder joint and act only to extend the elbow joint. The *anconeus muscle* also extends the elbow joint.

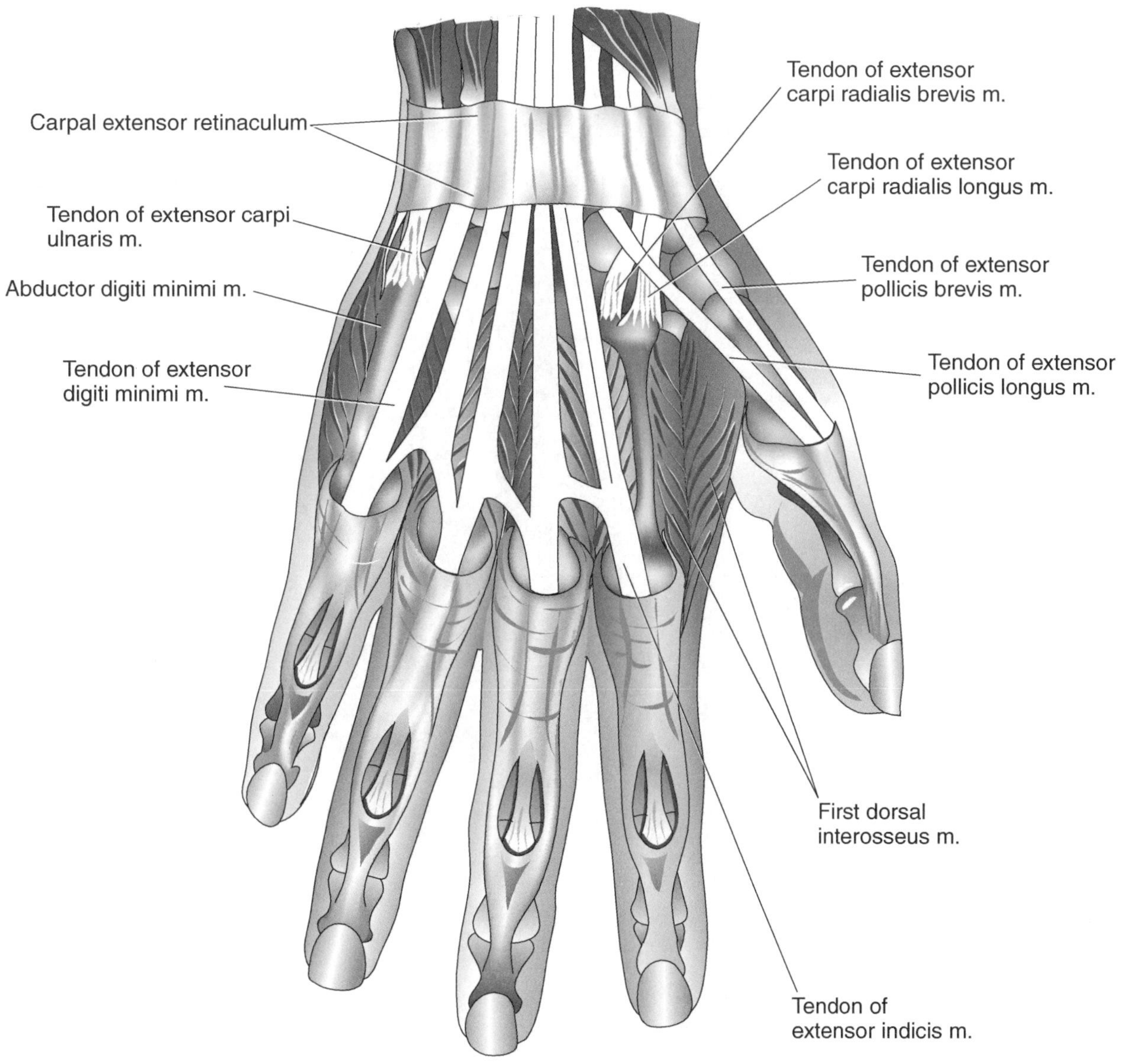

Figure 8-20A
Muscles of the Hand, Posterior Aspect

The nine **anterior muscles of the antebrachium** occupy an anteromedial position on the antebrachium. They include six muscles which flex the carpal and digital joints and three muscles which rotate the antebrachium. Even though several of these muscles originate from the medial epicondyle of the humerus, their action on the elbow joint is so minimal that it is usually ignored.

The six antebrachial flexor muscles consist of radial and ulnar carpal flexors, superficial and deep digital flexors, and two "other" flexors (Figure 8-18A). The *flexor carpi radialis muscle* is the most lateral of the anterior antebrachial muscles. Immediately medial to it is the smaller *palmaris longus muscle* which is absent on one or both sides in a small percentage of the population. Medial to the palmaris longus muscle is the *superficial digital flexor muscle* whose tendons extend down to the mid-

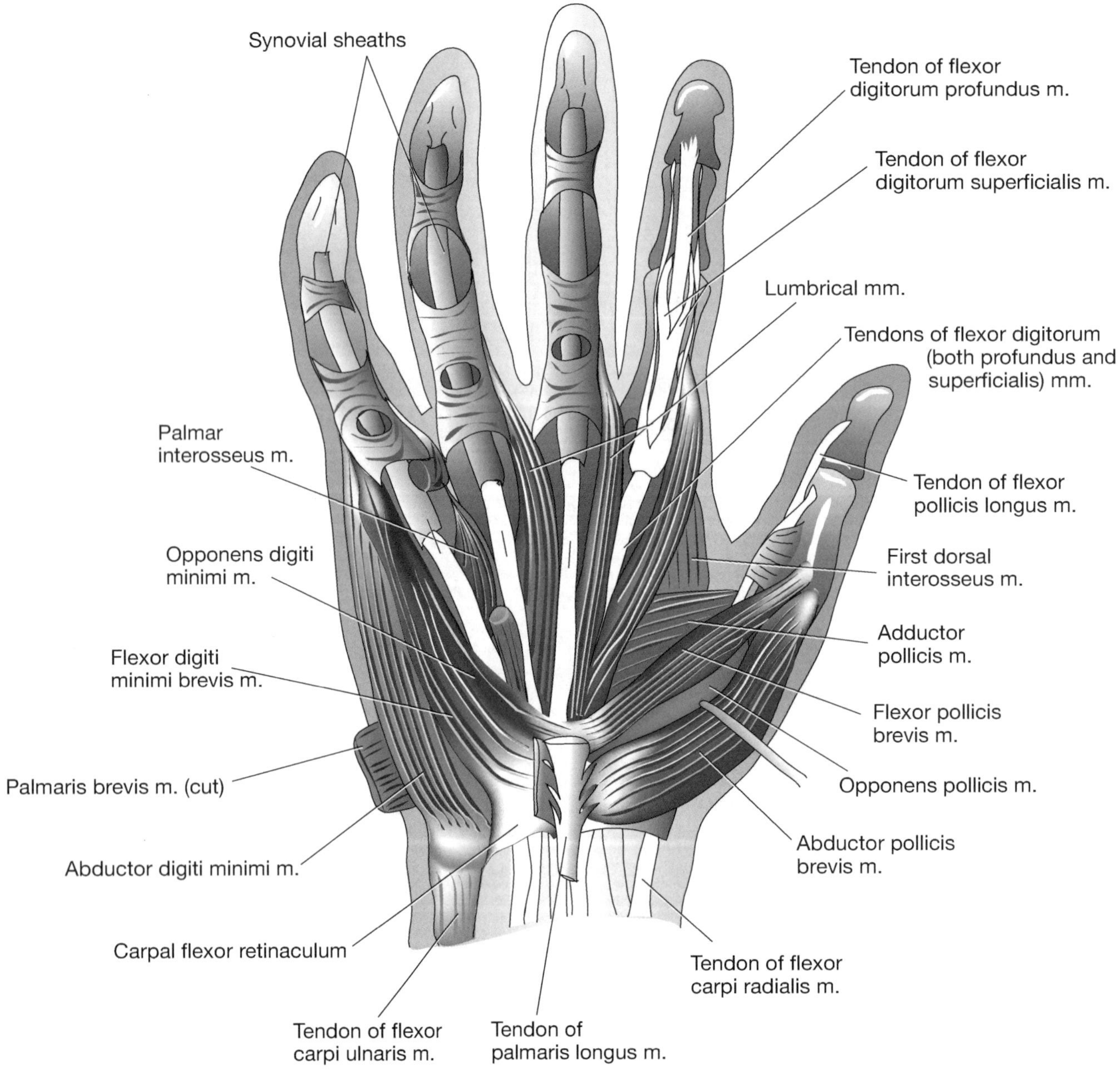

Figure 8-20B
Muscles of the Hand, Anterior Aspect

dle phalanges of the principal digits (2-5). The *flexor carpi ulnaris muscle* is the medial-most muscle in the anterior antebrachial group. It inserts on the pisiform, hamate, and fifth metacarpal bones. Deeper muscles of the anterior antebrachium include the *deep digital flexor muscle* whose tendons extend to the distal phalanges of the principal digits and the *flexor pollicis longus muscle* whose single tendon inserts on the distal phalanx of the thumb. At the carpus, the tendons of the six flexor muscles pass through the *carpal canal*. This passageway is formed by the carpal bones posteriorly and by the transversely oriented *flexor retinaculum* of the carpus (anteriorly). Note that the tendon

Table 8-5 Muscles Acting on the Thumb

Muscle	*Subgroup*
Abductor pollicis longus m.	Posterior antebrachial mm.
Abductor pollicis brevis m.	Thenar mm.
Flexor pollicis longus m.	Anterior antebrachial mm.
Flexor pollicis brevis m.	Thenar mm.
Extensor pollicis longus m.	Posterior antebrachial mm.
Extensor pollicis brevis m.	Posterior antebrachial mm.
Adductor pollicis m.	Intermediate mm. of manus
Opponens pollicis m.	Thenar mm.

of the palmaris longus muscle, which is the most superficial (anterior) of the muscles bound by the flexor retinaculum, actually passes through (splits) the retinaculum itself. The actions of the three antebrachial rotators are pronation (medial rotation) and supination (lateral rotation) of the antebrachium. Two of them are located near the cubital joint: *supinator muscle* (laterally) and *pronator teres muscle* (medially). The *pronator quadratus muscle*, so named because it is "four-sided", is located near the carpus (Figure 8-19).

The nine **posterior muscles of the antebrachium** are primarily extensors of the carpal and digital joints (Figure 8-18 B). In fact, all but one of them (abductor pollicis longus muscle) have "extensor" in their names (three "carpal", two "digital", two "pollicis", and one "indicis" extensors). Most of them originate on or near the lateral epicondyle of the humerus, but like their anterior antebrachial counterparts, they have no significant action on the elbow joint. At the posterior aspect of the carpus, the tendons of the posterior antebrachial muscles are bound in place by the *extensor retinaculum*.

The *extensor carpi radialis longus muscle* is the most lateral posterior antebrachial muscle and the *extensor carpi radialis brevis muscle* lies right next to it. Their tendons attach to the bases of the second and third metacarpal bones, respectively. The fact that the base of the second metacarpal bone is slightly distal to the base of the third one gives the muscles their differentiating names (the "longus" must course further distally to insert). The *digital extensor muscle* (m. extensor digitorum) lies medial to the extensor carpi radialis brevis and its tendons course distally to the distal phalanges of digits 2-5. Slender individuals can visualize these tendons on the posterior metacarpal region by forcefully extending their digital joints. The diminutive *extensor digiti minimi muscle* lies medial to the digital extensor. Its tendon fuses with the tendon of the digital extensor that courses to the little finger. The *extensor carpi ulnaris muscle* is the most medial of the posterior antebrachial muscles and lies adjacent to the ulna. The *extensor indicis muscle* lies deep to other muscles and its tendon of insertion courses distally to attach to the proximal phalanx of the index finger. The remaining three muscles in the posterior antebrachial group all act on the thumb and are partially covered by other antebrachial muscles. The most lateral one is the *abductor pollicis longus muscle*, the middle one is the *extensor pollicis brevis*, and the medial one is the *extensor pollicis longus muscle*. When the joints of the thumb are forcefully extended and the thumb is abducted, these tendons can be visualized. The depression bounded by the tendons of the extensor pollicis longus and brevis muscles is unofficially called the "anatomic snuffbox".

The **intrinsic muscles of the hand** (manus) are divided into three subgroups: *thenar muscles*, *hypothenar muscles*, and *intermediate muscles* (Figure 8-20). The three thenar muscles form the fleshy bulb at the base of the thumb termed the **thenar eminence**. They act on the thumb (Table 8-5). The four hypothenar muscles form the smaller fleshy bulb termed the **hypothenar eminence** on the palmaromedial aspect of the metacarpus. They act on the little finger. The four intermediate muscles of the manus are those located between the thenar and hypothenar eminences. The remarkable dexterity of the thumb results from the fact that eight different muscles (belonging to four different subgroups) act on it. These include short and long flexors, short and long extensors, short and long abductors, and two "adductors" (adductor pollicis and opponens pollicis muscles) (*see Appendix II*).

Objectives

21. Divide the muscles of the superior limb into six regional groups and state the general actions of each group.

Muscles of the Inferior Limb

The muscles of the inferior limb are divided into nine groups: (1) anterior muscles of the hip; (2) posterior muscles of the hip; (3) medial muscles of the hip; (4) anterior muscles of the thigh; (5) medial muscles of the thigh; (6) posterior muscles of the thigh; (7) anterolateral muscles of the crus; (8) posterior muscles of the crus; and (9) intrinsic muscles of the pes (*see Appendix I, Part G*).

The **anterior muscles of the hip** are the *iliacus* and *psoas major muscles* (Figure 8-23). These fuse to form the *iliopsoas muscle.* The latter courses across the anterior aspect of the hip to flex the joint and rotate the limb laterally. Roughly 40 of every 100 people have a *psoas minor muscle* located adjacent to the psoas major muscle.

The **posterior and lateral muscles of the hip** include the three *gluteal muscles* (posteriorly) (Figures 8-15 and 8-23) and the *tensor fasciae latae muscle* (laterally) (Figure 8-21, 8-22). The gluteus maximus muscle is the largest muscle in this group and forms the rounded contour of the buttock (along with a variable deposit of fat). The smaller gluteus medius and gluteus minimus muscles lie deep to it. The gluteal muscles extend the hip joint, and abduct and rotate the limb. The tensor fasciae latae muscle has a relatively small belly on the lateral aspect of the coxal region but it has an extensive aponeurosis called the **fascia lata** which lies superficially on the lateral aspect of the thigh. The name tensor fasciae latae is derived from the fact that contraction of the muscle belly pulls the fascia lata taut. An especially dense band about 2 cm wide within the fascia lata is called the **iliotibial tract.**

The six **medial muscles of the hip** are the *external* and *internal obturators, superior* and *inferior gemelli, quadratus femoris* and *piriformis muscles* (Figure 8-21). These muscles are relatively small and deeply located. They rotate the thigh laterally.

The **anterior muscles of the thigh** include the sartorius and quadriceps femoris muscles (Figure 8-24). The slender *sartorius muscle* has the longest muscle belly in the body. It courses obliquely across the thigh from anterior (in the coxal region) to medial (near the knee). The *quadriceps femoris muscle* forms the large muscle mass on the anterior aspect of the thigh. It has four named heads (*rectus femoris, vastus medialis, vastus lateralis, vastus intermedius muscles*) which originate from various loci on the os coxae and femur bone and then fuse to form a common tendon which contains the patella. The distal continuation of the tendon of the quadriceps femoris muscle from the patella to the tibial tuberosity is called the patellar ligament. The quadriceps femoris muscle extends the genual joint and the rectus femoris portion also flexes the hip joint. When the knee joint is locked firmly in extension, the vastus lateralis and vastus medialis muscles form obvious bulges on the thigh several centimeters above the patella.

The six **medial muscles of the thigh** are the gracilis, pectineus, and the four adductor muscles (Figures 8-23, 8-24). The *gracilis muscle* has a slender belly that adducts and medially rotates the

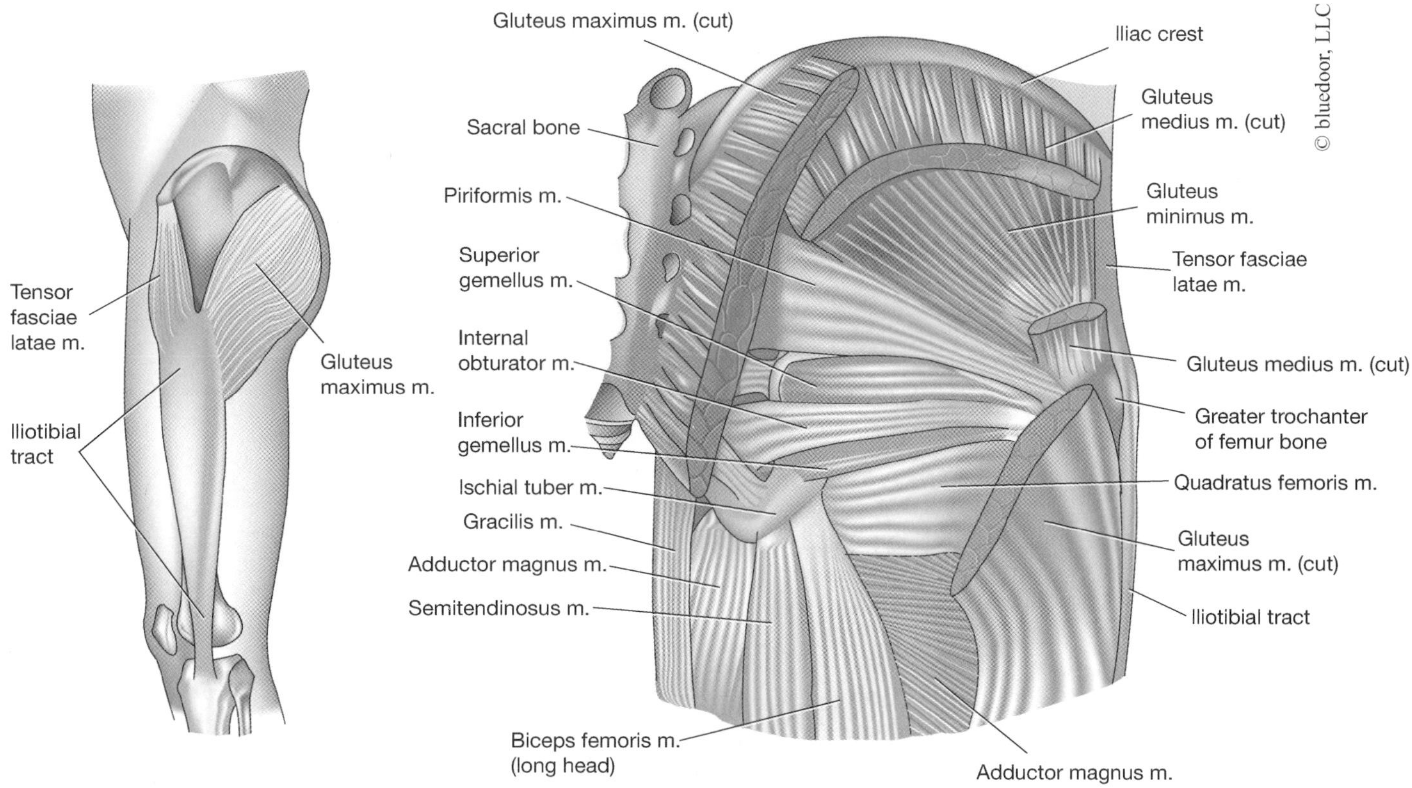

Figure 8-21
Selected Muscles of the Coxal Region

inferior limb and flexes the knee joint. The small *pectineus muscle* has similar actions. The four adductor muscles (longus, brevis, minimus, magnus) are named for their action on the hip joint (adduction) and for the relative size and configuration of their bellies. Together they form a significant muscle mass on the medial side of the thigh.

The three **posterior muscles of the thigh** are the biceps femoris, semitendinosus, and semimembranosus muscles (Figure 8-25). These muscles are known as the "hamstring" muscles because their well-developed distal tendons were used by butchers to hang hams over hooks and nails. They extend the hip joint, flex the genual joint, and rotate the inferior limb. The *biceps femoris muscle* originates as two heads that fuse to form a single belly. Its tendon of insertion forms the palpable cord-like structure on the lateral aspect of the posterior surface of the thigh just above the knee. The *semitendinosus muscle* lies medial to the biceps femoris muscle. Its name is derived from the fact that its tendon of insertion is several centimeters long and makes the muscle, in effect, half (*semi*) tendinous. This tendon forms the medially palpable band on the posterior thigh near the knee. The *semimembranosus muscle* lies between the biceps femoris and semitendinosus muscles. Its distal extent is more fleshy than cord-like and is positioned medial to the semitendinosus tendon.

The six **anterolateral muscles of the crus** lie on the lateral aspect of the tibia and fibula (Figure 8-29). They include the *anterior tibial, long digital extensor,* and *extensor hallucis longus muscles* as well as three *peroneus muscles* (*longus, brevis, tertius*). All six of these muscles have action on the tarsal joint (variously extending or flexing it) and two of them extend the digital joints as well. The *anterior tibial muscle* is the strongest of the tarsal joint flexors. Its large tendon can be visualized and palpated on the anterior aspect of the distal crus and the ankle when the tarsal joint is markedly

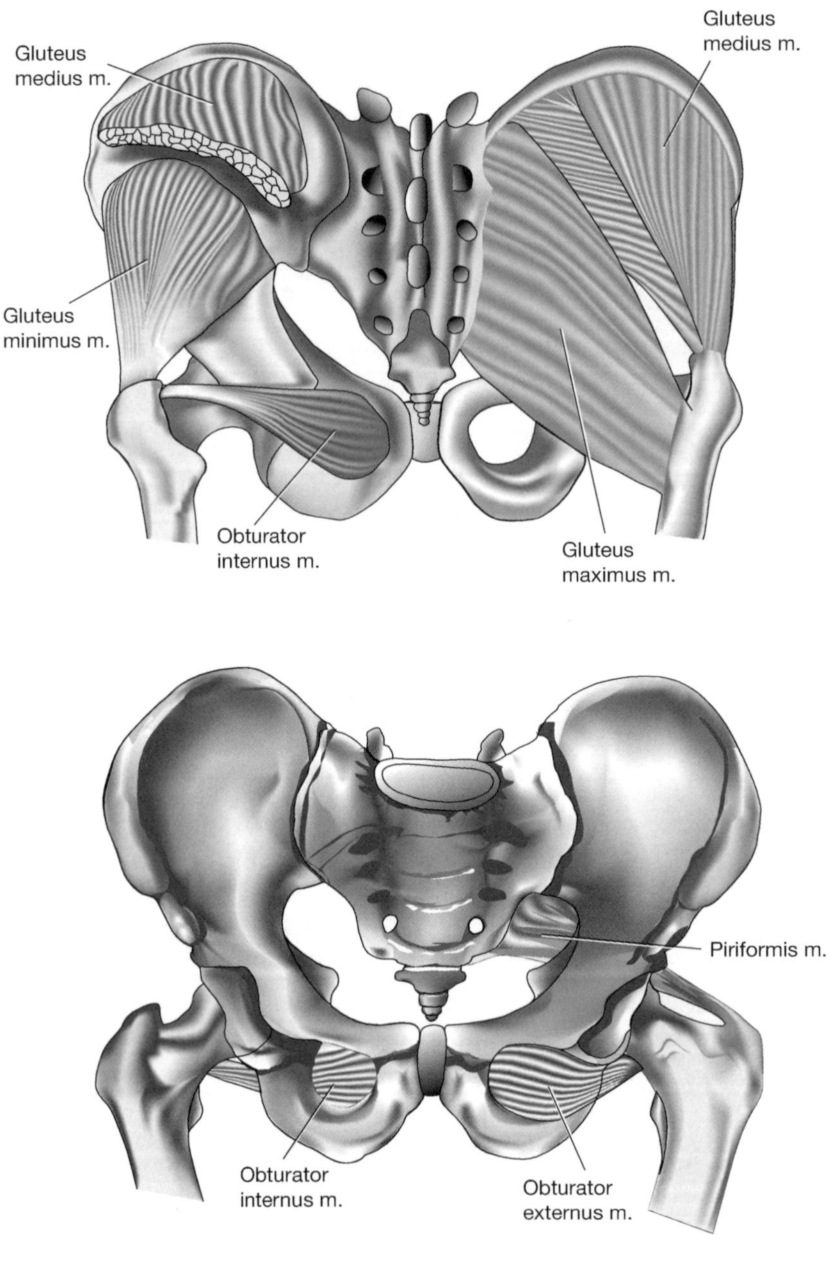

Figure 8-22

Selected Muscles of the Coxal Region (Posterior above, anterior below)

flexed. The belly of the *extensor hallucis longus muscle* lies adjacent to and behind that of the anterior tibial muscle. Its tendon courses down the anterior aspect of the tarsus just lateral to that of the anterior tibial muscle. The tendon can be visualized in its subcutaneous position along the dorsum of the first metatarsal bone, especially when the tarsal joint is flexed. The *long digital extensor muscle* corresponds to the digital extensor muscle of the superior limb. Its easily visualized tendons course across the dorsal metatarsus to insert on the distal phalanges of digits 2-5 (see Figure 8-29). The tendons of the long and short peroneus (fibularis) muscles (*peroneus longus* and *peroneus brevis*) course distally in the malleolar groove of the fibula. Since this groove is posterior to the center

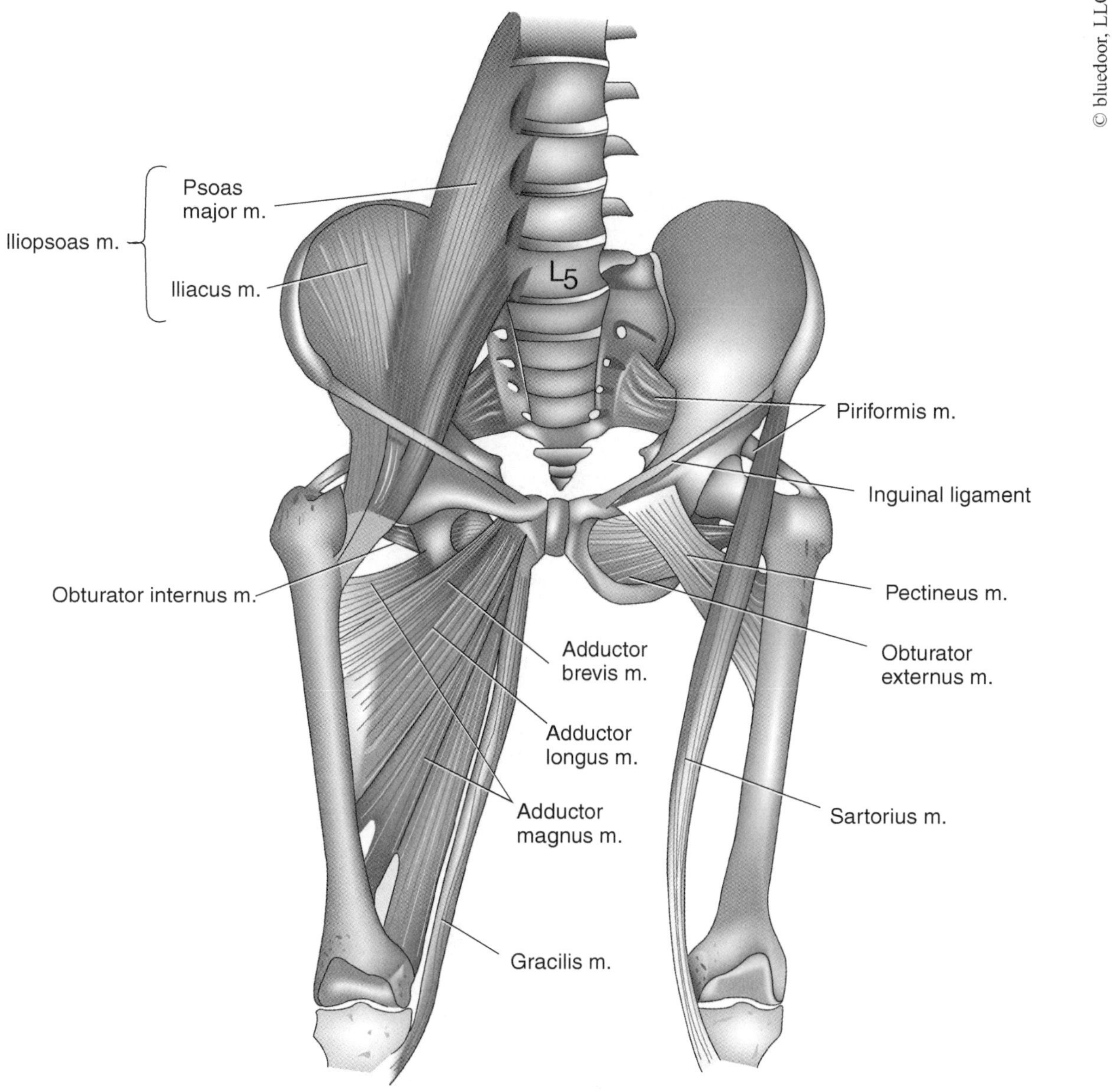

Figure 8-23
The Iliopsoas and Adductor Muscles

of rotation of the tarsal joint, contraction of the muscles causes extension (plantar flexion) of the joint. They also evert the foot. The *peroneus tertius* (third peroneus muscle) courses down the crus adjacent and deep to the long digital extensor muscle. It inserts on the base of the fifth metatarsal bone, flexes the tarsal joint and everts the foot.

The seven **posterior muscles of the crus** are the *gastrocnemius, soleus, plantaris, popliteus, flexor hallucis longus, flexor digitorum longus* and *posterior tibial muscles* (Figures 8-26, 8-27). These form the flesh of the calf of the leg. Most of them extend the tarsal joint and the two "flexors" flex the digital joints. Some (gastrocnemius and popliteus muscles) have flexor action on the genual joint. The *gastrocnemius* is the most superficial of these muscles. Its two heads partially fuse with

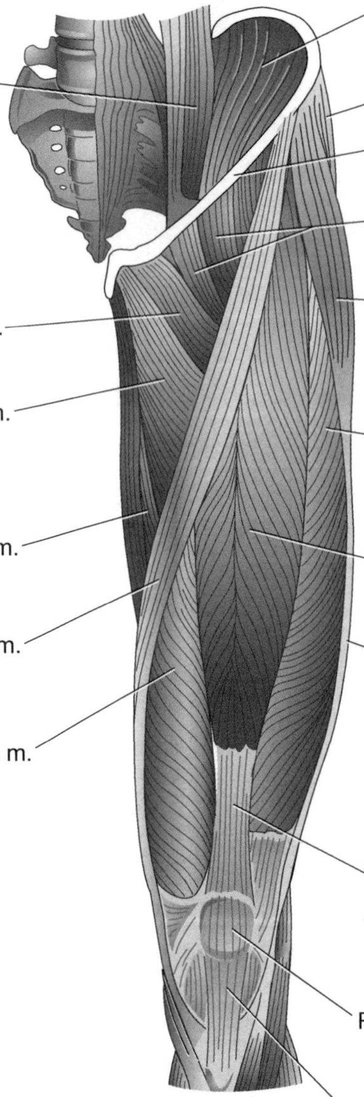

Figure 8-24
Muscles of the Thigh, Anterior View

the deeper *soleus muscle* to form the *triceps surae muscle.* The combined tendons from the three bellies coalesce to form the *calcanean tendon* which inserts on the tuber calcanei and can be easily palpated on the posterior aspect of the tarsal region. The belly of the diminutive *plantaris muscle* is positioned between those of the gastrocnemius and soleus muscles. Its slender tendon courses distally along the medial border of the calcanean tendon and also inserts on the tuber calcanei. The *popliteus muscle* is deeply located in the posterior aspect of the proximal crus (deep to the triceps surae muscle). It originates from the lateral epicondyle of the femur bone and slants down and medially to insert on the posterior side of the tibia. It and the triceps surae muscle are the only posterior crural muscles which are considered to flex the genual joint. None of the other muscles in this

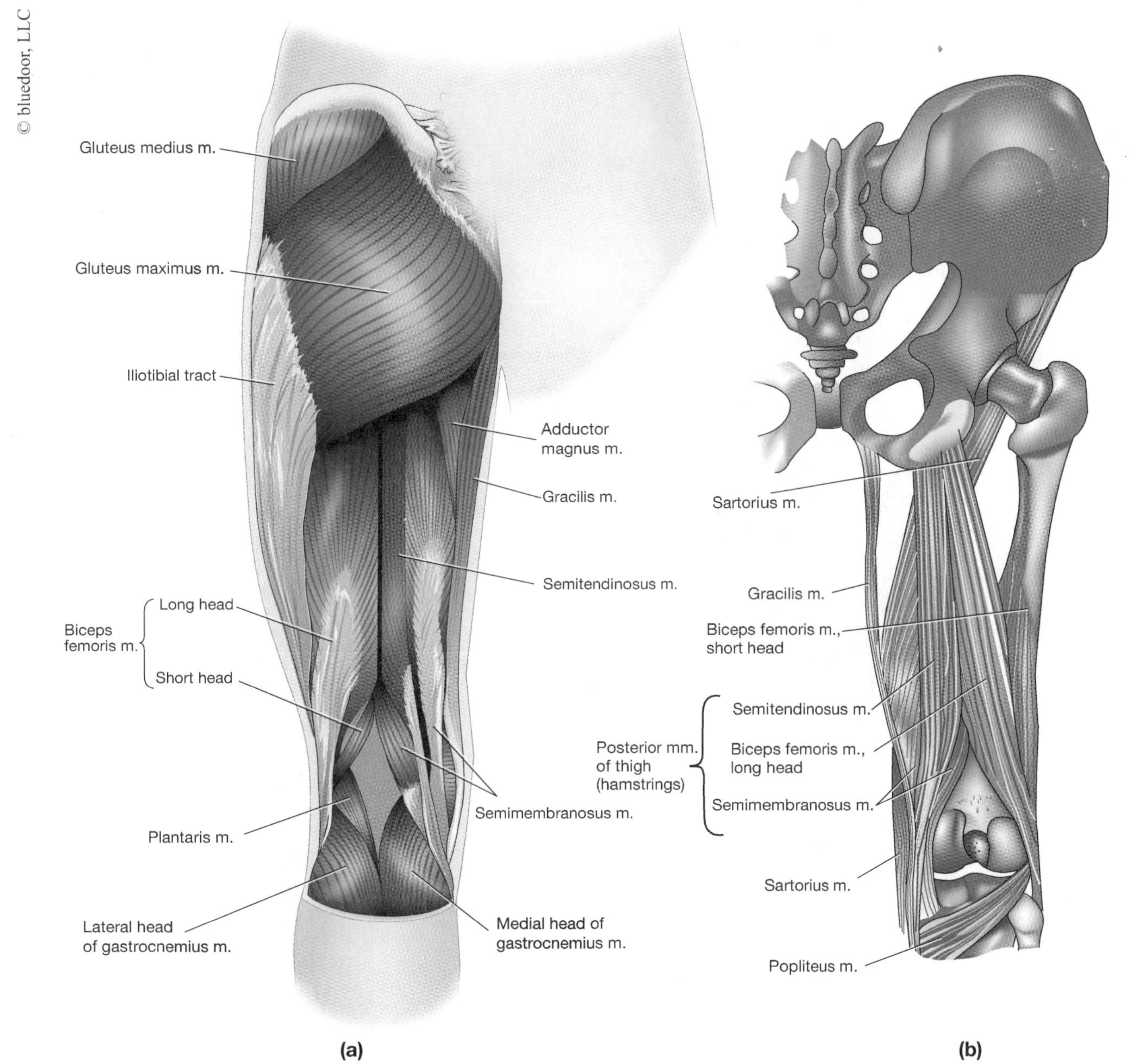

Figure 8-25

Posterior Muscles of the Thigh (a) Superficial View (b) Deep View

group bridge (cross) the genual joint except the plantaris muscle and the latter has such poor mechanical advantage for genual joint flexion that its flexor action is ignored. The remaining three muscles in the posterior crural group are largely hidden by the triceps surae muscle. They all have tendons which course distally just posterior to the medial malleolus of the tibia. The tendon of the *posterior tibial muscle* is the most anterior of the three and divides to insert on all of the tarsal bones except the talus and on the second through fourth metatarsal bones. The middle of the three tendons just posterior to the medial malleolus is that of the *long digital flexor muscle*. This muscle is homologous to the deep digital flexor muscle of the superior limb and inserts on the distal phalanges

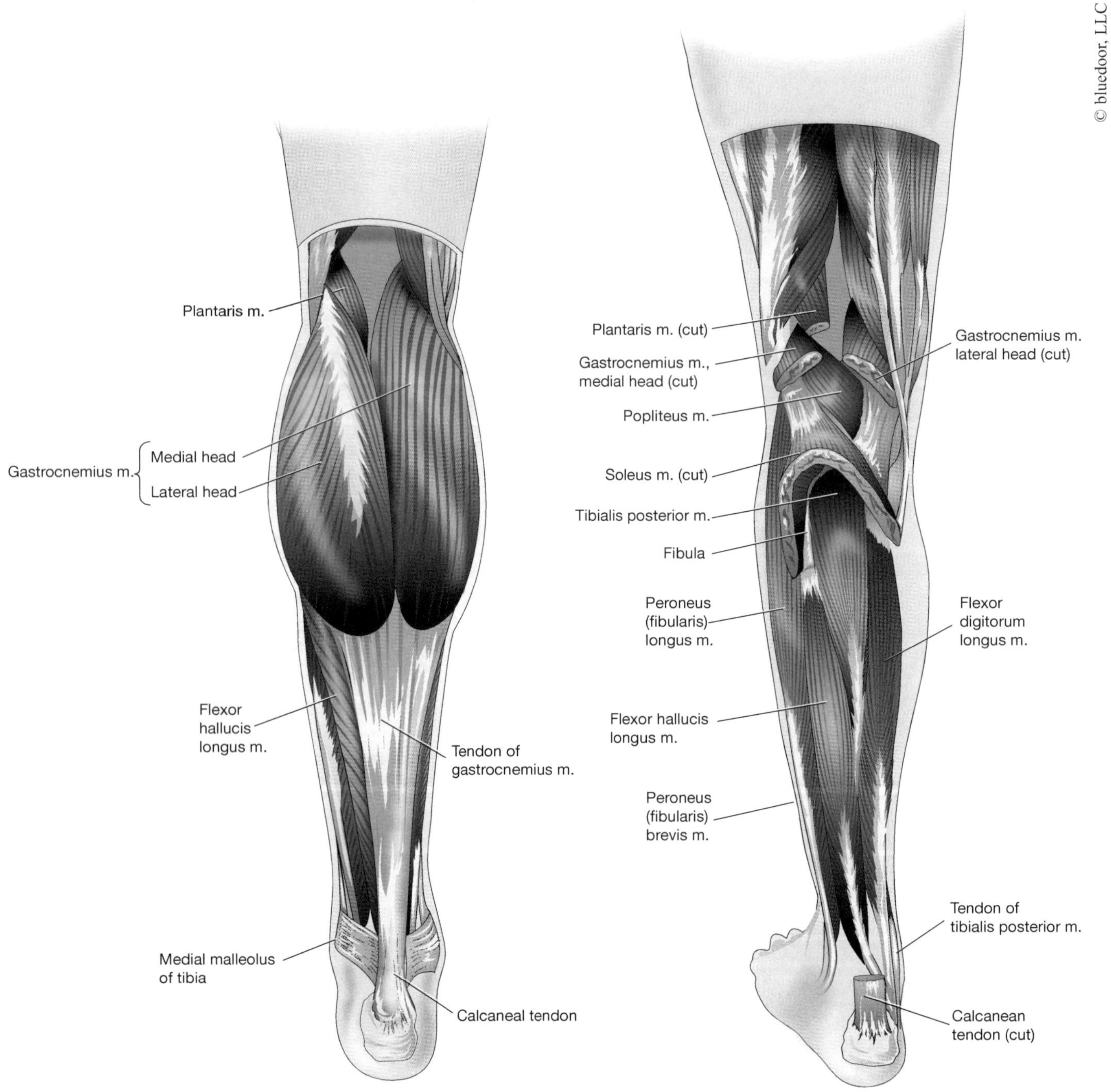

Figure 8-26

Posterior Muscles of the Crus (Superficial View)

of digits 2-5. The *flexor hallucis longus muscle* corresponds functionally to the flexor pollicis longus muscle of the superior limb. Its tendon lies posterior to those of the long digital flexor and posterior tibial muscles.

The **intrinsic muscles of the pes** are divided into three subgroups: special muscles of the big toe, special muscles of the little toe, and muscles common to several digits (Figures 8-30). The four special muscles of the big toe are an *abductor, adductor, short flexor* and *short extensor muscles.* The two

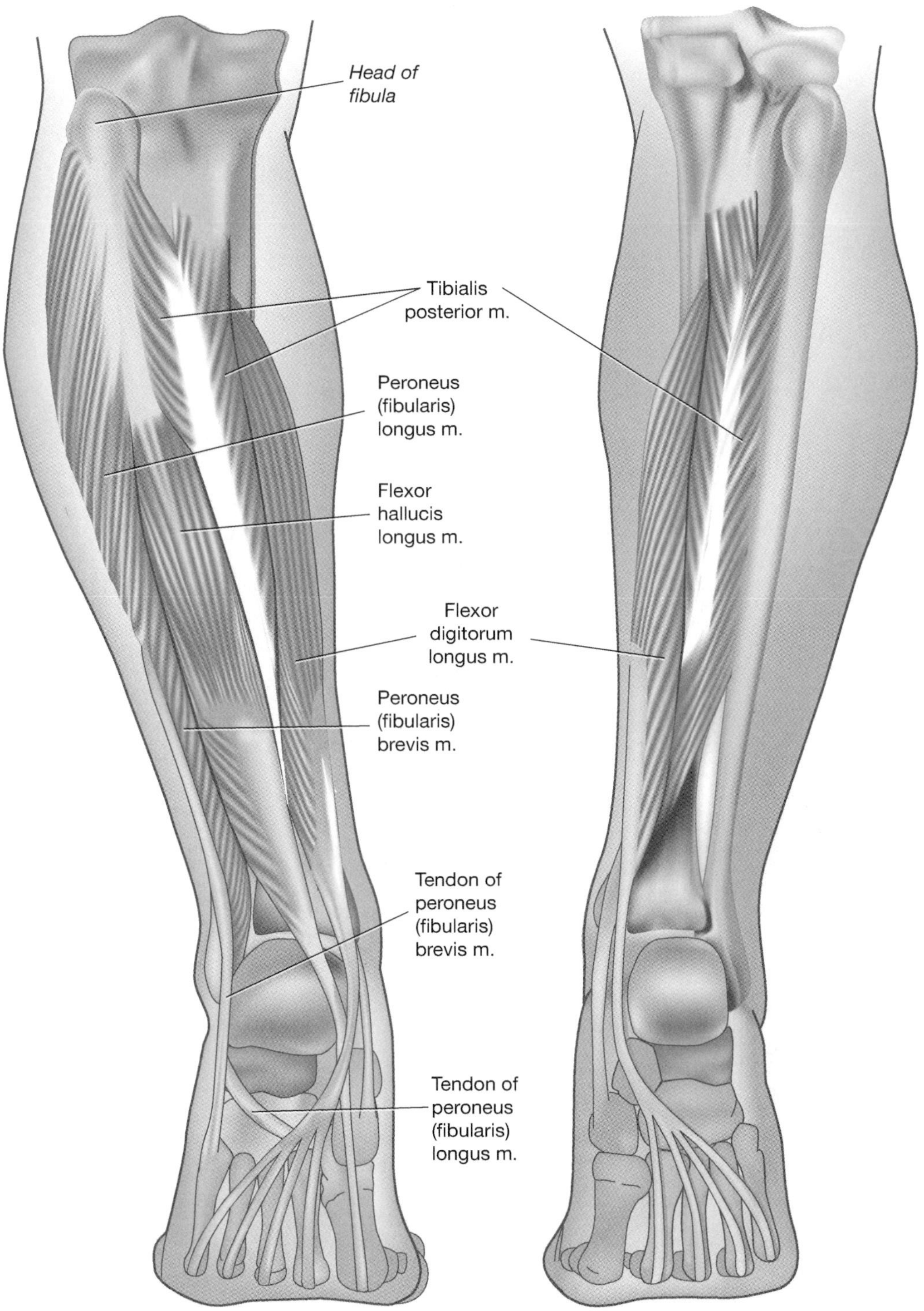

Figure 8-27

Posterior Muscles of the Crus (Deep View)

special muscles of the little toe include a *short flexor* and an *abductor*. Some individuals also have an identifiable opponens ("adductor") muscle associated with the little toe. The six intrinsic muscles common to several of the digits include digital extensors and flexors as well as muscles that adduct and abduct the toes.

Objectives

22. Divide the muscles of the inferior limb into nine regional groups and state the general actions of each group.

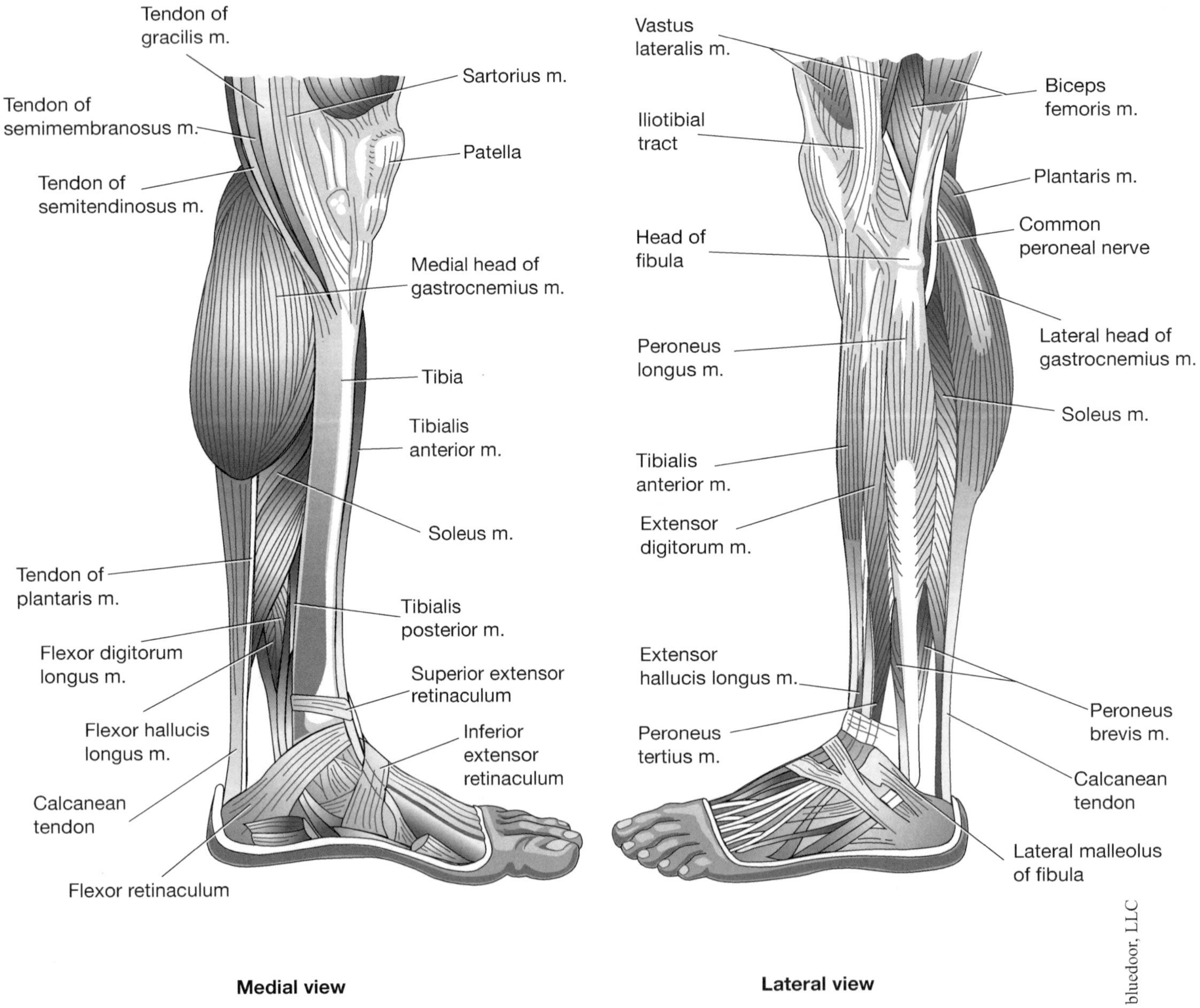

Figure 8-28

Anterolateral and Posterior Muscles of the Crus

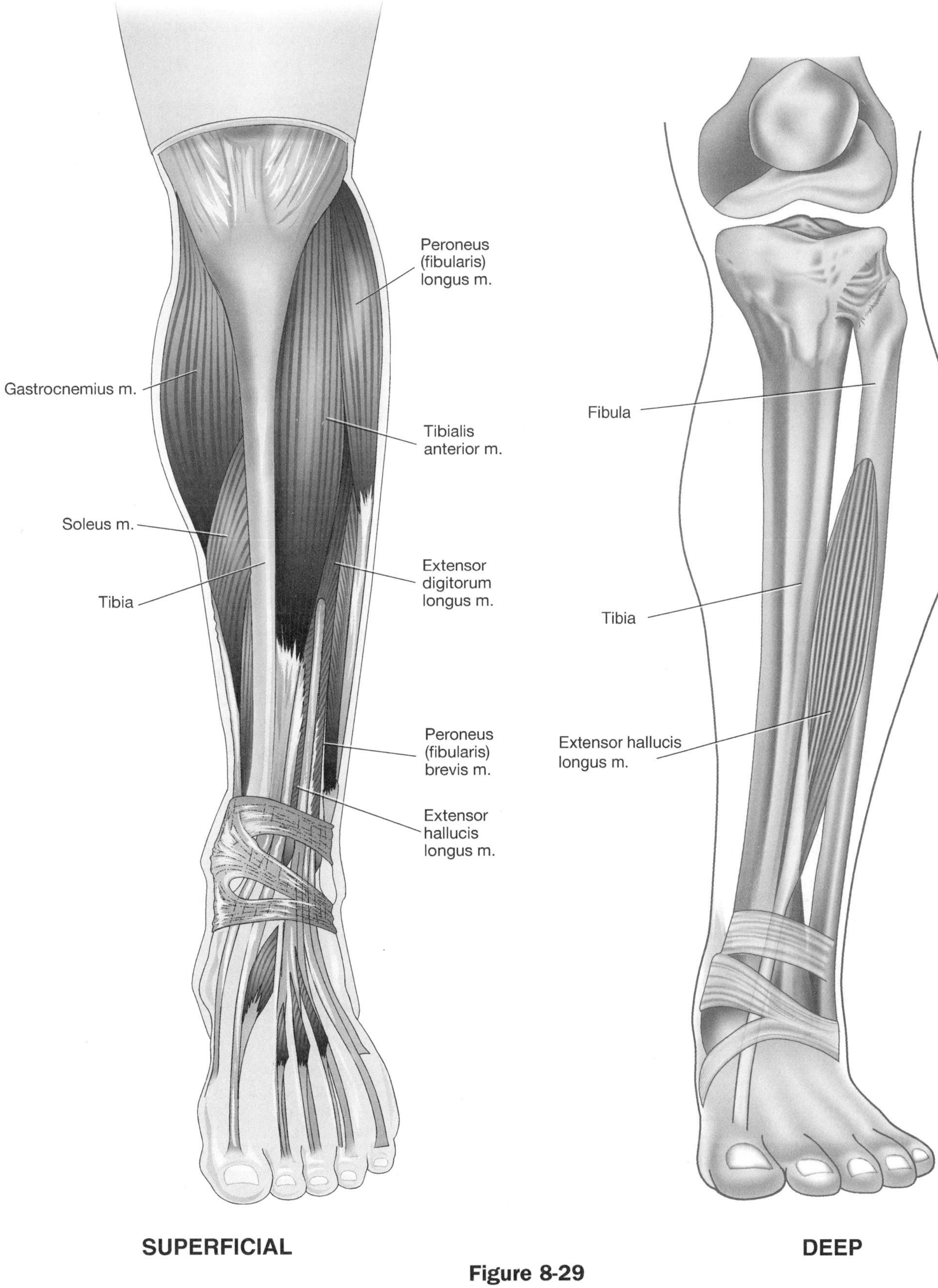

Figure 8-29

Anterolateral Muscles of the Crus (Anterior View)

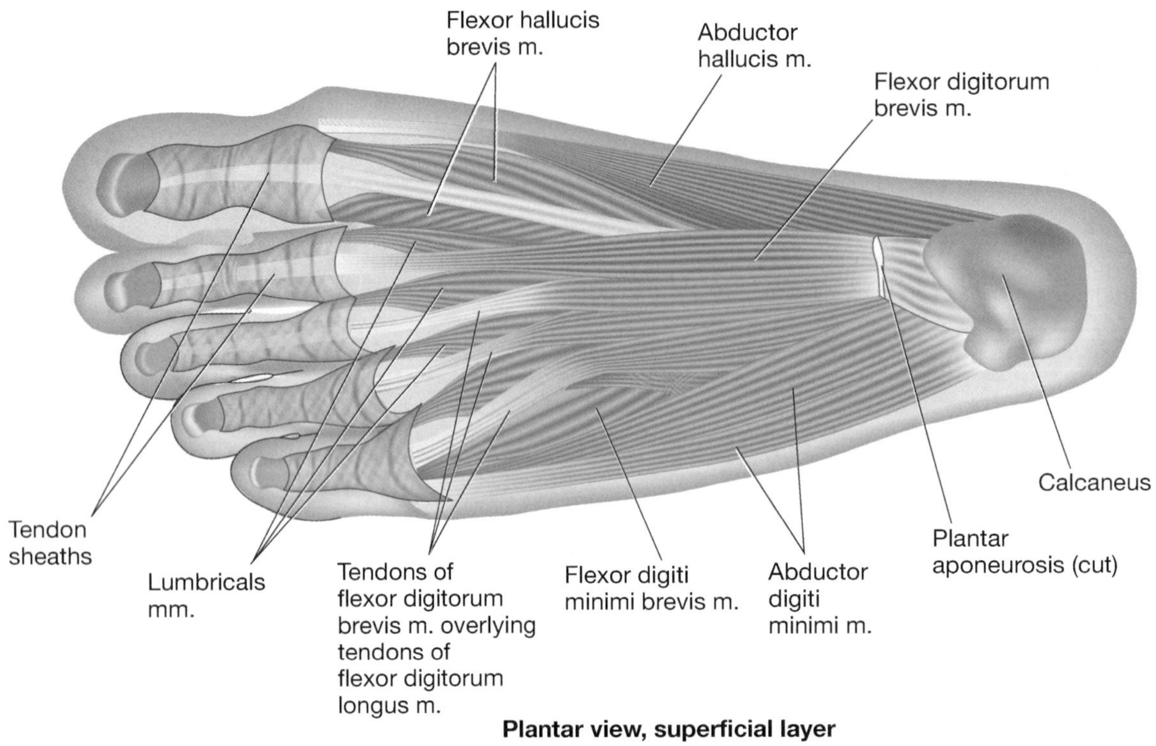

Plantar view, superficial layer

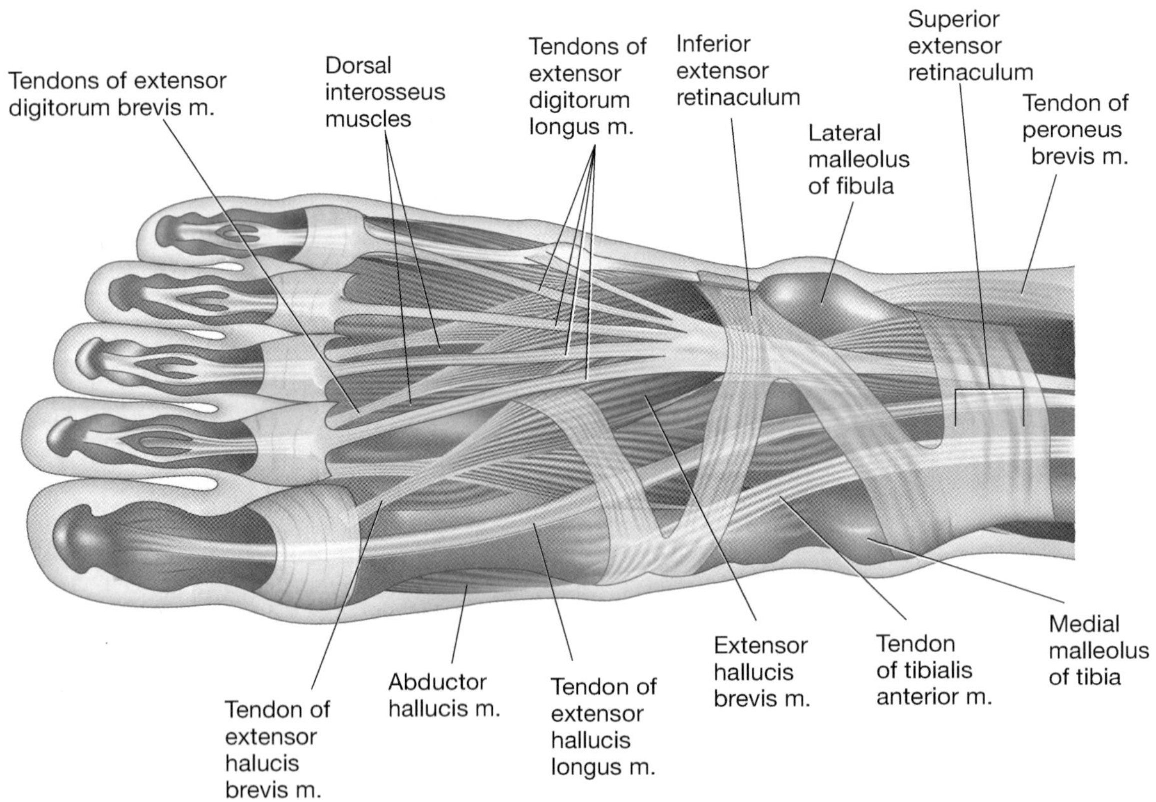

Dorsal view

Figure 8-30A

Muscles of the Pes

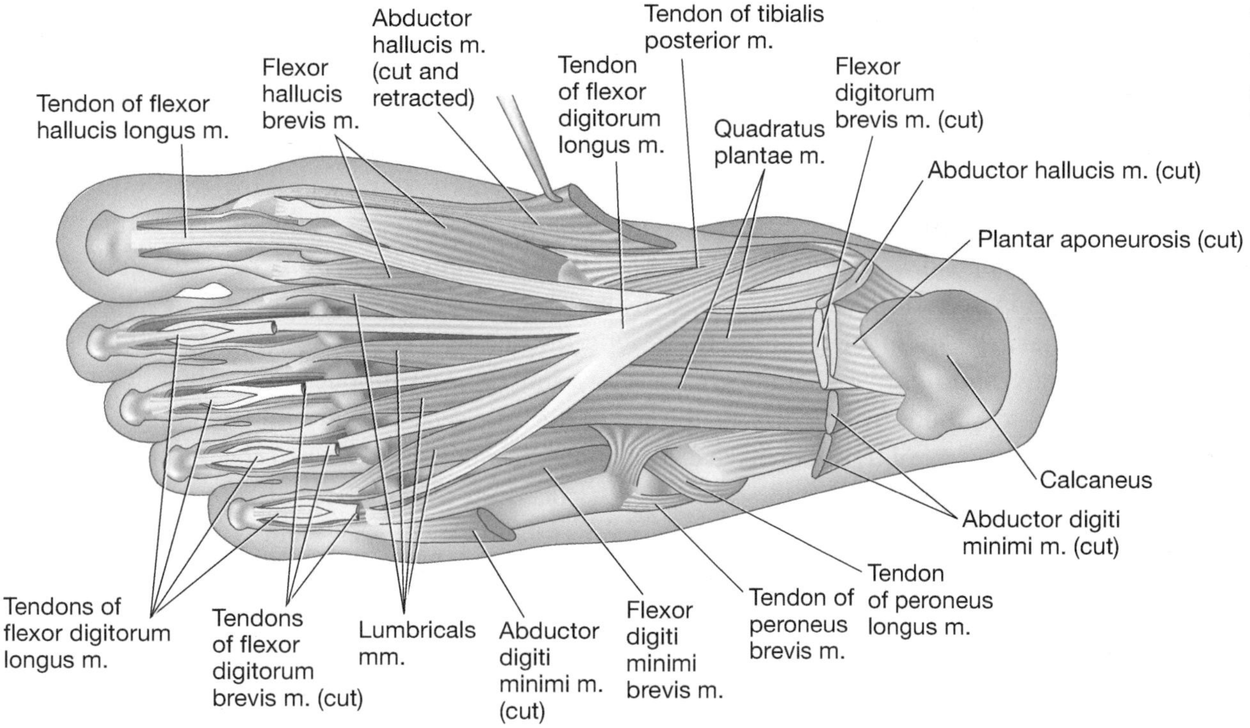

Plantar view, deeper layer

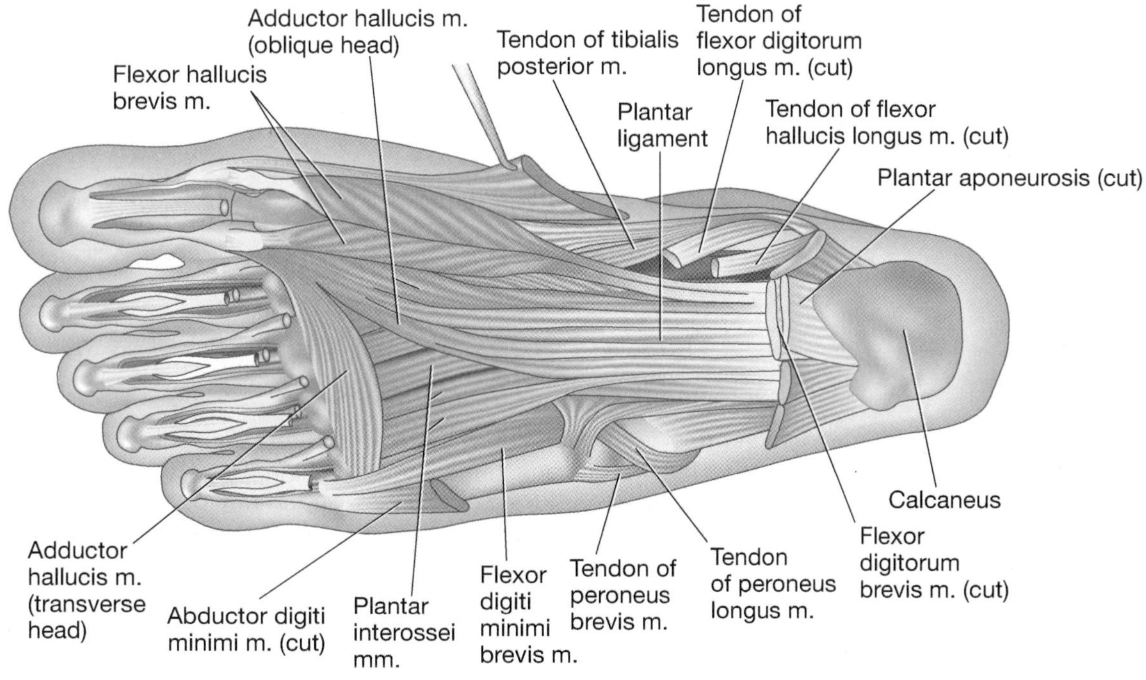

Plantar view, deepest layer

Figure 8-30B

Muscles of the Pes

Development of Skeletal Muscles

Skeletal muscles develop from **mesoderm**, the middle one of the three primary germ layers. At about three weeks of gestation the mesoderm located on each side of the notochord can be divided into three regions. The portion immediately adjacent to the notochord is called paraxial mesoderm, that furthest from the notochord is called the lateral plate mesoderm, and these are joined together by intermediate mesoderm. The **intermediate mesoderm** (**mesomere**) in some parts of the embryo forms the excretory units of the kidney (*see Chapter 19*). The **lateral mesoderm** (**hypomere**) splits into two layers (somatic and visceral) which contribute to the body wall and internal organs, respectively.

The **paraxial mesoderm** (**epimere**) is soon divided by transverse clefts into paired block-like masses called **somites**. Each somite gives rise to a muscle mass supplied by a spinal nerve and each pair of somites produces a vertebra. By the end of the fifth week there are 42-44 pairs of somites: four occipital, eight cervical, 12 thoracic, five lumbar, five sacral, and eight to 10 coccygeal pairs. The first occipital pair and the last five to seven pairs of coccygeal somites later disappear. Each remaining somite differentiates into a sclerotome, a dermatome, and a myotome (Figure 8-31). The **sclerotome** differentiates into connective tissue proper, cartilage, and bone. The **dermatome** forms the dermis and subcutaneous tissue. The mesodermal cells of the **myotomes** differentiate into **myoblasts** (Figure 8-32). These spindle-shaped cells fuse together to form multinucleated syncytial **myotubes** (a syncytium is a multinucleated mass of protoplasm produced by the merging of cells). As the myofilaments develop within the cytoplasm of the myotubes, they form the segregated organelles called myofibrils. The latter are so numerous that they force the nuclei peripherally. Myoblasts are added to the developing myofibers throughout most of gestation. By birth the myofibers are fully formed. Increase in muscle mass during growth is primarily a result of hypertrophy from the development of additional myofibrils within each muscle cell.

Objectives

23. Name the three divisions of mesoderm on each side of the notochord and state which one gives rise to myoblasts.

Figure 8-31 (Right)

Development of the Muscular System

Mesoderm (the middle germ layer) divides into a paraxial portion (adjacent to the notochord), lateral (hypaxial) mesoderm, and some intervening intermediate mesoderm. The paraxial mesoderm segments by four weeks to form somites (a) and each somite forms a dermatome, myotome, and a sclerotome. The lateral mesoderm on each side does not segment into somites but does split lengthwise into a lateral somatic (or parietal) part which contributes muscle tissue and connective tissue to the body wall and a medial (visceral) part, which contributes muscle tissue and connective tissue to internal organs. The space created between the parietal and visceral portions of the lateral plate forms the coelom (body cavity). This is divided by the diaphragm into the abdominal and thoracic cavities.

Cells from the somatic (parietal) parts of the mesoderm and the adjacent somites migrate laterally to form the limb buds (a, b). Mesoderm within the limb buds forms the various appendicular muscle groups (c). Somite mesoderm forms the epaxial muscles which lie posterior to the vertebral column. The hypaxial muscles of the body wall form from the lateral (somatic) part of the lateral plate mesoderm as noted above.

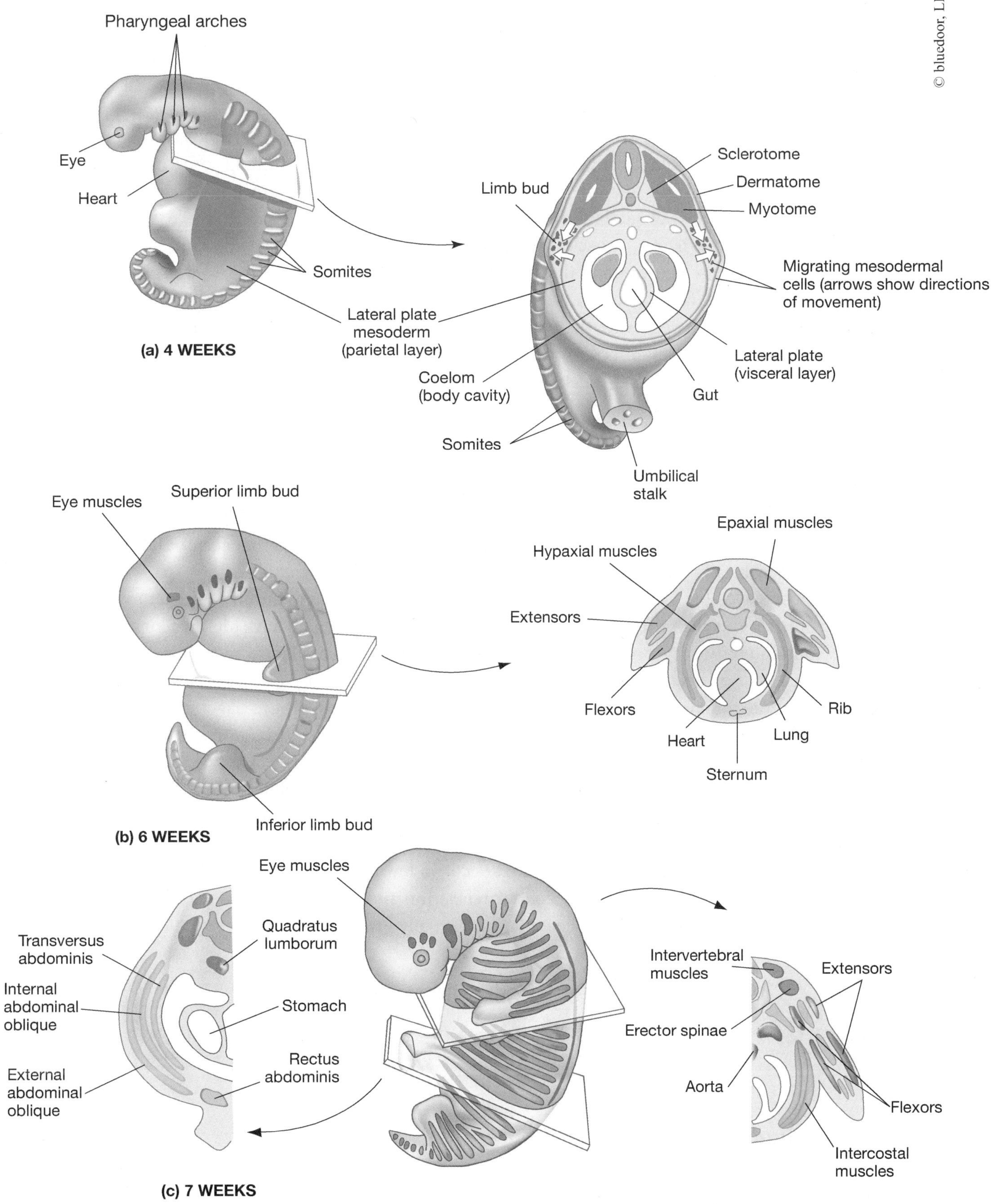

Pharyngeal arches
Eye
Heart
Somites
Lateral plate mesoderm (parietal layer)
Sclerotome
Limb bud
Dermatome
Myotome
Migrating mesodermal cells (arrows show directions of movement)
Lateral plate (visceral layer)
Coelom (body cavity)
Gut
Somites
Umbilical stalk
(a) 4 WEEKS
Eye muscles
Superior limb bud
Epaxial muscles
Hypaxial muscles
Extensors
Flexors
Rib
Heart
Lung
Sternum
Inferior limb bud
(b) 6 WEEKS
Eye muscles
Transversus abdominis
Quadratus lumborum
Internal abdominal oblique
Stomach
Rectus abdominis
External abdominal oblique
Intervertebral muscles
Extensors
Erector spinae
Aorta
Flexors
Intercostal muscles
(c) 7 WEEKS

Clinical Considerations

Muscles are subject to a number of clinical syndromes and conditions. Loss of innervation resulting in flaccid **paralysis** has already been mentioned. This typically occurs as a result of traumatic injury which disrupts a peripheral nerve. Muscles which lose their nerve supply undergo rapid **atrophy** (loss of muscle mass). That is the reason that the paralyzed limbs of invalids are so small.

Blunt trauma to a muscle belly causes bruising (**contusion**) by disrupting some muscle cells and causing hemorrhage within the muscle tissue. Tearing of muscle cells can also occur if a muscle is stretched beyond its physiological limit or if excessive antagonistic force is applied while it is contracting.

Myasthenia gravis is a muscle condition related to defective transmission of the nervous impulses between the neurons and the skeletal muscle cells. It is a chronic, progressive disease that usually begins in the face and cervical region. Women are affected more often than men. **Muscular dystrophy** is another progressive disease involving muscle atrophy. There are several types and the most common one is a sex-linked form affecting males. Affected boys usually die before maturity.

Body builders increase their muscle mass by inducing compensatory **hypertrophy** of individual muscle cells. The physical change that occurs is related to an increase in the number of myofibrils in the cytoplasm as well as to an increase in the thickness of the associated fibrous connective tissue ensheathments (epimysium, perimysium, endomysium). Muscle **cramps** are painful involuntary contractions that are believed to be related to alterations of the normal levels of certain electrolytes (especially calcium and potassium). The muscle "burn" and later soreness caused by heavy exercise are related to local changes in pH caused by the high levels of lactic acid that accumulate when muscles are anaerobically contracted.

Because skeletal muscle tissue has an extremely low regenerative capacity, injuries to it are generally more serious than those to connective tissues or epithelia which have high regenerative capacities. Consequently, surgeons avoid, when possible, making incisions directly across muscle bellies. Such incisions not only disrupt muscle cells but also sever the tiny nerve branches which course throughout the muscle belly. Orthopedic surgeons make every attempt to pass between muscle bellies when exposing bones and joints for internal fracture fixation. If large muscle bellies directly block their approach, surgeons will divide a muscle longitudinally (*i.e.*, pass *between* its fibers) or even detach its origin or insertion before they will consider transecting its belly.

Contraction of muscle tissue requires input energy at the end of the contraction/relaxation cycle. This energy is needed to effect relaxation and to "re-cock" the muscle cells for the next contraction. **Rigor mortis** is the stiffness of the body that occurs a few hours after death. This happens because the muscle tissue lacks the energy needed for relaxation and therefore remains in a contracted state for a period of time until chemical degradation partially breaks it down.

Objectives

24. Explain what causes rigor mortis, cramps, and paralysis.

Clinical Case Studies

Case 1—A 15-year-old boy playing "touch" football with several friends in his backyard, drove his hand through a bedroom window when he was tackled. A shard of glass severed several tendons on the anterior aspect of his antebrachium just above his wrist. The attending emergency room physician referred the patient to a surgeon for reconstruction of the damaged muscles. Which muscles would likely have been involved?

Case 2—A high school soccer player, involved in a pick-up game without shin guards, suffered a deep bruise to the muscles in her lower crus when she was firmly kicked on the lateral aspect of her limb several centimeters above her ankle. The resulting pain grew steadily worse over the next few hours and by midnight she was in agony with the injured area swollen and very "tight" to palpation. She underwent emergency surgery. Why?

Case 3—A body builder, doing "concentration curls" to increase the size and strength of his biceps brachii, was working with a heavier dumbbell than usual. He felt a sharp twinge of pain in the anterior aspect of his brachium accompanied by an audible but muffled ripping sound that he "felt" as well as heard. Afterward, the normal contour of his anterior brachium was significantly altered with less tissue mass than normal in the lower part and more tissue mass than normal in the upper part. What would explain these observations?

Points to Ponder

Since skeletal muscle cells in an adult do not divide, muscle mass increases in weight-lifters is not caused by hyperplasia of the myocytes. Instead, the cells undergo hypertrophy due to the exercise by increasing the number of myofibrils (contractile organelles) that they contain. Essentially everyone can increase their muscle mass and tone with exercise programs. Not everyone, however has the potential to develop a "Charles Atlas" type of body. Some individuals simply have more muscle cells than others.

When muscle bellies are traumatically severed, the ruptured ends heal back together by the proliferation of fibrous connective (scar) tissue. Some muscle cells invariably die due to the trauma and some may have their motor nerve supply disrupted. Consequently, the healed muscle is typically weaker than it was prior to the injury. When surgeons are forced to transect a muscle during an approach to bones or joints, they try to make the cut at one end or the other to minimize damage to the contractile cells and reduce the chance of permanent damage due to interruption of the blood or nerve supply. In some cases, surgeons may even elect to detach a muscle from its origin or insertion by cutting (a piece of) bone at its point of attachment. Bone tissue (once screwed or pinned back into position at the end of the procedure) often heals faster and with less chance of permanent dysfunction than might occur if the muscle belly or tendon had been transected.

Suturing the severed ends of a ruptured or transected muscle belly back together presents some technical difficulties related to the fact that the muscle tissue itself has little "holding" power (the sutures pull out easily). This is not quite as difficult but similar to sewing a couple of pieces of Jell-O® together. To combat this problem, surgeons typically don't try to suture the muscle tissue, but instead, place their sutures in the much tougher epimysium that surrounds the belly. Severed tendons also present special problems for reconstruction. Because they are mainly composed of dense regular fibrous connective tissue, suturing them is somewhat akin to trying to sew the business ends of two straw brooms together! Special techniques and suture placement patterns have been developed to counteract the tendency of the sutures to pull out of the tissue.

The muscle "burn" that often occurs during strenuous and repetitive muscle contraction is due to the accumulation of lactic acid— an end product of glucose metabolism under low oxygen conditions. When this occurs, cessation of the exercise for a few seconds will typically provide immediate relief because the lactic acid enters the blood stream, and is carried to the liver where it is converted back into pyruvic acid (and perhaps all the way back to glucose) by a "reverse glycolysis" series of chemical reactions called the Cori cycle that only hepatocytes have the metabolic machinery to perform.

Like liver cells, skeletal muscle cells can polymerize glucose to form and store intracellular glycogen. (They can also bind some oxygen in a hemoglobin-like compound called myoglobin). Endurance athletes try to preserve their muscle glycogen during competitions by maintaining a steady intake of high energy material. Once muscle glycogen is depleted, physical exhaustion is imminent.

Physical exercise that can be sustained for a considerable time (over 10 minutes) is often classified as an aerobic exercise. The implication is that oxygen intake is keeping up with the rate the muscles are using it in their contractions. Exercise that is more vigorous and cannot be sustained (lifting heavy weights, running up stairs, *etc.*) is often called anaerobic to imply that the oxygen intake is not keeping up with the oxygen needs of the contracting muscles.

Slang and Obsolete Nomenclature

UNOFFICIAL TERM	OFFICIAL DESIGNATION
deltoid muscle	deltoideus muscle *[musculus deltoideus]*
SDF	superficial digital flexor muscle *[m. flexor digitorum superficialis]*
DDF	deep digital flexor muscle *[m. flexor digitorum profundus]*
biceps muscle (brachium)	biceps brachii muscle *[m. biceps brachii]*
triceps muscle	triceps brachii muscle *[m. triceps brachii]*
H zone	H band *[stria H]*
sarcomere	myomere *[myomerum]*
sarcoplasm	cytoplasm *[cytoplasma]*
sarcolemma	cell membrane *[membrana cellularis]*, myolemma *[myolemma]*
sarcoplasmic reticulum	endoplasmic reticulum *[reticulum endoplasmaticum]*
Achilles tendon	calcanean tendon *[tendo calcaneus]*
quadriceps ligament	tendon of insertion of the quadriceps femoris muscle
hamstrings	posterior muscles of the thigh
biceps muscle (thigh)	biceps femoris muscle *[m. biceps femoris]*
external oblique m.	external abdominal oblique m. *[m. obliquus externus abdominis]*
internal oblique m.	internal abdominal oblique m. *[m. obliquus internus abdominis]*
triangularis m.	depressor anguli oris m. *[m. depressor anguli oris]*
tendinous inscription	tendinous intersections *[intersectiones tendineae]* of the rectus abdominis m.
frontalis m.	frontal belly *[venter frontalis]* of epicranius m.
occipitalis m.	occipital belly *[venter occipitalis]* of epicranius m.

Review Questions

1. A(n) ______________________ is composed of (contains) thin myofilaments plus interconnecting proteins.
   A. H band
   B. I band
   C. A band

D. M line
E. myomere

2. Which of the following statements is incorrect?
   A. Mastication typically follows prehension and deglutition typically follows mastication.
   B. The origin of a muscle is the attachment(s) that moves the least during muscle contraction.
   C. Muscle fasciculi are enveloped by c.t. proper ensheathments called endomysium.
   D. Retinacula are bands of dense regular collagenous connective tissue that bind tendons into groups and hold them in certain locations.
   E. The basic unit of skeletal muscle structure from Z line to Z line is called a myomere.

3. During muscular contraction, which of the following does not shorten (narrow)?
   A. myomere
   B. A band
   C. I band
   D. H band
   E. Choose this response if all the above (A-D) become shorter during muscle contraction.

4. Which of the following is not true?
   A. There are seven major groups of muscles in the body.
   B. The muscles of the head are subdivided into six subgroups.
   C. The muscles of the superior limb are subdivided into six subgroups.
   D. The muscles of the neck are subdivided into eight subgroups.
   E. Choose this response if all the above (A-D) are true.

5. Find the false statement.
   A. Epaxial muscles are the muscles located anterior to the transverse processes of the vertebrae.
   B. There are two anatomic forms of muscular attachment.
   C. The rotator cuff is actually a group of four muscles that traverse the shoulder joint superiorly, inferiorly, posteriorly, and anteriorly.
   D. Single-actioned muscles can be fixators but they cannot have fixators.
   E. When muscles contract, no movement may occur or even the motion opposite to their stated action(s) may occur.

6. Which of the following is part of a skeletal muscle?
   A. ligament
   B. retinaculum
   C. tendon
   D. bursa
   E. Choose this response if more than one of the above (A-D) are part of a muscle.

7. A muscle, "*musculus hypotheticus*," originates on the anterior aspect of the inferior angle of the scapula and inserts on the anterior aspect of the body of the humerus (just medial to the deltoid tuberosity of the humerus). Find the truth.
   A. It can flex the shoulder joint.
   B. It can abduct the superior limb at the shoulder joint.

C. It can flex the elbow joint.
D. It can internally rotate the free part of the superior limb.
E. It can protract the superior limb.

8. Find the correct match.
A. brachialis muscle—single action—anterior mm. of the antebrachium
B. orbicularis oculi muscle—single action—mm. of face
C. pectoralis minor muscle—multi-action—mm. of thorax
D. levator scapulae muscle—multi-action—mm. of back
E. rectus femoris muscle—multi-action—anterior mm. of hip

9. Find the correct statement.
A. The muscular system is the second largest body system.
B. Most muscles attach via broad flat tendons termed aponeuroses.
C. The sliding filament mechanism is essentially identical in all three types of muscle tissue.
D. Myofibers are composed of myofilaments and are located within myofibrils.
E. Choose this response if none of the above (A-D) are true.

10. Which item is false?
A. A given muscle may act as an agonist in one situation and function as a synergist, antagonist, or fixator in other situations.
B. Elastic recoil and gravity of certain body parts can produce body movement.
C. Large motor units are often found in the eye muscles of hypnotists.
D. The word "levator" in levator palpebrae superioris muscle refers to an action of the muscle.
E. The aponeuroses of three different abdominal muscles contribute to the linea alba.

Thought Questions

1. Does a muscle have to cross more than one joint to have more than one action? Explain.

2. Why can weight-lifters lift more weight or do more repetitions after "warming up" with lighter weights and fewer repetitions?

3. What are the advantages of midline abdominal incisions for surgical invasion of the abdomen *vs.* paramedian or paracostal approaches?

4. Most skeletal muscles in the limbs are involved in third class lever systems. Since third class levers always lose mechanical advantage, of what benefit is this design?

5. The carpal flexor retinaculum is a band of connective tissue that stabilizes the tendons of the anterior antebrachial muscles which continue distally into the manus. Tendons of which anterior antebrachial muscles are held in place by this retinaculum?

6. Muscle A is said to be a fixator muscle in regard to a certain action of muscle *B*. What does this imply about muscle *A?* About muscle *B?*

7. To which three groups of muscles of the superior limb do the eight "pollicis" muscles belong?

8. What is wrong with each of the following descriptions of muscle actions?
   A. extend the brachium.
   B. abduct the shoulder.
   C. flex the biceps brachii muscle.

9. Using your own body (or that of a *real* good friend) identify the following muscles:
   A. Most of the tendons visible subcutaneously on the back of the metacarpus.
   B. The one bruised by a law enforcement officer who discovers that the door he is trying to break down with his shoulder is solid oak.
   C. The one whose tendon bulges forward on the front of the ankle when the tarsal joint is forcefully flexed.
   D. The one responsible for the rippled appearance of the anterior abdomen in a thin, well exercised individual.
   E. The ones accentuated by wearing high-heeled shoes.

10. Where does the superficial digital flexor muscle go deep and the deep digital flexor muscle become superficial?

11. Bo and Jo (meat cutters) severed their second (Bo) and third (Jo) digits through the proximal interphalangeal joints. Discuss the antebrachial muscles they injured.

12. What is wrong with the statement..."skeletal muscles are composed of skeletal muscle tissue"?

13. What is the difference between a tendon and an aponeurosis? Between a tendon and a ligament? Between a ligament and a retinaculum?

14. What are the possible consequences of a muscle contracting with a force greater than the body's structure can withstand?

15. Why do men generally have bigger and stronger muscles than women?

16. Some extremely fit individuals have a negative specific gravity (*i.e.*, their bodies sink instead of float in water). Why?

17. The contraction of a muscle cell is "all or none" but a named muscle can contract with varying force. Explain.

18. Name two muscles that have inherently antagonistic actions (actions that are antagonistic to themselves).

19. The connective tissue band joining the patella to the tibial tuberosity has two acceptable names. What are they?

20. What do bursae, tendon sheaths, and sesamoid bones have in common?

21. Why do various sources cite different totals for the number of bones in the skeleton?

Answers to Clinical Case Studies

Case 1—Tendons on the anterior aspect of the distal antebrachium include those of the superficial and deep digital flexor muscles, radial and ulnar carpal flexor muscles, palmaris longus muscle, and flexor pollicis longus muscle. Any of these could have been injured but the deeply located ones are less vulnerable.

Case 2—This unfortunate individual suffered compartment syndrome wherein swelling from an injury (often caused by extravasation of blood) is limited by fascial encasements. As the pressure rises, pain results. In severe cases, like this one, surgery may be necessary to relieve the pressure and prevent permanent damage to the muscles involved. In these cases, the pressure can rise so high that blood flow through the involved structures is restricted and ischemic necrosis can result.

Case 3—This patient tore his biceps brachii muscle near its insertion. The contracted belly of the muscle caused the anterior bulge in his upper brachium. Absence of the muscle in the lower brachium resulted in the paucity of tissue mass in that region.

Answers to Review Questions

1. B. The I bands are caused by the presence of lighter-staining, thin myofilaments between the darker staining, thick myofilaments which cause the A bands.
2. C. Fasciculi are encased by perimysium.
3. B.
4. D. Cervical muscles are divided into six subgroups.
5. A. Hypaxial muscles are located anterior to the transverse process of the vertebrae.
6. C.
7. D.
8. B.
9. C.
10. C. Eye muscles have small motor units.

Answers to Thought Questions

1. In theory, every joint a muscle spans can be acted on by the muscle but in some cases the positions of the attachments are such that the force produced at the joint is minimal or negligible.

However, the number of actions can exceed the number of joints crossed if more than one action can be produced at a given joint. The biceps brachii muscle, for example, crosses only the shoulder and elbow joints but it has three actions since it can cause both flexion and rotation of the elbow joint (as well as flexion at the shoulder joint).

2. The warm up increases the blood flow to the exercised muscles which, in turn, facilitates removal of lactic acid during the subsequent, more vigorous exercise.

3. Midline abdominal incisions pass through the linea alba and avoid the bellies of the abdominal muscles altogether. Sutures in the linea alba have more holding power and form a more secure (stronger) abdominal closure than those placed (by necessity) in the bellies of the muscles when the other types of abdominal incisions are closed. The other surgical approaches to the abdomen *do* have advantages in certain procedures and they *are* used.

4. Although third class levers lose mechanical advantage, they gain total distance moved (or speed of movement) at the insertion *vs.* the origin. Thus, contraction of the biceps brachii muscle may cause the significant motion at the elbow joint even though the muscle belly itself may shorten only a few centimeters.

5. All of them except the three antebrachial rotators. Those whose tendons are held in place by the retinaculum are the flexor carpi radialis and ulnaris muscles, superficial and deep digital flexor muscles, palmaris longus muscle, and flexor pollicis longus muscle.

6. Muscle A must be antagonistic to one (or more) actions of muscle B (but A is *not* antagonistic to the specific action of B under discussion). Muscle B must be a multi-actioned muscle.

7. One of them is an anterior antebrachial muscle, three are posterior antebrachial muscles, and four are intrinsic muscles of the hand (three in the thenar group and one in the intermediate group).

8. A. Extension and flexion are terms applied to joints. Rigid body parts like the brachium, antebrachium, and thigh cannot be extended or flexed.
   B. Abduction/adduction are terms describing the movement of body parts in frontal (coronal) planes. The shoulder is not abducted—the superior limb is abducted at the shoulder joint.
   C. Muscles are contracted. The term *flex* should be reserved for joints.

9. A. Digital extensor muscle
   B. Deltoideus muscle
   C. Anterior tibial muscle
   D. Rectus abdominus muscle
   E. Gastrocnemius and soleus muscles (collectively called triceps surae m.)

10. They trade superficial/deep positions near the metacarpophalangeal joints. The four tendons of the SDF form loops or "holes" through which the four tendons of the DDF pass. Those of the SDF (now in the deep position) attach to the middle phalanges of digits 2, 3, 4, and 5, and those of the DDF (now in the superficial position) attach to the distal phalanges of digits 2, 3, 4, and 5.

11. Bo severed tendons of the superficial and deep digital flexors, the tendon of the digital extensor muscle, and the tendon of the extensor indicis muscle. Jo severed other tendons of these same muscles except for the extensor indicis muscle.

12. This statement ignores the fact that many other tissues are found in skeletal muscles. These include (a lot of) connective tissue proper, smooth muscle tissue, blood and epithelium (in vessels), and nervous tissue.

13. Aponeuroses are broad, flat tendons. Thus, all aponeuroses are tendons but not all tendons are aponeuroses. Tendons are subparts of muscles, whereas ligaments (of the skeletal system) are bands of connective tissue that stabilize the skeletal components around joints. Retinacula group tendons together and hold them in certain locations.

14. At least four things can happen. The muscle belly can rupture, one of its tendons can rupture, a tendon can be pulled loose (avulsed) from its attachment, or a bone can be fractured. A tendinous avulsion may involve tearing away a small bone fragment while leaving most of the bone intact.

15. Testosterone (which women produce but in lesser quantities) promotes skeletal muscle development and strength.

16. Fat floats in water, but skeletal muscle tissue sinks. This is due primarily to the iron containing myoglobin (an oxygen binding muscle pigment similar to the hemoglobulin in red corpuscles). Very fit individuals have a low fat content in their bodies.

17. When a skeletal muscle cell is stimulated by a nervous impulse, it contracts. Thus, the muscle cell is either contracted or relaxed (there are no gradations or intermediate states). Skeletal muscles, however, contain many skeletal muscle cells. The strength of contraction depends on how many skeletal muscle cells within a named muscle contract.

18. The deltoideus muscle (can both extend and flex the shoulder joint) and the brachioradialis muscle (can both pronate and supinate the manus/antebrachium).

19. Patellar ligament or tendon of insertion of the quadriceps femoris muscle. One should not call this structure the patellar tendon or the quadriceps femoris ligament.

20. They all share a functional purpose of protecting tendons from frictional degradation.

21. Some authors do not count the small sesamoid bones associated with tendons at the bases of the thumbs and big toes. These sources list a total of 206 bones in the skeleton. When totalling the bones, the os sacrum is counted as only one bone, even though the five sacral vertebrae fuse to form it. Similar logic is used when counting the four fused coccygeal vertebrae (they form one bone). In like manner, each os coxae is counted as a single bone in spite of the fact that an ilium, ischium and pubis fuse to form it.

CHAPTER 9

Introduction to the Nervous System and CNS

Chapter Outline and Key Concepts

INTRODUCTION

The nervous system has two major anatomic divisions: central nervous system (CNS= brain and spinal cord) and peripheral nervous system (PNS= nerves, ganglia, and sensory receptors).

The autonomic nervous system (ANS) includes those parts of the CNS and PNS that are motor to smooth muscle tissue, cardiac muscle tissue, and glandular epithelium.

FUNCTIONS OF THE NERVOUS SYSTEM

The nervous system and the rest of the body communicate via electrochemical phenomena called nervous impulses.

Impulses going from the central nervous system *to* the body are called efferent (motor) impulses.

Impulses *from* the body to the CNS are called afferent (sensory) impulses.

The PNS converts physical stimuli to sensory impulses, conducts sensory impulses to the CNS, and distributes motor impulses to muscle tissue and glandular epithelium.

The CNS receives sensory impulses, sends motor impulses, and processes and stores information.

NEURONS

Neurons are the impulse conducting cells of the nervous system.

Neurons have processes called axons (conduct impulses away from the cell body) and dendrites (conduct impulses toward the cell body).

Neurons are anatomically classified as pseudounipolar, bipolar, or multipolar based on the number of dendrites and the dendrite/ cell body/ axonal arrangement.

Neurons are functionally divided into four groups based on the source of their sensory impulses or the destiny of their motor impulses.

Nerves are bundles of neuron processes in the PNS and fiber tracts are neuronal bundles in the brain and spinal cord.

Ganglia are groups of neuron cell bodies in the PNS and nuclei are groups of neuron cell bodies in the CNS.

NEUROGLIA

Neuroglia (glial cells) are cells of the nervous system that support the neurons.

There are several types of glial cells and each one has a specific function.

Functions of neuroglia include forming myelin sheaths (neurolemmocytes and oligodendrocytes), forming the blood/brain barrier (astrocytes), and phagocytosis (microglia).

NERVE IMPULSE TRANSMISSION

The cytoplasm of neurons is negatively charged (due, primarily to a preponderance of negatively charged protein ions) and has a relatively high potassium ion and low sodium ion content compared to the extracellular fluid.

The sodium/potassium concentration gradients are established by an active transport mechanism called the sodium-potassium pump.

An impulse occurs when there is a sudden increase in permeability of the cell membrane to sodium ions.

The inrush of sodium ions (due to simple diffusion), followed by an out-rush of potassium ions (due to simple diffusion), causes the sudden change in neuronal voltage that constitutes an impulse.

When impulses reach the ends of axons, they cause the release of chemicals called neurotransmitters that diffuse across the synaptic clefts and interact with the cell membranes of the next cells.

The next cell (gland cell, muscle cell, or another neuron) is either stimulated or inhibited (depending on which of several kinds of neurotransmitters it receives).

DEVELOPMENT OF THE NERVOUS SYSTEM

Nervous tissue develops from the outer primary germ layer called ectoderm.

The ectoderm over the notochord thickens to form a neural plate.

The neural plate folds downward over the notochord to make a neural groove which closes to form the neural tube.

The neural tube becomes the brain (anteriorly/superiorly) and the spinal cord (posteriorly/inferiorly).

The primitive brain forms three vesicles that subdivide into the five vesicles that form the definitive parts of the brain.

MAJOR PARTS OF THE BRAIN

The cerebrum (largest part of the brain) is divided into two cerebral hemispheres and a few other portions.

Each cerebral hemisphere has five lobes and the lobes have specific functions.

The diencephalon has three major components: epithalamus, thalamus, and hypothalamus.

The thalamus is a relay center for most general sensory impulses that ascend the spinal cord.

The hypothalamus produces several hormones and contains several special centers that involve thermoregulation, hunger, thirst, sex, and emotional states.

The mesencephalon serves as a relay center for visual and auditory reflexes, and it contains motor nuclei for cranial nerves 3 and 4.

The pons contains nuclei for cranial nerves 5, 6, 7, and 8, and has two respiratory centers.

The cerebellum (second largest part of the brain) coordinates skeletal muscle activity.

The medulla oblongata is the most inferior part of the brain and serves as a decussation site for many of the ascending and descending fiber tracts.

MAJOR PARTS OF THE SPINAL CORD

The spinal cord is the direct inferior continuation of the medulla oblongata.

Thirty-one to 33 pairs of spinal nerves originate from the spinal cord.

The spinal cord has a tiny central canal surrounded by "X" ("H") shaped gray matter which is, in turn, surrounded by fiber tracts forming the white matter.

In most parts of the spinal cord, the gray matter forms (paired) anterior and posterior gray columns (horns).

The white matter of the spinal cord consists of ascending and descending fiber tracts grouped into (paired) anterior, lateral, and posterior funiculi.

CONNECTIVE TISSUE ENSHEATHMENTS OF THE CNS (MENINGES)

The outermost and strongest meninx is the dura mater.

The arachnoid mater (deep to the dura) has web-like strands that extend inwardly to the pia mater.

The spaces between the arachnoid filaments make up the subarachnoid space.

The delicate pia mater adheres to the brain and spinal cord.

PRODUCTION AND FLOW OF CEREBROSPINAL FLUID

CSF occupies the ventricles of the brain, subarachnoid space, and central canal of the spinal cord.

CSF is secreted by choroid plexuses at a rate of about 800 ml/day.

Only about 175 ml (total) of CSF is present at any given time.

CLINICAL CONSIDERATIONS

Concussions are "bruising" of brain tissue caused by trauma.

Cerebrovascular accidents (CVA's) are often called "strokes."

Paralysis includes several defined subtypes (quadriplegia, paraplegia, hemiplegia).

Electroencephalography measures the electrical activity of the brain.

Many CNS disorders have no observable anatomic alterations.

A number of infectious diseases affect the nervous system.

Selected Definitions

Anatomic (morphologic) types of neurons—the categories of neurons based on the number of dendrites and the physical relationship of the cell body to the axon and dendrite. Three types are described: pseudounipolar, bipolar, and multipolar.

Autonomic nervous system (ANS)—those parts of the nervous system that are motor to involuntary effectors. The ANS includes some parts of both the CNS and the PNS.

Axon—the single process of a neuron that carries an impulse away from the cell body. At the terminal end(s) of axons, impulses are synaptically transmitted to other neurons or to effectors.

Central nervous system (CNS)—the brain and spinal cord. The CNS receives sensory impulses, processes and stores information, and sends motor impulses out to effectors.

Cerebellum—the second largest part of the brain. It has two hemispheres united by a cerebellar vermis and functions in the coordination of skeletal muscle activity.

Cerebrospinal fluid (CSF)—the water based medium which occupies the ventricles and interconnecting channels of the brain, the central canal of the spinal cord, the subarachnoid space, and the osseous labyrinth of the temporal bone.

Cerebrum—the largest part of the brain. The cerebrum includes the left and right cerebral hemispheres and some intervening structures.

Dendrite—a neuronal process that carries an impulse toward the cell body of a neuron. Multipolar neurons have multiple dendrites, but bipolar and pseudounipolar neurons have one dendrite each.

Depolarization—a physiological term indicating an elevation in the intracytoplasmic voltage. If depolarization reaches the threshold potential, an action potential is triggered, consisting of rapid further depolarization followed by repolarization to re-establish the resting voltage.

Functional types of neurons—the categories of neurons based on the origin and destination of their impulses. Four types exist: somatic efferent, somatic afferent, visceral efferent, and visceral afferent neurons.

Gray matter—those parts of the brain and spinal cord that are darker in color than white matter (see below). The gray matter owes its pigmentation to the presence of large numbers of neuronal cell bodies, which, with their complement of organelles, impart the darker color.

Meninx (pl. **meninges**)—one of the three connective tissue proper encasements of the brain and spinal cord. Trabecular space between the innermost meninx (pia mater) and the middle one (arachnoid mater) contains cerebrospinal fluid and is called the subarachnoid space.

Motor impulse/neuron—a nervous impulse emanating from the brain or spinal cord/a neuron that carries such an impulse. Motor impulses are destined for glandular epithelium or muscle tissue.

Myelin—a lipid material manufactured by neurolemmocytes and oligodendrocytes. This substance is the insulating medium in myelinated neurons.

Neurotransmitter—a chemical involved in synaptic impulse transmission. Neurotransmitters, manufactured by neurons and sensory receptors, are released under appropriate stimulation.

Peripheral nervous system (PNS)—nerves, ganglia, and sensory receptors. The PNS generates sensory impulses and carries sensory and motor impulses to and from the CNS.

Repolarization—that part of an action potential consisting of a rapid drop in voltage after the potential has been raised by depolarization. Repolarization is effected by a rapid out-rush of potassium ions from the cytoplasm.

Sensory impulse/neuron—an impulse destined for the CNS/a neuron that carries such an impulse. Sensory impulses are generated by sensory receptors and then are conducted to the brain or spinal cord.

Sodium-potassium pump—the active transport mechanism found in most types of body cells that moves three sodium ions out of and two potassium ions into the cell for each ATP expended. These pumps are especially important in muscle cells and neurons.

Synapse—the junction of a neuron or sensory receptor with another cell. Sensory receptors synapse with neurons, and neurons synapse variously with other neurons, with muscle cells, or with glandular epithelial cells.

White matter—those parts of the brain and spinal cord that are notably whiter in color than the remainder (gray matter). White matter consists mainly of myelinated axons, and myelin is a white-colored lipid material.

Etymology *Scientia est potentia*—"Knowledge is power."

afferens (L), *to bring to*—afferent
arachn (L), *spider*—arachnoid mater
arbor (L), *tree*—arbor vitae
astro (L), *star*—astrocyte
automonia (G), *dependent*—autonomic
callosus (L), *callous skin*—corpus callosum
cauda (L), *tail*—cauda equina
conus (L), *cone*—conus medullaris
dia (L), *through*—diencephalon
durus (L), *hard*—dura mater
dys (L), *difficult*—dyslexia
efferens(L), *to carry outward*—efferent
enkephalos (G), *brain*—rhombencephalon
ependyma (G), *upper garment*—ependymal
epilepsia (G), *to seize, attack*—epileptic
equus (L), *horse*—cauda equina
gyrus (L), *circle*—gyrus
intumescere (L), *to swell, rise*—intumescence
lemma (G), *husk, rind*—neurolemmocyte
lexia (L), *word, speech*—dyslexia
mater (L), *mother*—dura mater
meninx (G), *membrane*—meninges
meta (L), *between*—metencephalon
multus (L), *much, many*—multipolar
myel (G), *marrow, spinal cord*—myelin
oblongus (L), *oblong*—medulla oblongata
oligos (G), *few*—oligodendrocyte
pia (L), *tender*—pia mater
pinea (L), *pine cone*—pineal
saltatorius (L), *relating to dancing*—saltatory
sulcus (L), *furrow*—sulcus
synapsis (G), *contact, point of juncture*—synapse
telos (G), *complete, mature*—telencephalon
thalamos (G), *room*—thalamus
vermis (L), *worm*—vermis
vitae (L), *life*—arbor vitae

Introduction

The nervous system exerts direct control over many organs of the body and indirectly influences most others. It is divided into the **central nervous system (CNS)** which consists of the brain and spinal cord and the **peripheral nervous system (PNS)** composed of the cranial nerves, spinal nerves, a number of ganglia, and some specialized sensory receptors. The **autonomic nervous system (ANS)** is a functional subdivision rather than an anatomic one. It consists of those parts of the CNS and PNS that control involuntary muscle tissue and glandular epithelium (*see Chapter 11*). The unofficial term "somatic nervous system" is sometimes used to refer to all parts of the nervous system except the ANS.

Objectives

1. Name the two major divisions of the nervous system and list the structures that comprise each one.
2. Define the ANS in terms of its relationship to the rest of the nervous system and its function.

Functions of the Nervous System

The nervous system communicates with the rest of the body and within itself by electrochemical energy in the form of **nervous impulses**. These impulses occur within individual nerve cells (neurons). Impulses which originate peripherally and are carried into the CNS within the cranial and spinal nerves are called **sensory** or **afferent** impulses. They convey both **general sensation** (heat, cold, touch, pressure, pain) as well as information related to the **special senses** (sight, hearing, smell, taste, body position, and balance). Impulses originating in the CNS and carried peripherally by the cranial and spinal nerves are called **motor** or **efferent** impulses. They are destined for muscle tissue (where they initiate contraction) and for glandular epithelium (where they control secretory activity).

The peripheral nervous system has three major functions and all are related to nervous impulses:

1. **Converting (transducing) various forms of energy to sensory impulses**. Specialized receptor cells are required for some of these conversions, including photoreceptors, thermoreceptors, chemoreceptors, and several kinds of mechanoreceptors.
2. **Conducting sensory impulses into the CNS via the cranial and spinal nerves**. These nerves serve as functional extensions of the brain and spinal cord. They consist of bundles of nerve cell processes.
3. **Distributing the motor impulses which originate in the brain and spinal cord to the muscle tissue and glands of the body**. These outgoing impulses travel within the same cranial and spinal nerves as the incoming sensory impulses but they are carried by different nerve cells.

The central nervous system also has three major functions:

1. **Receiving the sensory impulses carried by the cranial and spinal nerves.**
2. **Processing and storing information** (*i.e.*, interpreting, thinking, and memory).
3. **Sending motor impulses to muscle tissue and glandular epithelium.**

The physiologic mechanisms involved in memory, thinking, and information interpretation are not well understood, but nervous impulses are involved. There is no physiological difference between a *motor* impulse *vs.* a *sensory* impulse. Nor is there a difference in the nervous impulse carried by a nerve cell involved in vision *vs.* ones involved with the senses of smell, hearing, taste, *etc.* The functions of the nervous system are summarized in Figure 9-1.

Objectives

3. List the functions of the CNS and the functions of the PNS.

Neurons

The functional cells of the nervous system are **neurons**. They are anatomically and physiologically specialized for the conduction of electrochemical energy commonly called nervous impulses. Neurons are highly modified cells with extremely long, slender processes called **axons** and **dendrites**. These processes extend from the **cell body** to allow contact with other neurons or with glandular epithelium or muscle cells. Dendrites conduct impulses toward the cell bodies of neurons and axons conduct impulses away from the cell bodies (*i.e.*, toward other cells). Three morphological types of neurons are identified on the basis of the number and arrangement of the axons and dendrites: multipolar, bipolar, and pseudounipolar (Figure 9-2). **Multipolar neurons** have several dendrites and a single axon (which may have numerous branches). All motor neurons and essen-

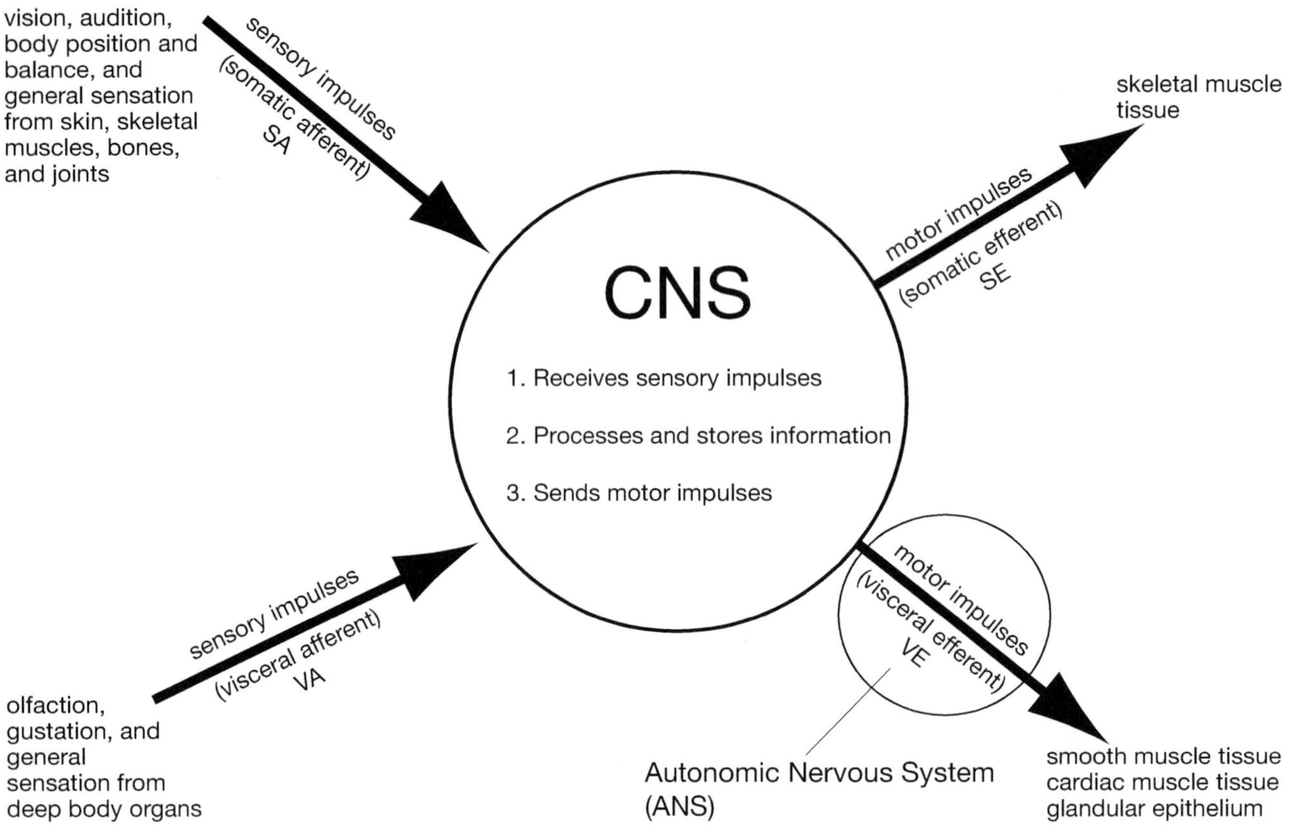

Figure 9-1

Schematic Representation of Sensory Input and Motor Output of the Nervous System

Note that even though the various sensory and motor pathways are physically separated in this schematic diagram, they are all distributed peripherally within the cranial and spinal nerves. Barring a few exceptions in the cranial nerves, grossly separate sensory and motor pathways in the peripheral nervous system do not exist (*i.e.,* essentially all nerves contain both motor and sensory pathways).

tially all of the neurons located totally within the CNS (**interneurons**) are multipolar. **Bipolar neurons** have a single dendrite and a single axon. They are the least numerous neuronal type and are found only in the retina of the eye, in the internal ear, and in the nasal mucosa where they carry sensory impulses interpreted by the CNS as vision, body balance/position, audition, and olfaction. (Bipolar neurons, incidentally, have nothing to do with the behavior disorder labeled "bipolar.") **Pseudounipolar neurons** resemble bipolar neurons except that the cell body is offset. This occurs because the axonal process fuses directly to the single dendritic process with a single combined connection making direct contact with the cell body. Pseudounipolar neurons carry all sensory information except for that relegated to bipolar neurons.

In addition to their morphological classification, neurons are functionally classified into four groups: somatic efferent, visceral efferent, somatic afferent, and visceral afferent. **Somatic efferent neurons** are the multipolar neurons which supply motor impulses to skeletal muscle. Their cell bodies are located in the brain and spinal cord and their axons are distributed to all of the skeletal muscles

Table 9-1 Functional Classification of Neurons

Functional Type	*Anatomical Type*	*Cell Body Location*	*Type/Distribution of Impulses*
Somatic Efferent (SE)	Multipolar	Brain: cranial nerve motor nuclei Spinal cord: anterior gray column	Motor to skeletal muscle
Visceral Efferent (VE)	Multipolar	Brain: motor nuclei of cranial nerves 3, 7, 9, 10 Spinal cord: lateral gray column in sacral region Autonomic ganglia	Motor to smooth m., cardiac m., and glandular epithelium
Somatic Afferent (SA)	Pseudounipolar (some bipolar)	Retina and sensory ganglia of cranial and spinal nerves	Sensory from retina (vision), internal ear (audition and balance), skin, skeletal muscle, bones, joints
Visceral Afferent (VA)	Pseudounipolar (some bipolar)	Nasal mucosa and sensory ganglia of cranial and spinal nerves	Sensory from nasal mucosa (smell), oral mucosa (taste), deep body organs

of the body. Skeletal muscle cells have no inherent contractility and thus require this innervation in order to shorten. **Visceral efferent neurons** are multipolar neurons which form a two neuron chain to smooth muscle cells, cardiac muscle cells, and glandular epithelium (*see Chapter 11*). The first neurons are called **preganglionic neurons** (cell bodies) and are located in the brain and spinal cord. The second neurons are called **postganglionic neurons** (cell bodies) and are located in autonomic ganglia in the peripheral nervous system. The visceral efferent neurons and the CNS centers which control them, comprise the autonomic nervous system which is discussed in Chapter 11. **Somatic afferent neurons** are those which carry sensory information from skin, skeletal muscles, bones, joints, and also from the retina (vision) and internal ear (audition and the sense of balance and body position). Their cell bodies are located in the sensory ganglia of the cranial and spinal nerves as well as in the retina. Most of them are pseudounipolar neurons but a few are bipolar (those in the retina and internal ear). **Visceral afferent neurons** carry sensory impulses from deep body systems as well as those involved in the special senses of smell and taste. Their cell bodies are located in the sensory ganglia of the cranial and spinal nerves as well as in the nasal mucosa. Like the somatic afferents, most visceral afferent neurons are pseudounipolar but those associated with the sense of smell are bipolar (Table 9-1).

Because neurons have such long processes, some parts of the nervous system consist almost entirely of bundles of processes (mainly axons) with few or no cell bodies present. Groups of processes within the brain and spinal cord are called (fiber) **tracts**. Those located outside the CNS are enclosed in connective tissue ensheathments and are called **nerves** (*i.e.*, cranial and spinal nerves). Groups of neuronal cell bodies within the CNS are called **nuclei** (singular: *nucleus*—not to be confused with the nucleus of a cell). Groups of neuronal cell bodies in the peripheral nervous system are called **ganglia** (singular: *ganglion*). There are two distinct types of ganglia: sensory and autonomic. **Sensory ganglia** are associated with the cranial and spinal nerves and are located near the attachment of these nerves to the brain and spinal cord. They contain the cell bodies of pseudounipolar neurons

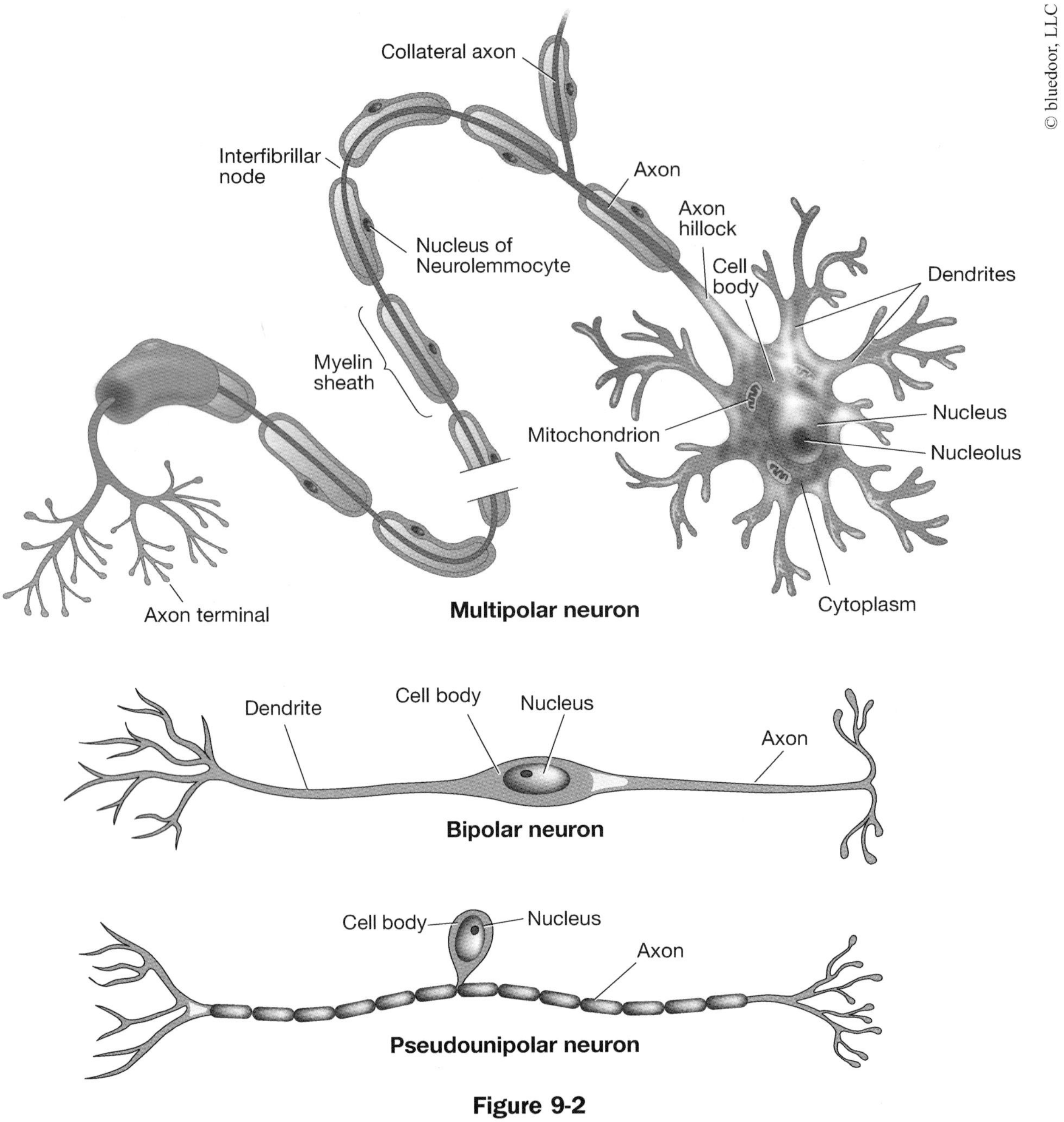

Figure 9-2

The Three Anatomic Types of Neurons

Multipolar neurons have multiple dendrites. Bipolar and pseudounipolar neurons have single dendrites (which may branch). A coating of neurolemmocytes ("Schwann cells") increases the speed of impulse conduction and is called a myelin sheath. Not all neurons are mylenated. Within the CNS, myelin sheaths are formed by oligodendrocytes.

(both SA and VA neurons) which convey general sensory impulses into the CNS. **Autonomic ganglia** contain the cell bodies of visceral efferent neurons and are found in many locations. There are three types of autonomic ganglia: terminal, sympathetic trunk, and named peripheral ganglia. They serve as synaptic sites between the first and second neurons in the two neuron chain of the autonomic nervous system and will be discussed in more detail in Chapter 11.

Objectives

4. Schematically represent the three anatomic types of neurons and state the functions of each.
5. Compare the four functional types of neurons in regard to their anatomic type, location of their cell bodies, and the structures that they are motor to or sensory from.

Neuroglia

Neurons are the only cells in the nervous system that are capable of transmitting nervous impulses. However, there are several other types of cells called **neuroglia** (or simply **glial cells**) that support and aid the function of neurons: neurolemmocytes, oligodendrocytes, astrocytes, microglia, satellite cells, and ependymal cells. **Neurolemmocytes** (formerly known as "Schwann" cells) are flattened cells that form electrically insulating layers around axons in the PNS called **myelin sheaths** (Figure 9-3). Their insulating property is derived from a lipid material in their cytoplasm called **myelin**. Each neurolemmocyte covers about a linear millimeter of axon by forming several snug wraps around it in a configuration similar to rolling a pencil up in a soft tortilla. Axons in the PNS that are surrounded by neurolemmocytes are said to be **myelinated** and those that lack neurolemmocytes are **unmyelinated**. Myelination affects the speed of nerve impulse conduction (see next section). **Oligodendrocytes** are cells which form myelin sheaths around axons within the CNS (Figure 9-4). **Astrocytes** are the largest and most numerous of the glial cells. They form a blood-brain barrier by being physically interspersed between the blood vessels and neurons within the brain. In this position they form a *final filter* for all materials that reach the neurons from the bloodstream. The **microglia** are phagocytic cells within the CNS. They are mobile and ingest foreign and degenerated material. **Ependymal cells** are cuboidally shaped cells that line the ventricles (fluid filled spaces) of the brain and the central canal of the spinal cord. In certain locations they are modified and secrete the cerebral spinal fluid (CSF) of the CNS. **Satellite cells** are supporting cells found in ganglia.

Objectives

6. State the function and location of each of the six types of glial cells. Differentiate myelin and myelin sheath.

Nerve Impulse Transmission

Neurons are able to conduct electrical (nervous) impulses because their cytoplasm is charged (negatively) compared to their extracellular environment (Figure 9-5). The potential difference is due to negatively charged protein ions in their cytoplasm and because of the excess of positively charged sodium ions (Na^+) that are actively transported out of the cells by a mechanism called the **sodium-potassium pump** (three sodium ions out of the cells and two potassium ions into the cells for each ATP used). This charge, called the **resting potential**, is about -65 millivolts (-65 one-thousandths of a volt). If a neuron is stimulated such that some of the positively-charged, extracellular sodium

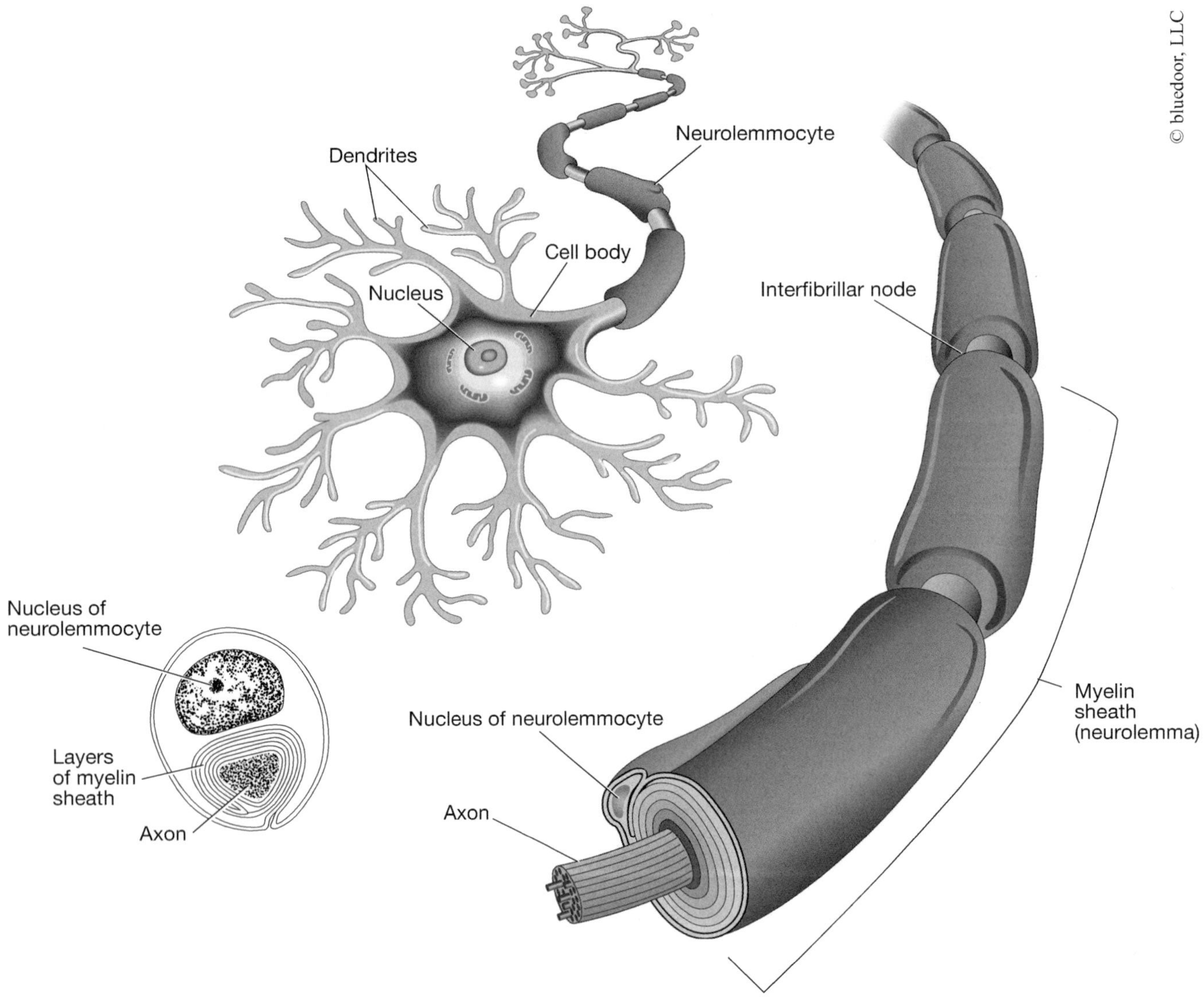

Figure 9-3
A Myelinated Axon

Neurolemmocytes are flattened glial cells that wrap themselves around axons in the PNS. Each neurolemmocyte covers only about a millimeter of axonal length, so many are required to cover a given axon. When impulse conduction occurs in a myelinated axon, the depolarization/repolarization occurs only at the gaps between neurolemmocytes called interfibrillar nodes ("nodes of Ranvier"). This "skipping" impulse conduction occurs faster than impulse conduction in unmyelinated axons and is called saltatory conduction.

ions readily diffuse back through the cell membrane, a measurable momentary change (reversal) in electrical potential occurs and this constitutes a local **depolarization** (charge reversal).

Once depolarization reaches a critical level called the **threshold** at any point on the cell membrane, the membrane becomes temporarily permeable to sodium. Sodium rushes in by simple diffusion due to the electrochemical gradient (large number of positively charged sodium ions outside the cell and a smaller number of sodium ions in the negatively charged cytosol). Enough sodium ions diffuse into the cell to cause a charge "reversal" or depolarization (positively charged cyto-

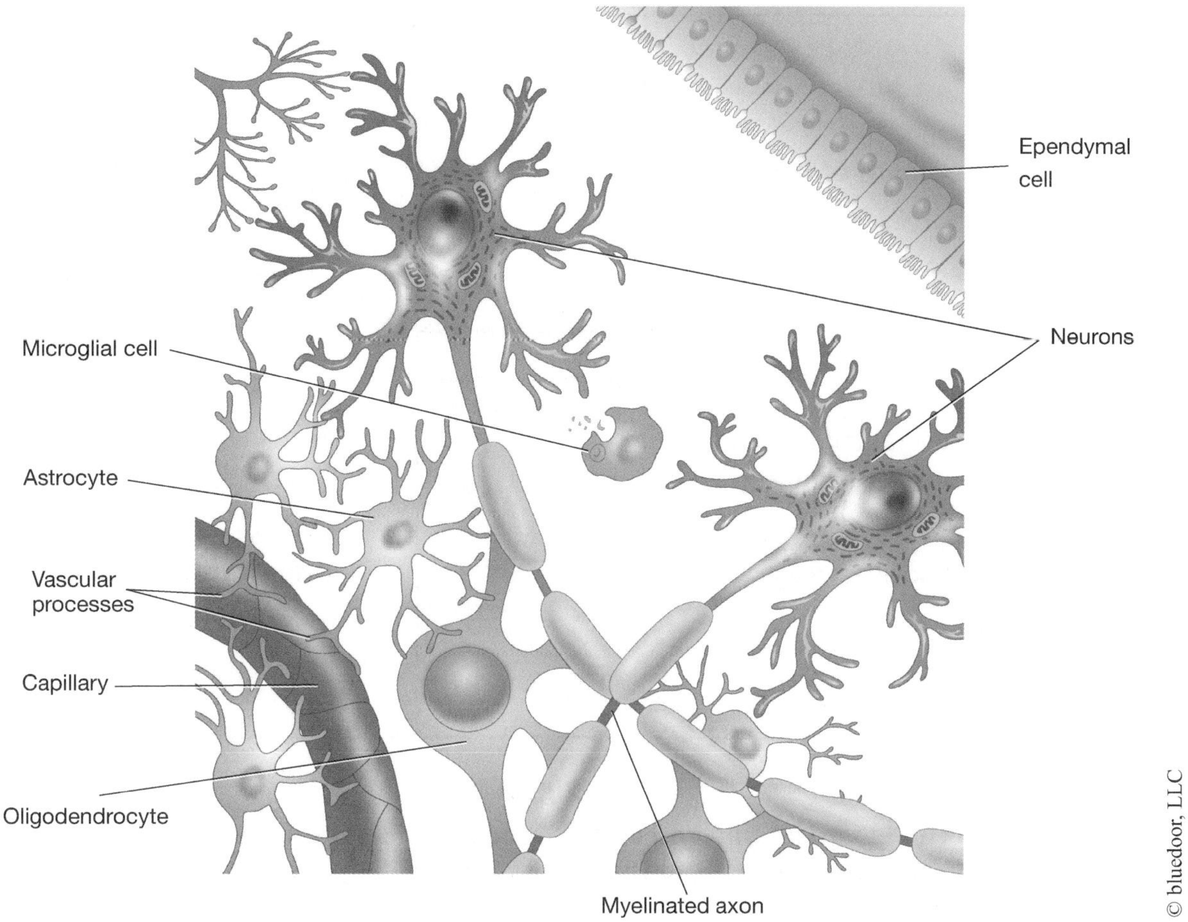

Figure 9-4

Glial Cells Found in the CNS

Ependymal cells line the ventricles of the brain and the central canal of the spinal cord. Microglia are wandering phagocytes. The vascular processes of astrocytes help them fulfill their role in the nutritional support of neurons. Oligodendrocytes form myelin sheaths in the CNS and are homologous to the neurolemmocytes found in the PNS. Each oligodendrocyte, however, participates in the myelinization of several adjacent axons.

plasm). This reversal makes the membrane temporarily permeable to potassium, and enough potassium (K^+) ions rush out of the cell (electrochemical gradient for K^+ is now strongly *out*) to re-establish the original resting voltage (**repolarization**). The cell membrane then becomes impermeable (once again) to both sodium and potassium until the next impulse occurs. Depolarization and repolarization last only a tiny fractional part of a second. As they move down a cell's membrane they constitute a **nervous impulse**.

Note that the sodium-potassium pump works continuously and has no *direct* role in a nervous impulse. However, *indirectly*, the pump plays a vital role by establishing the resting differences in sodium and potassium concentrations inside and outside the cell membrane. It is important to remember that a resting neuron's cell membrane is relatively impermeable to the simple diffusion of both sodium and potassium ions. Otherwise, the effects of the sodium-potassium pumps would be futile and we would be....dead!

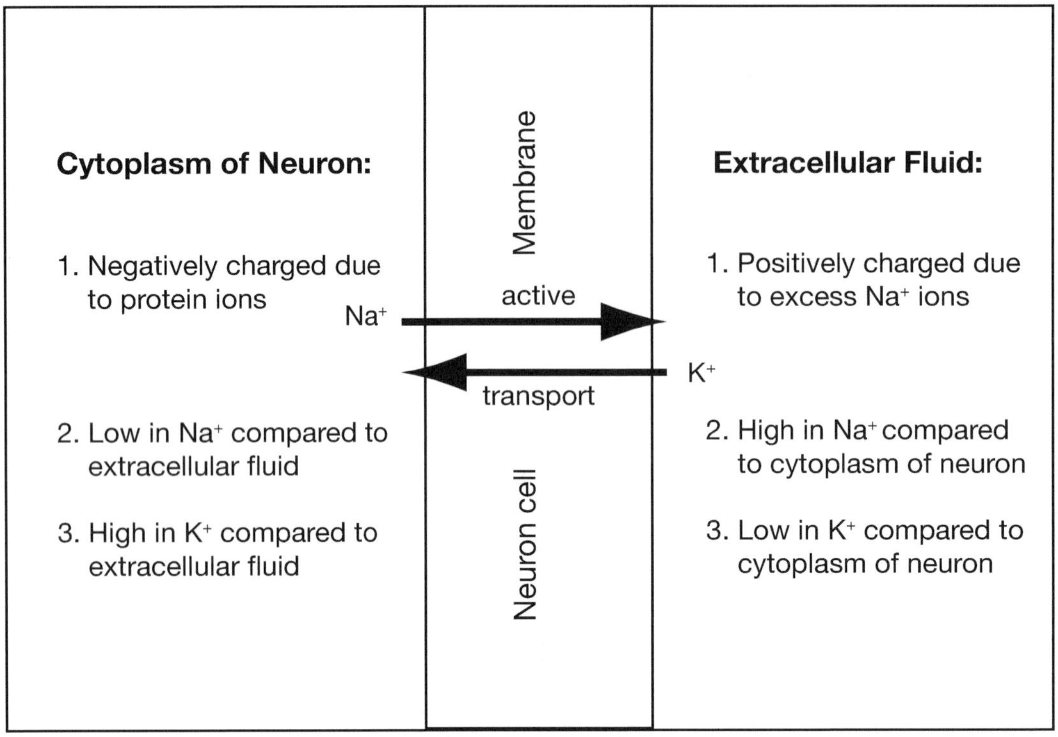

Figure 9-5

The Electrical Charge and Ion Concentration in the Cytoplasm of a Neuron Compared to that in the Surrounding Extracellular Fluid

Regardless of whether a neuron is sensory or motor, and if sensory, regardless of the type of sensory information ultimately interpreted by the brain (light, cold, heat, touch, *etc.*), the nature of the nervous impulse is the same. The speed at which the impulse is conducted through the cell varies from less than a meter per second in small unmyelinated neurons to over 100 meters per second in large myelinated ones. Myelinated neurons conduct impulses faster because the depolarization (*i.e.*, the electrical reversal) occurs only at the junctions of the ensheathing neurolemmocytes. In other words, it "skips" over the neurolemmocytes themselves by a process which physiologists call **saltatory conduction**.

Neurons pass impulses to other neurons or to muscle or glandular epithelial cells through special junctions called **synapses** (Figure 9-6). Those between two neurons consist of a narrow gap between the axon of the first neuron and usually the dendrite or the cell body of the second one. When the electrical impulse in the first neuron reaches the synapse, it initiates the release of a chemical substance called a **neurotransmitter**. This chemical diffuses across the synaptic gap, interacts with the cell membrane of the next neuron, and (if enough is released) either initiates an impulse therein (excitatory neurotransmitter) or inhibits an impulse in the next cell (inhibitory neurotransmitter). Rapid enzymatic decomposition of the neurotransmitters prevents them from initiating additional impulses. A number of different neurotransmitters have been identified. The most common ones in the PNS are **acetylcholine** and **norepinephrine**. Neurotransmitters are also released at the synapses between neurons and muscle or gland cells. Their interactions with these cells initiate contraction or control secretory activity.

Table 9-2 Derivations of the Definitive Parts of the Brain

Three Vesicle Stage	Five Vesicle Stage	Definitive Brain
Prosencephalon (forebrain)	Telencephalon	Cerebrum
	Diencephalon	Epithalamus Thalamus Hypothalamus
Mesencephalon (midbrain)	Mesencephalon	Mesencephalon
Rhombencephalon (hindbrain)	Metencephalon	Pons Cerebellum
	Myelencephalon	Medulla Oblongata

Objectives

7. Explain the phenomenon of nervous impulse transmission including depolarization, repolarization, threshold, the role of the sodium-potassium pump, and the role of neurotransmitters.
8. State how saltatory conduction differs from regular nervous impulse conduction.
9. Name the three basic types of cells with which a neuron can synapse.

Development of the Nervous System

Nervous tissue develops from the outer one of the three primary germ layers (ectoderm). Early in development, the area of the ectoderm overlying the notochord thickens to form a **neural plate** (Figure 9-7). A few days later the neural plate invaginates longitudinally to form a **neural groove**. Within the next few days this groove deepens and finally pinches off from the surface ectoderm to become a **neural tube** (dorsal hollow neural tube). The neural tube develops into the brain (anteriorly) and spinal cord (posteriorly). Groups of cells on each side of the neural tube separate from it to form **neural crests** which develop into sensory neurons, autonomic neurons, neurolemmocytes, melanocytes, and chromaffin cells.

The anterior end of the neural tube develops three bulges called **vesicles** which are destined to form the brain: **prosencephalon** (forebrain), **mesencephalon** (midbrain), and **rhombencephalon** (hindbrain). With further development, the prosencephalon divides into the **telencephalon** and **diencephalon**, and the rhombencephalon divides into the **metencephalon** and **myelencephalon**. The mesencephalon does not undergo further subdivision. Further development of these five vesicles forms the major parts of the brain (Table 9-2).

Several developmental disorders of the CNS can occur. Sometimes the brain simply fails to develop (**anencephaly**) or develops incompletely (**microencephaly**). Sometimes the brain appears grossly normal but fails to function properly, resulting in mental retardation. The spinal cord may be exposed near the surface of the body by failure of the surrounding vertebral column to properly enclose it (**spina bifida**).

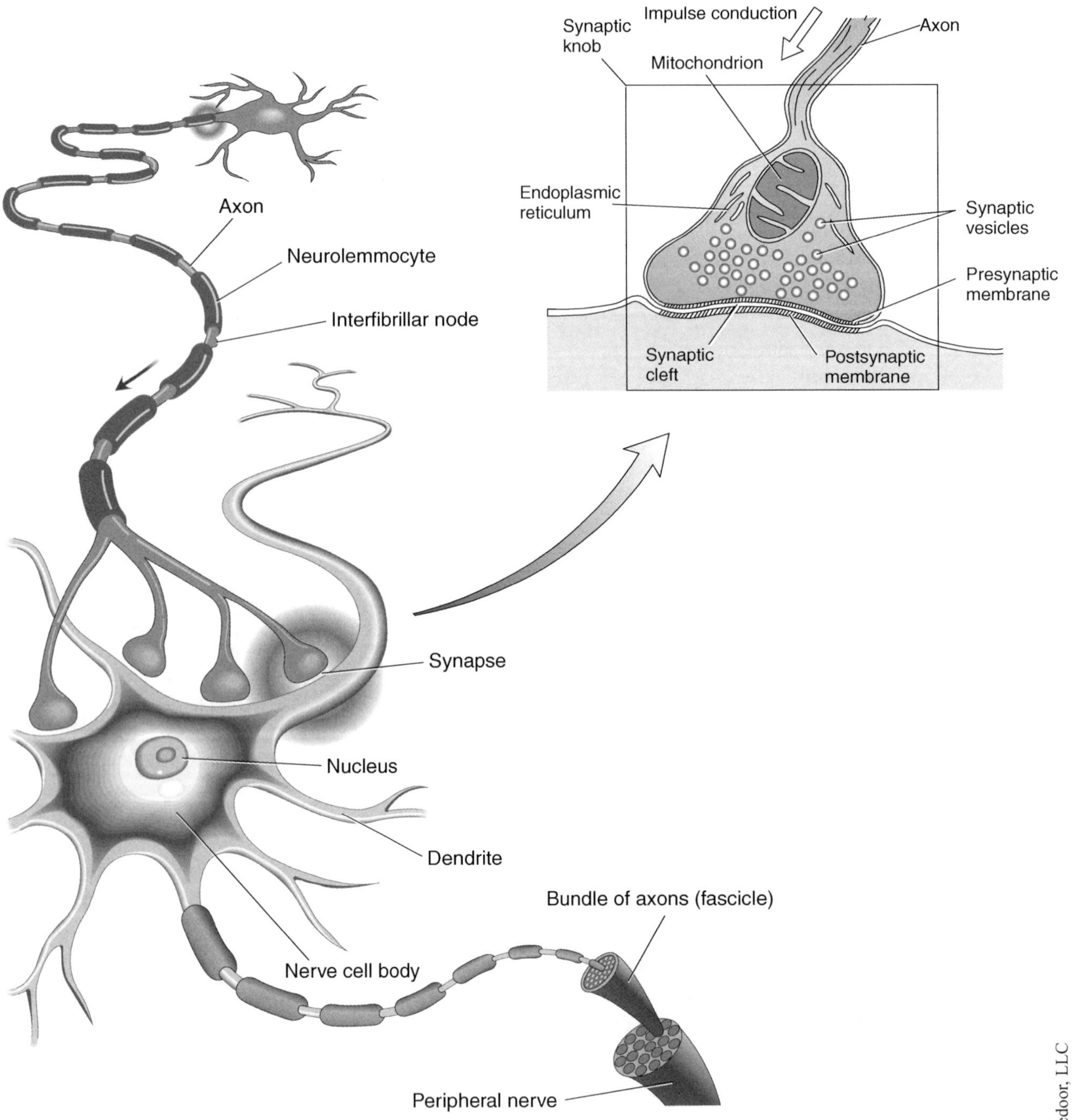

Figure 9-6

Microstructure of a Synapse

At synapses, chemicals called neurotransmitters are released from synaptic vesicles stored in the ends of axons. These chemicals diffuse across the synaptic cleft and interact with the cell membrane (postsynaptic membrane) of the next cell (another neuron, a muscle cell or a glandular epithelial cell). Neurotransmitters are divided into two general categories: excitatory and inhibitory.

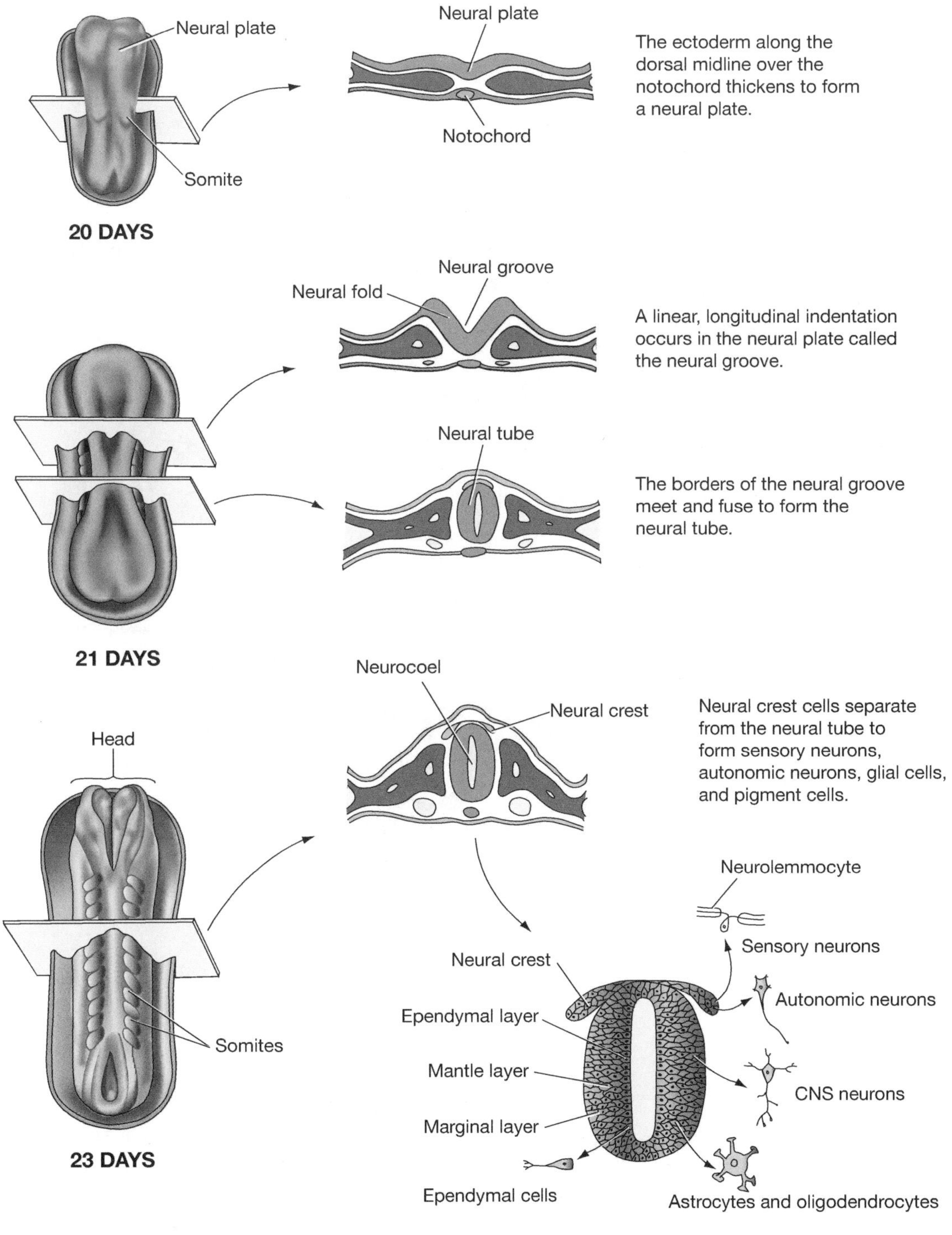

Figure 9-7

Development of the Central Nervous System

The ectoderm over the notochord forms a neural plate, then a groove, and finally a neural tube. Most of the length of the tube forms the spinal cord but the anterior (superior) end forms the brain. Further development of the brain is illustrated in Figure 9-15.

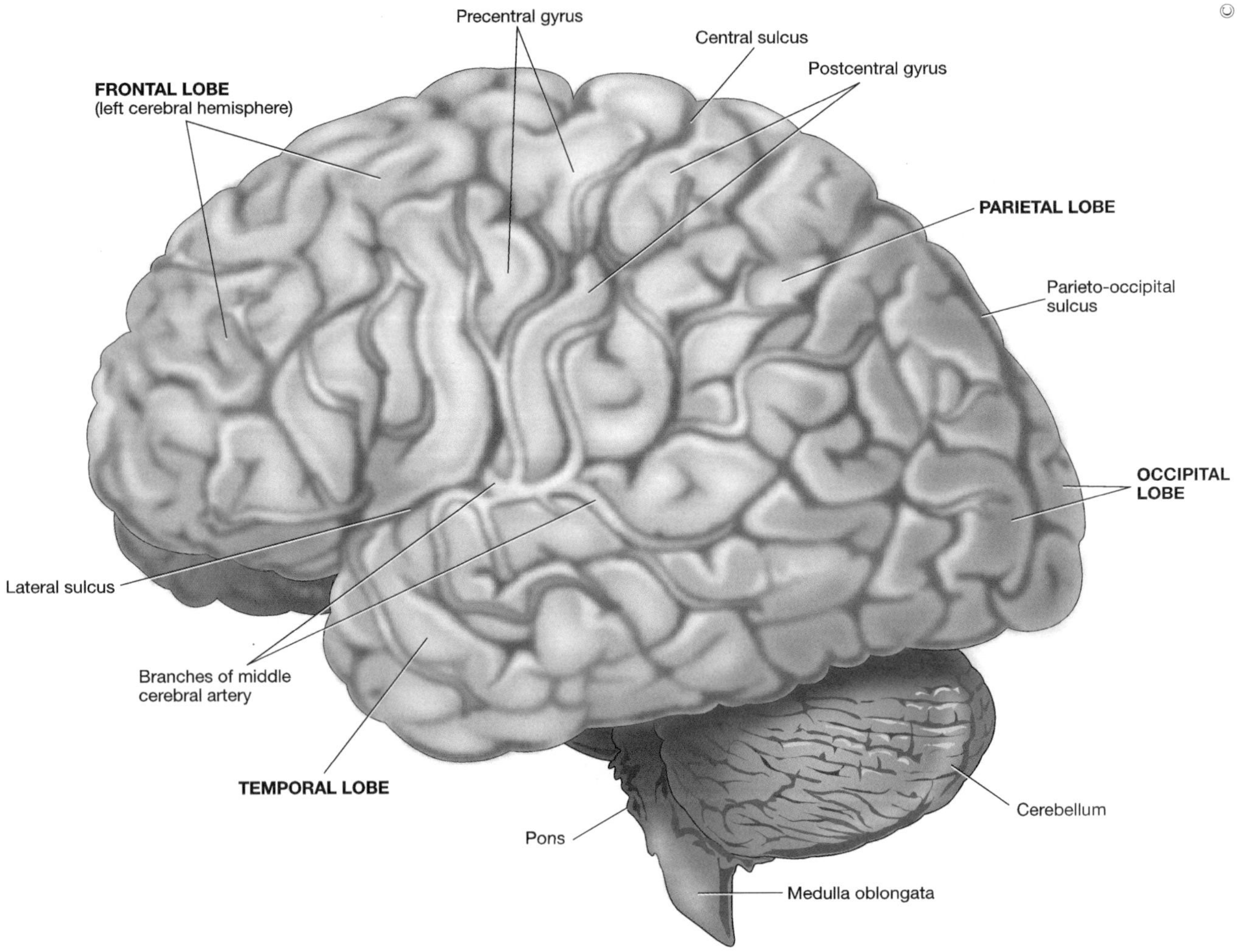

Figure 9-8

Landmarks of the Cerebrum

The cerebrum consists of two (right and left) cerebral hemispheres as well as several other components. Each hemisphere has five lobes. The insular lobe (insula) is not visible unless the frontal and temporal lobes are retracted from each other.

Objectives

10. Discuss the development of the nervous system including: neural plate, neural groove, neural tube, neural crests, the three vesicle stage, the five vesicle stage, and the derivatives of each vesicle.

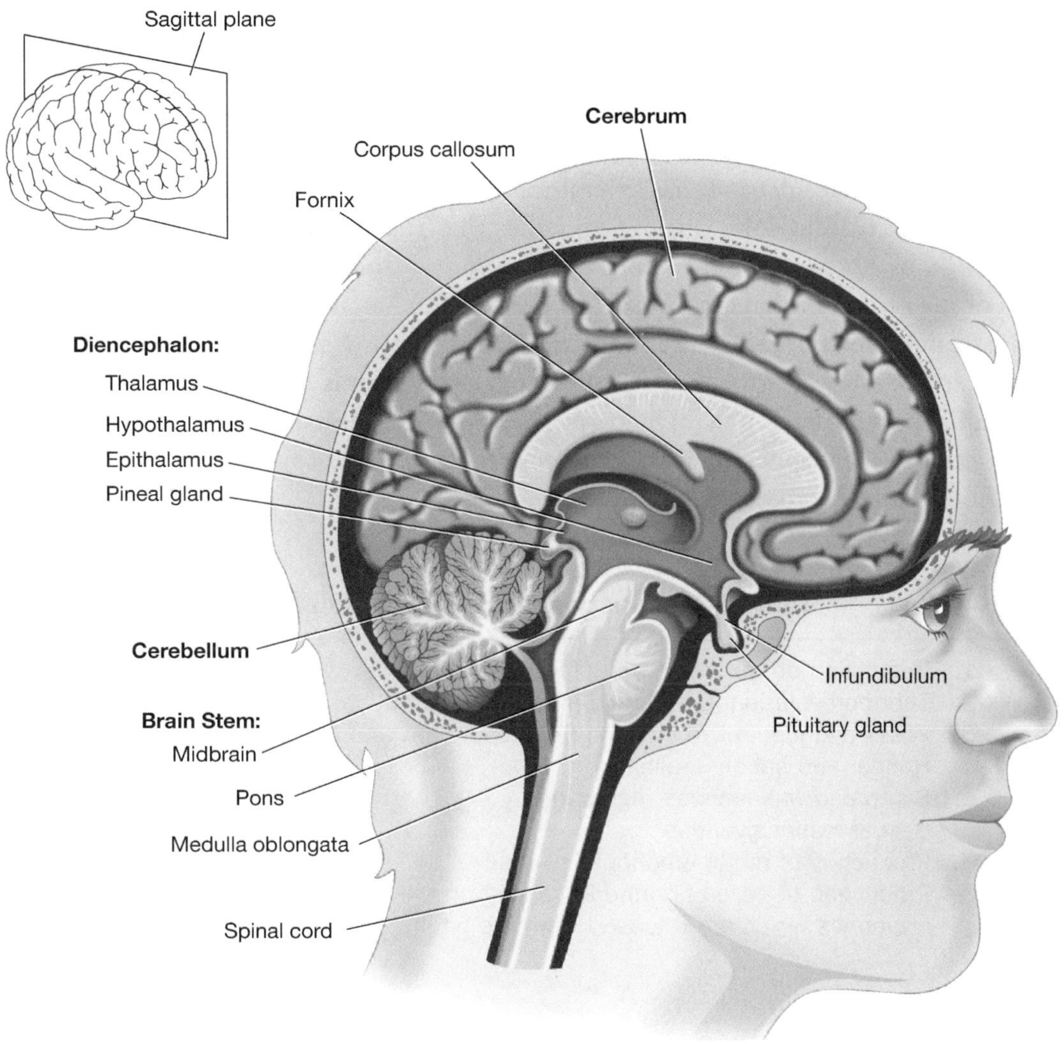

Figure 9-9
Midsagittal Section Through the Brain

Major Parts of the Brain

The largest part of the brain (encephalon) is the cerebrum (Figure 9-8). It has over 1,000 named parts and is the major center of sensory perception, thought, memory, and motor output. The outer portion of the cerebrum consists of numerous rounded ridges called **cerebral gyri** (singular = *gyrus*) separated by grooves called **cerebral sulci** (singular = *sulcus*) and **fissures**. These landmarks are relatively constant from one individual to another and have all been named. The major part of the cerebrum is divided into the left and right **cerebral hemispheres**. Each hemisphere is further divided into five lobes: frontal, parietal, temporal, occipital, and insular lobes. The **frontal lobe** is anteriorly situated (deep to the frontal bone and part of the parietal bone). Its major function is voluntary control of skeletal muscle activity, but it also has roles in verbal communication and thought.

Behind the frontal lobe and separated from it by the central sulcus is the **parietal lobe** (deep to the parietal bone). Its major function is general sensory perception. The **temporal lobe** is inferior to the frontal and parietal lobes and separated from them by the lateral sulcus. It is involved with the interpretation of sound and the sense of body position and balance. The **occipital lobe** forms the posterior portion of the cerebral hemisphere. Its anterior aspect is separated from the parietal lobe by the parieto-occipital sulcus. It has several roles in visual interpretation and coordination of eye movements. The **insular lobe** (insula) underlies the frontal, parietal, and temporal lobes. It is believed to be at least one of the centers of "memory" and integrates other cerebral activities. Portions of the cerebrum that are not part of the cerebral hemispheres include the rhinencephalon and the **corpus callosum**. The paired rhinencephalon consists primarily of the olfactory bulb and the medial and lateral olfactory gyri. The olfactory bulb extends forward and the fibers of the first pair of cranial nerves attach to it. The corpus callosum is a large interconnection between the left and right cerebral hemispheres. Each hemisphere surrounds a space called the **lateral ventricle** which is filled with cerebrospinal fluid (CSF).

Table 9-3 Functions of the Hypothalamus

1. Regulation of heart rate and blood pressure
2. Thermoregulation (sweating, shivering, vasomotion)
3. Water and electrolyte balance (ADH secretion and thirst center)
4. Hunger and satiety feelings
5. Sleep and wakefulness regulation
6. Sexual responsiveness
7. Production of major emotional states
8. Production of several hormones acting on the pituitary gland as well as two hormones which are released from the pituitary gland (ADH and oxytocin)

The diencephalon includes the epithalamus, thalamus, and the hypothalamus (Figure 9-9). These surround the single, cerebrospinal fluid-filled **third ventricle**. The thin **epithalamus** forms the roof of the third ventricle. Its posterior-most part is the **pineal body** (gland) which produces the hormone melatonin. The **thalamus** forms the lateral walls of the third ventricle and serves as a relay center for most general sensory impulses originating below the head. The floor of the third ventricle is formed by the **hypothalamus**. This relatively small part of the brain plays a number of very important functional roles (Table 9-3). These include centers for thirst, hunger, satiety, sleep, wakefulness, sexual responsiveness, and cardiovascular control. The hypothalamus also produces several hormones including two (antidiuretic hormone and oxytocin) that are ultimately released by the posterior lobe of the pituitary gland (*see Chapter 14*). The pituitary gland hangs from the underside of the hypothalamus by a slender stalk called the infundibulum. The **optic chiasm**, which continues anteriorly as the optic nerves, projects forward from the hypothalamus.

The **mesencephalon** is the smallest of the major parts of the brain. It serves as a reflex center for audition and vision and also contains the motor nuclei for the oculomotor and trochlear (third and fourth cranial) nerves. The mesencephalon surrounds the CSF-filled **mesencephalic aqueduct** (**cerebral aqueduct**) which connects the third ventricle to the **fourth ventricle**. The latter lies between the pons and medulla oblongata, anteriorly, and the cerebellum, posteriorly.

The **pons** lies anterior to the mesencephalon and forms a rounded bulge on the underside of the

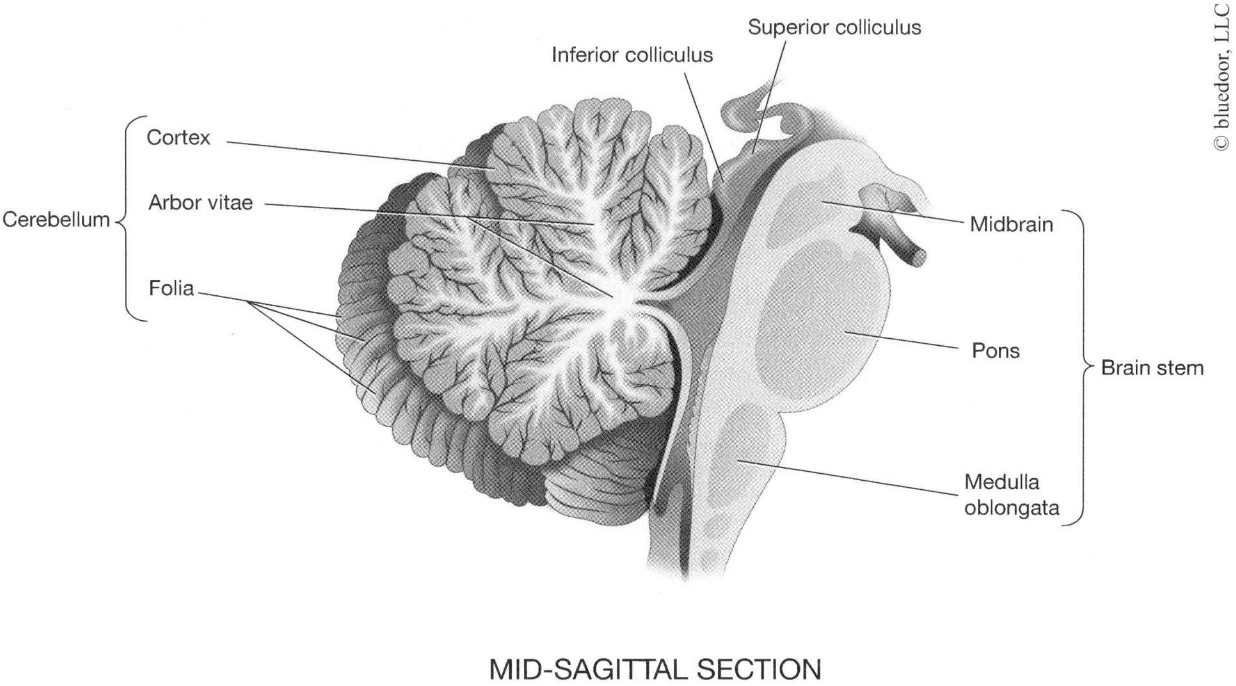

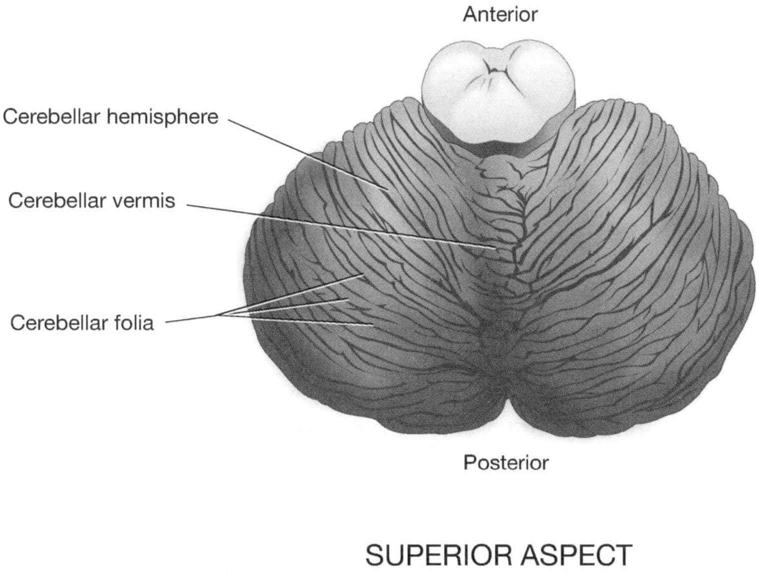

Figure 9-10
The Cerebellum

brain. It contains motor nuclei for cranial nerves 5, 6, 7 (trigeminal, abducens, facial nerves), sensory nucleus for cranial nerve 8 (vestibulocochlear nerve), and serves as a bridging connection between the medulla oblongata and mesencephalon. It also has connections to the cerebellum, and contains two respiratory centers.

The **cerebellum** is the second largest subdivision of the brain and occupies the posterior cranial fossa. It forms a distinctive rounded mass inferior to the occipital lobes of the cerebral hemispheres (Figure 9-10). White matter within the cerebellum appears to be shaped like a tree in a median section and is called the **arbor vitae**. The left and right **cerebellar hemispheres** are joined at the centrally located body by a "worm-shaped" structure called the **cerebellar vermis**. A number of cerebellar fissures divide the cerebellum into ten cerebellar lobules. The cerebellum coordinates the motor impulses to skeletal muscles. These impulses originate in the frontal lobes of the cerebral hemispheres. It is connected to the rest of the nervous system by three pairs of fiber bundles called superior, middle, and inferior **cerebellar peduncles**.

The **medulla oblongata** is the inferior-most portion of the brain and lies between the pons and spinal cord (Figure 9-9). The medulla contains nuclei that contribute fibers to cranial nerves 8, 9, 10, 11, and 12. It also has a cardiac center with inhibitory and excitatory functions, a vasomotor center which can elevate the blood pressure by causing vasoconstriction, and a respiratory center that controls the rate and depth of breathing. A major feature of the medulla is the decussation (crossing over from right to left and vice-versa) of sensory and motor fiber tracts passing to and from the spinal cord. This results in the fact that the left half of the brain is sensory and motor to the right half of the body and vice-versa.

Objectives

11. State the general function(s) of each of the major parts of the brain: cerebrum, epithalamus, thalamus, hypothalamus, mesencephalon, pons, cerebellum, medulla oblongata.
12. State the major function of each named lobe of a cerebral hemisphere.

Major Parts of the Spinal Cord

The **spinal cord** is the direct, inferior continuation of the medulla oblongata (Figure 9-11). It passes through the foramen magnum of the occipital bone and extends inferiorly through the vertebral canal. The spinal cord contains ascending (sensory) and descending (motor) fiber tracts, cell bodies of motor neurons, and cell bodies of interneurons (neurons between neurons). It is enclosed within connective tissue encasements (meninges) that are continuous with those around the brain. The spinal cord has few exterior landmarks. It is indented anteriorly by the **anterior median fissure** and posteriorly by the **posterior median sulcus**. It tapers as it courses inferiorly but has two subtle swellings called the **cervical** and **lumbosacral intumescences**. These enlargements occur because of the increased number of neurons and fiber tracts in those areas which are associated with the limbs. Inferiorly, the spinal cord ends as a conical projection termed the **conus medullaris** at the level of L1/L2.

The **spinal nerves** emerge from the spinal cord as anterior and posterior rootlets that coalesce to form the roots of the 31 to 33 pairs of nerves. These pass through the intervertebral foramina and are distributed segmentally to the body. Those that originate from the lower part of the spinal cord and continue beyond its L1/L2 termination form the **cauda equina** (so named because of its resemblance to a horse's tail). The structure and distribution of the spinal nerves will be discussed in Chapter 10.

A sectional view of the spinal cord (Figure 9-12) reveals that it consists of a centrally located "X" or "H" shaped region of **gray matter** surrounded by **white matter**. The gray matter contains a large number of neurons which impart a darker color than the surrounding white matter. The latter consists mainly of myelinated axons in ascending (sensory) or descending (motor) fiber tracts. The gray matter surrounds a tiny **central canal** which contains cerebrospinal fluid. Each half of the gray matter is divided into an **anterior** ("ventral") **gray column** and a **posterior** ("dorsal") **gray column**. In

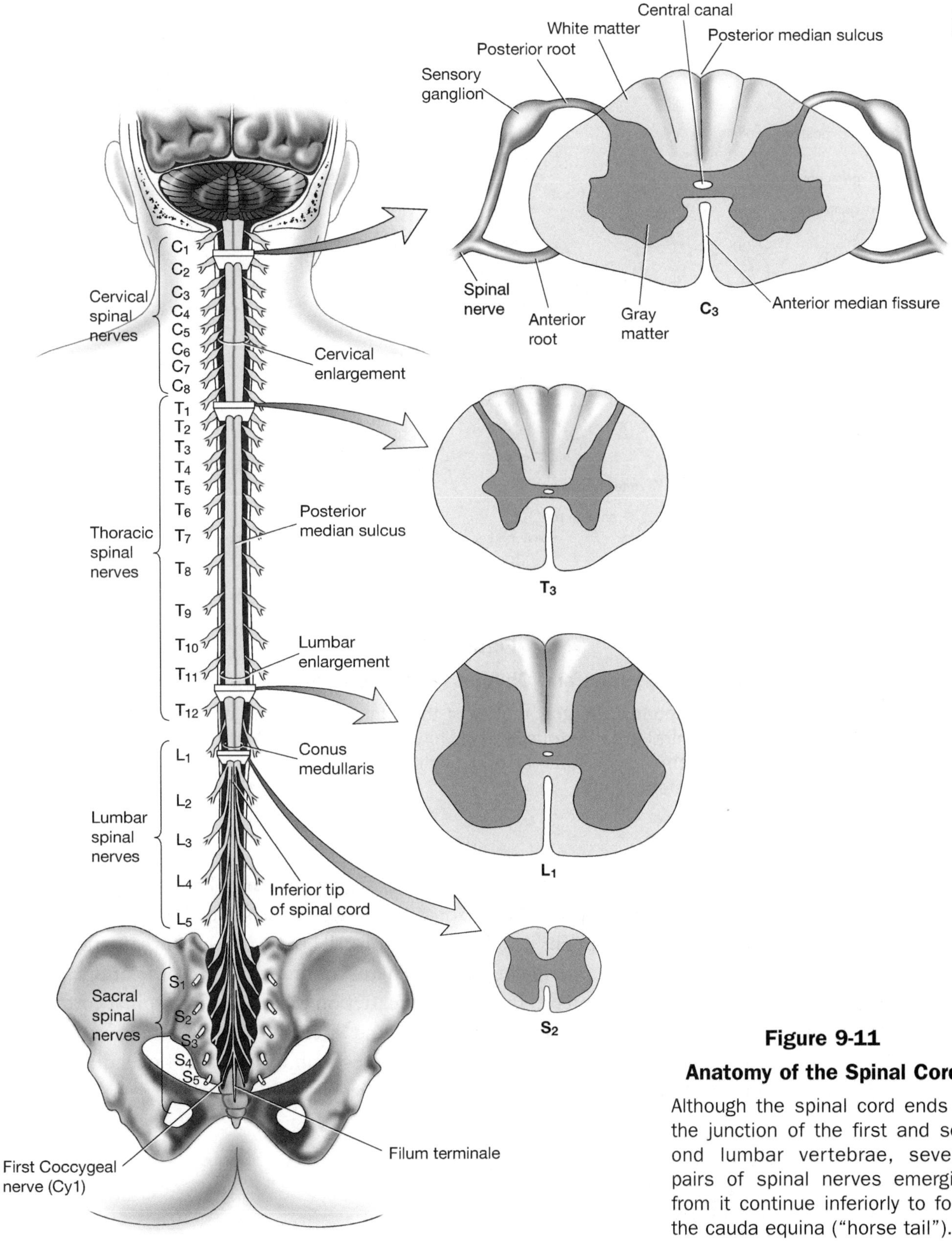

Figure 9-11
Anatomy of the Spinal Cord

Although the spinal cord ends at the junction of the first and second lumbar vertebrae, several pairs of spinal nerves emerging from it continue inferiorly to form the cauda equina ("horse tail").

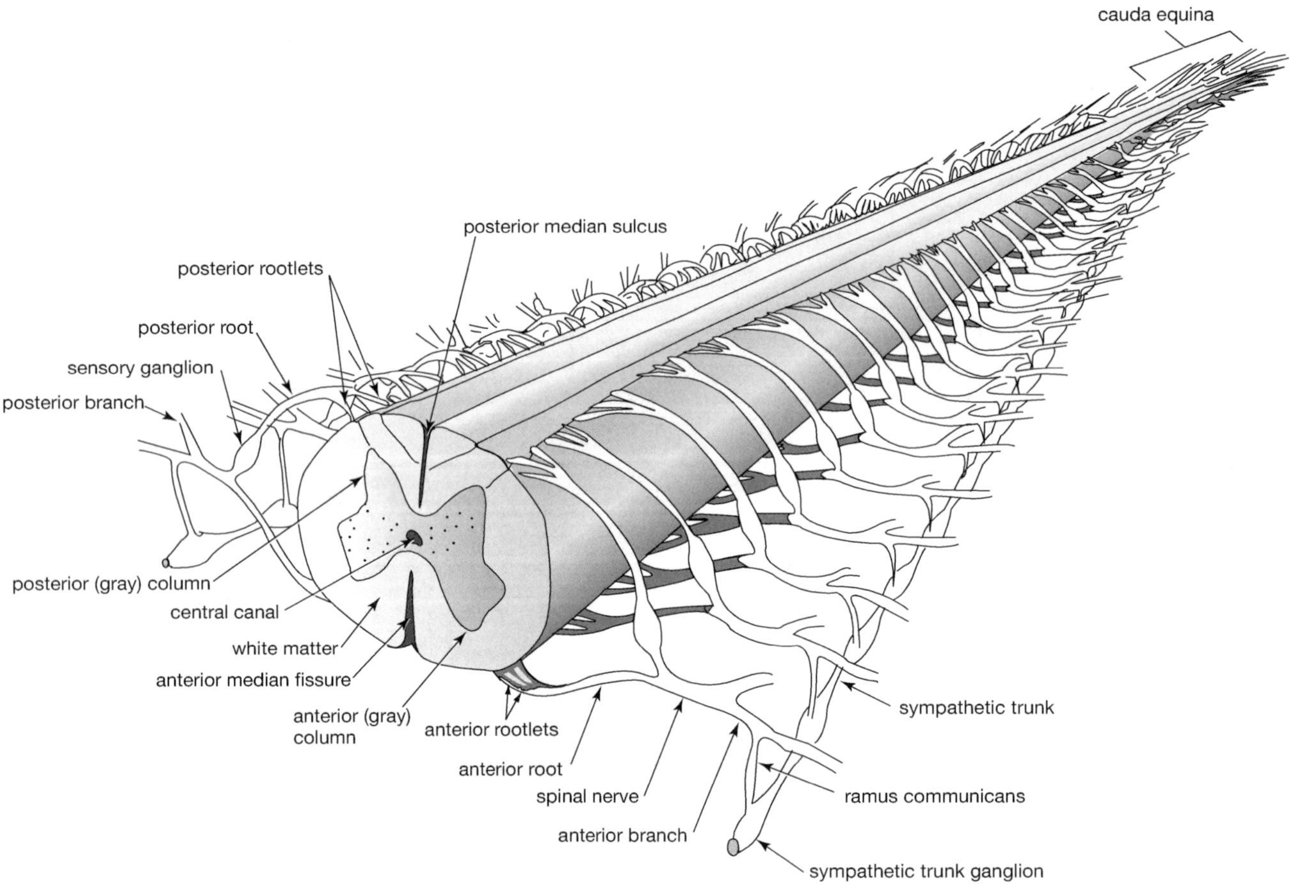

Figure 9-12

Transverse Section and Oblique Perspective of the Spinal Cord

In transverse sections, the gray matter of the spinal cord forms a central "X" or "H" shaped central area surrounded by white matter. The paired (left and right) spinal nerves emerge as anterior and posterior rootlets that coalesce to form anterior and posterior roots.

the thoracic region there is also a small, identifiable **lateral gray column**. The anterior column contains mostly somatic efferent neurons whose axons are carried to the skeletal muscles by the spinal nerves. The posterior column contains mostly interneuron cell bodies involved in somatic reflex arcs or in relaying sensory impulses up to the brain. The lateral column contains some of the presynaptic sympathetic neurons (see Chapter 11). The white matter on each side of the spinal cord is divided into three areas called **funiculi**: **anterior**, **posterior**, and **lateral**. These funiculi consist of named bundles of axons (fiber tracts) that transmit sensory impulses up to the brain (ascending tracts) or carry motor impulses down from the brain (descending tracts).

Objectives

13. Schematically diagram and label a transverse section of the spinal cord.
14. Explain why the spinal cord widens in two places.

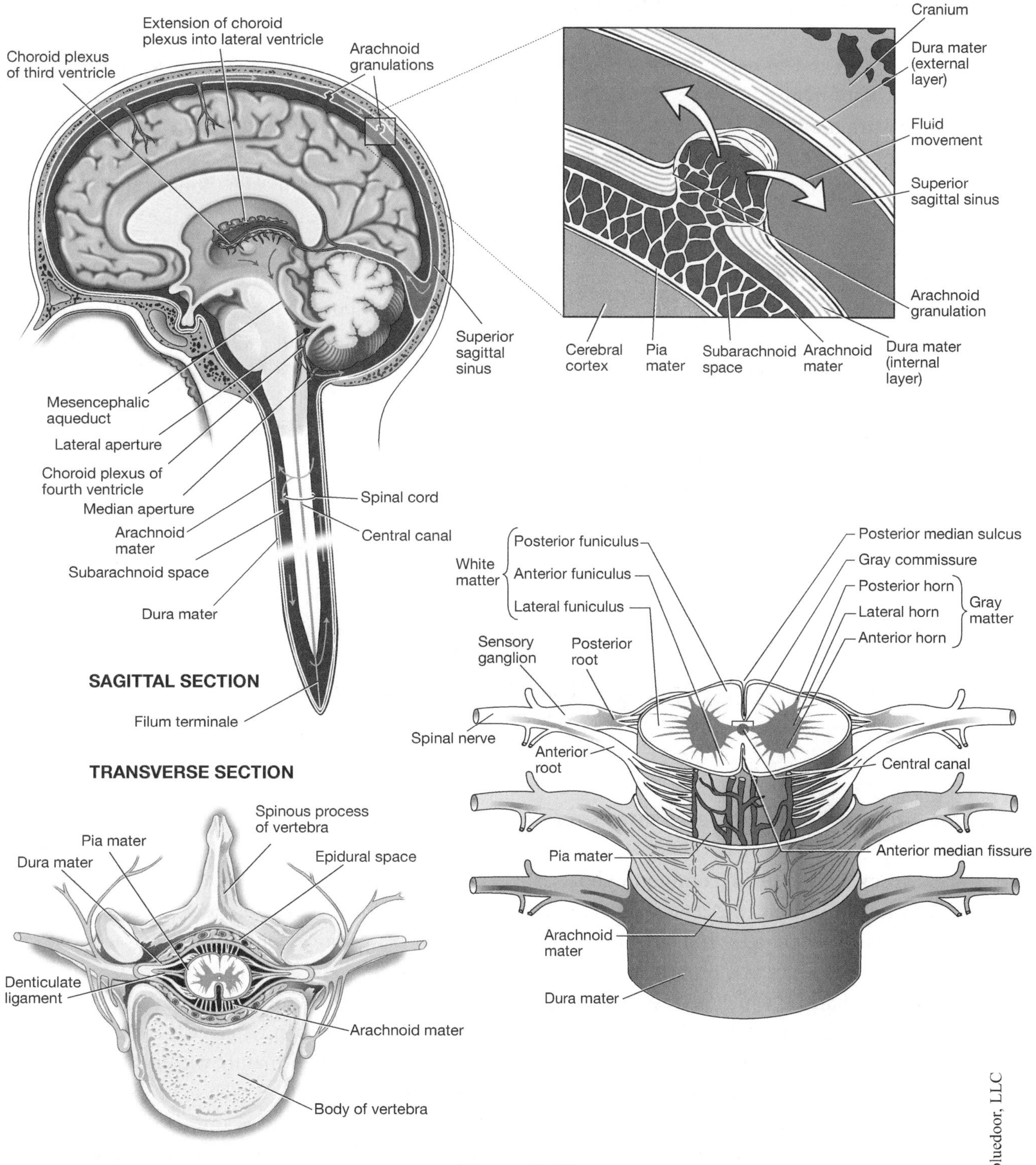

Figure 9-13

Meninges and Circulation of CSF

The three meninges (dura, arachnoid, and pia maters) form protective, connective tissue proper encasements around the spinal cord and brain. Cerebrospinal fluid which is manufactured by the choroid plexuses in the ventricles of the brain, flows into the subarachnoid space (between the arachnoid and pia maters) from whence it is absorbed into the bloodstream through arachnoid granulations. The venous channels, called sinuses, into which the CSF is absorbed occur between two layers of the dura: external and internal.

Connective Tissue Ensheathments of the CNS

The brain and spinal cord are encased by three connective tissue proper coverings called **meninges** (singular: meninx) (Figure 9-13). The outermost and thickest one is a relatively heavy layer termed the **dura mater** ("tough mother"). The dura mater around the brain is in contact with and fused to the brain case to form, in effect, the periosteum on the inner side of the cranial bones. In some places it has named folds which form partitions extending into the surface invaginations of the brain (Table 9-4). Large venous channels within the cranial dura mater are called dural sinuses, not to be confused with the air-filled *paranasal sinuses* of the upper respiratory system. The spinal dura mater is not fused to the inner side of the vertebral canal. In fact, a small epidural space exists in that location which is filled with highly vascularized areolar and adipose tissue. Deposition of local anesthetic can be made into the epidural space and constitutes "spinal" or "epidural" anesthesia.

The **arachnoid mater** ("spider mother") is the middle meninx and is adherent to and positioned just deep to the dura mater. This layer is named for its delicate web-like strands that extend inward to contact and fuse to the pia mater. The space between these strands is filled with cerebrospinal fluid and is called the **subarachnoid space**.

The **pia mater** ("tender mother") is the thinnest and innermost meninx. It is attached directly to the brain and spinal cord. It also lies adjacent to the ependymal cells lining the medial walls of the lateral ventricles and contributes vessels that form part of the choroid plexus (*see cerebrospinal fluid*).

Objectives

15. Sketch and label the relationship of the three meninges to the brain and spinal cord.

Production and Flow of Cerebrospinal Fluid

Cerebrospinal fluid (commonly abbreviated **CSF**) is a colorless, watery fluid that occupies the ventricles of the brain, the central canal of the spinal cord, mesencephalic aqueduct, subarachnoid space within the meninges, and surrounds the internal ear. Its position within the subarachnoid space allows it to serve as a protective hydro-cushion for the CNS. The specific gravity of CSF is slightly greater than 1.0 which is very close to that of the brain and spinal cord. Consequently the latter are almost "free floating". CSF is continually secreted by specialized ependymal cells overlying capillaries to form structures termed **choroid plexuses**. These are located mainly within the ventricles of the brain (Figure 9-14) and produce several hundred milliliters of CSF each day. The total volume within the CNS at any given moment averages about 175 ml. The excess is absorbed by draining into modified capillaries at specialized structures within the meninges termed **arachnoid granulations**.

CSF produced in the lateral ventricles within the cerebral hemispheres flows into the third ventricle by passing through two narrow openings called **interventricular foramina**. From the third ventricle, within the diencephalon, it flows through the **mesencephalic aqueduct** to the fourth ventricle located between the pons and medulla (anteriorly) and the cerebellum (posteriorly). Here it is joined by CSF flowing superiorly out of the central canal of the spinal cord. From the fourth ventricle, CSF enters the subarachnoid space by flowing through two lateral apertures and a third one located on the median plane.

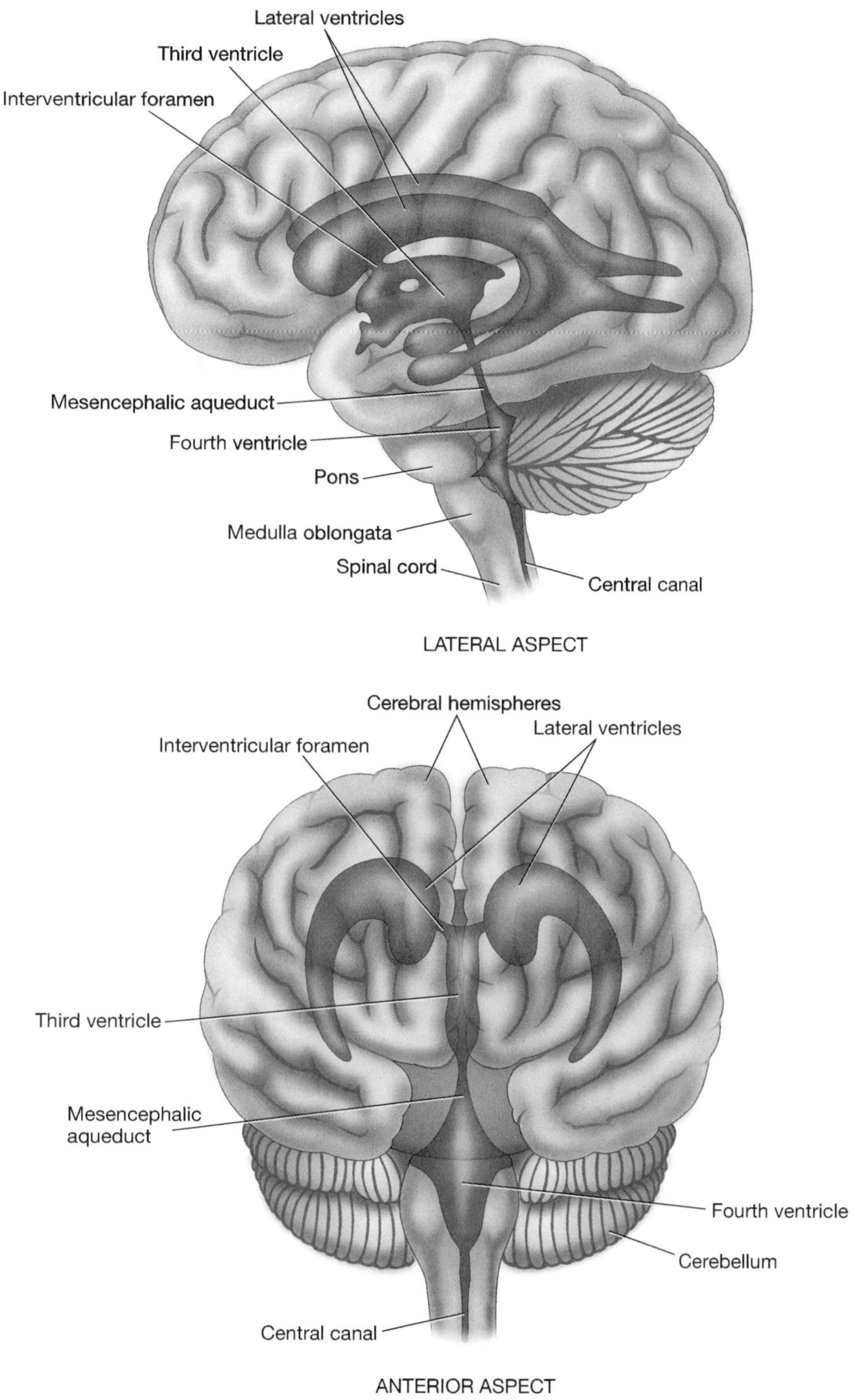

Figure 9-14

Ventricles of the Brain

The ventricles of the brain are spaces filled with cerebrospinal fluid (CSF). The two lateral ventricles are located within the left and right cerebral hemispheres. They are joined to the third ventricle (within the diencephalon) by interventricular foramina. The third ventricle is connected to the fourth one by the mesencephalic aqueduct. The fourth ventricle lies between the cerebellum (posteriorly) and the pons and medulla oblongata (anteriorly). It is continuous inferiorly with the central canal of the spinal cord.

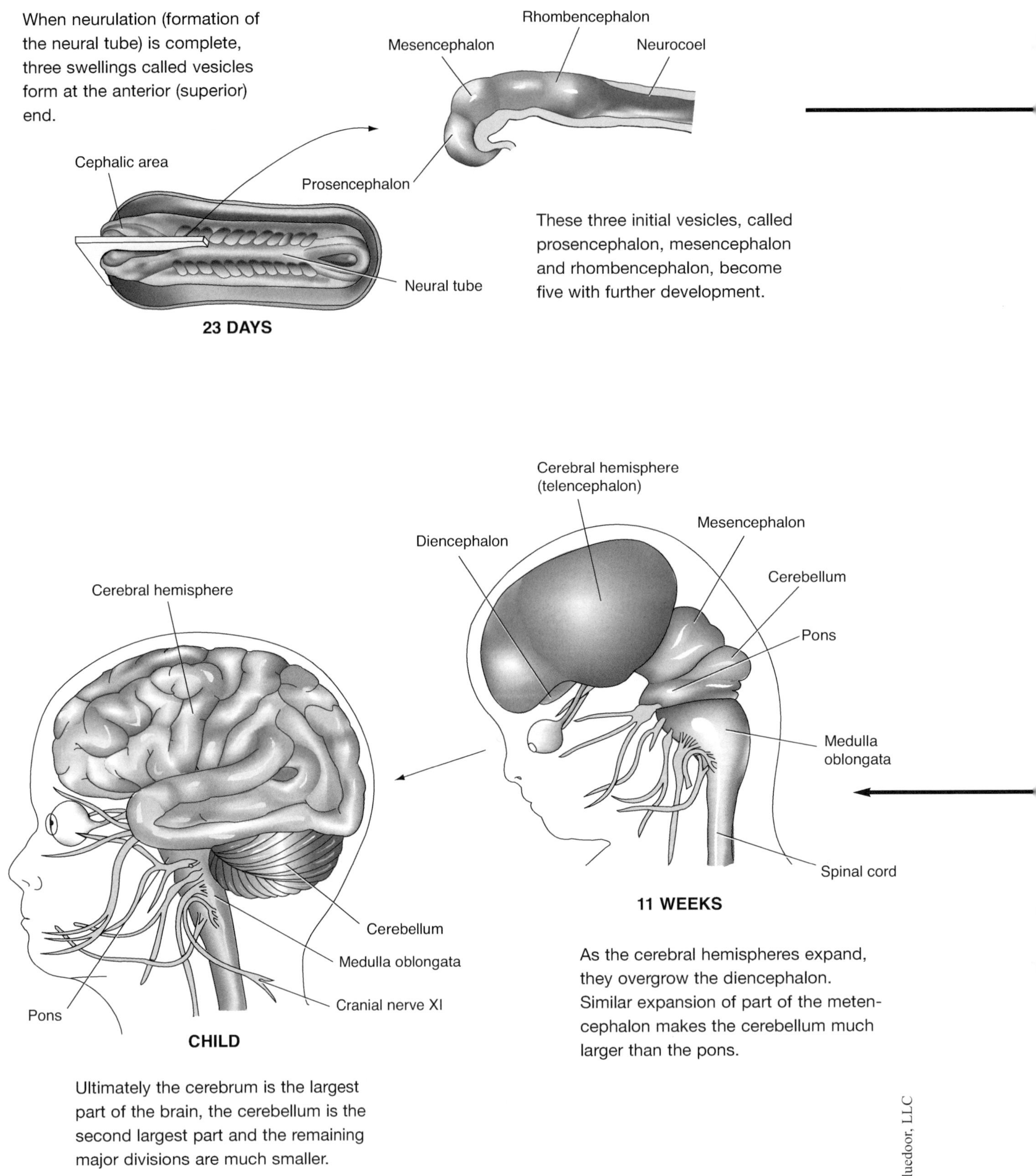

Figure 9-15
Development of the Brain and Spinal Cord

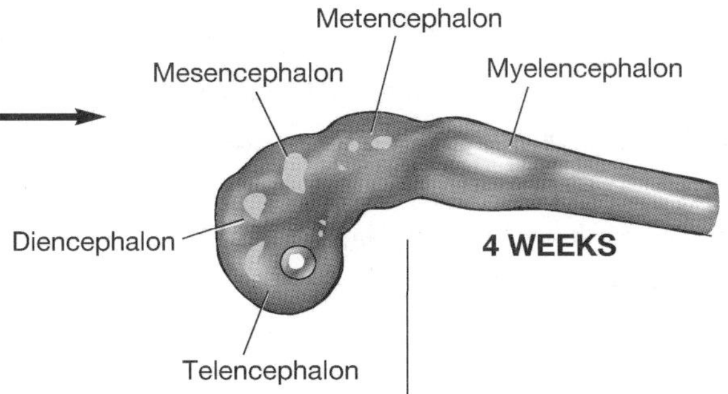

The prosencephalon subdivides to form the telencephalon and diencephalon. The rhombencephalon subdivides to form the metencephalon and myelencephalon. The mesencephalon does not subdivide.

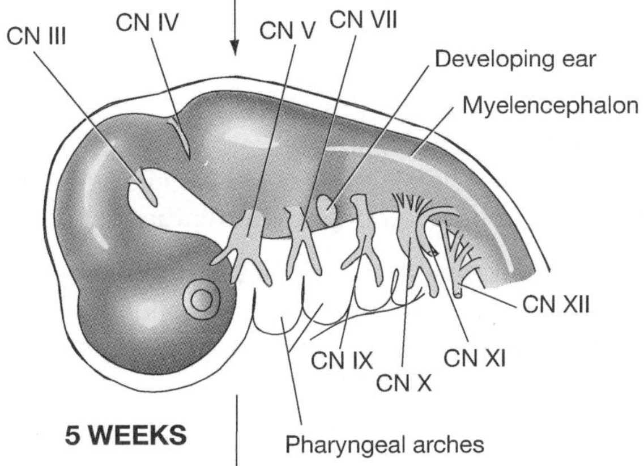

Crainial nerves develop in association with different parts of the primitive brain.

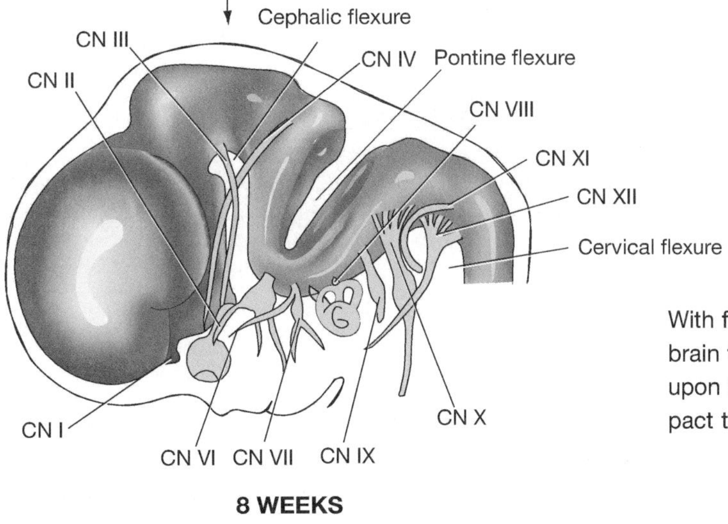

With further development, the brain folds inward or telescopes upon itself, giving it a more compact topography.

Figure 9-15 (continued)

If the flow or reabsorption of CSF is blocked at some point, excess CSF may collect to produce a condition called **hydrocephalus**. This sometimes requires surgical intervention to relieve the pressure. Otherwise, brain damage may result. Samples of CSF may be withdrawn for analysis in evaluating certain types of disorders. In the lumbar area it is often withdrawn from the subarachnoid space by a needle puncture between L3 and L4. There is no danger of hitting the spinal cord at this location because the latter ends at about L1/L2. The meninges, however, continue inferiorly for several vertebral segments. CSF may also be withdrawn by a similar (but more risky) puncture at the base of the skull. At that location the objective is to withdraw it from the cisterna magna. This is an enlargement of the subarachnoid space which occurs where the meninges reflect off the inferior aspect of the cerebellum to join the spinal cord.

Table 9-4 Named Partitions Formed by the Dura Mater

Partition	*Location*
Falx cerebri	Extends deeply into the longitudinal cerebral fissure on the median plane between the right and left cerebral hemispheres. It is anchored anteriorly to the crista galli of the ethmoid bone and posteriorly to the tentorium cerebelli.
Tentorium cerebelli	Extends transversely and deeply into the invagination separating the temporal and occipital lobes of the cerebrum from the cerebellum. It is anchored to the temporal and occipital bones and forms a roof over the posterior cranial fossa except for the tentorial notch [incisura tentorii] through which the mesencephalon passes.
Falx cerebelli	Divides the right from the left cerebellar hemispheres. It is anchored to the internal occipital crest.
Diaphragma sellae	Located between the hypothalamus and the pituitary gland. It is perforated in its center for the passage of the infundibulum (by which the pituitary gland is suspended from the hypothalamus)

Objectives

16. State where CSF is produced and reabsorbed, name the spaces that it occupies, and indicate the total volume produced each day as well as the volume present at any given moment.

Clinical Considerations

The position of the brain within the skull offers it substantial protection from traumatic injury. Nonetheless, a severe blow to the head, even without resulting in a skull fracture may cause a **concussion**. This is a "bruising" of brain tissue which may result in temporary unconsciousness or an extended coma. Temporary or permanent loss of memory (amnesia) and delirium (irrational consciousness) may also occur and may be accompanied by various degrees of temporary or permanent sensory and motor dysfunction. Traumatic injuries to the spinal cord nearly always involve fractures of vertebrae or luxations of the intervertebral articulations (such as "whiplash"). Because nervous tissue has such a low regenerative capacity, these types of injuries are quite serious. If the spinal cord is severed, it simply will not regenerate and this results in loss of all motor and sensory functions from that level inferiorly. Severence of the spinal cord in the upper cervical region will cause death because the motor output to the muscles of respiration is obliterated.

Cerebrovascular accidents (CVA, "stroke") are caused by blockages or ruptures of cerebral vessels which result in lack of blood flow to parts of the brain. The specific symptoms which result vary according to the location and extent of brain damage. Some patients recover completely. Others suffer permanent brain deficits which may cause paralysis, speech deficits, and loss of sensation.

Paralysis is a loss of motor (skeletal muscle) function which is usually caused by an injury to the brain, spinal cord, or peripheral nerve(s). Severe paralysis which results in loss of ability to move all limbs is called **quadriplegia**. If only the inferior limbs are involved it is called **paraplegia** and if the superior and inferior limb on the same side of the body are paralyzed, the condition is called **hemiplegia**.

The electrical activity of the brain can be monitored by **electroencephalography**. This involves electrodes that are attached to the scalp and the production of a brain wave pattern called an **electroencephalogram** (**EEG**). Deviations from the typical EEG patterns occur in various CNS diseases and conditions. Loss of brain waves is sometimes used to determine that death has "legally" occurred.

Many disease conditions of the CNS occur with little or no alterations in structure. Included are dyslexia, epilepsy, and other mental disorders. **Dyslexia** is a malfunction of the language center in which individuals reverse the order of syllables and words, especially when reading. **Epilepsy** involves periodic, temporary loss of consciousness and varying degrees of convulsive seizures. Affected individuals can often be medically controlled and lead normal lives. **Mental illness** involves a broad spectrum of CNS disorders. Historically, many of these have been grouped into **neuroses** (contact with reality is maintained) and **psychoses** (contact with reality is lost). The *Diagnostic and Statistical Manual of Mental Disorders* (DSM-IV) published by the American Psychiatric Association currently categorizes and classifies over 300 mental disorders that lack gross anatomic changes. These range from mental retardation and substance abuse to a number of thought and mood disorders.

The CNS is affected by a number of infectious diseases including polio, infectious meningitis, and syphilis. **Poliomyelitis** is a viral disease that destroys motor neurons in the anterior column of gray matter in the spinal cord. Because these are S.E. neurons, paralytic deficits occur in the skeletal muscles supplied by them. In this and many other parts of the world, polio has been controlled by immunization. **Meningitis** is caused by a bacterial or viral infection involving the meninges. It may be limited to the meninges of the spinal cord or it may also affect those covering the brain and cause *encephalitis*. Some cases are fatal. **Syphilis** is a sexually transmitted disease caused by a spirochete bacterium. It has a large number of physical manifestations including several that affect the brain and spinal cord.

Some diseases of the CNS result from degenerative conditions of myelin ensheathments. **Tay-Sachs** disease is a heritable condition caused by excess accumulation of one of the lipid components in myelin. It causes progressive symptoms that culminate in death in early childhood. Parents can be screened to determine if they are genetic carriers. **Multiple sclerosis** is a chronic progressive disease that destroys myelination. The affected areas are invaded by fibrous connective tissue which forms scars called *scleroses*. Affected individuals have a wide variety of symptoms depending on the areas in the body affected by the disease. They often have periods of clinical remission but eventually suffer permanent paralysis and then death.

Degenerative diseases of the CNS primarily affecting the elderly include Parkinson's disease and Alzheimer's disease. **Parkinson's disease** involves destruction of neurons within the basal nuclei of the brain resulting in muscular tremors, speech deficits, and other symptoms. Some patients can be improved pharmacologically by drugs which affect neurotransmitter metabolism. **Alzheimer's disease** is a progressive mental deterioration of unknown etiology (cause) that begins in middle age. Some evidence indicates that it may be related to a reduced ability of neurons in the brain to produce acetylcholine. Victims of this disorder begin to forget minor things and then more substantive information (names, addresses, *etc.*).

Objectives

17. Discuss hydrocephalus.
18. Define CVA and state its causes
19. Differentiate the various types of paralysis involving whole limbs.
20. Name several diseases that occur with no detectable change in brain or spinal cord and several that have CNS lesions.

Clinical Case Studies

Case 1—A newborn baby, normal in all other respects, was noted to have an unusually large head. In the first few days after birth, the infant's head enlarged even more and surgery was performed. What was the purpose of the surgery?

Case 2—A professional baseball pitcher, 29 years old, began losing control of his fastball and slowly developed loss of strength in his pitching (right) arm over a six month period. In the off season, his arm continued to atrophy in spite of a rigorous exercise program. Nerve function studies in the affected limb were normal and a radiographic study of the spinal cord revealed no abnormalities. When the pitcher began to develop intractable headaches, the team physician suspected a brain tumor might be present. If a tumor caused the problems, where would it likely be located?

Case 3—A few months after having a lumbar puncture at L2-L3 to retrieve a sample of cerebrospinal fluid, a meningitis patient developed paralysis of the muscles in her left inferior limb. She filed a legal suit against the physician who performed the puncture alleging that his faulty technique had damaged her spinal cord. Did she have a case?

Points to Ponder

The brain. When we see one in the lab sometimes we forget that it was once part of a person-good person or bad, black or white, Republican or Democrat, male or female—the brains are all similar, same parts in the same places. Same dips and folds, curves and bumps, gyri and sulci. Of the 10,000 (±) human body parts listed in the *Nomina Anatomica,* about 10 percent are landmarks of the brain. Strange that this most complex of all body structures is so poorly understood. Strange that sometimes major physical damage results in little physical dysfunction and vice-versa.

And then there's memory or (unfortunately) the lack of it. What is memory, how does it work, why is it so often fleeting? We can name a thousand brain parts but we can't explain how memory works or why it doesn't. And yet we measure the current strength of memory with tests and quizzes and score the owners with grades and even award degrees that reflect something we do not understand and cannot explain.

The brains of hard-core criminals have been analyzed in hopes of finding some defect to explain their behavior. The results have been essentially negative. To give neuroscience a handle on this disappointment the term "organic brain disorder" has been coined. There, we feel better. We've named something that we cannot explain. Makes it less ominous, puts it in a less distorted perspective. Science is like that. Needs garbage cans in which to jam all the stuff that doesn't neatly fit the artificial categories that we create. The brain seems to be a square peg and the pigeon-holes of its function are round. We hate it when that happens. Makes us look bad. Students, especially, have a hard time accepting that we know so much about so many things and yet so little about so much of the brain. A few decide, when facing this enigma, that they will do research. They will clarify the brain for all of us. Neurocrusaders bent on setting the record straight for all time. Some change their tune after a few months or a few years of clarifying nothing. Others add to the plethora of confusion already there. But a few do manage to push the shroud of ignorance further back and so we know more today than we did yesterday and we'll be further enlightened tomorrow.

The spinal cord is simpler. It could be compared to a telephone cable—a group of "wires" insulated from each other going to and from the brain and body. Just as the skull protects the brain from routine damage, the vertebral column surrounds and protects the spinal cord. The joints between the vertebrae allow some motion so that the spinal cord can be angled in all directions in degrees from negligible to Little Egypt—who could bend in ways that defied the realities of anatomical structure. The vertebral column has paired, lateral openings to allow the emergence of spinal nerves—those bundles of neuron processes that go to muscles and glands and come from sensory receptors. Sometimes these openings can pinch or pressure emerging nerves when the body is in certain positions causing pain or even paralysis. This may be related to problems with an invertebral disc—those shock absorbing spacers between vertebral bodies that can rupture or degenerate. Enter the neurosurgeon or sometimes orthopod to create more space or sometimes fuse adjacent vertebrae. The loss of motion at a few intervertebral joints does not significantly affect life as we know it (each one moves such a small amount anyway)!

If neurons can regenerate severed axons why can't a severed spinal cord heal? Well... if we could keep the scar tissue from invading a severed area, and if the traumatic incident that severed the cord in the first place could always be a neat, surgeon-like transection rather than the bone crushing incidents that often occur, and if one could juxta-position the severed ends of the spinal cord extremely accurately and hold it precisely there so that no movement occurred for months while the axons regenerated, then maybe transected spinal cords could heal successfully. (Don't hold your breath).

Slang and Obsolete Nomenclature

UNOFFICIAL TERM	**OFFICIAL DESIGNATION**
fissure of Sylvius	lateral sulcus *[sulcus lateralis]*
Schwann cell	neurolemmocyte *[neurolemmocytus]*
node of Ranvier	neurofibrillar node *[nodus neurofibrae]*
aqueduct of Sylvius	mesencephalic (cerebral) aqueduct *[aqueductus mesencephali/cerebri]*
ventral/dorsal gray columns	anterior/posterior *[anterior/posterior]* gray columns
longitudinal fissure	longitudinal cerebral fissure *[fissura longitudinalis cerebralis]*

foramen of Munro	interventricular foramen *[foramen interventriculare]*
foramen of Magendie	median aperture *[apertura mediana]* of fourth ventricle
foramen of Luschka	lateral aperture *[apertura lateralis]* of fourth ventricle
arachnoid villi	arachnoid granulations *[granulationes arachnoidea]*
arachnoid	arachnoid mater *[arachnoidea mater]*
dorsal (posterior) root ganglion	sensory ganglion *[ganglion sensorium]*
sympathetic chain	sympathetic trunk *[truncus sympatheticus]*
Nissl body	chromatophilic substance *[substantia chromatophilia]*

Review Questions

1. Find the truth.
   A. The occipital lobes of the cerebrum are involved with interpretation of taste.
   B. The prosencephalon gives rise to the telencephalon and diencephalon.
   C. The spinal cord ends in a conical projection called the conus medullaris at approximately T11/T12.
   D. Pia mater is directly superficial to arachnoid mater and is adherent to the cerebral cortex.
   E. Choroid plexuses produce several hundred milliliters of CSF each day, but the CNS contains only about 375 ml of CSF at any given moment.

2. Which of the following is mismatched with its function?
   A. temporal lobe of the cerebrum—interpretation of sound
   B. insular lobe of the cerebrum—integration of the other cerebral lobes
   C. parietal lobe of the cerebrum—general motor perception
   D. frontal lobe of the cerebrum—verbal communication and thought
   E. occipital lobe of the cerebrum—coordination of eye movements

3. Which of the following is not part of the spinal cord?
   A. anterior gray column
   B. lumbosacral intumescence (enlargement)
   C. ramus communicans
   D. central canal
   E. lateral funiculus

4. Which of the following statements is true?
   A. When electrical impulses pass from neuron to neuron, saltatory conduction has occurred.
   B. Myelin is the lipid found in myelin sheaths that surround many of the axons in the PNS and CNS.
   C. Groups of neuronal processes within the brain and spinal cord are called nerves.
   D. Hemiplegia is a condition where the contralateral limbs are paralyzed.
   E. CVA's are caused by blockage or rupture of coronary vessels.

5. Find the truth.
   A. One of the functions of the CNS is transducing various forms of energy to motor impulses.
   B. Bipolar neurons have one dendrite, one axon, and are found in the retina of the eye, in the middle ear, and in the oral mucosa.

C. Pseudounipolar neurons are the least numerous afferent neurons.
D. Multipolar neurons have a single dendrite and numerous axons.
E. The ANS is formed by parts of the PNS and CNS.

6. Which of the following major parts of the brain is mismatched with a function(s)?
A. thalamus—relay center for most sensory information
B. mesencephalon—a reflex center for audition and vision and contains motor nuclei for the oculomotor and trochlear nerves.
C. cerebellum—coordination of smooth muscle activity
D. pons—a bridging connection between the medulla and mesencephalon
E. medulla (oblongata)—decussation (crossing over) of motor and sensory fiber tracts passing to and from the spinal cord

7. Which of the following statements is false?
A. The gray matter of the spinal cord is penetrated by the central canal (of the spinal cord).
B. The spinal cord widens in the cervical and lumbosacral regions.
C. Neurons pass neurotransmitters to other neurons, to muscle cells, or to glandular epithelium.
D. Acetylcholine and norepinephrine are common neurotransmitters in the PNS.
E. Choose this response if all the above (A-D) are true.

8. Find the false statement.
A. Nasal mucosa and deep body organs contain visceral afferent (VA) fibers.
B. The majority of SA and VA neurons are bipolar neurons.
C. Somatic afferent (SA) neurons carry impulses from the internal ear, skin, joints, and muscles to the CNS.
D. Visceral efferent (VE) neurons are multipolar neurons which form a two neuron chain to smooth and cardiac muscle tissues and glandular epithelium.
E. Somatic efferent (SE) neurons are multipolar neurons that carry impulses to skeletal muscle tissue.

9. Which item is false?
A. An out-rush of potassium ions causes repolarization which re-establishes the resting charge of a neuron and the neuron once again becomes relatively impermeable to both sodium and potassium ions.
B. Sufficient stimulation of neurons allows sodium ions to diffuse back into their cytoplasm and causes a momentary rise in the electrical potential called depolarization.
C. When depolarization reaches a critical level called threshold, an impulse travels throughout the neuron.
D. The sodium-potassium pump uses active transport to move sodium ions into neurons.
E. Choose this response if all the above (A-D) are true.

10. Find the false statement.
A. Microglia are phagocytic cells within the brain and spinal cord.
B. Astrocytes form the blood/brain barrier.
C. Oligodendrocytes form myelin sheaths around axons within the CNS.
D. Ependymal cells line the ventricles of the brain and the central canal of the spinal cord.
E. Satellite cells are associated with ganglia located in the brain.

Thought Questions

1. Why is the spinal cord somewhat thicker in two areas than in the adjacent portions?

2. Nervous tissue develops from the outermost of the three germ layers (ectoderm). Explain why so few nervous system structures are located at the body surface.

3. Why is gray matter (light) gray and white matter whiter?

4. Explain how axons of myelinated neurons conduct impulses faster than those which are not myelinated.

5. How does synaptic transmission of nervous impulses occur?

6. Name the three kinds of cells which receive nervous impulses.

7. Nerve impulse transmission involves a rapid depolarization followed immediately by a repolarization. What causes the depolarization? The repolarization?

8. Significant trauma to the cerebral hemispheres may have relatively little effect on brain function. Why?

9. Where is local anesthetic deposited in "epidural" anesthesia?

10. Why are concussion type injuries closely monitored for several hours after their occurrence?

11. Explain why a severed spinal cord cannot heal back together and function.

12. Why can the vertebral canal be penetrated with a needle at L2-L3 with no concern about damage to the spinal cord?

13. Why do many sensory and motor tracts decussate at the medulla oblongata?

14. There are dozens of different neurotransmitters. Some are excitatory and some are inhibitory. How do inhibitory neurotransmitters work?

15. If the prosencephalon were damaged during early embryogenesis, what definitive part of the brain might be defective?

16. Once complex locomotor skills like serving a tennis ball or skating backwards have been mastered, an individual can do them without "thinking" about what is involved. How is this handled by the CNS?

17. Why is nerve impulse transmission described as an electrochemical phenomenon? Where is cerebrospinal fluid (CSF) found?

18. What disease syndrome can result from blockage of flow of CSF?

19. What is the difference between a motor impulse and a sensory impulse?

20. Do neurons function as "2-way streets" for impulse transmission?

21. Sensory neurons always synapse with . . .

Answers to Clinical Case Studies

Case 1—This infant suffered hydrocephalus. In some cases, the normal drainage channels from the lateral ventricles of the brain to the subarachnoid space do not develop properly and with continued production, the cerebrospinal fluid collects and causes cephalic enlargement. Most cases are easily corrected by installing a tiny plastic tube to bypass the blocked area. The tube is buried in the tissues of the neck and the free end of the tube is inserted into a large vein in the neck such that the CSF drains back into the blood.

Case 2—Frontal lobe of the left cerebral hemisphere. This part of the brain is motor to the right superior limb.

Case 3—No. First, the spinal cord ends at L1-L2, so this puncture was performed below its termination. Second, spinal cord damage, if present, would be evident immediately after the puncture. It would not develop several months later.

Answers to Review Questions

1. B.

2. C. Parietal lobes interpret sensory impulses.

3. C. The ramus communicans is a derivative of a spinal nerve.

4. B.

5. E.

6. C. The cerebellum coordinates *skeletal* muscle activity.

7. E.

8. B. Most are pseudounipolar.

9. D. The sodium-potassium pump moves sodium out of the neurons.

10. E. There are no ganglia in the brain.

Answers to Thought Questions

1. The two thickened areas (cervical and lumbosacral intumescences) occur because there are more neurons in those locations. The increased number occurs because the spinal nerves supplying the limbs originate there and more neurons are needed because there are more "things" that need a nerve supply.

2. During development, the ectoderm that forms nervous tissue forms a plate, a groove and then a tube that separates from the rest of the ectoderm and assumes a position buried in the underlying mesoderm.

3. The gray ("dirty" white) results from a higher concentrations of neuron cell bodies (where the organelles are concentrated) and the white results from the color of the myelin within the oligodendrocytes.

4. The phenomenon of impulse conduction is similar in myelinated and unmyelinated axons. In unmyelinated neurons, the depolarization/repolarization must occur along the whole extent of the axonal cell membrane. In myelinated neurons, depolarization/repolarization "skips" across the insulating cells (neurolemmocytes or oligodendrocytes) and only occurs at the minute gaps (nodes) between them. This phenomenon can be likened to two individuals racing up a stair with one having to take every step and the other taking two or three steps at a time.

5. Synaptic transmission of nervous impulses occurs by chemicals called neurotransmitters. These chemicals are released when an impulse reaches the end of an axon. They diffuse across a minute gap (called a synaptic cleft) and interact with the cell membrane of the next cell which may be a glandular epithelial cell, a muscle cell, or another neuron. Depending on its chemical composition, a given neurotransmitter may excite the next cell (initiate an impulse) or inhibit it (prevent an impulse).

6. The only cells which receive impulses are muscle cells, glandular epithelial cells, and neurons.

7. Depolarization (rising voltage) occurs due to a rapid diffusion of sodium ions (Na^+) into the cytoplasm through the suddenly (sodium) permeable cell membrane. Repolarization (falling voltage) occurs due to a rapid outflux of potassium ions (K^+).

8. Large parts of the brain (especially the cerebral cortex) do not appear to have significant functions. For example, most of the motor output from the frontal lobes occurs in the precentral gyri and other parts of the frontal lobes are relatively inactive. Similarly, most of the sensory perception in the parietal lobes is concentrated in the postcentral gyri with the remaining portions having little activity.

9. The anesthetic is deposited on the surface of the dura mater. It reaches nervous tissue by diffusion.

10. The trauma may have ruptured blood vessels. Extravasation of blood can put pressure on the brain since the skull is not expandable.

11. Axonal regeneration occurs very slowly and the severed ends cannot be held in correct apposition for the months required. In addition, scar tissue (connective tissue proper) tends to invade the injury and prevent regeneration.

12. Because the spinal cord ceases growing before the vertebral column, it is shorter (by several centimeters) than the vertebral canal. The cord itself ends at the level of the junction of the first and second lumbar vertebrae in a conical projection termed the conus medullaris. The last several pairs of spinal nerves (including those that originate from the lower lumbar, the sacral, and the coccygeal segments of the spinal cord) arise segmentally from their homonymous cord segments above this termination. They then continue inferiorily below the end of the the spinal cord and leave the vertebral canal at the appropriate intervertebral foramina. This bundle of nerves below the spinal cord is called the cauda equina ("horse tail").

13. No one knows why. This is the anatomic phenomenon that explains why the left part of the brain deals with sensory and motor impulses involving the right side of the body (and vice versa).

14. Inhibitory neurotransmitters hyperpolarize the next cell by lowering its resting voltage. This inhibits impulse initiation because the cell's voltage must be elevated to the threshold level to start an impulse.

15. The cerebrum and all derivatives of the diencephalon (epithalamus, thalamus, and hypothalamus).

16. The cerebellum is heavily involved in the coordination of skeletal muscle activity. It must first be "taught" what to do, but once these motor patterns are learned, the cerebellum allows an "auto-pilot" sort of control wherein an individual can perform complex motor tasks without much conscious involvement.

17. The impulse itself is produced by the diffusion of ions (charged sodium and potassium atoms). At synapses, chemicals (neurotransmitters) are involved. Cerebrospinal fluid is found in the ventricles of the brain, mesencephalic aqueduct, central canal of spinal cord, subarachnoid space, and between the osseus and membranous labyrinth.

18. Hydrocephalus. It can sometimes be treated by surgical installation of bypasses (shunts) that allow CSF to flow around blockages.

19. There is no difference in the impulses, themselves. Motor impulses are destined for muscles and glands. Sensory impulses are directed toward the spinal cord and/or brain.

20. No. A given neuron transmits in one direction only. Thus, a particular neuron is only involved with outgoing (motor) or incoming (sensory) impulses.

21. . . . other neurons. Some motor neurons, on the other hand, synapse with muscle cells, some synapse with glandular epithelial cells, and some synapse with other neurons.

CHAPTER

10 *Peripheral Nervous System*

Chapter Outline and Key Concepts

INTRODUCTION

The peripheral nervous system includes cranial nerves, spinal nerves, ganglia, and sensory receptors.

GENERAL STRUCTURE OF A NERVE

A nerve is a bundle of neuronal processes in the PNS.

Connective tissue proper encasements include epineurium (around a whole nerve), perineurium (around groups of fibers within a nerve), and endoneurium (around individual fibers).

Nerves are classified as cranial or spinal depending on whether they originate from the brain or spinal cord.

CRANIAL NERVES

The twelve pairs of cranial nerves (numbered and named) are sensory and motor primarily to cephalic structures.

The cranial nerves pass through several different foramina of the skull enroute to their destinations.

Three cranial nerve pairs are sensory only (CN 1, 2, and 8), five pairs are considered to be primarily motor (CN 3, 4, 6, 11, and 12), and the others are mixed.

Some cranial nerve pairs are relatively simple in that they have a single function (CN 1, olfaction; CN 2, vision.

A few cranial nerves are quite complex because they are sensory and motor to numerous body structures.

All cranial nerves carry some sensory fibers, but in the five cranial nerves that are considered to be primarily motor (CN 3, 4, 6, 11, 12), the only sensory fibers are proprioceptive (body position sense).

SPINAL NERVES

The 31± pairs of spinal nerves attach directly to the spinal cord.

Spinal nerves originate as anterior and posterior rootlets that coalesce segmentally to form anterior and posterior roots.

A spinal nerve is formed when an anterior root joins the ipsilateral posterior root at the same level.

Spinal nerves have three major branches: anterior branch (to structures primarily anterior to the vertebral column), posterior branch (to structures primarily posterior to the vertebral column), and ramus communicans (to ipsilateral sympathetic trunk).

Most spinal nerves supply body structures near their horizontal levels of origin.

The anterior branches of ipsilateral spinal nerves C5, C6, C7, C8, and T1 exchange fibers in a complex network called the brachial plexus.

There are fifteen named nerves that originate from each (left and right) brachial plexus and they supply structures primarily in the superior limbs.

The anterior branches of the ipsilateral lumbar and sacral spinal nerves exchange fibers to form the lumbosacral plexus.

There are seventeen named nerves that originate from each (left and right) lumbosacral plexus and they supply structures primarily in the inferior limbs.

GANGLIA

Ganglia are collections of neuron cell bodies in the PNS.

Sensory ganglia contain the cell bodies of pseudounipolar or bipolar neurons, are found near the origins of nerves, and do not serve as the site of synapses.

Motor (autonomic) ganglia contain the cell bodies of VE (postganglionic) neurons, are found in several loci, and are the site of the only neuron-to-neuron synapses in the PNS.

Motor ganglia can be divided positionally into three groups: those along the sympathetic trunks, those within the walls of the organs innervated, and those located along nerves and plexuses in the PNS.

SENSORY RECEPTORS

Sensory receptors are neurons or other specialized cells that convert various stimuli into nervous impulses.

Many sensory receptors are multicellular structures that contain support cells as well as impulse generating cells.

The numerous specific kinds of sensory receptors can be grouped into five categories depending on the type of stimuli to which they respond: mechano-, chemo-, photo-, thermo-, and nociceptors.

Based on the location of the inciting stimuli, receptors can be grouped as exteroceptors, visceroceptors, and proprioceptors.

Within physiologic limits, receptors are very stimulus specific.

CLINICAL CONSIDERATIONS

Severance of a nerve disrupts all of its sensory/motor functions beyond the point of injury.

Some dysfunctions of nerves occur with enough frequency that they are given specific names (*i.e.*, Bell's palsy).

A spinal reflex may be elicited during a physical exam to evaluate the nerves involved in its impulse transmission as well as the integrity of the spinal cord at that level.

Referred pain is pain perceived in one area of the body that is actually caused somewhere else.

Phantom pain is pain that is perceived to be "in" body parts that have been removed.

Selected Definitions

Ascending/descending fiber tract—a fasciculus of neuronal fibers in the spinal cord. Ascending tracts carry sensory impulses up to the brain and descending tracts carry motor impulses down from the brain to be distributed by spinal nerves.

Brachial plexus—the network of neuronal fibers formed initially on each side by the ipsilateral anterior branches of spinal nerves C5, C6, C7, C8, and T1. As these five roots converge and re-divide to form three trunks, six divisions, and three cords (fasciculi), they give rise to fifteen named nerves that are distributed to the ipsilateral superior limb and upper trunk.

Branches of a spinal nerve—the major fasciculi into which a spinal nerve divides after its formation via convergence of anterior and posterior roots. These include an anterior branch, posterior branch, and a ramus communicans (which typically arises from the anterior branch).

Cranial nerve—a nerve that originates directly from the brain. There are twelve pairs of cranial nerves and each pair has specific motor and/or sensory functions (mainly in the cephalic region).

Cutaneous receptor—a sensory receptor associated with the skin. These include various kinds of mechanoreceptors, thermoreceptors, and nociceptors, but no chemoreceptors or photoreceptors.

Epineurium—the outer connective tissue proper encasement of a nerve. When severed nerves are surgically rejoined, the sutures are placed (to the degree possible) in the epineurium.

Lumbosacral plexus—the network of neuron fibers formed initially by the ipsilateral anterior branches of the lumbar and sacral spinal nerves (and usually T12 and Cy1, as well). The lumbosacral plexus gives rise to 17 named nerves that are distributed to the ipsilateral inferior limb and pelvic region.

Ganglion—a collection (physical group) of neuron cell bodies in the peripheral nervous system. Such a collection in the brain or spinal cord is called a nucleus.

Motor (autonomic) ganglion—a ganglion composed of the cell bodies of postganglionic visceral efferent neurons. Such ganglia are located along the sympathetic trunks, in the walls of various organs, and as discrete entities in the head, neck, and trunk.

Nerve—a discreet bundle (fasciculus) of neuronal processes in the peripheral nervous system. Such a bundle within the substance of the brain or spinal cord is called a (fiber) tract.

Paralysis—loss of motor abilities related to nervous or muscular dysfunction. Slight (partial) paralysis is termed paresis.

Phantom (limb) pain—perceived pain in a part of the body that has been removed (amputated). This is apparently caused by continued firing of sensory neurons that have been disrupted by the surgery.

Proprioceptor—a sensory receptor located in a muscle, joint capsule, or the internal ear that generates impulses in response to body position and/or movement. They include neuromuscular spindles, neurotendinous spindles, stretch receptors in joint capsules, and the hair cells in the utricle, saccule, and semicircular ducts of the internal ear.

Sensory ganglion—a ganglion composed of the cell bodies of somatic afferent neurons and/or visceral afferent neurons. Such ganglia are located on the posterior roots of spinal nerves and near the origins of the cranial nerves.

Spinal nerve—a nerve that originates from the spinal cord. These paired entities are named for the region of the spinal cord from whence they arise and are sequentially numbered within each region.

Referred pain—pain perceived in a locus other than where the noxious stimulus actually occurs. Pain in viscera is often referred to other, more superficial, areas.

Roots of a spinal nerve—the two bundles of neuronal fibers (anterior and posterior) that join to form a spinal nerve. Each root is formed by the convergence of numerous rootlets that emerge from the spinal cord.

Sensory receptor—any of those structures that generate sensory impulses. Sensory receptors often contain supporting cells as well as those that generate impulses, and they may be divided into categories based on the types of stimuli to which they respond (thermoreceptors, photoreceptors, *etc.*), the location of such stimuli (exteroceptors, visceroceptors, *etc.*), and various other criteria (cutaneous receptors, phasic receptors, *etc.*).

Spinal reflex—the sum total of involuntary motor activity initiated by sensory inputs coursing through spinal nerves into the spinal cord (*vs.* a cranial reflex which involves cranial nerves and the brain). Spinal reflexes are called monosynaptic if they only involve one synapse in the spinal cord and disynaptic if they involve two.

Thermoreceptor—a sensory receptor that responds to temperature changes. Organs of Ruffini generate impulses when they are warmed and bulbs of Krause generate impulses when they are cooled.

Tonic receptor—a sensory receptor that continues to generate impulses as long as the stimulus is present. Those receptors (such as olfactory cells) that reduce or discontinue impulse generation when continually stimulated are called phasic receptors.

Etymology *Sine mora*—**"Without delay."**

abducere (L), *to lead away*—abducens
cochlea (L), *snail shell*—cochlea
colliculus (L), *small hill*—colliculus
communicare (L), *to share*—communicans
con, com (L), *with, together*—convergent
fasciculus (L), *small bundle*—fasciculus
ganglion (G), *mass of nerve tissue*—ganglion
geniculatus (L), *small knee, knot*—geniculate
glossa (G), *tongue*—glossopharyngeal
gustare (L), *to taste*—gustatory
kinesis (G), *motion*—kinesthetic
nocere (L), *to hurt, harm*—nociceptors
olfactorius (L), *to smell*—olfactory
ophthalmos (G), *eye*—ophthalmic
otikos (G), *relating to the ear*—otic
pharynx (L), *throat*—glossopharyngeal
strabismos (G), *squinting*—strabismus
trigeminus (L), *threefold, triple*—trigeminal
trochos (G), *wheel*—trochlear
vagari (L), *to wander*—vagus
vergent (L), *to bend, incline*—convergent
vestibulum (L), *a passage, hall*—vestibulocochlear
xero (L), *dry*—xerophthalmia

Introduction

The peripheral nervous system (PNS) is the portion of the nervous system that consists of cranial nerves, spinal nerves, sensory and autonomic ganglia, and sensory receptors. It includes all nervous system structures except the brain and spinal cord. As noted in Chapter 9, the functions of the PNS include converting various forms of energy into sensory impulses, conducting these sensory impulses into the CNS, and conducting motor impulses from the CNS to effector organs (muscles and glands).

Objectives

1. Review the components and functions of the PNS.

General Structure of a Nerve

A *nerve* is a bundle of **nerve fibers** (typically axons) in the peripheral nervous system. The connective tissue proper encasement surrounding the whole structure is termed the **epineurium** (Figure 10-1). Partitions of connective tissue proper inside the epineurium, called **perineurium**, subdivide the axons into groups called **fasciculi**. Each individual axon is surrounded by a connective tissue proper encasement termed **endoneurium**. These connective tissue ensheathments are analogous and partially homophonous to the epimysium, perimysium, and endomysium of skeletal muscle. Nerves, *per se*, do not exist in the CNS because groups of nerve fibers in the brain and spinal cord are called **nerve (fiber) tracts**.

Nerves which originate directly from (attach to) the brain are called **cranial nerves** (*see Table 10-1*) and those which join the spinal cord are called **spinal nerves**. Nearly all nerves consist of both efferent and afferent fibers and are therefore classified as **mixed nerves**. A few of the cranial nerves contain only afferent fibers and are classified as **sensory nerves**. There are no purely motor nerves although several of the cranial nerves are commonly classified as motor because the only sensory fibers that they contain are proprioceptive (*see Sensory Receptors*).

Objectives

2. Define nerve and differentiate it from nerve (fiber) tract.
3. Sketch a nerve in transverse section and label the epineurium, perineurium, and endoneurium.

Cranial Nerves

The 12 pairs of **cranial nerves** (Figure 10-2) are numbered 1-12 (using arabic or roman numerals) and are also named (Table 10-2). They are distributed mainly to the head and neck with the exception of the vagus (and to a lesser extent, the accessory) nerves which supply a number of structures

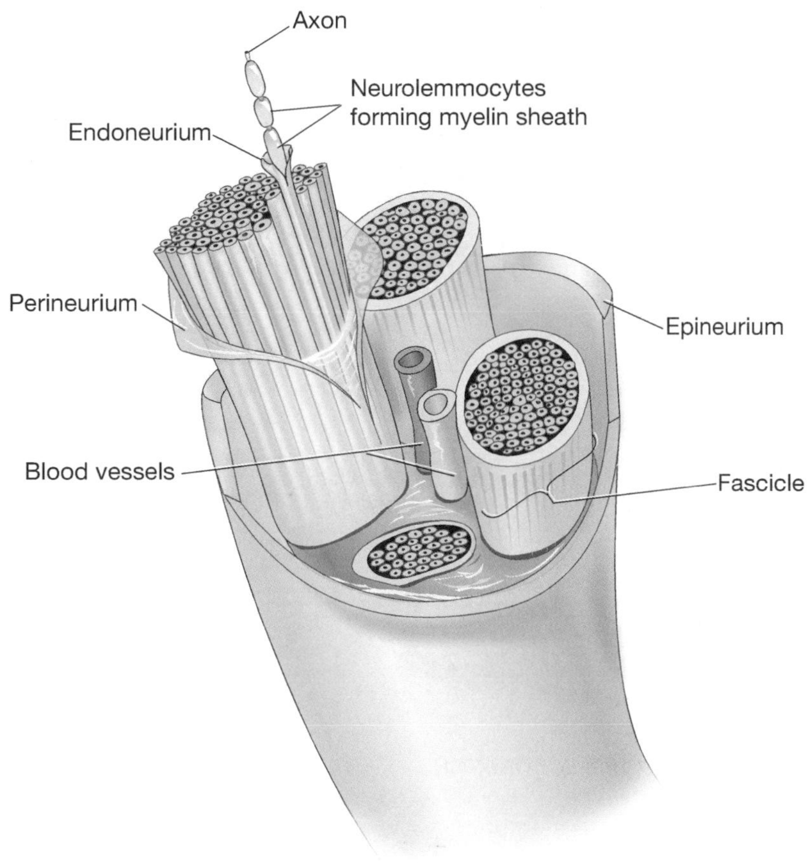

Figure 10-1

Structure of a Nerve

A nerve is a bundle of neuronal fibers (mostly axons) in the peripheral nervous system. The connective tissue encasements around individual nerve fibers, groups of fibers, and a whole nerve are called endoneurium, perineurium, and epineurium, respectively. The endoneurium is formed primarily by neurolemmocytes ("Schwann cells").

in the trunk. The cell bodies of the motor fibers carried by the cranial nerves are found in groups (nuclei) primarily within the mesencephalon, pons, and medulla oblongata of the brain. The cell bodies of the sensory fibers carried by the cranial nerves are located primarily in named sensory ganglia located along the course of the nerves near the brain. Students often employ a memory aid (mnemonic) to help them remember the names of the twelve pairs of cranial nerves: *On old Olympus' towering top a fine Victorian gentleman viewed a hawk.* The first letter of each word in this nonsense statement is identical to the first letter of the name of the numerically corresponding cranial nerve (*see Appendix III*).

After leaving the brain, the cranial nerves pass through foramina in the skull to reach the organs that they innervate. All of them carry sensory fibers and all but three pairs carry motor fibers as well. Several of the cranial nerves carry mostly motor fibers resulting in the fact that five pairs of them (oculomotor, trochlear, abducens, accessory, and hypoglossal nn.) are often considered to be primarily

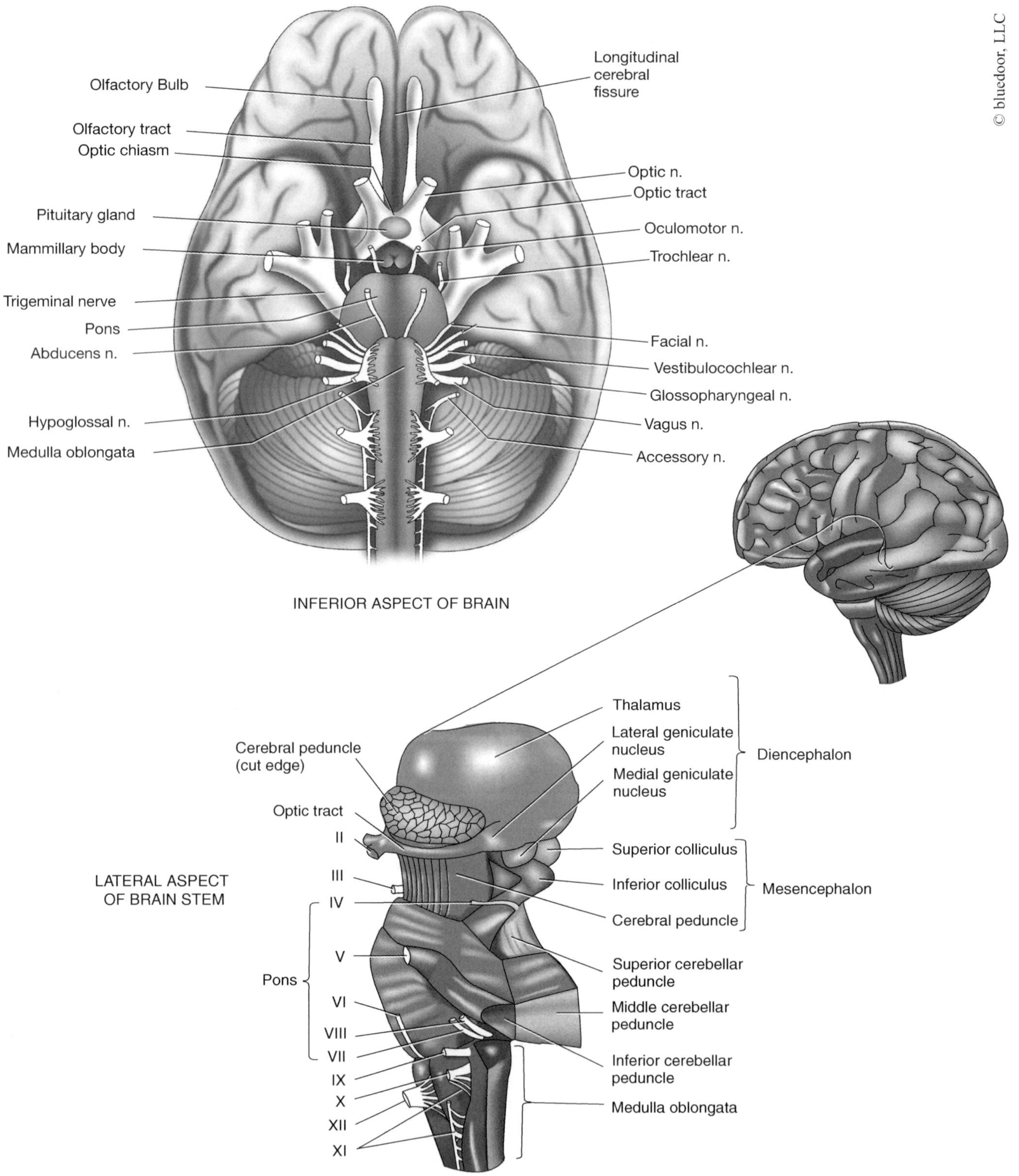

Figure 10-2

Cranial Nerves

The olfactory nerves (CN I) emerge from the olfactory bulbs and are such tiny bundles that they are not shown here (*see Figure 10-3*). The trochlear nerves (CN IV) are the only cranial nerves that do not emerge from the anterior aspect of the brain stem.

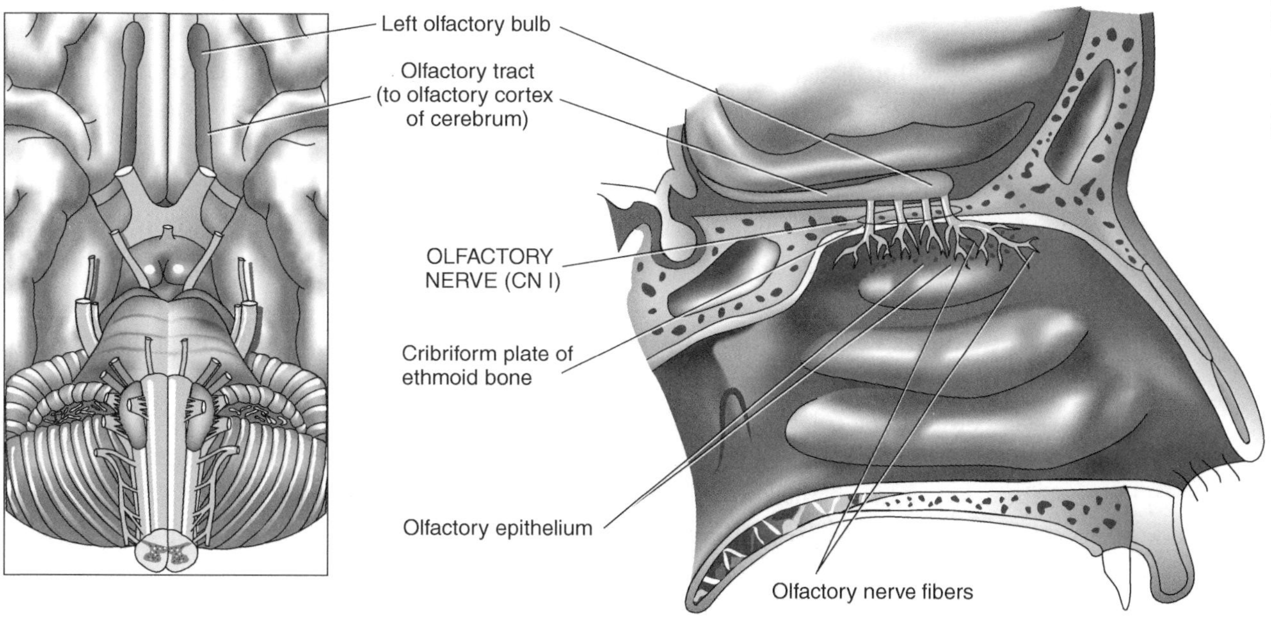

Figure 10-3
Distribution of Olfactory Nerve

Each olfactory nerve consists of about 20 bundles of fibers that penetrate the cribriform foramina of the ethmoid bone to be distributed to the nasal mucosa.

motor in function. Four pairs are considered to be **mixed**, (trigeminal, facial, glossopharyngeal, and vagus nn.), and three pairs are **sensory** only (olfactory, optic, and vestibulocochlear nn.). Students often employ another memory aid to help them remember the major roles of the cranial nerves as sensory, motor, or both (containing both sensory and motor fibers): *Six sailors made merry but my brothers said bad business, my man*. Note that the "s" implies sensory *only* and the "m" implies motor *mainly* ("b" = both). A number of criteria for comparing cranial nerves are listed in Table 10-3.

The **olfactory nerves (CN I)** carry olfactory (VA) impulses from the olfactory epithelium of the nasal cavity to the olfactory bulbs of the brain (Figure 10-3). The **olfactory epithelium** is a specialized part of the respiratory epithelium covering the superior third of the nasal septum and most of the superior nasal conchae of the ethmoid bone. The epithelial layer of this mucosa contains **olfactory cells** which are bipolar neurons whose cell bodies are scattered among the regular columnar epithelial cells and goblet cells. Only a very small percentage of inhaled air comes in contact with the olfactory mucosa (most passes inferior to it), but the olfactory cells are extremely sensitive chemoreceptors and trained individuals can distinguish thousands of different odors. Moisture in the form of mucus provided by goblet cells increases this sensitivity. Axons of the olfactory cells are collected into about twenty bundles from each half of the olfactory mucosa. These bundles collectively constitute the olfactory nerves. They course through the **cribriform foramina** of the ethmoid bone and synapse within the **olfactory bulb** of the rhinencephalon. The axons of these subsequent neurons form the **olfactory tracts** which terminate in the olfactory areas on the medial aspects of the temporal lobes of the cerebral cortex (Figure 10-2). There, the impulses are interpreted as odors.

The **optic nerves (CN II)** carry visual (SA) impulses from the retinae of the eyes to the optic chiasm of the brain (Figure 10-4). The photoreceptor cells **(rods and cones)** in the retina of each eye initiate nervous impulses in response to light. These synapse on **bipolar neurons** which in turn synapse on **ganglion cells** (all within the retina—*see Chapter 12*). Axons of the ganglion cells leave the back of each eyeball just medial to the posterior pole as the optic nerve which courses posteromedially through the orbit and then passes through the **optic canal** of the sphenoid bone. The orbital portion of the optic nerve is about 30 mm long and is slack enough to accommodate movement of the eyeball. It is surrounded by orbital fat, the rectus muscles of the eye, and is encased by meningeal extensions from the brain. After coursing through the optic canal, the optic nerves join at the midline to form the **optic chiasm** on the anterior aspect of the hypothalamus. Here the fibers from the medial half of each retina cross over (decussate) to the opposite side. This results in the fact that the **optic tracts** which continue posteriorly are composed of fibers carrying impulses from the lateral part of the ipsilateral retina and the medial part of the contralateral retina. The fibers in the optic tracts course posterolaterally and synapse primarily on neurons in the **lateral geniculate bodies** of the thalamus. Axons from these neurons continue to the visual cortex located in the occipital lobes of the cerebral hemispheres. A smaller percentage (20-30%) of the fibers in each optic tract course to the ipsilateral **superior colliculus** of the mesencephalon where they synapse on neurons involved in reflexes related to body/eye coordination.

Table 10-1 Attachment of Cranial Nerves to the Brain Stem *(See Figure 10-2)*

CN I	— Olfactory tract (from anteroinferior aspect of cerebrum)
CN II	— Optic tract (from the hypothalamus)
CN III	— Oculomotor sulcus (between hypothalamus and pons)
CN IV	— Base of inferior colliculus of mesencephalon
CN V	— Lateral aspect of pons
CN VI	— Anteromedial aspect of bulbopontine sulcus
CN VII	— Lateral aspect of bulbopontine sulcus
CN VIII	— Just lateral to facial nerve (see above)
CN IX	— Posterolateral sulcus of medulla oblongata (superior aspect)
CN X	— Posterolateral sulcus of medulla oblongata (just inferior to glossopharyngeal nerve)
CN XI	— Posterolateral sulcus of medulla oblongata (inferior to vagus nerve) and spinal cord
CN XII	— Emerges as a series of rootlets between the olive and the pyramid (anterolateral sulcus) of the medulla oblongata

The **oculomotor nerves (CN III)** innervate a number of muscles associated with the eyes (Figure 10-4). Each oculomotor nerve emerges from the oculomotor sulcus adjacent to the pons, courses through the **superior orbital fissure**, and divides into superior and inferior branches within the orbit. The **superior branch** carries multipolar (SE) fibers to the superior rectus muscle which rotates the eyeball superiorly and to the levator palpebrae superioris muscle which raises the upper eyelid to open the eye. The **inferior branch** supplies multipolar (SE) fibers to the medial rectus, inferior rectus, and inferior oblique muscles of the eye which rotate the eyeball in various directions. The SE fibers have cell bodies in the nucleus of the oculomotor nerve within the mesencephalon. Multipolar (VE) fibers which supply smooth muscles within the eyeball have their cell bodies in the accessory nucleus of the oculomotor nerve (also in the mesencephalon). They are carried by nerves to the **ciliary ganglion** located behind the eyeball. Axons from postganglionic fibers continue to the eyeball within **short ciliary nerves** and supply the ciliary muscle (a smooth muscle in the ciliary body which controls lens thickness) and the pupillary sphincter muscle (a smooth muscle in the iris which causes constriction of the pupillary aperture).

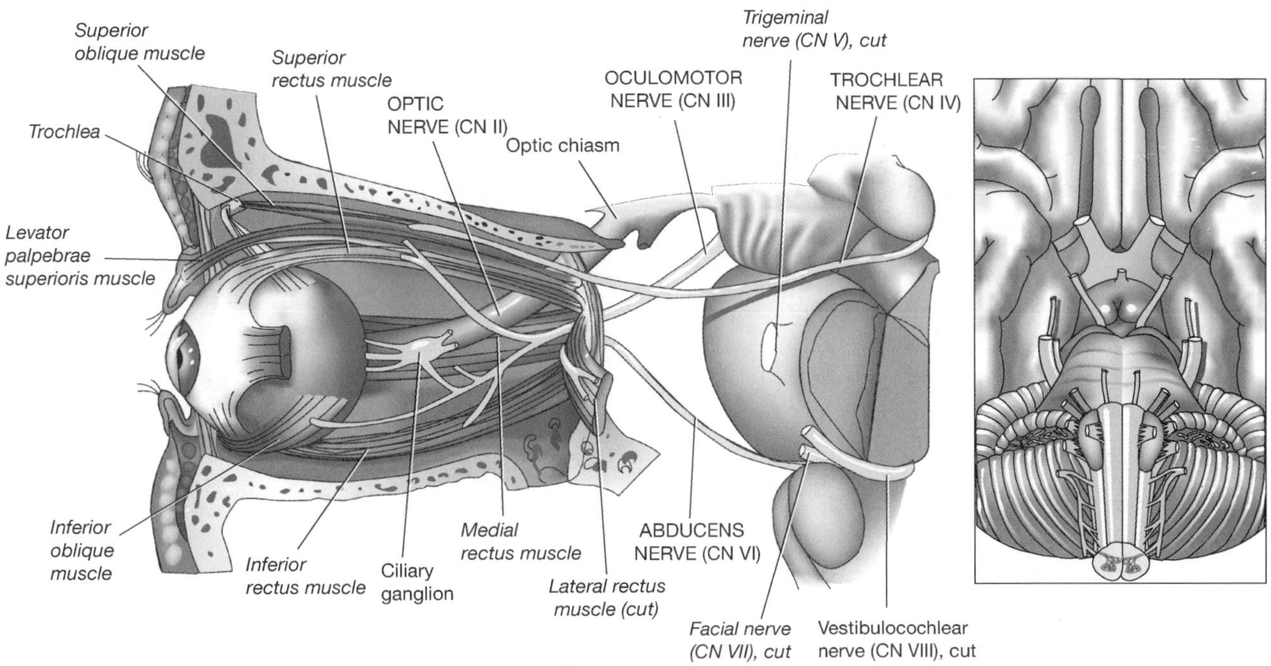

Figure 10-4

Distribution of Cranial Nerves 2, 3, 4, and 6

The optic nerves carry sensory impulses interpreted as vision. General sensory impulses from the eye (those interpreted as hot, cold, pressure, pain, touch) are carried by the ophthalmic nerve (not shown) from the trigeminal nerve (Figure 10-6). The trochlear, oculomotor, and abducens nerves are distributed to the ocular muscles.

The **trochlear nerves (CN IV)** are the smallest cranial nerves and the only pair that arise from the posterior (superior) aspect of the brain (Figure 10-5). Each one emerges from the posterolateral base of the ipsilateral **inferior colliculus** of the corpora quadrigemina. It then courses around the brainstem, penetrates the tentorium cerebelli, and courses anteriorly, adjacent to the oculomotor nerve. It passes through the **superior orbital fissure** and continues to the superior oblique muscle of the eye which it supplies with multipolar (SE) fibers (Figure 10-4). The cell bodies of these neurons are located in the nucleus of the trochlear nerve within the mesencephalon.

The **trigeminal nerves (CN V)** are the largest cranial nerves (in diameter) and are the principal sensory nerves of the head (Figure 10-6). Each one emerges from the inferolateral aspect of the pons as a larger sensory root and a smaller motor root. The sensory root is enlarged by the **trigeminal ganglion** which contains the cell bodies of its pseudounipolar (SA) neurons. Three named subdivisions of the trigeminal nerve attach to this ganglion: ophthalmic, maxillary, and mandibular nerves (Table 10-4). The **ophthalmic nerve** courses through the superior orbital fissure into the orbit. There it divides into several named sensory branches which are distributed to the nose, eye, upper eyelid, forehead, and vertex. The **maxillary nerve** courses through the foramen rotundum of the sphenoid bone. It divides into several named branches which are distributed to the upper lip, upper teeth, palate, cheek, and lower eyelid (Figure 10-7). The **infraorbital nerve** is the branch of the maxillary nerve that continues through the infraorbital foramen to be distributed to the face.

Table 10-2 Cranial Nerves

Number	*Name*	*Transmitting Foramen*	*Function*	*Neuron Type and Location of Cell Bodies*
I	**Olfactory nerve**	Cribriform foramina of ethmoid bone	VA neurons: sense of smell (olfaction)	Bipolar neurons in nasal mucosa (olfaction)
II	**Optic nerve**	Optic canal of sphenoid bone	SA neurons: vision	Bipolar neurons in retina
III	**Oculomotor nerve**	Superior orbital fissure	SE neurons: motor to superior, medial and inferior rectus mm., inferior oblique m., levator palpebrae superioris m. of the eye	Multipolar neurons in nucleus of oculomotor nerve in mesencephalon
			VE neurons: motor to ciliary m. of eye and pupillary sphincter m. of the iris	Multipolar neurons in accessory oculomotor nucleus within mesencephalon (pre-ganglionics), and within ciliary ganglion (post-ganglionics)
IV	**Trochlear nerve**	Superior orbital fissure	SE neurons: motor to superior oblique m. of the eye	Multipolar neurons in motor nucleus of trochlear n. within mesencephalon
V	**Trigeminal n.:**			
	Ophthalmic nerve	Superior orbital fissure	SA neurons: sensory from and around the eye (general sensation)	Pseudounipolar neurons in the trigeminal ganglion of the trigeminal nerve
	Maxillary nerve	Foramen rotundum of sphenoid bone	SA neurons: sensory from upper lip and surrounding skin, upper teeth and gums, and palate	Pseudounipolar neurons in the trigeminal ganglion of the trigeminal nerve
	Mandibular nerve	Foramen ovale of sphenoid bone	SA neurons: sensory from lower lip and surrounding skin, lower teeth and gums, tongue, and floor of oral cavity	Pseudounipolar neurons in the trigeminal ganglion of the trigeminal nerve
			SE neurons: motor to mm. of mastication	Multipolar neurons in the motor nucleus of the trigeminal nerve within the pons
VI	**Abducens nerve**	Superior orbital fissure	SE neurons: motor to lateral rectus m. of the eye	Multipolar neurons in the nucleus of the abducens n. within the pons
VII	**Facial nerve**	Passes through both the internal acoustic meatus and stylomastoid foramen of temporal bone	VA neurons: taste sensation (gustation) from anterior two-thirds of tongue	Pseudounipolar neurons in geniculate ganglion of the facial nerve
			VE neurons: motor to lacrimal, sublingual, and submandibular glands (lacrimation and salivation)	Multipolar neurons in the nucleus salivarius superior within the pons (pre-ganglionic) and the pterygopalatine, submandibular, and sublingual ganglia (post-ganglionic)
			SE neurons: motor to mm. of facial expression and the stapedius m.	Multipolar neurons in the nucleus of the facial nerve within the pons

Number	*Name*	*Transmitting Foramen*	*Function*	*Neuron Type and Location of Cell Bodies*
VIII	**Vestibulocochlear nerve**	Internal acoustic meatus of temporal bone (does not emerge from skull)	SA neurons: sensory from cochlear part of internal ear (audition) and vestibular part of internal ear (balance and body position)	Bipolar neurons in cochlear ganglion (audition) and vestibular ganglion (body balance and position)
IX	**Glossopharyngeal nerve**	Jugular foramen	VA neurons: taste sensation (gustation) from posterior one-third of tongue, general sensation from back of tongue and pharyngeal region	Pseudounipolar neurons in inferior ganglion of the glossopharyngeal nerve
			VE neurons: motor to parotid gland (salivation)	Multipolar neurons in nucleus salivarius inferior within medulla (pre-ganglionics) and in otic ganglion (post-ganglionics)
			SA neurons: sensory from a small cutaneous area behind the ear	Pseudounipolar neurons in the superior ganglion of the glossopharyngeal nerve
			SE neurons: motor to some skeletal mm. of the pharynx	Multipolar neurons in the nucleus ambiguus within the medulla oblongata
X	**Vagus nerve**	Jugular foramen	VA neurons: sensory from respiratory and digestive systems, and a few taste fibers from the tongue	Pseudounipolar neurons in the inferior ganglion of the vagus nerve
			VE neurons: motor to heart and to smooth muscle and glands of the respiratory and digestive systems	Multipolar neurons in the dorsal nucleus of the vagus n. within the medulla (pre-ganglionics) and in many ganglia throughout abdomen and thorax (post-ganglionics)
			SA neurons: sensory from skin in back of ear and posterior wall of external acoustic meatus	Pseudounipolar neurons in the superior ganglion of the vagus nerve
			SE neurons: motor to muscles of the larynx and pharynx	Multipolar neurons in the nucleus ambiguus within the medulla oblongata
XI	**Accessory nerve**	Jugular foramen	SE neurons: motor to trapezius and part of sternocleidomastoid muscles	Multipolar neurons within C1-C5 segments of spinal cord (spinal part) and within the nucleus ambiguus of the medulla
XII	**Hypoglossal nerve**	Hypoglossal canal of occipital bone	SE neurons: motor to muscles of the tongue and infrahyoid muscles	Multipolar neurons in the nucleus of the hypoglossal n. within the medulla

Note that any cranial nerve that supplies skeletal muscles (*i.e.*, all of them except the olfactory, optic, and vestibulocochlear nerves) also carries some SA proprioceptive fibers from those same muscles which are involved with body positional sense (proprioception). Proprioceptive fibers carry impulses generated in muscle bellies, tendons, and joint capsules interpreted as body position, *etc.* Sometimes the sensory fibers in the vestibular apparatus of the internal ear are also classified as proprioceptive. These SA neurons were intentionally left off of this chart for brevity on cranial nerves 3, 4, 6, 11, and 12. In other words, if the *only* sensory fibers carried by a cranial nerve are SA proprioceptives, no table entry was made. SA entries were made in the table for all other (non-proprioceptive) somatic afferent pathways.

Table 10-3 A Comparison of Cranial Nerves Using Various Criteria

Criterion	*Cranial Nerves*
Carry SE fibers (supply skeletal muscle)	All except CN I, II, and VIII
Carry SA proprioceptive fibers	All except CN I, II, and VIII
Carry SA fibers other than proprioception (vision, audition, and general sensation from skin, muscles, bones, and joints)	CN II, V, VIII, IX, and X
Carry VE fibers (autonomic fibers to involuntary muscle and glands)	CN III, VII, IX, and X
Carry VA fibers (olfaction, gustation, and sensation from deep body systems)	CN I, VII, IX, and X
Distributed to the tongue	CN V (mandibular n.), VII, IX, X, XII
Carry gustatory fibers	CN VII, IX, and X
Carry fibers distributed to the oral cavity (other than gustatory fibers)	CN V (maxillary and mandibular nerves), IX, and XII
Transmitted by jugular foramen of skull	CN IX, X, and XI
Transmitted by superior orbital fissure	CN III, IV, V (ophthalmic n.), and VI
Supply the muscles of the eyeball	CN III, IV, and VI
Carry sensory fibers from the eyeball	CN II (vision only) and V (ophthalmic n.)
Originate from superior aspect of brain	CN IV
Distributed to cervical, thoracic, and abdominal viscera	CN X
Do not emerge from the skull	CN VIII
Carry visual information	CN II
Carry olfactory information	CN I
Carry auditory information	CN VIII
Carry equilibrium information	CN VIII
Supply muscles of mastication	CN V (mandibular n.)

The largest and lateral-most branch of the trigeminal nerve is the **mandibular nerve**. It is joined by the small motor root of the trigeminal nerve and together they course through the foramen ovale of the sphenoid bone. Outside the skull, the mandibular nerve divides into a number of named branches which supply sensory fibers to the skin on the side of the head, mandibular regions, lower lip, tongue, and inferior teeth. One of these, the **inferior alveolar nerve**, enters the mandibular foramen to supply the inferior teeth with sensory fibers and then re-emerges at the mental foramen as the **mental nerve** to supply the lower lip. The motor (SE) fibers carried by the mandibular nerve supply the muscles of mastication, stapedius, mylohyoideus, and the anterior belly of the digastricus muscles. Their cell bodies are in the motor nucleus of the trigeminal nerve within the pons. The mandibular nerve also receives a branch of the facial nerve called the **chorda tympani** which includes the axons of taste fibers and the parasympathetic preganglionic fibers destined for the sublingual and submandibular (salivary) glands (see *facial nerve*).

The **abducens nerves (CN VI)** emerge from the brain within a groove called the **bulbopontine sulcus**. This is located between the posterior border of the pons and the anterior border of the

Table 10-4 Distribution of Components of the Trigeminal Nerve

Branches of the Ophthalmic Nerve:
Lacrimal n.—sensory from upper eyelid, lacrimal gland, and adjacent conjunctiva
Frontal n.—sensory from upper eyelid, forehead, and scalp (has supraorbital and supratrochlear branches)
Nasociliary n.—(several named branches) sensory from eyeball, ethmoidal sinus, nasal cavity, and upper eyelid
Branches of the Maxillary Nerve:
Nasopalatine n.—sensory from mucosa covering most of nasal septum and anterior part of the hard palate
Pharyngeal n.—sensory from mucous membrane of the nasal part of the pharynx posterior to the auditory tube
Major palatine n.—sensory from palate
Minor palatine nn.—sensory from soft palate and palatine tonsil
Superior alveolar nn.—sensory from superior teeth, maxillary dental alveoli, and adjacent oral mucosa
Infraorbital n.—sensory from upper lip, side of nose, and adjacent face
Branches of the Mandibular Nerve:
Masseteric n.—motor to masseter muscle and sensory to temporomandibular joint
Deep temporal nn.—motor to temporal muscle
Lateral pterygoid n.—motor to lateral pterygoid muscle
Medial pterygoid n.—motor to medial pterygoid muscle
Buccal n.—sensory from skin and mucous membrane of cheeks and gums
Auriculotemporal n.—(several named branches) sensory from the tympanic membrane, external acoustic meatus, parotid gland and skin of the scalp anterior to ear
Lingual n.—sensory from tongue (general sensation); the gustatory (taste) fibers from the facial n. join the lingual nerve through the chorda tympani
Inferior alveolar n.—motor to mylohyoid muscle; sensory from mandibular dental alveoli, inferior teeth, and adjacent gums
Mental n.—(anterior continuation of the inferior alveolar n.) sensory from skin of chin and lower lip

Note: In addition to these branches, each of the three major parts of the trigeminal nerve has a meningeal branch and there are numerous named branches associated with the pterygopalatine ganglion of the maxillary nerve and with the otic ganglion of the mandibular nerve. Because branches of the facial and glossopharyngeal nerves anastomose with the trigeminal nerve, some branches in this chart contain parasympathetic fibers to glandular structures.

medulla oblongata (see Figure 10-2). Each one courses anteriorly through the dura mater lining the anterior wall of the posterior cranial fossa. It then enters the cavernous sinus (a large venous channel) and finally exits the skull through the **superior orbital fissure.** Within the orbit, the abducens nerve courses anteriorly to supply the lateral rectus muscle of the eye with multipolar (SE) fibers (*see Figure 10-4*). Cell bodies of these axons are located in the nucleus of the abducens nerve within the pons. The abducens nerve is frequently traumatized resulting in an inability to rotate the eyeball laterally. This causes **convergent strabismus** ("crossed eyes").

The **facial nerves (CN VII)** emerge from the bulbopontine sulcus, lateral to the abducens nerves and medial to the vestibulocochlear nerves. Each facial nerve originates from the brain as a large root and a smaller root (intermediate nerve). These course laterally with the vestibulocochlear nerve into the internal acoustic meatus of the temporal bone. Within the meatus these two components fuse and enter the facial canal. There, the facial nerve widens at its **geniculate** (sensory) **ganglion** and gives off several named branches. The smallest of these is the stapedial nerve which supplies the stapedius muscle (*see Middle Ear*). Another branch, the nerve of the pterygoid canal, is joined by

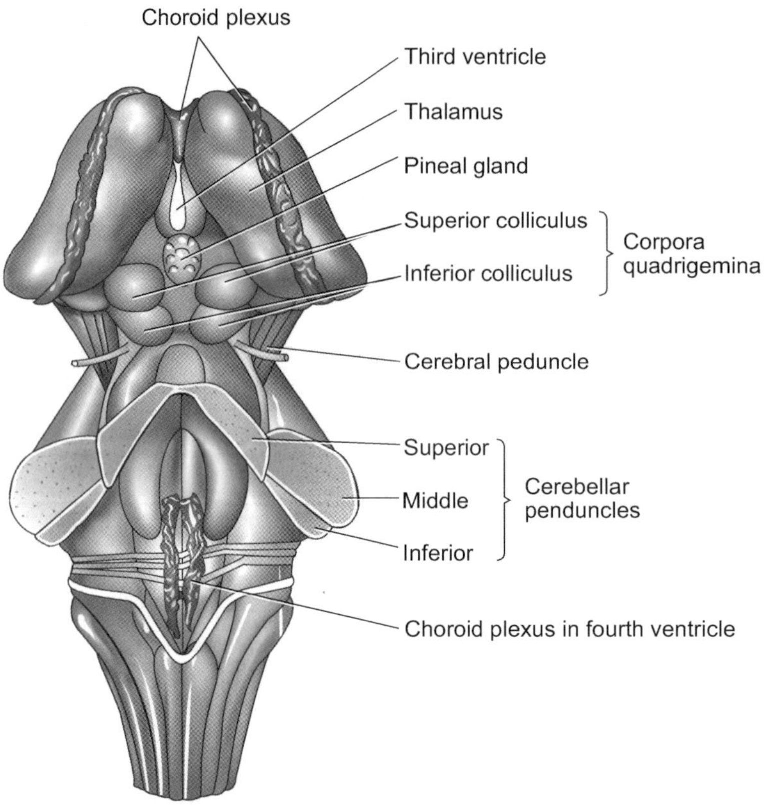

Figure 10-5

Posterior View of Brain Stem (with cerebellum removed)

The left and right trochlear nerves are the only cranial nerves that emerge from the posterior aspect of the brain. They attach just below the inferior colliculi of the corpora quadrigemina of the mesencephalon.

branches of the maxillary nerve at the pterygopalatine ganglion. The **chorda tympani** is a branch of the facial nerve which courses across the medial side of the tympanic membrane to ultimately join and be distributed with the lingual nerve (a branch of the mandibular nerve). The main continuation of the facial nerve exits the skull through the stylomastoid foramen of the temporal bone (Figure 10-8). It supplies motor fibers (SE) to the muscles of the face via several named branches. Sensory fibers (VA) in the chorda tympani carry taste sensation from the anterior two-thirds of the tongue. Some autonomic fibers (VE) of the facial nerve are distributed to the lacrimal gland and small named glands in the nasal mucosa and palate. These synapse on their postganglionic neurons in the **pterygopalatine ganglion**. Other VE fibers supply the sublingual and submandibular (salivary) glands. These synapse in the **sublingual** and **submandibular ganglia**.

The **vestibulocochlear nerves (CN VIII)** attach to the brain at the junction of the pons and medulla oblongata just lateral to the origin of the facial nerve. Each one enters the ipsilateral internal acoustic meatus of the temporal bone adjacent to the facial nerve (Figure 10-9). Within the meatus the vestibulocochlear nerve divides into the **cochlear nerve** and the **vestibular nerve**. These carry sensory (SA) information from the cochlear (auditory) and vestibular (equilibrium) portions

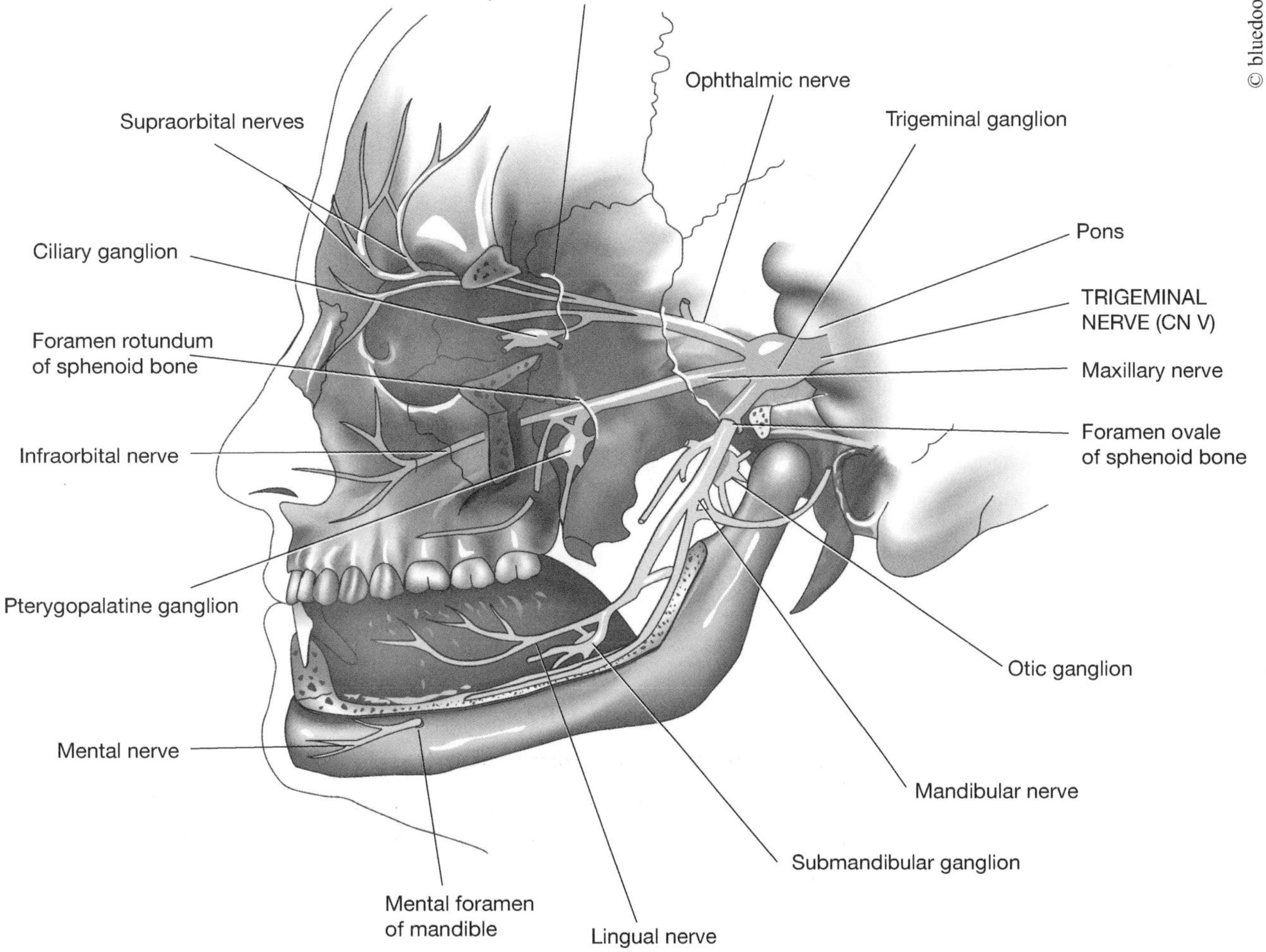

Figure 10-6
Trigeminal Nerve Distribution

of the internal ear. The fibers within the vestibulocochlear nerves are bipolar neurons and their cell bodies are located along the course of the nerves in the cochlear and vestibular ganglia. The vestibulocochlear nerves are the only pair of cranial nerves which do not emerge from the skull.

The **glossopharyngeal nerves (CN IX)** arise from the anterior portion of the **posterolateral sulcus** of the medulla oblongata. Their origins are sandwiched between those of the facial nerves (above) and the vagus and the accessory nerves (below). Each one leaves the cranial vault through the jugular foramen and divides into several branches which are distributed to the skeletal muscles of the pharynx (SE neurons), to the parotid (salivary) gland (VE neurons), to the posterior third of the tongue (VA neurons-taste), and to a small cutaneous area behind the ear (SA neurons) (Figure 10-10). The autonomic fibers to the parotid (salivary) gland synapse in the **otic ganglion**. The sensory fibers have their cell bodies in the **superior** (SA) and **inferior** (VA) **ganglia** of the glossopharyngeal nerve. These form small enlargements on the nerve as it emerges from the jugular foramen.

The **vagus nerves (CN X)** are the longest cranial nerves and are distributed throughout the cer-

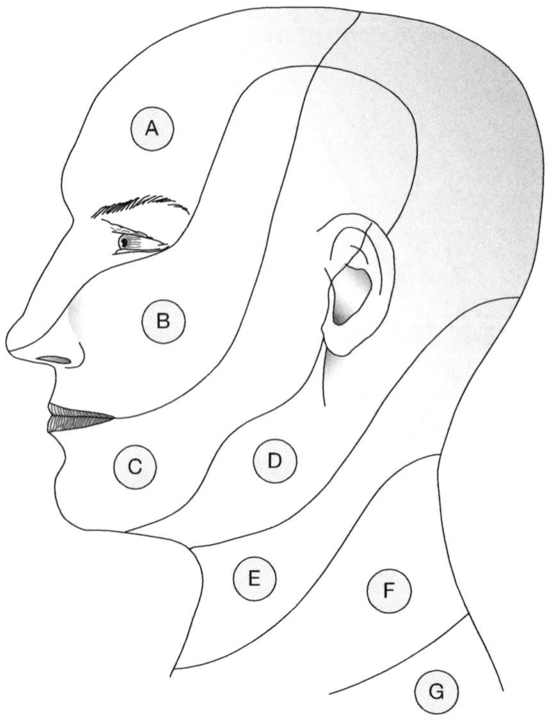

Figure 10-7

Cutaneous Innervation of the Head

Most cutaneous innervation in the anterior head is via the ophthalmic (A), maxillary (B), and mandibular (C) nerves. Areas D–G are innervated by cervical nerves C2, C3, C4, and C5, respectively.

vical, thoracic, and most of the abdominal regions (Figure 10-11). Each one arises from the lateral aspect of the medulla oblongata just below the ipsilateral glossopharyngeal nerve. It courses through the jugular foramen and continues inferiorly through the cervical region where it supplies branches to the pharynx as well as the superior laryngeal nerve to the laryngeal muscles. Within the thorax, the vagus nerve supplies branches to the heart, lungs, and esophagus as well as another branch (recurrent laryngeal nerve) which courses superiorly back to the larynx. It then follows the esophagus through the diaphragm and is distributed to the abdominal viscera. The vagus nerve supplies muscles of the pharynx and larynx (SE) fibers and also carries some general sensory (SA) fibers from the skin in the back of the ear and the wall of the external acoustic meatus. Branches of the vagus nerve also supply most of the motor (VE) fibers to the involuntary muscle and glands in the thoracic and abdominal cavities. The preganglionic/postganglionic synapses for these occur in numerous autonomic ganglia throughout those regions. About 80% of the fibers in each vagus nerve are sensory (VA) fibers from the cervical, thoracic, and abdominal viscera. The sensory fibers carried by the vagus nerve have fibers in the **superior** and **inferior ganglia** of the vagus nerve. These form small enlargements on the nerve near its emergence from the jugular foramen.

The **accessory nerves (CN XI)** supply branches primarily to the sternocleidomastoideus and trapezius muscles (Figure 10-12). Each one originates as two roots: one from the medulla adjacent to the origin of the vagus nerve and the other from the cervical spinal cord. These unite, pass

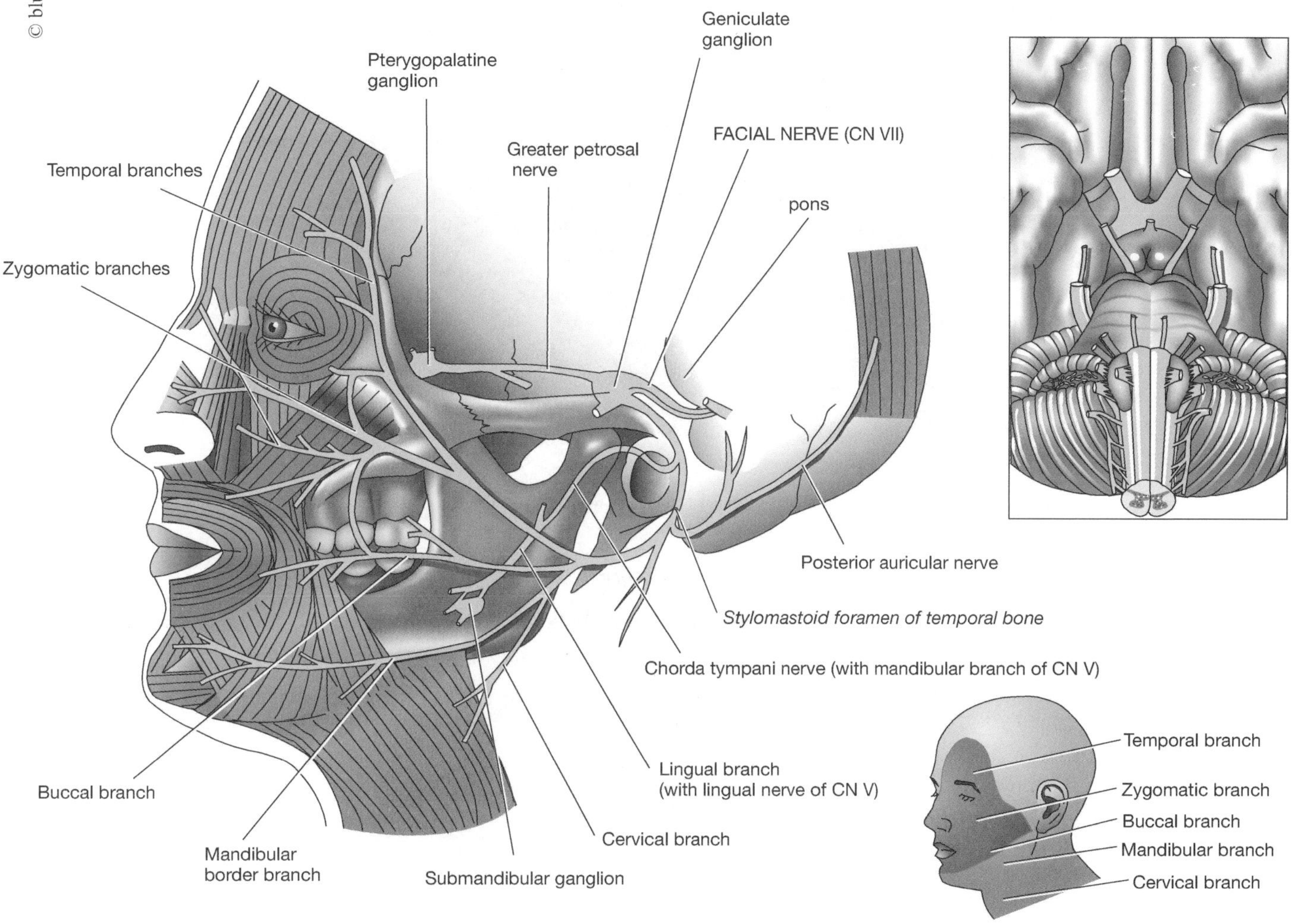

Figure 10-8
Distribution of Facial Nerve

through the jugular foramen and then divide into several branches for distribution.

The **hypoglossal nerves (CN XII)** are distributed to the lingual and infrahyoid muscles (Figure 10-12). Each one emerges as a series of 10 to 15 rootlets from the anterolateral sulcus between the olive and pyramid of the medulla oblongata. These fuse to form the hypoglossal nerve which passes through the ipsilateral hypoglossal canal in the occipital bone. In addition to the SE fibers, the hypoglossal nerves carry some SA (proprioceptive) fibers as do all cranial nerves which supply skeletal muscles (*see footnote at the bottom of Table 10-2*).

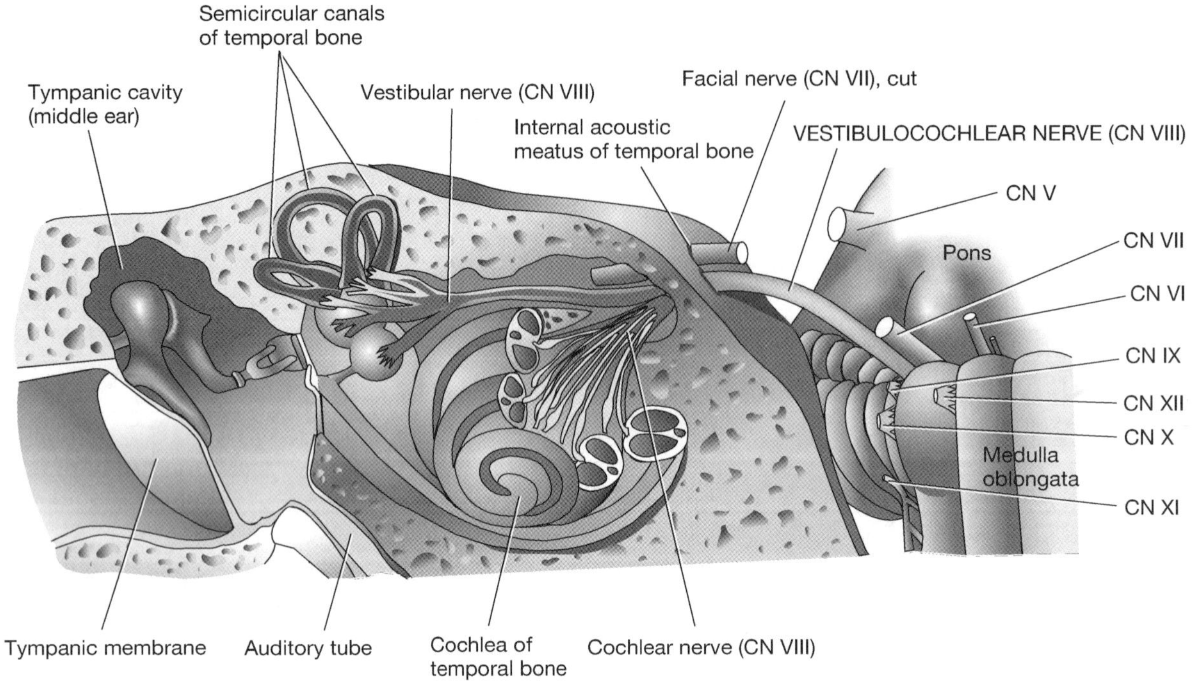

Figure 10-9

Vestibulocochlear Nerve Distribution

The vestibulocochlear nerve (CN VIII) is the only cranial nerve that does not emerge from the skull. It is distributed entirely to the internal ear (membranous labyrinth) which is found within the petrous part of the temporal bone.

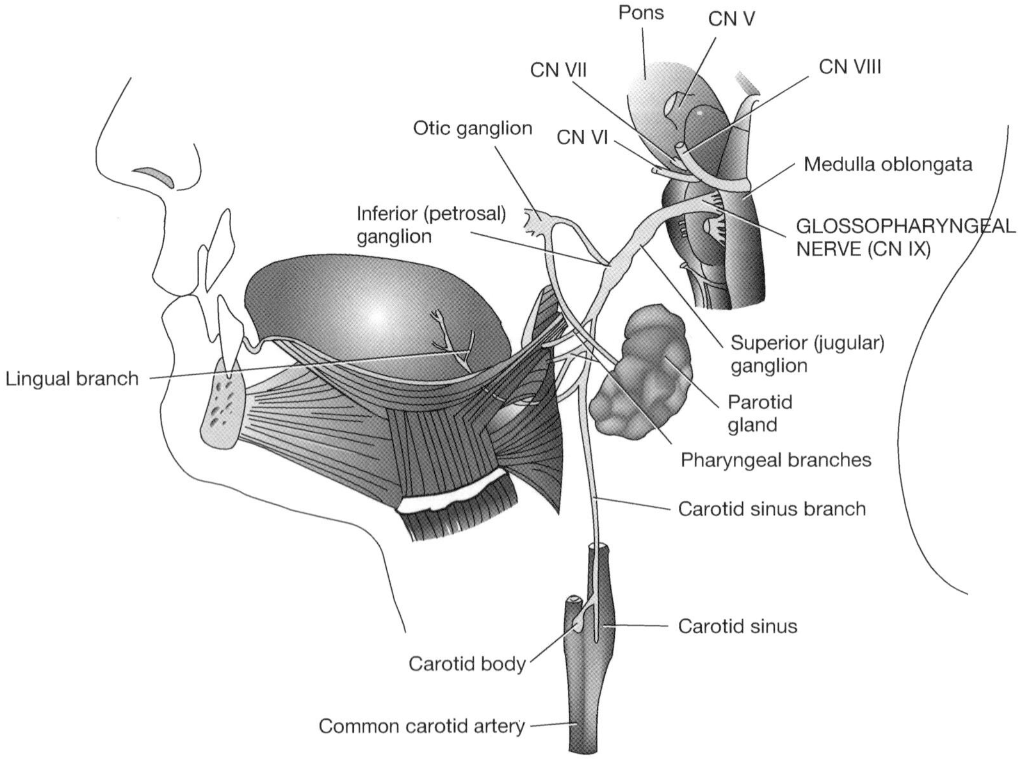

Figure 10-10

Distribution of Glossopharyngeal Nerve

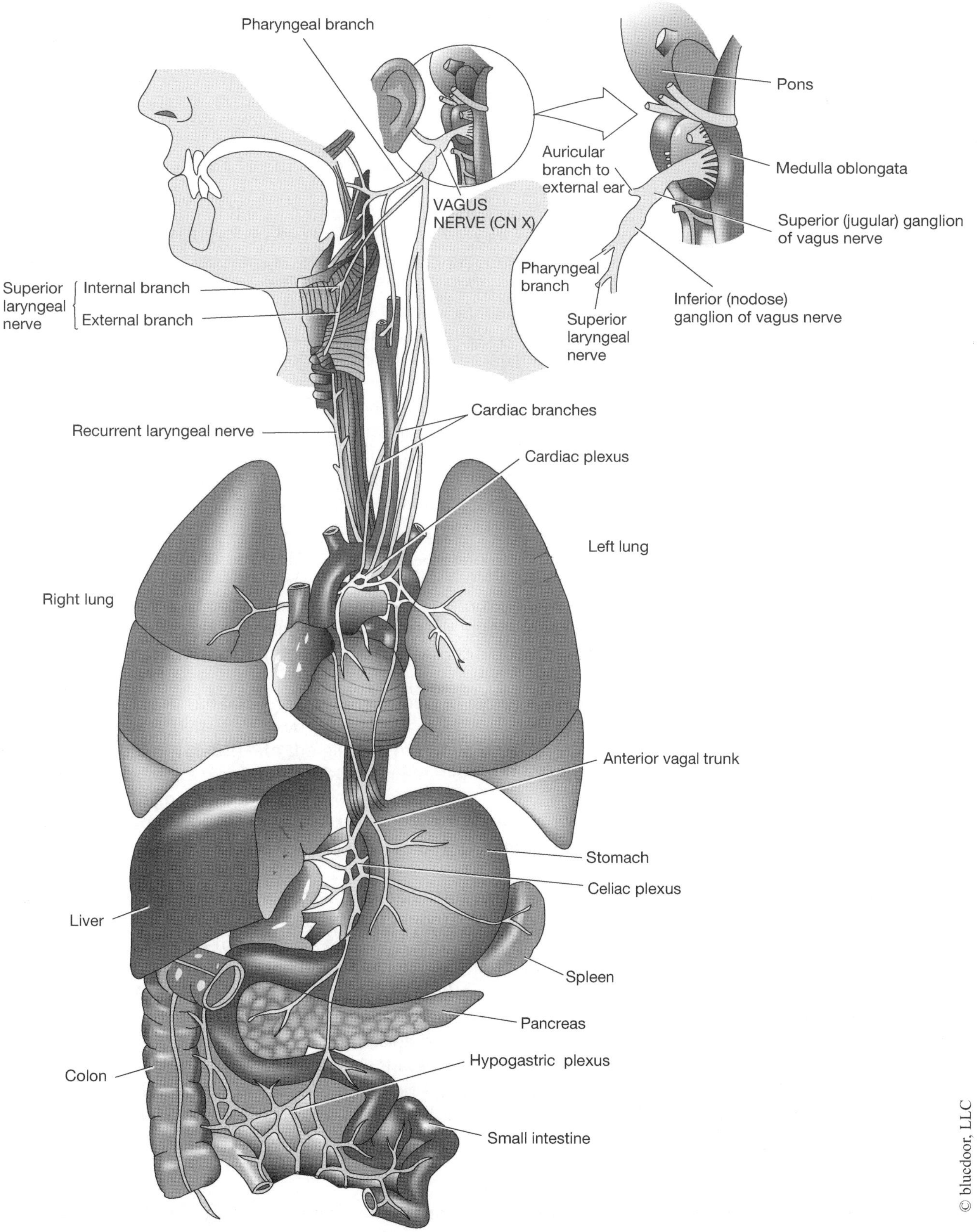

Figure 10-11

Distribution of the Vagus Nerve

The vagus nerve is widely distributed to the glandular epithelium and involuntary muscle within the thoracic and abdominal cavities.

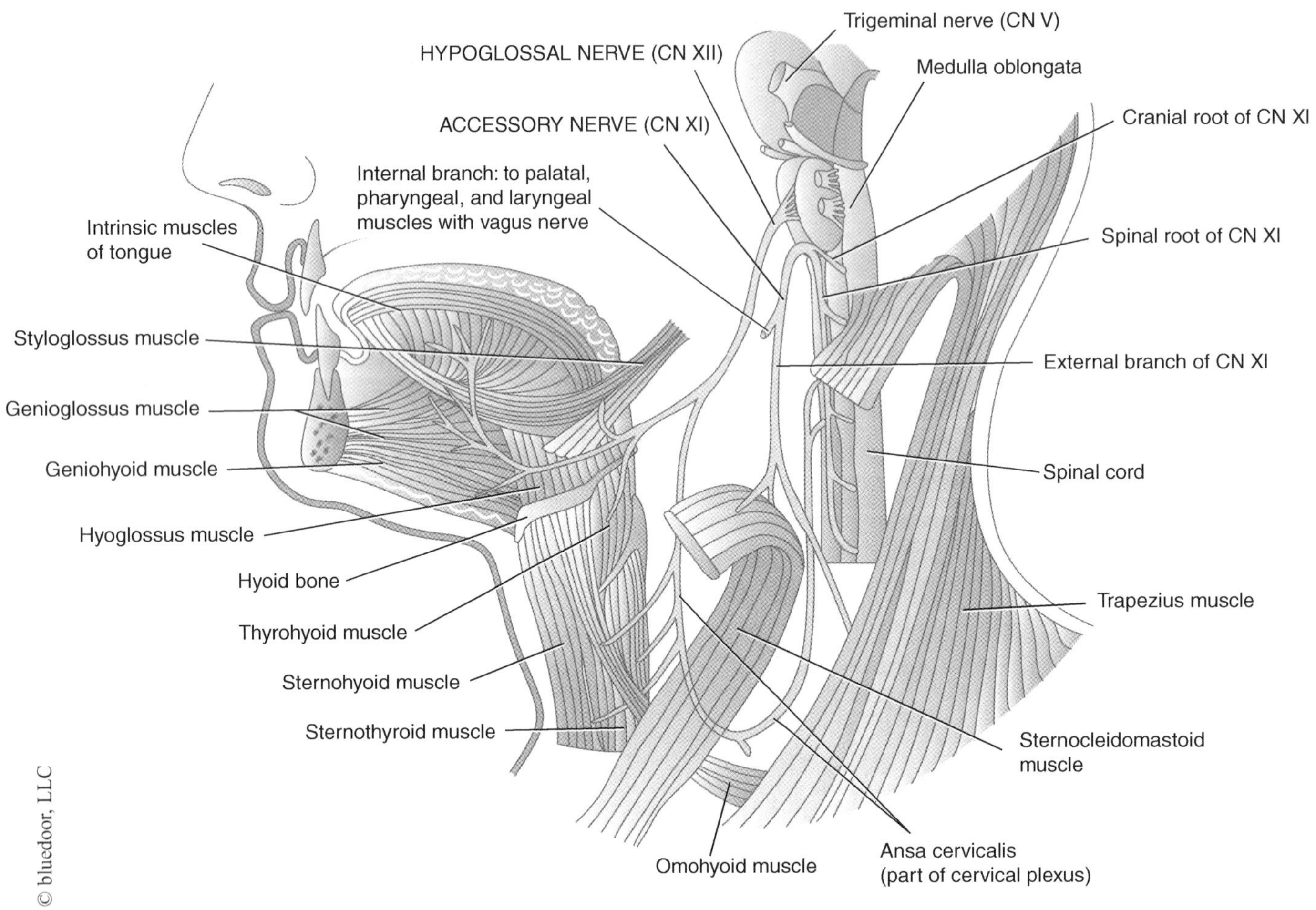

Figure 10-12
Distribution of Accessory and Hypoglossal Nerves

Objectives

4. For each cranial nerve, state its name, number, foramen of exit (from the skull), functional fiber type, and function.
5. Indicate which cranial nerves are sensory only, supply skeletal muscles, carry gustatory fibers, do not emerge from the skull, supply involuntary effectors, supply muscles that move the eyeball, originate from the superior (posterior) aspect of the brain, carry impulses interpreted as sound, emerge from the jugular foramen, carry impulses interpreted as sight, emerge from the superior orbital fissure, are distributed to the tongue, carry VA fibers that are distributed beyond the head.

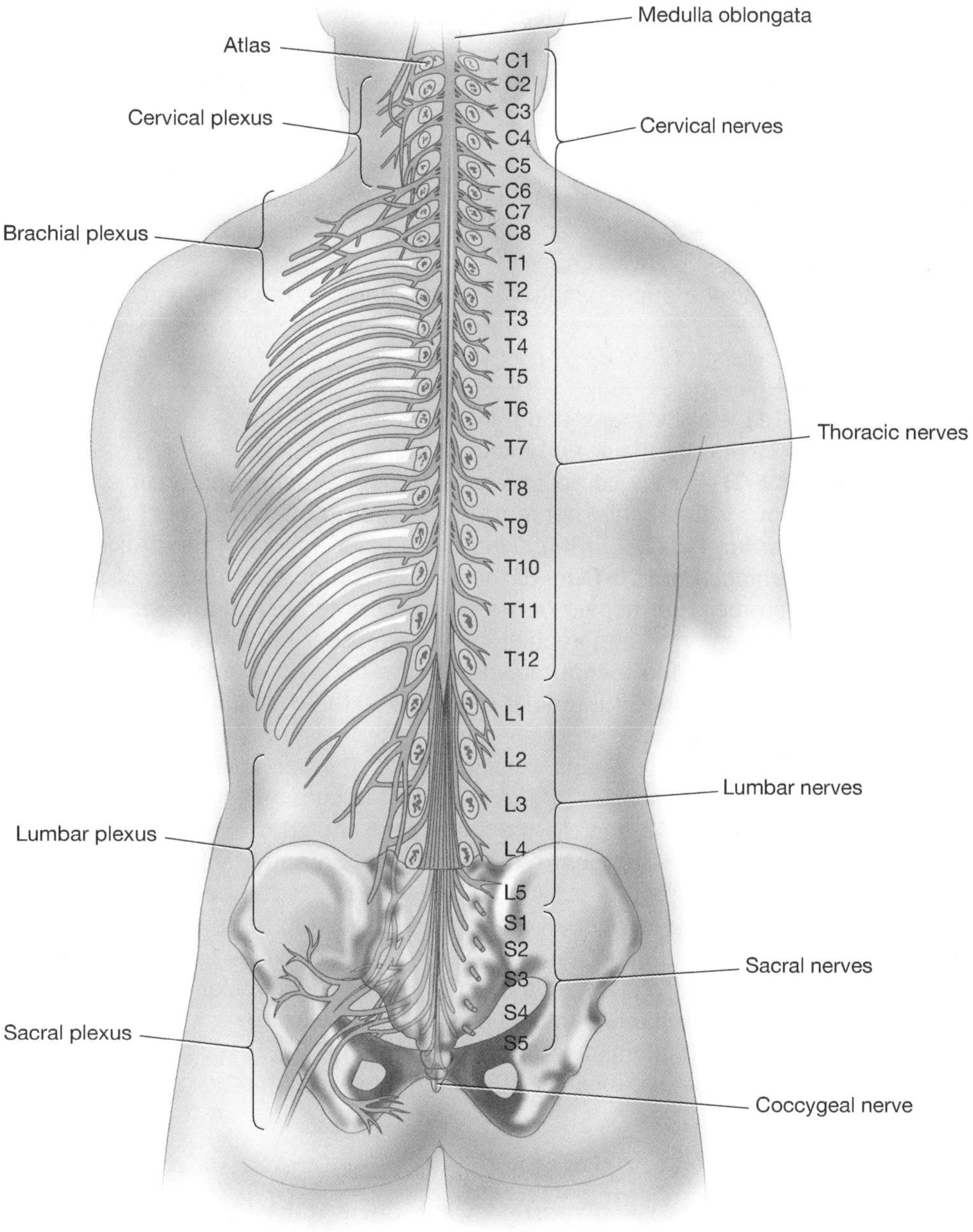

Figure 10-13

Posterior View of Spinal Cord and Spinal Nerves

Note that the spinal cord terminates at the level of vertebrae L1/L2. Spinal nerves continuing down the vertebral canal form the cauda equina.

Spinal Nerves

There are 31± pairs of **spinal nerves**: eight pairs originate from the cervical part of the spinal cord, 12 pairs from the thoracic part and five pairs from the lumbar portion. The number of sacral pairs is typically five but is reduced to four in those individuals that have only four sacral vertebral segments. One or two pairs of coccygeal spinal nerves is/are present (Figure 10-13). Each spinal nerve is formed by the mergence of a **posterior root** (carrying mostly sensory fibers into the spinal cord)

Table 10-5 Nerves of the Superior Limb

Named Nerve (Spinal Nerve Contribution)—Distribution
Supraclavicular Part of Brachial Plexus:
Dorsal scapular n. (C5-7)—to the levator scapulae, major rhomboideus, and minor rhomboideus muscles
Long thoracic n. (C5-7)—to the scalenus and serratus anterior muscles
Subclavian n. (C5-6)—to the subclavius muscle
Suprascapular n. (C5-6)—to the supraspinatus and infraspinatus muscles and to the shoulder joint
Infraclavicular Part of the Brachial Plexus:
Medial pectoral n. (C8-T1)—to the major and minor pectoral muscles
Lateral pectoral n. (C5-7)—to the major and minor pectoral muscles
Musculocutaneous n. (C5-7)—to the coracobrachialis, biceps brachii, and brachialis muscles; continues as the lateral cutaneous antebrachial nerve to the skin on the radial aspect of the antebrachium
Medial cutaneous brachial n. (T1-2)—to the skin on the ulnar aspect of the proximal brachium
Medial cutaneous antebrachial n. (C8-T1)—to the skin on the anterior aspect of the antebrachium (anterior branch) and skin on the ulnar aspect of the posterior antebrachium (posterior branch)
Median n. (C6-T1)—to the anterior antebrachial muscles (except the flexor carpi ulnaris m. and part of the deep digital flexor m.) and to the thenar muscles of the hand; it is cutaneously distributed to the palmar aspect of the manus (except the medial part) and to the dorsum of the distal half of digits 1-3 and the lateral aspect of digit 4
Ulnar n. (C7-T1)—to the flexor carpi ulnaris muscle, part of the deep digital flexor muscle, the hypothenar and many of the intermediate muscles of the manus; it is cutaneously distributed to the medial third of the manus including all of digit 5 and the medial aspect of digit 4
Radial n. (C5-8)—to the posterior muscles of the brachium and antebrachium (*i.e.,* the extensors of the elbow, carpal, and digital joints); it is cutaneously distributed to the central part of the posterior aspect of the antebrachium (posterior cutaneous antebrachial branch) and to the dorsum of the manus except for digit 5, the ulnar aspect of digit 4, and the distal halves of digits 1-4
Subscapular nn. (C5-7)—to the subscapularis muscle (upper subscapular n.) and to the teres major, teres minor and part of the subscapularis muscle (lower subscapular n.)
Thoracodorsal n. (C6-8)—to the latissimus dorsi muscle
Axillary n. (C5-6)—to the deltoideus muscle; it is cutaneously distributed over much of the deltoid region

and an **anterior root** (carrying mostly motor fibers out of the spinal cord) (*see Figure 9-12*). **Sensory ganglia** contain cell bodies of pseudounipolar neurons (no bipolar neurons in the spinal nerves) and are located on the posterior roots. After emerging from the vertebral canal through intervertebral foramina (except for the first cervical spinal nerves which course between the skull and the atlas), each spinal nerve is distributed as three branches: posterior branch, anterior branch, and ramus communicans (communicating branch). The **posterior** ("dorsal") **branch** consists of sensory and motor fibers that are distributed primarily to epaxial structures (*i.e.*, structures posterior to the vertebral column). It is typically smaller than the **anterior** ("ventral") **branch** which carries sensory and motor fibers that are distributed hypaxially. The diminutive **ramus communicans** (plural: rami communicantes) consists of pre- and postganglionic fibers of the autonomic nervous system. The **sympathetic trunk** is composed of two long nerve strands, one located on each side of the vertebral column, that extend from the base of the skull to the coccyx. The two nerve strands are interconnected and form cervical, thoracic, lumbar, and sacral ganglia. These receive preganglionic fibers from thoracic and upper lumbar anterior roots via the white rami communicantes and send

Table 10-6 Nerves of the Inferior Limb

Named Nerve (Spinal Nerve Contribution)—Distribution
Nerves derived from the Lumbar Plexus:
Iliohypogastric n. (T12-L1)—to the muscles of the abdominal wall and to a narrow band of skin superior to the buttock
Ilio-inguinal n. (L1)—to the skin of the scrotum, labia majora pudendi, and adjacent part of the thigh
Genitofemoral n. (L1-2)—divides into genital branch and femoral branch; the genital branch supplies the skin of scrotum, labia majora, and adjacent thigh and the femoral branch supplies the skin over part of the anterior, proximal aspect of thigh
Lateral cutaneous femoral n. (L2-3)—to skin over fibular aspect of the thigh
Obturator n. (L2-4)—distributed by anterior, posterior, and muscular branches to the skin over the medial aspect of the thigh, to the medial muscles of the thigh (except pectineus m.), and to the external obturator muscles
Accessory obturator n. (L2-4)—an inconstantly present nerve (present in over 30 percent of the population); it is distributed to the pectineus muscle and the coxal joint
Femoral n. (L2-4)—to pectineus, sartorius, and quadriceps femoris muscles; branches from these muscular rami supply coxal and genual joints; major cutaneous branch of femoral nerve is the saphenous nerve which supplies the skin over medial aspect of crus
Nerves derived from the Sacral Plexus:
Nerve of the internal obturator muscle (L5-S2)—to the internal obturator and superior gemellus muscles
Nerve of the piriformis muscle (S1-2)—to the piriformis muscle
Nerve of the quadratus femoris muscle (L3)—to the quadratus femoris and inferior gemellus muscles and the coxal joint
Superior gluteal n. (L4-S1)—to the tensor fasciae latae, gluteus medius, and gluteus minimus muscles and the coxal joint
Inferior gluteal n. (L5-S2)—to the gluteus maximus muscle
Posterior cutaneous femoral n. (S1-3)—to the skin of the buttock, external genitalia, and the posterior aspect of thigh and upper calf
Perforating cutaneous femoral n. (S1-4)—to a small area of skin over the inferior, medial aspect of the buttock; it may arise with the pudendal nerve or the gluteal branches of the posterior femoral cutaneous nerve
Pudendal n. (S2-4)—to the external anal sphincter and the skin of the labia/scrotum, and the penis/clitoris through its major branches: the inferior rectal nerves and the perineal nerves
Coccygeal n. (S3-5)—to the coccygeus and levator ani muscles
Sciatic n.—largest nerve in the body, divides into the tibial nerve and the common fibular nerve
Tibial n. (L4-S3)—to the semitendinous and semimembranous muscles, long head of the biceps femoris, and the adductor magnus muscles (these branches arise before the sciatic nerve divides); to the genual joint, muscles and skin of the calf; at the foot, it divides into medial and lateral plantar nerves which supply the sole of the foot and toes
Common fibular n. (L4-S2)—to the short head of the biceps femoris muscle (this branch arises before the sciatic nerve divides); to the genual and tibiofibular joints, and the tibialis anterior muscle

postganglionic fibers to anterior branches via the gray rami communicantes. Branches from the sympathetic trunk extend to adjacent viscera and blood vessels.

Anastomoses of the anterior branches of the first five cervical nerves (C1-C5) form the **cervical plexus** (Figure 10-14). This net-like structure innervates the skin of the scalp, neck, and superior aspects of the shoulder and chest, muscles of the neck, and the diaphragm.

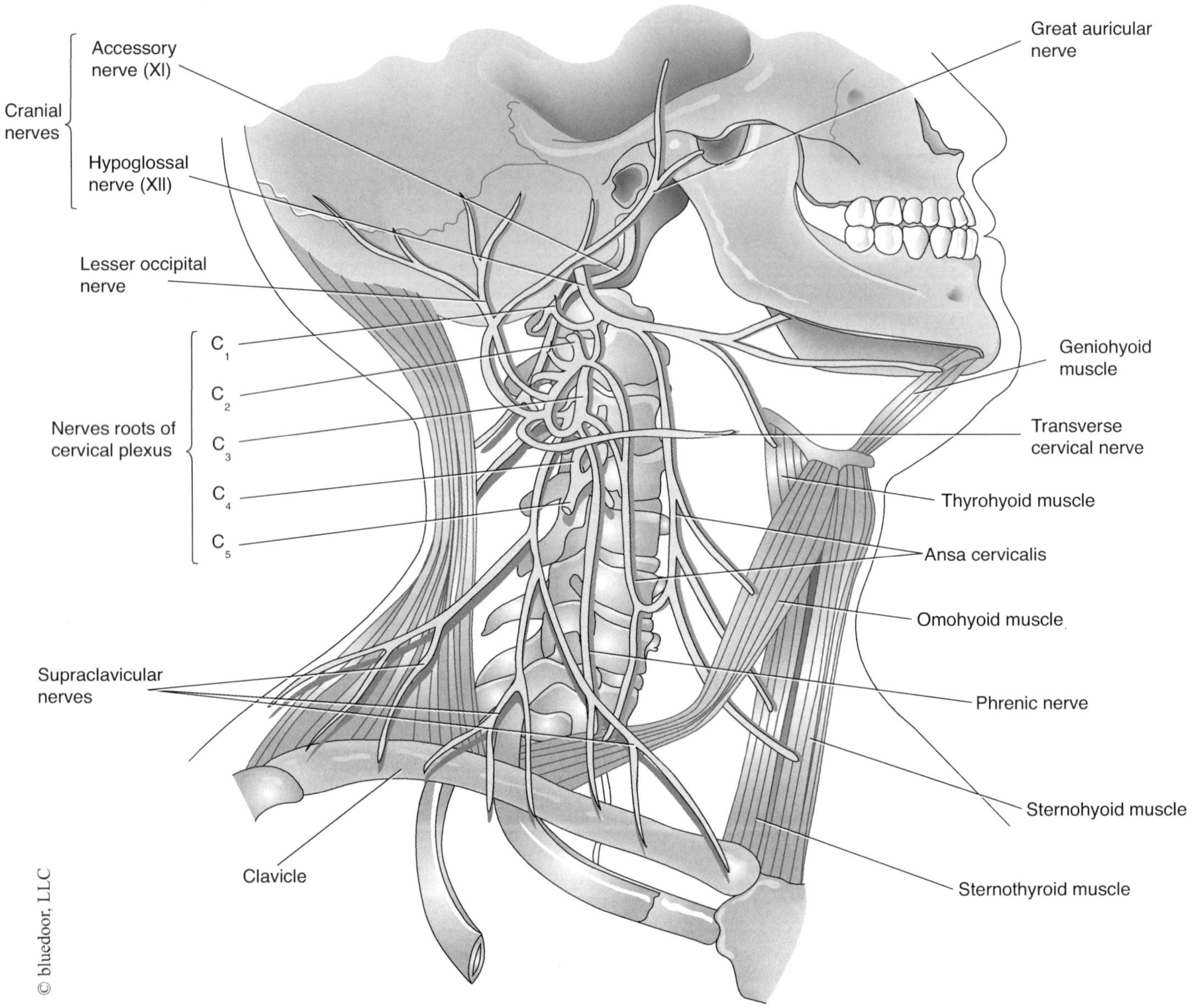

Figure 10-14
Cervical Plexus (and Accessory and Hypoglossal Nerves)

The nerves that supply each superior limb are branches of the ipsilateral **brachial plexus**. The latter consists of a complex exchange of fibers involving the anterior branches of the last four cervical and the first thoracic spinal nerves (C5, C6, C7, C8, T1). In some individuals, C4 and/or T2 also contribute to the plexus. The five principle roots (C5-T1) unite to form three named trunks after they emerge from the vertebral canal through their respective intervertebral foramina. The **upper (superior) trunk** is formed by a fusion of the anterior branches of C5 and C6. The **middle trunk** consists of the anterior branch of C7, and the **lower (inferior) trunk** is formed by a fusion of the anterior branches of C8 and T1. The trunks are located in the cervical region above the clavicle and each one divides into **anterior** and **posterior divisions**. The posterior divisions of all three unite to form a **posterior cord.** The anterior divisions of the upper and middle trunks form the **lateral cord**, and the anterior division of the lower trunk forms the **medial cord** (Figure 10-15).

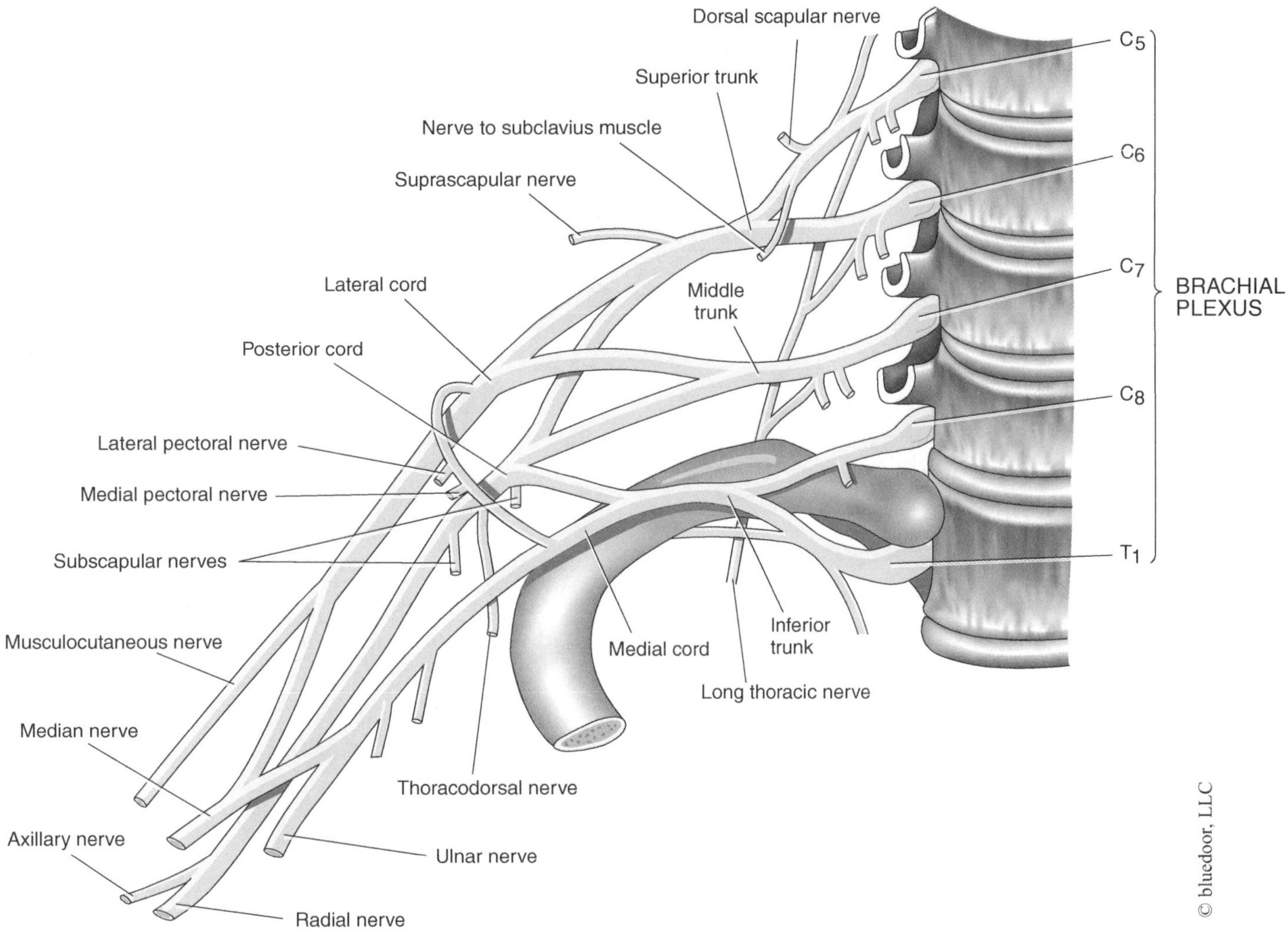

Figure 10-15

The Brachial Plexus

The brachial plexus is the network of neuronal fibers derived from the anterior branches of spinal nerves C5, C6, C7, C8, and T1. These anterior branches (called roots of the brachial plexus) unite to form the three trunks (superior, middle, inferior) as shown above. Each trunk divides into anterior and posterior divisions which, in turn form three cords (medial, lateral, posterior). The 15 named nerves that supply the superior limb are derived from this plexus (Table 10-5).

The 15 named derivatives of the brachial plexus that supply the superior limb are illustrated in Figure 10-15 and listed in Table 10-5. Most of these arise from the three terminal cords of the brachial plexus but some (suprascapular and long thoracic nerves) arise from more proximally located portions of the plexus. The brachial plexus branches of most significance are the musculocutaneous, median, ulnar, and radial nerves because they supply most of the muscles located in the free part of the limb. The **musculocutaneous nerve** supplies the coracobrachialis, biceps brachii, and brachialis muscles. It is also sensory to the skin on the anterior aspect of the forearm and most of the skin on the lateral half of the posterior forearm. The **median** and **ulnar nerves** supply the anterior antebrachial muscles and the muscles of the manus. They are also sensory to the skin of the manus (median nerve to the lateral two-thirds of the hand and ulnar nerve to the medial third). The **radial nerve** supplies the posterior muscles of the brachium and antebrachium (*i.e.*, the extensors

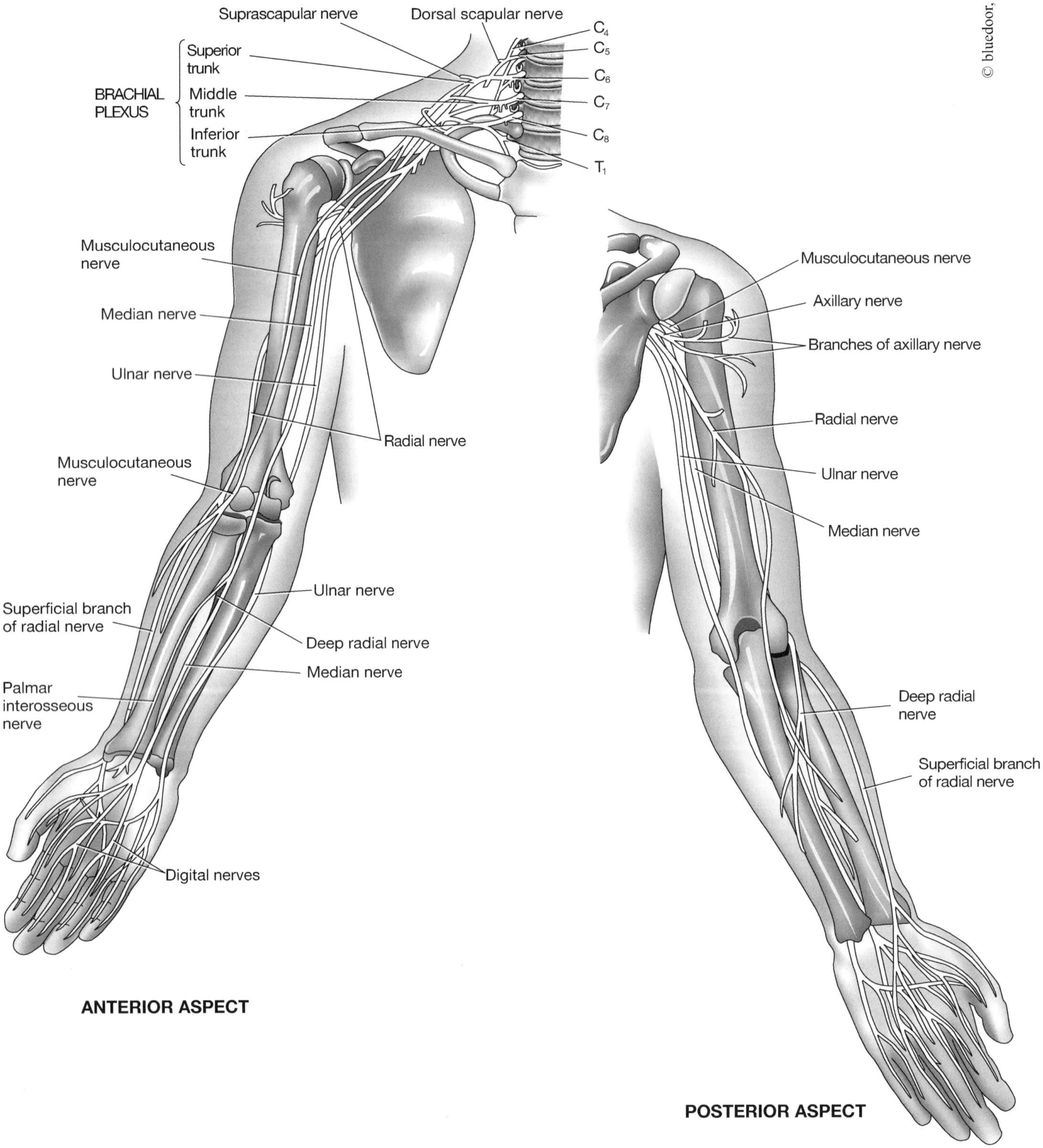

Figure 10-16

Major Named Nerves of the Superior Limb

of the elbow, carpal, and digital joints). It is cutaneously distributed to the posterior antebrachium (central part) and to the posterior manus (except for digit 5 and parts of digits 1-4).

The nerves that supply the inferior limbs are branches of the **lumbosacral plexus.** This consists of the lumbar plexus combined with the sacral plexus (Figure 10-17). The **lumbar plexus** is an exchange of fibers formed by the anterior branches of spinal nerves L1, L2, L3 and part of L4 (T12 usually contributes as well). The **sacral plexus** consists of fiber exchanges among the anterior branches of (part of L4) L5, S1, S2, S3, S4. The nerves of most significance that are derived from the lumbosacral plexus are the femoral, obturator, sciatic, tibial, and common fibular nerves (Table 10-6). They supply the muscles and most of the skin in the free part of the limb. The **femoral nerve** supplies the pectineus and sartorius muscles, and most significantly, the quadriceps femoris muscle. Its dysfunction results in inability to extend the knee joint. It is cutaneously distributed to the medial crus via a branch named the saphenous nerve. The **obturator nerve** supplies the medial muscles of the thigh and the external obturator muscle. It is sensory to skin on the medial aspect of the thigh. The **sciatic nerve** is the largest nerve in the body. It supplies the posterior thigh muscles and then divides into the **tibial nerve** (to the posterior muscles of the crus and most of the muscles of the pes) and the **common fibular nerve** (to the anterior muscles of the crus and a few muscles of the pes). The tibial and common fibular nerves also supply the skin of the foot and most of the skin on the anterior, lateral, and posterior aspects of the crus (Figures 10-17, 10-18).

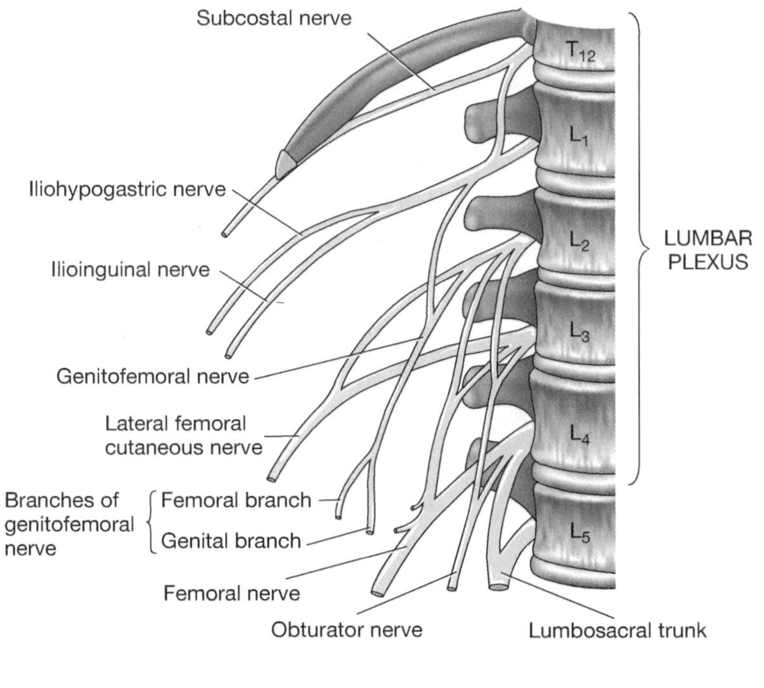

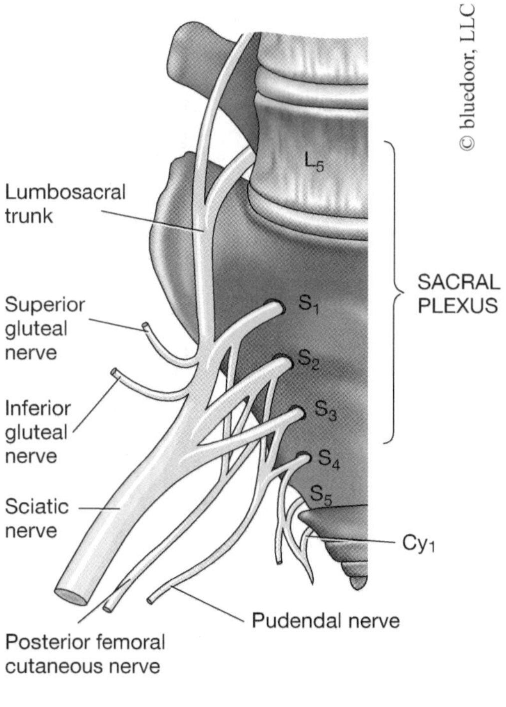

Figure 10-17

Lumbosacral Plexus

The lumbosacral plexus is the network of neuronal fibers derived from the anterior branches of the lumbar and sacral spinal nerves as well as the last thoracic and (sometimes) the first coccygeal spinal nerves. From it, the 17 named nerves that supply the inferior limb are derived (Table 10-6).

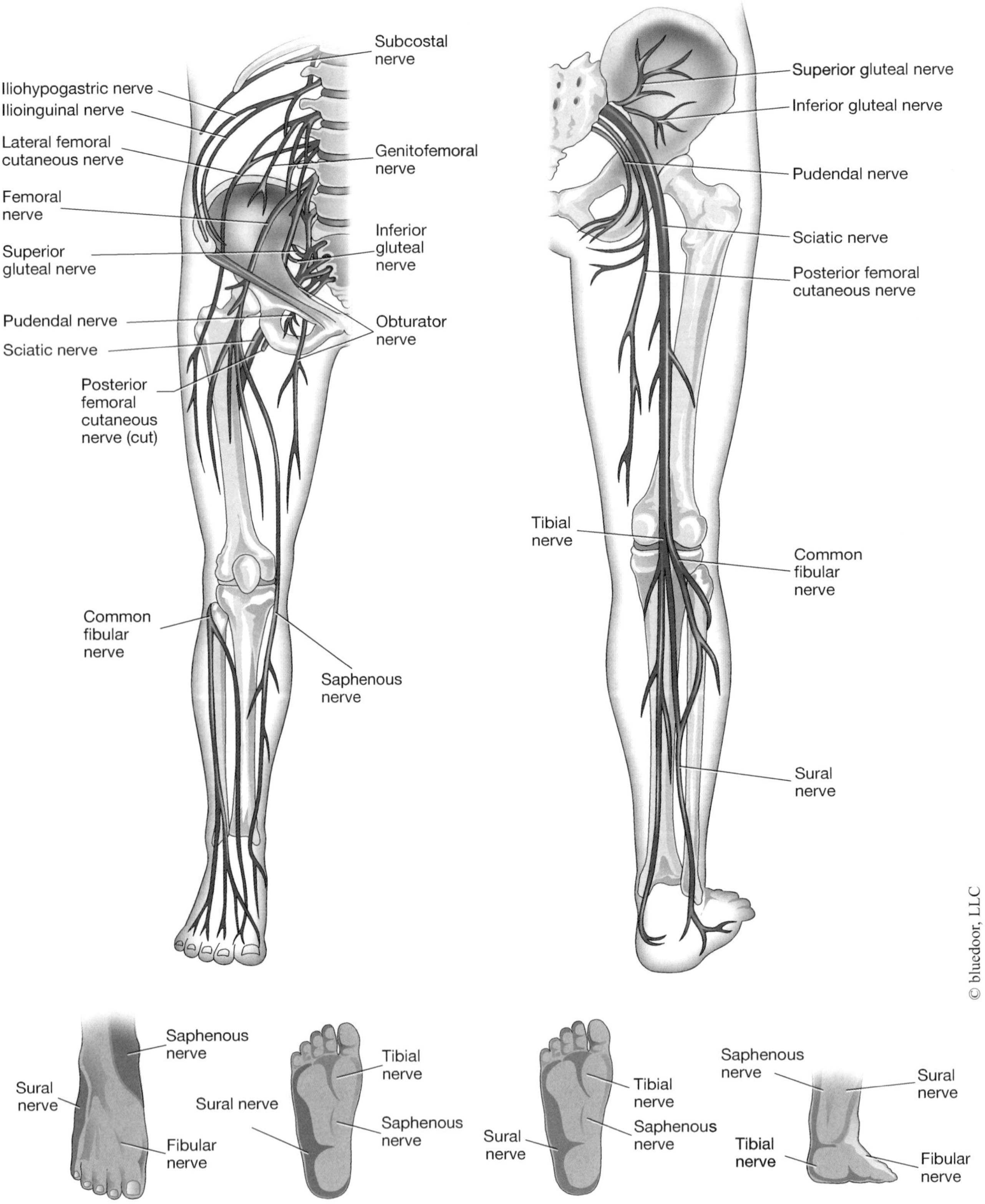

Figure 10-18

Major Nerves of the Inferior Limb and Their Cutaneous Distributions

Objectives

6. Sketch the origin of a spinal nerve from the spinal cord and label the rootlets, roots, branches, and sensory ganglion.
7. List the general kinds of information (sensory from, motor to) carried by: anterior branches of spinal nerves, posterior branches of spinal nerves, anterior roots of spinal nerves, posterior roots of spinal nerves.
8. Explain why severance of a nerve at a given location does not disrupt the functions of the nerve proximal to the site of injury.
9. Explain why nerve damage may be permanent.
10. Define the brachial plexus and state the sensory and motor functions of its four most significant derivatives: musculocutaneous, radial, median, and ulnar nerves.
11. Define lumbosacral plexus and state the sensory and motor functions of its largest derivatives: femoral, obturator, and sciatic nerves. Include the two named branches of the latter.

Ganglia

Ganglia are collections of neuron cell bodies in the peripheral nervous system. There are two types: sensory and autonomic. **Sensory ganglia** contain the cell bodies of pseudounipolar or bipolar neurons. They are found on the posterior roots of the spinal nerves and in association with most of the cranial nerves. Some of those associated with cranial nerves are individually named (Table 10-7). **Autonomic** (**motor**, **visceral**) **ganglia** are formed by groups of neuron cell bodies in the autonomic nervous system. In contrast to sensory ganglia where no synapses occur, autonomic ganglia serve as the synaptic sites between the pre- and postganglionic neurons in the two neuron motor chain of the ANS (*see Chapter 11*). Three general groups of autonomic ganglia occur: sympathetic trunk ganglia, named peripheral ganglia, and terminal ganglia. **Sympathetic trunk** ("**paravertebral**") **ganglia** occur segmentally along the sympathetic trunks and serve as synaptic sites for pre- and postganglionic sympathetic neurons. **Named peripheral** ("**prevertebral**") **ganglia** include those associated with cranial nerves 3, 7, 9, and 10, as well as named ganglia within the thoracic and abdominal cavities (Table 10-7). Some of these are strictly parasympathetic and some contain both sympathetic and parasympathetic neurons. **Terminal** (**intramural**) **ganglia** are autonomic ganglia located within the walls of the organs innervated. They are typically too small to be grossly observed. Autonomic ganglia will be covered in more detail in Chapter 11.

Objectives

12. Compare sensory and autonomic ganglia in regard to the presence of synapses, the functional types of neurons present, and the cranial nerves which have them.

Sensory Receptors

Before sensory information can be transported to the CNS, it must be transduced or converted to nervous impulses. In some cases, this transformation is accomplished by free nerve endings (*i.e.*,

Table 10-7 A Comparison of Sensory and Autonomic Ganglia

Criterion	***Sensory Ganglia***	***Autonomic Ganglia***
Synapses	None	Between pre-and post- ganglionic neurons
Composition	Cell bodies of pseudounipolar and some bipolar neurons (SA and VA)	Cell bodies of multipolar neurons (VE) whose axons are distributed to involuntary muscles and glands
Cranial nerve association	Trigeminal ganglion (CN 5) Geniculate ganglion (CN 7) Cochlear (spiral) ganglion (CN 8) Vestibular ganglion (CN 8) Inferior and superior ganglia of CN 9 Inferior and superior ganglia of CN 10	Ciliary ganglion (CN 3) Pterygopalatine ganglion (CN 7) Sublingual ganglion (CN 7) Submandibular ganglion (CN 7) Otic ganglion (CN 9) Terminal ganglia (CN 10)
Spinal nerve association	Posterior root of each one	Sympathetic trunk ganglia via rami communicantes of T1-L2, pelvic and terminal ganglia associated with sacral nerves
Named entities not associated with particular nerves	None	Numerous structures such as the celiac, superior, and inferior mesenteric ganglia

dendrites) which respond directly to touch or certain kinds of pain inducing stimuli. However, most sensory information is transduced by multicellular receptors that contain supporting cells as well as the specialized cells that generate the impulses. Most receptors are very stimulus specific. For example, the pressure receptors in the skin do not transmit impulses when subjected to heat, cold, or other stimuli (within physiological limits). Likewise the taste receptors on the tongue do not respond to heat, light, or pressure. Sensory inputs can be loosely grouped as special senses and general senses. The **special senses** include vision, audition, equilibrium, olfaction, and gustation. The **general senses** encompass touch, pressure, pain, heat, and cold.

There are many kinds of sensory receptors and they are often grouped into categories. One classification scheme divides them into five groups according to the general type of stimulus to which they respond (Table 10-8). These include photoreceptors, thermoreceptors, mechanoreceptors, chemoreceptors, and nociceptors. **Photoreceptors** are found only in the retina of the eye. When exposed to light, they form the impulses interpreted as vision. **Thermoreceptors** occur primarily in the skin and in the mucosal linings of some of the visceral body systems. Some of them respond to heat and other types respond to cold. **Mechanoreceptors** are a large and varied group of highly specialized receptors that transduce pressure, movement, stretching motions, and touch. **Chemoreceptors** respond to specific chemical stimuli and include cells within the taste buds in the oral cavity as well as the olfactory cells in the olfactory mucosa of the nasal cavity. **Nociceptors** respond to stimuli interpreted as pain. They are thought to actually be chemoreceptors in most cases because some of them have been shown to respond to the chemicals released when tissues are damaged.

Sensory receptors can also be grouped by the general location in the body where the impulses originate. These categories include exteroceptors, visceroceptors, and proprioceptors. **Exteroceptors** respond to stimuli from the external environment. They include all of the receptors in the skin as well

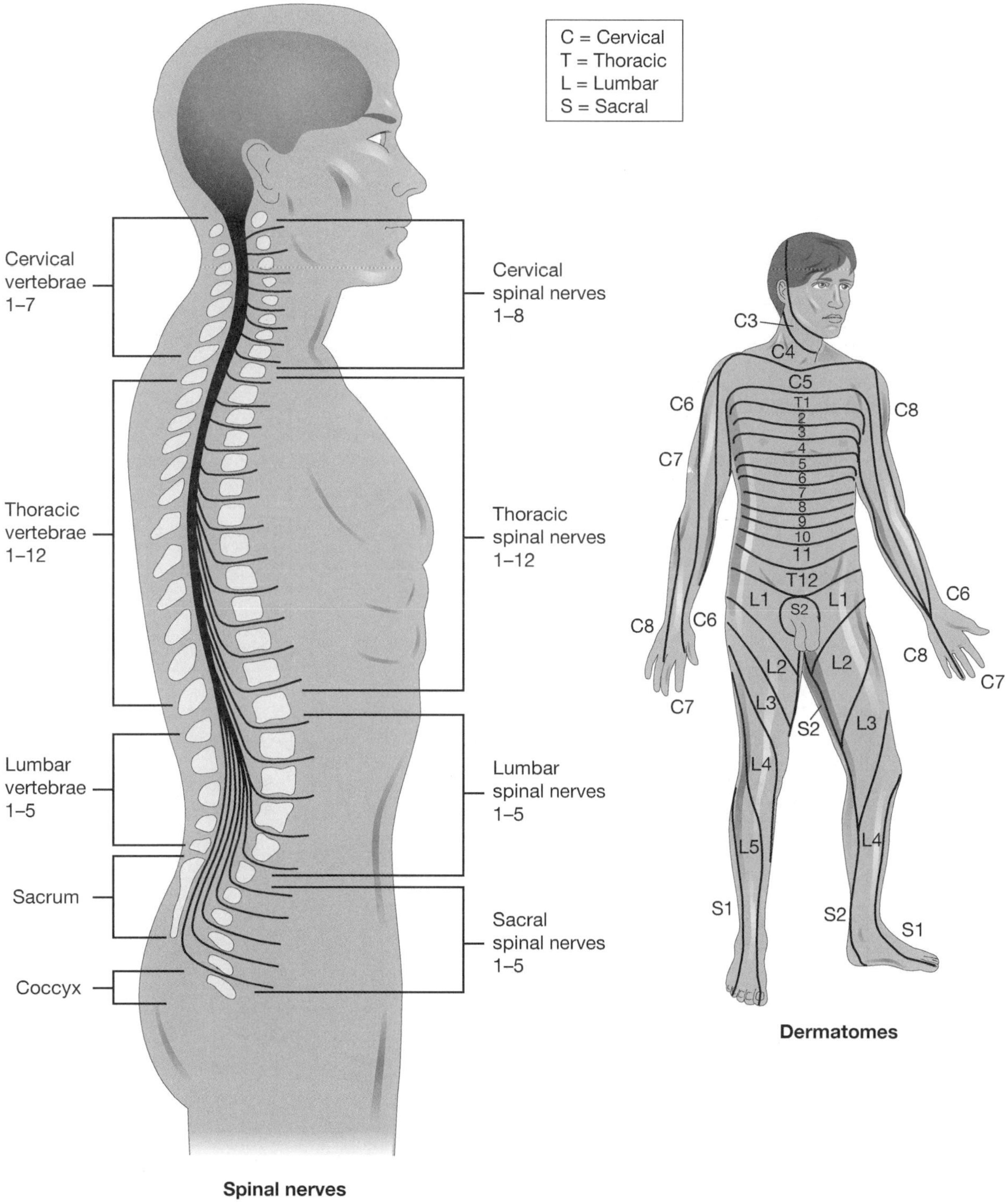

Figure 10-19

Dermatomes

Desensitization of skin can be used to help evaluate nerve injuries. Nerve damage close to the spinal cord results in the loss of sensation from one or more specific spinal nerve dermatomes. A dermatome is an area of skin supplied by a particular spinal nerve. Damage to a named nerve further peripherally (*i.e.*, distal to the brachial or lumbosacral plexus) results in loss of skin sensation over the areas supplied by that named nerve. Note: the artist did not render a coccygeal spinal nerve.

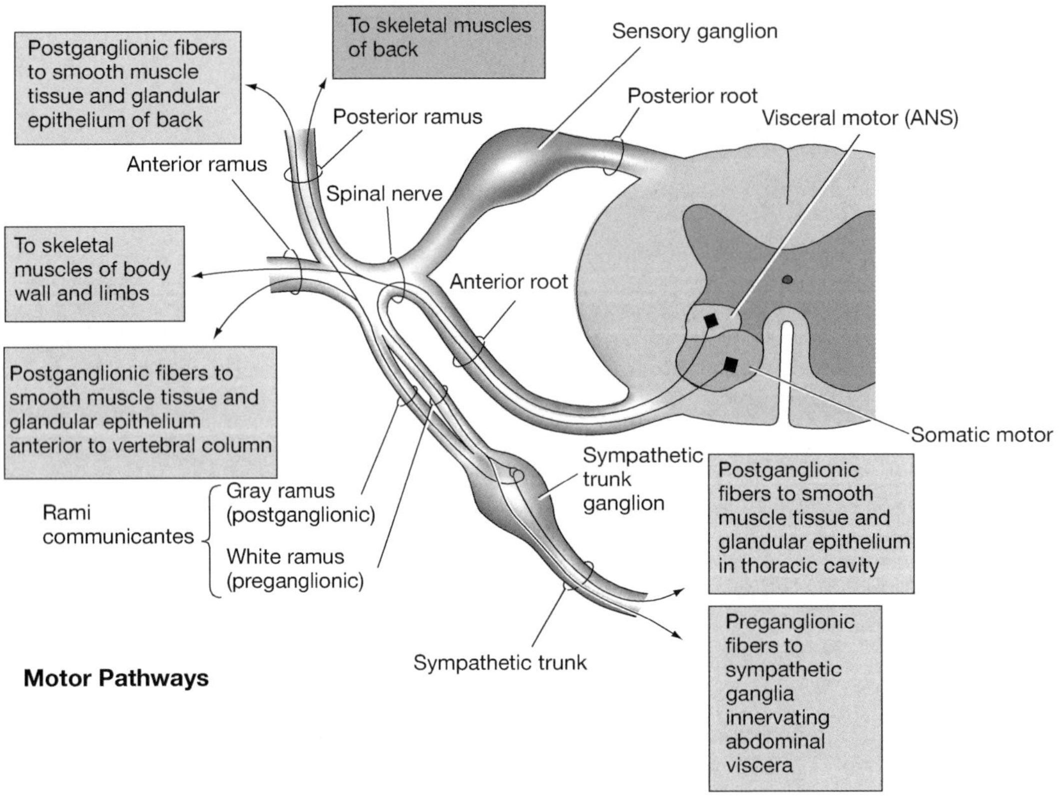

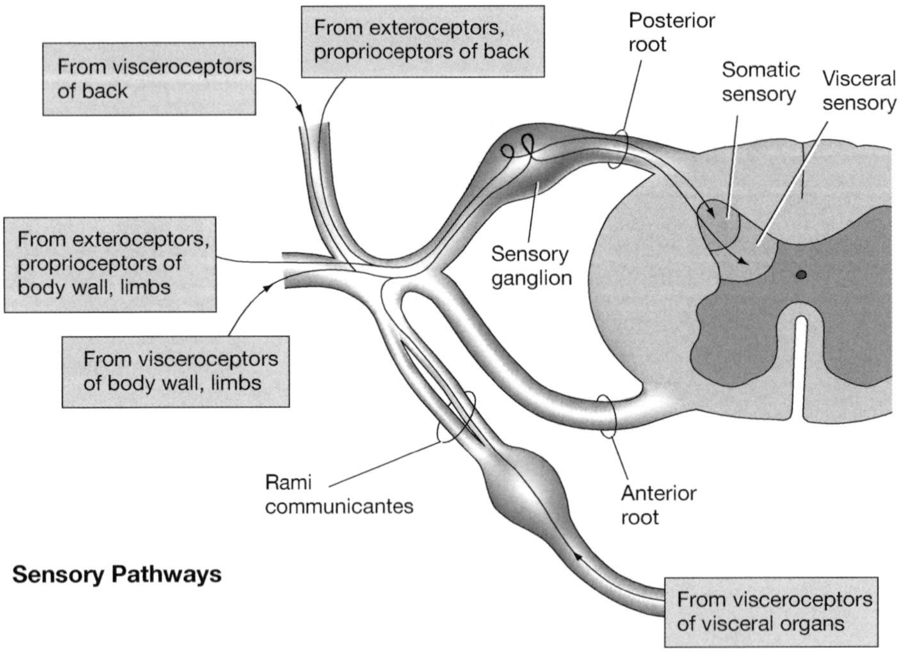

Figure 10-20

Motor and Sensory Pathways in a Spinal Nerve

Note that motor fibers form the anterior root of a spinal nerve and sensory fibers form the posterior root. The anterior and posterior branches of the spinal nerves contain both motor and sensory fibers.

Table 10-8 Classification of Sensory Receptors

Type of Energy Transduced:
Mechanoreceptors—pressure, vibration, touch, stretch, hair movement **Chemoreceptors**—activated by specific chemicals **Photoreceptors**—light **Thermoreceptors**—heat, cold **Nociceptors**—pain receptors, respond to chemicals released during tissue damage
Locus of Sensory Information:
Exteroceptors—external environment **Visceroceptors** (interoceptors)—visceral organs **Proprioceptors**—joints, tendons, muscle bellies and internal ear (vestibular apparatus)
Miscellaneous Categories of Receptors:
Cutaneous receptors—those located in the skin **Encapsulated receptors**—those which are surrounded by supporting cells **Free nerve endings**—unadorned neuronal dendrites **Kinesthetic receptors**—receptors that sense changes in angles of joints **Tonic receptors**—those which send impulses as long as a stimulus is received **Phasic receptors**—those which reduce their firing rate with time (when continuously stimulated)

as those associated with vision, hearing, taste, and smell. **Visceroceptors** (interoceptors) respond to stimuli in the deep body organs and carry sensations related to pain, hunger, thirst, fatigue, nausea, as well as fullness of the urinary bladder, stomach, *etc.* **Proprioceptors** initiate impulses related to body position, balance, and movement. They are located in the vestibular portion of the internal ear and within muscle bellies, tendons, and joint capsules.

There are several other terms used to describe some receptors or groups of receptors. **Cutaneous receptors** are those found in the skin (Figure 10-21). **Kinesthetic receptors** are the proprioceptors whose impulses are consciously perceived (impulses from some proprioceptors initiate reflexes at the subconscious level). **Encapsulated receptors** are those which are encased by supporting cells. **Free nerve endings** consist of unadorned neuronal dendrites.

Free nerve endings (terminatio neuralis libra) are the simplest receptors (Figure 10-21). They extend superficially into the deep layers of cells in the epidermis and respond to touch and pain. Some form plexuses around the base of hair follicles and respond to movement of the hair shaft. These are called **hair root endings** (terminatio folliculi pili). Another form of free nerve endings called **menisci tacti** (Merkel's cells) also convey touch sensations.

Several kinds of sensory receptors consist of dendritic endings that are encapsulated by connective tissue sheaths (Figure 10-21). **Pacinian corpuscles** are large encapsulated pressure receptors that are located in the skin and a few other places in the body (Table 10-9). They respond to vibrations as well as pressure. Other specialized pressure receptors called **baroreceptors** are found in vessel walls where they respond to changes in blood pressure. **Organs of Ruffini** (Ruffini corpuscles) are similar structurally but respond to heat. Both of these receptors are officially termed **lamellated corpuscles** (corpusculum lamellosum). Other encapsulated receptors include **corpusculi tactili** (Meissner's corpuscles) which are located in the skin and respond to light touch and **corpusculi bulboidea** (bulbs of Krause) which are integumentary receptors that respond to cold.

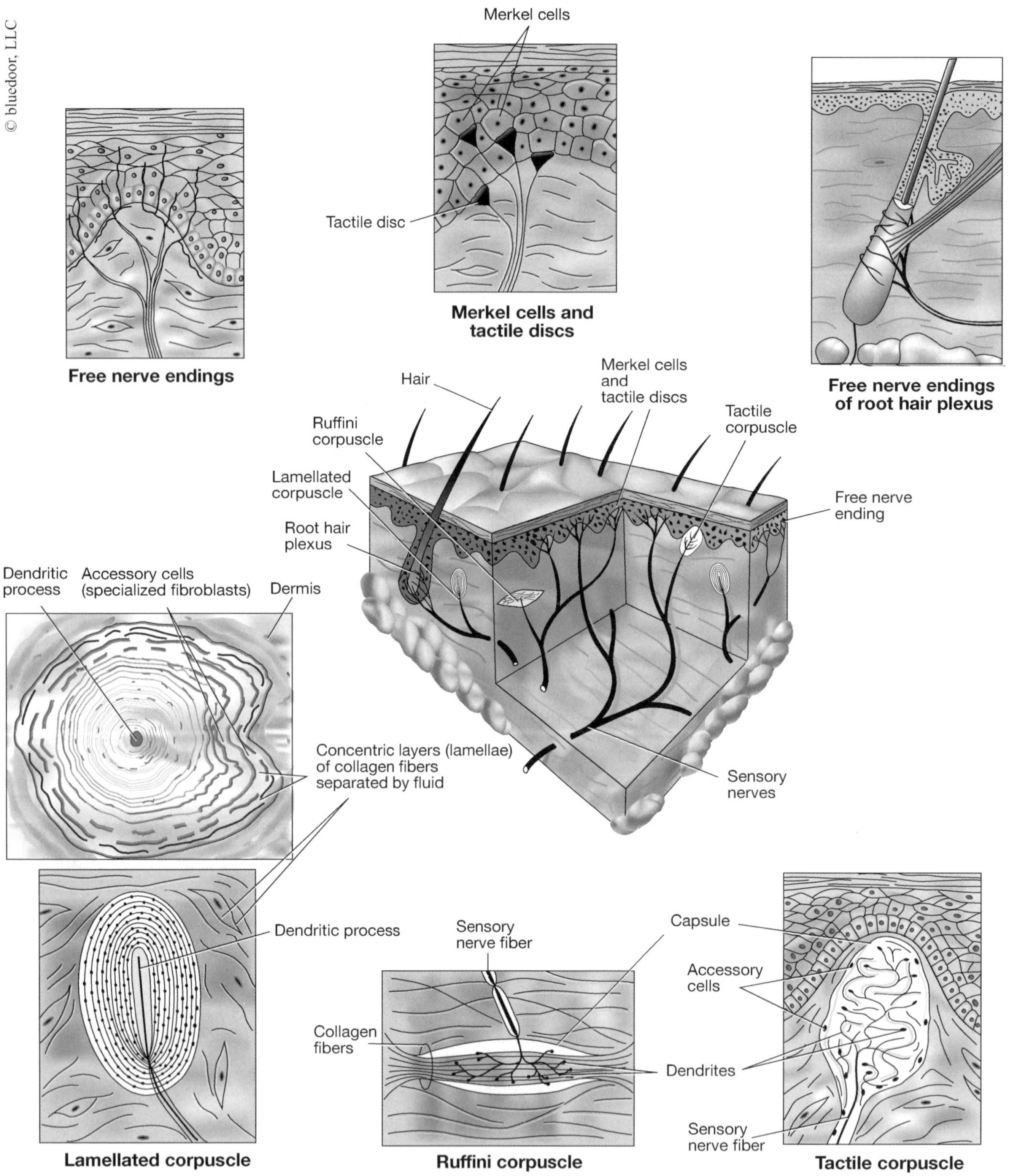

Figure 10-21

Sensory Receptors Found in the Skin

Note that eponymous nomenclature is often still used for various sensory receptors (Merkel cells, Pacinian corpuscles, Ruffini corpuscles).

Neuromuscular spindles (fusi neuromuscularis) are complex proprioceptors that are found in skeletal muscles. They contain some specialized skeletal muscle cells that contract to various degrees to adjust the length of the spindle to a certain tension, depending on the degree of contraction of the whole muscle belly. The spindles are stimulated by the stretching of the muscle belly and initiate a spinal reflex that results in subsequent contraction. Their role is to monitor the degree of belly contraction and to initiate contraction when the muscle belly is suddenly and unexpectedly stretched. **Neurotendinous spindles** (Golgi tendon organs) are also relatively complex structures associated with skeletal muscles. They are also activated by stretching, and under extreme circumstances initiate spinal reflexes that inhibit contraction of their parent skeletal muscle. Their role is a protective one designed to prevent a muscle from contracting with more force than it can structurally withstand.

The photoreceptors in the retina of the eye (rods and cones) are markedly specialized cells that respond to light. **Rods** (epitheliocyti bacillifer) are activated only by dim light and actually become nonfunctional in bright light. They are more numerous than cones (100 million *vs.* less than 10 million) and are concentrated in the peripheral aspects of the retina. Impulses generated by rods are interpreted as black and white vision (no color). The **cones** (epitheliocyti conifer) are more concentrated in the central region of the retina. They are responsible for color vision (including the "colors" of black and white). Their impulses result in sharper visual images than those produced by rods.

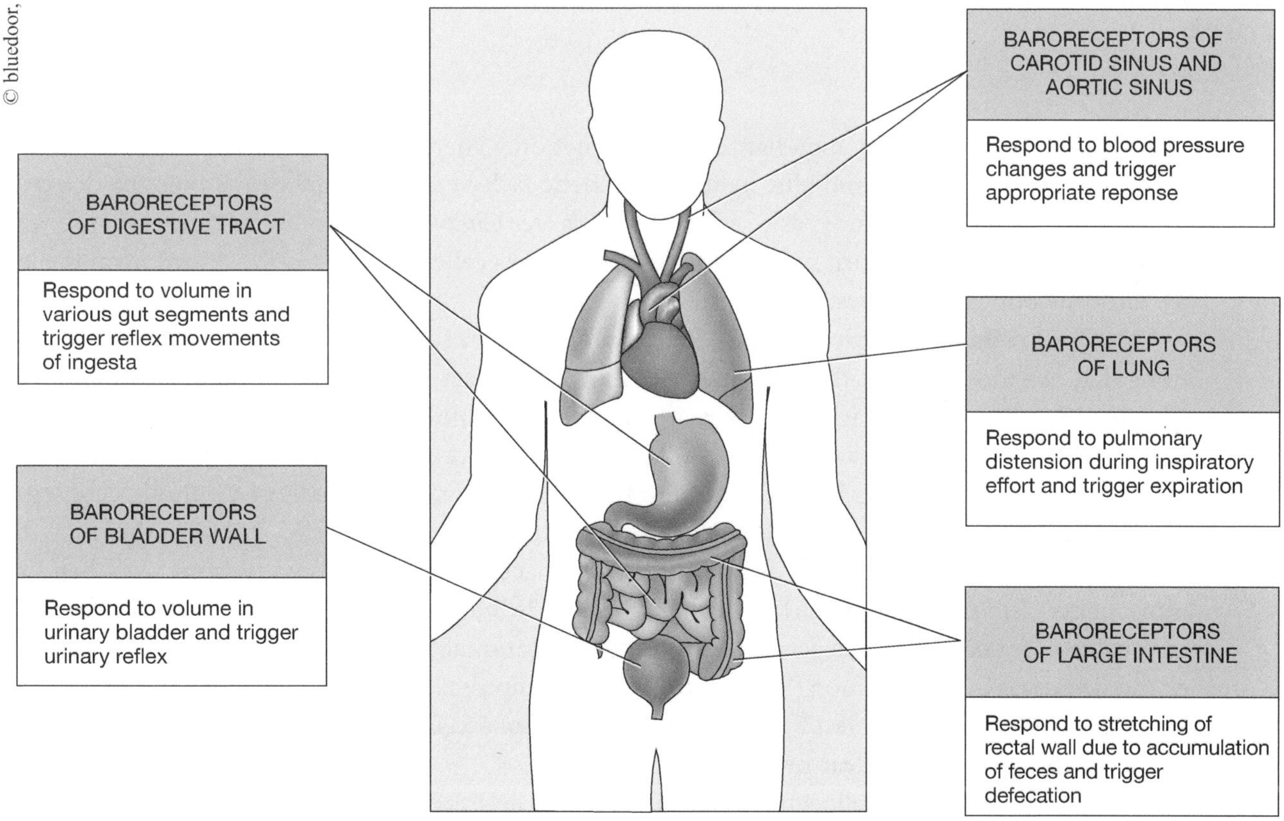

Figure 10-22

Baroreceptors and the Regulation of Involuntary Effectors

Baroreceptors generate sensory impulses important in the regulation of respiration, digestion, micturition, and defecation.

Table 10-9 Sensory Receptors

Common Name	*Location*	*Stimulus*
Free nerve endings	skin	pain, touch
Hair root endings	skin	movement of hair
Menisci tacti (Merkel's cells)	skin	touch
Corpuscula lamellosa (Pacinian corpuscles)	skin, synovial membrane, perimysium	pressure
Organs of Ruffini	skin	heat
Corpuscula tactili (Meissner's corpuscles)	skin	light touch
Corpuscula bulboidea (Bulbs of Krause)	skin	cold
Neuromuscular spindles	skeletal muscle bellies	stretch
Neurotendinous spindles (Golgi tendon organs)	tendons	stretch
Rods of retina	retina of eye	dim light
Cones of retina	retina of eye	bright light
Hair cells of spiral organ	internal ear	vibrations in fluid
Hair cells of crista ampullaris	internal ear	fluid movement (flow)
Hair cells of macula	internal ear	gravitational/inertial forces
Gustatory cells	taste buds of oral cavity	chemicals
Olfactory cells	olfactory mucosa of nasal cavity	chemicals
Baroreceptors	several organs	pressure

Cones must have reasonably high light levels to function. There are three types of cone cells (those that respond to red, green, and blue light), and genetic lack of one or more of the types or defective functioning results in certain types of color blindness (*see Chapter 12*). Rods and cones synapse with bipolar neurons which, in turn synapse with other neurons called ganglion cells. Axons from the latter form the optic nerve of each eye.

The **hair cells of the spiral organ** ("organ of Corti") in the internal ear have hair-like projections that are moved when the fluid in the internal ear is set in motion by sound vibrations (*see Chapter 13*). This initiates impulses that are conveyed to bipolar neurons whose cell bodies are in the cochlear ganglion of the cochlear nerve. When conveyed centrally and interpreted, these impulses result in audition. Similar **hair cells** are also found in the crista ampullaris of the fluid-filled semicircular ducts and the maculae of the utricle and saccule of the internal ear. Those in the ducts are stimulated by relative movement of the fluid which occurs during turning, twisting, and bending movements (angular acceleration) of the head/neck. The hair cells in the macula and saccule of the internal ear are embedded in a gel and respond to gravitational forces as well as straight-line increases and decreases in body motion (linear acceleration). Impulses generated by these hair cells are conveyed to bipolar cells in the vestibular ganglion. The bipolar cells in the cochlear and vestibular ganglia form the vestibulocochlear nerve.

Gustatory cells (epitheliocytus sensorius gustatorius) are located in the taste buds that are embedded in the fungiform and vallate papillae of the tongue as well as in the mucosa of the soft palate and oropharynx. A **taste bud** is a microscopic structure consisting of several gustatory cells surrounded by supporting cells (Figure 10-21). When the gustatory cells are stimulated by the appropriate chemicals, sensory neuron fibers at their bases generate impulses conveyed to the brain by the facial, glossopharyngeal, and to a lesser extent, the vagus nerves. There are four basic modal-

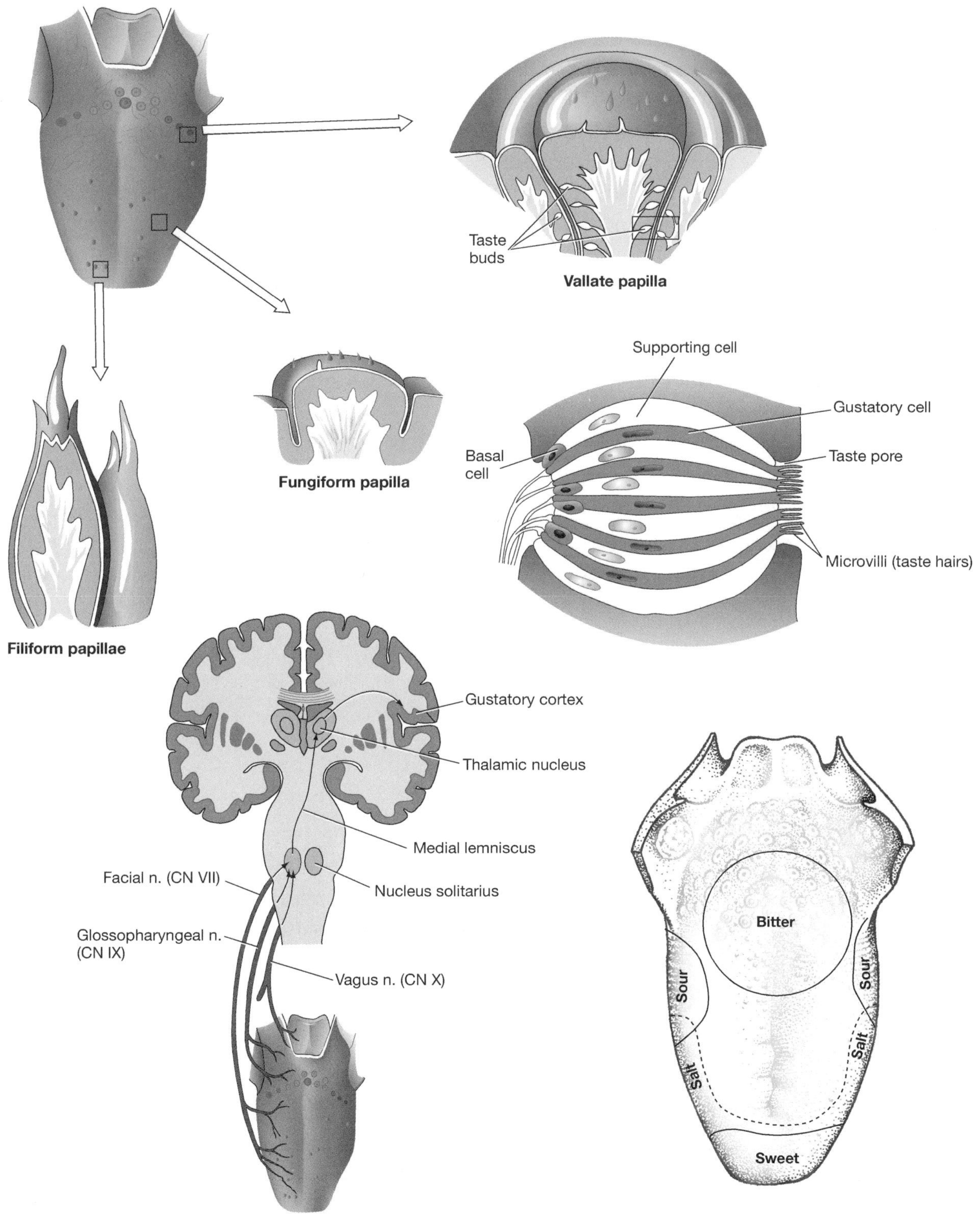

Figure 10-23

Gustatory Reception

The four modalities of taste are sweet, sour, salt, and bitter. Taste buds consist of groups of gustatory cells and supporting cells and can be found in the epithelium of vallate and fungiform papillae of the tongue. The distribution of taste buds that respond to the various taste modalities is shown.

ities of taste (salt, sour, sweet, and bitter) and their detection is concentrated over certain areas of the tongue surface (Figure 10-23). Pure salty sensations are produced by common table salt (NaCl) and are sensed over most of the tongue with the lateral and anterior aspects being most sensitive. Other salts such as potassium chloride (KCl) also taste salty but have a bitter flavor, as well. Sour taste is produced by hydrogen ions, thus all acids have a sour taste. Sour receptors are concentrated on the lateral aspects of the tongue. Sweet receptors are concentrated on the anterior aspect of the tongue. Most organic molecules have a "sweet" taste. Bitter sensations are evoked by quinine and a number of other unrelated compounds and have their receptors concentrated on the posterodorsal aspect of the tongue.

Olfactory cells (epitheliocytus neurosensorius olfactorius) are bipolar neurons whose dendritic endings are located in the olfactory mucosa of the nasal cavity. When stimulated by appropriate chemicals, these cells generate impulses which are conveyed to the brain in their axons. The latter comprise the olfactory nerves.

Objectives

13. Divide the senses into general and special categories.
14. Define sensory receptor and categorize receptors using the following criteria: type of energy transduced, locus of sensory input, cutaneous receptors, tonic vs. phasic receptors, encapsulated *vs.* "free" receptors.
15. Given a named sensory receptor, state its location and the type of stimulus to which it responds.
16. Describe the lingual locations of the four basic gustatory modalities: sweet, sour, salt, bitter.

Clinical Considerations

Individual cranial and spinal nerve dysfunctions can occur due to trauma, neoplasia, or localized infectious processes. Functional losses can be evaluated by monitoring various aspects of the normal sensory and motor roles of the nerves. Some of the methods used to evaluate the cranial nerves are summarized in Table 10-10. Dysfunction of an individual spinal nerve may be overlooked unless it results in desensitization of a noticeable area of skin or results in significant weakening or total loss of specific skeletal muscle contraction. The specific area of skin surface whose sensory neurons are carried by a particular spinal nerve (C2, C3, C4, *etc.*) is called a **dermatome**. Dermatome maps (*see Figure 10-19*) are helpful in evaluating nerve injuries.

The cranial nerves have considerable clinical significance. **Facial nerve paralysis** produces ipsilateral immobility of the facial musculature on the affected side resulting in facial distortion, inability to purse the lips or close the ipsilateral eye, and **xerophthalmia** (dry eye). If the cause of the paralysis cannot be traced to traumatic incident, the condition is classified as **Bell's palsy**. **Trigeminal neuralgia** is a condition characterized by severe pain when a sensory branch of the fifth cranial nerve is stimulated. The cause remains unknown. Various branches of the terminal nerve can be blocked with anesthetic to temporarily desensitize specific areas of the head. Dentists anesthetize an inferior alveolar nerve to desensitize the ipsilateral inferior teeth. The terminal branch of this nerve (mental nerve) emerges from the mental foramen of the mandible and supplies the lower lip. Thus, blockage of the inferior alveolar nerve also desensitizes the lower lip. The latter can also

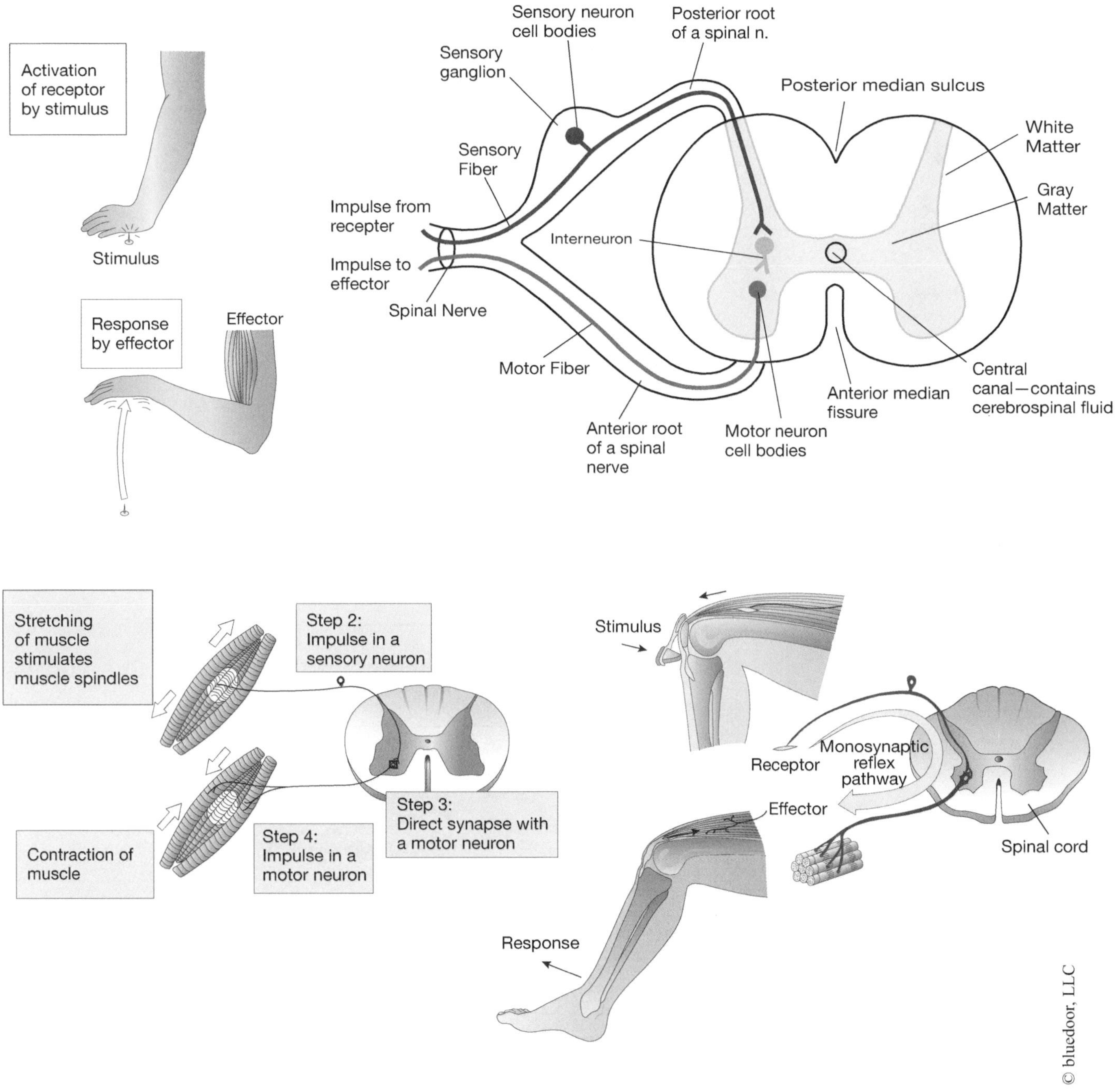

Figure 10-24

Spinal Reflexes

The basic components of a reflex arc are a sensory pathway (sensory receptor and sensory neuron), a motor pathway (motor neuron), and an effector (muscle tissue or glandular epithelium). Most spinal reflexes involve at least three neurons (the second one, called an interneuron, is located entirely within the brain or spinal cord). These reflexes, with two synapses between the three neurons, are called disynaptic reflexes. The patellar (knee jerk) reflex has only two neurons involved and is an example of a monosynaptic reflex. Note that a disynaptic reflex typically has four synapses and a monosynaptic reflex has three because the names (di- and mono-) do not include the synapse between the sensory receptor and the sensory neuron nor the one between the motor neuron and effector.

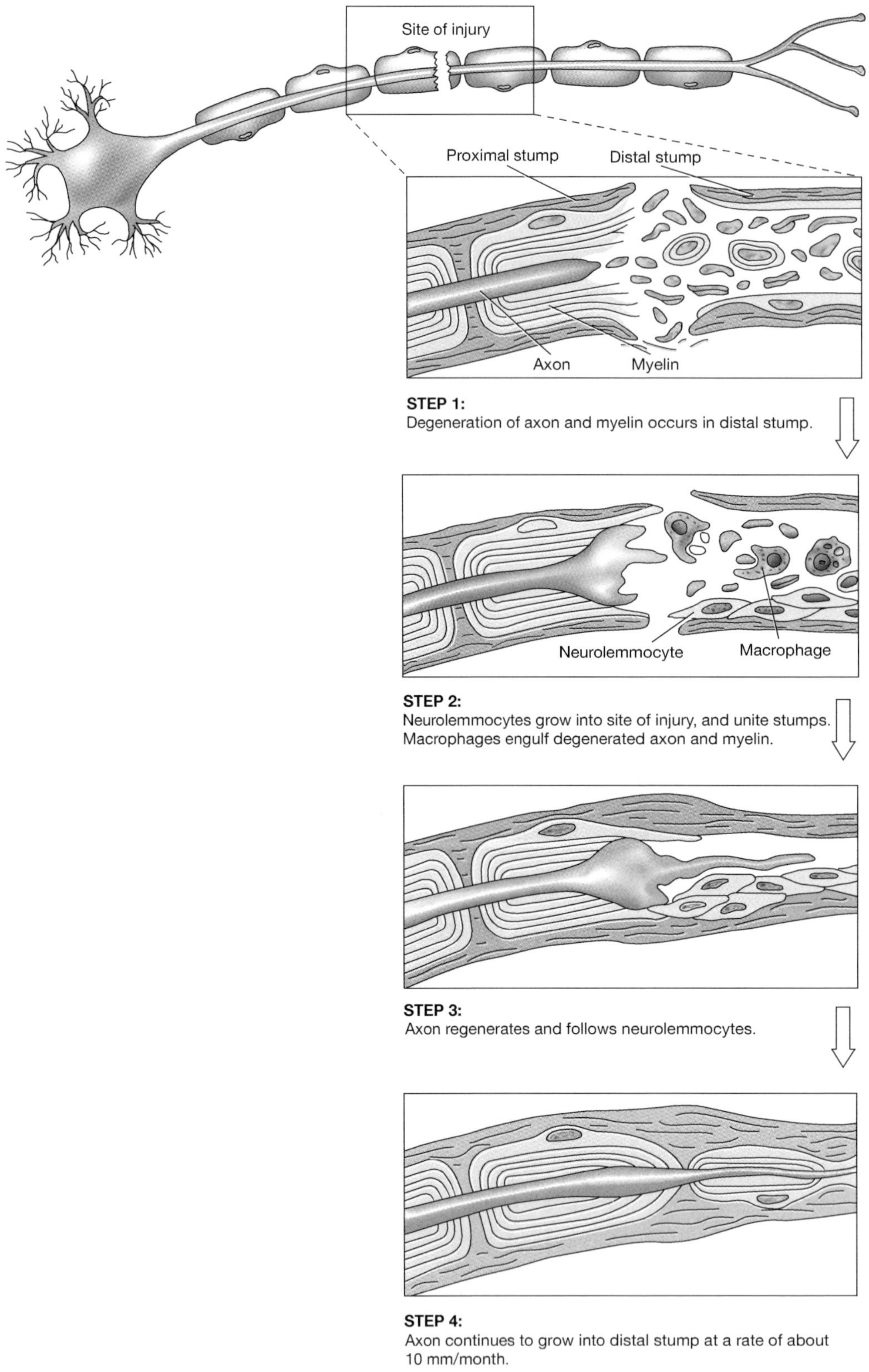

Figure 10-25

Neuronal Regeneration

When a nerve is disrupted, the neurons do not necessarily die. Under ideal conditions they can regenerate their severed processes. Regrowth of an axon is very slow, however, and can be inhibited by ingrowth of scar tissue.

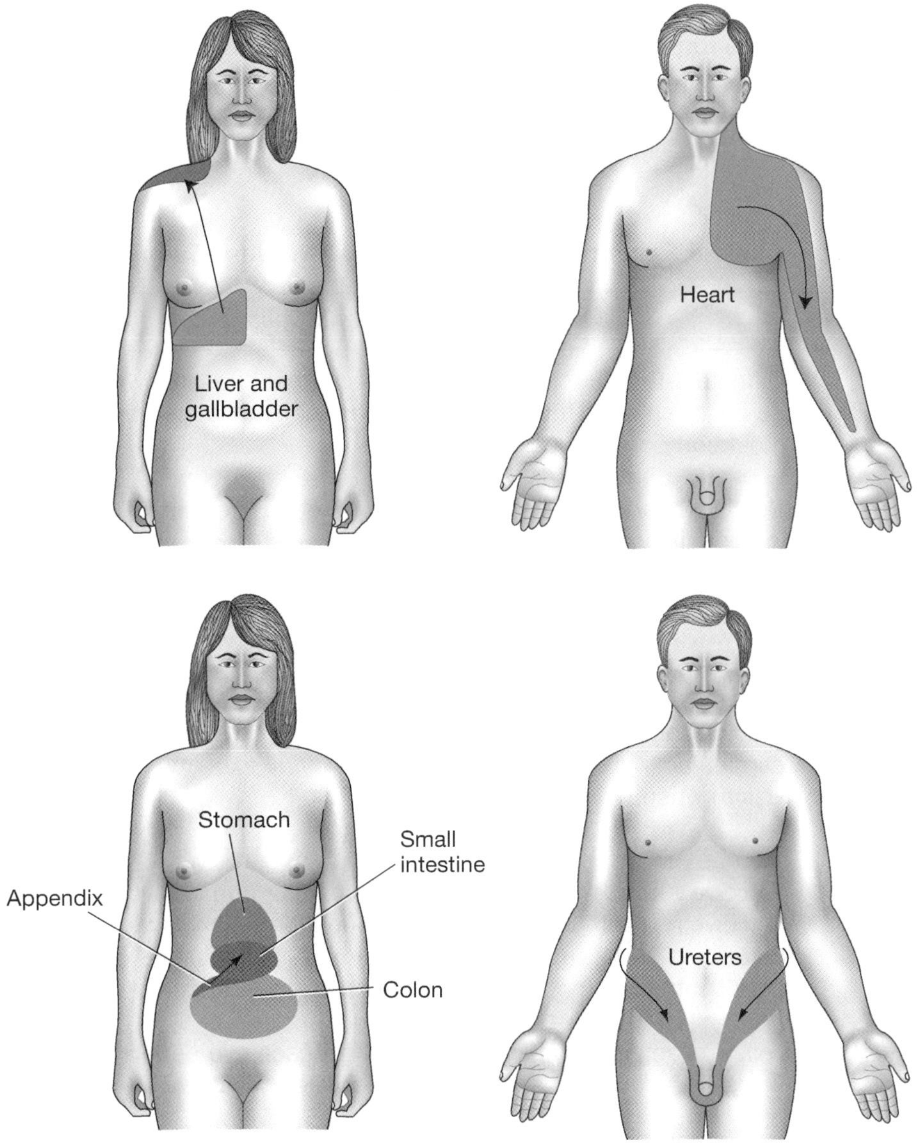

Figure 10-26

Referred Pain

Referred pain involves painful sensations arising in areas that are perceived as originating in other regions. Phantom pain is pain "perceived" to be in a body part that has been removed (*i.e.,* amputated foot).

be desensitized by injection of anesthetic at the mental foramina. The upper lip is supplied by the terminal portion of the maxillary nerve which emerges from the infraorbital foramen. Blockage of this nerve can be effected by anesthetic deposition at the infraorbital foramen of the maxilla.

The brachial plexus can be affected by trauma or disease in the cervical or axillary regions. These injuries are quite serious because they result in loss of function of various nerves that supply the superior limb. Injury to the upper part of the brachial plexus usually results from marked separation of the neck and shoulder (*i.e.*, motion in which the shoulder is forced downward while the neck is bent laterally toward the contralateral side). These injuries most commonly involve damage to spinal nerves C5 and C6. Lower brachial plexus injuries may occur when the limb is pulled forcefully superiorly (as when improperly disciplining a child by jerking a superior limb upward). These two types of injuries may avulse the roots of the inferior components of the brachial plexus from the spinal cord (C8 and T1).

Table 10-10 Clinical Examination of the Cranial Nerves *(See Figure 10-27)*

Nerve	*Procedure and Commentary*
Olfactory n.	Differentiate different odors using each nasal passageway separately. Loss of sense of smell is termed *anosmia* and may be caused by fractures of the ethmoid bone or neoplasia.
Optic n.	Use eye chart to test visual acuity with each eye separately and together. Total loss of vision is termed blindness and is usually related to retinal or optic nerve dysfunction. Partial losses may be related to other eye problems.
Oculomotor n.	Follow examiner's finger movement with each eye separately. Dysfunction prevents upward, downward, or medial (inward) movement of visual axis.
Trochlear n.	Follow examiner's finger movement with each eye separately. Dysfunction causes medial and downward deflection of visual axis and causes *diplopia* (double vision) when looking straight downward.
Trigeminal nerve:	
Ophthalmic n.	Perceive a touch to upper forehead, nose, or cornea.
Maxillary n.	Perceive a touch to superior gums, superior lip, or palate.
Mandibular n.	Perceive a touch to inferior gums, inferior lip, or tongue. Clench teeth and palpate contracted temporalis and masseter muscles.
Abducens n.	Follow examiner's finger movement with each eye separately. Dysfunction prevents abduction of visual axis and causes *convergent strabismus* ("cross-eyed").
Facial n.	Whistle, elevate eyebrows, and puff out cheeks; identify the taste of sugar, salt, vinegar, and quinine placed on the tip of the tongue. Facial paralysis results in flaccid paralysis of the facial muscles on the affected side.
Vestibulocochlear n.	Walk a straight line; test each ear separately with a tuning fork. Vestibular nerve dysfunction causes loss of equilibrium and cochlear nerve dysfunction results in hearing loss.
Glossopharyngeal n.	Note salivation and swallowing process. *Dysphagia* (difficult swallowing) and *xerostomia* (dry mouth) may occur with nerve dysfunction.
Vagus n.	Note swallowing and vocalization. Dysphagia and partial or complete loss of voice may occur with nerve dysfunction.
Accessory n.	Shrug shoulders and rotate head against resistance. Dysfunction results in flaccid paralysis and atrophy of the ipsilateral trapezius and sternocleidomastoideus muscles.
Hypoglossal n.	Protrude tongue against resistance. Dysfunction results in flaccid paralysis of the tongue on the affected side.

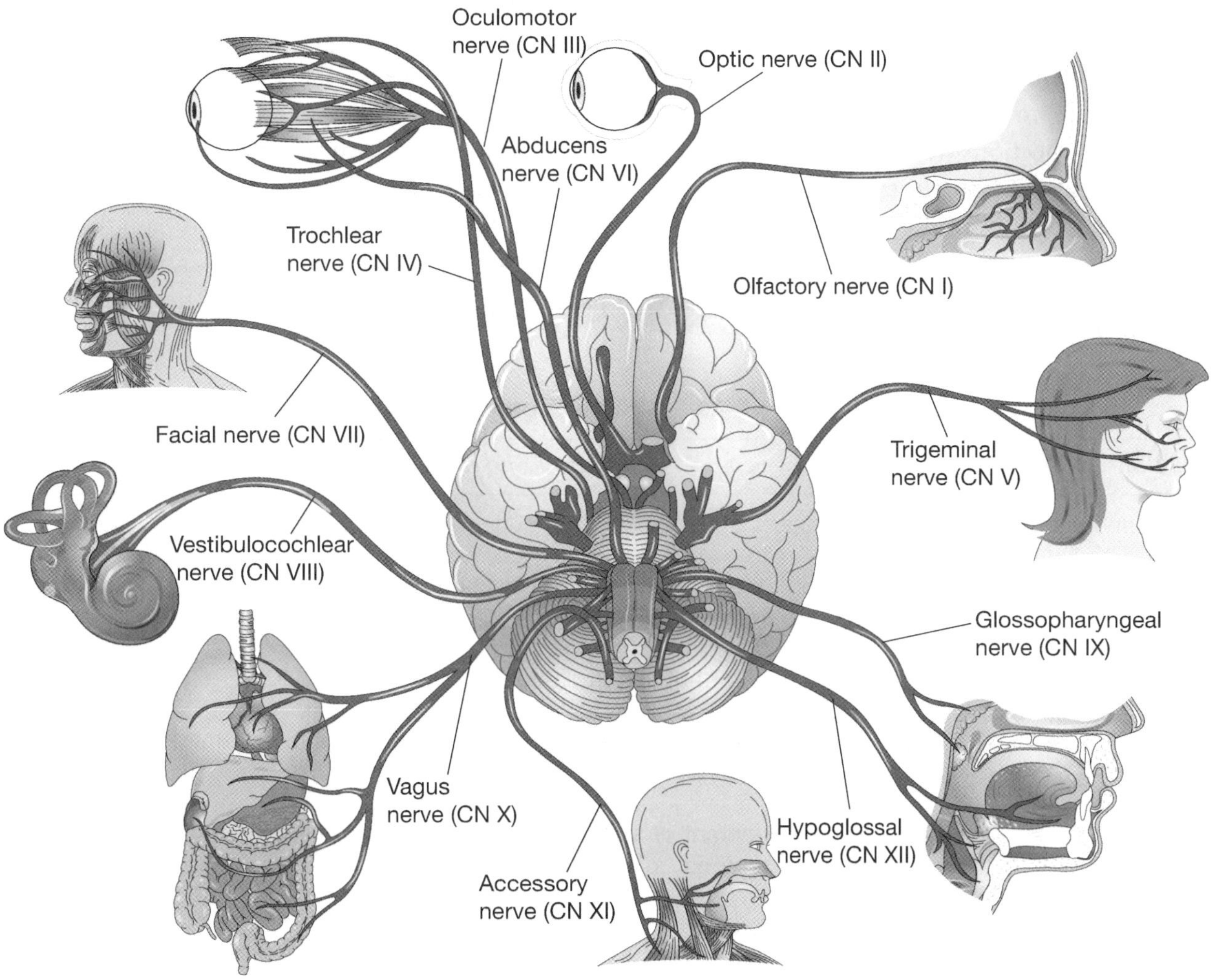

Figure 10-27
Distribution of Cranial Nerves

Spinal nerves and the functional integrity of segments of the spinal cord can be evaluated by certain spinal reflexes. The knee jerk or **patellar reflex**, for example, is elicited by sharply tapping the patellar ligament of a partially flexed and totally relaxed genual joint. A normal response is an immediate, involuntary, partial extension of the knee joint. This indicates that the spinal nerve components of the femoral nerve (L1, L2, L3) and the corresponding part of the spinal cord are functionally intact. This particular reflex is a **monosynaptic** one in which the sensory information generated by neuromuscular spindles is carried by pseudounipolar neurons to the spinal cord (Figure 10-24). These neurons synapse directly on motor neurons in the anterior column of the gray matter. Axons of these motor neurons then course out of the spinal cord to supply the quadriceps femoris muscle and effect extension of the knee joint. Similar reflexes in other areas are used by physicians to evaluate other nerves and spinal cord segments. Most reflexes involve additional (third) neurons, called **interneurons**, within the spinal cord that join the sensory neurons to the motor neurons. These reflexes are called **disynaptic** (since two synapses occur within the CNS).

Injury to a peripheral nerve that supplies limb musculature can be serious since dysfunction of these nerves can result in loss of ability to move the limb in certain ways. Sometimes a severed nerve will regain partial function if it is sutured back together. However, the sensory and motor axons must regrow (which they do at a very slow rate) and many of them fail to make proper and successful connections with their receptors and effectors. Amputees sometimes experience **phantom pain** in body parts that they no longer have. This occurs because sensory neurons that supplied amputated portions of the body sometimes continue to send impulses. **Referred pain** is pain that is perceived in certain areas or organs of the body but is actually caused in another location (Figure 10-26, Table 10-11). Usually, the area of referred pain is supplied by the same spinal nerve component as the actual site of the pain.

Table 10-11 Sites of Referred Pain

Actual Site of Pain	*Referred Site of Pain*
Lung/Diaphragm	Inferior aspect of the collum and superior portions of the deltoid regions.
Heart	Left pectoral area, ulnar aspect of superior limb, and area of first several thoracic vertebrae posteriorly.
Pancreas	Upper left quadrant of abdomen near the midline.
Stomach	Both upper quadrants of abdomen along midline and middle third of thoracic vertebrae posteriorly.
Liver	Upper right quadrant of abdomen near midline, inferior aspect of right side of collum, and inferior to right scapula posteriorly.
Small Intestine	Peripherally from umbilicus.
Vermiform Appendix	Right half of pelvic region.
Colon	Superior portion of pelvic region along midline.
Ovary	Bilateral to umbilicus.
Kidney	Superolateral aspects of thighs, anteromedial aspect of thighs, pelvic region, and inferior aspect of dorsum.
Ureter	Anteromedial aspect of thighs and pelvic region.
Urinary Bladder	Pubic area anteriorly, midpelvic region, superior aspect of natal cleft, and inferior to each buttock.

Objectives

17. Define dermatome and explain its clinical value.
18. Explain the functional losses related to dysfunction of each one of the cranial nerves.
19. List the components of a spinal reflex and differentiate monosynaptic *vs.* disynaptic reflexes.
20. Differentiate referred pain and phantom pain.

Clinical Case Studies

Case 1—A construction worker suffered a crushing fracture of his distal humerus when his elbow was trapped beneath a large I beam that was being hoisted off a semi-trailer bed. He noticed a loss of sensation to the hypothenar region of his hand and the strength of his grip was significantly weakened. Explain these latter observations.

Case 2—A 27-year old nurse complained of a weak left elbow and loss of sensation on the back of her hand that had been getting steadily worse. After noting that her upper arm on the affected side was significantly smaller in diameter than her right one (especially on the posterior aspect), the attending neurologist ordered a detailed radiographic study of the lower cervical part of the spinal cord. What was his tentative diagnosis?

Case 3—An eight-year-old girl, playing with her friends in her Tucson, Arizona backyard, suffered a deep puncture wound just below her right ear when she fell into the stiff leaves of a yucca plant. A painful abscess developed a few days later and she suffered a series of unusual symptoms that included a drooping cheek and flaccid lips on the right side and an inflamed right eye that seemed dry and difficult to close. Could there be a connection to the abscess?

Points to Ponder

A nerve—a group of nerve fibers in the peripheral nervous system. The term *nerve fiber* can imply a whole neuron, an axon or dendrite, or sometimes an axon only depending on the context in which it is used. This is a more liberal use of fiber than when one talks of a muscle fiber (which always implies a muscle cell) or a connective tissue fiber (which always implies an extracellular strand of protein). Bundles of nerve fibers in the brain or spinal cord are called fiber tracts instead of nerves. This is partly to demonstrate the locus (CNS *vs.* PNS) and partly because there are no significant physical demarcations that separate many of the adjacent tracts from each other.

Although both sensory (afferent, incoming) and motor (efferent, outgoing) impulses can be carried by a nerve or fiber tract, different neurons are involved. Neurons are one-way-streets as far as impulses are concerned. A given neuron is involved in a sensory pathway or a motor pathway—never both. We can interfere with impulse transmission—and do quite regularly in clinical medicine with anesthetic agents.

Local anesthetic agents, many of them cocaine derivatives, interfere with impulse transmission along the axons of neurons. These can be applied directly to exposed surfaces or (more commonly) injected into tissues where they contact the local nerve fibers by diffusion. General anesthetics cause a state of unconsciousness (with its accompanying loss of pain sensation over the entire body) and can be administered intravenously, intramuscularly, by inhalation, or via the digestive system (depending on the drug). An interesting variation of local *vs.* general anesthesia is intravenous regional anesthesia wherein part of a limb is anesthetized by i.v. administration of a local anesthetic. Using tourniquets to prevent the drug from "escaping" into the systemic circulation, this technique is useful in situations where complete loss of sensation from an area is needed but a general anesthetic is undesired. I had anesthesia of this type when I had screws and pins removed several months after surgical repair of a trimalleolar fracture of the ankle. First, the anesthetist started an i.v. in one of the dorsal metatarsal veins in my foot. Next, my limb was tightly wrapped in an elastic bandage to force out excess venous blood. One of two pneumatic tourniquets placed around my thigh was tightened, the elastic bandage was removed, and local anesthetic (lidocaine) was administered via the pre-placed i.v. After a few minutes, the surgeon cut and I watched and kibitzed. The tourniquet kept the anesthetic localized and the alternate one was inflated every few minutes as the pressure from the active one became unbearably uncomfortable. The most memorable event was when both tourniquets were released at the end of the procedure. The rush from that local anesthetic going systemic was significant. I could think, hear, see, and understand—but I couldn't talk! (My wife asked the anesthetist for a few take-home doses!)

Working by a different mechanism than local anesthetic (but also accomplishing an interruption of impulse transmission) is curare—the active chemical in the poison arrow blowgun darts used by the natives of the Orinoco River area in South America (when they are not watching TV). Curare blocks impulse transmission at neuromuscular junctions (motor end plates in skeletal muscle tissue) by competing for the receptors used by acetylcholine, the neurotransmitter. In smaller doses curare temporarily paralyzes. In larger doses curare is deadly because the muscles of respiration are paralyzed, and the individual dies of asphyxiation.

Slang and Obsolete Nomenclature

UNOFFICIAL TERM	OFFICIAL DESIGNATION
ophthalmic (mandibular/maxillary) branch of CN V	ophthalmic (mandibular/maxillary) nerve *[nervus ophthalmicus/maxillaris/mandibularis]*
ventral/dorsal root of spinal nerve	anterior/posterior root *[radix anterior/posterior]*
Meissner's corpuscles	tactile corpuscles *[corpuscula tactili]*
Bulbs of Krause	bulbar corpuscles *[corpuscula bulboidea]*
Pacinian corpuscles	lamellated corpuscles *[corpuscula lamellosa]*
Golgi tendon organs	neurotendinous spindles *[fusus neurotendineus]*
muscle spindles	neuromuscular spindles *[fusus neuromuscularis]*

Review Questions

1. Which of the following is not directly connected (attached) to the structure named?
   A. anterior root of a spinal nerve—sensory ganglion
   B. anterior branch of a spinal nerve—ramus communicans
   C. posterior branch of a spinal nerve—spinal nerve
   D. anterior rootlet of a spinal nerve—anterior root
   E. ramus communicans of a spinal nerve—sympathetic trunk ganglion

2. Find the false statement.
   A. Neuromuscular spindles are located in neurons and respond to stretching.
   B. Rods and cones are located in the eyeball and respond to light.
   C. Hair cells of the spiral organ are located in the internal (inner) ear and respond to vibrations.
   D. Organs of Ruffini are located in the skin and respond to heat.
   E. Gustatory cells are located in the taste buds and respond to chemicals.

3. Which of the following classes of sensory receptors is mismatched with the type of stimulus to which it may respond or with a location in which it may be found?

A. thermoreceptor—cold
B. photoreceptor—light
C. nociceptor—pressure
D. exteroceptor—heat
E. mechanoreceptor—tendon

4. Find the mismatch.
A. musculocutaneous n.—brachialis m.—skin of lateral (radial) aspect of forearm
B. median n.—palmaris longus m.—skin of lateral aspect of manus
C. radial n.—triceps brachii m.—skin of posterior antebrachium
D. obturator n.—gracilis m.—skin of medial thigh
E. femoral n.—pectineus m.—skin of lateral crus

5. Which item is false?
A. Three pairs of cranial nerves innervate the muscles that move the eyeballs.
B. Only two pairs of cranial nerves carry gustatory fibers.
C. Cranial nerve VIII does not emerge from the skull.
D. Only one cranial nerve pair innervates muscles of mastication.
E. Cranial nerve pairs V, VII, IX, X, and XII are distributed to the tongue.

6. Find the error.
A. Nerve (fiber) tracts are located in the CNS and nerves are located in the PNS.
B. All cranial nerves originate anteriorly on the brain.
C. Bipolar neurons are found in cranial nerves I, II, and VIII.
D. Two pairs of cranial nerves contain all four functional types of neurons, one contains only three, two contain only two, and seven contain only one type of functional neuron (disregarding SA proprioception).
E. Three cranial nerves pass through each jugular foramen.

7. Which of the following nerves is mismatched with either its sensory or motor function?
A. median nerve—innervates muscles of the anterior antebrachium
B. musculocutaneous nerve—innervates the coracobrachialis muscle and biceps brachii muscle
C. radial nerve—innervates posterior muscles of the brachium
D. femoral nerve—innervates the posterior muscles of the thigh
E. tibial and fibular nerves—sensory from the skin of the foot and most of the anterior, posterior and lateral aspects of the crus

8. Find the incorrect statement.
A. To test the functionality of the facial nerve, a patient can be asked to whistle, elevate the eyebrows, puff out the cheeks, and identify the taste of sugar and vinegar.
B. Only four of the 12 pairs of cranial nerves supply smooth muscle tissue, cardiac muscle tissue or glandular epithelium.
C. Cranial nerves III, IV, and VI supply muscles of the eyeball.
D. Cranial nerve VII is transmitted through the stylomastoid foramen of the temporal bone.
E. The vestibulocochlear nerves and vagus nerves contain all four functional types of neurons.

9. Which of the following cranial nerves is not a mixed (motor and sensory) nerve?
   A. vagus n.
   B. glossopharyngeal n.
   C. optic n.
   D. trigeminal n.
   E. facial n.

10. Which of the following is not true about cranial nerve III?
    A. it is sensory only
    B. carries SE fibers
    C. carries VE fibers
    D. supplies muscles of the eye
    E. emerges from the superior orbital fissure

Thought Questions

1. When a nerve is severed, some function can often be restored by suturing the severed ends back together. However, several months are required for recovery and recovery is typically only partial. Why?

2. If a patellar reflex ("knee jerk reflex") is normal, what can a medical practitioner conclude?

3. Which cranial nerves are involved in eating a pizza?

4. How does the optic chiasm assist the brain in interpreting the impulses associated with visual images?

5. The 4 taste modalities (sweet, sour, bitter, salty) do not explain the large variations in the tastes of different foods. What does?

6. What are the differences in sensory impulses involved in a hearing pathway, a visual pathway, or any other kind of sensory information?

7. Why is it that most spinal nerves carry fibers of all four functional modalities but the majority of cranial nerves carry only one, two, or three functional neuronal types?

8. How can a physician use a combination of loss of muscle function and loss of sensation to dermatomes to assess nerve damage?

9. Two men suffered complete severance of the radial nerve. One could still extend his elbow joint after the injury, but the other one could not. Explain.

10. Which named branches of the brachial plexus are the most significant in carrying impulses to and from superior limb structures?

11. Which named branches of the lumbosacral plexus are the most significant in carrying impulses to and from inferior limb structures?

12. A named appendicular nerve carries fibers from several segments of the spinal cord. How does this occur?

13. Why are posterior branches of spinal nerves usually much smaller in diameter than anterior branches?

14. Severance of left spinal nerve C7 is much more debilitating than severance of left spinal nerve T7. Why?

15. Loss of function of a certain spinal nerve will not necessarily deprive the patient of all sensation from its dermatome because...

16. Which of the five groups of sensory receptors (based on the type of stimulus which incites an impulse) has the most specific receptor types?

17. What do all sensory receptors have in common?

18. Severance of the spinal cord at a fairly high level can cause quadriplegia but may not interfere with respiration. Why?

19. Why are sensory nerve, motor nerve, and mixed nerve misleading terms?

20. Which two cranial nerve (pairs) have the most extensive areas of fiber distribution?

21. Which cranial nerve (pair) is shortest?

Answers to Clinical Case Studies

Case 1—The symptoms in this patient indicate damage to the ulnar nerve. This nerve courses between the medial epicondyle of the humerus and the olecranon where it would be vulnerable to the crushing injury that this patient suffered. The ulnar nerve is the structure that is responsible for the "funny bone" that people say is struck when they bang their elbow in a certain manner.

Case 2—Loss of sensation on the back of the hand, "weak elbow", and atrophy of the posterior brachial muscles all indicate dysfunction of the radial nerve. The physician ordered the radiographic study to see if the problem was caused by intervertebral disc disease or some other vertebral malady.

Case 3—The symptoms are compatible with dysfunction of the ipsilateral facial nerve. It emerges from the stylomastoid foramen of the temporal bone and the abscess was located in this general area.

Answers to Review Questions

1. A. The sensory ganglion is on the posterior root.

2. A. They are located in skeletal muscles.

3. C. Nociceptors respond to pain.

4. E. The femoral nerve is cutaneously distributed to the medial crus.

5. B. There are three (VII, IX, X).

6. B. The trochlear nerve is an exception to this.

7. D. The femoral nerve innervates the anterior muscles to the thigh.

8. E. The vestibulocochlear nerve has somatic afferent fibers only.

9. C. The optic nerve is sensory only.

10. A.

Answers to Thought Questions

1. Regeneration of the severed nerve processes is very slow (about 1 cm/month). In addition, for regeneration to occur, the severed processes must grow into the myelin sheaths of the severed distal parts of their fibers. Many regenerating fibers may fail to "find" a myelin sheath or get blocked by the ingrowth of fibrous connective (scar) tissue.

2. The sensory pathway (within the femoral nerve) is intact, the spinal cord segments involving the femoral nerve are functional, and the motor pathway within the femoral nerve is normal.

3. Looking at it involves the second pair of cranial nerves for vision and CN 3, 4, and 6 for eye movements. Smelling and tasting involves cranial nerves 1, 7, 9 (and perhaps 10). Chewing and savoring it involves cranial nerve 5 for the muscles that close the mouth in masticatory motions, cranial nerves 5 and 7 for opening the mouth (digastricus m.), and cranial nerve 12 for movements of the tongue. Cranial nerve 7 is involved in manipulations of the lips required during prehension and both 7 and 9 are required for salivation.

4. Some visual sensory fibers decussate at the optic chiasm and these pathways are destined for the occipital lobe of the contralateral cerebral hemisphere. Those that do not cross-over are destined for the occipital lobe on the ipsilateral side. Axons that do not decussate at the chiasm are mostly those carrying impulses generated by photoreceptors in the lateral aspects of the retinae. Those that do decussate are those carrying impulses from the medial aspects of the retinae. For this reason the impulses generated by retinal images of left peripheral vision objects end up in the left occipital lobe and then those generated by retinal images of right peripheral vision objects are sent to the right occiptial lobe (*see Figure 12-5*).

5. A significant portion of what we call taste is actually olfaction. This is supported by the fact that individuals with severe nasal congestion usually experience significant anosmia (reduction in their ability to taste).

6. The impulses are all the same. In fact, motor impulses are identical to them as well. The differences in sensations are determined by where the impulses go in the brain.

7. Spinal nerves are distributed to regional segments of the neck and trunk and to the limbs. These areas all contain skeletal muscle tissue (SE neurons), smooth muscle in vessel walls and glandular epithelium in sweat glands (VE neurons), all have cutaneous receptors and sensory neurons from bones, muscles, and joints (SA neurons) and all have sensory receptors in vessel walls (VA neurons). Many cranial nerves are much more limited in their distribution (CN 1, for example, is distributed to the nasal mucosa only).

8. Skeletal muscles have definitive nerves that supply them with motor impulses and loss of nerve supply is accompanied by paralysis of those muscles. Likewise named nerves carry sensory impulses from certain areas of the skin. Loss of sensation can be mapped and will indicate dysfunction of certain nerves.

9. The location (level) of the injury is significant. The one who could still extend his elbow joint (contract his triceps brachii muscle) must have had his radial nerve transected distal to the origin of the radial nerve branches to the triceps brachii muscle. In the other individual, the radial nerve was transected above the origin of these muscular branches.

10. Most of the muscles in the free part of the superior limb are supplied by the radial, ulnar, median, and musculocutaneous nerves.

11. Most of the muscles in the free part of the inferior limb are supplied by the sciatic nerve and its two terminal branches (tibial and common fibular nn.), obturator nerve and femoral nerve.

12. The numbered spinal nerves exchange fibers at the brachial and lumbosacral plexuses such that the named nerves continuing distally from the plexuses contain fibers from several numbered spinal nerves.

13. Nerve fibers in the posterior branches of the spinal nerves are primarily distributed to structures posterior to the frontal plane containing the vertebral canal. Fibers in the anterior branches supply structures in front of this plane. There is simply more "body" anterior to the plane than posterior to the plane and so anterior branches are larger than their posterior counterparts.

14. The seventh cervical spinal nerves supply fibers to the brachial plexus and thence to the superior limb. Disruption will leave parts of the limb dysfunctional. The seventh thoracic spinal nerves supply motor fibers to a regional segment of the thoracic wall. Loss of this innervation is much less debilitating.

15. There is considerable overlap in the cutaneous distribution of sensory pathways.

16. Mechanoreceptors.

17. An ability to generate a nervous impulse if supplied with the right type of stimulus (and sometimes even when supplied with the wrong type of stimulus).

18. The impulses controlling respiration (via the phrenic nerves to the diaphragm) leave the spinal cord within cervical spinal nerves C4 and C5. Transection of the spinal cord above the C4/C5 segments results in death by asphyxiation. Transection just below that level results in a quadriplegic individual (who can still respire).

19. Essentially all nerves are mixed (contain both motor and sensory fibers). Only a few of the cranial nerves are sensory only (CN 1, 2, 8). No nerves are motor only.

20. The vagus and accessory nerves (CN 10 and 11).

21. The olfactory nerves. Each one arises as 15-20 bundles of fibers from the ipsilateral olfactory bulb, passes through the cribriform foraminae of the ethmoid bone, and is distributed to the olfactory mucosa of the nasal cavity.

CHAPTER

11 Autonomic Nervous System

Chapter Outline and Key Concepts

INTRODUCTION

The ANS is that part of the nervous system that is motor to involuntary effectors.

Some parts of the CNS and some parts of the PNS are involved in the ANS.

The ANS has two divisions based on anatomic, pharmacologic, and functional criteria.

THE TWO NEURON CHAIN OF THE ANS

Motor pathways to voluntary effectors (skeletal muscles) involve single neurons extending from the CNS to the effector.

All involuntary (ANS) motor pathways involve a two-neuron chain.

First (preganglionic) neurons have cell bodies in the CNS (brain or spinal cord) and synapse on second (postganglionic) neurons in autonomic ganglia.

The two neuron chain allows a "multiplication" effect as well as excitatory/inhibitory influences on the postganglionic neurons.

THE ANS EFFECTOR ORGANS

ANS impulses to smooth muscle tissue influence blood pressure and distribution, peristalsis, luminal evacuation, piloerection, pupillary diameter, and thickness of the lens of the eye.

Autonomic impulses to cardiac muscle tissue influence heart rate and the strength of cardiac contraction.

Glandular epithelium can be stimulated to secrete or it can be inhibited by the ANS.

THE TWO DIVISIONS OF THE ANS

The sympathetic ("fight/flight") division of the ANS is sometimes called the "thoracolumbar" division because of the location of its preganglionic neurons (spinal cord—T1-L2).

The parasympathetic ("homeostatic") division of the ANS is sometimes called the "craniosacral" division because its preganglionic neurons are located in the brain and in the sacral part of the spinal cord.

Both divisions use (mostly) acetylcholine as a neurotransmitter at ganglia.

At effector organs, sympathetic pathways usually utilize norepinephrine as a neurotransmitter and parasympathetic pathways use acetylcholine.

Most involuntary effectors receive impulses from both divisions of the ANS but some are sympathetic only and some are parasympathetic only.

STRUCTURE OF THE SYMPATHETIC PART OF THE ANS

Preganglionic neuron cell bodies are located in the lateral columns (horns) of the gray matter in the T1-L2 segments of the spinal cord.

Axons of preganglionic neurons leave the T1-L2 part of the spinal cord and pass into the (paired) sympathetic trunks.

Pathways to peripheral effectors usually synapse in the sympathetic trunk ganglia and postganglionic axons are distributed with spinal nerves.

Pathways to centrally located effectors usually pass through the sympathetic trunk (without synapsing) and join their postganglionic neurons in centrally located ganglia.

STRUCTURE OF THE PARASYMPATHETIC PART OF THE ANS

Preganglionic neuron cell bodies are located in the brain (in motor nuclei of cranial nerves 3, 7, 9, and 10) and in the sacral part of the spinal cord.

Preganglionic axons of the cranial part of the parasympathetic division leave the brain via cranial nerves 3, 7, 9, and 10.

After synapsing within named autonomic ganglia in the cephalic region, parasympathetic fibers are distributed to salivary and lacrimal glands, smooth muscle of the eye, and (via the vagus nerves) to the smooth muscle and glands of the respiratory and digestive systems, and to the heart.

Preganglionic axons of the sacral part of the parasympathetic division synapse in ganglia located in the walls of the colon and urogenital organs.

HIGHER CENTERS WHICH CONTROL ANS OUTPUT

The brain contains centers in the medulla oblongata and hypothalamus that influence ANS output.

CLINICAL CONSIDERATIONS

Many drugs stimulate parts of the sympathetic or parasympathetic divisions of the ANS.

Neurogenic shock is a precipitous drop in blood pressure due to lack of sympathetic impulses to smooth muscle in vessel walls.

Selected Definitions

Acetylcholine—a neurotransmitter released in autonomic ganglia by the preganglionic neurons of both divisions of the ANS. It is also released by parasympathetic postganglionic neurons at their synapses with involuntary effectors.

Craniosacral—a term referencing the parasympathetic division of the ANS. It reflects the fact that the parasympathetic preganglionic neurons have their cell bodies in the brain and spinal cord and leave the CNS in (some of the) cranial and sacral nerves.

Effector—a tissue that responds to motor impulses. Effectors include muscle tissue and glandular epithelium.

Fight or flight—a phrase applied to the physiologic responses expected when the sympathetic division of the ANS is stimulated. These are the kinds of responses that occur when one is angered or scared.

Involuntary effector—an effector that is not under conscious control. Involuntary effectors include smooth muscle tissue, cardiac muscle tissue, and glandular epithelium.

Neurogenic shock—cardiovascular shock related to emotional states. The drop in blood pressure is caused by generalized vasodilation.

Norepinephrine—a neurotransmitter utilized by the postganglionic neurons in the sympathetic division of the ANS. It and the related neurotransmitter, epinephrine, are also released into the bloodstream by the adrenal medulla and induce a generalized sympathetic response.

Parasympathetic part ("division") of the ANS—The portion of the autonomic nervous system that produces reactions generally antagonistic to those considered to be "fight or flight". It is often called the "homeostatic" division of the ANS (= "rest and digest").

Paravertebral ganglion—an alternative name for any sympathetic trunk ganglion. These ganglia are synaptic sites for most of the sympathetic pathways distributed to peripherally located involuntary effectors.

Postganglionic neurons—visceral efferent neurons located in autonomic ganglia. They are the second neurons in the "two neuron chain" of the ANS and their axons are distributed to involuntary effectors.

Preganglionic neurons—visceral efferent neurons located in the brain or spinal cord. Their axons are distributed to autonomic ganglia where they synapse on postganglionic neurons.

Prevertebral ganglion—any of those autonomic ganglia that are big enough to see but are not located along the sympathetic trunk. Most of these have names and are sometimes collectively called named peripheral ganglia.

Ramus communicans—the small fasciculus of nerve fibers that connects the anterior branch of a spinal nerve to the ipsilateral sympathetic trunk or vertebral nerve. A typical ramus includes gray (unmyelinated) and white (myelinated) rami.

Splanchnic nerves—the nerves that leave the sympathetic trunks and course to abdominal and pelvic viscera. They include major, minor, lumbar, and sacral splanchnic nerves.

Sympathetic part ("division") of the ANS—that portion of the autonomic nervous system that produces "fight or flight" reactions. These include such things as increased heart rate, pupillary dilation, decreased salivation, and piloerection.

Sympathetic trunk ganglion—any of the autonomic ganglia located along the left or right sympathetic trunk. These ganglia serve as synaptic sites for most of the sympathetic pathways destined for peripheral ANS effectors (and even some of those distributed centrally).

Sympathomimetic drug—any pharmaceutical agent that induces responses typical of those of the sympathetic division of the ANS. These agents have been abused by professional athletes because of their performance enhancing properties.

Thoracolumbar—a term referencing the sympathetic division (part) of the ANS. It reflects the fact that the cell bodies of the sympathetic preganglionic neurons are located in the thoracolumbar parts of the spinal cord and their axons are carried by spinal nerve pairs T1-L2.

"Two neuron chain"—a phrase referring to the fact that the distribution of an impulse from the CNS to an involuntary effector requires two neurons. The first neuron is called the preganglionic neuron and the second one is termed the postganglionic neuron.

Visceral efferent (VE) neuron—any motor neuron that is part of the "two neuron chain" of the ANS. Those with cell bodies in the brain or spinal cord are called preganglionic neurons and those with cell bodies in motor (autonomic) ganglia are postganglionic neurons.

Voluntary effector—an effector that is under conscious (voluntary) control. The only voluntary effector is skeletal muscle tissue.

Etymology *Sine praeiudicio*—**"Without prejudice."**

mimicus (L), *mime*—parasympathomimetic
para (L), *near, beside*—parasympathetic
pharmacia (L), *drug, medicine*—pharmacologic
post (L), *hind, after*—postganglionic
soma (G), *body*—somatic
sympatheia (G), *sympathy*—sympathetic
synapsis (L), *contact*—synaptic cleft
viscus (L), *an internal organ*—visceral

Objectives

1. Review the definition of the ANS and compare it to the rest of the nervous system.

Introduction

The **autonomic nervous system (ANS)** is the portion of the nervous system that is motor to smooth muscle, cardiac muscle, and glands. It is a functional entity rather than an anatomic one and includes some parts of the CNS and some parts of the PNS. The ANS may be functionally contrasted with the rest of the nervous system (somatic nervous system) which not only has a different effector (skeletal muscle tissue) but also includes sensory neurons (Table 11-1). The ANS is divided into two parts (**sympathetic** and **parasympathetic**) by some anatomic, pharmacologic, and functional criteria.

Table 11-1 A Comparison of the ANS and the Somatic Nervous System

Criterion	*Autonomic Nervous System*	*Somatic Nervous System*
Effector organs	Smooth m., cardiac m., and glandular epithelium	Skeletal muscle
Number of neurons between the CNS and effector organ	Two (pre- and postganglionic)	One
Location of neurons (cell bodies)	Presynaptic: brain and spinal cord Postsynaptic: autonomic ganglia	Brain and spinal cord
Functional type of motor neurons	Visceral efferent (VE)	Somatic efferent (SE)
Sensory neurons	Absent	Present
Type of ganglia present	Autonomic (synapses occur)	Sensory (synapses do not occur)

The Two Neuron Chain of the ANS

In contrast to the somatic nervous system which uses only one neuron to reach its peripheral effector, the ANS uses a two neuron chain peripherally (Figure 11-1). The first neurons, called **preganglionic neurons**, have cell bodies in the brain or spinal cord and their axons course peripherally within cranial and spinal nerves (Figure 11-2). The axons of the preganglionic neurons synapse on the second neurons, called **postganglionic neurons,** at the various autonomic ganglia within the PNS. The axons of the postganglionic neurons continue on to their effector organs (smooth muscle tissue, cardiac muscle tissue, or glandular epithelium) by coursing within the named peripheral nerves or in some cases by following the vascular network. Both the preganglionic and the postganglionic neurons of the ANS are visceral efferent (VE) neurons.

The reason for having a two neuron chain in the ANS appears to be two-fold. First, each preganglionic neuron can synapse on several postganglionic neurons. This allows a "multiplication" effect whereby a relatively small output of impulses from the CNS can cause a relatively large peripheral response. The net effect is that the ANS operates at a subconscious (non-voluntary) level. The second purpose of the two neuron chain is to allow some PNS interaction between pre-ganglionic excitatory ("go ahead and do it") impulses and inhibitory ("not now") impulses. Postganglionic neurons must be stimulated to a certain level by excitatory preganglionic impulses before they will fire (transmit an impulse). If they receive a significant number of inhibitory impulses during a given time period they will not reach what is called **threshold potential** and will not fire.

Objectives

2. Diagram an ANS pathway and label the brain, spinal cord, preganglionic neuron, ganglion, postganglionic neuron, and effector organ.
3. Explain the functional value of the "two neuron chain."

The ANS Effector Organs

The effectors of the ANS are scattered throughout the body. **Smooth muscle tissue** is found within the walls of most of the organs of the visceral body systems, within the walls of blood vessels, at the base of hair follicles and within the iris and ciliary body of the eye. Some smooth muscle tissue

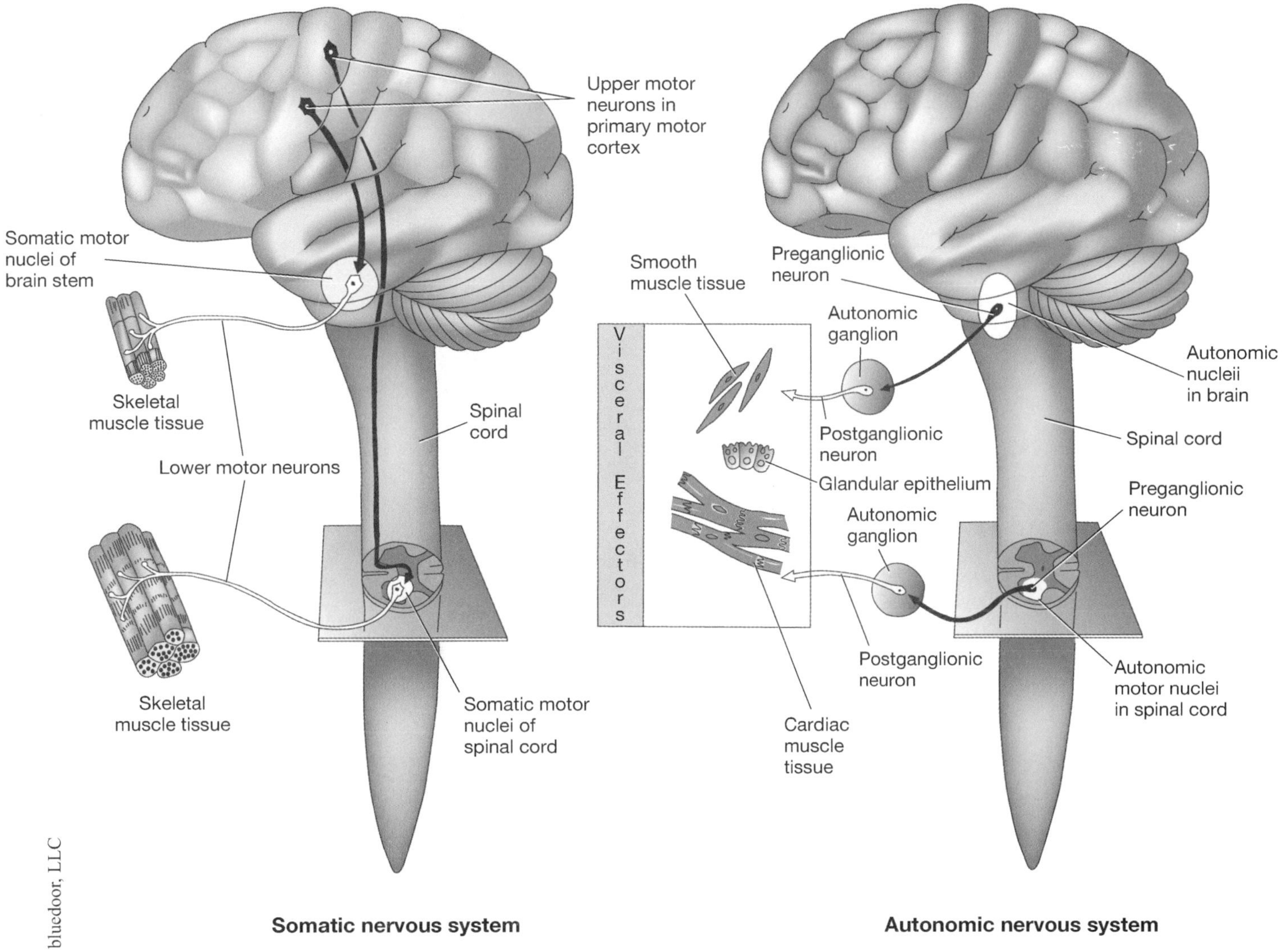

Figure 11-1

Comparison of the Somatic and Autonomic Nervous Systems

The effectors of the somatic nervous system are skeletal muscle cells and only a "one neuron chain" is present peripherally. In the ANS a "two neuron chain" is present with the cell bodies of the second (postganglionic or "ganglionic") neurons located in autonomic ganglia. The principal effectors of the ANS are involuntary muscle tissue (smooth and cardiac muscle tissue) and glandular epithelium (see *Table 11-1*).

has inherent rhythmicity (contraction/relaxation) which ANS impulses can facilitate or inhibit. Other smooth muscle tissue requires direct impulses from the ANS in order to contract. In the visceral organs, smooth muscle tissue helps propel material through the lumen (digestive, urinary, and reproductive systems) or helps control the size of the lumen (respiratory system). Smooth muscle within the vessel walls can be contracted or relaxed to increase or decrease the blood pressure. Smooth muscle sphincters in the arterioles determine which capillaries are open (patent) or closed at any given moment. Smooth muscle at the base of hair follicles allows the piloerection which is both an alarm mechanism and a vestigial thermoregulatory response. In the iris of the eye, smooth

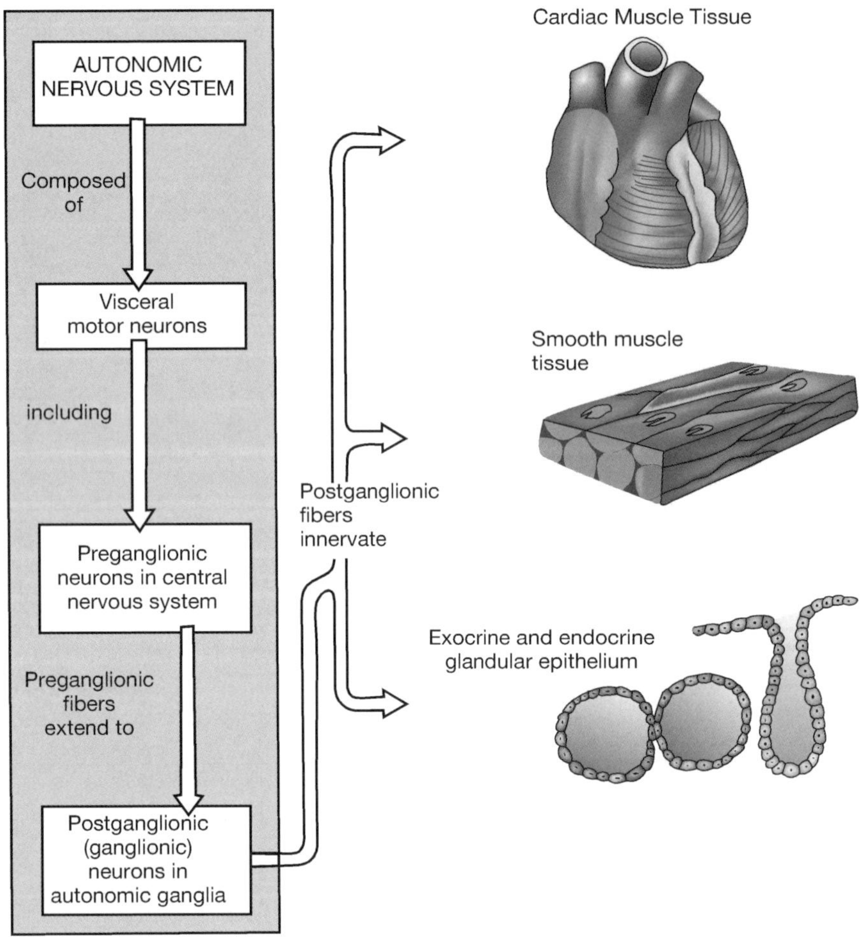

Figure 11-2

An Overview of the Autonomic Nervous System

muscle tissue forms the pupillary dilator and pupillary sphincter muscles which determine the sizes of the pupils which, in turn, determine the amount of light that strikes the retina of each eye. The smooth muscle tissue forming the ciliary muscle of the eye controls the thickness of the lens which must be altered to properly focus images of nearby *vs.* further away objects on the retina.

Cardiac muscle tissue is found within the heart and it also extends for a short distance into the pulmonary trunk and aorta. Like some smooth muscle tissue, it has inherent rhythmicity, but the ANS can speed or slow its frequency of contraction.

Glandular epithelium can be stimulated to secrete or can be inhibited from secreting by the ANS. Both exocrine glands and endocrine glands receive autonomic innervation. When the adrenal medulla is stimulated by the sympathetic division, it releases catecholamines which travel through the bloodstream and stimulate sympathetic effectors all over the body.

Objectives

4. Name the ANS (involuntary) effectors and state their locations.

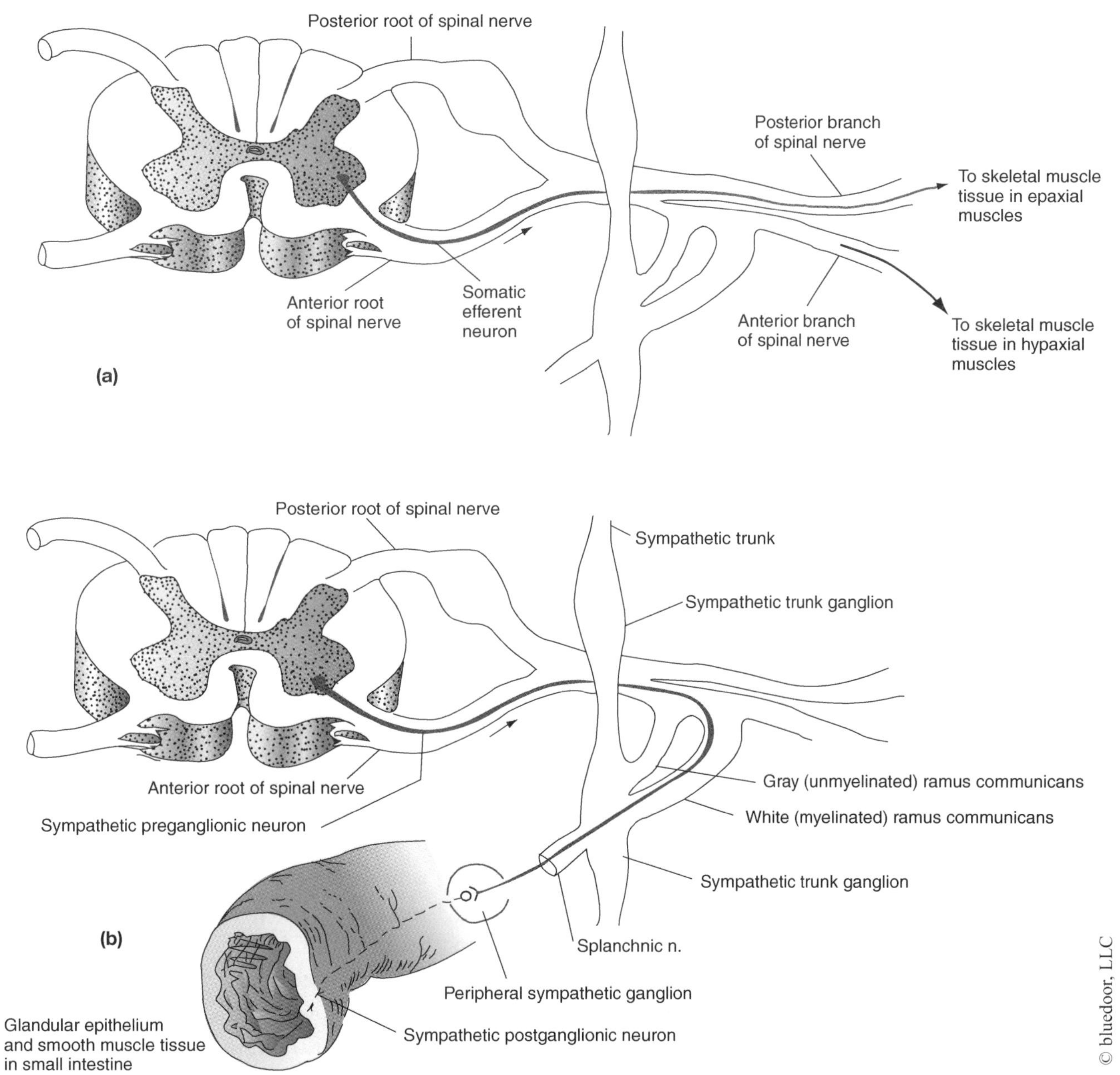

Figure 11-3

A Comparison of a Somatic Efferent Pathway (a) and a Visceral Efferent Pathway (b)

Somatic efferent neurons (A) supply skeletal muscle tissue. The neuron cell bodies are located in the brain (in motor nuclei of cranial nerves 3, 4, 5, 6, 7, 9, 10, 11, 12) or in the anterior gray columns of the spinal cord (as shown here). These neurons travel all the way to their effectors without synapsing on second neurons. They are distributed to epaxial muscles via the posterior branches of the spinal nerves and hypaxial muscles via the anterior branches. Visceral efferent neurons (B) supply smooth muscle tissue, cardiac muscle tissue, and glandular epithelium. They are distributed to their effectors by a two neuron chain. The cell body of the first neuron (preganglionic neuron) is located in the brain (motor nuclei of cranial nerves 3, 7, 9, 10), in the thoracic part of the spinal cord (anterior gray column as shown here), or in the sacral part of the spinal cord. They synapse on postganglionic neurons in autonomic ganglia. The postganglionic neurons are then distributed to their effector organs.

Table 11-2 A Comparison of the Two Divisions of the ANS

Criterion	*Sympathetic*	*Parasympathetic*
Location of preganglionic neuron cell bodies	T1-L2 segments of spinal cord	Brain and sacral part of spinal cord
Location of postganglionic neuron cell bodies	Sympathetic trunk ganglia, prevertebral ganglia, terminal ganglia	Autonomic ganglia of CN 3, 7, 9, 10 and terminal ganglia
Distribution of effectors	Throughout the body	Head, neck, thorax, and abdomen
Neurotransmitter secreted by preganglionic neurons	Acetylcholine (Ach)	Acetylcholine (Ach)
Neurotransmitter secreted by postganglionic neurons	Norepinephrine (NE)	Acetylcholine (Ach)
Changes in the body induced by effector organs	Fight/flight	Homeostasis

The Two Divisions of the ANS

The autonomic nervous system is divided into **sympathetic** and **parasympathetic parts** on the basis of anatomic, pharmacologic, and functional criteria (Table 11-2). The sympathetic portion is sometimes called the "*fight or flight*" division because it causes the changes in smooth muscle tissue, cardiac muscle tissue, and glandular epithelium that one would expect during the emotional states of anger or fear. It is also called the "*thoracolumbar*" division because its preganglionic neurons are located in those parts of the spinal cord. The parasympathetic portion is sometimes called the "*feed or breed*" ("rest and digest") division and induces changes in the effectors related to homeostatic states (internal dynamic equilibrium). It is also known as the "*craniosacral*" division because its preganglionic neurons are located in the brain and in the sacral parts of the spinal cord.

The specific **anatomic differences** between the sympathetic and parasympathetic parts of the ANS are based primarily on the locations of the cell bodies of the preganglionic and postganglionic neurons. Sympathetic preganglionic neurons are located in the T1 to L2 segments of the spinal cord (within the lateral gray column). Parasympathetic preganglionics are located in the brain (within motor nerve nuclei of cranial nerves 3, 7, 9, and 10) and in the sacral region of the spinal cord (in an area corresponding to the lateral gray column). Sympathetic postganglionic neurons are located in sympathetic trunk ganglia as well as in named ganglia primarily in the neck, thorax, and abdomen. Parasympathetic postganglionic neurons are located primarily in named ganglia in the head (associated with cranial nerves 3, 7, and 9), in the sacral region, and in terminal ganglia within the walls of the thoracic and abdominal organs (primarily associated with cranial nerve 10). In general, sympathetic effectors are found throughout the body and the parasympathetic effectors are limited to the head and to the viscera of the thorax, abdomen, and pelvis.

The **pharmacologic differences** between the two divisions of the ANS are based on the specific neurotransmitters used at different locations. Both divisions use *acetylcholine* at the ganglia (between pre- and postganglionic neurons). The parasympathetic division also uses *acetylcholine* as the postganglionic (neuron-to-effector-organ) neurotransmitter. In the sympathetic division, *norepinephrine* is the neurotransmitter released by the postganglionic neurons (Figure 11-5).

The **functional differences** between the two divisions of the ANS relate to the "fight/flight" *vs.* homeostatic roles of the two parts. Most of the changes in the body induced by stimulation of the sympathetic part can be deduced by considering what happens in an anger/fear situation. Parasympathetic responses can be logically deduced by considering a resolution from anger/fear (Table 11-3). Note that most ANS effectors receive both sympathetic and parasympathetic innervation and that the effect of stimulation is usually opposite for the two divisions. A few effectors receive sympathetic innervation but no parasympathetic inputs. These include sweat glands, smooth muscle in most vessel walls, the pupillary dilator muscle, arrector pili muscles at the base of hair follicles, and the adrenal medulla. The only effectors which receive exclusively parasympathetic innervation are the ciliary muscle of the eye which controls the thickness of the lens and the pupillary sphincter muscle which limits the amount of light entering the posterior and vitreous chambers of the eyeball.

Objectives

5. Differentiate the two divisions of the ANS using anatomic, functional, and pharmacologic criteria.
6. List some effectors that are stimulated only by the sympathetic part of the ANS and make another list for parasympathetic only.

Structure of the Sympathetic Part of the ANS

The sympathetic preganglionic neurons leave the spinal cord through the anterior rootlets of spinal nerves T1-L2 (Figure 11-4). The sympathetic preganglionic neurons course into the anterior branches of those spinal nerves and then enter the white (myelinated) **rami communicantes** (communicating branches) and course to the ipsilateral sympathetic trunk. They may travel up or down the sympathetic trunks some distance before synapsing. The left and right **sympathetic trunks** extend along each side of the vertebral column. Each trunk consists of a series of **sympathetic trunk ganglia** joined to each other by interganglionic rami and joined to the anterior branches of the spinal nerves by rami communicantes as noted above. After reaching the sympathetic trunk, the fate of a sympathetic preganglionic axon depends on whether it is part of a pathway to peripherally or centrally located effectors (Figure 11-7).

Objectives

7. Outline the structure of the sympathetic part of the ANS and state the effect of its stimulation on common ANS effectors.
8. Explain why the sympathetic pathways to peripheral effectors usually involve synapses in the sympathetic trunk ganglia. State where the synapses occur in sympathetic pathways to central effectors.

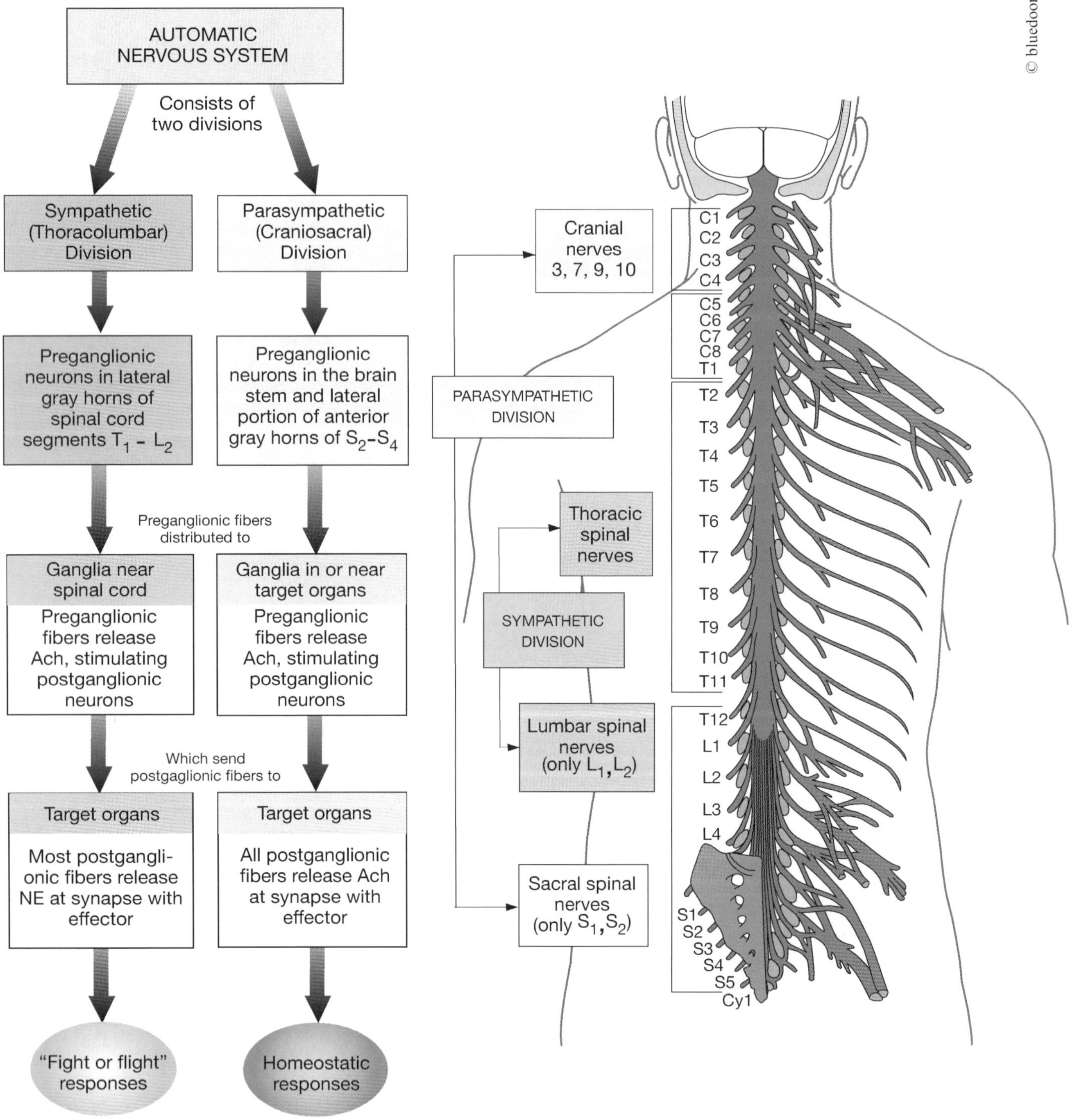

Figure 11-4

The Two Divisions of the ANS

Although similar in their two neuron chain, the two divisions of the ANS have several differences (*see Table 11-2 and Figure 11-5*).

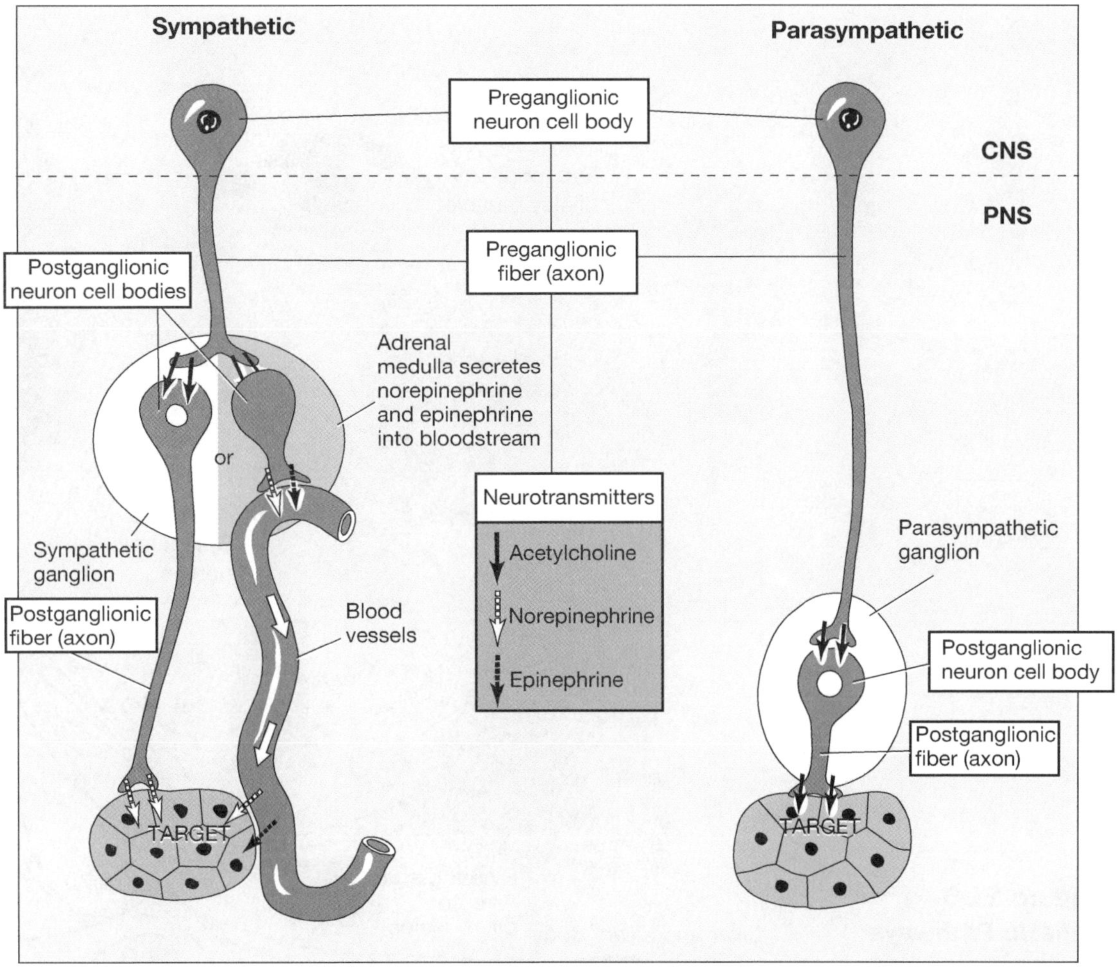

Figure 11-5

Neurotransmitters Used in the ANS

Both divisions use acetylcholine in the ganglia and the parasympathetic division also uses acetylcholine between the postganglionic ("ganglionic") neuron and the effector organ ("target"). The sympathetic division typically uses norepinephrine at the effector organ.

Structure of the Parasympathetic Part of the ANS

The parasympathetic preganglionic neurons leave the CNS through cranial nerves 3, 7, 9, 10, (the oculomotor, facial, glossopharyngeal, and vagus nerves) and through the sacral segments of the spinal cord. They synapse at autonomic ganglia in the head, thorax, abdomen, and pelvis (rarely at the sympathetic trunk ganglia). The postganglionic neurons are distributed to the heart as well as to smooth muscle and glands in the head, neck, thorax, and abdomen.

The parasympathetic fibers associated with the **oculomotor nerve** are distributed to the pupillary sphincter muscle of the iris and to the ciliary muscle of the eye. The pre/post synapses occur at the **ciliary ganglion** which is located within the orbit adjacent to the eyeball (Figure 11-8). Parasympathetic impulses carried by the oculomotor nerve result in constriction of the pupil of the eye and a change in the thickness of the lens.

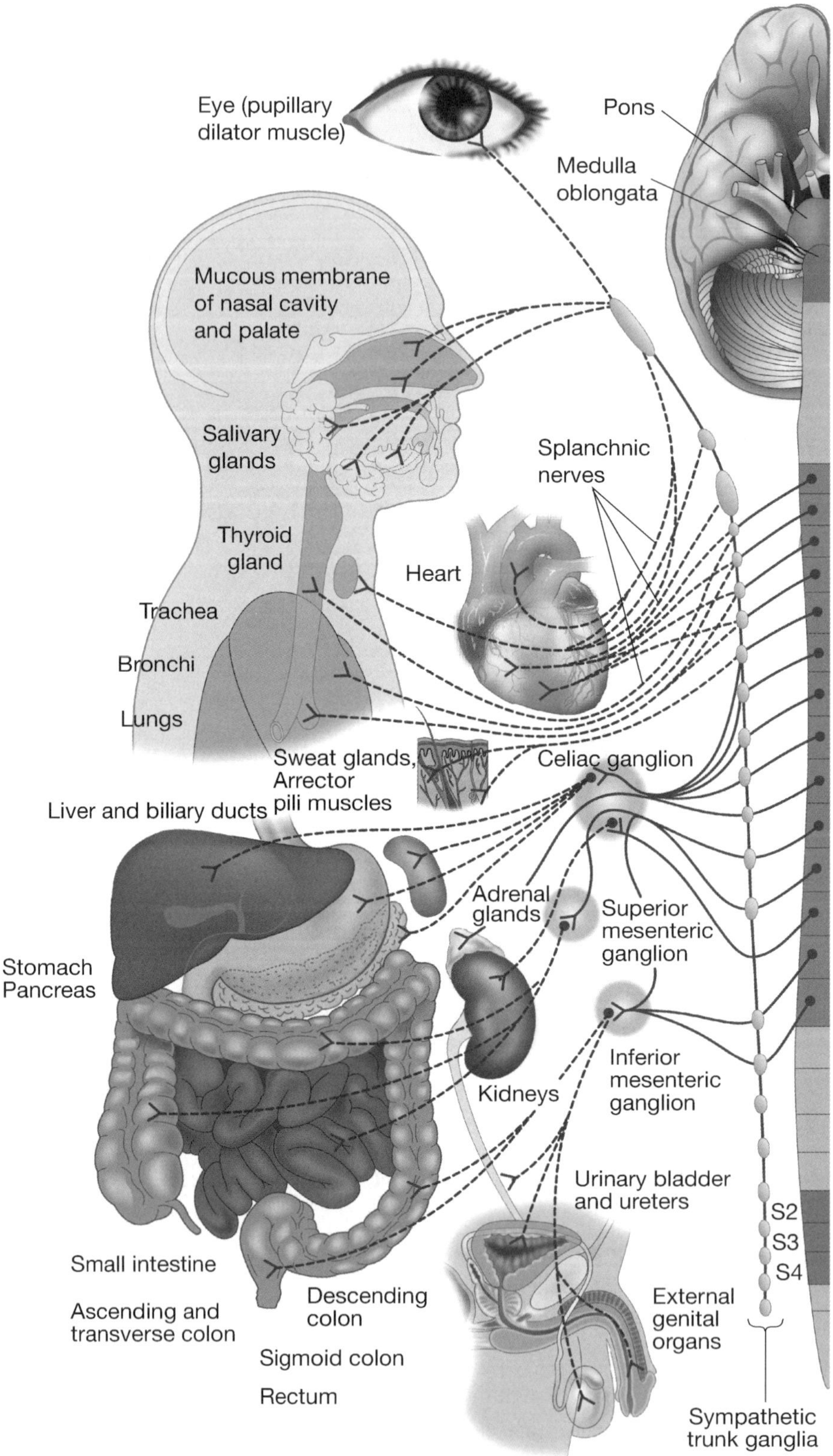

Figure 11-6
Sympathetic Pathways

Preganglionic neuron cell bodies are located in the spinal cord (lateral gray columns) from T1 - L2. Their axons travel to the sympathetic trunks via the white rami communicantes of the spinal nerves. Once in the sympathetic trunk, the axons either synapse on their second (postganglionic) neurons in sympathetic trunk ganglia or travel to other ganglia to synapse. Postganglionic axons to peripheral effectors (sweat glands, arrector pili muscles, smooth muscle in peripheral vessels) travel back up the gray rami communicantes to be distributed with other fibers of the spinal nerves (*see Figure 11-7A*). The axons of all postganglionic neurons synapse on involuntary effectors (smooth muscle cells, cardiac muscle cells, glandular epithelium).

Figure 11-7

Comparison of Sympathetic Pathways to Peripheral Effectors *vs.* Central Effectors

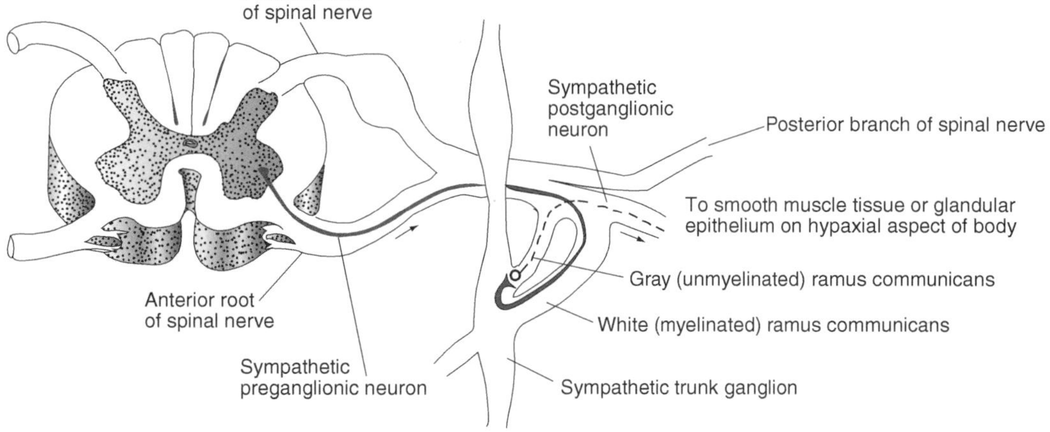

In sympathetic pathways destined for the head or other peripheral effector organs (to sweat glands, arrector pili muscles, smooth muscle in vessel walls, etc.), preganglionic neurons synapse on postganglionic neurons within the sympathetic trunk ganglia. Axons from the postganglionic neurons course back up the rami communicantes and are distributed by the branches of the spinal nerves to the various peripheral effector organs. Since the preganglionic axons are typically myelinated and the postganglionics are usually not, each ramus communicans is divided into a **white ramus** (preganglionic axons) and a **gray ramus** (postganglionic axons).

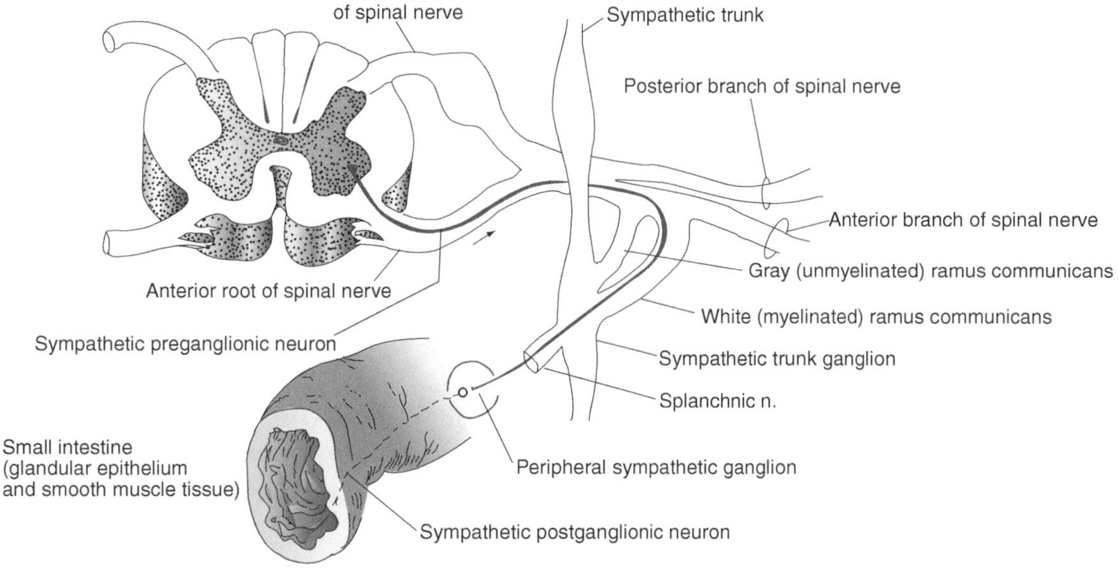

Most of the sympathetic preganglionic neurons which are part of pathways destined for centrally located effector organs (cardiac muscle, smooth muscle, and glandular epithelium in visceral organs) do not synapse in the sympathetic trunk. Instead, they pass on through the sympathetic trunks without synapsing and leave via a number of pathways including the splanchnic nerves. They continue on to other named peripheral ganglia (**celiac, superior mesenteric, inferior mesenteric,** and others) where they synapse on their postganglionic neurons. The axons of the postganglionic neurons in these pathways usually follow blood vessels to the various central effector organs.

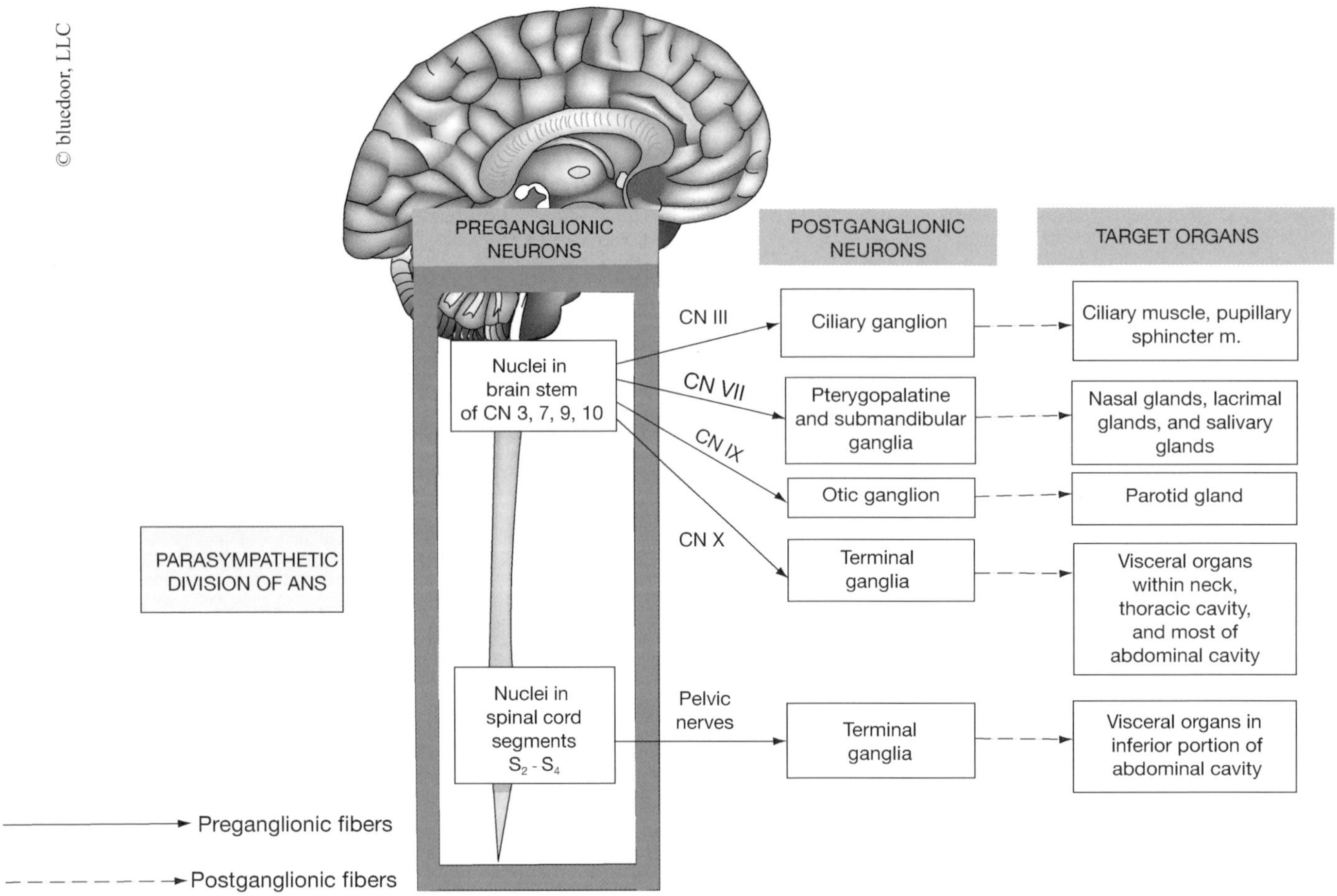

Figure 11-8

Functions of the Parasympathetic Division

Note: numerous other named ganglia occur (*see Table 11-4*).

The parasympathetic fibers associated with the **facial nerve** are distributed to smooth muscle and glands in the nasal mucosa, pharynx, and palate, to the sublingual and submandibular glands, and to the lacrimal gland in the orbit (Figure 11-8). The pre/post synapses occur in the **pterygopalatine ganglion** and the **submandibular ganglion**. Parasympathetic impulses carried by the facial nerve result in salivation, lacrimation, and secretion by the exocrine glands in the nasal and oral mucosae. The parasympathetic fibers associated with the **glossopharyngeal nerve** are distributed to the parotid gland (Figure 11-8). The pre/post synapses occur in the **otic ganglion** and the impulses result in salivation.

The parasympathetic fibers associated with the **vagus nerve** are distributed to the heart and to the smooth muscle and glands in the lower respiratory organs, and most of the digestive organs (Figure 11-8). Most of the pre/post synapses occur within the organs innervated. These autonomic ganglia, which are too small to see without magnification and are not individually named, are called **terminal (intramural) ganglia**. Parasympathetic impulses carried by the vagus nerves decrease the heart rate, stimulate peristalsis in the alimentary canal and ureters, cause bronchoconstriction, and stimulate secretion by the various glands in the lower respiratory system and in the alimentary canal.

Figure 11-9
Parasympathetic Pathways

Parasympathetic preganglionic neurons are located in the brain (in motor nuclei of cranial nerves 3, 7, 9, 10) and in the sacral part of the spinal cord. Some postganglionic neurons are located in named ganglia and some are located in unnamed terminal ganglia. Note that parasympathetic pathways are distributed centrally to deeper structures in the head, neck and trunk. There are no parasympathetic pathways to the pathways to the limbs or to superficial effectors.

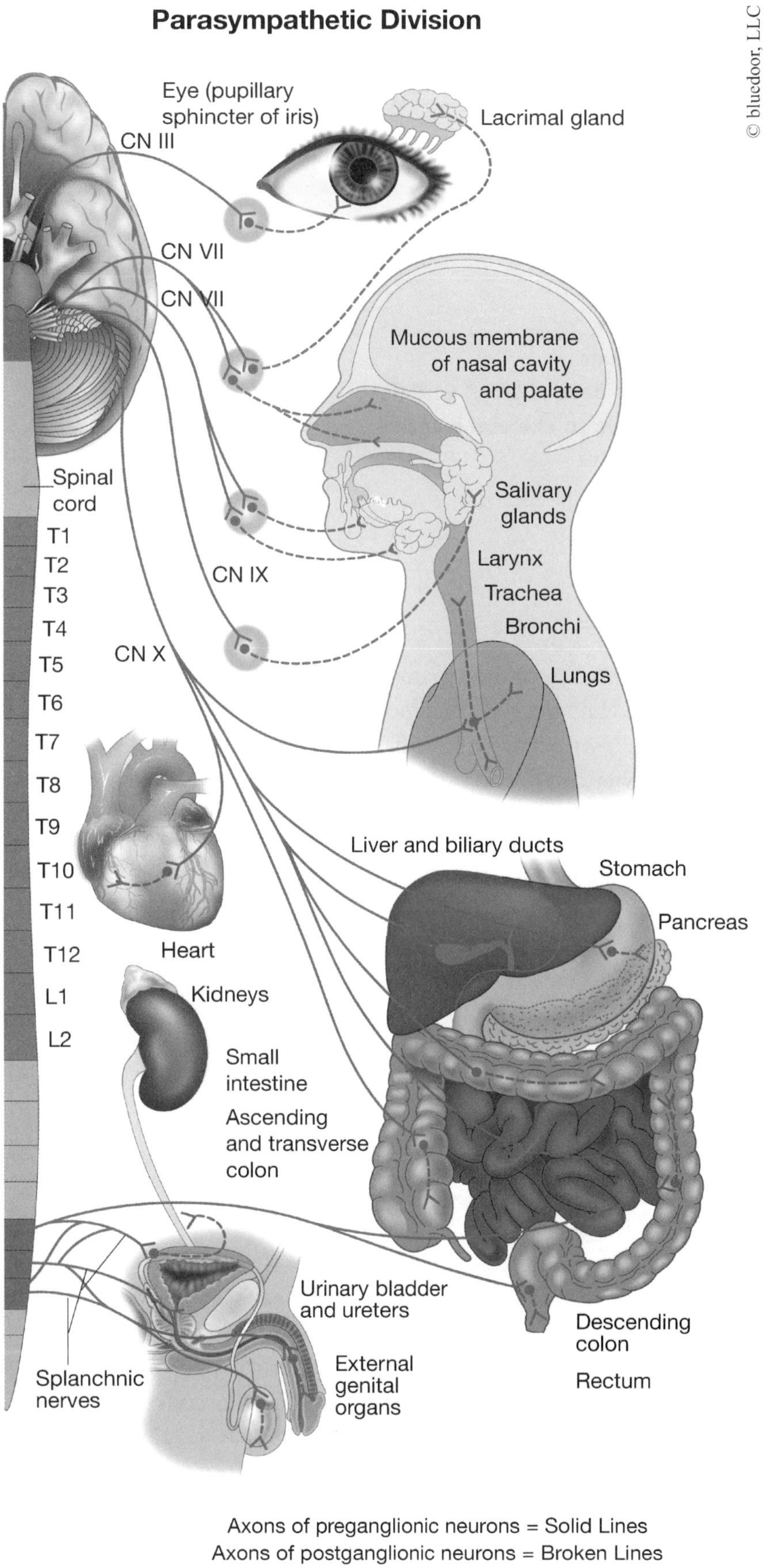

Table 11-3 Effects of ANS Stimulation on Various Effector Organs

Structure	*Sympathetic Stimulation*	*Parasympathetic Stimulation*
Pupillary dilator muscle	Contracts (pupil dilates)	Absent
Pupillary sphincter muscle	Absent	Contracts (pupil constricts)
Ciliary muscle of eye	Absent	Controls tone
Bronchi and bronchioles	Dilates	Constricts
Mucous glands	Inhibits secretion	Stimulates secretion
Heart	Increases heart rate	Decreases heart rate
Sweat glands	Stimulates secretion	Absent
Salivary glands	Inhibits secretion	Stimulates secretion
Surface and central blood vessels	Constricts	Dilates those to penis
Blood vessels to skeletal muscles	Dilates	Absent
Urinary bladder	Changes muscle tone	Stimulates contraction
Arrector pili muscles	Stimulates contraction	Absent
Intestine	Decreases motility	Increases motility
Adrenal medulla	Stimulates release of catecholamines	Absent
Penis	Ejaculation	Erection

The autonomic pathways originating in the sacral portion of the spinal cord are carried by the pelvic nerves to the sigmoid colon, rectum, urinary bladder, and reproductive viscera. The pre/post synapses occur in terminal ganglia within the walls of these organs. Stimulation of these parasympathetic pathways results in contraction of the wall of the urinary bladder, peristaltic waves which empty the rectum, and various sexual responses.

Objectives

9. List the cranial nerves that carry parasympathetic preganglionic fibers.
10. Outline the structures of the parasympathetic part of the ANS and state the effect of its stimulation on common ANS effectors.

Autonomic Ganglia

Autonomic (motor) ganglia are localized groups of postganglionic VE neurons found in the PNS. They should be distinguished from **sensory ganglia,** which are groups of cell bodies of sensory (SA and VA) neurons. Sensory ganglia are all associated with spinal and cranial nerves and are close to the brain and spinal cord. Autonomic ganglia are scattered in specific locations in the head, neck, and trunk. For purposes of discussion it is convenient to divide them into three groups: sympathetic trunk ganglia, terminal ganglia, and named ganglia. **Sympathetic trunk ganglia** are located along the left and right sympathetic trunks. Since the sympathetic trunks lie parallel and close to the vertebral column, they are often called paravertebral ganglia (= "near the vertebrae"). They are associated with sympathetic pathways—especially those distributed to peripherally located effectors. **Terminal ganglia** are autonomic ganglia found in the walls of the organs innervated. For this rea-

Table 11-4 Major Named Ganglia of the ANS

Cardiac ganglion—any of several small ganglia associated with the cardiac plexus (also known as "Wrisberg's ganglia")

Celiac ganglion—either of two sympathetic/parasympathetic ganglia found in the celiac plexus near the diaphragmatic crura. They receive fibers from the greater and lesser splanchnic nerves.

Superior mesenteric ganglion—a sympathetic ganglion closely associated with the superior mesenteric artery and with the celiac ganglion (sometimes multiple).

Inferior mesenteric ganglion—a sympathetic ganglion in the inferior mesenteric plexus near the origin of the inferior mesenteric a.

Phrenic ganglion—a small sympathetic ganglion within the phrenic plexus near the celiac plexus.

Renal ganglia—small sympathetic ganglia in the renal plexus near the origin of the renal arteries.

Pelvic ganglia—small sympathetic/parasympathetic ganglia found within the pelvic plexus.

Superior cervical ganglion—the most superior ganglion on each sympathetic trunk. Fibers from it innervate the heart, pharynx, larynx and head.

Middle cervical ganglion—a ganglion on the sympathetic trunk at the level of the cricoid cartilage of the larynx. Fibers from it innervate the heart, neck, and superior limb.

Cervicothoracic (stellate) ganglion—a ganglion at the level of vertebrae C7-T1. It consists of the inferior cervical and first thoracic sympathetic trunk ganglia and its fibers are distributed to the head, neck, heart and superior limb.

Ciliary ganglion—a parasympathetic ganglion in the posterior orbit. Preganglionic fibers from the oculomotor nerve carry impulses to it and the postganglionic fibers supply the ciliary and pupillary sphincter muscles.

Pterygopalatine ganglion— a parasympathetic ganglion located in the pterygopalatine fossa. Preganglionic fibers are from branches of the facial nerve and postganglionics are distributed to the lacrimal, nasal, and palatine glands.

Otic ganglion—a parasympathetic ganglion located in the the infratemporal fossa. Preganglionic fibers are supplied by the glossopharyngeal nerve and postganglionics are distributed to the parotid gland.

Submandibular ganglion—a parasympathetic ganglion located near the submandibular gland. Its preganglionic fibers are derived from the facial nerve (via the chorda tympani and lingual nerve). Postganglionic fibers supply the sublingual and submandibular glands.

son they are also called **intramural ganglia**. They are often microscopic but even those large enough to be seen are not obvious because they become incorporated into the structure of the organs in which they are found. Terminal ganglia are involved in both sympathetic and parasympathetic pathways. **Named ganglia** are those autonomic ganglia that are large enough to see, are structurally independent of major organs, and are not located along the sympathetic trunks. They are given unique names related to location or function (Table 11-4). Like terminal ganglia, named ganglia are involved in both sympathetic and parasympathetic pathways.

Irrespective of their categorization as terminal, sympathetic trunk ganglia, or named ganglia, all autonomic ganglia consist of groups of postganglionic neuron cell bodies along the "two neuron chain" of the ANS. These are the VE motor neurons whose axons continue on to synapse directly with smooth muscle cells, cardiac muscle cells, or glandular epithelium.

Higher Centers Which Control ANS Output

The peripheral "two neuron chain" of the ANS which extends to the various autonomic effector organs is under the control of a number of autonomic centers in the brain. The medulla oblongata has nuclei that control motor output to the effectors in the cardiovascular, respiratory, digestive, urinary, and reproductive systems. Nuclei within the hypothalamus also have control over autonomic output as do the neurons within the so-called limbic system, a group of nuclei and fiber tracts around the brainstem that includes the hypothalamus, fornix, and several other structures.

Objectives

11. Name the higher centers which control ANS output.

Clinical Considerations

The functional interactions of the two divisions of the ANS are dynamic and complex. Many pharmaceutical preparations affect one or both divisions to some degree. Some drugs which are administered for a particular effect have numerous other "side" effects on other organs and systems of the body. Agents such as *epinephrine, ephedrine, etc.* which stimulate the sympathetic division of the ANS (or block the parasympathetic division) are called **sympathomimetic drugs** because they evoke some of the fight/flight types of responses. This type of drug can be instilled into the eye, for example, to dilate the pupil so that a physician can better examine the retina with an ophthalmoscope. Asthmatic individuals use sympathomimetic drugs to dilate the bronchial passageways. Some professional athletes have been known to overdose Sudafed®, an over-the-counter sympathomimetic which is intended to relieve some of the symptoms of the common cold. It increases their heart rate, blood flow to skeletal muscles, and general aggressiveness. **Parasympathomimetic drugs** are those which cause physiologic changes that mimic stimulation of the parasympathetic part of the ANS.

Neurogenic shock is a precipitous drop in blood pressure mediated by temporary inhibition of the sympathetic pathways (due to extreme emotional disturbance) which stimulate the normal tone of the smooth muscle in vessel walls. It is one of the several types of circulatory shock and can be precipitated by psychological (emotional) states.

Objectives

12. Define sympathomimetic and parasympathomimetic.

Clinical Case Studies

Case 1—A 30-year-old secretary suffering from a severe head cold, took two Contac® cold tablets to relieve her runny nose. When those failed to have any noticeable effect she took three more two hours later and another two within another hour. She soon began to have visual difficulties, became so "cotton-mouthed" that swallowing was difficult, and noticed that her heart was racing and pounding in her chest for no apparent reason. Alarmed, she sought medical attention. Explain her various symptoms.

Case 2—A 60-year old grandmother with a history of hypersensitivity to bee stings was stung by a hornet during a morning walk through the woods behind her house. Feeling somewhat disoriented, she returned to her house and laid down. When discovered a few minutes later by her husband and son, she was gasping for air and was terrified at her inability to breathe properly. On the way to an emergency medical facility, she passed out from hypoxia (inadequate oxygen levels). Emergency medical personnel revived her with multiple injections of epinephrine (adrenaline) and she recovered uneventfully within an hour. What caused her hypoxia?

Case 3—A world class weightlifter was disqualified from a competition after traces of ephedrine® (a sympathomimetic agent) were discovered in his urine. What edge would this banned pharmaceutical give him in competition?

Points to Ponder

Some effectors (skeletal muscle tissue) are said to be voluntary. This means that we have conscious control over them. The others (cardiac muscle tissue, smooth muscle tissue, and glandular epithelium) are involuntary—implying that we are not directly (consciously) involved in their control. These involuntary effectors are the ones controlled by the ANS, the ones we don't have to think about. And thank goodness! How inconvenient if one had to consciously remember to salivate, secrete, change heart rate, *etc.* Given our irresponsible stewardship over mundane responsibilities (like the location of the car keys and billfolds), it's fortunate for us that the ANS requires so little conscious input. Otherwise, we'd continually find ourselves pushing the limits of life's biological variables. Can you imagine feeling sluggish and bloated, having gained a few pounds in a few days just because you forgot to peristalse!

The two divisions of the ANS allow easy test questions but that was probably not His intent. Sympathetic and parasympathetic—often working in opposition, but sometimes cooperatively and/or complementarily. Mostly both acting on the same organs but sometimes not. The basics are simple... two neuron chain... smooth muscle, cardiac muscle, glandular epithelium... different neurotransmitters... The distribution network is a bit complex (diagrams are complicated—almost intimidating) and the higher brain centers that are involved remain somewhat mysterious.

And why this two neuron chain? George Burns, playing God (in the movie "Oh, God!") admitted that a couple of his creations needed improvement. He cited the ostrich as an example of a silly looking bird and somewhat apologetically admitted that the seeds in avocados are too large. A single neuron from the CNS to the effector requires direct (conscious) involvement of the CNS. Because of the multiplication effect (wherein first neurons interact with numerous second neurons), a two neuron chain promotes significant response at the effectors with the minimal CNS output.

And there are the over generalizations that we make—that the parasympathetic part moves variables toward set points/ranges—is the homeostatic or craniosacral division. The sympathetic tending to move away from the status quo— "fight or flight" or thoracolumbar is what we all memorize. Pat answers to always asked questions. Sometimes the ANS plays tricks that annoy, frustrate, or even threaten life. A new groom, so excited on his wedding night that he can't consummate (bummer). A little boy, first time alone in a public restroom, has to urinate, but can't. An individual gets stung by a bee, goes into anaphylactic shock—can't breathe, dies.

The ANS interactions with urinary bladders are interesting. Bladders have different capacities. Many men can forget theirs for several hours. Some women all day (unless they are pregnant). Many of us ignore ours all night and then dump the whole collection in a brief (satisfying) moment about dawn. As bladders normally fill, slowly, continuously, a reasonable distention is required before the owner is even alerted to the situation. Even then, the voluntary over-ride allows us to ignore. More collects, more messages of greater urgency, are sent. Emphatic, if the volume is five hundred milliliters, urgent if six hundred, imperative if seven hundred. Sooner or later the owner has to relent and allow the ANS to empty the thing. First, the voluntary, conscious relaxation of the skeletal muscle sphincter. Then the involuntary smooth muscle sphincter must be relaxed. Finally, the contraction of smooth muscle in the bladder wall. Takes a few seconds. Can be hurried, if really necessary, by added pressure from a good abdominal press. But who would really want to rush a good thing! Unless, of course, someone else is beating on the bathroom door, or one hears a car approaching an isolated site selection on a back road.

Slang and Obsolete Nomenclature

UNOFFICIAL TERM	OFFICIAL DESIGNATION
sympathetic chain	sympathetic trunk *[truncus sympatheticus]*
thoracolumbar division of the ANS	sympathetic part *[pars sympathetica]* of the ANS
craniosacral division of the ANS	parasympathetic part *[pars parasympathetica]* of the ANS
homeostatic division of the ANS	parasympathetic part *[pars parasympathetica]* of the ANS
fight or flight division of the ANS	sympathetic part *[pars sympathetica]* of the ANS
feed or breed division of the ANS	parasympathetic part *[pars parasympathetica]* of the ANS
rest and digest division of the ANS	parasympathetic part *[pars parasympathetica]* of the ANS

Review Questions

1. Which one of the following does not have parasympathetic stimulation?
   A. ciliary muscle of eye
   B. sweat glands in limbs
   C. heart
   D. penis
   E. bronchi

2. Find the error.
   A. The effector organs of the somatic nervous system are skeletal muscles.
   B. In the ANS, there is a two neuron "chain" between the CNS and the effector organ.
   C. Both motor and sensory neurons are present in the somatic nervous system but not in the ANS.
   D. The neurotransmitters released by postganglionic neurons interact with neurons, muscle cells, or glandular epithelium.
   E. The brain and spinal cord serve as locations for cell bodies of neurons in both the somatic nervous system and the ANS.

3. Which item is false?
   A. Norepinephrine is secreted by sympathetic preganglionic neurons.
   B. Effectors of the parasympathetic division of the ANS are located in the head, neck, and trunk.
   C. Homeostasis is associated more with the parasympathetic division than with the sympathetic division of the ANS.
   D. The location of the parasympathetic preganglionic neuron cell bodies is the brain and sacral part of the spinal cord.
   E. Acetylcholine is secreted by parasympathetic preganglionic and postganglionic neurons.

4. Find the false statement.
   A. Sympathetic pathways to deep effectors pass through rami communicantes only once (along their course).
   B. The "multiplication effect" is one of the benefits of a two neuron chain in the ANS.
   C. There is no parasympathetic stimulation of arrector pili muscles.
   D. There are four subgroups of autonomic ganglia.
   E. The ANS is composed of parts of both the CNS and PNS.

5. Which of the following cranial nerves do not carry parasympathetic fibers?
   A. CN III
   B. CN VII
   C. CN IX
   D. CN X
   E. CN XI

6. Which statement is false?
   A. The effector organs of the ANS include cardiac muscle, skeletal muscle, and glandular epithelium.
   B. Sensory neurons are present in the somatic nervous system and absent in the autonomic nervous system.
   C. SE neurons are not found in the ANS.
   D. Synapses occur in autonomic ganglia but not in sensory ganglia.
   E. Several effectors receive sympathetic but no parasympathetic inputs.

7. Find the incorrect statement.
   A. Inhibitory impulses can prevent postganglionic neurons from reaching threshold.
   B. Smooth muscle is found within the walls of most visceral body systems, within the walls of blood vessels, at the base of hair follicles, and within the iris and ciliary body of the eye.
   C. Cardiac and smooth muscle have inherent rhythmicity, but the ANS can speed or slow its frequency of contraction.
   D. The parasympathetic division of the ANS is sometimes called the fight or flight division.
   E. Acetylcholine is secreted by the preganglionic and postganglionic neurons of the parasympathetic division of the ANS.

8. Which of the following is not a sympathetic response?
   A. sweating
   B. dilation of pupils of eyes
   C. increased salivation
   D. bronchodilation
   E. increased blood flow to skeletal muscles

9. A sympathetic pathway to a sweat gland would probably not involve...
   A. the sympathetic trunk.
   B. a named peripheral nerve.
   C. the anterior branch of a spinal nerve.
   D. the superior mesenteric ganglion.
   E. the spinal cord from T1 to L2.

10. Gray (*vs.* white) rami communicantes would best be described as consisting of ...
    A. preganglionic parasympathetic fibers.
    B. postganglionic sympathetic fibers.
    C. preganglionic sympathetic fibers.
    D. axons of SE neurons.
    E. postganglionic parasympathetic fibers.

Thought Questions

1. Why does the ANS not constitute a third part of the nervous system (along with the PNS and CNS)?

2. Why (how) does the ANS function at a subconscious level?

3. Explain what is meant by prevertebral, paravertebral, and terminal ganglia.

4. What are the differences between sensory ganglia and motor (autonomic) ganglia?

5. Most autonomic effector organs are innervated by both divisions of the ANS. How are those effectors which are innervated by only one division controlled?

6. What are the pharmacologic differences between the two divisions of the ANS?

7. Would a drug that stimulated acetylcholine receptors cause sympathetic or parasympathetic responses?

8. Since all preganglionic sympathetic neurons are located in the thoracic part of the spinal cord (T1-L2), how do sympathetic neurons get distributed to other parts of the body?

9. Do skeletal muscles receive any sympathetic neurons?

10. What is the difference in the two divisions of the ANS in regard to general areas of distribution?

11. What would be the general effect of a parasympathetic blocking agent (such as atropine)?

12. Explain why rami communicates in the thoracic region include both white and gray rami, but those in the cervical region are gray only.

13. What is wrong with the statement "The only synapses in the peripheral nervous system are those occurring in the autonomic ganglia."?

14. Is the sympathetic division of the ANS "excitatory" or "inhibitory"?

15. Which cranial nerves carry sympathetic preganglionic neurons?

16. Are there any sensory pathways found in autonomic structures?

17. Drugs like ephedrine are called sympathomimetics because they stimulate sympathetic effectors. What types of body responses would you expect after taking a drug of this type?

18. What is the basis for the saying... "I was so mad that I couldn't see (straight)"?

19. Most of the effects of the two divisions of the ANS are antagonistic to each other. Give an example where the two divisions work together cooperatively.

20. Some parasympathomimetic drugs, like muscarine, stimulate acetylcholine receptors at parasympathetic effector organs. Others, like nicotine, stimulate ganglionic transmission and also stimulate skeletal muscle cells. Compare the types of autonomic responses you would expect from these two drugs.

21. Why are parasympathetic blocking agents considered to be sympathomimetic drugs?

Answers to Clinical Case Studies

Case 1—Contac® contains scopolamine which is a parasympathetic blocking agent. By overdosing on this across-the-counter cold remedy, this patient severely reduced the output of her salivary glands, caused pupillary dilation, and blocked the ciliary muscle's role in accommodation (focusing of the eyes). With the parasympathetic input to the heart blocked, the sympathetic input caused her high heart rate (tachycardia). Scopolamine is, thus, a sympathomimetic drug.

Case 2—This individual suffered anaphylactic shock which caused severe bronchial constriction. The bronchi constrict so strongly that normal respiration cannot occur. The epinephrine injections caused bronchial dilation and allowed the patient to breath normally again. After this incident, the patient began to keep Allergin® emergency kits with her at all times and had the opportunity to use one three weeks later when she was stung by a wasp. By injecting the epinephrine immediately, she was able to prevent the bronchial constriction and averted dyspnea (difficult breathing) altogether.

Case 3—This sympathomimetic drug is closely related to the "adrenalins" and would increase blood flow to skeletal muscles as well as increase the strength of their contractions. In short, the drug is a performance enhancer.

Answers to Review Questions

1. B. Parasympathetic pathways are limited to deeper organs in the head, neck, and trunk.

2. D. Postganglionic neurons do not interact with other neurons.

3. A. Preganglionic neurons in both divisions secrete acetylcholine.

4. D. There are only three: sympathetic trunk (paravertebral) ganglia, named peripheral (prevertebral) ganglia, and terminal ganglia.

5. E.

6. A. Smooth muscle, but not skeletal.

7. D. The sympathetic division is "fight or flight".

8. C.

9. D.

10. B. The preganglionic axons are usually myelinated (white ramus).

Answers to Thought Questions

1. All of the components of the ANS are part of either the CNS or the PNS. The ANS is a functional subdivision rather than a third anatomic one.

2. The total CNS output required is very small due to the "multiplication" effect whereby each preganglionic neuron synapses with numerous postganglionic neurons. The total CNS output can be so small (because of this multiplication) that it is not even noticed—thus "subconscious."

3. These terms apply to various groups of autonomic ganglia. Those within the sympathetic trunks are also called paravertebral ganglia since they are positioned along each side of (near) the vertebral column. Prevertebral ganglia are named ganglia anterior to ("pre") the vertebral column. Terminal (intramural) ganglia are those located in or close to the walls of the organs innervated.

4. Sensory ganglia contain cell bodies of VA or SA neurons, are located near the origins of cranial or spinal nerves, and synapses do not occur within them. Motor ganglia contain the cell bodies of postganglionic VE neurons, are located in numerous places (see item 3, above) and synapses between pre-and postganglionic neurons occur within them.

5. Effector organs having only sympathetic or parasympathetic inputs are controlled by the number of impulses they receive.

6. Oversimplified, both divisions use the same neurotransmitter at the ganglia (acetylcholine), but they use different ones at their effector organs. There, the sympathetic division uses norepinephrine and the parasympathetic division uses acetylcholine.

7. In theory, both divisions would be stimulated because both use ACh as a neurotransmitter in ganglia. In reality, there are different kinds of Ach receptors (muscarinic, nicotinic) and various pharmaceuticals may stimulate both or only one.

8. Sympathetic nerve fibers extend the sympathetic trunks into the pelvis inferiorly and the vertebral nerves extend them superiorly into the head. Postganglionic sympathetic neurons are carried by all of the spinal nerves. Cephalic distribution follows the major arterial channels in the head.

9. Yes, but not to the skeletal muscle cells, themselves. The sympathetic pathways are destined for the smooth muscle tissue within the blood vessel walls.

10. The sympathetic division is distributed to essentially all parts of the body. The parasympathetic pathways are limited to the head, neck, and trunk.

11. Since the output of the parasympathetic division is blocked, the sympathetic responses would be more obvious. This is due to the fact that most involuntary effectors receive antagonistic input from the two divisions of the ANS.

12. The white rami are bundles of axons of preganglionic sympathetic neurons. All of these exit the spinal cord from T1-L2. The gray rami are bundles of postganglionic axons leaving the sympathetic trunks (and vertebral nerves) to rejoin the spinal nerves for distribution with them.

13. Those synapses are the only ones between neurons in the PNS but there are also synapses between the motor neurons and effector organs and between sensory receptors and sensory neurons.

14. Some pathways are excitatory and others are inhibitory. Sympathetic fibers to salivary glands and smooth muscle in the intestinal wall, for example, are inhibitory.

15. None of them (all sympathetic preganglionics originate in the spinal cord). The oculomotor, facial, glossopharyngeal, and vagus nerves (CN 3, 7, 9, 10) carry parasympathetic preganglionic neurons.

16. Yes, many sensory neurons follow autonomic pathways, but they are not considered to be part of the ANS, *per se.*

17. Typical sympathetic responses like increased heart rate, pupillary dilatation, *etc.*

18. Anger causes a generalized sympathetic response including marked dilation of the pupils of the eyes. This may allow so much light to reach the retinae that the photoreceptors are over driven and vision is impaired.

19. In the male reproductive system the parasympathetic division controls erection of the penis and the sympathetic division is responsible for ejaculation.

20. Nicotine should increase both sympathetic and parasympathetic output since it stimulates ganglionic transmission. Muscarine should result in only parasympathetic responses.

21. Most involuntary effectors receive both sympathetic and parasympathetic innervation and their effects are usually antagonistic to each other. Thus, a parasympathetic blocker would enhance sympathetic responses.

CHAPTER 12 *The Eye*

Chapter Outline and Key Concepts

INTRODUCTION

The eye includes the eyeball, optic nerve, ocular muscles, and lacrimal apparatus, all of which are housed in the orbit.

ORBIT

The bony hollow that houses the ocular structures is called the orbit.

Seven bones contribute to the formation of the orbit, with the largest portions contributed by the maxilla, zygomatic, and frontal bones.

GENERAL STRUCTURE OF THE EYEBALL

The eyeball is spheroidal with anterior and posterior poles, an imaginary axis connecting them, an equator, and three major layers.

The outer coat (fibrous tunic) of the eyeball includes the sclera and cornea.

The middle coat (vascular tunic or uveal tract) of the eyeball includes the iris, ciliary body, and choroid.

The internal coat (internal tunic) of the eyeball includes the lens, retina, and three chambers (anterior, posterior, and vitreous).

The retina has ten named layers and three named regions (optical, iridial, and ciliary).

The photoreceptors called rod cells respond to dim light, are associated with black and white vision (only), and do not allow crisp vision.

The photoreceptors called cone cells require moderate to bright light, are associated with all color vision (including black and white) and allow sharp visual images.

Most of the retina is a mixture of rods and cones (with a preponderance of rods).

The fovea centralis is a small central retinal area (almost all cones) where most images are projected.

The lens is suspended from the edges of the ciliary body by proteinaceous strands called zonular fibers.

The large space behind the lens, filled with vitreous humor, is called the vitreous chamber.

The aqueous-humor-filled spaces in front of and behind the iris are the anterior and posterior chambers.

CONTROL OF LENS THICKNESS (ACCOMMODATION) AND PUPILLARY DIAMETER

The lens is an elastic structure that has a natural tendency to thicken.

Contraction of the ciliary muscle allows the lens to thicken.

Relaxation of the ciliary muscle allows the lens to be pulled back into its thin configuration.

The diameter of the pupil (hole in the center of the iris) determines the amount of light that reaches the photoreceptors.

Contraction of the pupillary dilator muscle is controlled by the sympathetic division of the ANS.

Contraction of the pupillary sphincter muscle is controlled by the parasympathetic division of the ANS.

MUSCLES OF THE EYE

Four rectus muscles and two oblique muscles control movements of the eyeball.

The rectus muscles rotate the eye superiorly, inferiorly, medially, and laterally.

The superior and inferior oblique muscles also rotate the eyeball.

PALPEBRAE

The eyelids are covered by skin externally and are lined on their ocular aspects by mucous membrane called conjunctiva.

The palpebral conjunctiva reflects onto the eyeball to form the bulbar conjunctiva which covers the front part of the eyeball.

LACRIMAL APPARATUS

The lacrimal apparatus of each eye includes the lacrimal gland and its ducts, lacrimal punctae, lacrimal canaliculi, lacrimal sac, and nasolacrimal duct.

DEVELOPMENT OF THE EYE

The eyes begin development as outgrowths of neuroectoderm from the prosencephalon (primitive brain) called optic vesicles.

The overlying surface ectoderm invaginates to form the lens. Surface ectoderm also forms the cornea, conjunctiva, and lacrimal gland.

The narrow optic stalk of this invagination becomes the optic nerve and the optic vesicle forms the retina.

Surrounding mesoderm invades these structures to form the sclera, vitreous body and most of the vascular tunic.

CLINICAL CONSIDERATIONS

Lens opacities are called cataracts and increased intraocular pressure (from aqueous humor) is called glaucoma.

If the lens focuses images in front of the retina, the condition is called myopia (and if behind the retina—hyperopia).

Strabismus is non-alignment of the visual axes and may be convergent or divergent.

Physicians specializing in eyes are called ophthalmologists and medical technicians who specialize in visual deficits and their corrections are called optometrists.

Keratitis and conjunctivitis (inflammations of the cornea and conjunctiva, respectively) are common maladies associated with ocular foreign bodies.

Selected Definitions

Accommodation—changing the thickness of the lens in order to keep images focused on the retina. Nearby objects necessitate that the lens is thicker, while distant objects require a thinner lens.

Anterior chamber of the eyeball—the space between the cornea and iris. The space between the iris and the lens is termed the posterior chamber (of the eyeball) and both spaces contain aqueous humor.

Aqueous humor—the watery fluid that occupies the anterior and posterior chambers of the eyeball. It is slowly but continuously secreted by some specialized cells in the posterior chamber and is reabsorbed from the anterior chamber.

Cilia—eyelashes (*vs.* supercilia which are eyebrows). The cilia embedded in superior palpebrae (eyelids) are longer that those in the inferior palpebrae.

Cone cell—a photoreceptor located in the optic part of the retina that generates impulses interpreted as color vision. The term "cone", often used synonymously with cone cell, technically refers only to the superficial, cone-shaped end of the cell where the visual pigment is located.

Conjunctiva—the mucous membrane that lines the deep (inner) surfaces of the eyelids (palpebral conjunctiva) and then reflects onto the anterior aspect of the eyeball (bulbar conjunctiva).

Eye—the visual organ. It includes the eyeball, eyelids, and lacrimal apparatus, has several associated muscles, and is partially housed within the orbit.

Fibrous tunic of the eyeball—the outer one of the three main layers of the eyeball. It is divided into the transparent cornea and the opaque, white sclera.

Fovea centralis of the retina—a small area near the center of the posterior aspect of the retina. Essentially all of the photoreceptors located within it are cones (in contrast to the mixture of rods and cones in other parts of the optic portion of the retina).

Internal tunic of the eyeball—the internal one of the three main layers of the eyeball. It includes the lens, retina, and the three fluid-filled chambers.

Lacrimal apparatus—the lacrimal gland and the channels that convey excess lacrimal secretion into the nasal cavity. The latter include superior and inferior lacrimal canaliculi, the lacrimal sac, and the nasolacrimal duct.

Myopia—a visual deficit in which the focal point is anterior to the plane of the retina. Often termed "nearsightedness," myopia can be caused by a lens that is too thick or an eyeball that is too "long" (egg-shaped from front to back).

Ophthalmologist—a physician specializing in medicine and surgery of the eye. Ophthalmologists often refer patients to optometrists for correction of visual deficits.

Optometrist—a biomedical professional specializing in visual deficits and their correction. Optometrists are highly trained professionals but are not physicians.

Presbyopia—loss of elasticity *(i.e.,* "stiffening") of the lens associated with aging. As this occurs, it is accompanied by visual deficits related to an inability to properly accommodate.

Retina—that part of the internal tunic of the eyeball that coats the back side of the iris, both sides of the ciliary body, and lines the vitreous chamber. The iridial and ciliary parts of the retina have no photoreceptors, but the optic (visual) part of the retina has several named layers including one in which the rods and cones are located.

Rod cell—a photoreceptor located in the optic part of the retina that generates impulses under dim light conditions resulting in black and white (only) visual images. The term "rod", often used synonymously with rod cell, technically refers only to the superficial rod-shaped end of the cell where the visual pigment is located.

Scleral venous sinuses ("canals of Schlemm")—the tiny channels near the junction of the iris and cornea through which aqueous humor leaves the anterior chamber of the eyeball. These join tiny venules that return the aqueous humor to the circulating bloodstream.

Strabismus—a condition in which visual axes fail to align properly. Convergent strabismus is often termed "cross-eyed" and divergent strabismus is sometimes called "lazy-eye."

Vascular tunic (uvea) of the eyeball—the middle one of the three main layers of the eyeball. It is divided into the iris, ciliary body, and choroid.

Vitreous humor—the clear, gelatinous fluid that occupies the vitreous chamber of the eyeball. Like aqueous humor, it helps maintain the shape of the eyeball and stabilizes the positional relationships of its various components.

Etymology *Lex talionis*—**"An eye for an eye."**

accommodare (L), *to make fit*—accommodation
aditus (L), *opening for entrance*—aditus orbitalis
cataracta (L), *portcullis (barrier)*—cataract
chori (G), *distinct*—choroid
corneus (L), *horny*—cornea
fornix (L), *arch, vault*—conjunctival fornix
glaucoma (L), *cataract (of eye)*—glaucoma
humor (L), *fluid*—aqueous humor
hyalos (G), *transparent, glassy*—hyaloid canal
iris (G), *rainbow*—iris
lacrimare (L), *to weep*—lacrimal gland
limbus (L), *border*—corneal limbus
macula (L), *spot, stain*—macula
ora (L), *orifice*—ora serrata
palpebra (L), *eyelid*—palpebral conjunctiva
presby (G), *older*—presbyopia
ptosis (G), *fall*—ptosis
rete (L), *net*—retina
serratus (L), *saw*—ora serrata
skleros (G), *hard*—sclera
stigma (G), *spot, mark*—astigmatism
vitreus (L), *glass*—vitreous humor
xero (G), *dry*—xerophthalmia
zona (L), *belt, girdle*—zonular fiber

Introduction

The eye is a highly specialized sensory organ that includes the eyeball, optic nerve, and a number of associated accessory structures including the eyelids, extra-ocular muscles, and the components of the lacrimal apparatus. It transduces light into nervous impulses interpreted by the brain as the special sense of vision. Significantly more complex than the organs involved in most of the other special senses, the eye is also subject to a number of unique disorders and diseases. The sensory losses from ocular dysfunctions are more debilitating than the losses of other sensory inputs.

Objectives

1. List the major structures included in the eye.

Orbit

The eye is housed in a bony structure called the **orbit** (Figure 12-1). The orbit houses the eyeball, lacrimal gland, and the extrinsic muscles of the eye. It protects the eye on all aspects except the anterior side. The anterior opening of the orbit is the **aditus orbitalis**. It is bordered by the **orbital margin** which is subjectively subdivided into supraorbital, infraorbital, medial, and lateral borders. Seven different bones contribute to the formation of the orbit. Major portions of the superior, lateral, inferior, and posterior walls are formed by the frontal, zygomatic, maxillary, and sphenoid bones, respectively. The medial wall is formed primarily by small portions of the lacrimal, ethmoid, and palatine bones. It has a small depression termed the **fossa for the lacrimal sac**. Three major openings are present at the posterior aspect of the orbit: optic canal of the sphenoid bone, superior orbital fissure, and inferior orbital fissure. The **optic canal** is a passageway in the sphenoid bone that transmits the optic nerve. The **superior orbital fissure** is a cleft between the greater and lesser wings of the sphenoid bone. It transmits the oculomotor, trochlear, ophthalmic, and abducens nerves (cranial nerves 3, 4, part of 5, and 6) as well as the ophthalmic veins. The **inferior orbital fissure** is a cleft between the greater wing of the sphenoid bone and the maxilla. It transmits parts of the maxillary branch of the trigeminal nerve and the infraorbital vessels.

Objectives

2. Name the bones which form the orbit and the four major openings into/out of the orbit.

General Structure of the Eyeball

The **eyeball** is a spheroid organ. The center of its anterior aspect is an unmarked reference point termed the **anterior pole** (Figure 12-2,3). The corresponding point on the posterior aspect is the **posterior pole**. An imaginary line connecting these poles is the **axis of the eyeball**. A plane perpendicular to the axis halfway between the two poles intercepts the surface of the eyeball at its **equator**.

Structurally the eyeball has three named layers: fibrous, vascular, and internal tunics (coats) (Figure 12-2). The **fibrous tunic** includes the sclera and cornea. The **sclera** forms the "white" of the eye, is composed of dense, irregular, fibrous connective tissue, and is less than 1.0 mm thick over most of its extent. The **cornea** is the transparent portion on the anterior aspect of the fibrous tunic. It bulges anteriorly with a smaller radius of curvature than the sclera. The junction between the cornea and sclera is termed the **limbus of the cornea**. Histologically, the cornea has five named lay-

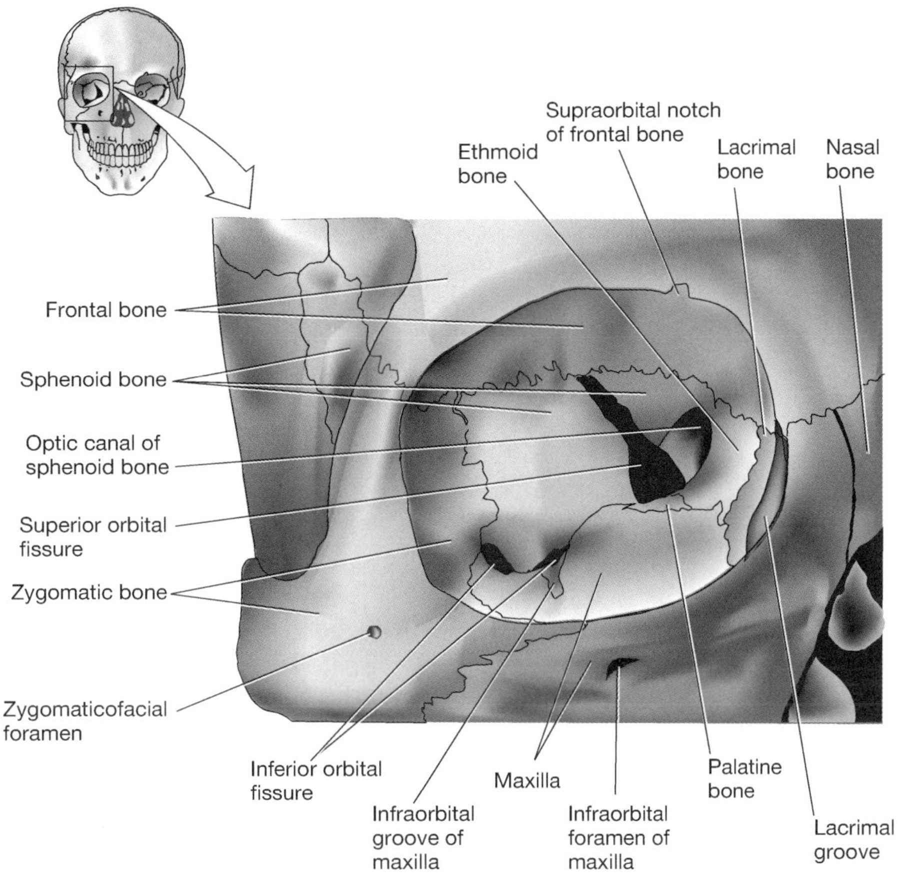

Figure 12-1
The Orbit

The orbit is formed by parts of seven bones and is penetrated by several foramina and fissures which serve as neurovascular passageways. The most significant of these are the superior orbital fissure, the inferior orbital fissure, and the optic canal of the sphenoid bone.

ers: anterior epithelium, anterior limiting layer, substantia propria, posterior limiting layer, and posterior epithelium. When viewed from the front, the cornea is slightly elliptical with a greater horizontal than vertical diameter (12 mm *vs.* 11 mm).

The **vascular tunic (uveal tract)** of the eyeball has three major components: choroid, ciliary body, and iris. The **choroid** forms the posterior part of the vascular tunic and lines most of the sclera. Histologically it has four identifiable layers: suprachoroid, vascular, choroidocapillary, and basal layers. The **ciliary body** forms a thickened ring-like structure slightly posterior to the junction of the cornea and sclera. The **zonular fibers**, which suspend the lens, attach to the margin of the ciliary body, and the ciliary body contains the **ciliary muscle** (a smooth muscle that controls the thickness of the lens). The **iris** is immediately anterior to the ciliary body. It is a circular, diaphragm-like structure with a central opening, the **pupil**, slightly medial to its anatomic center. The size of this aperture is controlled by two sets of smooth muscles (*see Accommodation*). The iris is the "colored" portion of the eye and its pigmentation varies among individuals from blue through various shades of green to brown and almost black.

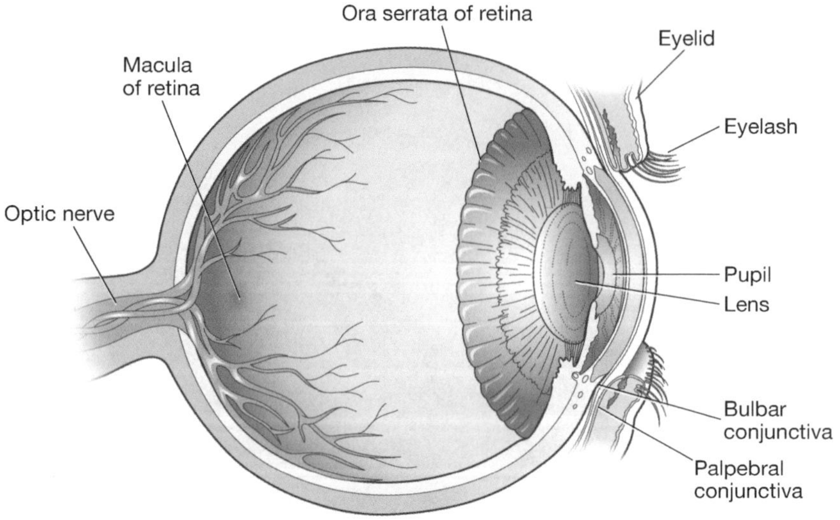

Sagittal section of left eyeball and eyelids

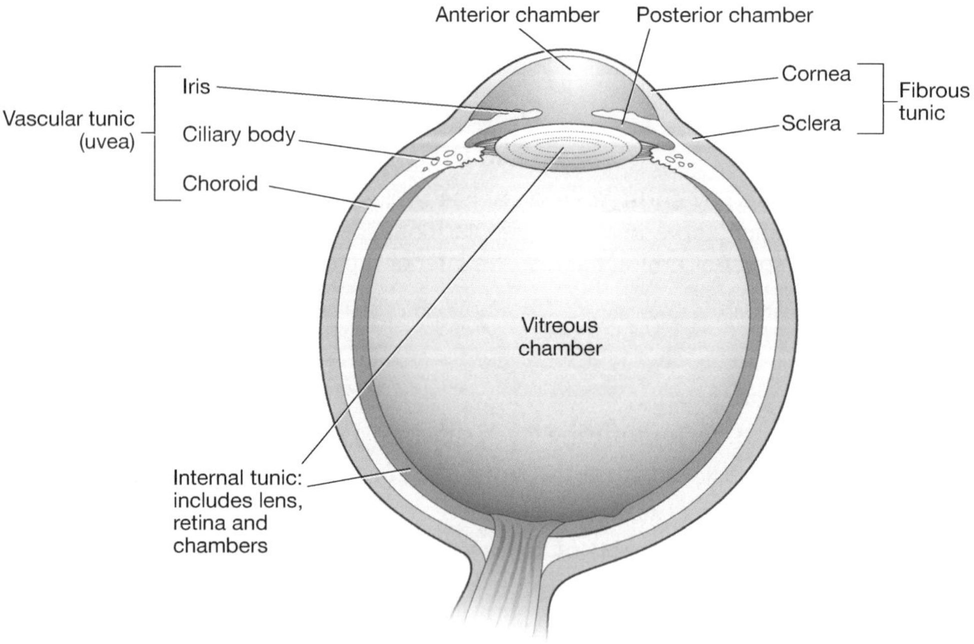

Horizontal section of right eyeball

Figure 12-2

Major Components of the Eyeball

Notice how large the vitreous chamber is in comparison to the anterior and posterior chambers.

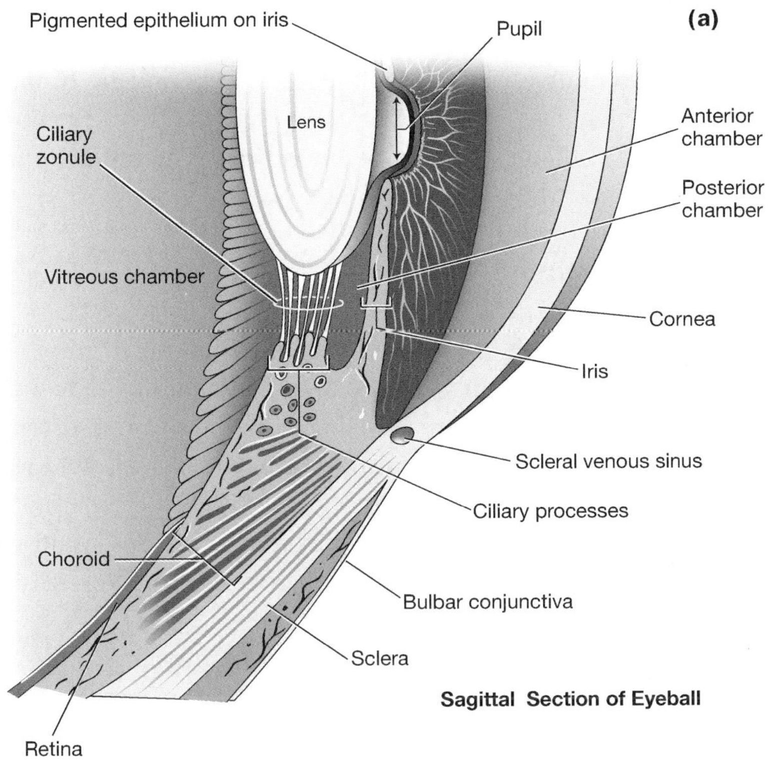

Figure 12-3
Sagittal and Transverse Sections of the Eyeball

Light must pass through several structures to reach the retina. In (a), note that aqueous humor, produced by cells on the posterior side of the iris, must flow through the pupil and into the anterior chamber before it is reabsorbed into the scleral venous sinuses ("canals of Schlemm"). In (b), note that the visual axis projects images onto the fovea centralis of the retina. Its junction with the cornea marks the anterior pole of the eyeball, and its junction with the back of the eyeball marks the posterior pole.

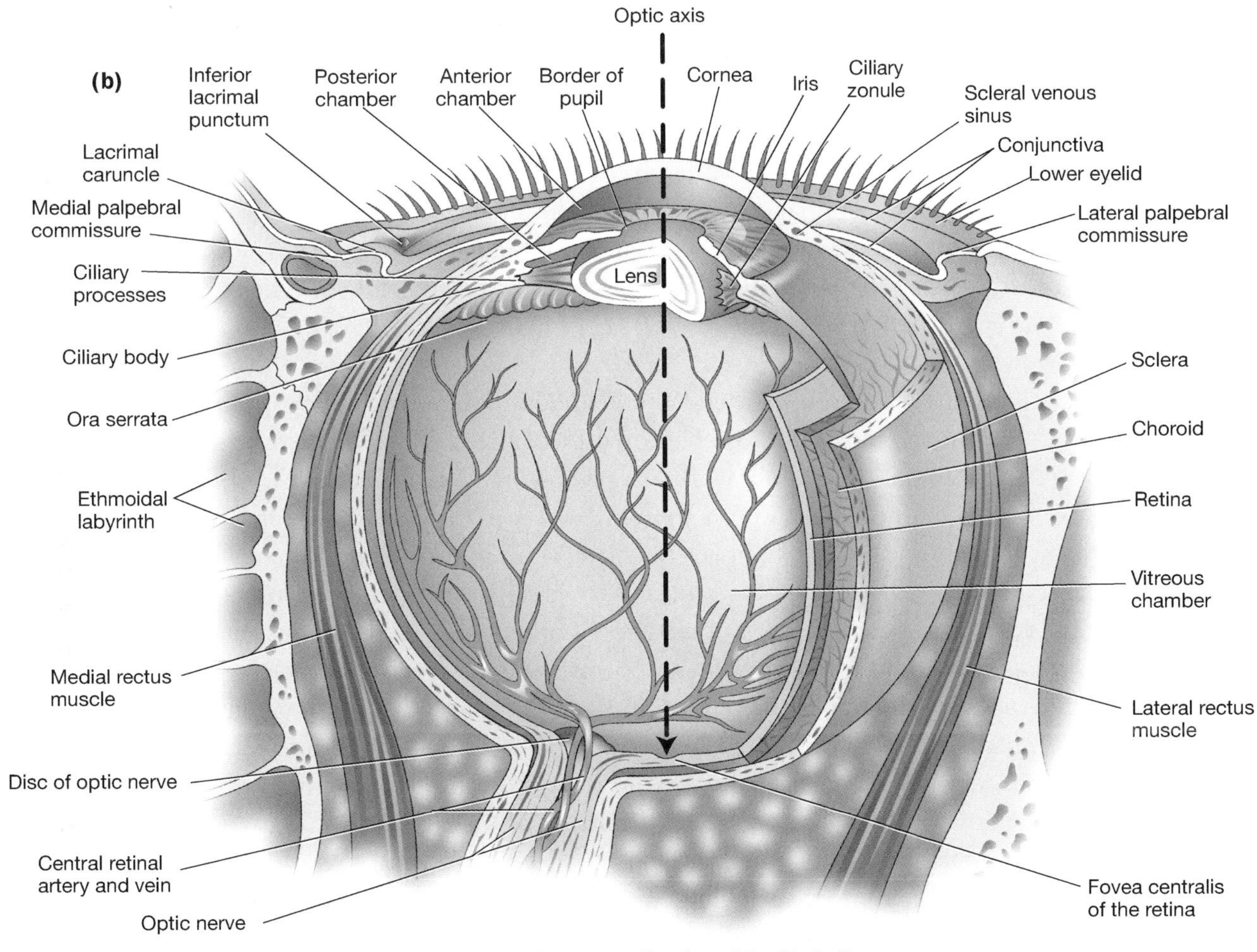

The **internal tunic** of the eyeball includes the retina, lens, and the chambers (internal spaces). The **retina** is the portion of the eyeball that lines the choroid, ciliary body, and the posterior aspect of the iris. The ciliary and iridial parts of the retina have no photoreceptor cells and are histologically termed the **blind part** of the retina. The blind part of the retina is separated from the optical part of the retina by an irregular margin called the **ora serrata of the retina**. The **optical part** of the retina consists of ten named layers from inward to outward (Figure 12-4):

1. ***Internal limiting layer:*** a membrane-like structure which lies adjacent to the vitreous body. It is formed by the bases of specialized cells called radial gliocytes ("Muller's cells"). These cells extend through almost the whole thickness of the retina and give it structural stability. The internal limiting layer is the deepest layer of the retina and the one that incoming light strikes first. (Note: as light rays pass through the retina, they are traveling from deep to superficial.)
2. ***Nerve fiber layer:*** axons of the ganglionic cells (plus specialized astrocytes, vessels, and radial gliocytes).
3. ***Ganglionic layer:*** nuclei of the multipolar neurons with which the bipolar neurons synapse.
4. ***Internal plexiform layer:*** processes of amacrine cells (*see 5 below*), axons of bipolar cells and dendrites of ganglion cells.
5. ***Internal nuclear layer:*** the nuclei of the bipolar cells, radial gliocytes (*see 1 above*), plus nuclei of some other cells (horizontal and amacrine cells) which interconnect various parts of the retina.
6. ***External plexiform layer:*** formed by the inner ends of the rod and cone cells synapsing with the dendritic ends of bipolar neurons.
7. ***External nuclear layer:*** the layer formed by the nuclei of the rod and cone cells. These form the outer one of three layers of nuclei (*see layers 3 and 5*).
8. ***External limiting layer:*** a membrane-like layer formed by the outer parts of radial gliocytes.
9. ***Layer of rods and cones (neuroepithelial layer):*** the outer, light-sensitive portions of the visual cells. Rods allow only black and white vision and function only in low light levels. Cones are responsible for color vision and require high light intensity.
10. ***Pigmented layer:*** a single layer of low cuboidal cells adjacent to the choroid that contain a pigment called fuscin. The pigmented layer of the retina is the most superficial retinal layer and is the last layer encountered by an incoming ray of light.

Light striking the retina must traverse the first eight layers (listed above) to strike the rods and cones (layer 9). The rods and cones are photoreceptors that initiate the nervous impulses ultimately responsible for vision. Rods only work at very low light levels and allow only black and white vision. Cones require more light to function, give sharper visual images than rods, are responsible for all vision at medium and high light levels, and all color vision. Three kinds of cone cells are present: some respond to red, some to blue, and some to green light. Lack or dysfunction of one or more of these cell types is responsible for various types of *color blindness*. Impulses generated by rods and cones next pass through the cells whose nuclei form the external nuclear layer, then those of the internal nuclear layer, and finally the cells of the ganglionic layer. Axons of ganglionic cells form the optic nerve which courses to the brain (Figure 12-6). These leave the retina by coursing to a central area on the posteromedial aspect that is devoid of visual cells and is termed the **disc of the optic nerve**. This is functionally a "blind spot." The **macula** of the retina is a small area (about 3 x 5 mm) located below and lateral to the optic disc near the posterior pole of the eyeball. Its central portion is the **fovea centralis** and provides the best visual acuity because it is composed almost entirely of cone cells and also because some of the inner layers of the retina are absent allowing more direct

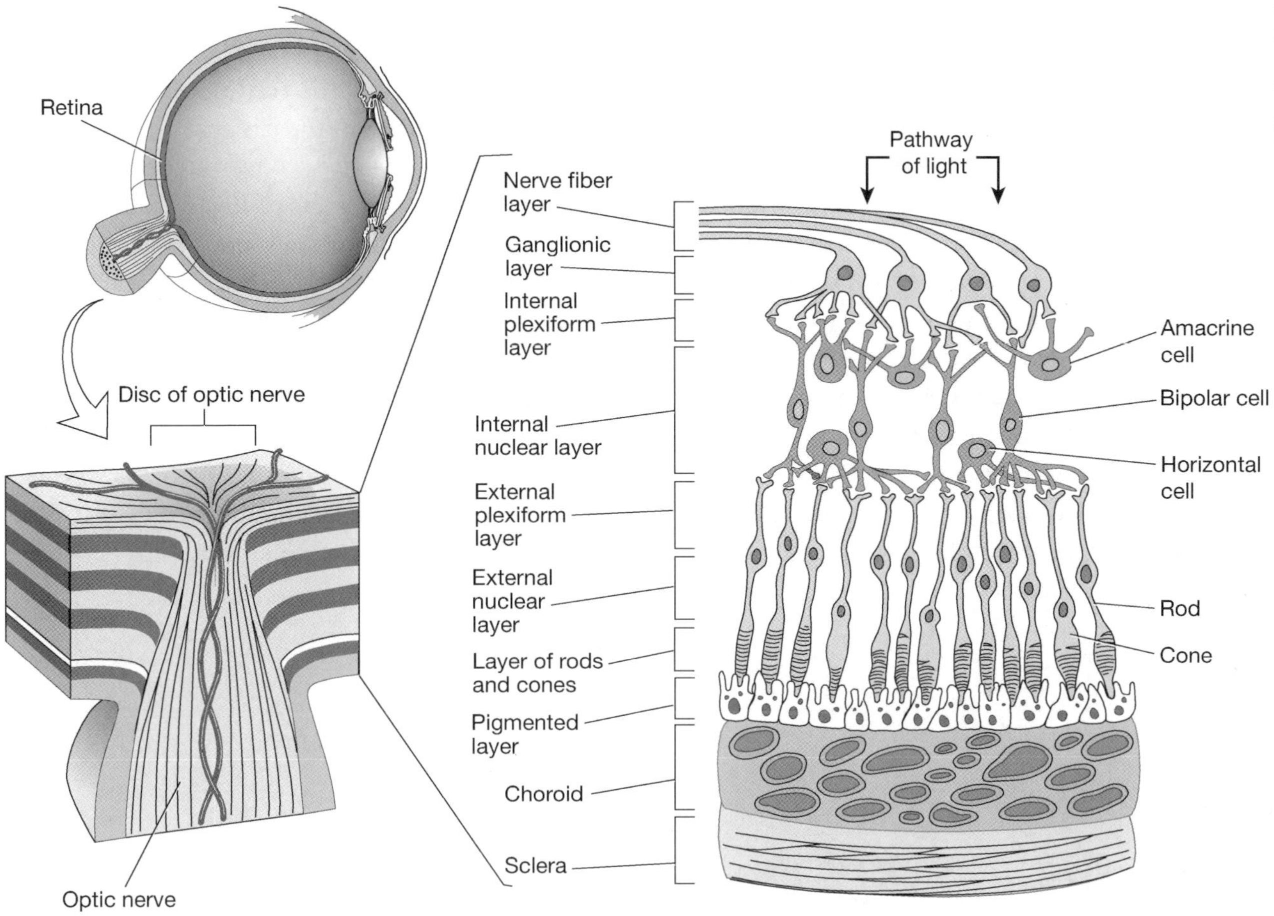

Figure 12-4

Layers of the Eyeball

Note that incoming light must pass through nine named layers of the retina before reaching the pigmented layer where it is reflected back into the rods and cones. Note that the deepest layer of the retina (internal limiting layer) and layer 8 (external limiting layer) are not represented here.

access of light to the photoreceptors. Direct (central vision) images are focused on this area of the retina. The retina is amply supplied with vessels from the choroid. These enter the posterior portion of the eye at the optic disc.

The **lens** is a transparent biconvex structure which refracts light and focuses inverted and reversed images onto the retina (Figure 12-5). It has a capsule, an anterior epithelial layer, and is composed primarily of **lens fibers** which are united by an amorphous ground substance. The fibers are formed by epithelial cells which lose their nuclei and become transparent. The outer ones are firmer and form the **lens cortex**. The inner fibers are softer and form the **lens nucleus**. For purposes of description, the lens has anterior and posterior poles, an axis (connecting the poles), and an equator. The equator of the lens is suspended from the inner edge of the ciliary body by a group of **zonular fibers** collectively called the **ciliary zonule** (Figure 12-3). These anchor to about 70 tiny projections from the ciliary body termed **ciliary processes**. The lens itself is somewhat elastic with a natural tendency to become thicker (front to back). Decreased tension on the suspending zonular fibers allows the lens to assume a thicker anterior/posterior profile (see next section). Opacity (clouding) of the lens is called a **cataract** and can be caused by a number of different factors.

The chambers of the eye include the anterior chamber, posterior chamber, and vitreous chamber. The **anterior chamber** is the space between the cornea and the iris. It is continuous through the pupillary aperture with the **posterior chamber** which is located between the iris and the lens. These chambers are filled with **aqueous humor**, a clear, watery fluid continually secreted by specialized cells on the posterior aspect of the iris. Aqueous humor keeps the anterior parts of the eyeball from collapsing. It is reabsorbed from the anterior chamber by flowing back into the venous system through a number of openings termed **scleral venous sinuses** ("canals of Schlemm"). These are located at the periphery of the anterior chamber near the iridocorneal angle. Interference with the reabsorption of aqueous humor causes increased intra-ocular pressure due to its continual production. This is clinically termed **glaucoma** and can lead to blindness if not medically or surgically corrected.

The **vitreous chamber** is significantly larger than the anterior and posterior chambers. It is located between the lens and the retina and is filled with an amorphous gelatinous material called **vitreous humor**. This is encapsulated by a transparent **vitreous membrane** to form the **vitreous body**. The vitreous body keeps the posterior portion of the eyeball from collapsing. It is not continuously produced and cannot be replaced if traumatically lost.

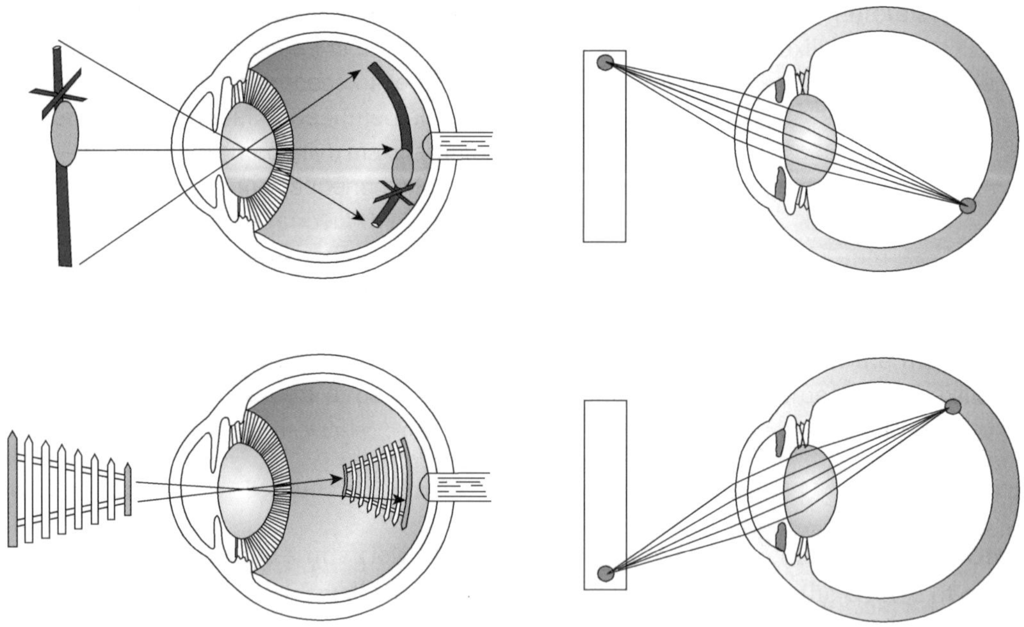

Figure 12-5

Image Inversion and Reversal by the Lens

Images that strike the retina are inverted and reversed by the lens.

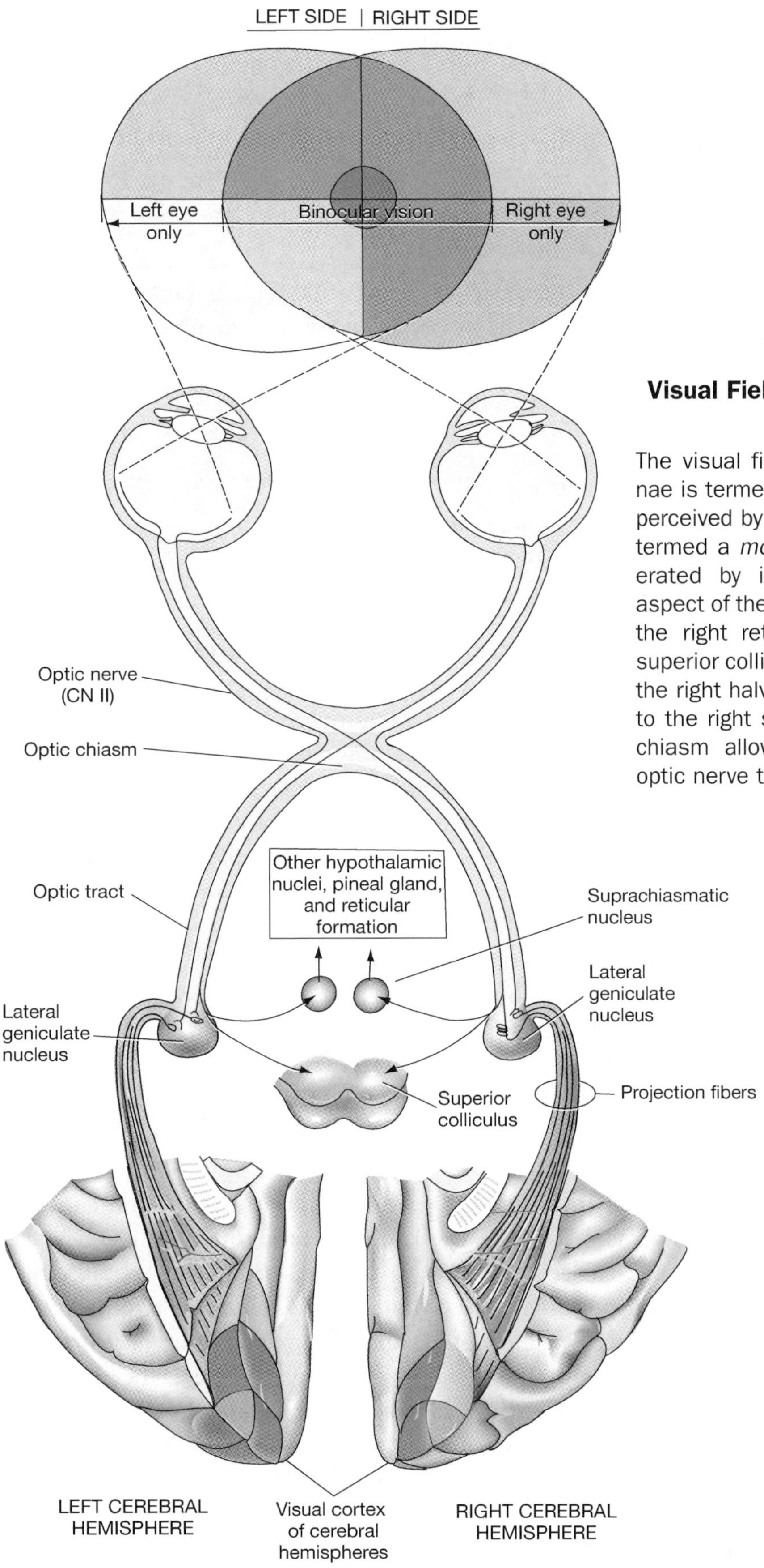

Figure 12-6

Visual Fields of the Left and Right Eyes

The visual field projected onto both retinae is termed the *binocular field* and that perceived by only one eye or the other is termed a *monocular field.* Impulses generated by images striking the lateral aspect of the left retina and medial half of the right retina are carried to the left superior colliculus. Impulses generated in the right halves of the retinae are carried to the right superior colliculus. The optic chiasm allows some fibers from each optic nerve to decussate ("cross over").

Objectives

3. Define the following ocular landmarks: anterior and posterior poles, axis of eye, equator of eyeball.
4. Name the three major layers of the eyeball, the major subparts of each and schematically represent and label them in a drawing of a sagittally sectioned eyeball.
5. Demonstrate an understanding of the retina including the number of layers that compose it and its regional peculiarities (disc of optic nerve, fovea centralis, *etc.*).
6. Compare rods and cones in regard to color sensitivity, visual acuity, and functionality at various light levels. Use this to explain why color vision does not occur in very dim light and why visual acuity is reduced at dusk.
7. Define fovea centralis and explain why looking directly at a small structure in poor light (*i.e.*, a dim star) may cause it to "disappear."
8. Discuss the production, flow, and reabsorption of aqueous humor and explain what happens in glaucoma.
9. Name the items that must be penetrated in order for incoming light to reach the rods and cones.

Control of Lens Thickness (Accommodation) and Pupillary Diameter

The lens changes anterior/posterior thickness in order to properly focus the images of nearby vs. distant objects on the retina. This process is called **accommodation** (Figure 12-7). To focus nearby objects, as in reading this text, the lens must be relatively thick. This increased thickness occurs by contraction of the ciliary muscle in the ciliary body which is innervated by postganglionic parasympathetic fibers carried by branches of the oculomotor nerve. The ciliary muscle consists of several bundles of smooth muscle fibers which form a functional sphincter muscle. When they contract, they decrease the overall diameter of the ring-like ciliary body. This reduces the tension on the suspending zonular fibers and allows the natural elasticity of the lens to cause it to "ball up" and thicken along its axis. To make the lens thinner in order to focus the images of distant objects on the retina, the ciliary muscle relaxes. When it does, the diameter of the ring formed by the ciliary body increases. This increase is due to the tension of the connective tissues initially stretched by the original ciliary muscle contraction. When these tissues assume their original position (due to elastic recoil), they cause increased tension on the zonular fibers which pulls the lens back into a thinner configuration.

If the accommodation mechanism fails to properly focus images onto the retina, a condition of **myopia** or **hyperopia** results (Figure 12-7, 8). In myopic (**nearsighted**) individuals, the image is focused anterior to the retina. This occurs because the lens gets too thick or because the eyeball is abnormally elongated in an anterior/posterior direction. Concave lenses are required for correction. Myopia is a common aging change related to elongation of the eyeball (from reabsorption of the fat located behind it). Hyperopic (**farsighted**) individuals focus images behind the retina. This occurs because the lens fails to thicken enough during accommodation or in cases where the eyeball is too short along its anterior/posterior diameter. Convex lenses correct hyperopia. Reduced ability to accommodate due to loss of lens flexibility is called **presbyopia**.

Pupillary diameter determines the amount of light that strikes the retina (Figure 12-9). To make the pupil smaller, the **pupillary sphincter muscle** of the iris contracts. This is a smooth muscle innervated by postganglionic parasympathetic fibers carried by branches of the oculomotor nerve.

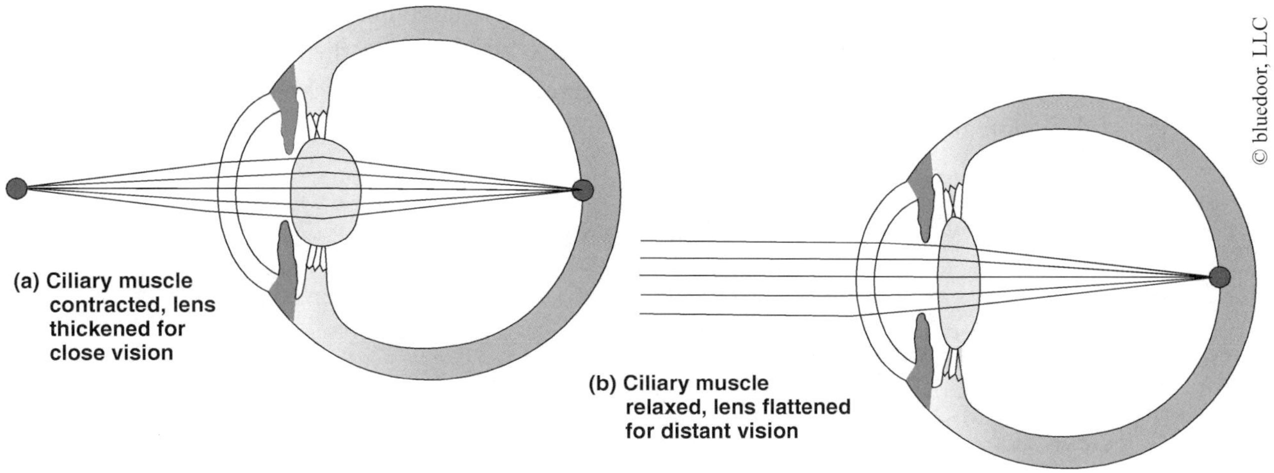

Figure 12-7

Accommodation

The lens has a natural (elastic) tendency to become spherical. When the ciliary muscle contracts, the ring of tissue in which it is embedded (ciliary body) becomes smaller in diameter. This releases tension on the zonular fibers and allows the lens to become thicker (a). When the ciliary muscle relaxes, the lens is stretched back out into a relatively thin (anterior to posterior) configuration (b) by elastic recoil of the tissues in the ciliary body. A thicker lens is necessary for viewing "close" objects (*i.e.,* reading) and a thinner lens is required to view distant objects.

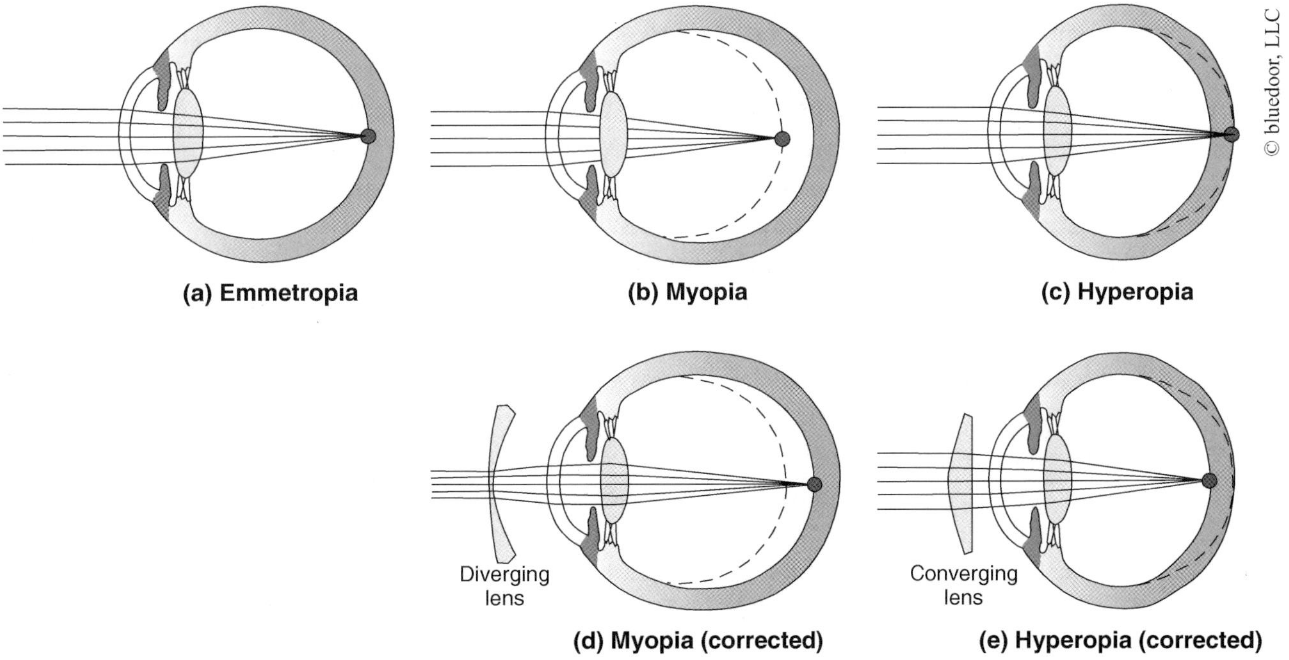

Figure 12-8

Hyperopia, Myopia, and Corrective Lenses

A normal eye (a) compared to ones exhibiting myopia (b) and hyperopia (c). Myopic (near-sighted) eyes focus the image in front of the retina and can be corrected with diverging (concave) lenses. In hyperopic (far-sighted) individuals, the image is focused behind the retina. This can be corrected with converging (convex) lenses.

It is embedded within the pupillary margin of the iris. Enlargement of the pupil is caused by contraction of the **pupillary dilator muscle** which is also embedded in the tissue of the iris. It consists of radially oriented fascicles of smooth muscle originating at the ciliary border of the iris and inserting at the pupillary margin.

Objectives

10. Explain the process of accommodation and relate it to myopia and hyperopia (and their correction with artificial lenses).
11. Show how the arrangement of smooth muscle fibers in the iris allows both dilation and constriction of pupillary diameter. Briefly discuss the influence of light level (bright/dim) on pupillary diameter.

Muscles of the Eye

The skeletal muscles associated with the eye include four rectus muscles, two oblique muscles, and the levator palpebrae superioris muscle (Figure 12-10). The **rectus muscles (superior, inferior, medial,** and **lateral)** originate via a common anular tendon near the posterior aspect of the orbit. They course anteriorly to insert into the sclera of the eye somewhat anterior to the equator. Their individual contraction rotates (tilts) the eyeball in the direction indicated by their name. The **superior oblique muscle** is the smallest of the eye muscles. After originating near the posterior aspect of the orbit, it courses anteriorly and passes through the *trochlea of the superior oblique muscle.* This is a cartilaginous loop attached to the superomedial aspect of the orbit. At this point, its tendon of insertion turns laterally, courses deep to the superior rectus muscle, and inserts on the superolateral aspect of the eyeball. Its contraction tilts the visual axis inferiorly and laterally. The **inferior oblique muscle** originates from the medial aspect of the orbit and inserts on the lateral aspect of the eyeball deep to the lateral rectus muscle. Its contraction moves the visual axis superiorly and laterally.

The **levator palpebrae superioris muscle** does not attach to the eyeball. It originates from the sphenoid bone near the posterior aspect of the orbit and inserts into the tissue of the superior eyelid. It opens the eye by elevating the upper eyelid. Closure of the eye is effected by contraction of the **orbicularis oculi muscle** (a facial muscle) which encircles the palpebral margins.

The muscles of the eye are innervated by the third, fourth, and sixth cranial nerves. The trochlear nerve innervates the superior oblique muscle, the abducens nerve innervates the lateral rectus muscle, and the oculomotor nerve supplies the remaining muscles of the eye. Students sometimes use the memory aid LR_6 SO_4Rest_3 to remember these relationships. In this formula *LR* stands for lateral rectus muscle, *SO* stands for superior oblique muscle, and *Rest* represents the other eye muscles. The orbicularis oculi muscle is a facial muscle and is innervated by the facial nerve.

Objectives

12. Name the extrinsic muscles of the eye and state the action and innervation of each.
13. State which muscle opens and which one closes the eye and state the innervation of each.

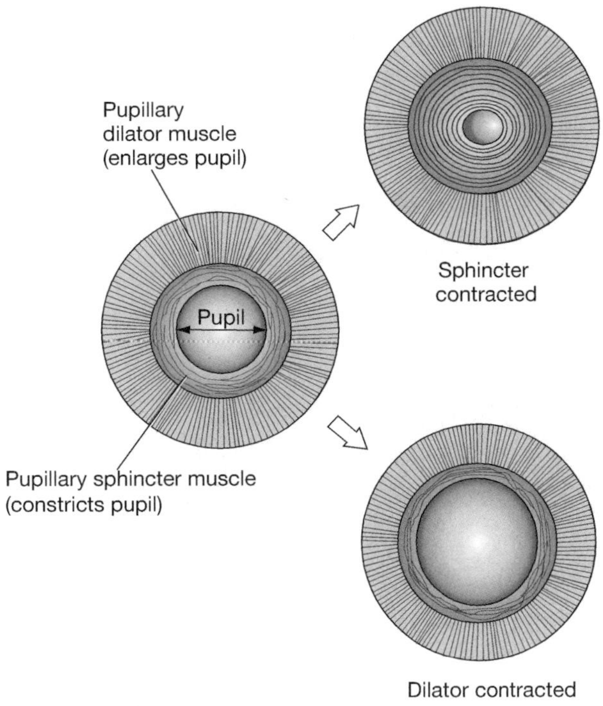

Figure 12-9

Dilation and Constriction of the Pupil

In dim light, sympathetic impulses cause contraction of the pupillary dilator muscle. These fibers are radially arranged and cause the pupil to enlarge. This increases the amount of light striking the retina. In bright light, the pupillary sphincter muscle is stimulated by parasympathetic neurons. This causes constriction of the pupil to reduce the amount of incoming light.

Palpebrae

The **palpebrae** are the superior and inferior eyelids. Dense fibrous connective tissue plates within each eyelid called superior tarsus and inferior tarsus impart some rigidity. The palpebral opening between the lids forms acute angles (canthi) medially and laterally. These are sometimes confused with the actual attachments of the lids to each other which are termed **medial** and **lateral palpebral commissures** (Figure 12-12). **Eyelashes** (**cilia**) are embedded in the anterior edges of each eyelid and those of the upper lid are characteristically longer than their lower counterparts. They have sudoriferous **ciliary glands** ("glands of Moll") and sebaceous glands ("glands of Zeis") associated with their follicles. **Tarsal** ("Meibomian") **glands** are sebaceous glands that discharge near the posterior edge of each eyelid (Figure 12-11). Their oily secretion helps to prevent lacrimal secretion from spilling over the palpebral margins.

The posterior aspect of each eyelid is covered by a modified mucous membrane called the **palpebral conjunctiva**. This reflects onto the sclera at a sharp angle called the **conjunctival fornix** to form the **bulbar conjunctiva**. On the front of the cornea, this conjunctiva forms the outer two of five named corneal layers: anterior corneal epithelium and anterior limiting layer. The potential space between the palpebral and bulbar conjunctiva is called the **conjunctival sac**. The presence of the conjunctiva and its reflection at the fornix prevents a contact lens from getting completely "lost" by wedging itself around behind the eyeball.

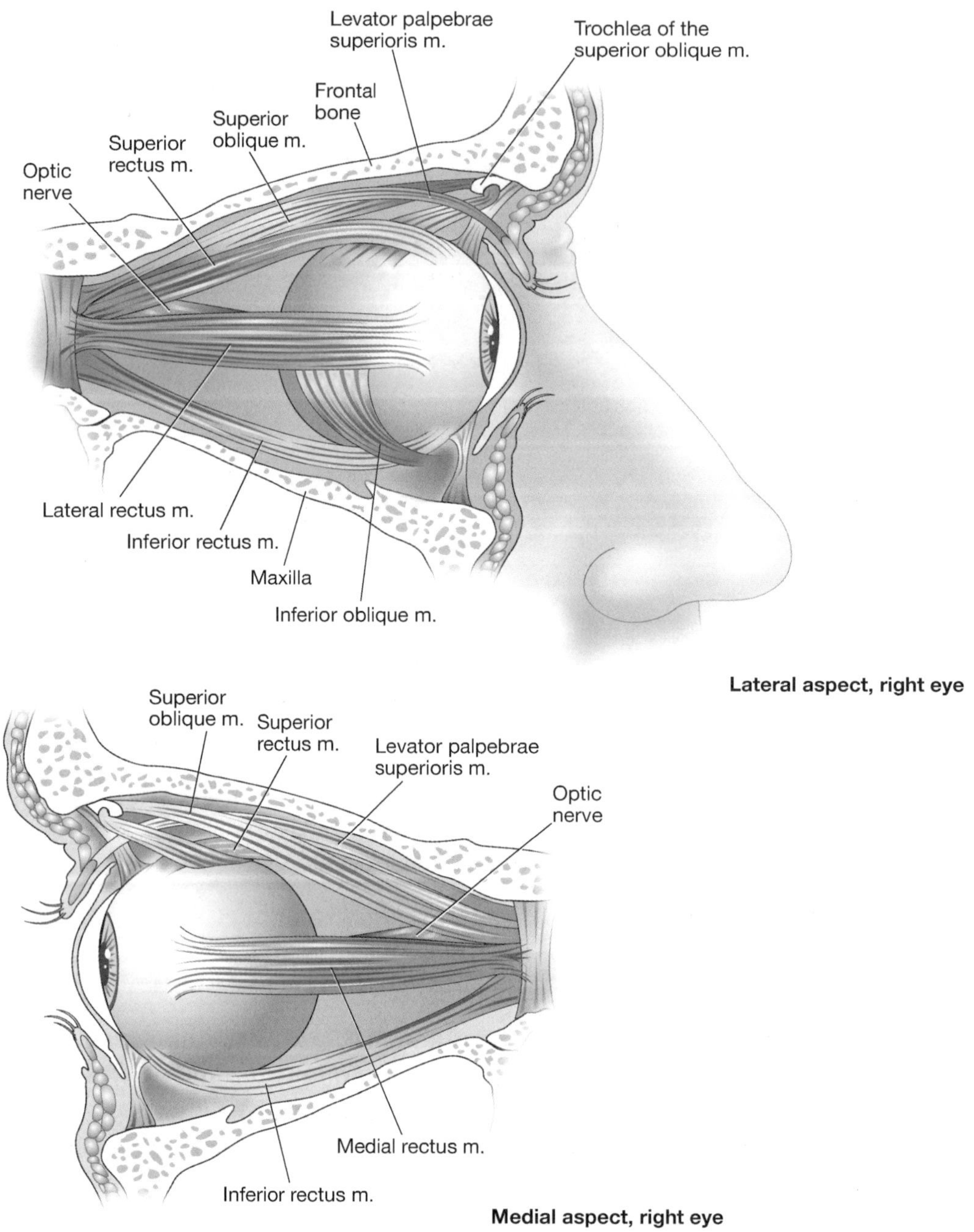

Figure 12-10

Extrinsic Muscles of the Eyeball

All of the eye muscles except the inferior oblique muscle originate from the posterior aspect of the orbit. They are innervated by the cranial nerves according to the formula $LR_6SO_4Rest_3$ (*see text*). Contraction of the various muscles rotates the visual axis in the direction implied by the muscle name (superiorly, inferiorly, medially, laterally). Contraction of the oblique muscles tilts the visual axis slightly.

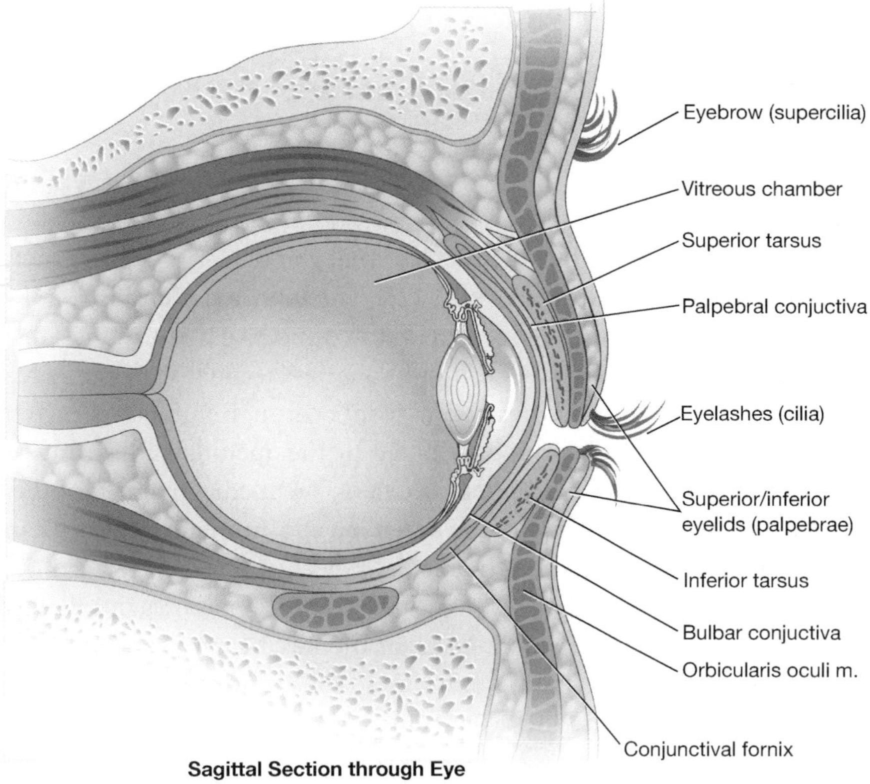

Sagittal Section through Eye

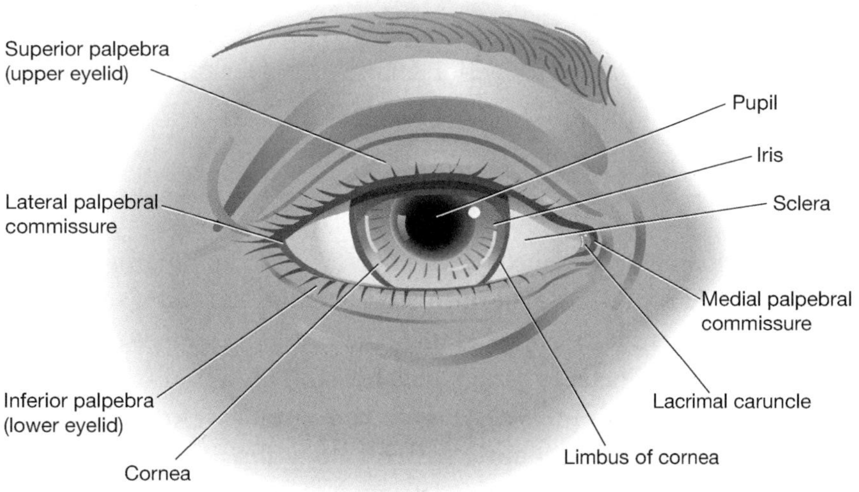

Anterior Aspect of the Eye

Figure 12-11

Palpebrae

The mucous membrane on the surface of the eyeball is called bulbar ("ocular") conjunctiva and it reflects onto the posterior aspect of the eyelids to become palpebral conjunctiva at the conjunctival fornix. The external surface of each palpebra is covered with skin. Shown but not labeled are fascicles of the orbicularis oculi muscle and the sebaceous glands called tarsal ("meibomian") glands. The superior and inferior tarsi are plates of connective tissue that stiffen the eyelids.

Objectives

14. Discuss conjunctiva and the various glands associated with the eyelids.

Lacrimal Apparatus

The **lacrimal apparatus** includes the lacrimal gland, lacrimal punctae, lacrimal canaliculi, lacrimal sac, and nasolacrimal duct (Figure 12-12). The **lacrimal gland** is a flattened exocrine gland roughly dime-sized in diameter. It is located in the connective tissue of the superolateral aspect of the orbit and continually secretes a watery fluid known as lacrimal secretion ("tears"). This fluid enters the superolateral aspect of the conjunctival fornix through numerous excretory ductules. It flows over the surface of the eyeball and is distributed by the opening and closing of the eyelids. It then enters the **superior** and **inferior lacrimal puncta** on the medial margins of the eyelids and drains into the lacrimal sac by flowing through the **superior** and **inferior lacrimal canaliculi.** The **lacrimal sac** occupies a small depression on the medial aspect of the orbit termed the fossa for the lacrimal sac. The sac drains into the inferior nasal meatus of the nasal cavity through the **nasolacrimal duct.** Lacrimation is normally evaporated from the nasal cavity. Irritation of the eye from trauma and some types of emotional states can overload the lacrimal drainage system such that tears spill over the palpebral margins and the nose "runs."

Objectives

15. Schematically represent the lacrimal apparatus and label: lacrimal gland, lacrimal puncta (superior/inferior), lacrimal canaliculi (superior/inferior), lacrimal sac, and nasolacrimal duct.

Development of the Eye

Each eye begins developing in the fourth week of gestation as an outgrowth of neuroectoderm from the prosencephalon (Figure 12-13). This protrusion is called an **optic vesicle** and remains attached to the prosencephalon by a narrow **optic stalk**. The overlying surface ectoderm thickens to form a **lens placode** and then invaginates to form a **lens fovea**. This invagination breaks free of the surface to form the **lens vesicle** and the optic vesicle invaginates around it forming **inner** and **outer layers of the optic cup**. A groove (called the **optic fissure**) along the underside of the optic cup/stalk surrounds the hyaloid vessels which supply the developing lens. The inner layer of the optic cup develops into the nervous layer of the retina and the outer layer forms the pigmented layer. The optic stalk becomes the optic nerve. The lens vesicle develops into the lens and mesoderm invades the developing eye to form the sclera, lens capsule, vitreous body, and parts of the iris, ciliary body, and choroid. Surface ectoderm forms the cornea, conjunctiva, and lacrimal gland. Mesoderm forms the muscles of the eye. The **hyaloid canal** is a remnant of the hyaloid vessels. It often breaks up to form "floaters" noticeable when the visual field has a light-colored background (as when looking at the sky).

Objectives

16. Indicate which major parts of the eyeball develop from neuroectoderm vs. surface ectoderm.

Clinical Ophthalmology

Nearsightedness, farsightedness, glaucoma, and cataracts have already been mentioned. **Strabismus** is a condition in which the visual axes do not converge on the same object. This is termed convergent strabismus in cross-eyed individuals and divergent strabismus (lazy eye) if the affected eye is rotated laterally. Surgical correction is often required and involves lengthening or shortening of eye muscles. **Retinal detachment** is caused by separation of the retina from the surrounding tissues. It may be caused by trauma, neoplasia, or degenerative changes and is sometimes surgically correctable. **Astigmatism** is an irregular curvature in the cornea or lens which results in distortion of the visual image. A number of different types have been identified depending on the locus of the irregular curvature and the type of resulting distortion. Astigmatism is often treated by corrective lenses. A **stye** is a localized infection involving the follicle of an eyelash. It is a painful but not serious condition that is readily treatable by medical intervention. **Blindness** is a reduced or lack of visual perception related to developmental anomalies, trauma, or diseases of the eyeballs, optic nerves, or occipital lobes of the cerebral hemispheres. **Total blindness** (complete absence of light

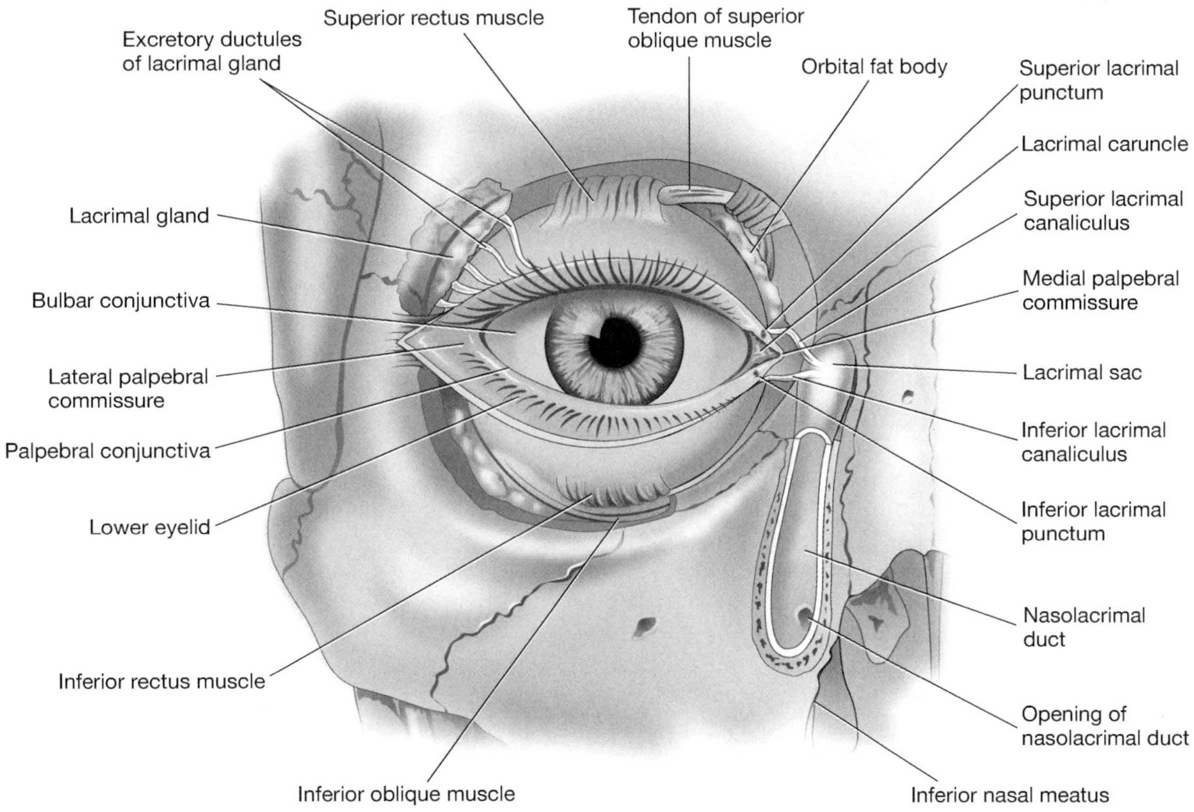

Figure 12-12

Lacrimal Apparatus

Tears (lacrimal secretions) produced by the lacrimal gland flow freely over the surface of the eyeball and enter the superior lacrimal punctum or the inferior lacrimal punctum. Lacrimation is then transported to the lacrimal sac via the superior and inferior lacrimal canaliculi. From the lacrimal sac, tears drain through the nasolacrimal duct into the inferior nasal meatus of the nasal cavity located below the inferior nasal concha.

perception) is distinguished from **legal blindness** which is quantitative loss of visual acuity defined by statute. In most parts of the United States, an individual is legally blind if neither eye has better than 20/20 vision (after correction) and the visual field is only 20 degrees or less. The term **night blindness** refers to abnormally poor vision in dim light conditions, and **snow blindness** is temporary partial blindness related to exposure to exceptionally bright light—often caused by the glare of the sun upon snow. **Color blindness** is due to a congenital lack of or nonfunction of one or more of the three types of cones in the retina. Individuals with normal color vision have all three types of cones and are called **trichromats.** Those with only two of the cone types are called **dichromats.** Dichromats who are missing red cones have **protanopia**, and those with dysfunctional green cones have **deuteranopia**. Both of these latter types of color blindness are X-linked traits affecting about one percent of males and rarely occurring in females. Dichromasy involving blue cones is called **tritanopia** and is very rare. Individuals with only one functional type of cones are called **monochromats** and perceive only black, white and shades of gray.

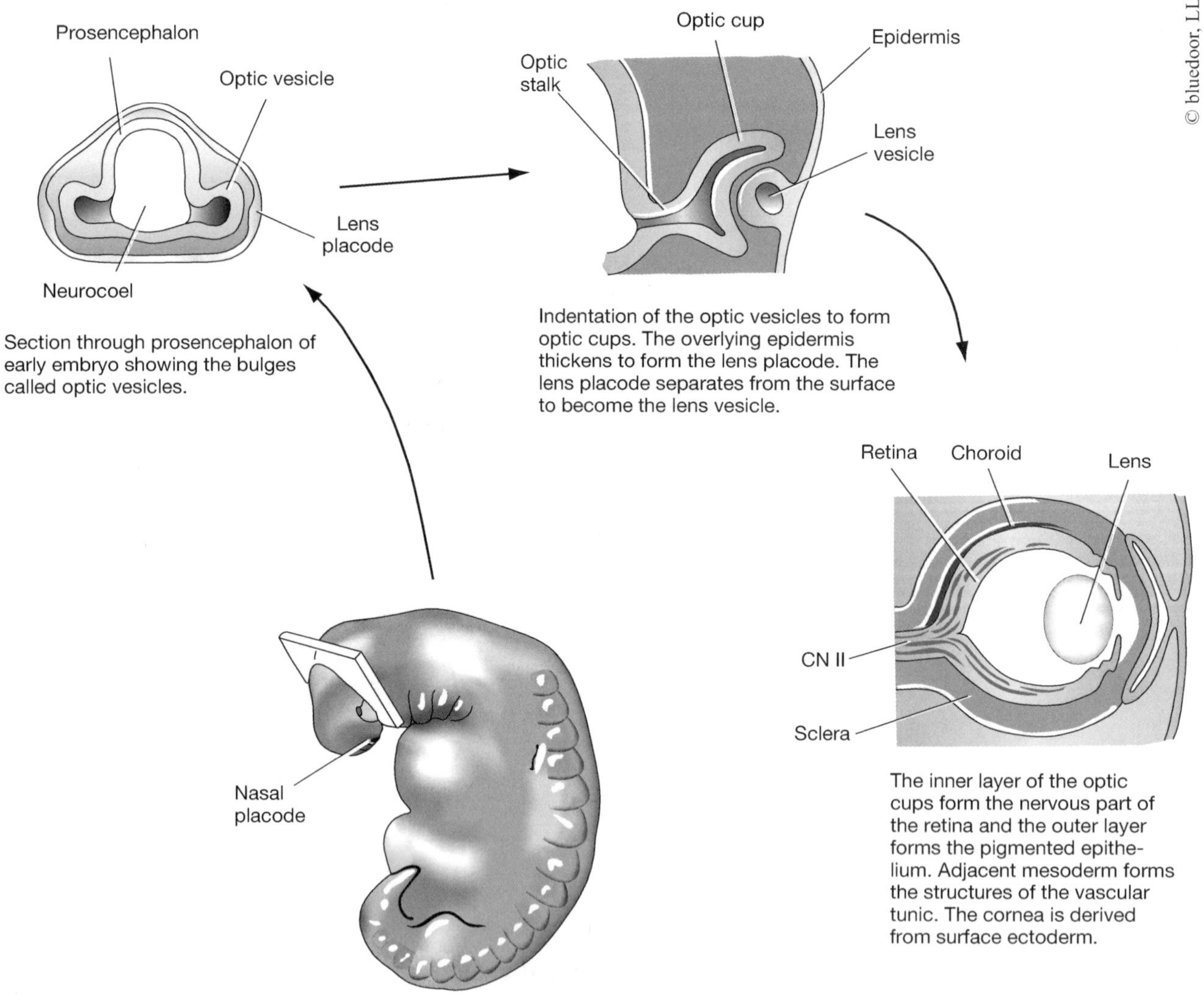

Figure 12-13

Development of the Eye

Inflammatory processes of various ocular structures are given specific names. **Conjunctivitis** is inflammation of the conjunctiva and may result from traumatic irritation ("something in" the eye), sunburn, or infectious organisms. If caused by microbial infection, conjunctivitis is often termed "pinkeye." **Keratitis** is an inflammation of the cornea. It may be caused by severe conjunctivitis and may also occur as a secondary complication of a systemic disease.

Radial keratotomy is a surgical procedure used to change the focal length of the eyeball as a treatment for visual deficits. Several shallow incisions are made into (but not through) the cornea with a laser beam to change its anterior convexity. The pattern of the incisions can be varied such that healing will either increase or decrease the corneal curvature. Whole corneas can be transplanted to replace those severely scarred by keratitis or keratoconjunctivitis.

Drooping of an upper eyelid (usually caused by dysfunction of the oculomotor nerve) is called **ptosis**. Damage to a facial nerve results in an inability to close the ipsilateral eye due to loss of innervation of the orbicularis oculi muscle. This leads to drying of the cornea (called **xerophthalmia** or **keratitis sicca**), irritation, and excessive lacrimation.

The medical speciality related to specialized training in diseases and surgery of the eye is called **ophthalmology**. Ophthalmologists must first go to medical school and then, after graduation, complete extensive (several years of) additional training. **Optometrists**, on the other hand, are concerned primarily with visual deficits and correction of them with lenses (glasses or contacts). Optometrists are not physicians, but ophthalmologists and other physicians often refer patients to them for corrective lenses. One of the instruments used to examine eyes is called an **ophthalmoscope**. In order to get a good view of the retina, the pupil must be enlarged by dilating it with sympathomimetic drugs. This allows a clear view of the retinal vessels. These are branches of the ophthalmic artery and vein that enter the back of the eyeball after coursing to it with the optic nerve. Since extensions of meninges surround the optic nerve (and these vessels), increased pressure in the cerebrospinal fluid inhibits venous return from the eyeball. This causes edema of the retina detected by swelling (bulging) of the disc of the optic nerve and is important in the evaluation of concussions.

Objectives

17. Define strabismus (convergent/divergent), astigmatism, ophthalmology, optometry, keratitis, cataract, presbyopia, conjunctivitis, and xerophthalmia.

Clinical Case Studies

Case 1—A three-year-old girl was taken to the emergency room after being struck in the eye by a spike nail thrown by her older brother. There was a visible hole at her corneoscleral junction and part of her iris protruded from it. She was rushed into emergency surgery where an ophthalmologist replaced her iris and closed the hole with tiny sutures. The wound healed uneventfully. What chance was the child given of having normal vision after an incident of this type?

Case 2—A college student woke up in severe pain after going to bed without removing his contact lenses. His vision was blurred and his pain was so severe that he sought medical help. What caused his pain?

Case 3—Two junior high school boys suffered severe pain in their eyes and visual impairment after playing at a construction site. No external trauma was evident and when questioned, they mentioned that they had watched a welder at work for several minutes. Could there be a connection between their clinical condition and the welding that they watched?

Points to Ponder

Man's retina has an estimated 125 million rods and 4-7 million cones. In the central retinal area called the fovea, the cones are solidly packed in at a concentration of about 120,000 per square millimeter. The rest of the visual part of the retina is a mixture of rods and cones. Rods function in dim light and cones work in moderate to bright light. When the photoreceptors are stimulated, we say that the rods give us black-and-white-vision and the cones give us color. In reality, of course, rods and cones simply initiate nervous impulses. The impulses, carried to the brain, are interpreted as black and white or color vision.

The chemical reaction that light invokes is the same in rods and cones. The reactive photochemical is called 11-cis-retinal (a derivative of beta carotene). Retinal is combined with proteins called opsins (scotopsin in rods and photopsin in cones) to form visual pigments. When struck by light, the cis-retinal is converted to trans-retinal, which initiates a chain of reactions resulting in the generation of a nervous impulse. The trans-retinal is then converted back to its cis form and reused (the eyes have been into recycling for millennia longer than the population as a whole).

So, back to the dim-light *vs.* bright-light and the black-and-white *vs.* color thing... Rods are considered to be more sensitive than cones because they do the cis-to-trans conversion at very low light levels. In bright light, the rods can't recycle the trans-retinal back to the cis form. Consequently, rods are said to be "bleached out" by bright light and become non-functional. Everyone knows from personal experience that upon entering a very dimly lit area, a few moments are required to become dark adapted. This time is required for the rods to recycle the trans-retinene back to the cis form (which they can do in a dimly lit environment). Unfortunately, in very dim light, the cones become non-functional. (They require higher light levels to trigger the cis-trans conversion). (Very) dim light vision is thus limited to rods and the brain interprets impulses initiated by rods as black-and-white images. (Incidentally, neither rods nor cones work in absolute darkness).

Cones contain the same photopigment as rods. They are less sensitive than rods in that they require higher light intensities to function. Additionally, in the bright light they need to trigger the cis-trans reaction, cone cells are still able to convert the trans form back to the cis. Therefore, cones continue to function in bright light (unlike the rods which fizzle). Cones are divided into three categories: blue, green, and red. Those that respond to blue light (optimally absorbing light in the blue region of the visible spectrum) are called blue cones. But those in the business recognize that the cones aren't blue and their impulses aren't blue either. Brain interpretation of the impulses they generate gives us the blue. Green cones and red cones absorb light in their namesake regions of the visible spectrum. The differences in the colors of light to which the three cone cell types respond is related to the particular proteins associated with the photopigment. These different proteins explain the three color categories of cone cells by determining which colors of light are absorbed by the cell and trigger the cis-trans conversion (to initiate the impulse).

"You have pretty eyes," he said. "Size, cilia, distance apart, how they sit in my orbits, or the color reflected through my contacts?" she queried back. Dejected, he went back to dating the girl next door and swore off pre-meds for good. So there it is—in black and white—and in color.

Slang and Obsolete Nomenclature

UNOFFICIAL TERM	OFFICIAL DESIGNATION
uvea	uveal tract *[tractus uvealis]*
canal of Schlemm	scleral venous sinus *[sinus venosus sclera]*
nervous (neural) tunic of eyeball	internal tunic of eyeball *[tunica interna bulbi]*
radial muscle of iris	pupillary dilator muscle *[musculus dilator pupillae]*
pupillary constrictor muscle of iris	pupillary sphincter muscle *[musculus sphincter pupillae]*
circular muscle of iris	pupillary sphincter muscle *[musculus sphincter pupillae]*
suspensory ligament of eye	zonular fibers/ciliary zonule *[fibrae zonulares/zonula ciliares]*
white of eye	sclera *[sclera]*
posterior cavity (chamber) of eye	vitreous chamber *[camera vitrea]*
fovea	fovea centralis *[fovea centralis]*
optic disc	disc of optic nerve *[discus nervi optici]*
blind spot	disc of optic nerve *[discus nervi optici]*
bony orbit	orbit *[orbit]*
orbital fat	orbital fat body *[corpus adiposum orbitae]*
macula lutea	macula *[macula]*
optic chiasma	optic chiasm *[chiasma opticum]*
ocular conjunctiva	bulbar conjunctiva *[tunica conjunctiva bulbaris]*
tear gland	lacrimal gland *[glandula lacrimalis]*
meibomian glands	tarsal glands *[glandulae tarsales]*
glands of Zeis	sebaceous conjunctival glands *[glandulae sebaceae conjunctivales]*
glands of Moll	ciliary conjunctival glands *[glandulae ciliares conjunctivales]*

Review Questions

1. Which item is not part of the vascular tunic of the eye?
   A. ciliary muscle
   B. lens
   C. iris
   D. choroid
   E. ciliary body

2. Which ocular muscle is mismatched with its function?
   A. ciliary muscle—contraction causes the lens to become thinner
   B. pupillary sphincter m.—contraction reduces the amount of light that strikes the retina
   C. lateral rectus muscle—contraction of the left one rotates the left eyeball to the left
   D. medial rectus muscle—vigorous simultaneous contraction of the left and right muscles causes (temporary) convergent strabismus
   E. If all of the above are correctly matched, choose this response.

3. Which statement regarding the retina is false?
   A. It has ten named layers and the photoreceptors are one of the outermost (superficial) layers.
   B. To read this question, the active photoceptors are rods.
   C. Most of the optic part of the retina contains a mixture of rods and cones.
   D. The retina extends onto the posterior aspects of the ciliary body and iris.
   E. The cones are less sensitive to light than rods.

4. Which statement regarding the lens is false?
   A. It has a natural tendency to thicken ("ball up").
   B. It is suspended from the edge of the iris by zonular fibers.
   C. It is positioned between the posterior chamber and the vitreous chamber.
   D. It is positioned between aqueous humor and vitreous humor.
   E. Opacity of the lens is called a cataract.

5. Which item does not have to be traversed by light passing into the eyeball enroute to the rods and cones?
   A. several layers of the retina
   B. aqueous humor
   C. cornea
   D. vitreous humor
   E. If all of the above are traversed by light enroute to the rods and cones, choose this response.

6. Aqueous humor is not found in the...
   A. anterior chamber of the eyeball.
   B. scleral venous sinuses.
   C. posterior chamber of the eyeball.
   D. pupil of the iris.
   E. If aqueous humor is present in all of the above, choose this response.

7. Which ocular condition is misdefined?
   A. glaucoma—increased extraocular pressure
   B. presbyopia—loss of elasticity of the lens
   C. diplopia—double vision
   D. hyperopia—farsightedness
   E. myopia—condition in which images are brought to a focal point anterior to the retina

8. Which structure belonging to the lacrimal apparatus would not have to be encountered by a droplet of lacrimal secretion enroute to the inferior nasal meatus?
   A. lacrimal gland
   B. conjunctiva
   C. lacrimal sac
   D. inferior lacrimal punctum
   E. nasolacrimal duct

9. Which cranial nerve has no ocular distribution?
   A. optic nerve
   B. CN I

C. trigeminal nerve
D. CN VII
E. abducens nerve

10. Which item would not be included in the internal tunic of the eye?
    A. pigmented layer of the retina
    B. photoreceptors
    C. anterior chamber
    D. disc of the optic nerve
    E. ciliary body

Thought Questions

1. Why are rod and cone cells oriented (pointed) away from the incoming light that enters the eye?

2. Explain how myopia can result from either an eyeball that is too "long" or a lens that remains too thick.

3. Why are periodic eye exams recommended even for individuals with no visual impairment or known eye problems?

4. Explain why a crying individual usually has a runny nose.

5. Why are images in one's peripheral vision not as sharp as those in the central visual field (at normal light levels)?

6. What keeps contact lenses in place and what prevents them from slipping all the way around behind the eyeball when they are displaced?

7. A very dim star often "disappears" when one gazes directly at it, but "reappears" in the peripheral visual field when one's visual axes are slightly shifted. Why?

8. Which two anatomic features of the fovea centralis contribute to the visual clarity of the images projected thereon?

9. Discuss the pupillary light reflex.

10. Why is loss of the vitreous humor more serious than loss of aqueous humor?

11. How does contraction of the ciliary muscle cause (allow) the lens to thicken?

12. Compare and contrast the roles of rod cells and cone cells in the visual process.

13. Discuss the functions of aqueous and vitreous humor.

14. Explain the phrase "so mad that he couldn't see straight."

15. In addition to the photoreceptors, how many other layers of cells are found in the 10 layers of the retina?

16. Is the retina limited to the vitreous chamber?

17. What is the physical relationship of the "blind spot" to the fovea centralis?

18. In theory, which eye muscles could be eliminated without seriously impairing eye movements?

19. How would unilateral dysfunction of an abducens nerve affect the eyes?

20. What special purpose do sebaceous glands located at the margins of the eyelids serve?

21. What three fluids must be traversed by light which reaches the retina?

Answers to Case Studies

Case 1—The iris was not damaged and since the wound occurred at the corneoscleral junction, the tiny scar that resulted was not in the patient's line of vision. This wound caused no long term effects and was not a factor in the child's less than perfect vision.

Case 2—Some kinds of contact lenses cannot be worn overnight because they interfere with the diffusion of oxygen into the superficial layers of the cornea. Without oxygen, some of the cells in these layers die. Chemicals released by the dead cells cause the pain.

Case 3—The ultraviolet wavelengths of light that are produced by a welding arc can "burn" the retina. That is why welders wear heavy, dark, eye shields when they work.

Answers to Review Questions

1. B. The lens belongs to the internal tunic.

2. A.

3. B. Rods are non-functional at moderate to bright light levels because they cannot regenerate cis-retinal.

4. B. The lens is suspended from the edge of the ciliary body.

5. E.

6. E.

7. A. Glaucoma is increased intra-ocular pressure.

8. D. The droplet could be transported to the lacrimal sac by the superior lacrimal punctum and superior lacrimal canaliculus.

9. B. CN I is the olfactory nerve.

10. E. The ciliary body is one of the three parts of vascular tunic (uveal tract).

Answers to Thought Questions

1. Light apparently passes through the layer of rods and cones, strikes the pigmented layer, and then is reflected back into the photoreceptors. It is not clear if the receptors get "double" stimulated by this process as some have suggested.

2. In myopia, the lens brings light rays to a focal point in front of the retina (rather than right on the retina). If the lens were not as thick, the focal point of the light rays would be further posterior (toward the retina). Likewise if the eyeball were "shorter" overall from front to back, the retina and focal point of the light rays could intersect. Elongation of the eyeball is a normal aging phenomenon due to loss of fat in the posterior aspect of the orbit. That is why so many older people are myopic.

3. Increased intra-ocular pressure (glaucoma) can cause serious eye damage before the individual is aware of the problem. Periodic eye exams include a check for this problem.

4. Tears from each eye normally enter the lacrimal punctae, drain through the lacrimal canaliculi to the lacrimal sac, and then flow inferiorly through the nasolacrimal duct into the inferior nasal meatus where they are evaporated by the air movements of respiration. During emotional stress, the ANS increases the secretion rate of the lacrimal glands. The excess lacrimation exceeds the evaporation rate and the nose runs.

5. The central visual field is projected onto the fovea centralis of the retina—an area entirely formed of cones. Peripheral vision images are projected onto adjacent parts of the retina where there is a mixture of rods and cones. At normal light levels the cones are functional but the rods are not. Thus, the lowered peripheral vision acuity is primarily due to a reduced number of functional photoreceptors in the peripheral visual field. Even at lower light levels (where the rods become functional) the visual acuity is reduced because they do not produce images as sharp as those from cones.

6. Contact lenses tend to stay centered on the corneas because their radii of curvature match. The part of the eyeball covered by sclera has a larger radius (*i.e.*, it is flatter). Contact lenses cannot get "behind" the eyeball because the bulbar conjunctiva on its surface is continuous with the palpebral conjunctiva lining the eyelids. A displaced contact lens is stopped by the conjunctival fornix where bulbar conjunctiva meets (and is continuous with) palpebral conjunctiva.

7. Looking directly at a very dim star projects its image on the fovea centralis of the retina. The photoreceptors in this area (entirely cones) do not function in very dim light and so the star cannot be seen. When the star's image strikes an adjacent part of the retina (as it does when the visual axes are slightly shifted) it activates the rods in that part of the retina (which do respond to dim light).

8. The fovea centralis is entirely cones which produce greater visual acuity than rods, and there are fewer retinal layers in the foveal region that light must pass through before activating the cones.

9. The pupillary light reflex refers to the changes in pupillary diameter induced by changes in light intensity. Its purpose is to allow adequate light to stimulate the photoreceptors but prevent higher levels that "overdrive" them. In bright light, the pupils get smaller due to parasympathetic stimulation of the pupillary sphincter muscle in the iris. In dim light the pupils get larger due to sympathetic stimulation of the pupillary dilator muscle of the iris.

10. Unlike aqueous humor, which is continuously secreted, vitreous humor (once formed) cannot be replaced by the body.

11. The lens is an elastic structure that has a natural tendency to become spheroid. When the ciliary muscle contracts, it causes the ring of tissue (ciliary body) from which the lens is suspended (by zonular fibers) to become smaller in diameter. This reduces tension on the zonular fibers and the lens becomes more spheroid (thicker).

12. Rods and cones are the functional parts of rod and cone cells. Rods function in very dim light, allow black and white vision only, and their impulses do not result in sharp visual images. Cones function in moderate to bright light, allow color images (including black and white), and their impulses result in crisp visual images. Neither rods nor cones are functional in complete darkness.

13. The humors keep the eyeball inflated to its proper shape. The aqueous humor probably serves as nutrient source for some of the living cells of the posterior and anterior chambers.

14. Anger causes a release of epinephrine from the adrenal medulla. This, in turn, results in a generalized sympathomimetic response including pupillary dilation. The pupil is actually dilated too much (by the emotional response) and allows too much light to strike the retina. This over drives the cones and reduces visual acuity.

15. Two. There are three layers of cells (total) in the retina. Their cell bodies make up the retinal layers termed *ganglionic layer, internal nuclear layer,* and *external nuclear layer.*

16. No. The back side of the iris is covered by retina, too. This iridial part of the retina, as well as the retina covering the back side of the ciliary body, has no photoreceptors.

17. The "blind spot" is the disc of the optic nerve. It is located slightly above and medial to the fovea-centralis.

18. One could logically produce all necessary eye movements with the rectus muscles alone. The two oblique muscles seem superfluous.

19. Unilateral dysfunction of an abducens nerve will paralyze the ipsilateral lateral rectus muscle. Tone in the medial rectus muscle of that eye will draw the visual axis medially. The individual will suffer convergent strabismus (*i.e.,* will be cross-eyed).

20. The oily secretion of these glands coats the palpebral margins (edges of the lids) and prevents tears from spilling over them (normally).

21. Lacrimal secretion, aqueous humor, and vitreous humor.

CHAPTER 13 *The Ear*

Chapter Outline and Key Concepts

INTRODUCTION

The ear is the principal receptor organ for hearing, equilibrium, and body position/motion detection.

The ear is divided into three major parts called the external, middle, and internal ear.

EXTERNAL EAR

The external ear includes the pinna (auricle) and the external acoustic meatus.

The pinna is flexible but maintains its form due to the auricular cartilage within it.

Numerous folds and indentations on the pinna are named.

The external acoustic meatus is the air-filled channel that conducts sound vibrations to the tympanic membrane.

Earwax produced by the ceruminous glands of the external acoustic meatus keeps the tympanic membrane pliable.

MIDDLE EAR

The middle ear includes the tympanic membrane, tympanic cavity (cavity of the middle ear), auditory tube, and the auditory ossicles.

The tympanic membrane is a thin connective tissue proper structure covered externally by skin and internally by mucous membrane.

The auditory ossicles are the smallest bones in the body and conduct sound vibrations across the tympanic cavity from the tympanic membrane to the fluid surrounding the internal ear.

The auditory ("eustachian") tube connects the cavity of the middle ear to the pharynx and allows pressure equalization on both sides of the tympanic membrane.

Two tiny skeletal muscles (stapedius and tensor tympani muscles) attach to two of the auditory ossicles to dampen vibrations during very loud noises.

INTERNAL EAR

The internal ear is housed within a series of fluid-filled channels in the temporal bone collectively called the osseous labyrinth.

The fluid within the osseous labyrinth (in which the internal ear is suspended) is called perilymph and is, in reality, cerebrospinal fluid.

The internal ear is a set of endolymph-containing structures suspended in the perilymph and collectively termed the membranous labyrinth.

The three main subparts of the internal ear and the names of the osseous labyrinth channels in which they are suspended are: cochlear duct (cochlea), semicircular ducts (semicircular canals), utricle and saccule (vestibule).

The cochlear duct of the internal ear is responsible for generation of impulses related to hearing via detection of vibrations by hair cells in the spiral organ.

The three semicircular ducts generate impulses in response to turning/twisting movements (angular acceleration) via endolymph movement which bends the hairs of hair cells.

The utricle and saccule generate impulses in response to straight line movements (linear acceleration) via gravitational and inertial forces which bend the hairs of hair cells.

DEVELOPMENT OF THE EAR

The internal ear develops from surface ectoderm which goes through otic placode, otic fovea, and otocyst stages.

The pinna develops from the first pharyngeal cleft.

The auditory ossicles form by mesenchymal condensations within the first and second branchial arches.

Endoderm forms the auditory tube and the lining of the tympanic cavity.

CLINICAL CONSIDERATIONS

Deafness is reduced or absent ability to detect sound.

Conductive deafness involves the external and middle ears; sensory deafness involves the internal ear, neural pathways, and/or the brain.

Otitis externa, media, and interna are inflammations of the major ear subdivisions.

"Tubes" are sometimes placed through the tympanic membranes of children's ears to allow drainage from recurring otitis media.

Vertigo (dizziness) can result from overstimulation of or inflammation of the semicircular ducts or the hair cells in the utricle and saccule.

Selected Definitions

Auditory ("eustachian") tube—the air-filled tubular channel joining the nasal part of the pharynx to the tympanic cavity. The auditory tube passively transports air to/from the tympanic cavity to equalize pressure therein with the atmospheric pressure.

Auditory ossicles—a collective name for the malleus, incus, and stapes. These diminutive bones conduct sound vibrations through the tympanic cavity and amplify them.

Cerumen—earwax. Cerumen is produced by the ceruminous glands in the skin of the external acoustic meatus and functions to keep the tympanic membrane soft and pliable.

Cochlear duct—that part of the membranous labyrinth located within the cochlea. It is the only part of the internal ear involved in audition.

Crista ampullaris—the dilation at one end of each semicircular duct. It contains a gelatinous structure called a cupula that has hair cells embedded in its base.

Deafness—reduced or lost ability to hear. It is commonly classified as conductive deafness (if the problem is related to the external or middle ears) and sensory deafness (if the problem is located in the internal ear, vestibulocochlear nerve, or the brain).

External ear—the part of the ear visible on the side of the head. It consists of the auricle (pinna) and the external acoustic meatus ("ear canal").

Hair cell—any of the sensory receptors in the spiral organ, statoconial membranes, or cupulae of the semicircular ducts. Hair cells are mechanoreceptors which generate impulses in response to movement of their cytoplasmic processes ("hairs").

Internal ear—a series of interconnected tubular channels within the osseous labyrinth of the temporal bone. These contain endolymph and include the cochlear duct, saccule, utricle, and three semicircular ducts.

Macula (of the utricle/saccule)—the sensory receptor organs of the utricle and saccule. A macula is a gelatinous structure with hair cells embedded into its basal side and statoconia attached to its free surface.

Membranous labyrinth—an alternative name for the internal ear. Its subdivisions are often confused with the names of the bony channels (parts of the osseous labyrinth) which surround them.

Middle ear—the part of the ear occupied by the tympanic cavity. It includes the tympanic membrane, the auditory ossicles, and the auditory tube.

Osseous labyrinth—the channels in the temporal bone that surround the various components of the internal ear. These channels include three semicircular canals, a vestibule, and a cochlea.

Saccule—the globular portion of the membranous labyrinth between the utricle and the cochlear duct. It is connected to them by short channels termed the utriculosaccular duct and ductus reunions, respectively.

Secondary tympanic membrane—the membrane stretched across the cochlear window of the osseous labyrinth. The secondary tympanic membrane separates air in the tympanic cavity from the perilymph in the membranous labyrinth and functions as a pressure relief valve for the vibrations occurring in the perilymph.

Semicircular duct—any of the three tubular portions of the membranous labyrinth that leave and return to the utricle. Each semicircular duct has a structure containing hair cells that respond to angular acceleration around a particular axis.

Spiral organ ("organ of Corti")—the specialized sensory structure located within the cochlear duct. Hair cells of the spiral organ generate impulses in response to sound vibrations.

Statoconia ("otoliths")—the calcium carbonate/protein complexes that are adherent to the free surfaces of the statoconial membranes of the utricle and saccule. Statoconia add mass to the membranes, making them more easily shifted by gravitational and inertial forces.

Tinnitus—continuous ringing in the ears. Tinnitus can be so prominent that it interferes with normal hearing.

Tympanic membrane ("eardrum")—the structure that is stretched across the deep end of the external acoustic meatus. It consists of a thin layer of connective tissue proper sandwiched between skin and mucous membrane.

Utricle—the globular portion of the membranous labyrinth to which the three semicircular ducts attach. The utricle is connected to the saccule by a tiny, tubular channel called the utriculosaccular duct.

Etymology *Arrectis auribus*—**"With ears pricked up."**

akoustikos (G), *to hear*—acoustic
auricula (L), *diminutive of ear*—auricle
cochlea (L), *snail shell*—cochlea
crista (L), *crest, ridge*—crista
cupula (L), *cup*—cupula
flaccidus (L), *flabby*—flaccid
heliko (G), *spiral*—helicotrema
helix (L), *spiral*—helix
konis (G), *dust*—statoconia
lympha (L), *water*—perilymph
miringa (L), *membrane*—myringotomy
peri (L), *around*—perilymph
scala (L), *ladder*—scala
statos (G), *standing*—statoconia
tectorius (L), *cover*—tectorial
tinnire (L), *to ring*—tinnitus
tragos (G), *a part of the ear*—tragus
trema (G), *hole*—helicotrema
vertigo (L), *action of whirling*—vertigo
vestibulum (L), *chamber*—vestibule

Introduction

The ear (vestibulocochlear organ) is the principal receptor organ for hearing, equilibrium, and body position. It has three major divisions: external ear, middle ear, and internal ear (Figure 13-1). The external ear is the only visible portion and has a number of vestigial auricular muscles that are so tiny that they are difficult to identify. The function of the external ear is to collect and funnel atmospheric vibrations to the tympanic membrane. Vibrations of the tympanic membrane are amplified by passing through the auditory ossicles (malleus, incus, and stapes) in the air-filled cavity of the middle ear. The fluid-filled internal ear occupies a number of channels in the petrous part of the temporal bone called the osseous labyrinth. It consists of a group of similarly shaped but smaller structures termed the membranous labyrinth. The latter is divided into a cochlear labyrinth which transduces sound vibrations to nervous impulses (for hearing) and a vestibular labyrinth which monitors body position and movement (for equilibrium).

External Ear

The **external ear** receives sound vibrations and channels them to the tympanic membrane. It consists of the auricle (pinna) and the external acoustic meatus. The **auricle** is the flexible structure that protrudes from the side of the head. It contains the elastic **auricular cartilage** which imparts most

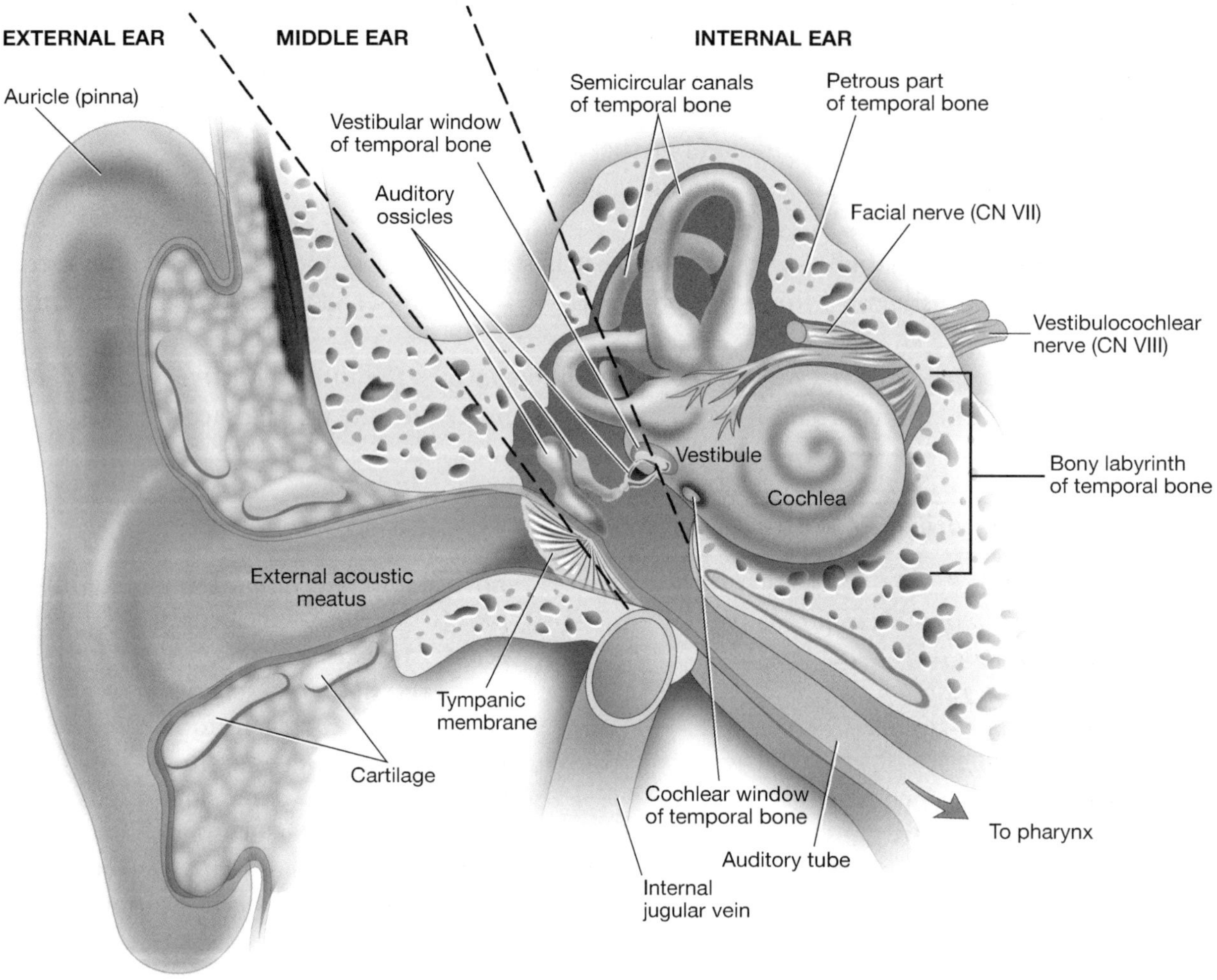

Figure 13-1

Major Features of the Ear

The ear is divided into three major divisions: external ear, middle ear, and internal ear. The external ear has only two major components: pinna (auricle) and external acoustic meatus ("external auditory canal"). The air-filled cavity of the middle ear (tympanic cavity) is connected to the pharynx by the auditory tube. Sound vibrations transmitted by the auditory ossicles are transmitted to fluid associated with the internal ear at the vestibular ("oval") window. A membrane across the cochlear ("round") window called the secondary tympanic membrane serves as a pressure relief valve. It bulges or sucks in as the baseplate of the stapes vibrates in and out. Note: the semicircular canals, vestibule, and cochlea are subdivisions of the bony labyrinth of the temporal bone. These house (surround) but are not part of the internal ear. Technically, none of the parts of the internal ear can be seen in this illustration.

of its form. The folded edge of the auricle is termed the **helix** and is divided into a tail, a spine, and a crus (Figure 13-2). The **tail of the helix** blends inferiorly into the earlobe. The **spine of the helix** is the posterior and superior portion and the **crus** is the downward continuation of the anterior part that ends near the middle of the pinna. The crus divides the invaginated hollow of the ear, termed

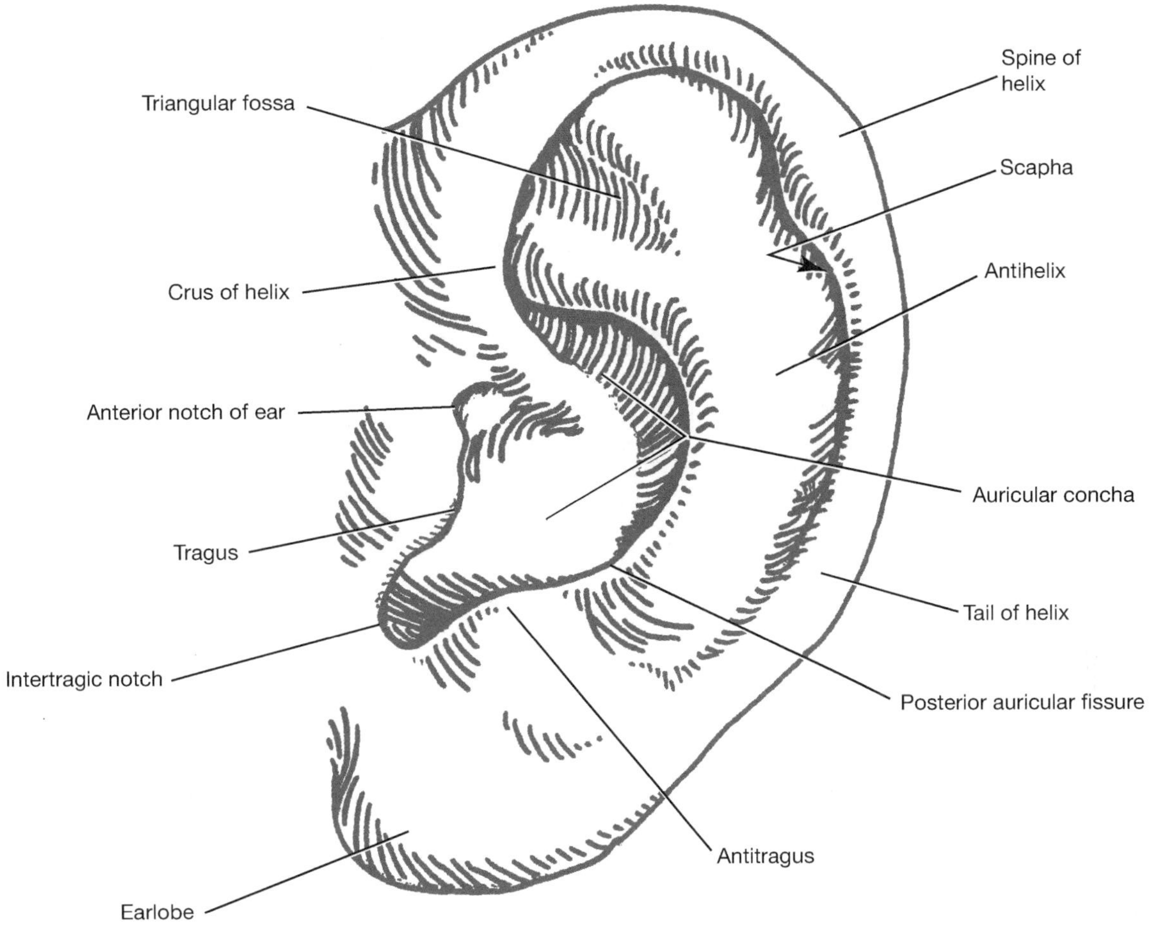

Figure 13-2
Landmarks of the Auricle

the **auricular concha**, into an upper, smaller part (cymba of the concha) and a larger, lower part (conchal cavity) which is continuous with the external acoustic meatus. The **antihelix** is the rounded undulation of the pinna that is anterior and roughly parallel to the spine of the helix. Its superior extent is indented by a finger-tip sized depression termed the **triangular fossa**. The longitudinal furrow between the helix and the antihelix is the **scapha**. The **earlobe** is the fleshy inferior projection of the auricle. It is not supported by cartilage and is therefore more easily pierced for earrings than other parts of the auricle.

The small tongue-like projection just anterior to the external acoustic meatus is the **tragus**. A similar projection from the superior margin of the earlobe is the **antitragus**. The deep indentation between the tragus and antitragus is termed the **intertragic notch**. The indentation above the tragus which separates it from the crus of the helix is the **anterior notch of the ear**. The indentation posterior to the antitragus is the **posterior auricular fissure**. It overlies a palpable depression in the auricular cartilage termed the **antitragohelicine fissure**. Three landmarks on the medial side of the pinna correspond to structures on the lateral side: **conchal eminence**, **eminence of the scapha**, and **eminence of the triangular fossa**.

The **external acoustic meatus** is the air-filled passageway that channels sound vibrations from the auricle to the tympanic membrane. Its external opening is called the **external acoustic pore**. The meatus has a lateral cartilaginous portion and a deeper osseous portion formed by the temporal bone. It is lined by skin containing specialized holocrine glands (**ceruminous glands**) that produce **cerumen** (earwax). This wax keeps the tympanic membrane soft and pliable. It may also serve as an insect repellent. Many individuals have had the experience of having a small insect fly into their ear, stomp around for a moment, and then quickly leave.

Objectives

1. List the two main components of the external ear and state the function of each.
2. Explain the purpose of ceruminous glands.
3. Sketch a pinna and label its parts.

Middle Ear

The **middle ear** consists of the tympanic membrane, tympanic cavity, auditory tube, and the auditory ossicles. The **tympanic membrane** is popularly called the "eardrum". It is a thin, skin-covered, connective tissue proper structure that completely separates the medial end of the external acoustic meatus from the tympanic cavity. The tympanic membrane vibrates in response to sound waves in the atmosphere. These movements have extremely small amplitudes (for "normal" volume sounds) on the order of the diameter of a molecule of hydrogen. The small, superoanterior portion of the tympanic membrane is termed the **flaccid part** and the remainder is termed the **tense part** (Figure 13-3). The tympanic membrane is not readily visible without instrumentation because of a gentle bend in the cartilaginous external acoustic meatus. With an otoscope, the profile of the **malleus** can be seen where its "handle" (manubrium) and lateral process attach to the medial side of the tympanic membrane. From a point near the flaccid part, it extends inferiorly and somewhat posteriorly about two-thirds of the distance across the membrane. At the inferior end of the malleus, the tympanic membrane is depressed at a landmark called the **umbo of the tympanic membrane**.

The **tympanic cavity** is the air-filled cavity of the middle ear. It is traversed by the three auditory ossicles and has six named walls: membranous, labyrinthine, tegmental, jugular, mastoid, and carotid. The **membranous wall** is the lateral side of the tympanic cavity formed primarily by the tympanic membrane.

The **labyrinthine wall** is on the medial side and separates the tympanic cavity from the structures of the internal ear. It has a rounded protuberance termed the **promontory** that corresponds to the first coil of the cochlea (on the other side of the wall). It has two openings of functional significance: the **vestibular** ("oval") **window** and the **cochlear** ("round") **window**. The base of the stapes fits into the vestibular window and is held in place by the tympanostapedial syndesmosis. The secondary tympanic membrane covers the cochlear window and assists in the dissipation of wave energy at the end of the scala tympani (*see Internal Ear*). The **tegmental wall** is the superior wall of the tympanic cavity. The space between it and the auditory ossicles is termed the **epitympanic recess**. The **jugular wall** is the inferior wall (floor) of the tympanic cavity. The **mastoid wall** at the posterior aspect is penetrated by an opening into the mastoid antrum of the temporal bone. This

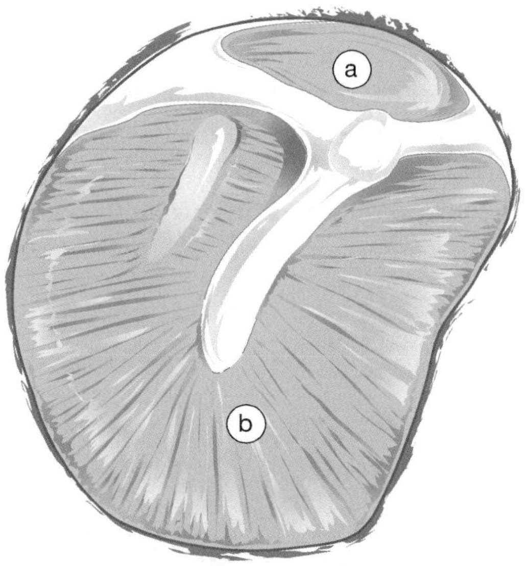

Figure 13-3

Right Tympanic Membrane (as viewed through an otoscope)

The profile of the manubrium ("handle") and lateral process of the malleus can be seen through the tympanic membrane. The flaccid part (a) of the tympanic membrane is superoanterior to the malleus and the remainder is the tense part (b).

communicates with the air-filled **mastoid cells** of the mastoid process of the temporal bone. The **carotid wall** at the anterior aspect of the tympanic cavity is penetrated by the tympanic opening of the auditory tube.

The **auditory tube** is the passageway connecting the tympanic cavity to the nasal part of the pharynx. It has osseous and cartilaginous portions which are lined by mucous membrane. The pharyngeal opening of the auditory tube is located in the lateral aspect of the nasal part of the pharynx ("nasopharynx"). The tube allows equalization of air pressure on both sides of the tympanic membrane by allowing air into or out of the otherwise closed tympanic cavity in response to changing barometric pressure.

The **auditory ossicles** are the three tiny bones within the tympanic cavity: malleus, incus, and stapes (Figure 13-4). They transmit sound vibrations from the tympanic membrane across the tympanic cavity to the internal ear. The **malleus** is attached to the medial side of the tympanic membrane and has a head, neck, anterior and lateral processes, and a manubrium ("handle"). It articulates with the incus at the tiny, synovial, **incudomallear joint**. The **incus** has a body, a long crus, and a short crus. The lenticular process projects from the long crus and articulates with the stapes at the **incudostapedial joint** (a synovial joint). The **stapes** is the smallest bone in the body and distinctly resembles a stirrup on an English riding saddle. It has a head, anterior and posterior crura, and a base. The oval-shaped **base of the stapes** fits into the vestibular window of the labyrinthine wall of the tympanic cavity and is secured there by a fibrous articulation termed the **tympanostapedial syndesmosis**. As it vibrates in response to sound waves, the base of the stapes moves in and out of the vestibular window like a plunger imparting hydrostatic waves to the perilymph surrounding the membranous labyrinth. The auditory ossicles are covered by the delicate mucosa which lines the tympanic cavity. This covering prevents their desiccation (drying).

The stapedius and tensor tympani muscles are two tiny skeletal muscles that attach to the auditory ossicles. Their contraction dampens vibrations of excessive amplitude and serves to protect the delicate structures of the internal ear from damage. The **stapedius muscle** originates from a small projection on the mastoid wall of the tympanic cavity. It inserts on the constricted portion of the stapes near the head (commonly called the "neck"). The **tensor tympani muscle** originates on the cartilaginous portion of the auditory tube. It inserts on the manubrium of the malleus.

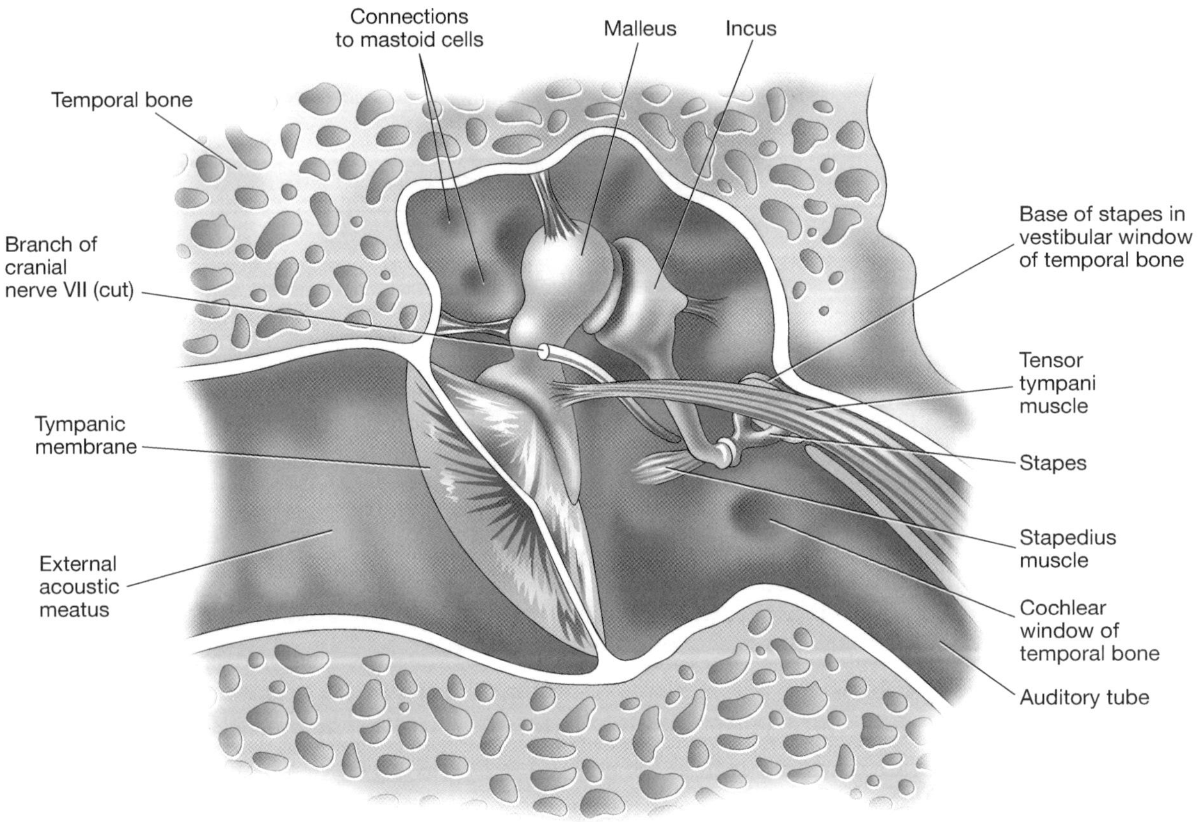

Figure 13-4
Middle Ear

The tympanic cavity is completely separated from the external acoustic meatus by the tympanic membrane. However, it is continuous with the pharynx via the auditory tube. The positional relationships of the auditory ossicles and the stapedius and tensor tympani muscles can be seen.

Objectives

4. List the components of the middle ear and state the purpose of each.
5. List the auditory ossicles in the order that sound vibrations pass through them and name the three joints involved.
6. State which direction air moves in the auditory tube in response to changing barometric pressure.
7. List the muscles associated with the auditory ossicles and state their function.

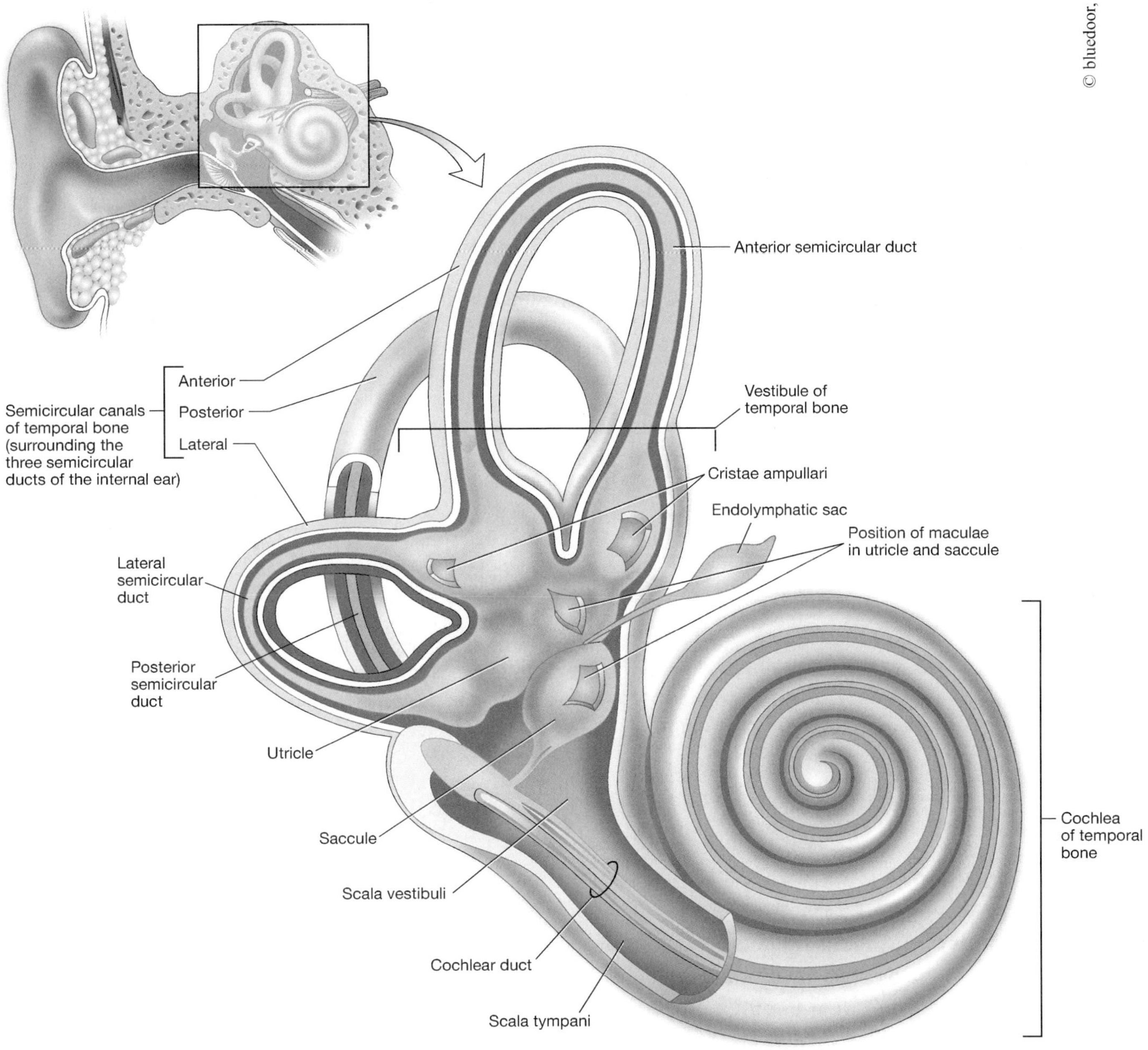

Figure 13-5
Structures of the Internal Ear

The internal ear (membranous labyrinth) is a set of interconnected endolymph containing membranous structures located within a slightly larger set of bony channels collectively called the osseous labyrinth. The narrow space between the osseous labyrinth and the membranous labyrinth (shown in black in the drawing) is filled with perilymph as are the scala vestibuli and the scala tympani which are continuous with that space. The loop-like semicircular canals are subdivisions of the osseous labyrinth which contain the three semicircular ducts. The bulbous enlargement of the osseous labyrinth, which surrounds the internal ear components called utricle and saccule, is the vestibule. The inner ear structure within the cochlea is the cochlear duct and the latter contains the spiral organ ("organ of Corti").

Table 13-1 A Comparison of the Three Main Components of the Membranous Labyrinth (Internal Ear)

Criteria	*Cochlear Duct*	*Utricle and Saccule*	*Semicircular Ducts*
Location in osseous labyrinth of temporal bone	Cochlea of temporal bone	Vestibule of temporal bone	Semicircular canals of temporal bone
Sensation resulting from impulses	Hearing	Detection of straight line motion	Detection of turning and twisting motions
Component where hair cells are located	Spiral organ ("Organ of Corti")	Statoconial membrane of macula	Cupula of crista ampullaris
Means by which hair cells are stimulated	Vibrations in endolymph	Gravitational and inertial forces	Movement (flow) of endolymph
Transmission of impulses	Cochlear nerve of cranial nerve VIII	Vestibular nerve of cranial nerve VIII	Vestibular nerve of cranial nerve VIII
Destination of impulses	Neurons in medulla oblongata, thence to inferior colliculus in mesencephalon, on to the thalamus, and then to the auditory cortex of the temporal lobes of the cerebrum.	Cerebellum and vestibular nuclei of medulla oblongata, thence to oculomotor center of brain (eye movement) and to the spinal cord (movement of head, neck, and limbs).	Cerebellum and vestibular nuclei of medulla oblongata, thence to oculomotor center of brain (eye movement) and to the spinal cord (movement of head, neck, and limbs).

Internal Ear

The **internal ear** is housed in a series of channels within the petrous part of the temporal bone termed the osseous labyrinth (Figure 13-5). The **osseous labyrinth** is a diverticulum of the cranial cavity and the two are connected by the internal acoustic meatus. The major parts of the osseous labyrinth are the cochlea, vestibule, and the three semicircular canals. The **cochlea** is a snail-shaped, coiled channel with a large **base** and a small **cupula** (apex). The **spiral canal of the cochlea** coils around approximately two and one-half times from the cochlear base to the apex. The **vestibule** of the osseous labyrinth is a globular cavity and the **osseous semicircular canals** are three channels which extend from and return to the vestibule. The semicircular canals are designated **anterior**, **posterior**, and **lateral** according to their relative positions and each one is oriented in a different plane. The **internal acoustic meatus** opens into the medial side of the osseous labyrinth and transmits the facial and vestibulocochlear nerves from the cranial cavity. The osseous labyrinth contains a watery fluid called **perilymph** which has been shown to be cerebrospinal fluid (CSF). Suspended within the perilymph is a membranous structure called the membranous labyrinth.

The **membranous labyrinth** (internal ear) (Figure 13-5) occupies the osseous labyrinth and has the same general shape, but its parts are much smaller (Table 13-1). It is filled with a fluid called **endolymph**. Endolymph is produced in the outer wall of the cochlear duct in the stria vascularis.

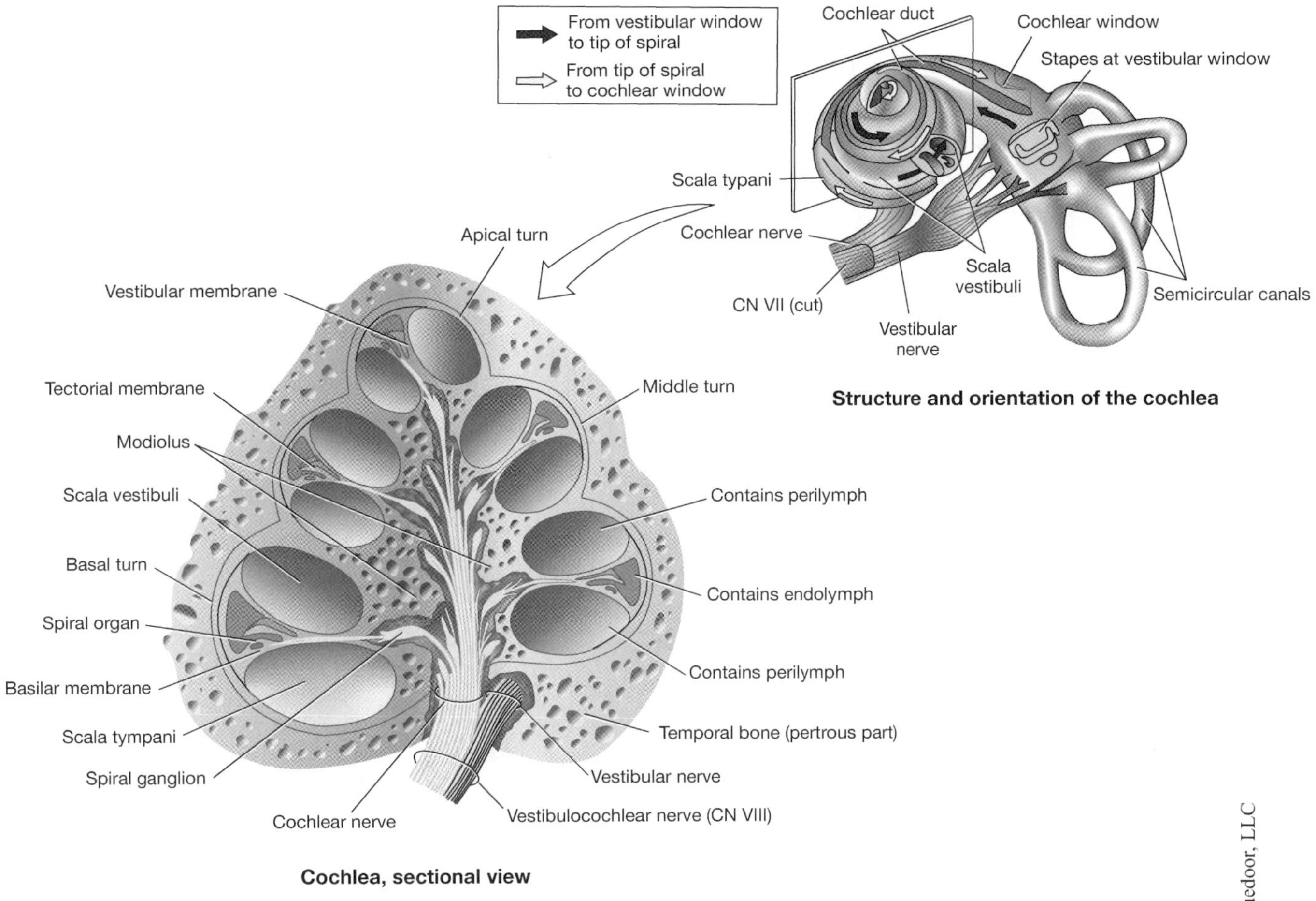

Figure 13-6

Cochlea and Cochlear Duct

The cochlea is a spiral-shaped, hollowed out space within the temporal bone. Within it, the small cochlear duct winds around accompanied by two perilymph-filled spaces called the scala vestibuli (above the duct) and scala tympani (below the duct). If the cochlear duct remained circular in transverse section and centered within the cochlea, the two scali would be continuous. However, the duct becomes wedge-shaped or triangular in transverse section and is attached to both "sides" of the surrounding cochlea. Consequently, the scala vestibuli and the scala tympani are separate, perilymph-filled spaces that join only at the tip (apex) of the cochlea.

As mentioned above, the space between the osseous labyrinth and the membranous labyrinth is filled with a fluid called perilymph. This perilymphatic space communicates with the subarachnoid space by a tiny channel termed the **perilymphatic duct (cochlear aqueduct)**.

The portion of the membranous labyrinth within the cochlea is called the **cochlear duct** (Figure 13-6, 7). It occupies the central portion of the spiral canal and spirals around two and a half times. The perilymph-filled spaces above and below the cochlear duct are called the **scala vestibuli** and the **scala tympani**, respectively. Although they are completely separated from each other throughout

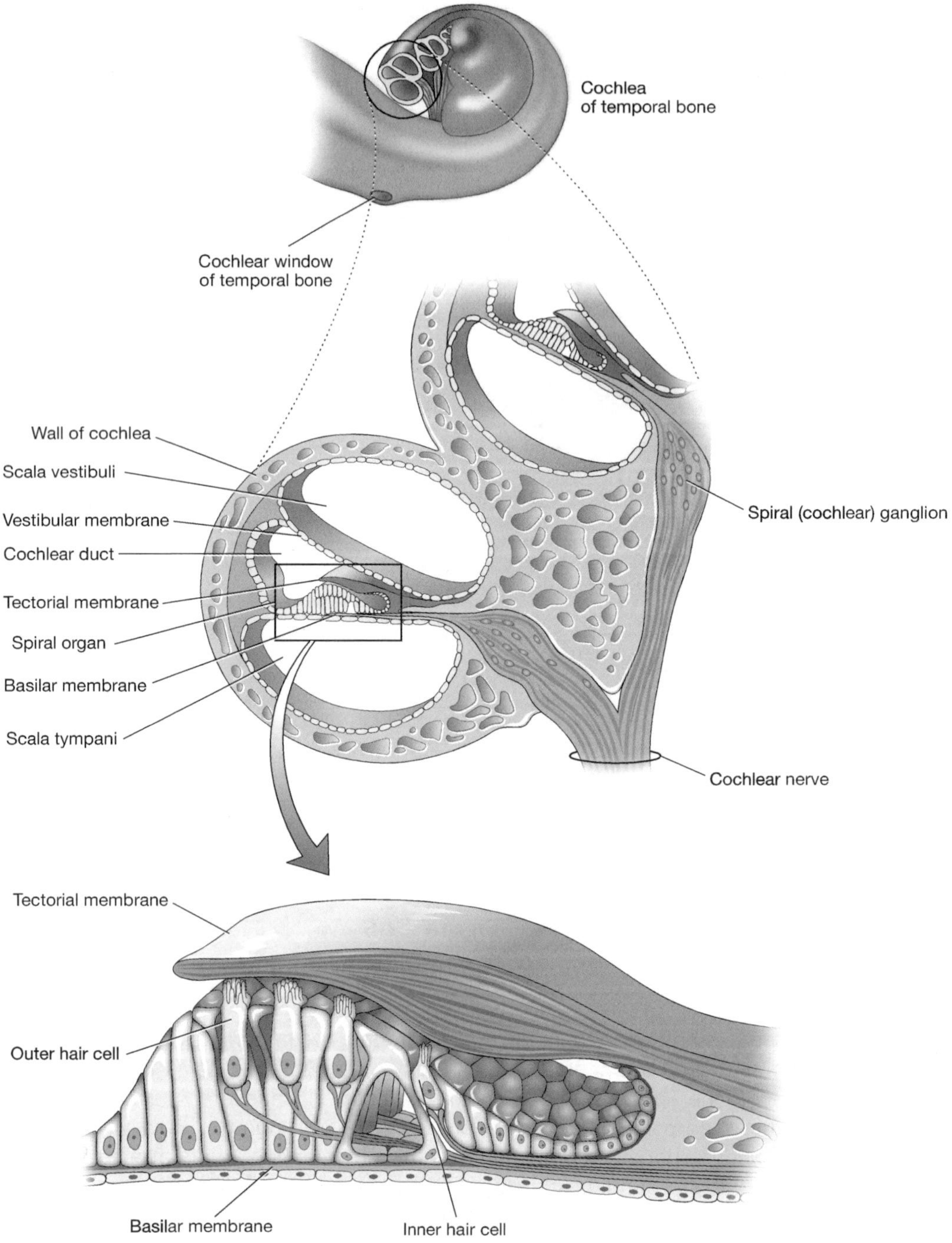

Figure 13-7
Cochlear Anatomy

The top and bottom walls of the cochlear duct are called the vestibular membrane and basilar membrane, respectively. The spiral organ contains hair cells interspersed among supporting cells which extend up to a "tongue-like" tectorial membrane projecting from the axial wall of the cochlear duct. Vibrations within the perilymph of the scala vestibuli and scala tympani pass through the walls of the cochlear duct and set up motion waves within the endolymph. Relative motion between the hairs of the hair cells and the tectorial membrane bends the hairs of the hair cells. This movement causes the hair cells to generate sensory impulses which are carried to the brain by the vestibulocochlear nerve and interpreted as sound.

most of the spiral canal by the cochlear duct, the scala vestibuli and scala tympani communicate with each other at the apex of the cochlea through an opening called the **helicotrema**. The perilymph within the scala vestibuli is set in motion by vibrations of the base of the stapes at the vestibular window. These hydrostatic waves move throughout the membranous labyrinth within the cochlea. A membrane across the cochlear window allows perilymph within the scala tympani to bulge out each time that the stapes vibrates "in" and vice-versa. This membrane is called the **secondary tympanic membrane**.

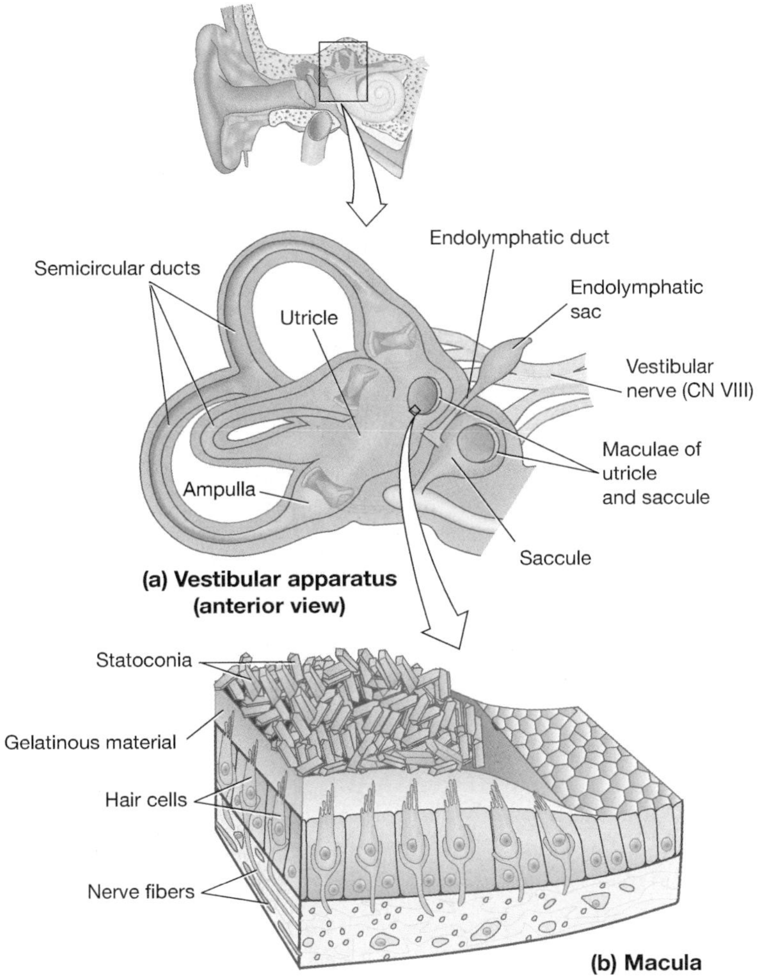

Figure 13-8

The Macula of the Utricle and Saccule

The utricle and saccule of the membranous labyrinth each contain a statoconial membrane attached to one wall (a). Statoconia ("otoliths") (b, c) embedded in the gelatinous material of the membrane give it enough mass that gravitational and/or inertial forces can shift it and stimulate the hair cells embedded in the deep side of the membrane. When the head is upright (normal anatomic position) the statoconial membrane of the utricle is in a horizontal position, so it responds (generates impulses) to forward/backward movement and to left/right movement but not to up and down motion. The statoconial membrane within the saccule is vertically oriented in a sagittal plane. Therefore, it responds to forward/backward and to up/down motion but not to left/right motion.

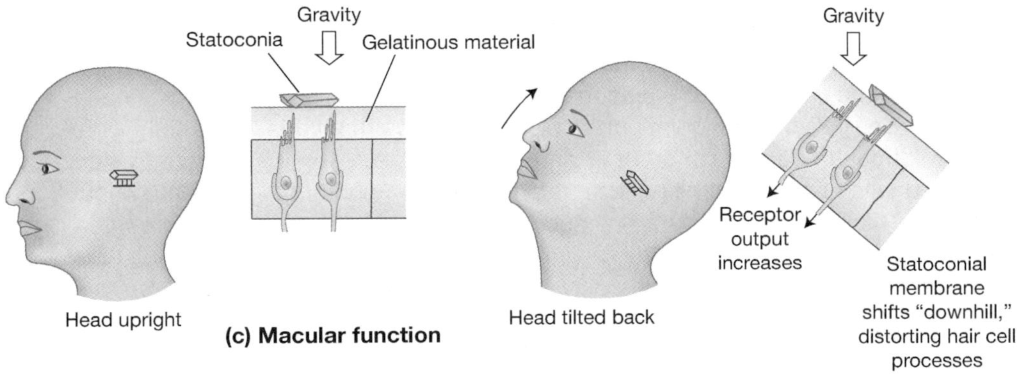

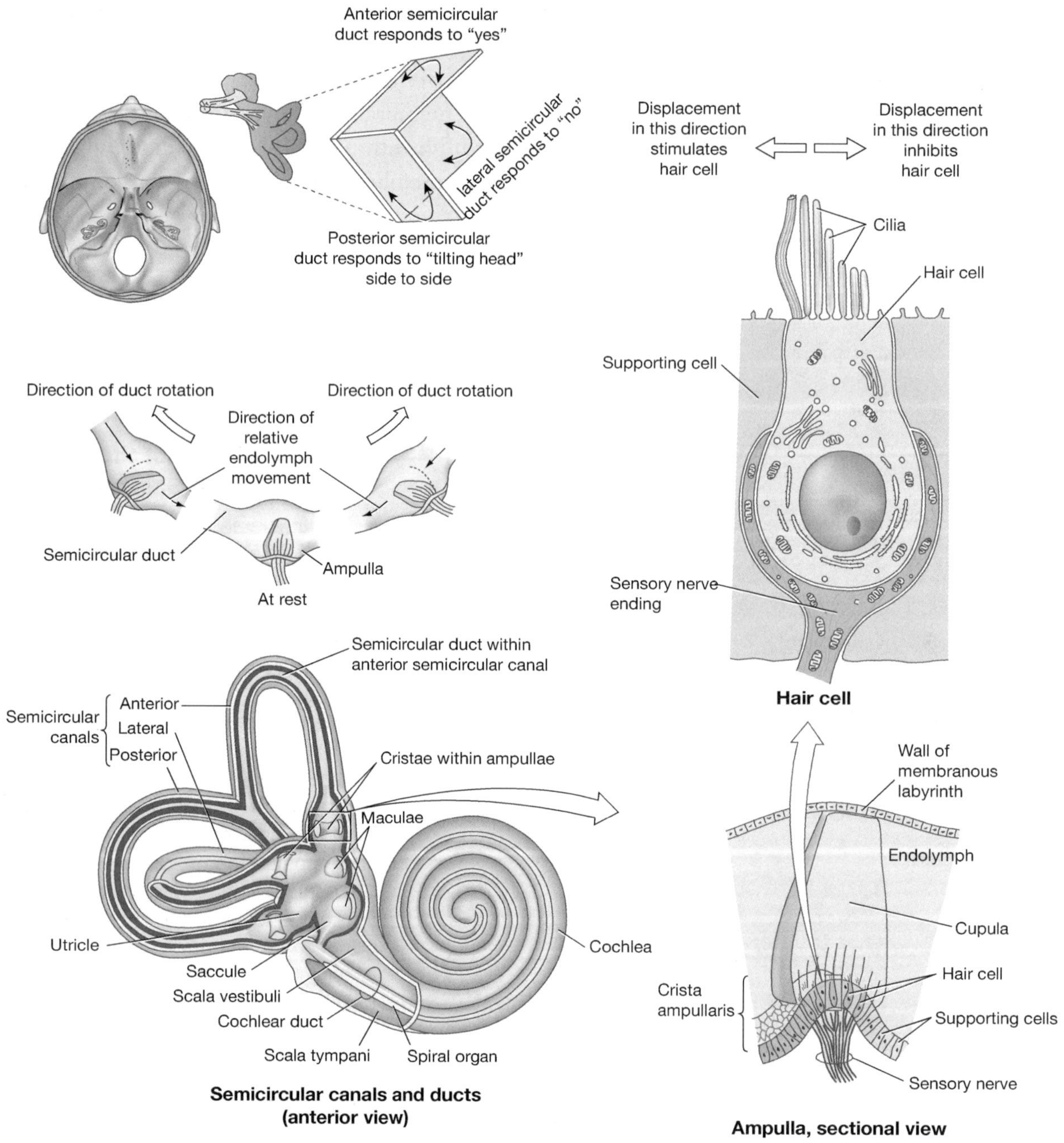

Figure 13-9

Semicircular Ducts and Detection of Angular Acceleration

The three semicircular ducts all circle away from and rejoin the utricle. Attached to the wall of the duct within the bulbous enlargement (ampulla) at one end of each duct is the specialized sensory receptor called a crista ampullaris. Hair cells within the gelatinous cupula of the crista ampullaris are sensitive to motion. When embedded cilia of the hair cells are bent by endolymph pushing against the cupula as the head is turned or twisted, sensory impulses are generated that are interpreted as turning or twisting motion (angular acceleration). Each of the three semicircular ducts is oriented in a plane perpendicular to those of the other two. This allows turning/twisting (angular acceleration) movements in any plane to be detected. Because of their spatial orientation, the anterior semicircular duct primarily detects nodding ("yes") movements of the head, the lateral one primarily detects rotational ("no") movements, and the posterior duct detects tilting of the head from one shoulder to the other.

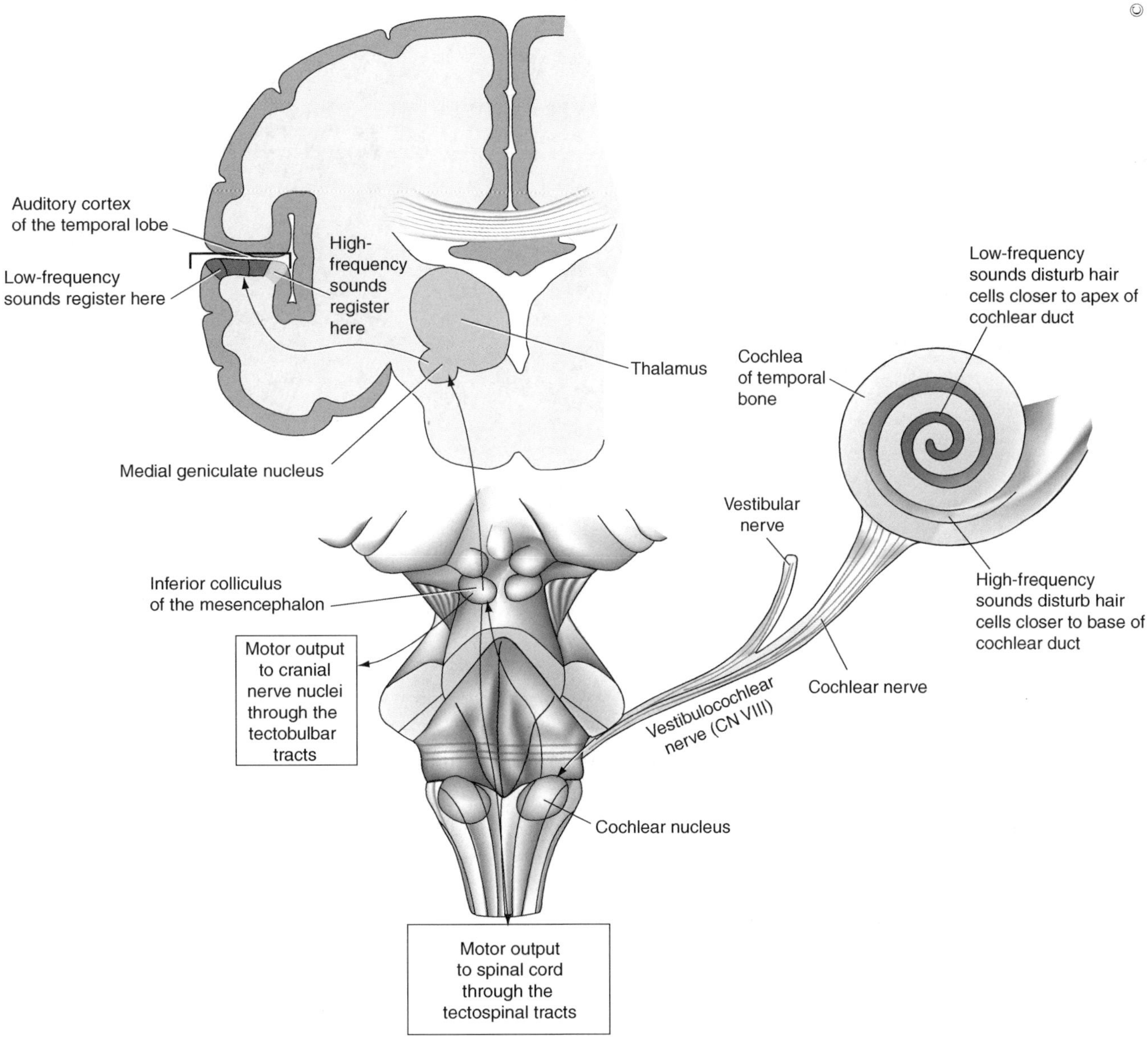

Figure 13-10

Neural Pathways for Audition

Impulses generated in the spiral organ of the cochlear duct are conducted to the cochlear nuclei within the brainstem. From there, they are sent to the inferior colliculi of the corpora quadrigemina which may generate motor impulses involved in an auditory reflex. From the inferior colliculi, impulses are sent through the thalamus to the auditory cortex of the temporal lobes of the cerebral hemispheres where they are interpreted as sound.

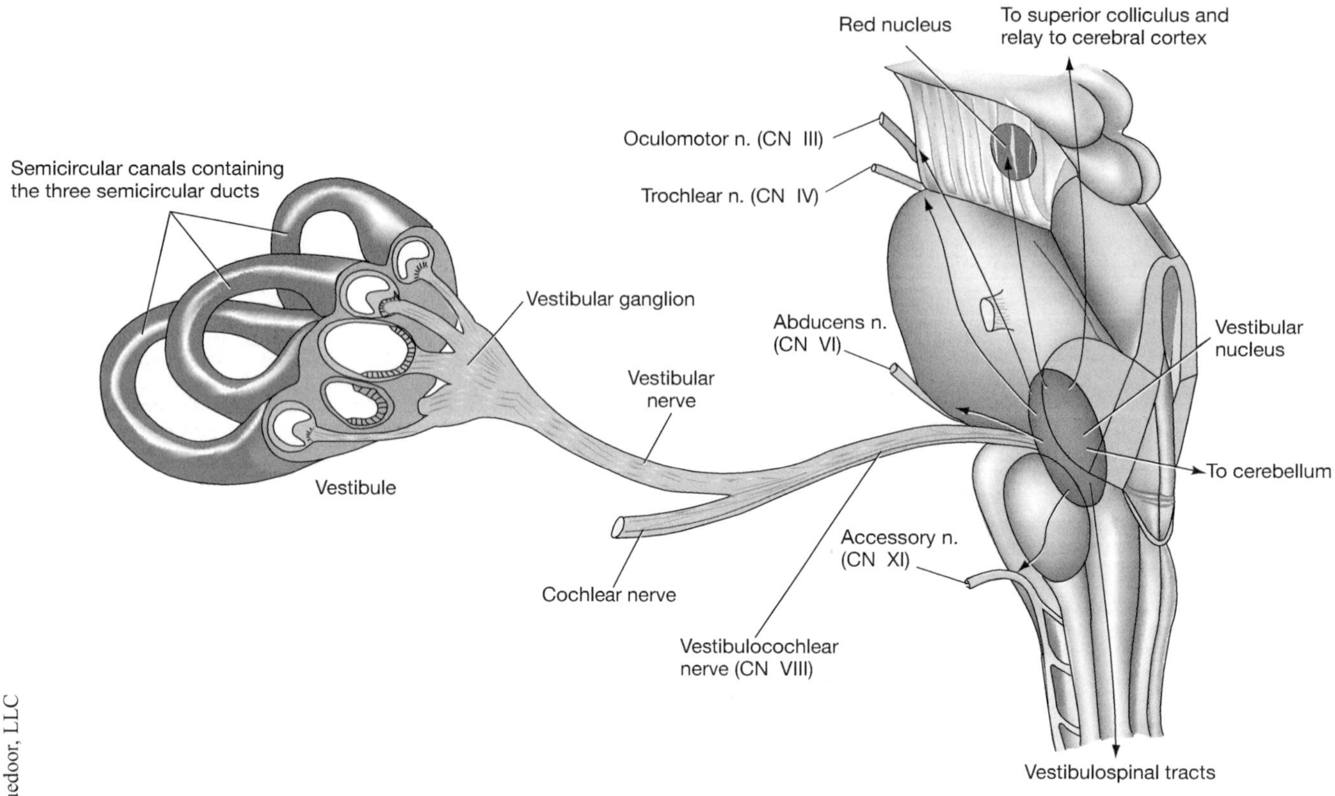

Figure 13-11

Neural Pathways for Equilibrium

Impulses generated within the semicircular ducts, utricle, and saccule are conducted via the vestibulocochlear nerve to the vestibular nucleus within the brainstem. Motor outputs to several cranial nerves can be initiated from this nucleus and impulses can be sent on up to the cerebral cortex as well.

The **cochlear duct** is somewhat triangular in transverse section. The membrane separating it from the scala vestibuli above it is termed the **vestibular membrane** (or **vestibular wall of the cochlear duct**). The membrane separating the cochlear duct from the scala tympani below it is officially termed the **spiral** (**basilar**) **membrane** (or **tympanic wall of the cochlear duct**). The external wall of the cochlear duct parallels the outer wall of the spiral canal. The **stria vascularis** forms the majority of this wall and produces endolymph.

The **spiral organ** ("organ of Corti") is the transducer (via hair cells) which converts motion in the fluid of the membranous labyrinth to nervous impulses interpreted by the brain as sound. It is positioned within the cochlear duct on the **basilar membrane**. The spiral organ is a complex structure containing four rows of **external hair cells** and one row of **internal hair cells**. Hair cells are specialized receptors that are piriform (pear-shaped) and each one has a cell membrane projection from its superior end called a "hair." These projections touch or are embedded in a thin **tectorial membrane** that extends from the axial aspect of the cochlear duct. When the "hairs" of the hair cells move due to hydrostatic waves (undulations) in the endolymph, the hair cells produce nervous impulses that are conducted centrally by the bipolar cells (SA) of the cochlear nerve (Figure 13-10).

The vestibular portion (equilibrium apparatus) of the membranous labyrinth includes the utricle, saccule, and the semicircular ducts. The utricle and saccule occupy the vestibule of the osseous labyrinth. The **utricle** is connected to the three semicircular ducts by five openings (the anterior and posterior ducts have one common "leg" into the utricle) and it (utricle) also has openings into the endolymphatic duct and saccule. The **saccule** is located between the utricle and cochlear duct and has openings into the endolymphatic duct, cochlear duct, and utricle. Thickened areas in the walls of the utricle and saccule called **maculae** contain hair cells whose cytoplasmic extensions are embedded in a gelatinous structure called the **statoconial membrane** (Figure 13-8). Adherent to the opposite side of the membrane within the endolymph are numerous crystals called **statoconia** ("otoliths"). These are formed of calcium carbonate and a protein, and they function to increase the mass of the membrane. The **cilia** ("hairs") of the hair cells initiate impulses when they are bent due to gravitational or inertial forces on the statoconial membrane. Because of the orientation of their maculae and hair cell processes, the utricle responds primarily to horizontal movement (left, right, forward, backward) and the saccule generates impulses in response to forward, backward, up, and down motions (see legend, Figure 13-8). Impulses generated in the maculae are conducted centrally by the bipolar cells in the vestibular nerve (Figure 13-11).

The three **semicircular ducts** (anterior, posterior, and lateral) are located within the homonymous semicircular canals. Each duct is enlarged near one of its two attachments to the utricle. This enlargement is called a **membranous ampulla**. Within each ampulla is a specialized structure called the **crista ampullaris** (Figure 13-9). This consists of a number of hair cells whose cilia are embedded in a gelatinous protein-polysaccharide mass termed a **cupula**. When turning/twisting movements of the head and neck occur, the endolymph within the semicircular ducts presses against the cupulae and bends the cilia of the hair cells. This initiates impulses which are sent to the brain through the bipolar cells of the vestibular nerve (Figure 13-11) and interpreted as turning/twisting motions (angular acceleration).

Objectives

8. Define osseous labyrinth, divide it into its three major components, and state which parts of the membranous labyrinth (internal ear) each one contains.
9. Define membranous labyrinth, divide it into its three major components, and indicate the sensation with which each one is associated.
10. State the location of perilymph and endolymph.
11. Sketch and label a section through the cochlea of the temporal bone.
12. Explain how gravity and inertial forces interact with the maculae in the saccule and utricle to cause impulses that allow us to detect linear acceleration.
13. Explain how endolymph in the semicircular ducts interacts with the cupula of a crista ampullaris to cause impulses that allow us to detect angular (turning, twisting) movements.
14. List, in order, all of the items that sound vibrations pass through to reach the hair cells in the spiral organ.

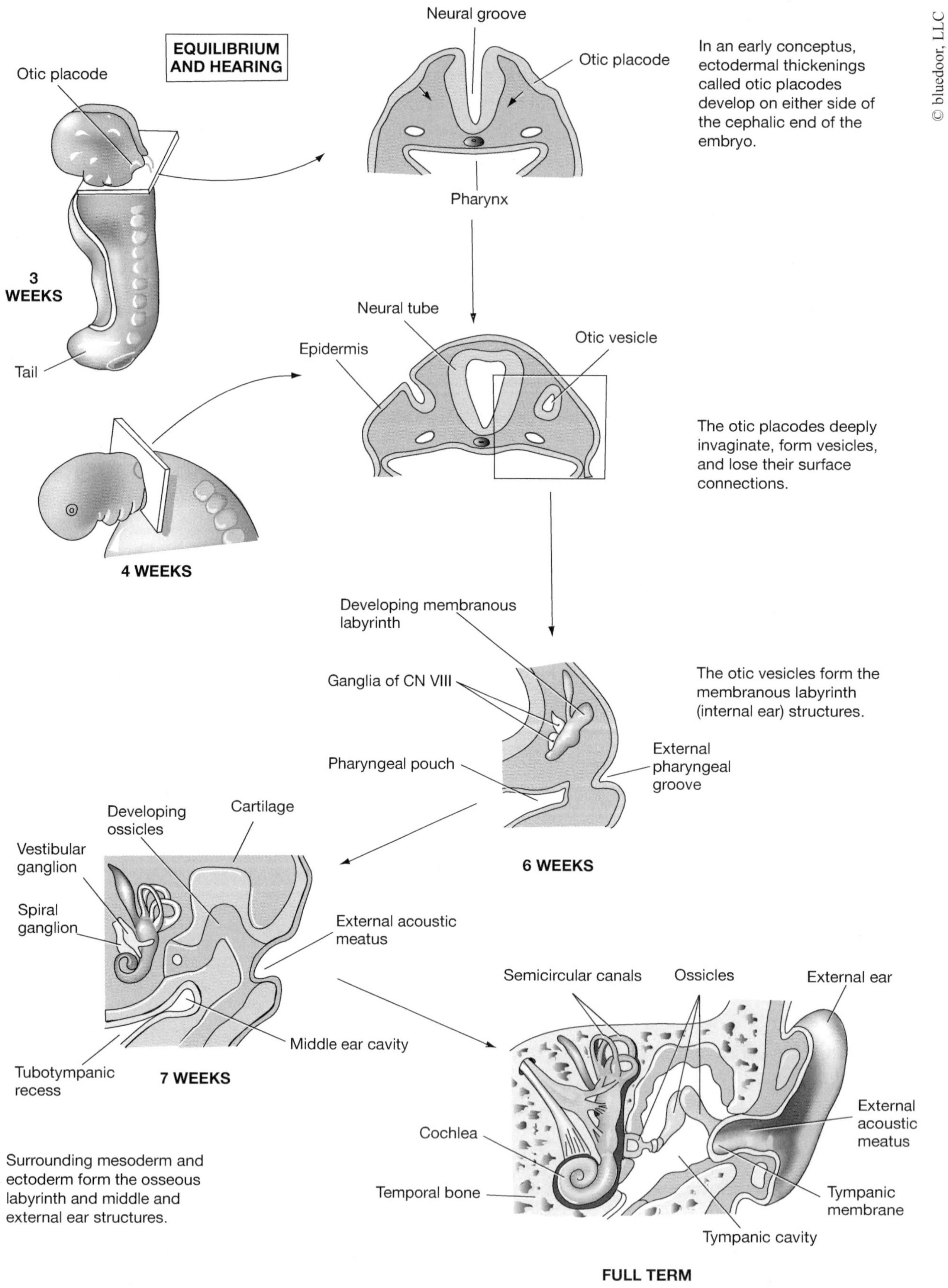

Figure 13-12
Development of the Ear

Development of the Ear

The ear begins developing during the first month of gestation at about the same time that the neural groove is enclosing to form the neural tube. Left and right thickenings in the surface ectoderm called **otic placodes** appear lateral to the developing hindbrain (Figure 13-12). Each placode invaginates to form an **otic fovea**. As the surface edges of the fovea meet, they fuse and the resulting **otocyst** (**otic vesicle**) pinches off from the surface ectoderm. Each otocyst forms the ipsilateral membranous labyrinth which is invaded by the neuroectodermally derived components of the vestibulocochlear nerve. The surrounding mesoderm differentiates into the osseous labyrinth and the perilymphatic space surrounding the membranous labyrinth.

The pinna (auricle) develops from the dorsal part of the first pharyngeal cleft. It is formed from surface ectoderm covering mesodermally-derived cartilaginous components (Figure 13-12). The external acoustic meatus forms as an invagination of surface ectoderm (Figure 13-12). This invagination approaches an evagination of the pharyngeal endoderm called the **tubotympanic recess** which occurs at the level of the first pharyngeal pouch. These tubes approach each other and fuse end-to-end to form the tympanic membrane. The auditory ossicles develop from mesodermal (mesenchymal) condensations derived from the first and second branchial arches. The malleus fuses to the inner aspect of the tympanic membrane and the stapes contacts the membranous labyrinth of the internal ear through the vestibular window. The enlarged end of the tubotympanic recess surrounds the auditory ossicles to form the tympanic cavity. The medial portion of the recess forms the auditory tube.

Objectives

15. Indicate which parts of the definitive ear are derived from each of the following: otocyst, mesoderm, neuroectoderm, first pharyngeal cleft, surface ectoderm, and tubotympanic recess.

Clinical Considerations

Loss of hearing is defined as **conductive deafness** when it is caused by interference in the transmission of sound waves from the air through the tympanic membrane and auditory ossicles. It impairs hearing at all sound frequencies and involves the external and/or middle ears only. Examples of conditions which would be classified as conduction deafness include accumulation of excess ear wax, ruptured tympanic membrane, accumulation of pus in the tympanic cavity, and synostosis of the joints associated with the auditory ossicles. **Sensory deafness** results from problems within the cochlear duct, within the pathways transmitting the impulses to the auditory cortex of the temporal lobe, or within the auditory centers of the temporal lobes. Sensory deafness may result in reduced ability to hear sounds of certain frequencies. This can be caused or aggravated by continuous exposure to sounds of certain pitches, especially if they are loud.

Pharyngitis associated with common colds can interfere with the function of the auditory tube by causing partial or complete blockage of its lumen. This results in reduced auditory acuity because the resulting pressure difference between the atmosphere and middle ear causes tension in the tympanic membrane as it bulges in or out. This tension reduces the ability of the membrane to vibrate freely. If severe, the condition can be quite painful. **Otitis media** (middle ear infections) can cause pain and temporary deafness for the same reasons.

The tympanic membrane can be ruptured by direct physical trauma (*i.e.*, poking it with a toothpick), by extremely loud noises (gunshot within an enclosed area), or by the accumulation of pus within it accompanied by impaired drainage through an inflamed auditory tube. It often heals in these situations with relatively little net loss of hearing. Physicians sometimes drain middle ear infections by a surgical incision through the tympanic membrane (**myringotomy**). In young children with chronic otitis media, physicians will often install tiny plastic drainage tubes directly through the tympanic membrane. These remain in place for several weeks until they are ultimately sloughed out (nearly always into the external acoustic meatus). Children typically outgrow the need for such tubes when their own auditory tubes develop sufficient diameter to serve as functional drains for their middle ears. The continuous ringing, whistling, clicking, or booming sounds that some individuals hear (especially in a very quiet environment) are called **tinnitus**. Some forms can even be heard by individuals other than the patient. There is little that can be done to correct this disorder.

Loss of normal function of the vestibular apparatus produces a condition called **vertigo** in which equilibrium is severely impaired. This can result from inflammation of the structures of the internal ear (**otitis interna**). Temporary vertigo can be induced by sustained spinning movements (whirling around several times on a barstool). These movements induce movement of the endolymph within the inner ear which continue after the individual has ceased turning. The relative motion of the endolymph within the semicircular ducts causes individuals to feel that they or the room are still spinning. Severe vertigo can induce nausea (motion sickness).

Accumulation of excess cerumen (earwax) can partially block the external acoustic meatus and thereby temporarily reduce auditory acuity. Accumulated wax which touches the tympanic membrane can inhibit its vibrations. Excessive accumulation may require professional medical assistance for removal. Inflammation of the external acoustic meatus and/or the pinna constitutes **otitis externa**.

Objectives

16. Differentiate sensory *vs.* conductive deafness.
17. Define tinnitus, myringotomy, otitis (externa, media, interna), and vertigo.

Clinical Case Studies

Case 1—A 45-year-old college professor suffered nausea and dizziness of sudden onset. Her only other symptoms were a fever and headache. Within two days she was unable to keep her balance enough to walk, and she suffered continuing nausea. She was diagnosed with a viral infection of the internal ear. How could such an infection be related to her symptoms?

Case 2—A 33-year-old construction worker complained of a "ringing" noise in his ears of several months duration that was very irritating in a quiet environment. Even with considerable background noise, the ringing was loud enough to be bothersome. What causes this?

Case 3—A college senior suffered a head cold about two weeks after a ski trip. After developing severe sinusitis as part of her overall syndrome, she developed an earache that became so unbearable that she made an appointment with a nurse practitioner. On the way to the appointment, her pain suddenly subsided. The nurse practitioner found pus tinged with blood in the young woman's external acoustic meatus. What happened?

Points to Ponder

The ears. Who comes to mind? Birds, reptiles, and amphibians forgot to pick up parts of theirs and the excess went to Dumbo—complete with airfoils. Shakespeare's Mark Antony, apparently aware of some shortage of ears, asked his friends and countrymen for theirs. Van Gogh, unable to visit his girlfriend in person, sent one of his (all by itself) just to show her his affection. According to an old country music song, "Rumor has it" that she sent it back with the message... "Here's a quarter, call someone who cares."

The parts of ears that we can see, the pinnas, are relatively unnecessary for hearing, and so birds lack them (for aerodynamic reasons) as do reptiles (pinnas would be a nuisance in the grass!). Pinnas vary considerably from person to person in size, shape, how far they stick out, etc. Women who uncover theirs know why and those who won't, know why too. Among other functions, pinnas are a useful place to park jewelry and a public place to perforate. They are said to be as unique as fingerprints. (Just press your ear against this ink pad, please!)

The process of hearing begins when sound vibrations (usually traveling in air) strike the tympanic membrane (known to everyone in the third grade class as the eardrum). Slight differences in the time required for sound vibrations to reach our left eardrum vs. our right allow us to locate the direction from whence a sound emanates. One tenth of a millimeter thick, it has skin on the outside and mucous membrane on the inside. It can be ruptured by Q-tips, paper clips, very loud noises, and pressure from the pus that collects during middle ear infections. After breaking, it usually heals with minimal loss of hearing acuity. Sometimes when it heals, a permanent hole remains—the unfortunate owner can usually hear adequately, but is very susceptible to recurring middle ear infections—especially subsequent to moisture accumulation after showers and swimming. As a consolation prize for this infirmity, these individuals can impress anyone who will watch by blowing smoke out of them—appearing to the uninitiated observer as though the brain must be on fire.

The middle ear is everyone's favorite. Contains three cute little bones—smallest in the body. Have known about them since third grade, too (same lesson as the eardrum). But we may not have learned that they enhance the minuscule amplitude of the tympanic membrane's vibrations—about 20 times, so it is said. The tympanic membrane vibrations are much too small to see. Twenty times bigger they are still much too small to see.

The stapes is given the responsibility of passing the vibration baton on to the perilymph in this air/membrane/bone/fluid relay. (Now we are deeper into the temporal bone than anyone normally goes). The vibrations pass through a fluid called perilymph and make the membranous labyrinth (containing endolymph) vibrate. The vibrating endolymph causes movements between the hairs of hair cells and a structure called the tectorial membrane. Moving the hairs of the hair cells is like touching the trigger of a set mouse trap. Things happen. In this case, nervous impulses are generated that are carried to the brain via the cochlear part of the vestibulocochlear nerve and interpreted as sound.

Detection of motion and body position involves some other specialized structures within the internal ear. Who among us did not whirl around during recess (playing helicopter) until we got our vestibular (equilibrium) apparatus so confused that it wouldn't allow us to stand up? The basis, of course, was getting fluid (endolymph) within the semi-circular ducts moving such that it didn't stop when we did. (Bar stools and circular piano stools work great, too). Unfortunately, many of us learned the hard way that over-stimulating the semi-circular ducts often excites the nausea center as well. So we quit doing the helicopter thing right after lunch and did it during morning recess, instead. (Phonics was going to make us sick anyway!)

Slang and Obsolete Nomenclature

UNOFFICIAL TERM	OFFICIAL DESIGNATION
external auditory meatus	external acoustic meatus *[meatus acusticus externus]*
ear canal	external acoustic meatus *[meatus acusticus externus]*
oval window	vestibular window *[fenestra vestibuli]* of temporal bone
round window	cochlear window *[fenestra cochleae]* of temporal bone
organ of Corti	spiral organ *[organum spirale]*
tympanic duct	scala tympani *[scala tympani]*
vestibular duct	scala vestibuli *[scala vestibuli]*
Eustachian tube	auditory tube *[tuba auditoria]*
footplate of stapes	base of stapes *[basis stapes]*
eardrum	tympanic membrane *[membrana tympanica]*
scala media	cochlear duct *[ductus cochlearis]*
otoliths	statoconia *[statoconia]*
otolith membrane	macula of the utricle/saccule *[macula utriculi/sacculi]*
bony labyrinth of cochlea	osseous labyrinth *[labyrinthus osseous]* of temporal bone
auditory nerve	cochlear nerve *[nervus cochlearis]*
statico-acoustic nerve	vestibulocochlear nerve *[nervus vestibulocochlearis]*
inner ear	internal ear *[auris interna]*
mastoid sinuses	mastoid cells *[cellulae mastoideae]* of temporal bone
membranous labyrinth of semicircular canal	semicircular duct *[ductus semicircularis]*

Review Questions

1. Which one of the following is not associated with the middle ear?
   A. incudomallear joint
   B. tensor tympani muscle
   C. auditory tube
   D. statoconia
   E. tympanic membrane

2. Which of the following is not a feature of the osseous labyrinth?
   A. semicircular canal
   B. cochlear duct
   C. cochlear window
   D. vestibule
   E. vestibular window

3. Which item is not found within the membranous labyrinth?
   A. perilymph
   B. tectorial membrane
   C. hair cells
   D. crista ampullaris
   E. statoconia

4. To stimulate hair cells in the spiral organ, sound vibrations do not typically pass through which of the following?
   A. bone(s)
   B. air
   C. skin
   D. perilymph
   E. a fibrocartilaginous joint
   F. a mucous membrane

5. Hair cells in the ____________________ are stimulated by ____________________ .
   A. cupula of the crista ampullaris—vibrations in endolymph
   B. statoconial membrane of the utricle—flow (movement) of endolymph
   C. spiral organ of the cochlear duct—gravitational and/or inertial forces
   D. saccule—vibrations in perilymph
   E. If none of the above correctly fill the blanks, choose this response.

6. The secondary tympanic membrane...
   A. serves as a "back up" for the primary tympanic membrane.
   B. covers the vestibular ("oval") window.
   C. gets pushed outward by endolymph whenever the stapes vibrates "in."
   D. vibrates at the same frequency as the malleus.
   E. completely closes off the end of the auditory tube.

7. Of the following seven membranes (tympanic membrane, vestibular membrane, mucous membrane, statoconial membrane, basilar membrane, secondary tympanic membrane, tectorial membrane), ________ (number) are found within or form boundaries of the cavity of the middle ear.
   A. 2
   B. 3
   C. 4
   D. 5
   F. 6

8. Which of the following is not a component of the membranous labyrinth?
   A. semi-circular duct
   B. cochlea
   C. utricle
   D. saccule
   E. If all of the above are parts of the membranous labyrinth, choose this response.

9. Which item does not separate (lie between) endolymph and perilymph?
   A. vestibular membrane
   B. wall of semicircular canal
   C. basilar membrane
   D. wall of utricle
   E. wall of saccule

10. Which statement is true?
    A. When descending, scuba divers must move air into their tympanic cavities through their external acoustic meatuses.
    B. The purpose of ear wax (cerumen) is to help keep the secondary tympanic membrane soft and pliable.
    C. Endolymph is CSF.
    D. The hair cells in the utricle respond only to horizontal motions and those in the saccule respond only to vertical motions (of the upright, normally positioned head).
    E. Lassie (the movie star) is (was) a male dog.

Thought Questions

1. What is the apparent purpose of statoconia?

2. Hair cells initiate impulses in all three major areas of the internal ear. Explain the differences in the types of stimuli to which they respond.

3. Before stimulating hair cells in the spiral organ, sound vibrations must pass through numerous structures. Name them in order.

4. Explain the "popping" of ears that occurs when driving up or down a mountain pass. Why is hearing more acute just after ears pop?

5. Why are middle ear infections often so painful?

6. Why do individuals with inner ear infections often suffer vertigo?

7. What kinds of noises are especially damaging to the ears?

8. What is the purpose of the "tubes" often placed through the tympanic membranes of children who have recurring middle ear infections? Why are these usually unnecessary after a few months (or years)?

9. Ear plugs reduce external noises (or prevent one from hearing them at all). They also alter but do not block the sound of one's own voice. Why?

10. What is the purpose of the secondary tympanic membrane?

11. The statoconial membrane in the utricle is horizontally oriented when the body is in the normal anatomical position. Of the three general directions of linear acceleration movements (anterior/ posterior, medial/lateral, superior/inferior), which one(s) should stimulate hair cells therein?

12. Spinning on a bar stool causes vertigo commonly called dizziness. Why does the associated disorientation continue for a few moments after the spinning has stopped?

13. What purpose do the auditory ossicles serve?

14. Why is conduction deafness easier to correct than sensory deafness?

15. What property of sound vibrations is related to pitch? To loudness?

16. Differentiate the two fluids associated with the internal ear.

17. Why is the osseous labyrinth not considered to be part of the internal ear? What are its three main divisions?

18. What purpose is served by having the three semicircular ducts all oriented in different planes?

19. What usually happens after a tympanic membrane is ruptured?

20. Why do insects (gnats, *etc.*) that wander into the external acoustic meatus usually beat a hasty retreat (after stomping around for a few moments)?

21. How are different pitches of sound perceived?

Answers to Clinical Case Studies

Case 1—The vestibular apparatus of the internal ear is involved with the sense of balance and equilibrium. When the areas of the brain that receive impulses from the vestibular apparatus are hyperstimulated, nausea, vertigo, and inability to maintain one's balance result.

Case 2—This condition, called tinnitus, is present in most individuals to some degree. It is typically so mild and is usually masked by background noise to the point that it goes largely unnoticed. The cause remains unknown.

Case 3—Her tympanic membrane, which had been bulging outward due to the pressure of a pus-filled tympanic cavity, ruptured. Since the eardrum was no longer stretched after the rupture, the pain was instantaneously relieved. Most ruptured tympanic membranes heal uneventfully with little or no loss of hearing acuity. Swelling in this patient's pharynx blocked the auditory tube and prevented the pus from draining into the pharynx.

Answers to Review Questions

1. D. Statoconia are calcium carbonate/protein structures that are part of the statoconial membrane. These membranes are part of the utricle and saccule of the internal ear.

2. B. The cochlear duct is the part of the membranous labyrinth (internal ear) involved in detection of sound.

3. A. Perilymph surrounds the membranous labyrinth.

4. E. There are two synovial joints and a fibrous joint (tympanostapedial syndesmosis) associated with the auditory ossicles, but no fibrocartilaginous joint.

5. E. B and D are both gravitational/inertial forces; A is flow (movement) of endolymph; C is vibrations in endolymph.

6. D. The problem with choice "C" is endolymph.

7. B. The tympanic membrane, secondary tympanic membrane, and the whole tympanic cavity is lined by a mucous membrane.

8. B. The cochlea is part of the osseous labyrinth. It houses the cochlear duct which is part of the membranous labyrinth.

9. B. The wall of the semicircular canal is the surface of the temporal bone adjacent to perilymph within the canal. The wall of the semicircular duct does lie between endolymph and perilymph.

10. E. Lassie was a male dog playing the part of a female. Several different collies have played Lassie over the years. All of them have been male dogs in real life (a hold-over from the Shakespearian age). I met Lassie once and asked him how he felt about playing a drag dog. He said the pay was good and that he got to wear his own coat. The part he hated most was passing up so many attractive fire hydrants. The problem with "A" is external acoustic meatus; the problem with "B" is secondary; in "C", perilymph is CSF but endolymph is not; in "D" the hair cells in the saccule respond to vertical movements and to forward/backward motion, but not to left/right movements.

Answers to Thought Questions

1. Statoconia ("otoliths") increase the mass of the statoconial membrane such that it is more easily influenced by gravitational and inertial forces. When these forces move the membrane, hair cells are stimulated, nervous impulses are generated, and the brain detects straight line motions (linear acceleration).

2. Those in the spiral organ of the cochlear duct respond to vibrations in the endolymph. Hair cells in the crista ampullaris of each semicircular duct respond to movements of the cupula. The

cupula reacts to fluid (endolymph) flow against it produced by turning and twisting movements (angular acceleration). Hair cells in the statoconial membranes of the utricle and saccule respond to gravitational and inertial forces which cause the whole membrane to shift during straight line motions (linear acceleration).

3. (Air), tympanic membrane (three layers), auditory ossicles (and associated joints), perilymph, vestibular membranes, endolymph, hairs of hair cells touching tectorial membrane.

4. The "popping" is caused by tiny bursts of air moving into or out of the cavity of the middle ear via the (normally collapsed) auditory tube. This allows the pressure on the medial side of the tympanic membrane to be the same as the pressure on the outside—assuring free movement when the membrane vibrates. Because the auditory tube tends to collapse (*i.e.*, is not continuously open) a slight pressure differential (inside/outside) must occur before movement of the air that causes the "pop". As soon as this happens, pressure is equalized (or at least more nearly equalized), the tympanic membrane can vibrate more freely, and hearing is more acute.

5. The inflammation that occurs often causes sufficient soft tissue swelling to functionally close the auditory tube. Accumulation of pus in the cavity of the middle ear stretches the tympanic membrane ("eardrum") and stimulates pain receptors.

6. The inflammatory process causes malfunction of the sensory receptors associated with the semicircular ducts as well as those in the utricle and saccule. These sensory receptors are responsible for balance and equilibrium.

7. Loud noises, especially those of constant pitch. These apparently damage the hair cells in the spiral organ of the cochlear duct.

8. The tubes act as artificial auditory tubes by allowing an equalization of pressure on the two sides of the tympanic membrane. In very young children, the auditory tubes are very small and swell shut quite easily. With growth, the auditory tubes enlarge and this becomes less of a problem.

9. The sound of an individual's voice normally reaches the owner's ears both through air vibrations as well as via transmission through the bones of the skull. Earplugs can block the air source but they do not block the pathway through the osseous structures.

10. The secondary tympanic membrane serves as a pressure relief valve. Every time the stapes vibrates in, the secondary tympanic membrane vibrates out, and vice-versa. This is necessary because fluids are relatively incompressible and the osseous labyrinth which surrounds the perilymph and internal ear components will not expand.

11. Anterior/posterior and medial/lateral. Superior/inferior motions should not stimulate hair cells associated with this membrane.

12. The dizziness occurs when endolymph within one (or more) of the semicircular ducts begins to flow and push continuously against the cupula of its ampulla. When one stops spinning the fluid movement does not immediately stop—therefore, the dizziness continues.

13. Auditory ossicles conduct the sound vibrations across the cavity of the middle ear (tympanic cavity) from the tympanic membrane to the perilymph within the osseous labyrinth surrounding the internal ear. In the process, the amplitude of the vibrations is increased about 20-fold.

14. Conduction deafness involves problems with the external and middle ears. These include relatively benign and easily correctable problems such as accumulation of ear wax (cerumen) in the external acoustic meatus. More difficult to manage problems with the auditory ossicles may require surgical installation of prosthetic devices. Sensory (internal ear) deafness cannot be medically managed because there are no prosthetic devices for the delicate internal ear structures. Even if there were, there is no way to connect such devices to the vestibulocochlear nerve.

15. Pitch depends on the frequency of sound vibrations (number of vibrations per second) and loudness is related to amplitude (strength of the vibrations).

16. Perilymph fills the space between the osseous and membranous labyrinths. It may be useful to consider that the membranous labyrinth is "floating" in or suspended in the perilymph. Perilymph has been shown to be cerebrospinal fluid. The perilymphatic space is connected to the subarachnoid space by a tiny perilymphatic duct. Discovery of this duct underscored the fact that perilymph is, in reality, cerebrospinal fluid. Endolymph is the fluid within the membranous labyrinth. It differs slightly in composition from perilymph. Endolymph is secreted by specialized cells in a part of the wall of the cochlear duct called the stria vascularis.

17. Just as the skull is not part of the brain (but does surround it), the osseous labyrinth surrounds but is not part of the internal ear. The three major parts of the osseous labyrinth are the cochlea (surrounding the cochlear duct), the semicircular canals (surrounding the semicircular ducts), and the vestibule (which contains the utricle and the saccule).

18. This arrangement allows detection of angular acceleration (turning/twisting) in any direction.

19. It usually heals with little or no loss of auditory acuity.

20. Cerumen (earwax) repels insects.

21. Sound vibrations of a certain frequency "disturb" (stimulate) hair cells only at certain locations in the 2½ turns of the spiral organ. Other pitches disturb hair cells at different loci. The temporal lobes somehow relate impulses generated in the different regions as different pitches.

CHAPTER

14 Endocrine System

Chapter Outline and Key Concepts

INTRODUCTION

The endocrine system includes the organs and tissues that produce hormones.

The hormone producing tissues are glandular epithelium which was developmentally derived from surface epithelium.

HORMONES

Hormones are chemicals that are produced at a particular site, transported by the bloodstream, and act at one or more other sites.

Any locus of action of a hormone constitutes (one of) its target(s).

Hormones can be divided into four chemical groups: proteins and polypeptides, steroids, catecholamines, and modified amino acids.

MECHANICS OF HORMONE ACTION

Hormones affect the rate of the body's chemical reactions by affecting enzyme production and/or activity.

THE ("TRUE") ENDOCRINE ORGANS

The "true" endocrine organs are those that have no known function other than hormone production (pineal, pituitary, thyroid, parathyroid, and adrenal glands).

The pineal gland (pineal body), located on the midline at the posterior aspect of the epithalamus, produces one hormone (melatonin).

The pituitary gland (hypophysis), suspended under the brain by a slender stalk of tissue called the infundibulum, is divided into anterior and posterior lobes.

The anterior lobe of the pituitary gland ("anterior pituitary") has three named subparts and produces seven known hormones: GH, TSH, ACTH, FSH, LH (called ICSH in males), LTH, and MSH.

The posterior lobe of the pituitary gland ("posterior pituitary") does not produce hormones but it stores and releases ADH and oxytocin which are manufactured by the hypothalamus.

The thyroid gland, located on the anterior aspect of the trachea just below the larynx, is divided into left and right lobes connected by an isthmus.

Hormones produced by the thyroid gland include T_3, T_4, and calcitonin.

The parathyroid gland consists of four islets of tissue embedded in the posterior aspect of the thyroid gland that produce one hormone (parathyroid hormone = PTH).

The paired adrenal glands cap the superior aspects of the kidneys and each is divided into a cortex and a medulla.

The adrenal cortex produces three groups of steroidal hormones: glucocorticoids, mineralocorticoids, and gonadocorticoids.

The adrenal medulla produces adrenalin (epinephrine and norepinephrine).

NON-ENDOCRINE ORGANS THAT PRODUCE HORMONES

The hypothalamus (the part of the brain just above the pituitary gland) produces more hormones than any other structure in the body.

At least eight hypothalamic hormones target the anterior lobe of the pituitary, reaching it by blood vessels constituting the hypothalamohypophysial portal system.

Two hypothalamic hormones (ADH and oxytocin) travel to the posterior lobe of the pituitary via bundles of axons of their neurosecretory cells collectively called the hypothalamohypophysial tract.

The pancreas is a digestive organ that produces two known hormones (insulin and glucagon) within groups of glandular epithelial cells called pancreatic islets.

The small intestine produces three known hormones: secretin, cholecystokinin, and enterogastrone (GIP).
The kidney is a urinary organ that produces renin and erythropoietin.
The ovary is a female reproductive organ that produces estrogen and progesterone.
The testis is a male reproductive organ that produces testosterone.
The thymus is a lymphatic organ that produces thymosin.
The placenta produces chorionic gonadotropin and somatomammotropin.
The chemical regulator produced by the stomach (gastrin) is an autocrine regulator rather than a hormone because it targets the organ where it is produced.

INTERNAL REGULATION OF THE ENDOCRINE SYSTEM

The general principle governing hormone secretion is negative feedback.
Many hormones regulate the production or release of other hormones by other organs.

DEVELOPMENT OF THE ENDOCRINE ORGANS

The anterior lobe of the pituitary gland develops from an upward evagination of oral ectoderm.
The posterior lobe of the pituitary gland develops from a downward extension from the primitive brain.
The thyroid gland develops from an outpouching of pharyngeal endoderm.
The parathyroid glands originate from ectoderm tissue in the third and fourth pharyngeal pouches.
The adrenal glands are formed from mesoderm (cortex) and from ectoderm (medulla) derived from the neural crests.
The pineal body develops from part of the primitive brain (diencephalon).

CLINICAL CONSIDERATIONS

Diseases can result from hypo- or hypersecretion of most any of the several dozen hormones.
Some endocrine disorders are relatively benign; others are serious and can result in death.

Selected Definitions

Adrenal medulla—the central part of each adrenal gland. It produces epinephrine and norepinphrine, and releases them into the bloodstream when stimulated by sympathetic preganglionic neurons.

Anterior lobe of the pituitary gland—the front part of the hypophysis, sometimes called the "anterior pituitary". This part of the pituitary gland produces at least seven hormones.

Beta cells of the pancreatic islets—those cells of the pancreatic islets that produce insulin. The pancreatic islets also have alpha cells that produce glucagon and other types of cells whose functions remain unclear.

Diabetes mellitus (sugar diabetes)—an endocrine disorder related to inadequate release of insulin from the beta cells of the pancreatic islets. It is clinically characterized by polydipsia (excessive thirst), polyuria (excessive urine production), and high blood sugar levels (hyperglycemia).

Follicles of thyroid gland—microscopic vesicular "sacs" of thyroid tissue consisting of simple cuboidal epithelium surrounding thyroglobulin. Thyroglobulin is a proteinaceous material to which thyroid hormone is temporarily attached before subsequent release by hydrolysis.

Glucocorticoid hormones—one of three groups of steroidal hormones produced by the adrenal cortex. The glucocorticoids stimulate gluconeogenesis by the liver and have anti-inflammatory properties.

Gonadocorticoid hormones—sex hormones produced by the adrenal cortex. These include some hormones of the opposite gender.

Hormone—a chemical regulator carried by the blood that produces an effect at a locus other than the organ where it was produced. Chemical regulators acting on the same organ that produced them are either autocrine or paracrine regulators.

Hypophysis—the pituitary gland. It is suspended below the hypothalamus by a stalk of tissue called the infundibulum of the pituitary gland and is divided into anterior and posterior lobes.

Hypothalamohypophysial portal system—a set of capillaries in the hypothalamus connected to a set in the anterior lobe of the pituitary gland by venules coursing down the outside of its infundibulum. It carries a number of hypothalamic hormones directly down to their target cells.

Hypothalamohypophysial tract—a bundle of axons of neurosecretory cells within the infundibulum of the pituitary gland. It transports ADH and oxytocin (produced in the supraoptic and paraventricular nuclei of the hypothalamus) down to the posterior lobe of the pituitary gland from whence they are released into the bloodstream.

Infundibulum of the pituitary gland—the stalk of tissue that connects the pituitary gland to the underside of the hypothalamus. The venules around the infundibulum are part of the hypothalamohypophysial portal system and the fasciculus of neuronal fibers within it constitutes the hypothalamohypophysial tract.

Isthmus of the thyroid gland—the thin portion of the thyroid gland that connects its left and right lobes. There is no functional significance related to the subdivisions of the thyroid gland.

Pancreatic islets—groups of endocrine cells scattered among the "regular" (exocrine) pancreatic cells (pancreatic acinar cells). Specific cell types in the islets include beta cells (which produce insulin) and alpha cells (which produce glucagon).

Paraventricular nucleus of the hypothalamus—a group of neurosecretory cells in the hypothalamus that produce oxytocin. Axons of these cells (and those of the supraoptic nucleus) form the hypothalamohypophysial tract which transports oxytocin (and ADH) down the infundibulum to the posterior lobe of the hypophysis.

Pineal body (gland)—a small structure forming the posterior aspect of the epithalamus. It produces melatonin.

Supraoptic nucleus of the hypothalamus—a group of neurosecretory cells in the hypothalamus that produce antidiuretic hormone (ADH). Axons of these cells (and those of the paraventricular nucleus) form the hypothalamohypophysial tract which transports ADH (and oxytocin) down the infundibulum to the posterior lobe of the hypophysis.

Target—the cells, tissues, or organ where a chemical regulator exerts its effects. Some chemical regulators have multiple targets.

Thyroxine (tetraiodothyronine, T_4)—a hormone produced by the thyroid gland that increases the basal metabolic rate. Thyroxine and T_3 (triiodothyronine) are collectively called thyroid hormone.

True endocrine organ—an organ that has no known functions except the production of chemical regulators. The true endocrine organs are the pineal, pituitary, thyroid, parathyroid, and adrenal glands.

Zona fasiculata of the adrenal cortex—the middle one of the three named layers of the adrenal cortex. It is sandwiched between the zona glomerulosa and the deeper zona reticularis of the adrenal cortex.

Etymology *aurea mediocritas*—"**Moderation in all things.**"

ad (L), *toward, adjacent to*—adrenal
adeno (G), *gland*—adenohypophysis
akros (G), *extremity*—acromegaly
anti (L), *against*—antidiuretic
cortex (L), *bark*—gonadocorticoids
diabetes (G), *siphon*—diabetes
diureticus (L), *to urinate*—diuretic
endemia (G), *action of swelling*—endemic
glucose (G), *sweet*—glucocorticoids
gonad (L), *primary sex gland*—gonadocorticoids
harmon (G), to stir up—hormone
hypophysis (L), *pituitary gland*—hypophysis
in (L), *not*—diabetes insipidus
infundibulum (L), *funnel*—infundibulum
isthmos (G), *thin connection*—isthmus
lacto (L), *milk*—prolactin
megas (G), *large*—acromegaly
mellitus (L), *honey, sweet*—diabetes mellitus
myx (L), *mucus, slime*—myxedema
oestrus (L), *frenzy*—estrogen
oxy (G), *quick*—oxytocin
porta (L), *gateway*—portal
renal (L), *kidney*—adrenal
sapidus (L), *savory*—diabetes insipidus
supra (L), *above*—suprarenal
thyroides (L), *shield-like*—thyroid
tokos (G), *childbirth*—oxytocin

Introduction

The endocrine system is a chemical control system which includes five relatively small, anatomically separate organs termed **endocrine glands** (Table 14-1, Figure 14-1) as well as groups of glandular epithelial cells within several organs that belong to other body systems (Table 14-2). The products secreted by these structures are called **hormones**. Hormones enter the bloodstream and are carried throughout the body, but they act only on specific cells, tissues, and organs which respond to them. These are called the **targets** of the hormones and respond because they contain specific **receptors**. The parenchyma of endocrine organs and the endocrine epithelial cells found in some other organs are all derived from membranous (surface) epithelium which invades the underlying connective tissue during development, loses all connection to the surface, and begins secreting chemical regulators.

Table 14-1 Hormones Released by the Five "True" Endocrine Organs

Pineal gland:

Melatonin—stimulates the release of some hormones from the hypothalamus and is involved in circadian rhythms

Pituitary gland (hypophysis):

Anterior lobe of the pituitary gland (adenohypophysis):

- Somatotropin (growth hormone/GH)—stimulates protein synthesis and general body growth
- Thyrotropin (TSH)—stimulates the thyroid gland to release thyroid hormone
- Adrenocorticotropic h. (ACTH)—stimulates production of hormones by the adrenal cortex
- Follicle stimulating h. (FSH)—promotes sperm production and follicle development
- Luteinizing h. (LH), interstitial cell stimulating hormone (ICSH)—promotes ovulation, corpus luteum formation, and testosterone production (same substance in males and females)
- Prolactin (PRL)—promotes milk production within mammary glands
- Melanocyte stimulating h. (MSH)—causes dispersion of melanin granules within melanocytes

Posterior lobe of the pituitary gland (neurohypophysis):

- Oxytocin (OXY)*—stimulates contraction of uterine musculature and myoepithelial cells in mammary glands
- Antidiuretic h.* (ADH)—reduces urine output by increasing renal resorption of water

Thyroid gland:

Tetraiodothyronine or thyroxine (T_4)—increases protein synthesis, basal metabolic rate, and growth
Triiodothyronine (T_3)—(same as above)
Calcitonin—lowers blood calcium by inhibiting its release from bone tissue

Parathyroid gland:

Parathyroid h. (PTH)—increases blood calcium by acting on bone tissue, intestine, and kidneys

Adrenal (suprarenal) gland:

Adrenal cortex:

- Glucocorticoids—increase liver glycogen concentration and reduce inflammation
- Mineralocorticoids—promote sodium and other electrolyte retention by acting at the renal tubules
- Gonadocorticoids—supplement the sex hormones produced by the testis and ovary

Adrenal medulla:

- Epinephrine—increases heart rate, constricts vessels, dilates respiratory passageways, increases blood glucose levels
- Norepinephrine—same as above

*Oxytocin and ADH are actually manufactured by neurosecretory cells in the hypothalamus but are stored in and released from the posterior lobe of the pituitary gland.

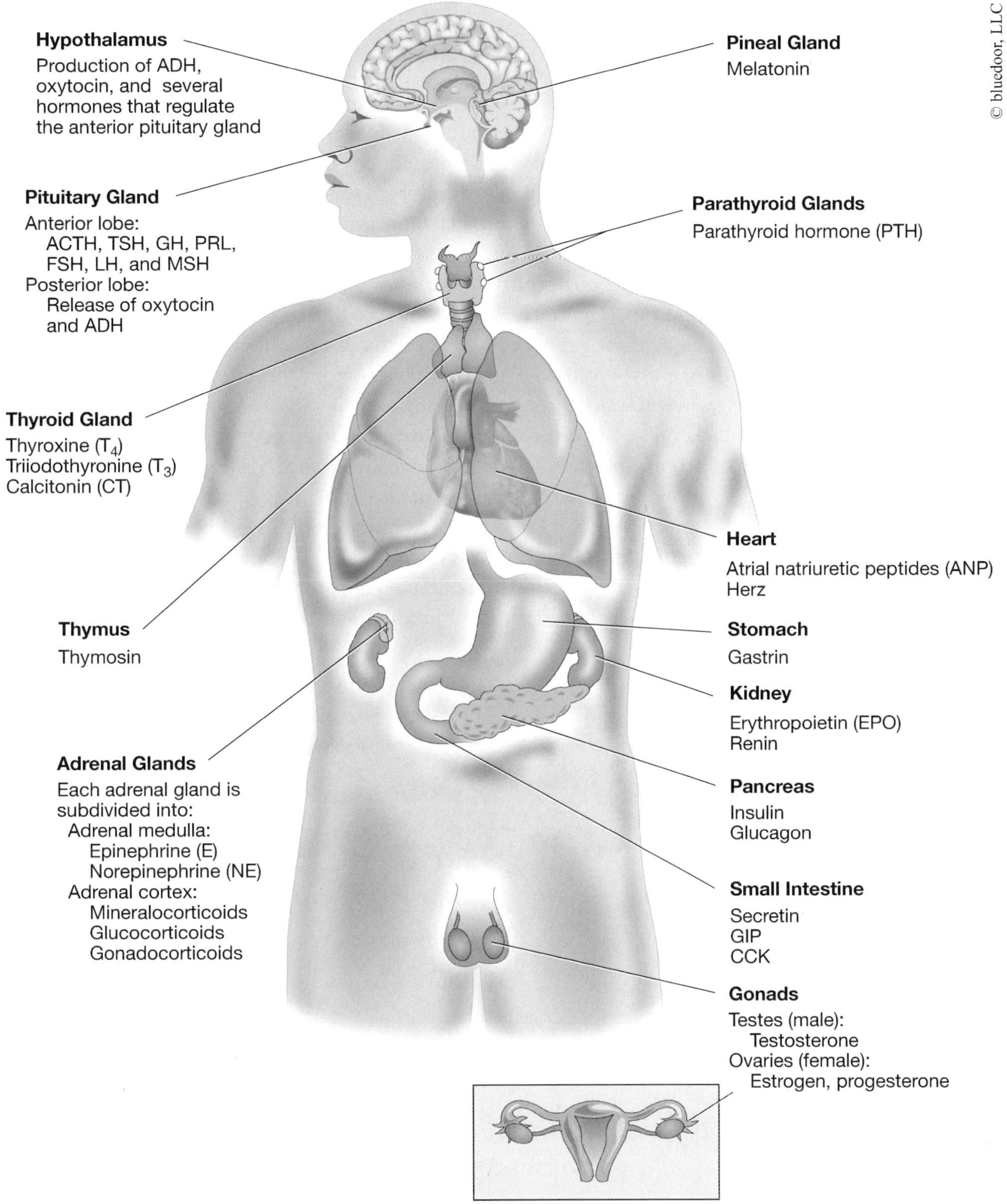

Figure 14-1

Hormone Producing Structures

Some of these have no other known functional roles in the body. They constitute the five "true"endocrine organs and "belong" (as organs) to the endocrine system (*see Table 14-1*). Others, like the heart, kidney, and pancreas, produce one or more hormones but actually "belong" to other body systems (*see Table 14-2*).

Hormones

The term *hormone* is derived from a Greek word meaning to excite or to arouse. A **hormone** is defined as a chemical substance produced at one location in the body, transported by the bloodstream, and exerting an effect at one or more locations other than its site of production. By these criteria, even carbon dioxide, which stimulates the respiratory centers in the brain, satisfies the definition of a hormone. However, the term is usually reserved for more complex compounds. Several dozen hormones have been identified. These fall into four basic chemical categories: steroids, polypeptides and proteins, catecholamines, and modified amino acids (Figure 14-2). **Steroid hormones** are chemically related to cholesterol and have a basic structure consisting of three 6-carbon rings linked to a five-carbon ring (Figure 14-2). They include the sex hormones (testosterone, progesterone, estrogen) as well as those produced by the cortex of the adrenal gland. The majority of hormones are **proteins** or **polypeptides.** These vary in size from those composed of several hundred amino acids, to ones with only three amino acids such as thyrotropin releasing factor (TRF) secreted by the hypothalamus. The **catecholamine hormones** (epinephrine and norepinephrine) are relatively simple 6-carbon ring compounds that have an amino (NH_2) group on a carbon side chain. The thyroid hormones are **modified amino acids** consisting of triiodothyronine (T_3) and tetraiodothyronine (T_4, thyroxine). In addition to hormones, a number of chemical regulators have been discovered that act on the organs that produce them. These substances, which include prostaglandins, have been termed autocrine or paracrine regulators to distinguish them from hormones (which target organs other than their site of production).

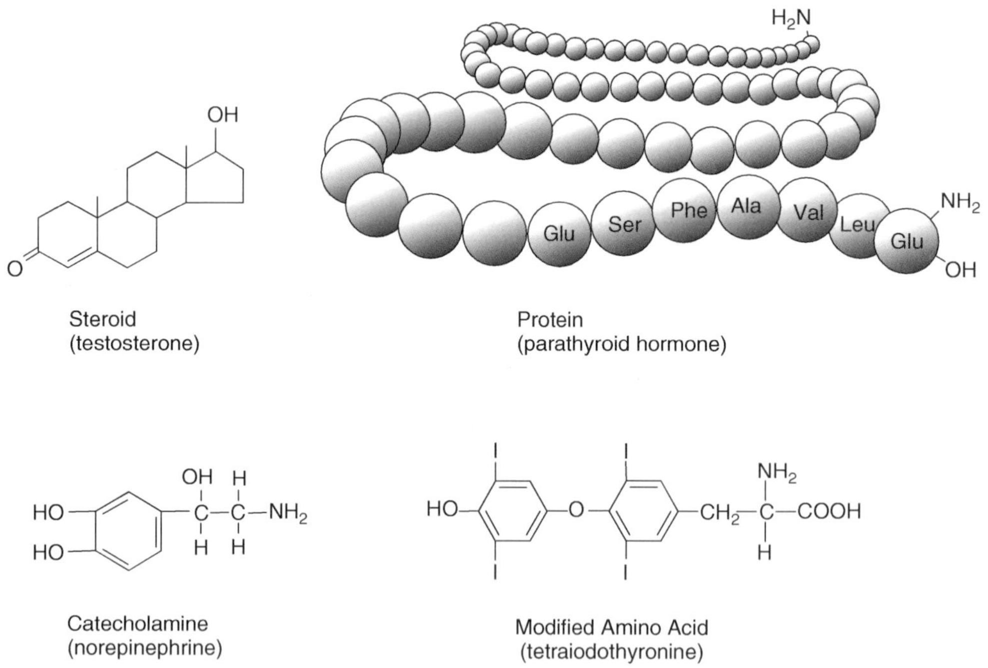

Figure 14-2

Examples of the Four Chemical Categories of Hormones

The majority of hormones are proteins or polypeptides. Steroid hormones include the sex hormones (estrogen, progesterone, and testosterone) as well as the hormones produced by the adrenal cortex. The only modified amino acid hormones are tetraiodothyronine (=thyroxine=T_4) and triiodothyronine (T_3). The major catecholamine hormones are epinephrine and norepinephrine.

Table 14-2 Hormones Produced by "Non-Endocrine" Organs

Hypothalamus:

Growth h. releasing factor (GRF)—stimulates release of GH from anterior lobe of pituitary gland
Growth h. release inhibiting factor (GR-IH)—inhibits release of GH
Thyrotropin releasing factor (TRF)—stimulates release of TSH from anterior lobe of pituitary gland
Corticotropin releasing factor (CRF)—stimulates release of ACTH from anterior lobe of pituitary gland
Gonadotropin releasing factor (GnRF)—stimulates release of LH (ICSH) and FSH from anterior lobe of pituitary gland
Prolactin release inhibiting factor (PR-IF)—inhibits release of PRL from anterior lobe of pituitary gland
Melanocyte stimulating hormone releasing factor (MRF)—stimulates release of MSH from anterior lobe of pituitary gland
Melanocyte stimulating hormone inhibiting factor (MIF)—inhibits release of MSH from anterior lobe of pituitary gland
(Oxytocin and antidiuretic hormone are produced by the hypothalamus but they are released from the posterior lobe of pituitary gland—*see Table 14-1*)

Pancreas:

Insulin—lowers blood sugar levels by facilitating transport of sugar into cells
Glucagon—raises blood sugar levels by stimulating hepatocytes to convert glycogen to glucose

Small intestine:

Gastric inhibitory peptide (GIP)—inhibits gastric motility and secretion, stimulates insulin release
Cholecystokinin (CCK)—stimulates contraction of gallbladder and secretion of pancreatic enzymes
Secretin—stimulates production of pancreatic juice

Stomach:

Gastrin—promotes hydrochloric acid production by parietal cells*

Kidney:

Renin—enzymatically helps convert angiotensinogen to angiotensin which raises the blood pressure
Erythropoietin—stimulates the production of red blood corpuscles by the bone marrow

Thymus:

Thymosin—stimulates the T-lymphocytes

Ovary:

Progesterone—keeps uterine lining conducive to implantation and placentation
Estrogen—promotes production of female secondary sex characteristics and functions in uterine cycle

Testis:

Testosterone—promotes production of male secondary sex characteristics

Heart:

Herz—augments cardiac contraction*
Atrial natriuretic peptide (ANP)—increases capillary filtration, salt and water secretion, decreases arterial pressure, secretion of renin, angiotensin, aldosterone, and ADH

Placenta:

Chorionic gonadotropin—assists progesterone in keeping uterine lining conducive to pregnancy
Somatomammotropin—stimulates development of mammary glands

---

* Because they act on the same organs that produce them, herz and gastrin qualify as autocrine regulators rather than hormones.

Objectives

1. Define hormone and target, and state what differentiates hormones from other kinds of chemical regulators (*i.e.,* autocrine and paracrine regulators).

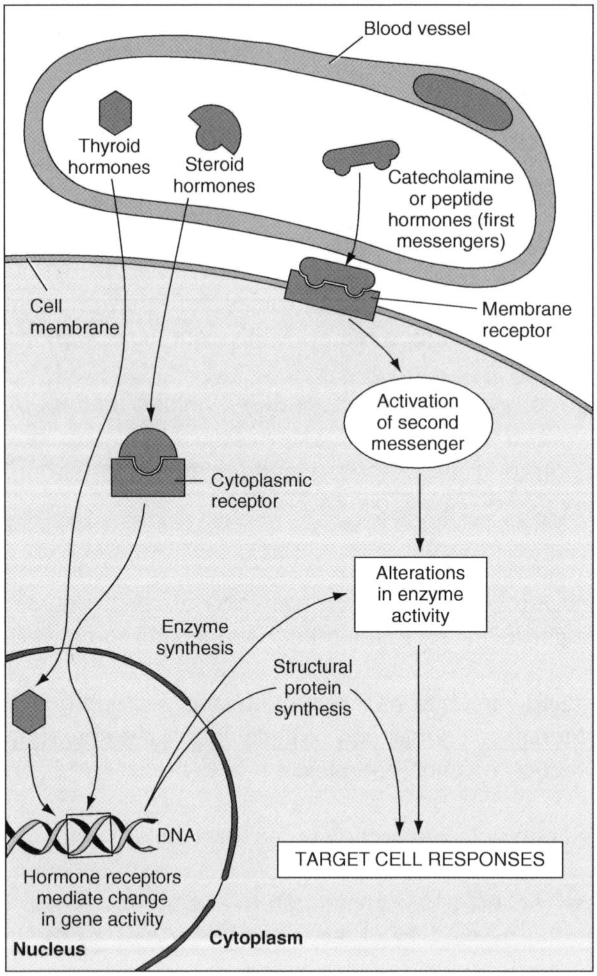

Figure 14-3

Mechanisms of Hormone Action

Tri- and tetraiodothyronine (thyroid hormones) diffuse directly into the nucleus to specific genes. Steroid hormones interact with their receptors in the cytoplasm. Catecholamine hormones and protein/polypeptide hormones bind with receptors on the cell surface (*see Table 14-3*).

Mechanisms of Hormone Action

Hormones do not initiate metabolic reactions, but they influence the rate at which reactions occur by affecting the rate of enzyme production or activity. The different classes of hormones have somewhat different mechanisms of action but the net result is similar: they alter cellular metabolism (Figure 14-3, Table 14-3). The small hormones, such as the thyroid hormones, can penetrate directly into the nucleus where they *activate specific genes* (Figure 14-3). The steroid hormones also readily diffuse through cell membranes and they interact with receptors in the cytoplasm of their target cells. These hormone/receptor complexes are then transferred to the cell nucleus where they activate specific genes. The polypeptide, protein, and catecholamine hormones do not readily cross cell membranes. Their receptors are located on the cell membranes of the target cells. Hormone/receptor interactions in these cases result in production of other chemical compounds which *activate enzymes* that have already been synthesized. Hormones function at low concentrations, and are continually produced at varying rates. Most of them have short physiological half-lives (minutes to hours) due to their rapid inactivation by metabolic transformations. When hormones are administered at very high (non-physiological) levels, abnormal responses may occur. These may be caused by their interacting with receptors of different (but related) hormones or by metabolic transformations of the hormones themselves. The latter occurs in bodybuilders who take high doses of steroid hormones.

Table 14-3 Mechanisms of Hormone Action

Hormone Type	*Location of Receptors*	*Effect of Hormone/Receptor Interaction*
Modified amino acid (T_3,T_4)	Nucleus of target cells	Direct activation of specific genes
Steroid hormones	Cytoplasm of target cells	Hormone/receptor complexes are transferred to nuclei where they activate specific genes
Catecholamines, polypeptides, and proteins	On the cell membrane	Hormone/receptor complexes cause production of other compounds which activate enzymes that have already been produced

Objectives

2. Differentiate the four chemical categories of hormones in regard to the location of the receptors on the target cells and the effect of hormone/receptor interactions.

The ("True") Endocrine Organs

The "true" **endocrine organs** are those hormone producing structures which have no other functions in the body. They include the pineal, pituitary, thyroid, parathyroid, and adrenal glands. These five organs belong to the endocrine system, *per se*, although at least 10 organs belonging to other body systems are known to produce hormones (*see Table 14-2 and footnote*).

The **pineal gland (pineal body)** is a small cone-shaped structure located on the midline at the posterior aspect of the epithalamus (Figure 14-4). Its name is derived from the Latin *pineus* which means pine cone. It contains lime concretions (inorganic masses) called "brain sand" which make it visible radiographically. The pineal gland secretes the hormone melatonin. Melatonin is involved in circadian rhythms and is believed to stimulate the production of certain hypothalamic hormones, most of which, in turn, control the secretion of hormones by the anterior pituitary gland. It is an interesting phenomenon that the pineal gland is attached to the brain but receives no direct innervation from it. Instead, it receives postganglionic fibers from the sympathetic division of the ANS.

The **pituitary gland (hypophysis)** is a rounded structure about 13 mm in diameter. It is suspended from the inferior aspect of the hypothalamus by a thin stalk of tissue (**infundibulum**) located

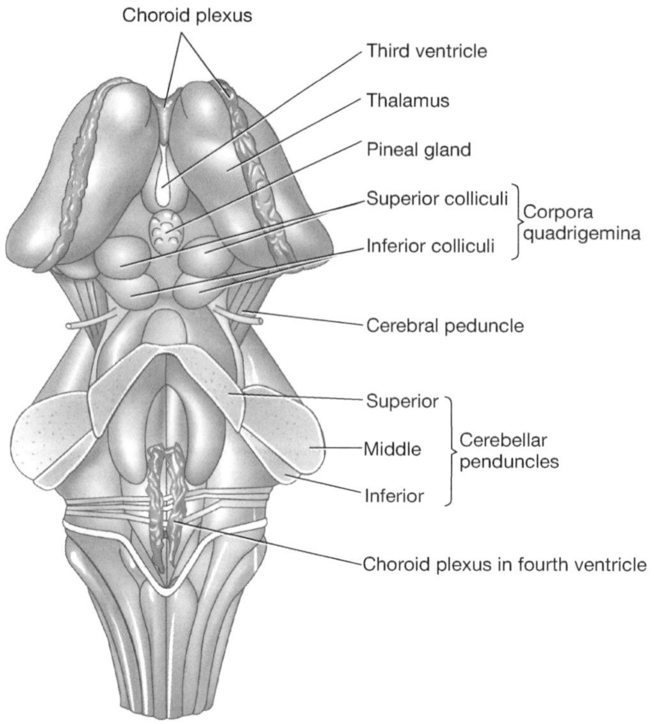

Figure 14-4

Posterior View of Brainstem and Pineal Gland (Body)

The pineal body forms the most posterior part of the epithalamus. It lies between and just superior to the superior colliculi of the corpora quadrigemina. The only hormone produced by the pineal body is melatonin.

behind the optic chiasm. The infundibulum penetrates a fold of dura mater termed the diaphragma sella to reach the hypophysis. The pituitary gland sits on the sella turcica of the sphenoid bone and is directly below the cerebral arterial circle (*see Cardiovascular System*). It is divided into an **anterior lobe (adenohypophysis)** and a **posterior lobe (neurohypophysis)**. To save space, these names are often shortened to the unofficial *anterior pituitary* and *posterior pituitary*. The anterior lobe develops as an out-pouching (evagination) of epithelium from the roof of the oral cavity which later loses all oral connections. It is divided into a bulbous portion (**pars distalis**), a slender portion adherent to the anterior aspect of the infundibulum (**pars tuberalis**), and a thin plate of tissue between the pars distalis and the neurohypophysis termed the **pars intermedia** (Figure 14-5). The **posterior lobe of the pituitary gland** is formed directly from part of the brain and is divided into the suspending infundibulum and the **pars nervosa** which lies directly behind the anterior pituitary. The pituitary gland releases nine known hormones. Seven of these are manufactured by various cells in the anterior pituitary and many of them exert controlling influences over the production of hormones by other organs (Table 14-1). The manufacture and release of hormones by the anterior lobe is controlled largely by the hormones released by the hypothalamus. The two hormones released by the posterior pituitary gland are **oxytocin** and **ADH.** These are actually manufactured in the supraoptic and paraventricular nuclei of the hypothalamus and travel through the axons of the neurosecretory cells down through the infundibulum to the pars nervosa of the posterior pituitary gland where they are stored until they are released

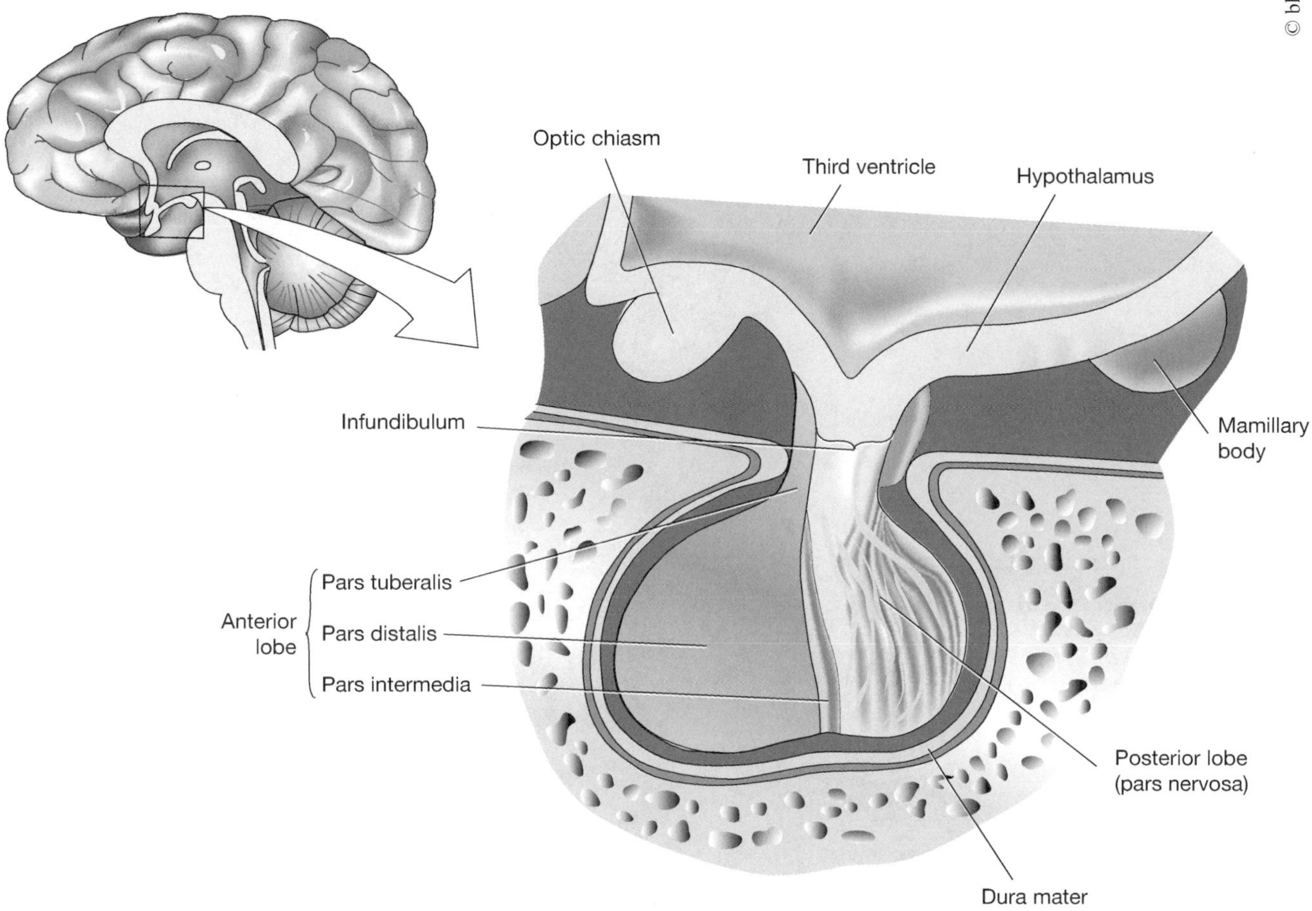

Figure 14-5
Pituitary Gland

The pituitary gland is suspended from the hypothalamus by a stalk of tissue called the infundibulum. The anterior lobe of the pituitary gland secretes/releases seven hormones. The posterior lobe of the pituitary gland produces no hormones but does store/release ADH and oxytocin. These hormones are produced by the supraoptic and paraventricular nuclei of the hypothalamus and they are transported to the posterior lobe of the pituitary gland via a bundle of axons of neurosecretory cells called the hypothalamohypophysial tract.

(Figure 14-5, 6). For many years, the pituitary gland was considered to be the "master gland" of the body because it produces so many different hormones that influence the activity of other body organs. However, the discovery that the hypothalamus produces even more hormones and that most of these influence pituitary activity disproved the "master gland" concept. More recent evidence suggests that the pineal gland may control some hypothalamic activity. The discovery of autonomic nerve fiber endings in the pineal gland have further discredited any "master gland" theories.

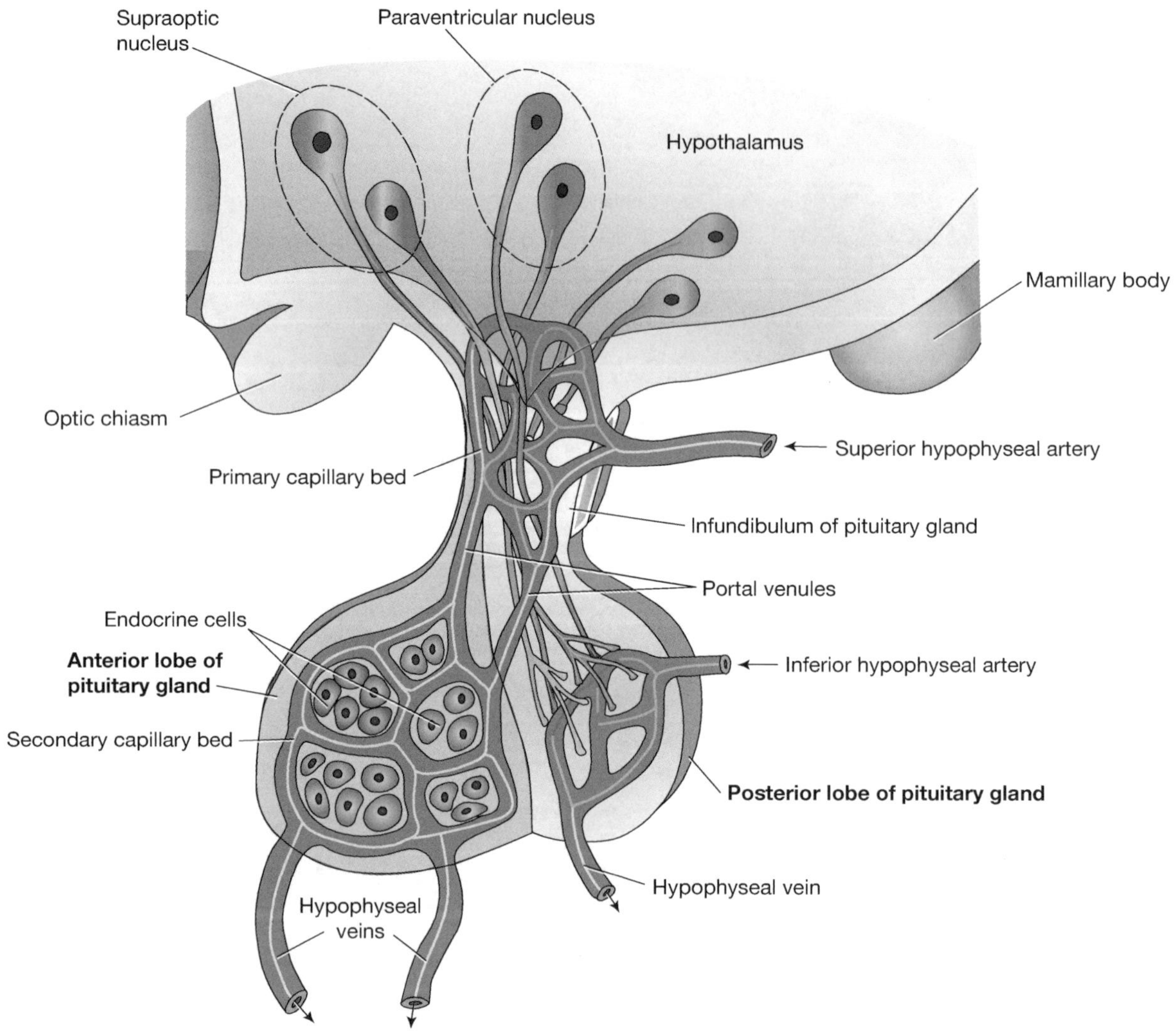

Figure 14-6

Hypothalamohypophysial Tract and Hypothalamohypophysial Portal System

The tract is a bundle of axons of the neurosecretory cells in the supraoptic and paraventricular nuclei of the hypothalamus. It carries ADH and oxytocin down the infundibulum to the posterior lobe of the pituitary gland for storage/release. The portal system is a set of venules that carry blood from a first capillary bed in the hypothalamus to a second one in the anterior lobe of the pituitary gland. This delivers several hypothalamic hormones to their target (anterior pituitary) in concentrations high enough to be effective (*see Hypothalamus*).

Objectives

3. Divide the hormone producing structures of the body into two groups: the "true" endocrine organs and the structures belonging to other body systems that produce hormones.

Several different cell types have been identified in the pituitary gland but attempts to match these with specific hormonal products have been unsuccessful. The various hormones released are summarized in Table 14-1 but will be considered more fully herein:

1. **Somatotropin** is also called **growth hormone (GH).** It promotes general body growth by promoting mitotic activity. Two hypothalamic hormones (GRF and GR-IH) control the secretion of somatotropin (*see Table 14-2*). Inadequate quantities of this hormone during childhood and adolescence result in a type of **dwarfism.** Hypersecretion in immature individuals results in **giantism.** If hypersecretion occurs in an adult, the condition called **acromegaly** results. Affected individuals have osseous enlargements involving the distal limbs, mandible, and nose.
2. **Thyrotropin** is also called **thyroid stimulating hormone (TSH)**. It increases the activity of the thyroid gland and is, in turn, under the influence of thyrotropin releasing factor from the hypothalamus. If the diet is deficient in iodine, the thyroid gland cannot manufacture enough thyroid hormone. This causes an increase in TSH release, enlargement of the thyroid gland, and is diagnosed as **endemic goiter** (*see Thyroid gland*).
3. **Adrenocorticotropic hormone (ACTH)** stimulates the production of the three groups of hormones produced by the adrenal cortex. It is released in response to corticotropin releasing factor (CRF) from the hypothalamus.
4. **Follicle stimulating hormone (FSH)** is responsible for stimulating the monthly ovarian cycle in females, and for stimulating spermatogenesis in males. The release of FSH and LH (*see below*) are partially controlled by gonadotropin releasing hormone from the hypothalamus.
5. **Luteinizing hormone (LH)** stimulates ovulation and formation of the corpus luteum in females. In males, the same hormone is known as **interstitial cell stimulating hormone (ICSH)** and stimulates the interstitial cells of the testis to produce testosterone.
6. **Prolactin (PRL)** is also known as **lactogenic hormone (LTH)**. It promotes lactation after parturition in females and has essentially no function in males. Its release is controlled by prolactin release inhibiting factor from the hypothalamus.
7. **Melanocyte stimulating hormone (MSH)** is known to increase skin pigmentation in some species of animals by affecting the dispersion of pigment granules in pigment cells (melanocytes). Whether this is true in mankind remains uncertain. Two hypothalamic hormones affect the secretion of MSH (*see Table 14-2*).
8. **Antidiuretic hormone (ADH)** is also known as arginine **vasopressin.** It acts on the renal tubules to increase the reabsorption of water from filtrate. This reduces the water lost in the urine. ADH also causes constriction of blood vessels which elevates the blood pressure. ADH is released in response to rising osmolality of the blood (*i.e.*, increasing electrolyte concentrations). Inadequate levels of this hormone cause a disease condition called **diabetes insipidus** which is characterized by excessive urination and thirst.
9. **Oxytocin (OXY** or **OXT)** targets the uterine musculature and the myoepithelial cells of the mammary gland causing uterine contraction and stimulating milk "let down". It has lesser functions in males. Both oxytocin and ADH are manufactured in the hypothalamus and then delivered to the posterior pituitary through the axons of neurosecretory cells (Figure 14-6). These two hormones are released from the posterior pituitary.

The **thyroid gland** is positioned just below the larynx at the superior end of the trachea (Figure 14-8). It consists of **left** and **right lobes** joined on the anterior midline by a connecting segment termed the **isthmus of the thyroid gland**. Sometimes isolated groups of thyroid cells called accessory thyroid

Table 14-4 A Comparison of Hormone Transport Mechanisms Associated with the Infundibulum of the Pituitary Gland

Criteria	*Hypothalamohypophysial Tract*	*Hypothalamohypophysial Portal System*
Composition	Axons of neurosecretory cells	Venules
Location	Within infundibulum	Around infundibulum
Destination	Posterior lobe of pituitary gland	Anterior lobe of pituitary gland
Transports...	ADH and oxytocin (neither of which target the pituitary gland)	Numerous hormones all of which target the anterior lobe of pituitary gland
Purpose	Remains an enigma	Deliver hormones to their target in concentrations sufficient to exert their effect

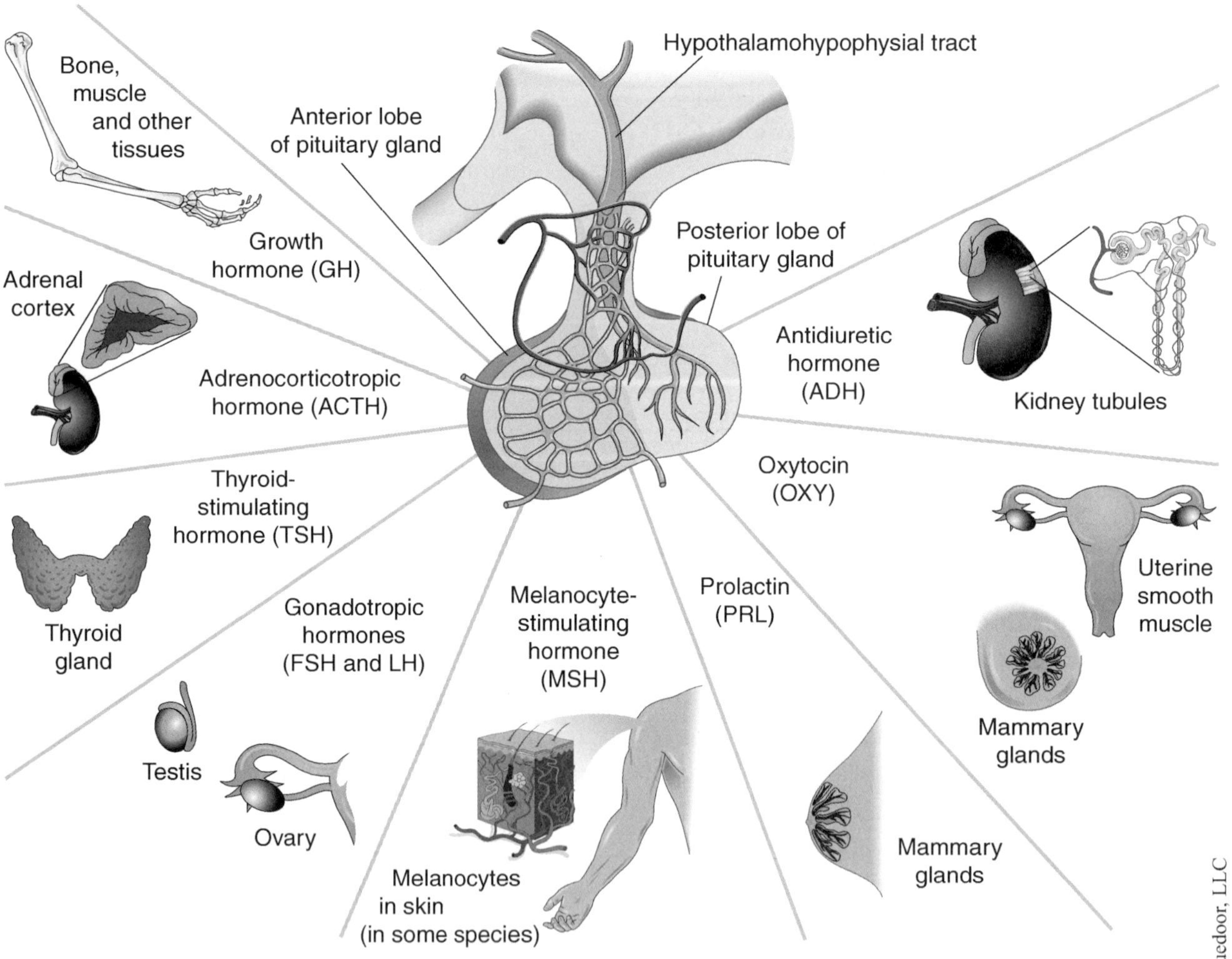

Figure 14-7

Pituitary Hormones and Their Targets

Note that in males, luteinizing hormone (LH) is called ICSH (interstitial cell stimulating hormone).

glands occur which are separated from the main thyroid mass. Microscopically, the thyroid gland consists of vesicular sacs formed by simple cuboidal epithelium called follicular cells which secrete and synthesize several forms of iodine containing amino acids. The two main ones are **tetraiodothyronine** (**thyroxine** or **T_4**) and **triiodothyronine** (**T_3**). These substances are collectively termed thyroid hormone and are stored within the vesicles as part of a protein material called thyroglobulin ("colloid"). Synthesis of this protein and its hydrolysis to release the thyroid hormones occurs continuously.

Thyroid hormone accelerates cellular reactions, increases the basal metabolic rate, and is essential for proper development of the central nervous system. If too little thyroid hormone is produced or released, **hypothyroidism** results with lethargy, lowered body temperature, and obesity. If this occurs at birth, infantile myxedema or cretinism results. If it occurs in adults the term myxedema is often used. Hypersecretion of thyroid hormones results in **Graves disease** (**toxic goiter**). Affected individuals have high metabolic and heart rates, lose body weight, and frequently have bulging eyes (exophthalmos) because of edema in the soft tissues around the eyeballs. **Endemic goiter** is an enlargement of the thyroid gland that occurs from inadequate dietary intake of iodine. In this disease, the thyroid gland secretes inadequate thyroid hormone and the anterior pituitary gland secretes excessive thyrotropin in response. This causes the thyroid gland to enlarge. In addition to thyroid hormone, the thyroid gland also produces a hormone called **calcitonin** (**thyrocalcitonin**). This polypeptide reduces blood levels of calcium and phosphorus by directly increasing their deposition into bone tissue. Calcitonin is secreted in response to hypercalcemia (high levels of blood calcium).

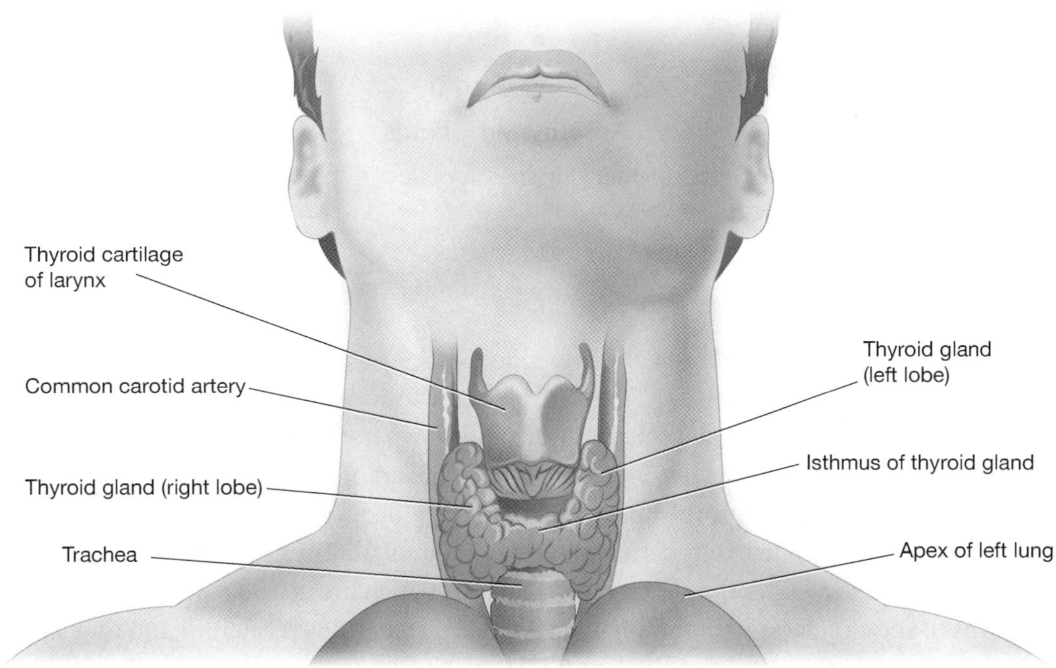

Figure 14-8

Thyroid Gland

The thyroid gland is positioned on the anterior aspect of the trachea just below the larynx. Grossly it consists of a left lobe, a right lobe, and a connecting isthmus.

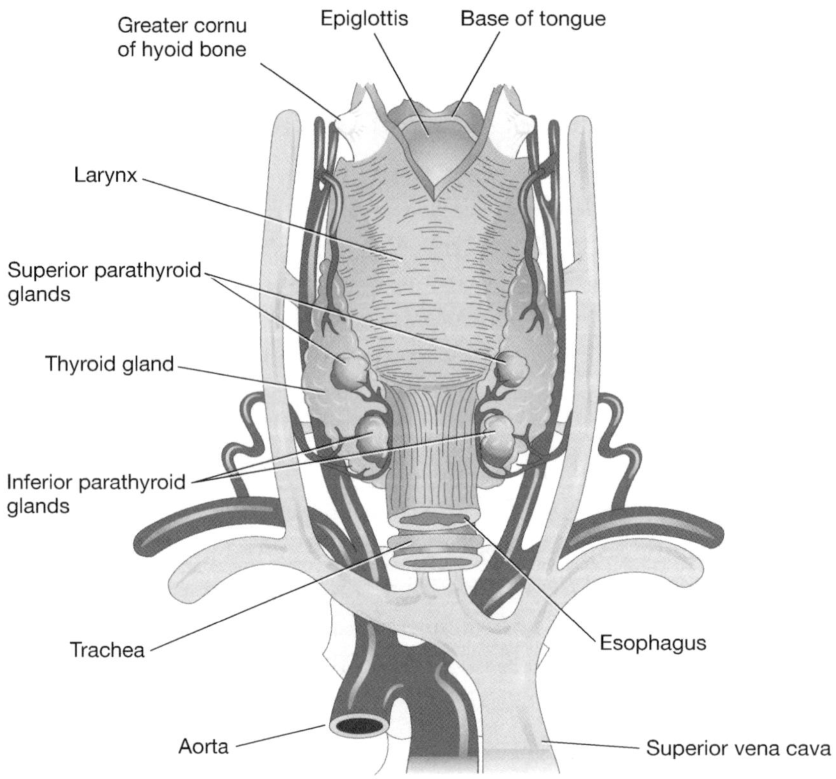

Figure 14-9
Parathyroid Glands

There are usually four parathyroid glands embedded in the posterior aspects of the left and right lobes of the thyroid gland.

The small **parathyroid glands** are embedded in the posterior aspect of the left and right lobes of the thyroid gland (Figure 14-9). There are typically four of them: left and right superior parathyroid glands (parathyroid III) and left and right inferior parathyroid glands (parathyroid IV). They are flattened ovoids measuring about 2 x 3 x 6 mm. Histologically, they contain principal ("chief") cells which produce **parathyroid hormone** (**PTH**) and oxyphil cells (function unknown). PTH increases blood calcium levels by acting on bone tissue, small intestinal mucosa, and the kidneys. In bone tissue, PTH stimulates the activity of osteoclasts which break down bone matrix and return calcium ions to the circulation. In the small intestine, PTH augments calcium and phosphorus absorption by stimulating the uptake of these materials by the columnar epithelial cells lining the intestinal lumen. In the kidney, PTH causes calcium retention and phosphaturia. The net effect of PTH is increased blood calcium levels. In fact, the secretion of PTH is regulated by and is inversely proportional to the serum calcium levels. **Hypoparathyroidism** from diseases of the parathyroid glands or loss of them during surgical procedures involving the thyroid gland can lead to hypocalcemia, convulsions, tetany, and death (in the absence of therapy). **Hyperparathyroidism** leads to hypercalcemia, hyperphosphatemia, increased renal excretion of calcium, and osteitis fibrosa cystica. This condition leads to pathological fracturing of the weakened bones.

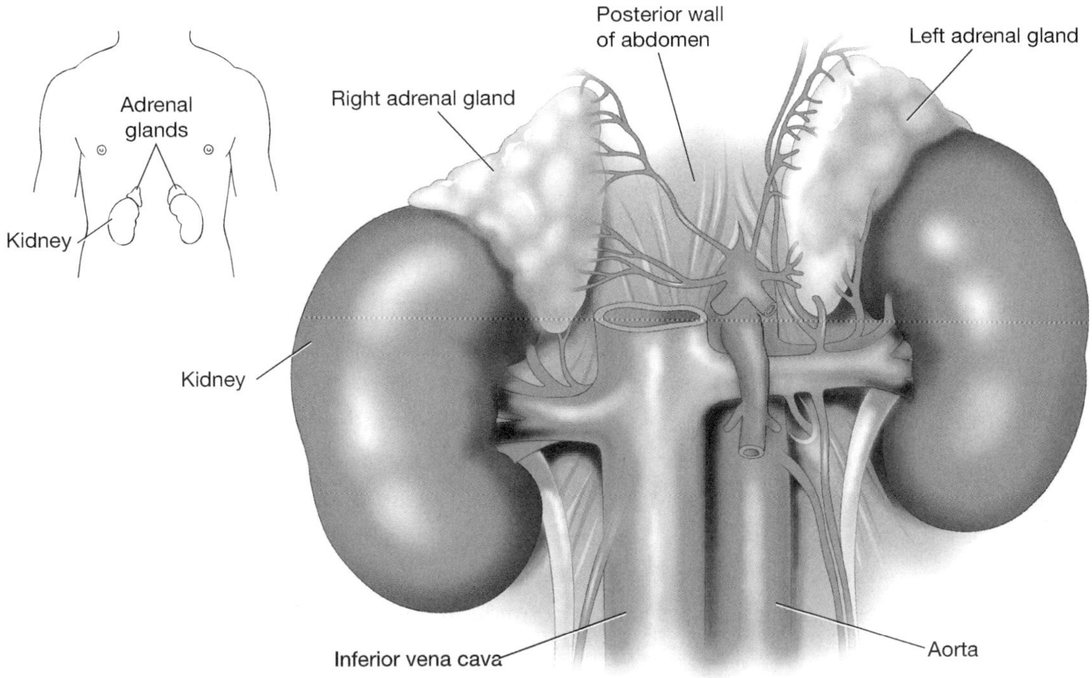

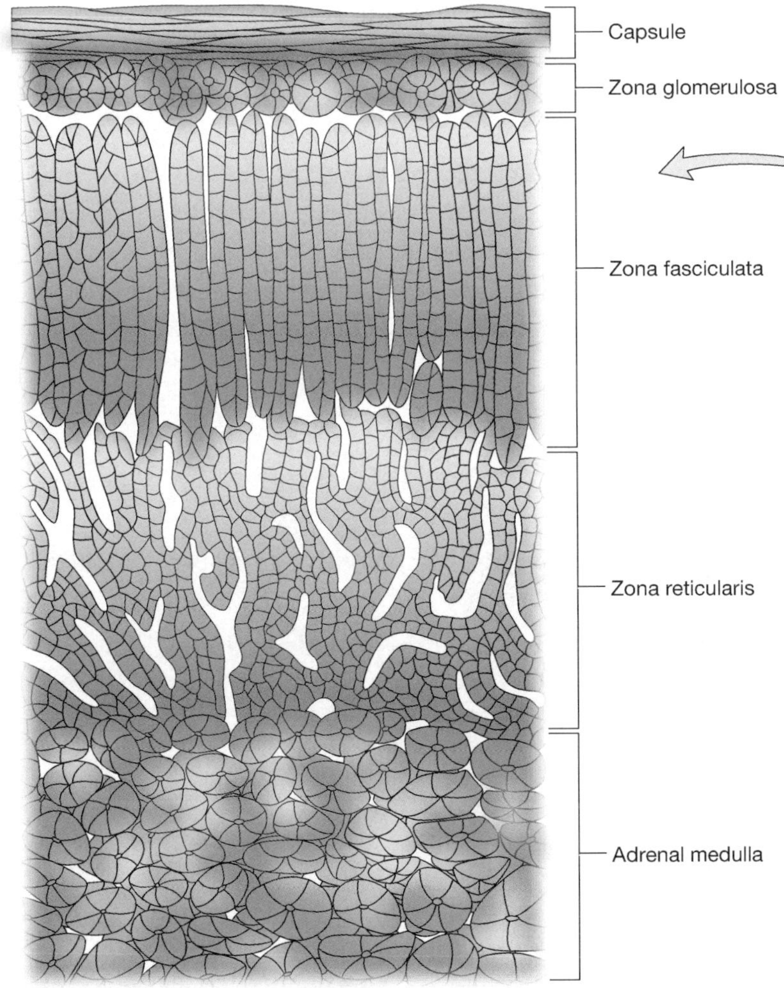

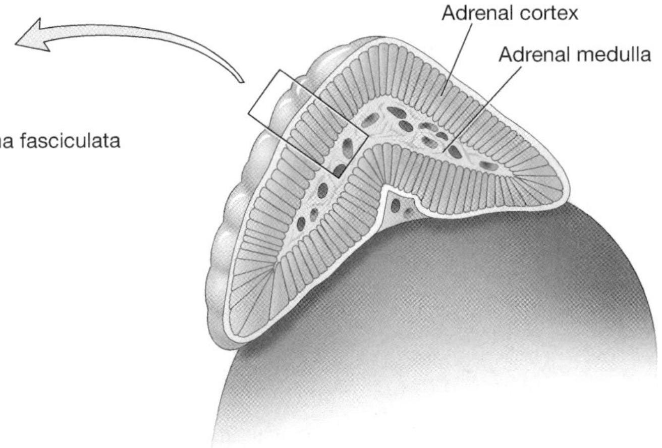

Figure 14-10

Adrenal Glands

The adrenal glands are positioned on the superior extremities of the kidneys. Each adrenal gland has an adrenal cortex that produces three groups of steroid hormones and an adrenal medulla that produces epinephrine and norepinephrine. Three layers of the adrenal cortex can be distinguished histologically.

The left and right **adrenal** (**suprarenal**) **glands** cap the superior ends of the kidneys (Figure 14-10). They are positioned in the posterosuperior aspects of the abdominal cavity adjacent to the musculature of the back. They measure about 1 x 3 x 5 centimeters and are somewhat cone-shaped with a triangular silhouette. The adrenal gland has two major layers: cortex and medulla. The **adrenal cortex** is divided into three named layers: zona glomerulosa (externally), zona fasciculata, and zona reticularis (internally). Cells within these zones manufacture the three groups of adrenocortical hormones. These include the glucocorticoids ("cortisones"), mineralocorticoids, and gonadocorticoids. The **glucocorticoids** are produced primarily by the zona fasciculata of the adrenal gland. They are anti-inflammatory and help maintain the integrity of capillary endothelium. They also promote gluconeogenesis and facilitate the formation of hepatic glycogen. Clinically they are administered to reduce inflammation. Their use after surgery is often contra-indicated because they suppress the regeneration of epithelial and connective tissue. Hypersecretion of corticosteroids (from an adrenal tumor or high secretion of ACTH) results in a disease termed **Cushing's syndrome**. With time, the metabolic changes that this causes may result in a hump-backed posture and a "moon-face". The **mineralocorticoids** are produced mainly by the zona glomerulosa of the adrenal cortex. One of these hormones, called aldosterone, augments the resorption of sodium from filtrate in the renal tubules which ultimately reduces urine volume and conserves water. Inadequate secretion of both glucocorticoids and mineralocorticoids results in hypoglycemia, dehydration, electrolyte imbalances and generalized weakness. Darkening of the skin also occurs because the high levels of ACTH have some MSH activity. The **gonadocorticoid hormones** are secreted mainly by the zona reticularis of the adrenal cortex. They have mainly androgenic characteristics and supplement the gonadal hormones.

The **adrenal medulla** contains cells which secrete **epinephrine** and **norepinephrine**. Secretion of these hormones stimulates the "fight or flight" responses of the sympathetic division of the ANS, except that the effect lasts longer. The sympathetic division of the ANS stimulates the secretion of these substances by the adrenal medulla in response to stress and/or fear. Individuals suffering continuous high stress and those with tumors of the adrenal medulla may have continuous secretion of epinephrine and norepinephrine by the adrenal medulla, resulting in total body fatigue and susceptibility to other diseases. This condition is called **generalized adaptation syndrome**.

Objectives

4. State the name, location, and secretory products of the five "true" endocrine organs.
5. Differentiate the hypothalamohypophysial tract from the hypothalamohypophysial portal system in regard to composition, specific location, destination, hormones transported, and purpose.
6. Name the two main parts of the pituitary gland, the three parts of the thyroid gland, and the two major components of each adrenal gland.

Non-Endocrine Organs that Produce Hormones

A number of organs that belong to other body systems produce one or more hormones. These include the hypothalamus, pancreas, small intestine, kidney, heart, ovary, testis, placenta, thymus, and stomach. These structures are not considered to be endocrine organs, *per se*, because they have other roles within their parent systems.

The **hypothalamus** is the inferior part of the diencephalon and physically forms the floor of the third ventricle within the brain. It has a number of important functions in the nervous system (*see Chapter 9*) and also produces at least 10 known hormones (Table 14-2). The majority of these polypeptides influence the rate of release of other hormones from the anterior pituitary. Included are hormones that stimulate the release of growth hormone, thyrotropin, ACTH, FSH, LH (ICSH), and MSH. The hypothalamus also produces hormones that *inhibit* the release of growth hormone, MSH, and LTH from the anterior pituitary. Very small amounts of these hormones are produced. They are absorbed by capillaries in the hypothalamus and carried directly to the anterior pituitary in the venules of the **hypothalamohypophysial portal system** (Figure 14-5, 6). These vessels deliver the hypothalamic hormones directly to the anterior pituitary in a small quantity of blood which prevents them from being diluted below active concentrations. The hypothalamus produces two other hormones, oxytocin and antidiuretic hormone, that are actually released from the posterior pituitary. These are produced by neurosecretory cells in the supraoptic nucleus (ADH) and paraventricular nucleus (oxytocin) of the hypothalamus. Axons from these cells form the **hypothalamohypophysial tract** which courses down through the infundibulum to the posterior pituitary where the hormones are stored and released (Figure 14-5, 6). This is the only known instance of hormones being produced in one location and then stored and released from another one.

The **pancreas** is an important digestive organ that produces pancreatic juice as an exocrine product. Scattered among the pancreatic acinar cells that secrete pancreatic juice are isolated groups of endocrine cells called **pancreatic islets** that produce insulin and glucagon (Figure 14-11). **Insulin** is secreted by the **beta cells** of the islets. It facilitates the movement of glucose out of the bloodstream and into the cells of the body, thereby lowering blood sugar. It is released in response to high levels of blood sugar. Lack of insulin or lack of *enough* functional insulin (low insulin levels) causes the high blood sugar disease called diabetes mellitus. Hypersecretion of insulin causes a condition called hypoglycemia (low blood sugar). The **alpha cells** of the pancreas produce **glucagon**. This hormone elevates blood sugar by stimulating the liver and skeletal muscles to break down (hydrolyze) their glycogen.

The **small intestine** is the most important organ in the chemical hydrolysis and absorption of ingested food materials. Its mucosal cells produce at least three different hormones which are released when the small intestine is full of ingesta: gastric inhibitory polypeptide, cholecystokinin, and secretin. **Gastric inhibitory polypeptide** (**GIP**) is also known as **enterogastrone**. This hormone inhibits gastric motility and secretions, and also stimulates insulin release from the pancreatic islets. **Cholecystokinin** (**CCK**) stimulates the contraction of the gallbladder and the secretion of pancreatic enzymes. This adds bile and digestive enzymes to the ingesta. **Secretin** causes the release of pancreatic juice and also sensitizes the pancreas to the effects of cholecystokinin.

The **kidney** is the principal organ of the urinary system and manufactures (secretes) urine through the processes of filtration, secretion, and selective reabsorption. It produces two different hormones: renin and erythropoietin. **Renin** is an enzyme which is produced by the juxtaglomerular cells of the renal tubules. It catalyzes the conversion of angiotensinogen to angiotensin, thereby raising the blood pressure. **Erythropoietin (EPO)** is a substance that stimulates the production of red blood corpuscles in the bone marrow.

The **ovary** produces the female sex cells (ova). It also produces the female sex hormones: estrogen and progesterone. **Estrogen** is produced by the cells around the developing ova. It is responsible for the development of the female secondary sex characteristics. Especially high levels are produced each month as a follicle matures. These levels stimulate some of the cyclical changes in the female reproductive system. Estrogen is a generic term that encompasses several estrus-producing steroids including estradiol, estrone, and estriol. **Progesterone** is produced in high levels after ovulation by the cells

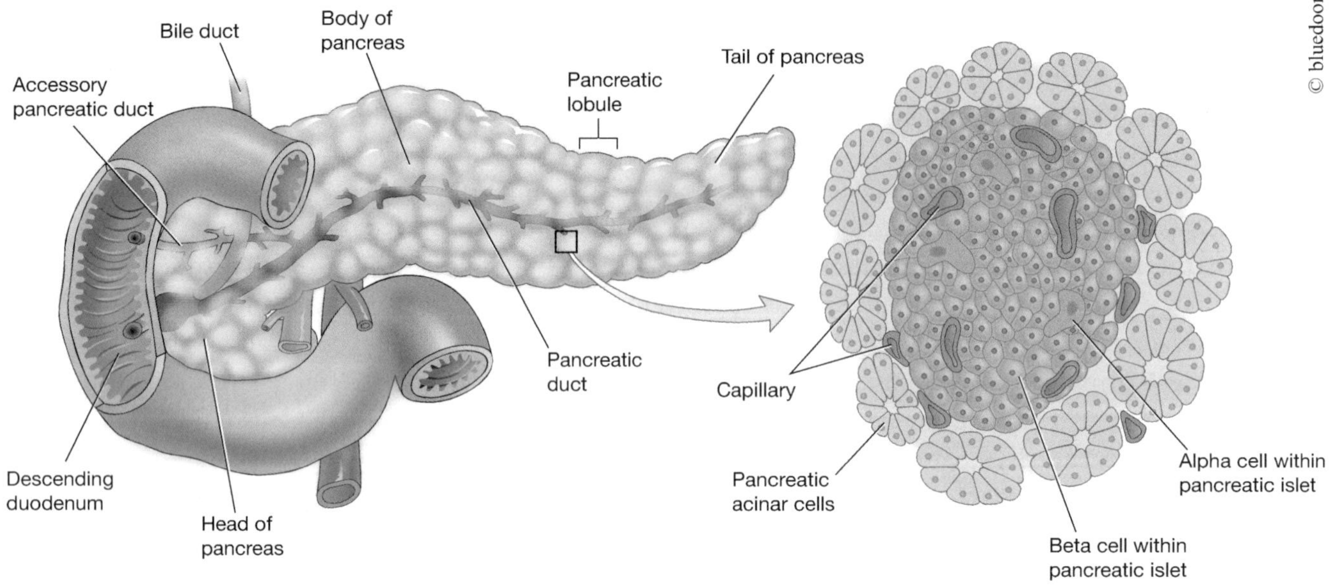

Figure 14-11

Pancreas

The pancreas is a digestive organ that produces pancreatic juice (via the pancreatic acinar cells) and glucagon and insulin (via the alpha and beta cells, respectively) within the pancreatic islets.

left behind in the ovary (forming the structure known as the corpus luteum). It induces changes in the uterine lining which are conducive to implantation and the maintenance of pregnancy. The low levels of female sex hormones present in men are derived from the cortices of their adrenal glands.

The **testis** produces male sex cells (spermatozoa) within microscopic channels called seminiferous tubules. It also produces the male sex hormone (testosterone). **Testosterone** is secreted by the interstitial cells of the testis which are located between the seminiferous tubules. Testosterone promotes the production of male secondary sex characteristics and is responsible for libido. The lower levels of testosterone found in females are produced by the cortices of their adrenal glands.

The **placenta** is the structure whereby the fetus is physically attached to the uterine wall. It is formed partly from fetal tissue and partly from the uterine lining. The placenta produces at least two hormones: chorionic gonadotropin and somatomammotropin. **Chorionic gonadotropin** is also known as **HCG** (**human chorionic gonadotropin**). It helps maintain the integrity of the corpus luteum and thereby assists in keeping the uterine lining conducive to pregnancy. **Somatomammotropin** has actions similar to growth hormone and promotes the development of the mammary glands.

The **thymus** is a lymphatic organ that is relatively large in newborns and decreases markedly in size with maturity. It produces lymphocytes (T cells) which produce cytokines (boost T-cell function). It also produces a hormone which stimulates T-lymphocytes (**thymosin**).

The **stomach** is a key organ in the digestive system. It produces a "hormone" called **gastrin** which promotes hydrochloric acid secretion by the parietal cells of the stomach. Actually, gastrin better fits the definition of an **autocrine regulator**. Such compounds are similar in general concept to hormones but target the same organ in which they are produced. Prostaglandin (one of the subtypes of lipids—*see Chapter 2*) is also an autocrine regulator.

The **heart** is more than just a pump, it also secretes **atrial natriuretic peptide** (**ANP**) and **herz**. ANP has actions opposite those of angiotensin. Natriuretic substances inhibit reabsorption of cations (in particular sodium) from urine. ANP inhibits aldosterone production, renin release, and vasopressin secretion. Herz augments cardiac contraction and is an autocrine regulator rather than a true hormone.

Objectives

7. Name the hormone producing structures that belong to "other" (non-endocrine) body systems and name the hormones that each one produces.

Internal Regulation of the Endocrine System

The general principle which regulates the secretion of all hormones is called **negative feedback**. The secretion of any given hormone is stimulated when the effect of that hormone is needed in the body. Conversely, when a hormone's effect is adequate (or excessive), its secretion/release is inhibited. The exact mechanism whereby negative feedback occurs varies from hormone to hormone. In some cases, these feedback pathways involve other hormones (Figure 14-7).

Objectives

8. Given the target and general effect (action) of a hormone, state the conditions that should cause an *increase* (and those that should cause a *decrease*) in the secretion/release of that hormone.

Development of the Endocrine Organs

The pituitary gland develops from two different primordia: an upward ectodermal outpouching from the oral cavity called the **hypophysial sac** ("Rathke's pouch") and a downward extension from the floor of the diencephalon called the **neurohypophysial bud** (Figure 14-12). The hypophysial sac appears at about three weeks gestation. It grows dorsally and loses its connection to the oral cavity by the end of the second month. It comes in close contact with the neurohypophysial bud growing down from the diencephalon and ultimately forms the anterior lobe of the pituitary gland. The neurohypophysial bud forms the posterior lobe of the hypophysis and the infundibulum ("stalk").

The thyroid gland begins its development during the third week of gestation as an endodermal proliferation on the floor of the primitive pharynx (Figure 14-12). These cells form the thyroid diverticulum which penetrates the underlying mesoderm and descends anterior to the pharyngeal gut as a bilobed diverticulum. This diverticulum continues downward to become the thyroid gland. It reaches its final position in front of the trachea in the seventh week. By this time it has formed its two lobes and connecting isthmus. During its early development, the thyroid gland remains connected to the pharynx by a stalk of tissue known as the **thyroglossal duct**. The latter disappears by the time the thyroid reaches the trachea. Its remnant on the floor of the pharynx forms the median landmark known as the foramen cecum of the tongue. Any thyroid tissue which separates from the migrating mass may form thyroglossal cysts.

The parathyroid glands develop from endodermal tissue in the third and fourth pharyngeal pouches. The dorsal parts of the left and right third pharyngeal sacs ("pouches") form the **inferior parathyroid buds** and the homologous portions of the left and right fourth pharyngeal sacs form the **superior parathyroid buds**. These four buds lose their contact with the pharynx, migrate with, and become embedded in, the thyroid gland.

Each adrenal gland is formed by two primordia: a mesodermal component that forms the cortex and an ectodermal portion that forms the medulla (Figure 14-12). During the fifth week of gestation, mesoderm above (anterior to) that which forms the ipsilateral kidney forms the primitive adrenal cortex. This tissue is later replaced by a second wave of migrating mesodermal cells. The cells which form the adrenal medulla are ectodermally derived from the neural crest cells which break free from the neural tube. These cells, initially called **chromaffin cells**, are encapsulated by the invading mesodermal cells which form the cortex. Adrenal development is not complete until a child is three years old.

The pineal gland (body) develops from the posterior portion of the upper part ("roof") of the diencephalon. It initially appears as an epithelial thickening on the midline and starts to evaginate by the seventh week of gestation.

Objectives

9. Review how endocrine glands develop from surface epithelium. (*See Figure 3-4*).
10. State the two origins of the pituitary gland and relate them to the definitive pituitary structures.

Clinical Considerations

Disease conditions can result from under production or over production of most any of the several dozen hormones. In some cases, these are difficult to diagnose because they produce very subtle symptoms. Other hormonal imbalances can produce serious and even life threatening conditions. Some endocrine diseases, such as diabetes mellitus (caused by hyposecretion of insulin) are easily controlled by hormone injections. Others such as those caused by hypersecretion of hormones from cancerous tissues may require surgery. Table 14-5 lists a number of disease conditions related to endocrine disorders.

Objectives

11. State the condition that should result from under or over-secretion of a particular hormone.

Table 14-5 Examples of Diseases Related to Endocrine Disorders

Condition	*Cause*	*Major Feature*
Diabetes mellitus	Hyposecretion of insulin	High blood sugar, glycosuria
Hypoglycemia	Hypersecretion of insulin	Low blood sugar, fatigue
Cushing's syndrome	Tumor of adrenal cortex or hypersecretion of ACTH	High levels of corticosteroids, "buffalo hump", "moon face"
Addison's disease	Hyposecretion of glucocorticoids and mineralocorticoids	Severe electrolyte imbalance, dehydration
Generalized adaptation syndrome	Stress induced hypersecretion by adrenal medulla	Fatigue and increased susceptibility to infectious diseases and cancer
Pituitary dwarfism	Hyposecretion of growth h.	Small stature
Giantism	Hypersecretion of growth h. during adolescence	Very large stature
Acromegaly	Hypersecretion of growth h. after adolescence	Elongated hands, feet, and face
Grave's disease	Hypersecretion of thyroid h.	High metabolic and heart rate, weight loss
Cretinism	Hyposecretion of thyroid h. in the newborn	Stunted growth, mental retardation, lethargy
Myxedema	Hyposecretion of thyroid h. in an adult	Low metabolic rate, obesity, lethargy
Primary hyperparathyroidism	Neoplasia of parathyroid gland	Demineralization of bones, pathological fractures
Hypoparathyroidism	Non-function of or surgical loss of parathyroid glands	Hypocalcemia, convulsions, tetany
Diabetes insipidus	Hyposecretion of antidiuretic hormone	Excessive thirst and urination, ion imbalance

Clinical Case Studies

Case 1—A young couple took their five-year-old son to a pediatrician because of concern about his physical stature. Although normal in overall outward appearance, he was very small for his age and was frequently mistaken for a three-year-old. What hormonal deficiency might have caused the boy's small size?

Case 2—A college co-ed visited an endocrinologist because of self-consciousness related to excessive body hair. She had thicker and more noticeable hair on her arms and legs than most females her age and also had noticeable hair on her upper lip and face. What could cause these symptoms?

Case 3—A high school cheerleader underwent a physical exam after she passed out twice for no obvious reason at basketball games. She also complained about sudden periods of extreme drowsiness—especially after eating. What condition would explain her symptoms?

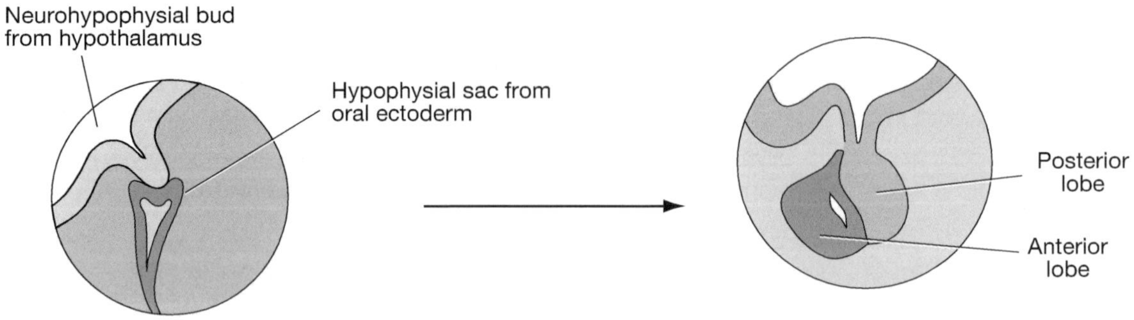

To form the pituitary gland, the neurohypophysial bud grows downward from the hypothalamus and forms the posterior lobe of the hypophysis and its infundibulum. The hypophysial sac grows upward from the roof of the oral cavity to form the anterior lobe.

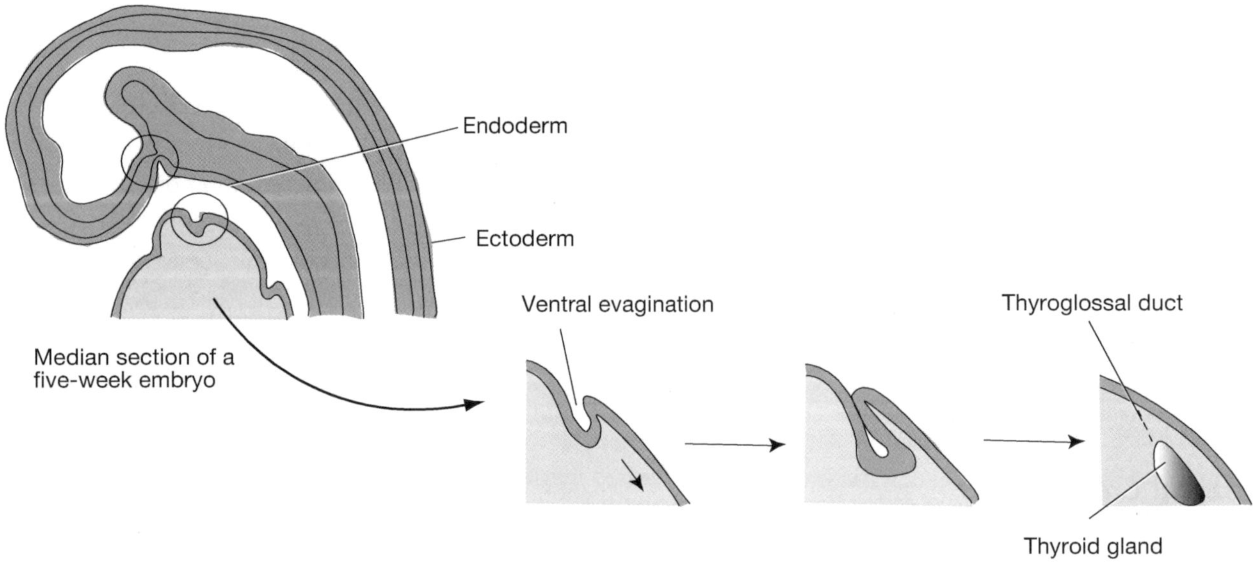

The thyroid gland forms from a ventral evagination of the pharyngeal endoderm. This diverticulum is bilobed and each lobe forms a lobe of the definitive thyroid. The thyroglossal duct connecting the evagination to the pharynx above it eventually disappears.

Figure 14-12

Development of the Pituitary, Thyroid, Adrenal, and Parathyroid Glands

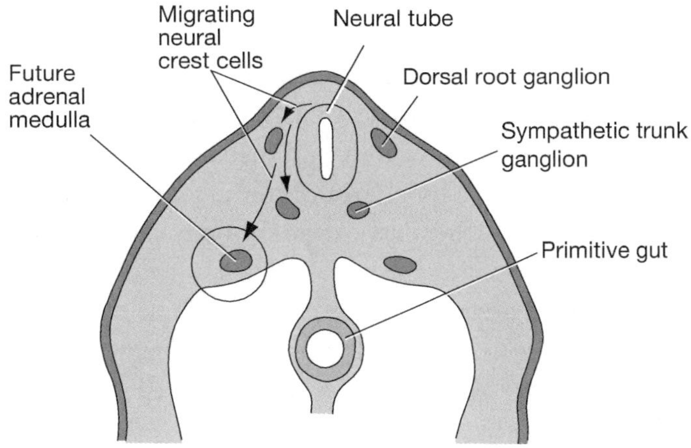

Transverse section of a five-week embryo

The neural crest cells which separate from the early neural tube form dorsal root (sensory) ganglia of spinal nerves as well as autonomic ganglia. Some of them migrate further down to form the adrenal medulla. Surrounding epithelial cells from the mesoderm form the adrenal cortex.

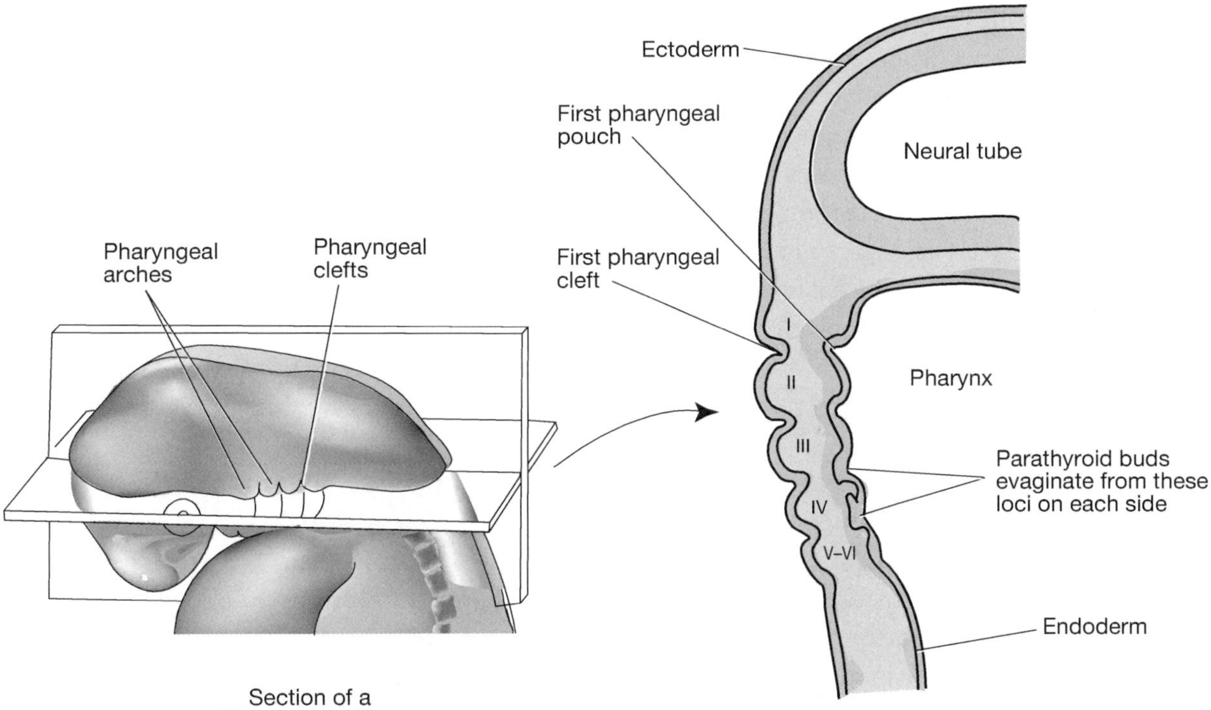

Section of a five-week embryo

Human embryos develop five (sometimes six) pharyngeal arches. The indentations between arches are called pharyngeal clefts externally and pharyngeal pouches (sacs) internally. The dorsal masses of the third and fourth pharyngeal arches form evaginating parathyroid buds. These buds lose their connections to the pharynx, and invade the developing thyroid gland to become the definitive superior and inferior parathyroid glands on each side.

Figure 14-12 (Continued)

Points to Ponder

Hormones are powerful chemicals that are capable of producing significant effects in very low concentrations. They are rapidly degraded and have fleeting effects unless continually secreted. They control numerous aspects of growth, reproduction, and metabolism in general. Several dozen hormones have been identified and studied. The list elongates continually. Together with other chemicals called paracrine and autocrine regulators, chemical control of body functions is much more prevalent than we realized a few decades ago.

What should be considered an endocrine organ? Anything that produces a chemical regulator? No, too long a list! Most organs would qualify under that scheme. So, we find ourselves reduced to a short list of true endocrine organs and a longer list composed of organs that produce one or more hormones but really belong to other systems.

Men often seem taken back to learn that they personally produce detectable amounts of estrogen and progesteroids (although they are not surprised that *what's-his-name* does). Likewise, women produce testosterone in varying amounts from individual to individual. Hormonally, we are not absolutely male and female. A given individual is chemically more (or less) male and less (or more) female. Add to all this a confused mental or emotional slant, various incidents in formative (or later) years and occasional individuals decide that they want to be the opposite gender even though their anatomy dictates otherwise.

Many folks are surprised to learn that the majority of hormones are proteins or polypeptides because the ones always in the news, the performance enhancing androgens that some athletes abuse and then get disqualified for using, are steroids. Unfortunately, some individuals have even died due to complications following steroid abuse.

Some endocrine disorders are so common that everyone is familiar with them. Diabetes mellitus (sugar diabetes) is a common example. The pancreas just fails to produce enough insulin to control blood levels of sugar (glucose). The solution seems easy (add insulin) but taking the right amount can be a delicate balancing act with the amount of dietary sugar intake. At the other end of the insulin spectrum is hypoglycemia which occurs when the pancreas secretes too much insulin.

What about that other diabetes (diabetes insipidus)? Antidiuretic hormone (ADH) is not produced in adequate levels. Increased urination (polyuria) and excessive thirst (polydipsia) are classic symptoms.

Endocrine disorders include a whole list of too much as well as a bunch of not enough diseases. Hyperthyroidism (too much thyroid hormone) results in hyperactive, thin individuals. Too much growth hormone (somatotropin) during development makes professional basketball centers but can lead to a number of specialized problems that such individuals face. Some endocrine disorders can be fatal while others seem unreasonably cruel. An especially noxious condition is the hirsutism (excessive body hair in a male pattern) suffered by some women. Typically caused by androgen excess related to the adrenal cortex, it has serious emotional and social consequences.

Hormones play critical roles even in prenatal development. Anatomic primordia destined to be several of the reproductive organs are identical in males and females. Under the influence of male sex hormones, these become male reproductive organs and under the influence of female sex hormones these primordia will develop into female organs.

In fraternal male/female twin calves, the hormones produced by the male fetus during gestation interfere with the proper development of the female's reproductive organs. The female born under such conditions is typically sterile and is called a freemartin— but that's in cattle!

Slang and Obsolete Nomenclature

UNOFFICIAL TERM	OFFICIAL DESIGNATION
islets of Langerhans	pancreatic islets *[insulae pancreaticae]*
thymus gland	thymus *[thymus]*
anterior pituitary	anterior lobe *[lobus anterior]* of pituitary gland
posterior pituitary	posterior lobe *[lobus posterior]* of pituitary gland
"C" cell of thyroid gland	parafollicular cell *[endocrinocytus parafollicularis]* of thyroid gland
intermediate lobe of the pituitary gland	intermediate part *[pars intermedia]* of the anterior lobe of the pituitary gland
Rathke's pouch	hypophysial sac *[saccus hypophysialis]*
interstitial cell of Leydig	interstitial cells *[endocrinocytus interstitialis]* of testis

Review Questions

1. Which one of the following is not a "true" endocrine organ?
   A. pineal body
   B. pituitary gland
   C. thymus
   D. adrenal gland
   E. parathyroid gland

2. Which one of the following is a mixed (endocrine/exocrine) organ?
   A. placenta
   B. hypothalamus
   C. thymus
   D. kidney
   E. heart

3. Which organ is matched with a hormone that it manufactures?
   A. adrenal gland—ACTH (adrenocorticotropic hormone)
   B. thyroid gland—thyrotropin
   C. posterior lobe of pituitary gland—oxytocin
   D. small intestine—secretin
   E. stomach—gastric inhibitory polypeptide

4. Which statement is true regarding the pituitary gland?
   A. It produces more hormones than any other structure in the body.
   B. It manufactures seven hormones and releases nine into the bloodstream.
   C. It is suspended from the mesencephalon by a stalk of tissue termed the infundibulum.
   D. It serves as a target for all of the hormones produced by the hypothalamus.
   E. If more than one of the above are true, choose this response.

5. Which statement is false regarding the thyroid gland?
   A. Its enlargement is called a goiter.
   B. It consists of two lobes connected by an isthmus.
   C. It produces T_3, thyroxine, and calcitonin.
   D. The parathyroid glands are embedded in it.
   E. It is positioned just above the larynx on the anterior aspect of the neck.

6. Parathyroid hormone elevates blood calcium levels by decreasing calcium loss in the urine, increasing the absorption of calcium from the small intestine, and by increasing the reabsorption of bone tissue by osteoclasts. Which one of the following is not a logical sequel to chronic hyperparathyroidism (secretion of too much parathyroid hormone)?
   A. increased release of calcitonin (a hormone that decreases blood calcium levels)
   B. weakened bone
   C. loose teeth
   D. hypercalcemia
   E. hyperphosphaturia (increased phosphate loss in urine)
   F. If all of the above are logical sequels, choose this response.

7. Which statement regarding the adrenal gland is false?
   A. Its cortex is divided into three named layers.
   B. It produces catecholamines and steroid hormones.
   C. Its medulla releases epinephrine and norepinephrine.
   D. Hyposecretion of adrenal cortex hormones produces a condition called Cushing's syndrome.
   E. Each adrenal gland is positioned on the superior end of a kidney adjacent to the muscles of the back.

8. Which statement regarding hormones is false?
   A. Most hormones are proteins or polypeptides.
   B. All hormones are carried to their targets by the bloodstream.
   C. Hormones are secreted in minute quantities and are rapidly inactivated (after release) by being converted to other compounds.
   D. Only the testis, ovary and adrenal gland produce steroid hormones.
   E. Autocrine and paracrine regulators are hormones.

9. The hypothalamohypophysial portal system...
   A. terminates in the posterior lobe of the pituitary gland.
   B. consists of axons of neurosecretory cells.
   C. carries a number of hypothalamic hormones to their target.
   D. is also known as the hypothalamohypophysial tract.
   E. begins in the hypophysis and consists of blood vessels.

10. Which structure produces more than one hormone?
    A. parathyroid gland
    B. pineal gland
    C. kidney
    D. thymus
    E. testis

Thought Questions

1. What is the criterion for distinguishing the five "true" endocrine organs from the numerous other hormone producing structures?

2. Which "hormones" listed in Table 14-2 defy the definition of a hormone?

3. All hormones affect the production of or activate what group(s) of biological macromolecules?

4. Compare and contrast the hypothalamohypophysial tract and portal system in regard to structure, location, destination, and hormones transported.

5. The hypothalamus releases fewer hormones than it manufactures and the pituitary gland releases a larger number than it manufactures. Explain this observation.

6. Why does the thyroid gland enlarge in response to low dietary intake of iodine?

7. What effect should hyperparathyroidism (hypersecretion of parathyroid hormone) have on the skeletal system?

8. Which non-endocrine system produces the largest number of hormones?

9. Why do hormones act only on certain cells, tissues, or organs? (*i.e.*, What makes a target a target?)

10. Explain how increasing the output of melatonin by the pineal body can result in an elevation of the basal metabolic rate (BMR).

11. Hypoglycemic individuals often suffer low blood sugar after ingestion of simple carbohydrates. Explain why.

12. Name the three organs known to secrete steroidal hormones.

13. Which two hormones can be found in women but are not normally present in men?

14. How can anger result in generalized increase in circulatory epinephrine?

15. What is the usual source of androgens in females who develop thick facial hair?

16. Discuss the general chemical characteristics of hormones including the names of the four major groups, the half-life (once released into the bloodstream), and the general concentrations needed to produce an effect.

17. What functional purpose does the hypothalamohypophysial portal system serve? Could not the hormones that it transports simply be released into the main part of the systemic circulation (and still reach their targets)?

18. Which of the five true endocrine organs have gross subdivisions? Name the subparts.

19. What do the word roots "tropin" and "statin" mean in the name of a hormone? What does "stimulating" mean? "Releasing"? "Inhibiting"?

20. In what form is thyroid hormone (T_3 and T_4) stored in the thyroid gland?

21. What hormones are acronymed T_1 and T_2?

Answers to Clinical Case Studies

Case 1—A deficiency of growth hormone (somatotropin) produced by the anterior pituitary gland is the likely cause of this child's small stature.

Case 2—Excessive body hair in a male distribution pattern is called hirsutism or hypertrichosis. It is usually produced by high levels of androgens (male sex hormones). The usual source of the hormone in women is the adrenal cortex.

Case 3—This young woman's symptoms are characteristic of classic hypoglycemia. The cause is related to overproduction of insulin by the pancreas. When individuals with this condition have any subtle blood sugar increase, too much insulin is released. Since it lowers blood sugar by facilitating the movement of sugar out of the bloodstream and into the cells, low blood sugar levels result.

Answers to Review Questions

1. C. The thymus produces a hormone (thymosin), but it belongs to the lymphatic system.

2. D. The kidney produces an exocrine product (urine) and two hormones (renin and erythropoietin).

3. D.

4. B. A is wrong because the hypothalamus produces more hormones than the pituitary gland. The problem with "D" is that ADH and oxytocin (produced by the hypothalamus), do not target the anterior pituitary gland.

5. E. The thyroid gland is just *inferior* to the larynx.

6. F. A and D would occur due to the abnormally high blood levels of calcium. B, C, and E would occur due to bone tissue reabsorption.

7. D. *Hyper*secretion of adrenal cortex hormones can cause it.

8. E. Autocrine and paracrine regulators are biochemicals that do not fit the definition of hormones because they act within the same organ that produced them.

9. C. A and B both refer to the hypothalamohypophysial tract and E is wrong because the portal system *ends* in the anterior lobe of the hypophysis (pituitary gland).

10. C. The kidney produces erythropoietin and renin.

Answers to Thought Questions

1. The five "true" endocrine organs have no other known functions except hormone production. The "other" hormone producing structures do have other functional roles.

2. Gastrin and herz. Since they act on the same organ that produces them, they are really autocrine regulators rather than hormones.

3. Proteins (enzymes).

4.

Criterion	Tract	Portal System
Structure	axons of neurosecretory cells	blood vessels
Location	within infundibulum	around infundibulum
Destination	posterior lobe of pituitary gland	anterior lobe of pituitary gland
Hormones transported	oxytocin and ADH	a bunch (*see Table 14-2*)

5. Two of the hormones manufactured by the hypothalamus are stored in and released from the posterior lobe of the pituitary gland.

6. Without iodine, functional T_3 and T_4 cannot be manufactured. In response to the low levels of these hormones, TSH (thyrotropin) levels increase and cause the thyroid gland to enlarge.

7. Parathyroid hormone (PTH) increases blood levels of calcium by acting on osteoclasts (bone reabsorption), kidney (calcium retention) and intestine (calcium absorption). Prolonged secretion of high levels of PTH can cause so much osteoclastic activity that bones can become quite weak and fractures can easily occur. Teeth may become so loose that they are lost.

8. Nervous system. The digestive system produces a large number, too.

9. Only certain cells/tissues/organs have the specific receptors to which a given hormone binds.

10. Melatonin stimulates the hypothalamus. One of the hypothalamic hormones is thyrotropin releasing factor which stimulates the anterior lobe of the pituitary gland to release TSH. The TSH targets the thyroid gland and increases its output of T_3 and T_4 which increase BMR.

11. The sugar intake increases blood sugar levels which (in hypoglycemic individuals) can stimulate an *over* release of insulin. The high levels of insulin result in subsequent low blood sugar levels because insulin facilitates movement of glucose from the blood into body cells.

12. Testis, ovary, adrenal gland.

13. Chorionic gonadotropin and somatomammotropin. Men do produce measurable amounts of progesterone and estrogen.

14. The sympathetic impulses produced by anger stimulate release of epinephrine from the adrenal gland. This hormone causes a generalized sympathomimetic response by stimulating sympathetic effectors.

15. The cortex of the adrenal gland.

16. Hormones include proteins and polypeptides, steroids, modified amino acids, and catecholamines. In general, hormones have a short half life (hours/days), but they are powerful chemicals as evidenced by the tiny quantities needed to produce an effect.

17. The hypothalamohypophysial portal system transports a number of hypothalamic hormones directly to their target (anterior lobe of the pituitary gland). If these hormones (which are produced in especially minute quantities) were released into the blood stream and carried at random to the anterior lobe of the pituitary gland, the dilution factor would render them ineffective due to the small quantities produced.

18. The pituitary gland has anterior and posterior lobes. Its anterior lobe has three subparts. The adrenal gland has a cortex and medulla and the cortex has three named (histological) layers. The thyroid gland has two lobes and a connecting isthmus. The pineal body has no gross subdivisions, but forms the posterior aspect of the epithalamus. The parathyroid gland is represented by four groups of cells embedded in the posterior aspects of the lobes of the thyroid gland. The upper two originate from the left and right third pharyngeal arches and are often designated parathyroid III. The lower two are derived from the fourth pharyngeal arches and are designated parathyroid IV.

19. "Tropin" and "stimulating" imply that the hormone acts on something in a positive (stimulatory) manner. "Releasing" means that the hormone in question causes the release of the hormone in its name. "Inhibiting" and "statin" imply that the hormone inhibits the action of the hormone in its name (usually by interfering with the release of the other hormone).

20. Thyroid hormone is stored in a form called colloid wherein the T_3 and T_4 are combined with a protein. At their release, T_3 and T_4 are cleaved from the protein by hydrolysis.

21. T1 refers to monoiodothyronine and T_2 is diiodothyronine. These substances are produced by the thyroid gland but have essentially no biological activity in comparison to their more highly iodinated counterparts (T_3 and T_4).

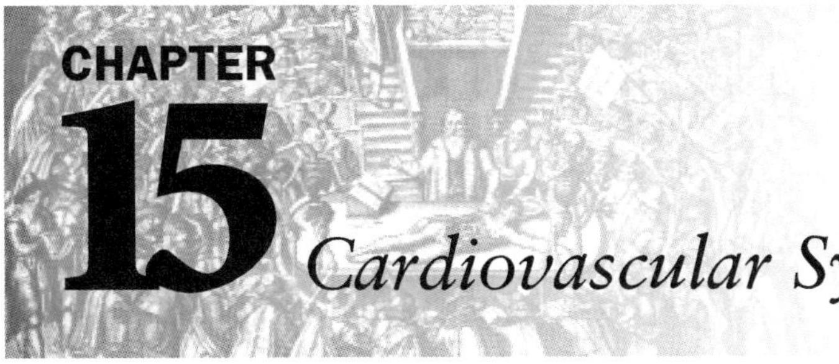

CHAPTER 15 Cardiovascular System

Chapter Outline and Key Concepts

INTRODUCTION

The components of the cardiovascular system include the heart, arteries, capillaries, veins, and blood.

Blood, the only liquid tissue in the body, is also the only tissue that serves as a major part of a system without being part of an organ.

FUNCTIONS OF THE CARDIOVASCULAR SYSTEM

The cardiovascular system transports wastes, nutrients, and hormones, helps regulate body temperature and pH, and is heavily involved in body defense.

HEART

The heart is a muscular pump composed primarily of cardiac muscle tissue and connective tissue proper.

The three layers of the heart wall are epicardium (visceral pericardium), myocardium, and endocardium (from without inward).

The four chambers of the heart include the left and right atria and the left and right ventricles.

The left and right sides of the heart are completely separated in a normal individual by the interatrial septum and the interventricular septum.

The left and right atrioventricular (AV) valves are located between their respective atria and ventricles.

The aortic and pulmonary valves separate the aorta and pulmonary trunk from the left and right ventricles, respectively.

The valves of the heart prevent backflow of blood and are passively opened and closed by blood flow.

Modified cardiac muscle cells called purkinje fibers initiate and distribute the electrical impulses responsible for cardiac contraction.

ARTERIES

Arteries transport blood away from the heart and have three named layers in their walls: tunica intima, tunica media, and tunica externa.

The largest arteries, called elastic arteries, modulate the systolic and diastolic blood pressure.

Most arteries visible to the naked eye are muscular arteries which regulate overall blood pressure.

The smallest arteries (arterioles) distribute blood into capillary beds.

CAPILLARIES

Capillaries join the smallest arteries to the smallest veins and are the only vessels with walls thin enough for nutrients and waste products to diffuse across.

Due to the rhythmic contraction/relaxation of precapillary sphincters, blood enters only some of the capillaries at any given moment.

All capillaries "leak" fluid due to their thin walls, and those in some organs are more porous than others.

VEINS

Veins receive blood from capillaries and return it toward the heart.

The smallest veins, called venules, drain into larger veins—the largest of which enter the left and right atria of the heart.

Some veins, especially those in the limbs, have valves which prevent backflow.

CIRCULATORY PATTERNS

The blood flow from the heart to the lungs and back to the heart is called the pulmonary circulation, and flow from the heart to the rest of the body and then back to the heart is called the systemic circulation.

In both the pulmonary and the systemic circulations the typical flow pattern is heart/ arteries/ capillaries/ veins/ heart.

Portal flow patterns differ from the norm by having blood flow through two different sets of capillaries (separated by venous channels) before it returns to the heart.

MAJOR SYSTEMIC ARTERIES

The aorta is divided into an ascending part, aortic arch, and descending part and these supply all of the blood to the (other) systemic arteries.

The ascending part of the aorta has only two branches: left and right coronary arteries.

The aortic arch has three branches: brachiocephalic trunk, left common carotid artery, and the left subclavian artery.

The descending part of the aorta is divided into thoracic and abdominal portions and has numerous branches.

MAJOR SYSTEMIC VEINS

The four largest systemic veins are the superior and inferior venae cavae, the hepatic portal vein, and the azygos vein.

The superior vena cava returns blood from the head, neck, thorax, and superior limbs to the right atrium of the heart.

The inferior vena cava returns blood from the abdomen, pelvis, and inferior limbs to the right atrium of the heart.

The azygos vein collects venous blood from the thoracic wall and empties into the superior vena cava.

The hepatic portal vein carries venous blood from the stomach, intestine, pancreas, and spleen to the liver.

BLOOD

Blood is about 55% plasma (fluid) and 45% formed elements.

Plasma is about 92% water and the remainder includes three major groups of proteins (albumins, globulins, and fibrinogen), as well as electrolytes, carbohydrates, and lipids.

Formed elements of blood include platelets, RBC's, and five types of WBC's.

FETAL CIRCULATION

Since fetal nutrient/waste exchange occurs at the placenta, and fetal lungs have a high resistance to blood flow, anatomic peculiarities are present in the fetal circulatory system.

Pulmonary flow resistance is bypassed via the foramen ovale and ductus arteriosus.

Blood is transported to/from the placenta by the paired umbilical arteries and the single umbilical vein.

The high oxygen content of blood entering the fetus via the umbilical vein is reduced by mixing with low oxygen blood at three loci: liver (hepatic vein), inferior vena cava, and right atrium of the heart.

At birth, most of the fetal specific structures close by contraction of smooth muscle related to higher oxygen levels in the blood (closure of the foramen ovale of the heart is an exception).

Failure of the foramen ovale or ductus arteriosus to close properly results in patent foramen ovale or patent ductus arteriosus.

DEVELOPMENT OF THE CARDIOVASCULAR SYSTEM

Blood vessels and blood cells develop from mesoderm in the early embryo.

Six pairs of aortic arches develop which form parts of the large arteries near the heart.

The heart begins developing at the end of the third week as a pair of tubular structures that fuse together.

The cardiac tube bends, and bulges form on it which develop into the heart chambers.

The left and right sides of the heart are separated by ingrowths which form the interatrial and interventricular septae.

CLINICAL CONSIDERATIONS

Sphygmomanometers are used to measure systemic blood pressure which is recorded as two numbers: systolic and diastolic pressure.

Circulatory shock results from a precipitous drop in blood pressure and may be caused by major blood loss, emotional trauma, sudden heart failure, or certain kinds of toxins.

The electrical activity of the heart can be monitored by an EKG.

A heart attack is caused by ischemic necrosis of cardiac muscle tissue—classically due to blockage of vessels supplying cardiac muscle tissue.

Cardiac murmurs are abnormal heart sounds related to the turbulent flow of blood.

Murmurs can be caused by valvular stenoses and insufficiencies, patent ductus arteriosus, interventricular septal defects, and even by severe anemia.

Blood transfusions can result in severe (even lethal) transfusion reactions if incompatible blood types are mixed.

Selected Definitions

Blood—the liquid tissue forced through blood vessels by the contractions of the heart. It transports nutrients, waste products, and chemical regulators, assists with thermoregulation and acid/base balance, and plays several roles in body defense.

Blood vessel—any of the tubular organs that transport blood including arteries, veins, and capillaries. Arteries and veins are transport tubes only, but capillaries have walls thin enough to allow diffusional exchange with the interstitial fluid.

Cardiac cycle—the repeating sequence of cardiac activity. It begins with atrial contraction, followed by ventricular contraction, followed in turn, by a short period of relaxation involving the whole heart.

Cardiac murmur—an abnormal heart sound. Any cardiac sound in addition to "lub" (first heart sound) and "dub" (second heart sound) constitutes a cardiac murmur.

Cardiac output (CO)—the total volume of blood entering the systemic circulation each minute. It is quantitated by CO = HR x SV where HR represents the heart rate (contractions/minute) and SV is the stroke volume (amount of blood pumped by each contraction).

Cardiogenic shock—a precipitous drop in blood pressure related to inadequate pumping by the heart. Other causes of shock include hypovolemia, endotoxemia, and generalized vasodilation.

Electrocardiogram (EKG, ECG)—a printout charting the electrical activity of the heart. EKG's require specialized monitoring and recording equipment collectively called an electrocardiograph.

First heart sound—the first of the two "normal" heart sounds. Often vocalized as "lub", it occurs just after the initiation of ventricular systole and is related to simultaneous closure of the two atrioventricular valves.

Heart—the muscular pump that forces blood through blood vessels. It has four valves, four chambers, three surfaces, two ends, and three named layers.

Myocardium—the thick, middle layer of the heart. It consists primarily of well-vascularized cardiac muscle tissue.

Pericardium—the serous membrane forming the closed body cavity into which the heart is invaginated. That portion forming the thin outer layer of the heart is the epicardium (visceral pericardium) which is separated from the surrounding parietal pericardium by a tiny volume of pericardial fluid in the pericardial cavity.

Plasma—the liquid part of blood constituting about 55% of its volume. Plasma is about 92% water and most of the rest is proteins, with smaller amounts of ions and small organic molecules.

Portal system—a portion of the systemic circulation where blood serially flows through two different capillary beds in different organs before it returns to the heart. The two present in mankind are the hepatic and hypothalamohypophysial portal systems.

Precapillary sphincter—a tiny ringlet of smooth muscle tissue around the initial segment of a capillary. Rhythmic contraction/relaxation of these sphincters based on oxygen levels in the surrounding tissues governs blood flow through most capillaries.

Pulmonary circulation—that part of the circulatory pathway involving blood flow to, through, and back from the lungs. It is considered to begin in the right ventricle of the heart and end in the left atrium.

Purkinje fibers—modified cardiac muscle cells that are specialized for impulse conduction. These cells form the electrical control system of the heart including the SA node, AV node, and atrioventricular fasciculus.

Systemic circulation—that part of the circulatory pathway from the heart to most of the body and then back to the heart. The systemic circulation begins in the left ventricle and ends in the right atrium.

Systole—that period of the cardiac cycle involving contraction of cardiac muscle tissue (*vs. diastole* which refers to the period of cardiac muscle tissue relaxation). Atrial systole occurs a split second prior to ventricular contraction.

Tunica media (of a vessel)—the relatively thick middle layer of an artery, vein, or lymphatic vessel. It is sandwiched between the lining layer (tunica intima) and the outer coat (tunica externa).

Valvular insufficiency—a valve that "leaks" because it does not form a "blood tight" seal when closed. Any of the four cardiac valves can be insufficient, and this typically causes a murmur as blood regurgitates through the improperly closed valve.

Vasa vasorum—those tiny vessels that penetrate the walls of other arteries, veins, and lymphatic vessels from without. They carry blood to and from the capillaries that permeate vessel walls.

Etymology ***Sursum corda*—"Lift up your heart."**

a (G), *without*—azygos
albus (L), *white*—albumin
anastomosis (G), *opening*—anastomoses
angei (G), *blood vessel*—angioblast
aorte (G), *to lift, heave*—artery
athere (G), *gruel*—atherosclerosis
auricula (L), *diminutive of ear*—auricle
basis (L), *base*—basophil
bifurcatus (L), *spit in two*—bifurcation
bradys (G), *slow*—bradycardia
capillus (L), *hair*—capillary
carn (L), *flesh*—carneae
cor (L), *heart*—coronary
diastole (G), *dilatation*—diastole
eosin (G), *rose colored*—eosinophil
fenestra (L), *window*—fenestrated
kardia (G), *heart*—electrocardiogram
karos (G), *heavy sleep*—carotid
koilia (G), *belly*—celiac
mano (G), *gas*—sphygmomanometer
mitra (L), *turban*—mitral
neutr (L), *neutral*—neutrophil
patere (L), *to be open*—patent
pectere (L), *to comb*—pectinate muscle
saphenes (G), *clearly visible*—saphenous
sino (G), *sinus*—sinoatrial
skleroun (G), *to harden*—arteriosclerosis
sphygmos (G), *pulse*—sphygmomanometer
stenosis (G), *act of narrowing*—stenosis
systole (G), *contraction*—systole
tachy (G), *rapid*—tachycardia
thrombo (G), *lump, clot of blood*—thrombocyte
vas (L), *vessel*—vasa vasorum
vena (L), *blood vessel*—vein

Introduction

The cardiovascular system consists of only five major components: heart, arteries, veins, capillaries, and blood. The **heart** is a muscular pump that propels blood throughout the vascular pathways. It contracts over 100,000 times and pumps about 2000 gallons of blood during each 24 hour period. Arteries, capillaries, and veins form a network of several thousand miles of passageways leading to virtually every part of the body. The few avascular structures include mature cartilage, membranous epithelium, some epidermal derivatives (hair and nails), and the cornea and lens of the eyeball. **Arteries** transport blood away from the heart and **veins** carry blood back toward the heart. **Capillaries** are the microscopic vessels between the arterial and venous channels. They are the functional vessels involved in the exchange of nutrients and wastes between blood and other body tissues. **Blood** is the only fluid tissue in the body and it serves as the transport medium of the cardiovascular system. It is the only tissue that functions as a major component of the body without being part of an organ.

Objectives

1. Name and define the components of the cardiovascular system.

Functions of the Cardiovascular System

The cardiovascular system has several distinctive functions including the exchange of oxygen and carbon dioxide, transportation of nutrients, wastes, and hormones, regulation of body pH and temperature, and it plays a number of roles in body defense:

1. **Oxygen/carbon dioxide exchange** involving the lungs and body tissues. The tissues of the body utilize oxygen and produce carbon dioxide as an end product of carbohydrate metabolism. Red blood corpuscles (cells) pick up oxygen at the lungs and transport it to the tissues of the body. Carbon dioxide is absorbed by the blood and carried back to the lungs where it is exhaled with expired air. Although oxygen is a nutrient and carbon dioxide is a waste product, O_2/CO_2 exchange is usually considered separately from nutrient/waste exchange (*see Item 2 below*) because of its singular importance.
2. **Nutrient/waste exchange** primarily involving the digestive and urinary organs. Nutrients are absorbed into the bloodstream from the digestive system (primarily from the small intestine). They are then carried throughout the body where they are utilized by various tissues as needed. Some metabolic wastes picked up by the bloodstream are eliminated by the kidneys as components of the urine.
3. **Hormone transport** from site of release to the various targets. Hormones are chemical substances produced at specific locations in the body. They are carried by the bloodstream throughout the body but act only on the cells, tissues, or organs that have specific receptors for them.
4. **Acid/base balance** involving buffers in the blood. The carbon dioxide produced by carbohydrate metabolism forms carbonic acid when dissolved in the water-based tissue fluids ($CO_2 + H_2O = H_2CO_3$). Hemoglobin and bicarbonate (HCO_3^-) buffers help absorb the excess hydrogen ions and prevent marked changes in pH. Blood pH must remain in the range of 7.35–7.45 to prevent coma or convulsions.
5. **Thermoregulation** of the body. Because essentially all parts of the body are permeated by blood vessels, blood flow tends to equalize the temperature of various body organs. When the core body temperature rises, a larger percentage of the blood is channeled to superficial vessels to help radiate the excess heat. Conversely, when the core body temperature drops, surface blood flow is reduced to lessen heat loss.
6. **Body defense** by several components of blood. First, blood contains gamma globulins in the form of antibodies that impart immunity and resistance to some potential pathogens. Some of the white blood cells are phagocytic and directly combat bacterial invaders. Finally, the clotting mechanism, which is activated by the chemicals released during tissue damage, typically prevents excessive blood loss in all but very severe traumatic injuries.

Objectives

2. List the functions of the cardiovascular system.

Heart

The **heart** serves as a muscular pump to propel blood throughout the body (Figure 15-1). It weighs about 300 grams and is composed primarily of cardiac muscle tissue and connective tissue proper. It has four chambers (two atria and two ventricles), four valves (that prevent reflux of blood), three named layers in its walls, and it is invaginated into a serous body cavity (pericardial cavity). The heart is located within the thoracic cavity between the lungs and is centered slightly to the left of the median plane. It forms part of the **mediastinum** which is a partition that separates the lungs from each other. The broad, superior end of the heart where the vessels attach is the **base** and the inferior, pointed end is the **apex**. The apex is directed slightly to the left and inferiorly (Figure 15-1). The anterior aspect of the heart is the **sternocostal surface**, and the inferior aspect is the **diaphragmatic surface**. The left side is called the **pulmonary surface** and the right side is called the **right border**. There are three subtle grooves on the surface of the heart. The **anterior** and **posterior interventricular grooves** mark the position of the interventricular septum that internally separates the left and right ventricles. The **coronary groove** is a fat-filled landmark between the atria (above) and the ventricles (below) (Figure 15-3).

The heart wall has three named layers: endocardium, myocardium, and epicardium (Figure 15-2). The **endocardium** consists of the thin lining layer formed by simple squamous epithelium and a layer of subepithelial fibrous connective tissue. The simple squamous epithelium is called **endothelium** and not only lines the heart but also extends into the vessels and forms the inner layer of their walls. The **myocardium** is the thick middle layer of the heart wall formed primarily by cardiac muscle and connective tissue proper. It is the contractile portion of the heart and also contains the specialized cardiac muscle cells called purkinje fibers that initiate and conduct the impulses for contraction. The **epicardium** is the thin outer layer of the heart wall. It consists of a thin fibrous connective tissue encasement with simple squamous epithelium called **mesothelium** on the surface. The epicardium forms the **visceral layer of the serous pericardium** and is often called the **visceral pericardium**. The latter forms the inner part of a closed sack into which the heart is invaginated with the visceral layer adherent to the surface of the heart and the **parietal layer** reflecting away from it at the base. This parietal layer is properly named **parietal layer of the serous pericardium**, but it is often called simply **parietal pericardium**. The small space between the parietal and visceral layers is called the **pericardial cavity**. The relationship between these can be understood by imagining the heart being pushed into the top of a soft balloon. The epicardium would be the part of the balloon in contact with the heart. The air-filled space inside the balloon would represent the pericardial cavity. The latter is only a small space containing a minuscule amount of serous fluid. The outer part of the balloon (continuous with the inner part) represents the parietal layer of the pericardium.

Objectives

3. Name the major external landmarks of the heart.
4. List and differentiate the three layers of the heart wall.

The four chambers of the heart are the left and right atria and the left and right ventricles (Figure 15-4). The atria are thin-walled chambers positioned above the ventricles. They are separated from each other by a partition of tissue termed the **interatrial septum**. The atria collect blood returning from the lungs (left atrium), and from the rest of the body (right atrium). The **right atrium** receives the superior vena cava, inferior vena cava, as well as the coronary sinus which returns blood from the heart muscle, itself. These vessels empty into a portion of the right atrium termed the **vena caval sinus**. The remainder of the right atrium forms an "ear-like" projection termed the **auricle of the right atrium**. The **left atrium** receives four pulmonary veins and has a projection termed the **auricle of the left atrium**. Small ridges extending into the lumina of the auricles of the right and left atria (and to a lesser extent into the rest of the atria) are called **pectinate muscles**. The ventricles have much thicker walls than the atria and are separated from the atria by a partition called the **atri-**

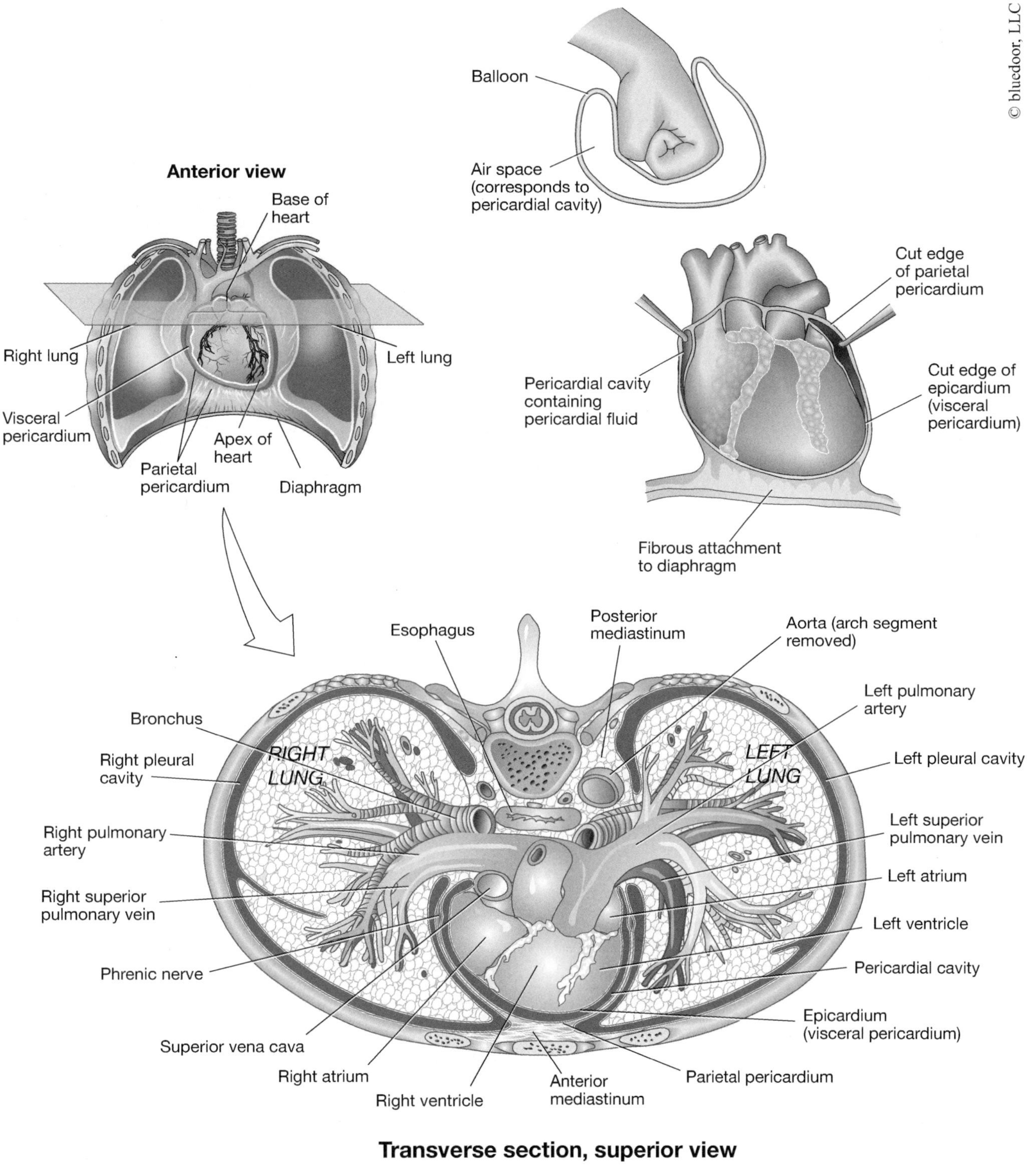

Figure 15-1

Position and Orientation of the Heart

The heart is centered slightly to the left of the median plane with its apex directed to the left and inferiorly. Along with the esophagus, trachea, and neurovascular structures, the heart forms part of the partition between the lungs called the mediastinum. The heart is invaginated into the pericardial cavity as shown by the schematic fist into the balloon. The pericardial membrane that adheres to the heart is called the epicardium (visceral pericardium) and that which reflects away is the parietal pericardium.

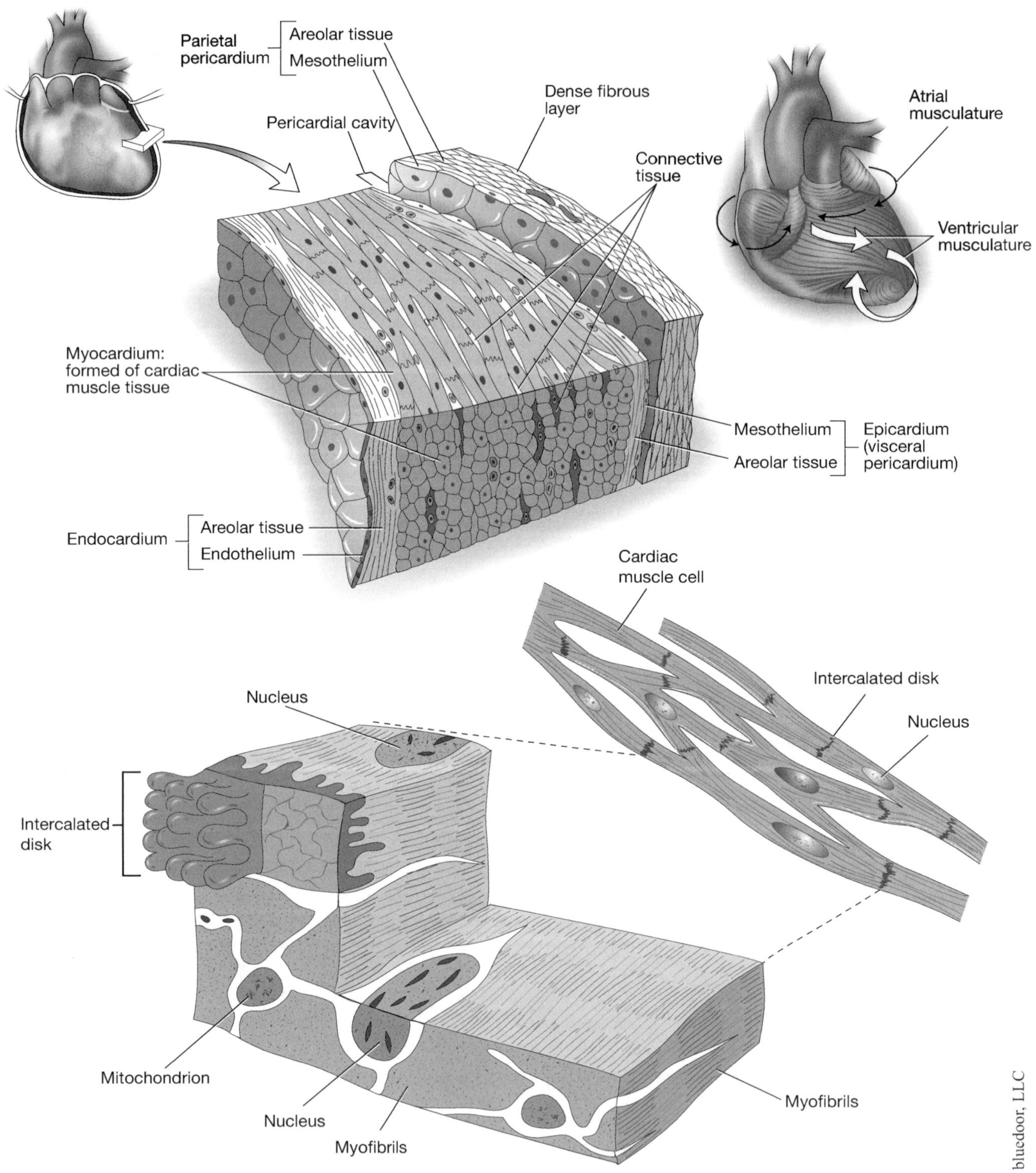

Figure 15-2

Heart Wall and Cardiac Muscle Tissue

The outer layer of the heart wall, called epicardium or visceral pericardium, consists of a layer of simple squamous epithelium called mesothelium, plus a thin layer of connective tissue proper. The middle layer of the heart wall (myocardium) is composed primarily of cardiac muscle tissue. The thin endocardium that lines the chambers of the heart consists of simple squamous epithelium called endothelium plus a thin layer of connective tissue proper.

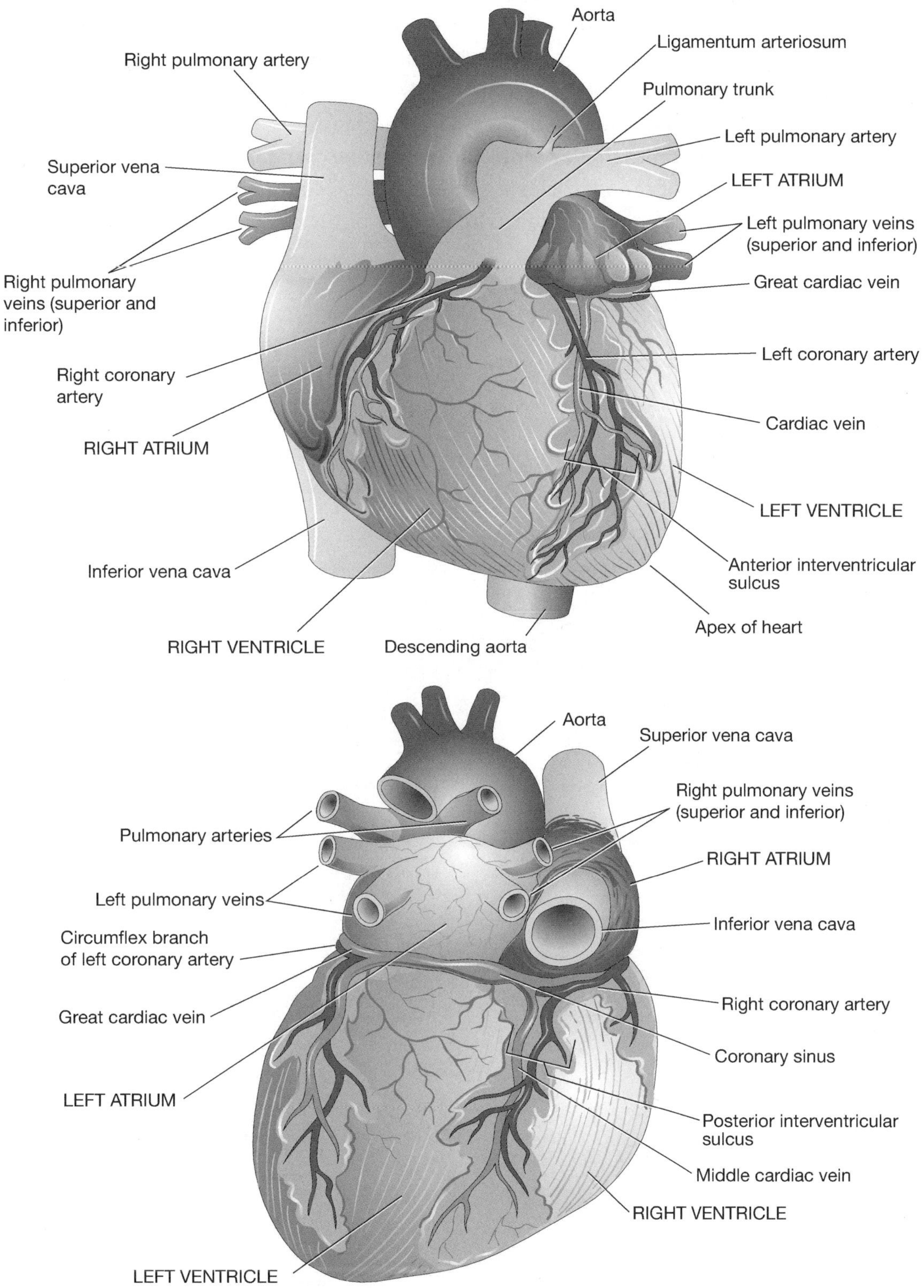

Figure 15-3

Surface Features of the Heart

Anterior (sternocostal) surface of the heart (above) and diaphragmatic (inferior) surface (below).

oventricular septum. The **right ventricle** receives blood from the right atrium through the right atrioventricular valve and pumps it into the pulmonary trunk through the pulmonary valve. The **left ventricle** receives blood from the left atrium through the left atrioventricular valve and pumps it into the aorta through the aortic valve. Its wall is almost twice as thick as that of the right ventricle because it pumps blood throughout the body. The ventricles are separated from each other by a partition called the **interventricular septum. Trabeculae carneae** are the ridges lining the ventricular walls. The cavities of the ventricles are similar in total volume, but the lumen of the left ventricle is almost round in transverse section, whereas that of the right ventricle is crescent (half-moon)

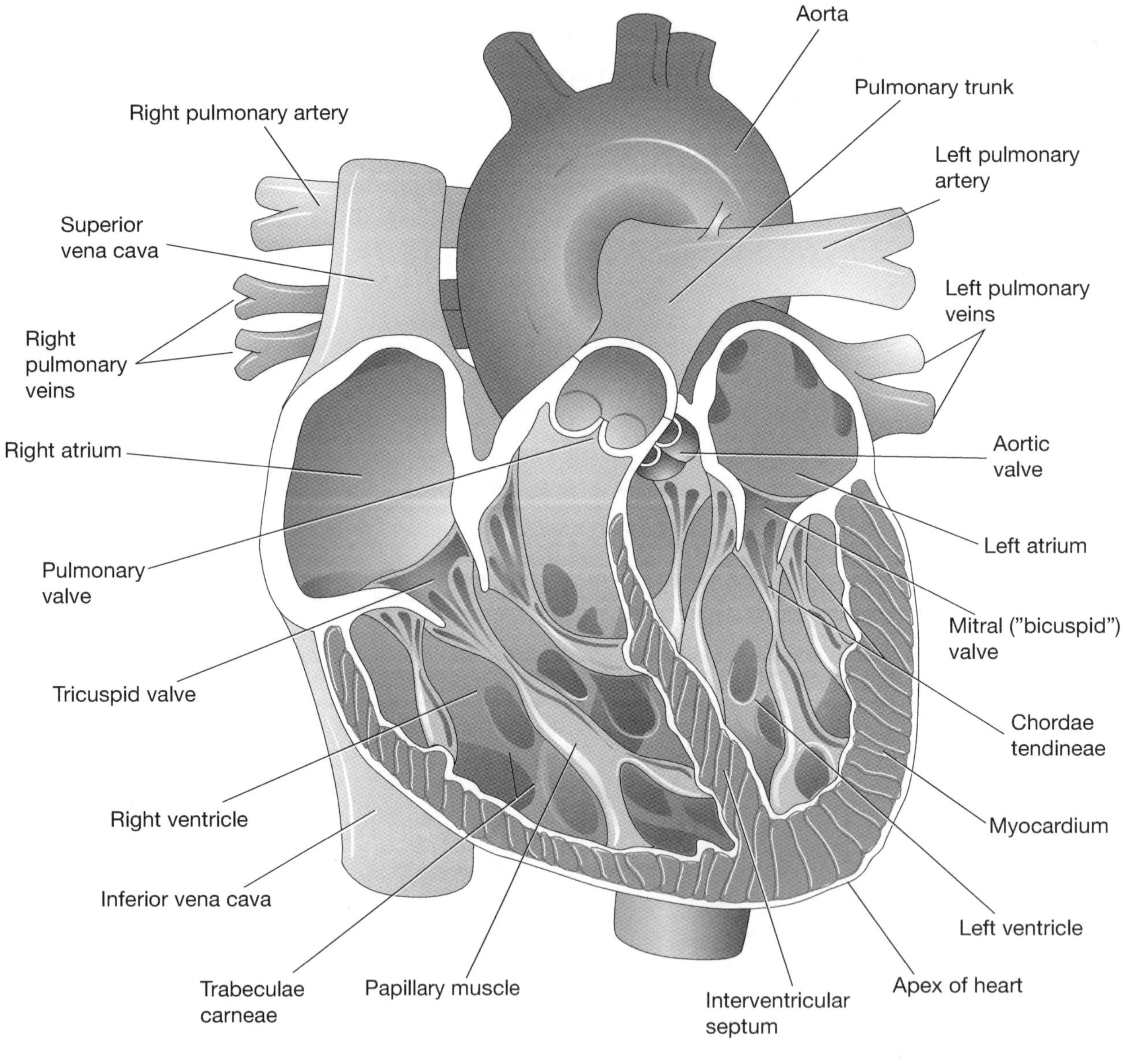

Figure 15-4

Internal Structure of the Heart

Note how thin the atrial walls are when compared to the ventricles and note that the left ventricular wall is much thicker than that of the right one.

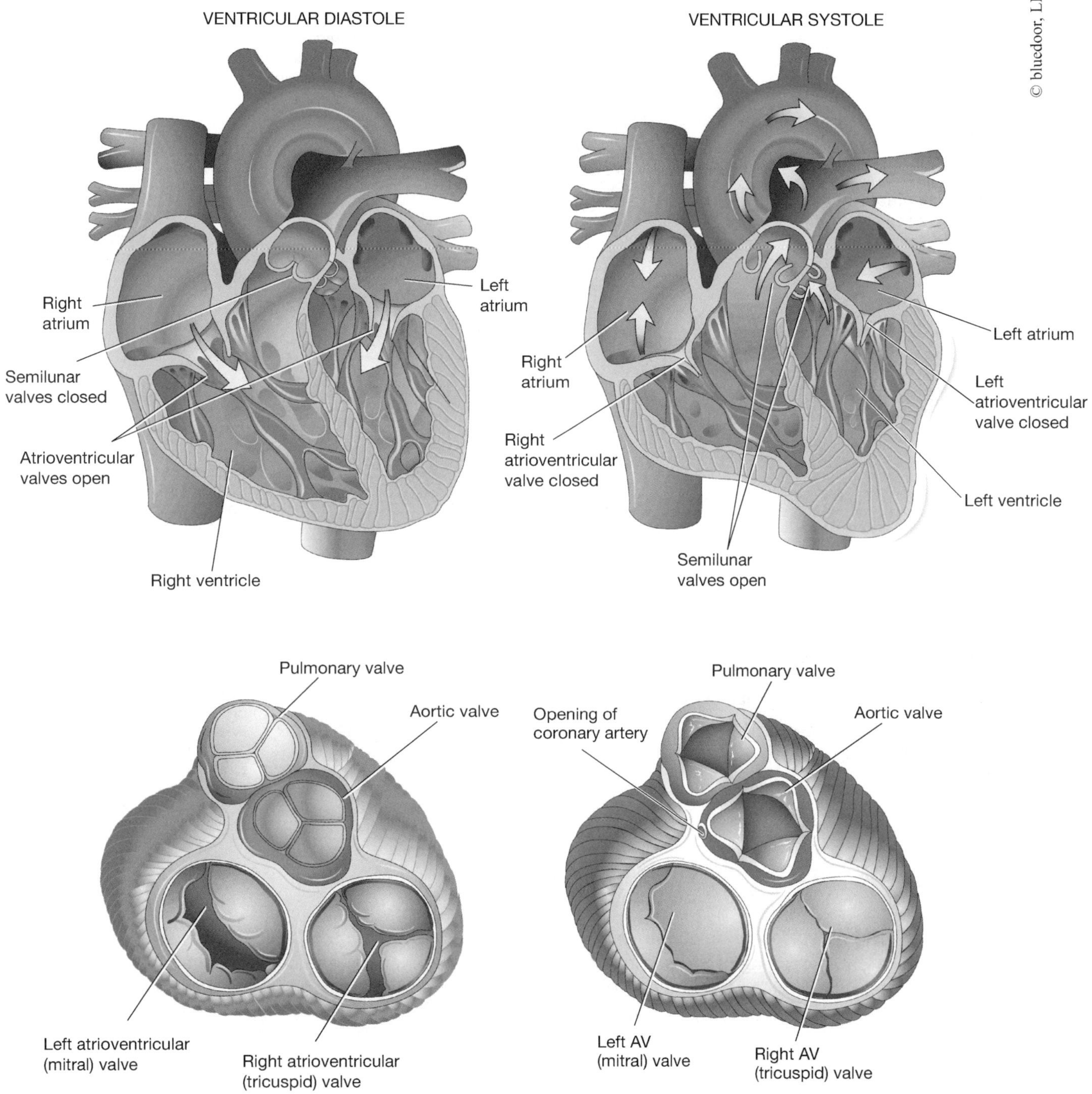

Figure 15-5

Valves of the Heart
(Frontal Sections Above/Transverse Sections Below)

During ventricular diastole (relaxation), the AV valves are open and the "semilunar" valves (aortic and pulmonary valves) are closed. When the ventricles are contracting (systole) the AV valves are closed and the "semilunar" valves are open. Note that "semilunar" is not part of the name of the aortic and pulmonary valves, but is often used to refer to them collectively (*i.e.,* the two semilunar valves).

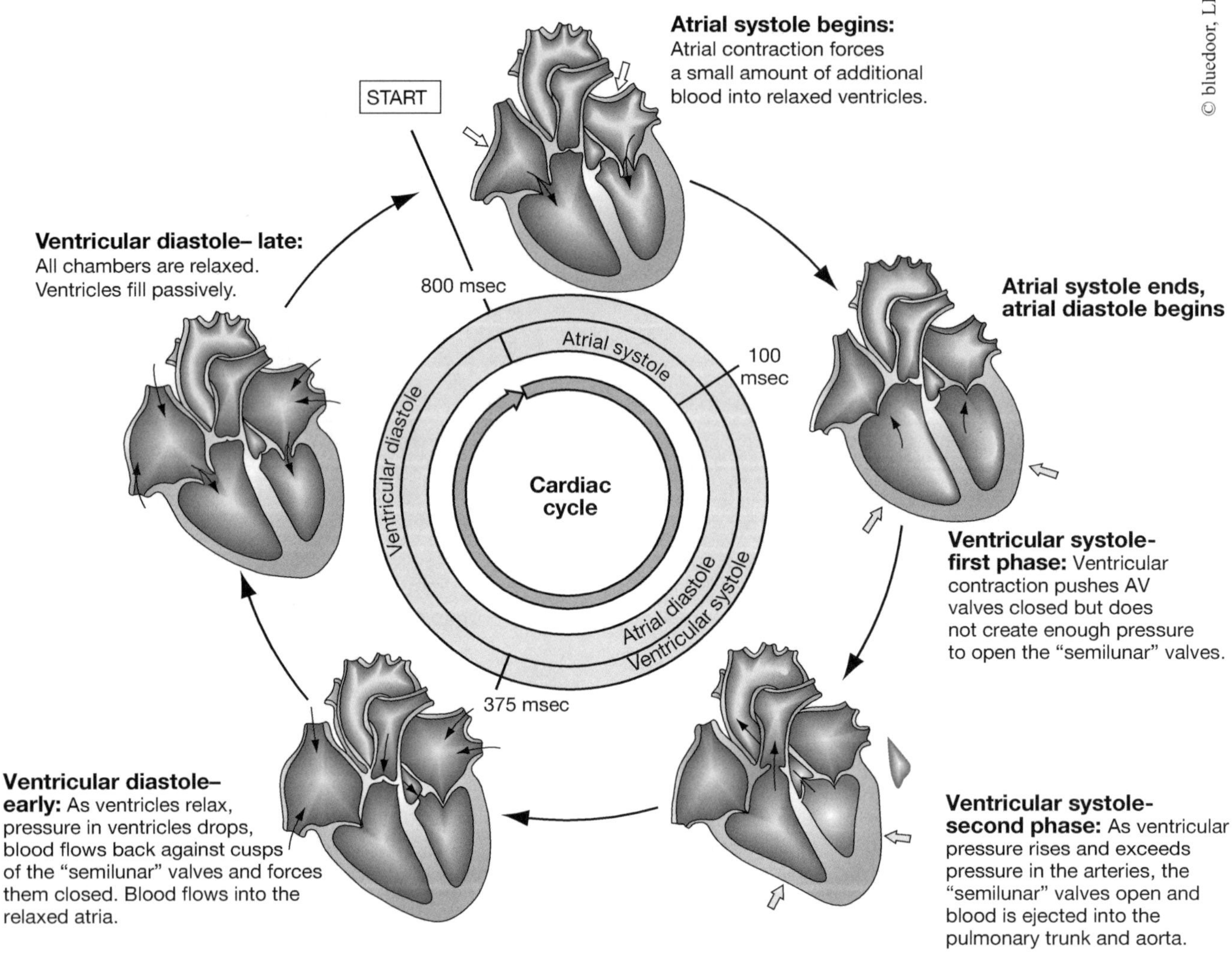

Figure 15-6
Cardiac Cycle

The AV valves close at the very beginning of ventricular systole, followed immediately by opening of the aortic and pulmonary valves. At the end of ventricular systole (beginning of ventricular diastole) the aortic and pulmonary valves close followed immediately by the opening of the AV valves.

shaped. The lumen of the right ventricle is crossed by a bundle of cardiac tissue called the **trabecula septomarginalis**. It contains conducting fibers and is part of the modified cardiac musculature involved in controlling the activity of the heart. The narrowed outflow portion of the right ventricle leading up to the valve of the pulmonary trunk is called the **conus arteriosus** or **infundibulum of the heart**.

The valves of the heart prevent backflow by allowing blood to flow only in the proper direction. They are passively opened by blood flowing through them in the correct anatomic direction and passively closed by the regurgitation of blood in the "wrong" direction. The left and right atrioventricular valves are somewhat more complex than the aortic and pulmonary valves (Table 15-1). The

Table 15-1 A Comparison of the Four Cardiac Valves

Criteria	*Right Atrioventricular Valve*	*Left Atrioventricular Valve*	*Pulmonary Valve*	*Aortic Valve*
Location	Between right atrium and ventricle	Between left atrium and ventricle	Between right ventricle and pulmonary trunk	Between left ventricle and ascending aorta
Aliases	Tricuspid valve	Mitral or "bicuspid" valve	"Semilunar" valve	"Semilunar" valve
Are open during	Ventricular diastole	Ventricular diastole	Ventricular systole	Ventricular systole
Are closed during	Ventricular systole	Ventricular systole	Ventricular diastole	Ventricular diastole
Stenosis causes:	Diastolic murmur	Diastolic murmur	Systolic murmur	Systolic murmur
Insufficiency causes:	Systolic murmur	Systolic murmur	Diastolic murmur	Diastolic murmur
Structure	Three cusps anchored by chordae tendineae to papillary muscles	Two large and two small cusps anchored by chordae tendineae to papillary muscles	Three leaflets, no chordae tendineae or papillary muscle anchor points	Three leaflets, no chordae tendineae or papillary muscle anchor points

right atrioventricular valve (also known as the **tricuspid valve**) (Figure 15-5) has three membranous leaflets called **anterior**, **posterior**, and **septal cusps**. These meet edge-to-edge in the center of the atrioventricular orifice when the valve is closed and fold downward against the ventricular walls when the valve is open. To anchor the edges of the cusps when the valve is closed and keep them from folding up into the atrium, fibrous cords called **chordae tendineae** attach along their margins. These are anchored to myocardial projections from the right ventricular walls called **papillary muscles**. The **left atrioventricular** (**mitral**) **valve** is similar structurally to the right AV valve except that it has only two major cusps (**anterior** and **posterior cusps**). There are smaller cusps at each end of these called **commissural cusps**. The **aortic valve** is positioned in the outflow passageway between the cavity of the left ventricle and the aorta. The **valve of the pulmonary trunk** (**pulmonary valve**) occupies a similar position in the wall of the right ventricle between the cavity of the right ventricle (specifically the conus arteriosus) and the pulmonary trunk. The aortic and pulmonary valves are sometimes called "semilunar" valves because each one of their three leaflets is somewhat half-moon shaped. The leaflet margins are not anchored by chordae tendineae, but the center of each one has a thickened area termed the **nodule of the semilunar leaflet**. The cusps or leaflets of all four heart valves normally close securely enough to prevent any backflow of blood.

The normal cardiac cycle includes alternating periods of contraction (called **systole**) followed by a longer period of relaxation (called **diastole**) (Figure 15-6). During diastole the AV valves are open (due to the gravitational force which pulls atrial blood down into the ventricles) and the aortic and pulmonary valves are closed due to the pressure in the aorta and pulmonary trunk. At the beginning of systole, the atria contract just before the ventricles. This empties the atria and fully fills the ventricles. When the ventricles begin to contract, the intraventricular pressure rises and the initial regurgitation of blood back toward the atria closes the atrioventricular valves by "ballooning" them back into the atrioventricular orifices. This prevents further reflux. As the pressure within the ventricles rises, it opens the aortic and pulmonary valves, and the ventricular blood is ejected through them into the aorta and pulmonary trunk. When the ventricles cease contracting (at the beginning of diastole), back pressure in the aorta and pulmonary trunk causes blood to begin to flow back through them. This closes the valves by ballooning the leaflets back toward the ventricles to prevent further backflow. When the heart is again in a relaxed (diastolic) state, the AV valves open and the cycle repeats itself.

There are two (major) normal heart sounds. The **first heart sound** ("lub") is associated with simultaneous closure of the right and left atrioventricular valves. This is followed in rapid succession by the **second heart sound** ("dub") which is associated with simultaneous closure of the aortic and pulmonary valves. The period of time between the first and second heart sounds corresponds to ventricular systole. The longer period of time between the second heart sound and the next first heart sound corresponds to ventricular diastole. Abnormal heart sounds are related to turbulent flow of blood and are called **cardiac murmurs**. They can be caused by several cardiac abnormalities including heart valves that do not open and close properly. Heart valves may not close securely enough to prevent leakage. Those that "leak" are said to be **insufficient** and the turbulent flow of blood regurgitating through them causes a murmur. Valves also cause murmurs if they fail to completely open. This condition, called **valvular stenosis** (narrowing), can be caused by certain types of infectious diseases that cause scarring and fusion of the edges of adjacent cusps. Since insufficient valves murmur only when they are closed and stenotic valves murmur only when they are open, physicians can use deductive reasoning to help them diagnose valvular cardiopathy. For example, a murmur that occurs only during ventricular systole could be caused by an insufficient atrioventricular valve (both of which are closed) or it might be due to a stenotic aortic or pulmonary valve (both of which are open). Deducing which valve is affected involves noting where on the chest wall the murmur is loudest (*see Figure 15-39*).

Objectives

5. Differentiate the four heart chambers in regard to what enters/leaves.
6. Differentiate the four heart valves in regard to their names (and aliases), location, general structure, and their open/shut position during the cardiac cycle.
7. Discuss the cardiac cycle.
8. State the names and causes of the normal heart sounds.
9. Explain the causes of cardiac murmurs.

Contraction of the heart muscle is controlled by modified cardiac muscle cells called **purkinje fibers**. These cells are specialized for the conduction of impulses rather than for contraction. A localized group of them in the wall of the right atrium, called the **sinoatrial (SA) node**, initiates the impulses that lead to systole (Figure 15-7, 8). These impulses travel throughout the atria in purkinje fibers. When the impulse reaches another group of cells near the top of the interventricular septum called the **atrioventricular (AV) node**, it is delayed for a fractional part of a second before being passed on to the ventricles. This allows the atria to empty before the ventricles contract. Excessive impulse delay at this point constitutes partial or complete heart block (*see Clinical Considerations*). From the atrioventricular node, the impulses continue down the **atrioventricular fascicle** (bundle) of purkinje fibers and are carried on to the ventricular walls by the **left** and **right crura** of this fascicle. To reach the external wall of the right ventricle, a fascicle of purkinje fibers travels through the **trabecula septomarginalis**. This is a well-developed trabecula carnea that extends from the interventricular septum to the outer wall of the right ventricle.

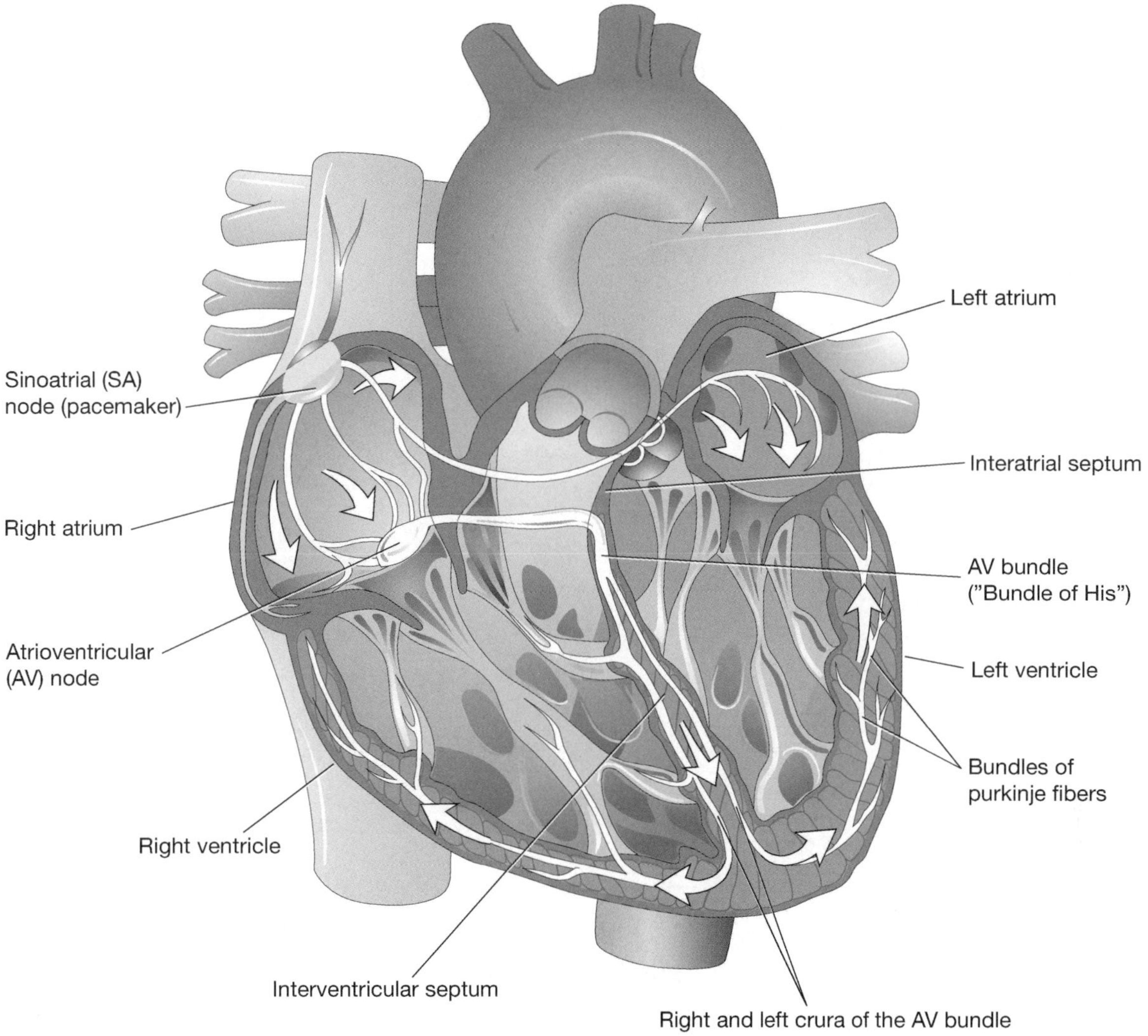

Figure 15-7

Conduction System of the Heart

The impulse for contraction is initiated in the SA node—a group of specialized cardiac muscle cells (purkinje fibers) located in the wall of the right atrium near the opening of the superior vena cava. The impulse spreads throughout both atria, is delayed 0.12–0.20 seconds at the AV node (at resting heart rates), and is then conducted by purkinje fibers making up the atrioventricular bundle. The latter splits into the left and right crura (left and right "bundle branches") which are distributed to the myocardium of the ventricular walls.

Objectives

10. Discuss the electrical conduction system of the heart.

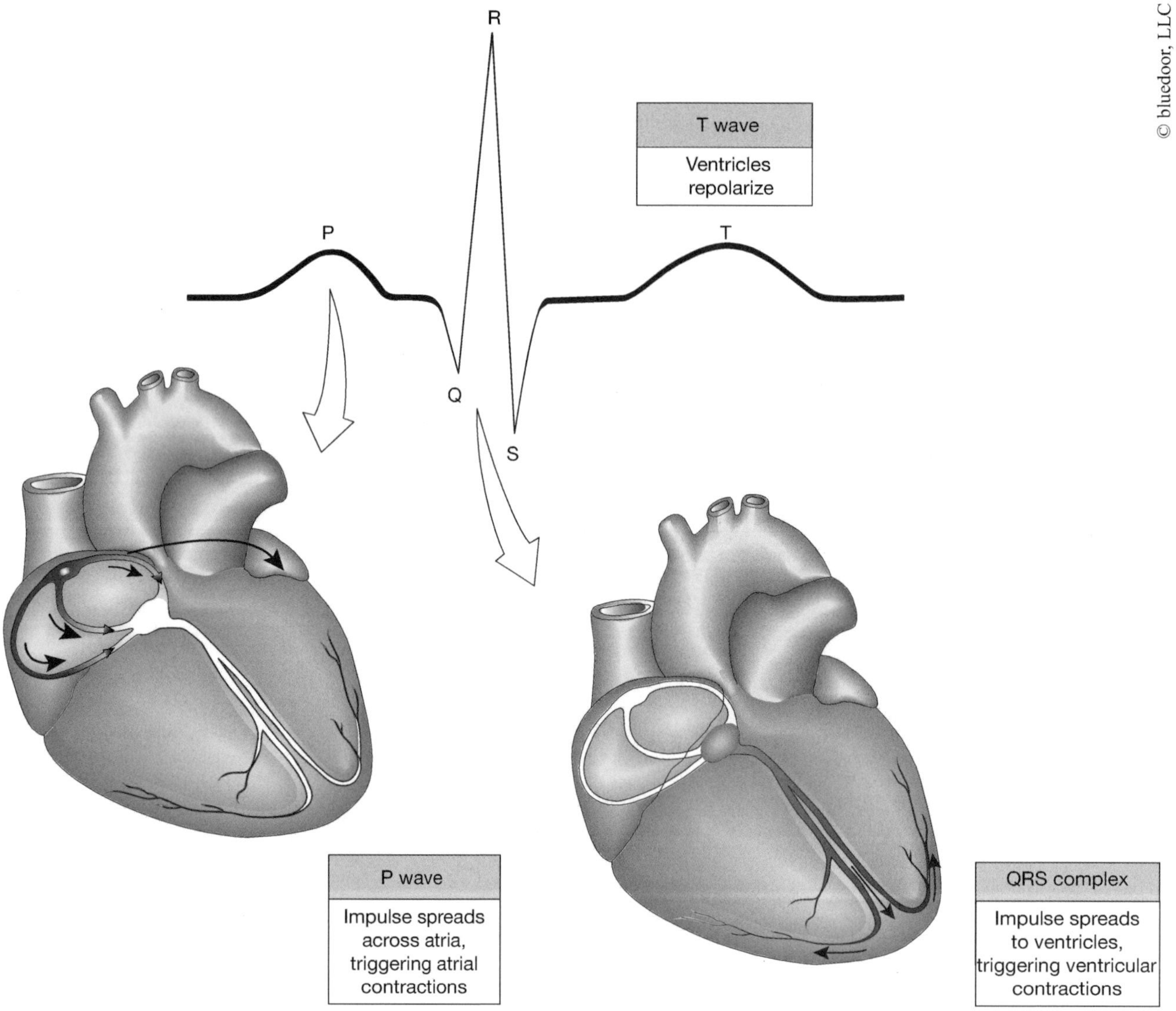

Figure 15-8

Electrocardiogram

An EKG monitors the electrical activity of the heart and can be used to detect some kinds of cardiac problems. The three major parts of a typical EKG signature are the P wave, QRS complex, and the T wave. The P wave represents depolarization of the atrial myocardium. The QRS complex is caused by depolarization of the ventricular myocardium. Repolarization of ventricles causes the T wave. Atrial repolarization is overshadowed by the QRS complex and does not register.

Arteries

Arteries are the vessels which carry blood from the heart to the capillaries. Three named layers form their walls: tunica intima, tunica media, and tunica externa. The **tunica intima** consists of a lining of simple squamous epithelial cells (endothelium), a small amount of subendothelial connective tissue proper, and a thin but distinct layer of elastic fibers termed the internal elastic membrane (Figure 15-9, 10). The **tunica media** consists primarily of smooth muscle tissue with variable amounts of elastic connective tissue, and is encased in a distinct layer of elastic fibers termed the external elastic

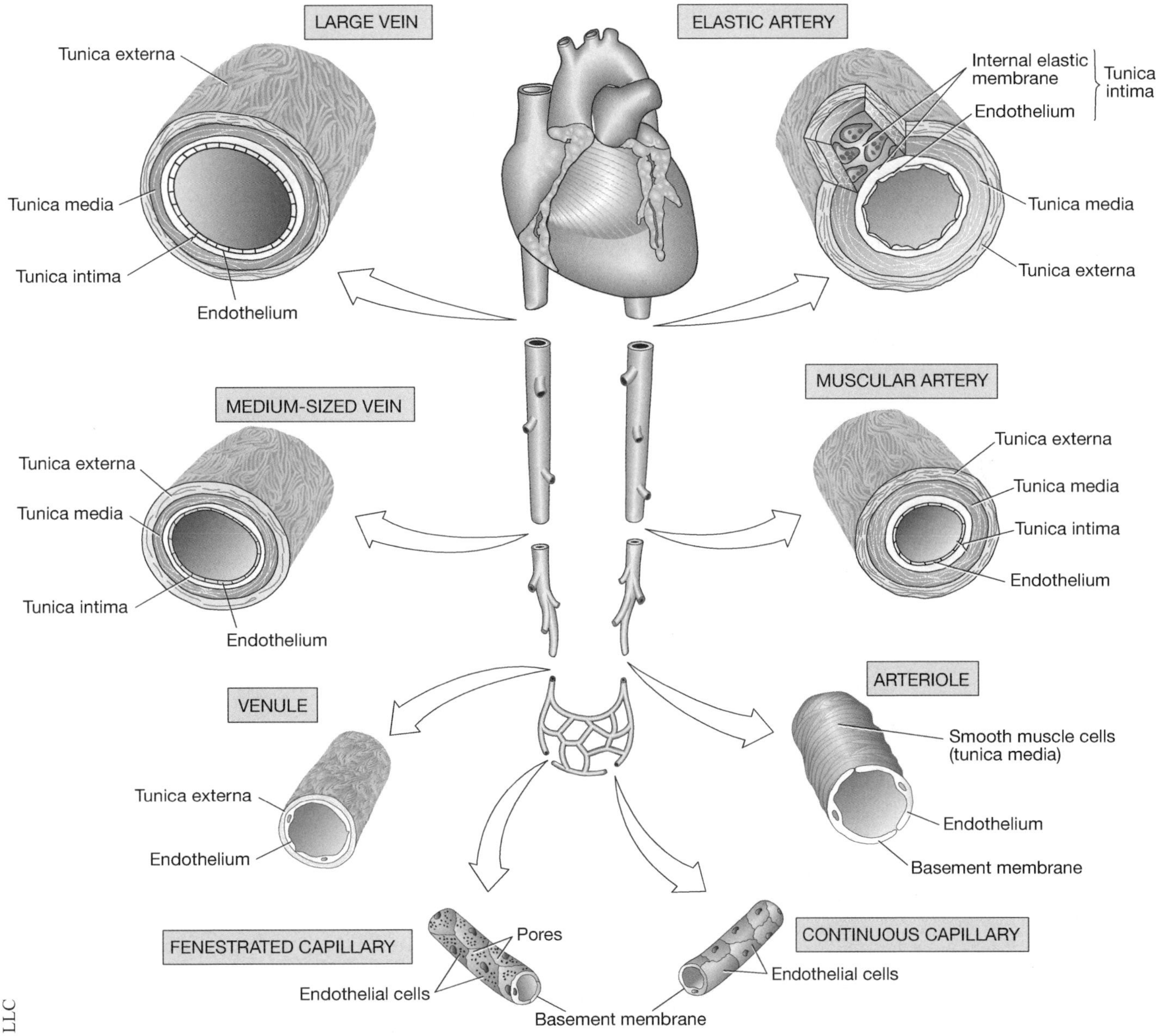

Figure 15-9

Blood Vessels

Arteries carry blood away from the heart and have thicker walls and smaller lumina than their venous counterparts. Capillaries are the only vessels with walls thin enough for diffusion of nutrients and waste products. The largest arteries are classified as elastic arteries, and they modulate (dampen) the blood pressure. Most arteries are muscular arteries which control overall blood pressure and allow differential flow to various organs as needed. The smallest arteries (arterioles) supply capillaries. Capillaries drain into venules which, in turn, drain into veins. All veins larger than venules are simply called veins, with no other official classification.

membrane. The **tunica externa** is dense, fibrous connective tissue which forms the outermost layer of the arterial wall.

The largest arteries (aorta, pulmonary trunk, and some of their branches) are termed **elastic arteries** because they have a significant amount of elastic connective tissue in their tunica media. When the heart contracts and forces blood into them, they expand. Then, while the heart is in diastole, the elastic fibers reduce the arteries back to their original diameters. This helps to smooth out the blood flow; otherwise, it would be extremely high during systole and very low during diastole. Most arteries in the body which can be seen with the naked eye are **muscular arteries**. These arteries include those down to about 100 microns in diameter, and are characterized by having mainly smooth muscle in their tunica media. This muscle can be involuntarily contracted by the ANS to elevate the blood pressure, or relaxed to lower it. The smallest arteries are called **arterioles** and average about 40 microns in diameter. Arterioles supply capillaries (several each) and in some cases empty directly into tiny veins (venules) in a pattern called **arteriovenous anastomoses** (shunts). These connections are mainly found near the surface of the skin where they are involved in thermoregulation.

It is important to realize that arteries are only transport channels and have walls much too thick to allow exchange of nutrients and wastes. Only the cells of the tunica intima are nourished by the blood in the arterial lumen. Consequently, blood in the peripheral arteries, such as those in the digits, has essentially the same oxygen concentration as that in the aorta. The tissues in the walls of arteries and veins are nourished by a set of vessels that enter from their external surfaces. These are called **vasa vasorum** (*vessels of the vessels*).

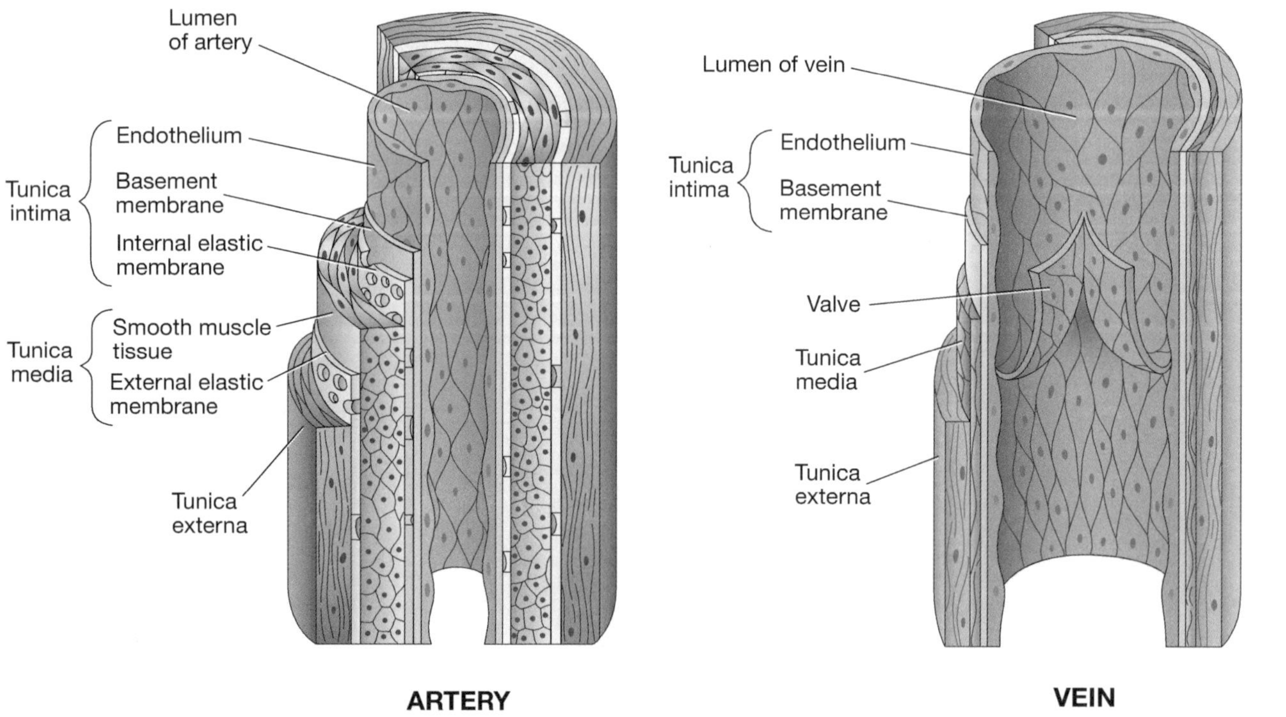

Figure 15-10

Structure of Vessel Walls

Arteries and veins both have three main layers in their walls: tunica externa, tunica media, and tunica intima. The specific components vary somewhat and the tunica media is much thicker in arteries. Many veins contain valves which allow blood to flow only toward the heart.

Objectives

11. Define arteries and differentiate the three size classes.

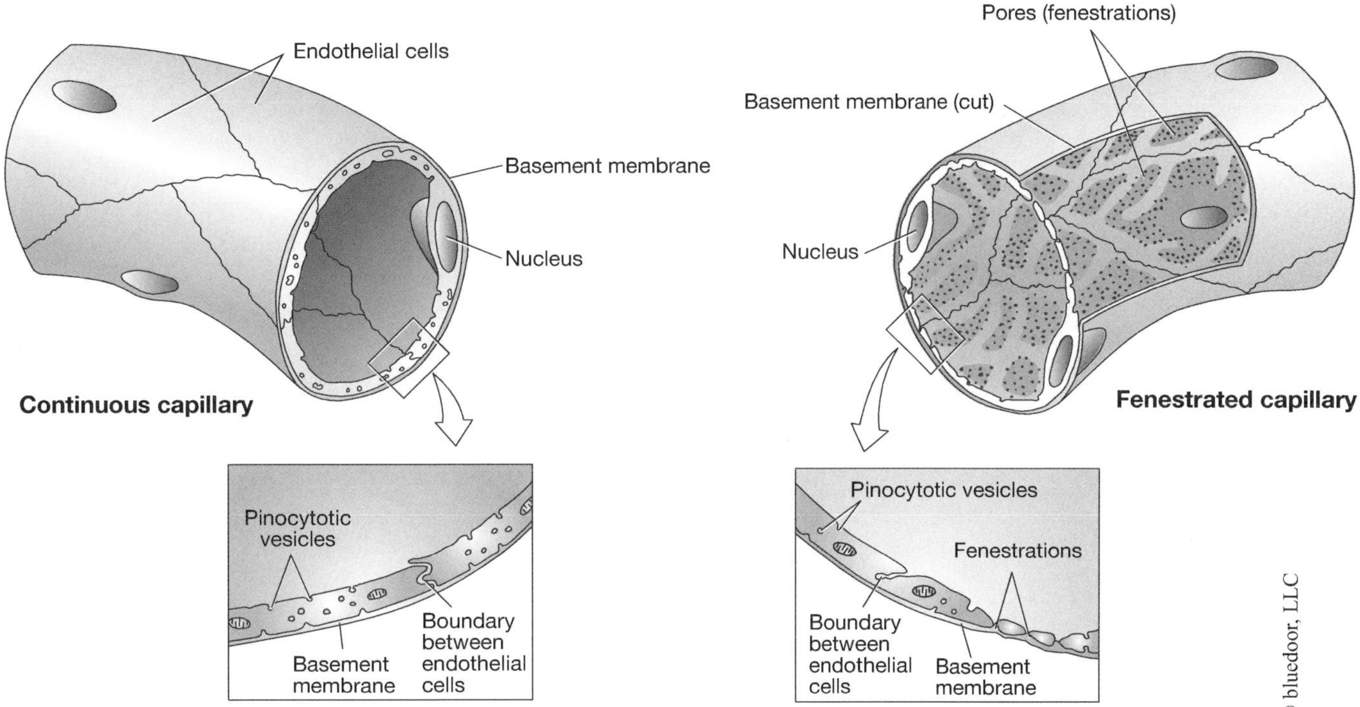

Figure 15-11
Capillaries

Capillaries have extremely thin walls to facilitate nutrient waste exchange. Those in most parts of the body are continuous, but fenestrated capillaries are found in some organs (choroid plexuses of brain, glomeruli of kidneys, some endocrine organs) to facilitate diffusion. In a few loci (liver, bone marrow, spleen) the capillaries have even larger pores and less basement membrane and are called sinusoids.

Capillaries

Capillaries are the smallest vessels and the only ones with walls thin enough to allow diffusion of nutrients and waste products. They are positioned between arterioles and venules (Figure 15-11, 12). A capillary wall consists of a single layer of simple squamous epithelium (endothelium) surrounded by a very thin layer of connective tissue proper. Typical capillaries are 10 μ or less in diameter. This is so small that red blood corpuscles are forced through them in single file. It is estimated that there are several billion capillaries in the body that provide a total surface area of several hundred square miles for exchange of nutrients and wastes. All cells in vascularized tissues of the body are believed to be located less than 100 μ from a capillary. The only avascular structures in the body are membranous epithelium, epithelial derivatives (hair, nails), structures composed of mature cartilage, and the cornea and lens of the eye.

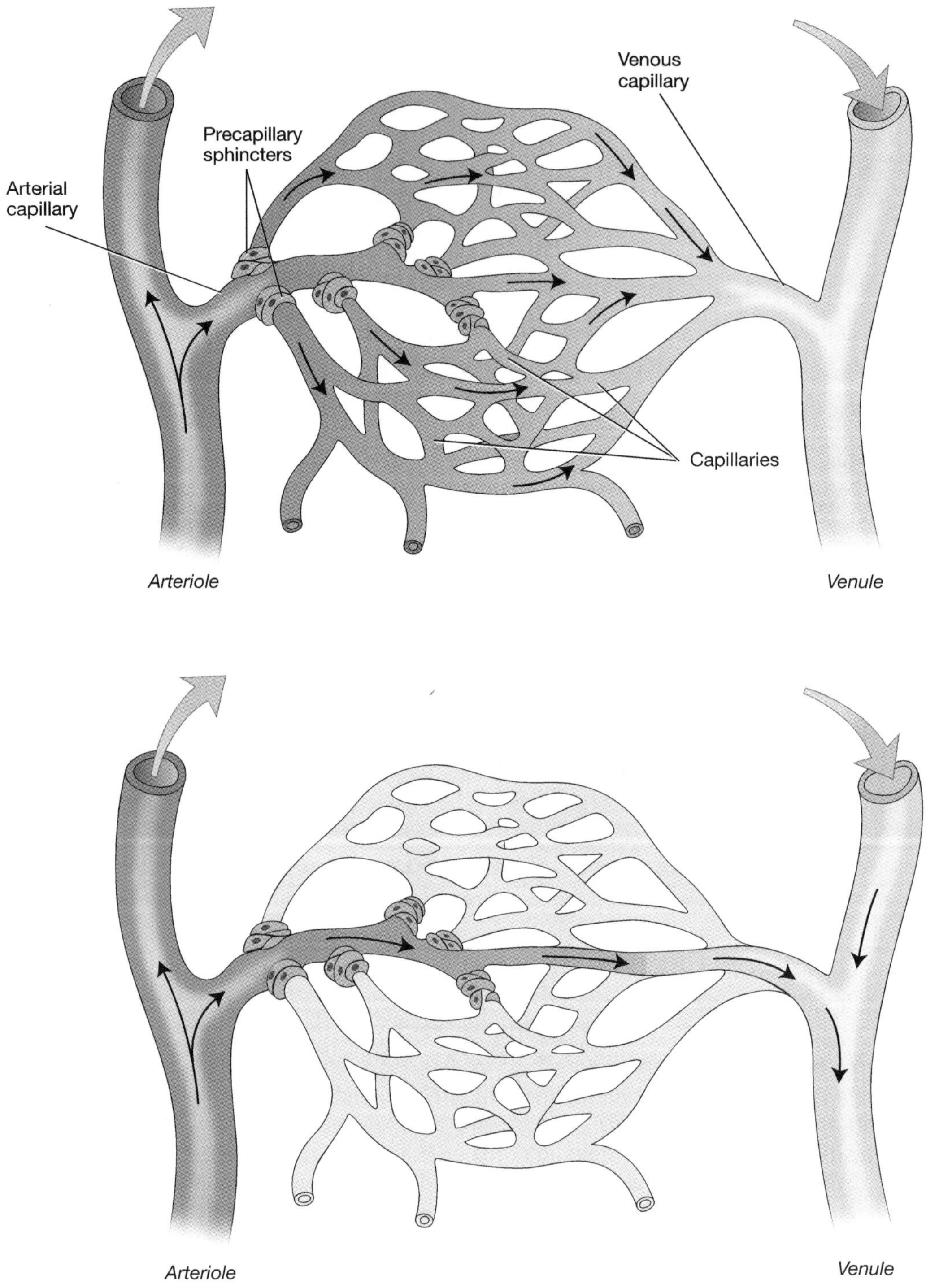

Figure 15-12

Microcirculation Through a Capillary Bed

Due to rhythmic contraction/relaxation of precapillary sphincters (which is dependent on the oxygen levels of adjacent tissues), only some of the capillaries carry blood at any given moment. Arterial capillaries (also called metarterioles, precapillary arterioles, and precapillaries) supply capillaries and venous capillaries (also called postcapillaries and postcapillary venules) drain the capillary beds.

Only about 5-7% of the total blood volume is in capillaries at any given moment (Figure 15-14). This is partially due to the fact that the largest percentage of the blood is located in venous channels. Another reason is that only some of the capillaries are open and functional at any given time. In skeletal muscles (at rest), blood flows through only 10-20 percent of the capillary beds present. This is controlled by the **precapillary sphincters** of arterioles. These tiny rings of smooth muscle encircle capillaries as they leave arterioles. They alternately and rhythmically open and close allowing blood to flow into only a fractional part of the capillaries during any one time. If these are paralyzed by a circulating toxin, too many capillaries will be open simultaneously resulting in a precipitous drop in blood pressure (*see the discussion of circulatory shock in Clinical Considerations*).

Capillaries in different organs vary in overall diameter and in the "tightness" with which the endothelial cells are joined. Most capillaries have intercellular pores that are about 40 angstroms (40×10^{-10} mm) in diameter and allow exchange of small molecules between blood and interstitial fluid. Those in the CNS do not have these channels and this may be a factor in the blood-brain-barrier. Capillaries in the kidney, endocrine glands, intestines, and choroid plexuses of the brain have **fenestrated endothelial cells**. The fenestrae are pores about 1000 angstroms in diameter which allow the passage of larger molecules. Modified capillaries in some locations (bone marrow, liver, spleen) are termed **sinusoids**.

The blood pressure in capillaries is very low. The systemic arterial pressure is reduced to only a few millimeters of mercury by the thinner-walled peripheral vessels which also dampen out all systemic/diastolic pressure difference at the capillary level. All capillaries lose a small amount of fluid from the blood that they carry due to "leakage." This fluid enters the extracellular space and the excess is absorbed into lymphatic capillaries as lymph (*see Chapter 16*).

Objectives

12. Explain why capillaries are the only blood vessels which can exchange nutrients and waste products with surrounding tissues, and list the avascular components of the body.
13. Discuss the normal function of pre-capillary sphincters and explain how (why) endotoxic shock occurs.

Veins

Veins are the vessels which collect blood from the capillaries and return it to the heart. The smallest veins attach directly to capillaries and are termed **venules** and all larger ones are termed veins. Venous channels have the same three named layers in their walls as arteries (tunica externa, tunica media, and tunica intima), but their walls are thinner overall and the tissue composition of the layers is somewhat different (fewer smooth muscle cells and elastic fibers) (*see Figure 15-10*). Most veins parallel arteries and are named after the arteries that they follow. The pressure in the veins is very low (averaging 1-2 mm Hg). Because of this low pressure, blood travels much more slowly in veins than it does in arteries. Nonetheless, a given vein carries almost as much blood volume per unit time as the artery that it follows. The only volume difference between the two is that which is lost into the extracellular fluid by "leaking" through the capillary walls. Some of the veins, especially those in the limbs, have **valves** that prevent backflow. The lower pressure in venous channels allows them to have thinner walls than their arterial counterparts, and the slower flow dictates that their overall diameters are larger than the arteries that they follow.

Objectives

14. Compare an artery to the vein that follows it (satellite vein) in regard to thickness of the wall, overall diameter, volume of blood transported/unit time, and the presence of valves.

Circulatory Patterns

The circulation of blood away from the heart and then back to it occurs in two separate sets of vessels (Figure 15-13). The flow of blood from the right ventricle to the lungs and then back to the left atrium (heart-lungs-heart) is termed the **pulmonary circulation** (Figure 15-15, 16). Its major function is to allow blood to exchange carbon dioxide for oxygen in the lungs. The flow of blood from the left ventricle to the (rest of the) body and back to the right atrium (heart-body-heart) is termed the **systemic circulation**. This portion of the circulation has a variety of functions as outlined previously. The normal systolic/diastolic pressures in the systemic circulation are higher than those in the pulmonary circulation. Higher systemic pressures are necessary due to the fact that a much larger percentage of the body is supplied by the systemic circulation. Blood within the systemic circulation must be moved further and against more resistance than blood in the pulmonary circulation.

The general flow schemes in the pulmonary circulation and systemic circulations are identical. Blood leaves the heart in a single artery which supplies smaller arteries. These supply a series of smaller arteries down to arterioles. Arterioles supply capillaries and the capillaries drain into venules. Venules drain into an increasingly larger series of veins that eventually drain back into the heart. This pattern (arteries-arterioles-capillaries-venules-veins) is the standard flow scheme for almost all sets of vessels in the body. Blood normally flows through only one set of capillaries before returning to the heart. There are two places, however, where blood courses through two different sets of capillaries in series (instead of only one) before returning to the heart. These are called **portal systems** and include the hypothalamohypophysial portal system and the hepatic portal system. The **hypothalamohypophysial portal system** ensures that the hormones released by the hypothalamus will reach the anterior pituitary gland in sufficient concentrations to exert their effects. It is discussed in Chapter 14 and illustrated in Figure 14-6. The **hepatic portal system** involves the venous drainage of the structures supplied by three unpaired branches of the abdominal aorta into the liver. It will be separately discussed after a consideration of major systemic vessels.

Most body structures receive only arterial (high oxygen) blood. The liver and pituitary gland are exceptions since they also receive blood of low oxygen tension via their portal systems. The only other organs with a *"dual"* blood supply are the lungs and heart.

Objectives

15. Compare a standard circulatory pattern to a portal pattern and name the two portal systems found in the human body.
16. Indicate what is meant by a "dual blood supply" and name the organs which have one.

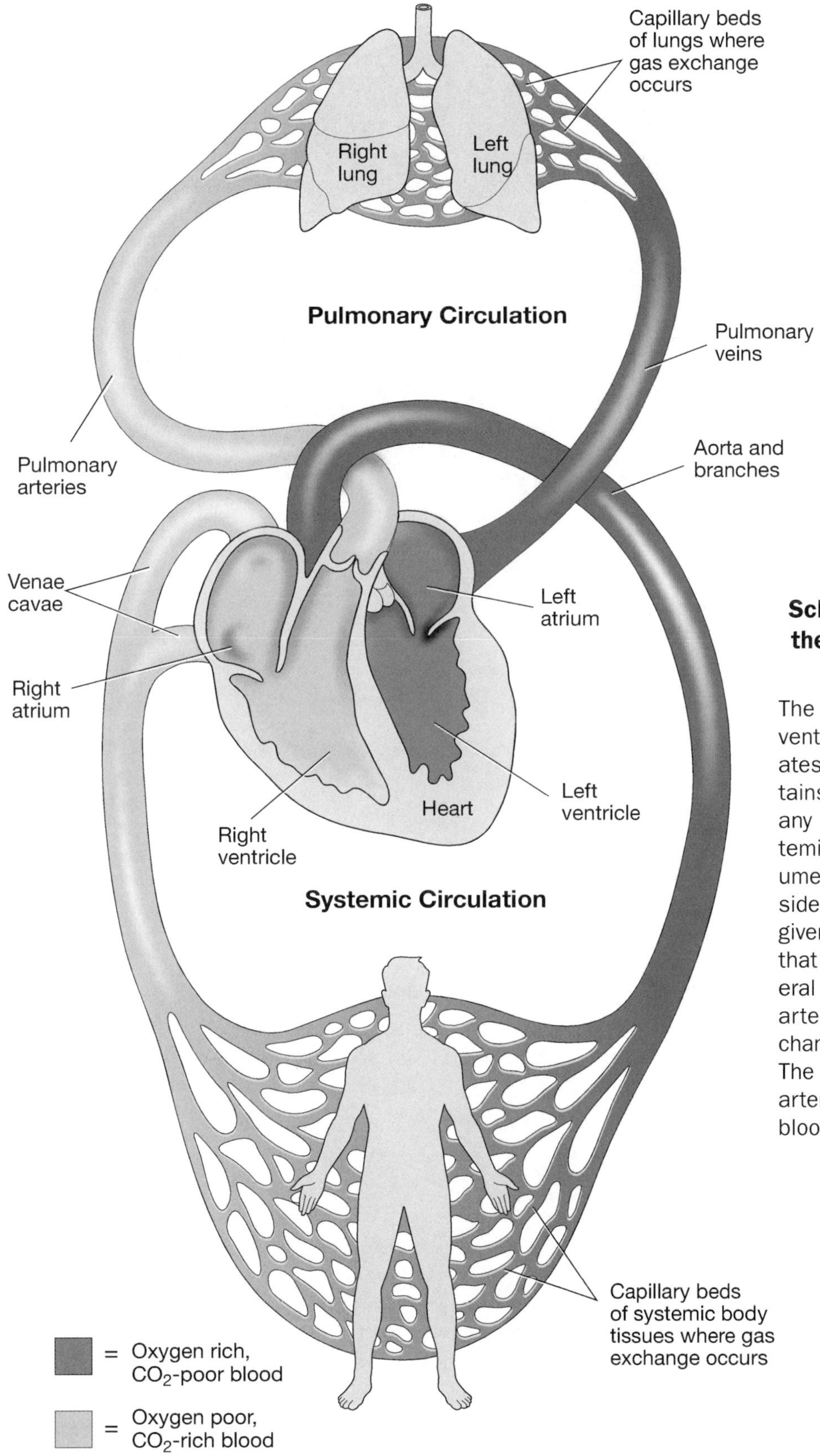

Figure 15-13

Schematic Representation of the Pulmonary and Systemic Circulatory Patterns

The pulmonary circulation (right ventricle – lungs – left atrium) operates at a lower pressure and contains less total blood volume at any given moment than the systemic circulation. However, the volume of blood passing through each side (right/left) of the heart at any given moment is normally equal to that passing through the contralateral side. Note that the systemic arteries and pulmonary venous channels carry oxygen-rich blood. The systemic veins and pulmonary arteries transport oxygen depleted blood.

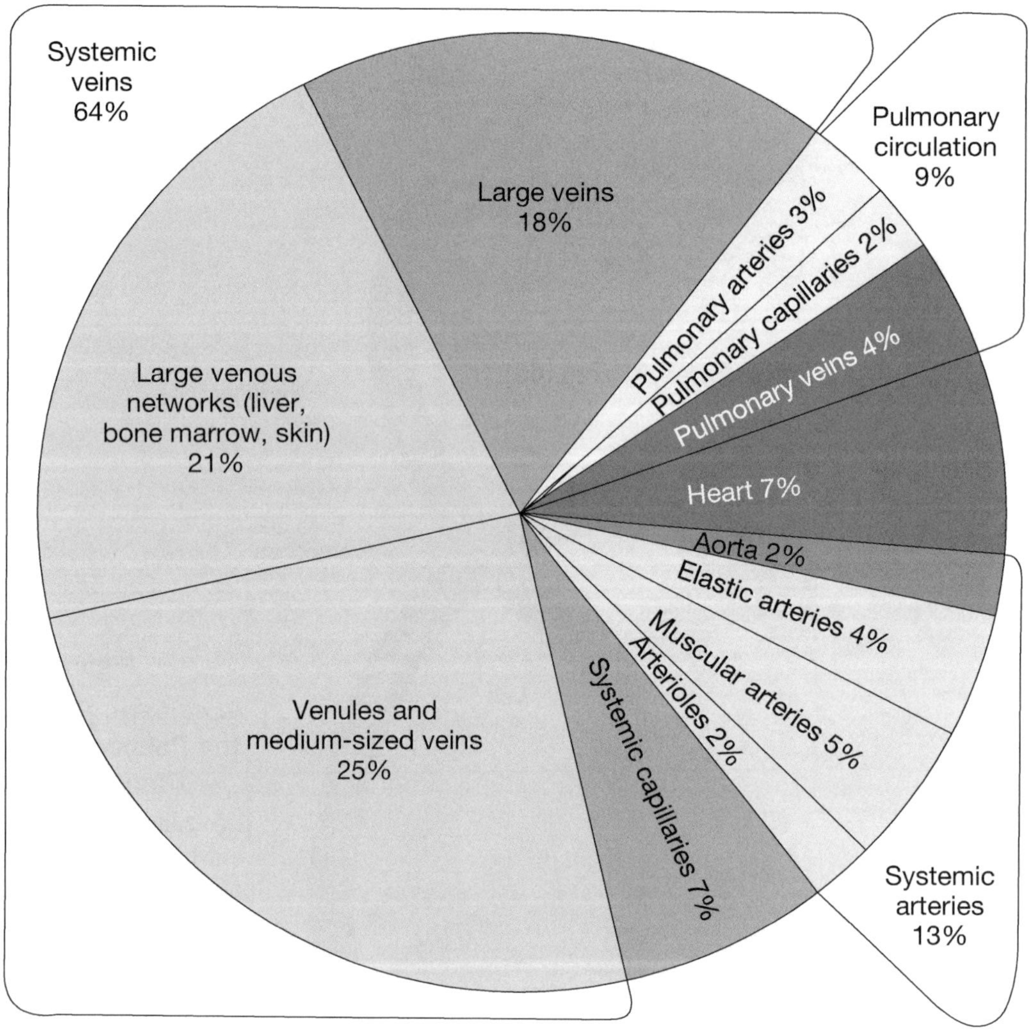

Figure 15-14

Distribution of Blood in the Cardiovascular System

Approximately 84% of the total blood volume is in the systemic circulation, 7% is in the heart, and 9% is in the pulmonary circulation. The systemic venous system accounts for about 64% of the blood in the human body and 21% of this venous blood is held in venous reservoirs.

Major Systemic Arteries

All of the systemic arteries are branches of the **aorta** or are supplied by its branches (Table 15-2, Figure 15-17). As the aorta leaves the left ventricle, it is directed superiorly as the **ascending** (**part of the**) **aorta**. It then turns 180° to the left and downward to form the **aortic arch**. The remainder of the aorta is termed the **descending** (**part of the**) **aorta** and is divided into a **thoracic part** and an **abdominal part**. To save time and space, the thoracic part of the descending aorta is often shortened to the unofficial term "*thoracic aorta*." Likewise, the abdominal part of the descending aorta is often unofficially called the "*abdominal aorta*." The descending aorta terminates in the lower lum-

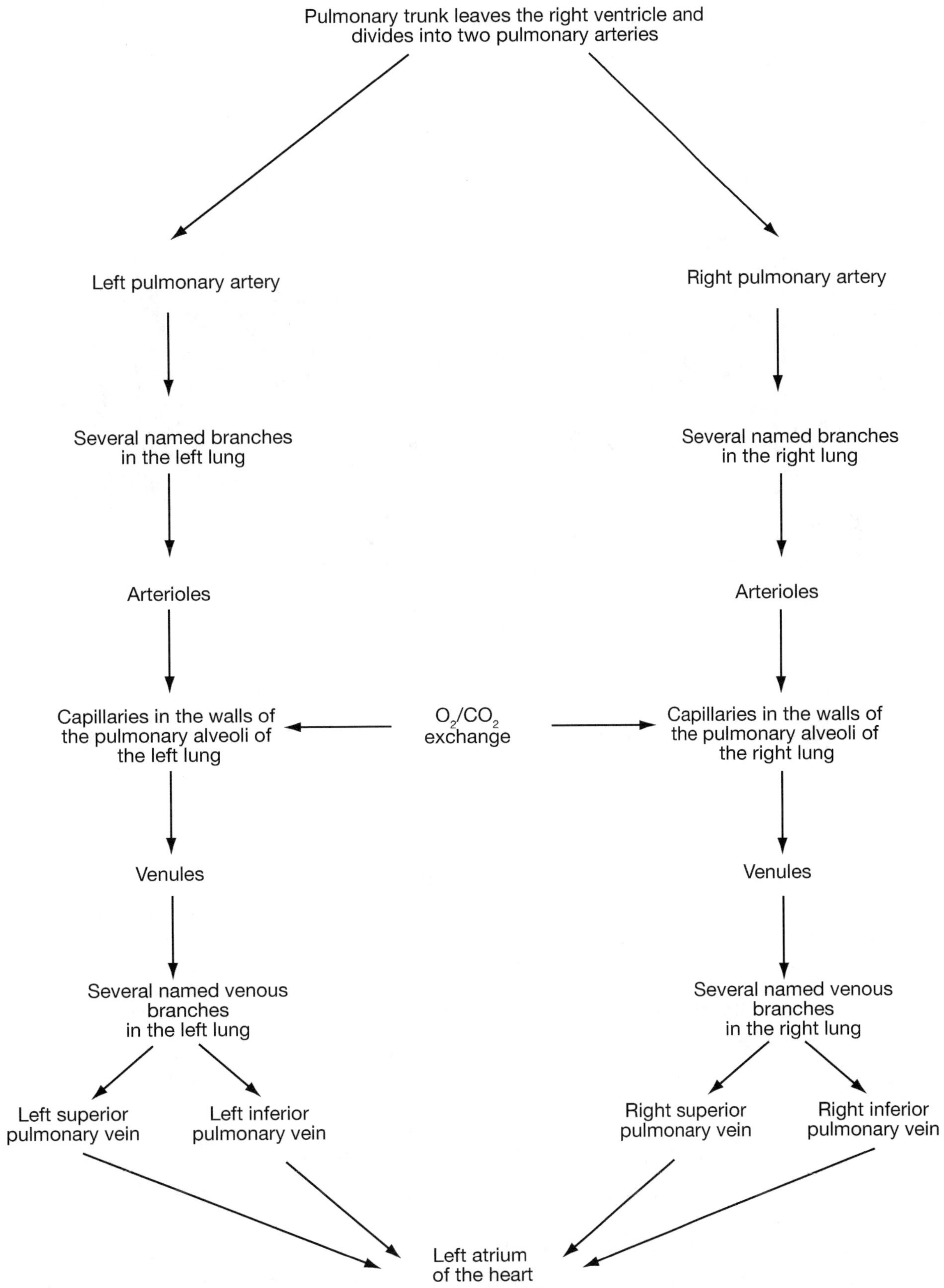

Figure 15-15

Schematic Representation of the Pulmonary Circulation

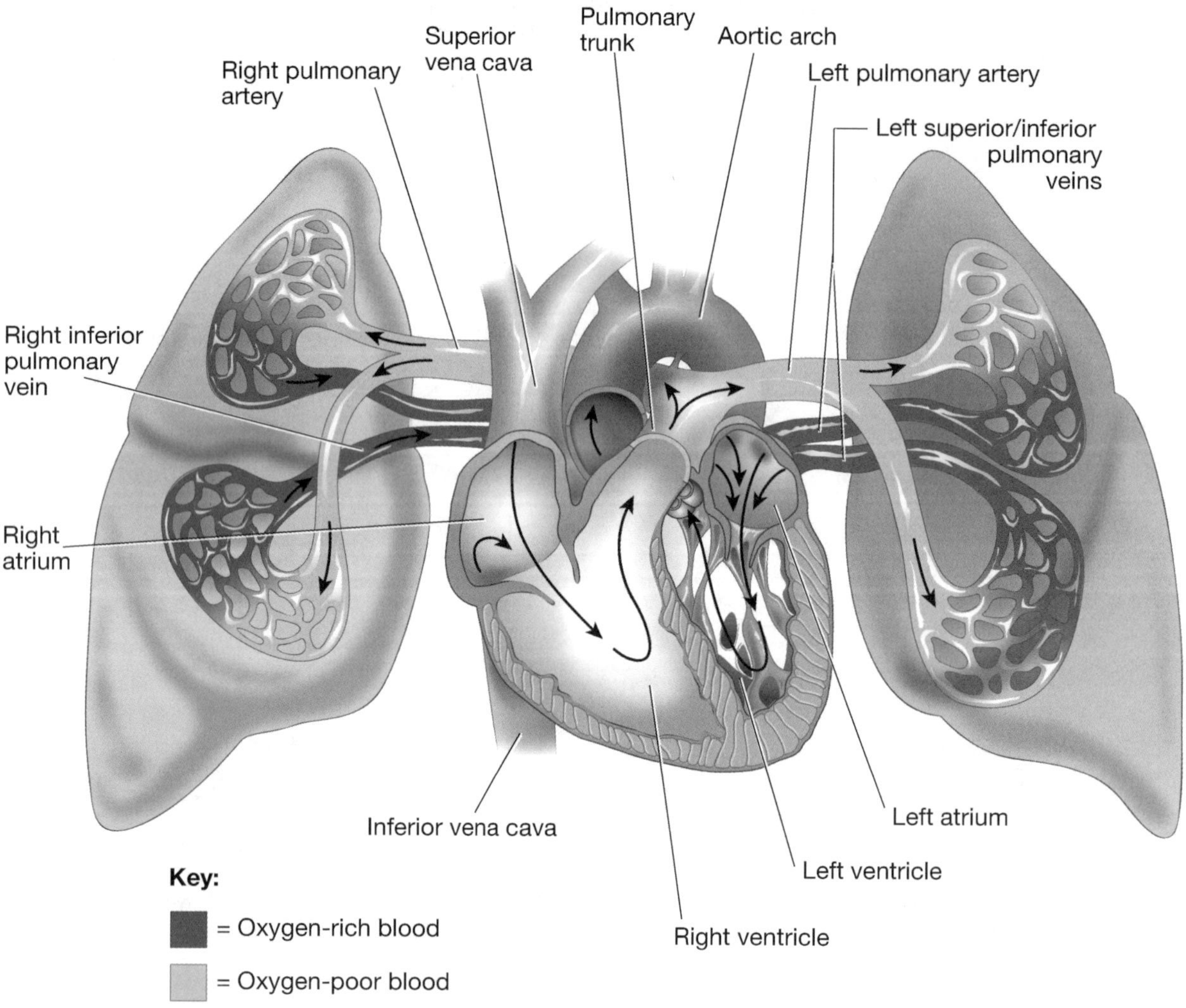

Figure 15-16
Pulmonary Circulation

Blood is pumped to the lungs through the left and right pulmonary arteries. Each pulmonary artery is a single vessel with numerous branches distributed to the various parts of each lung. After flowing through capillary beds in the lungs, blood is returned through an ever larger series of venous channels which ultimately enter the left atrium of the heart as the left and right superior and inferior pulmonary veins (*see Figure 15-15*).

bar region by dividing into the left and right common iliac arteries at the **aortic bifurcation**. Throughout its course, the descending aorta is located in the posterior aspects of the thoracic and abdominal cavities.

The ascending part of the aorta has only two branches: the right and left coronary arteries. The **right coronary artery** courses around the right side of the heart in the coronary groove and supplies numerous branches to the heart. The **left coronary artery** is larger than the right one and divides into an anterior interventricular branch and a circumflex branch. Each of these supplies several named branches to the heart.

Table 15-2 Branches of the Aorta

Ascending Part of the Aorta (two branches):
- Right coronary a.—to the right atrium and right ventricle
- Left coronary a.—to the left atrium and left ventricle

Aortic Arch (three branches):
- Brachiocephalic trunk—to the right side of the head and neck and the right superior limb
- Left common carotid a.—to the left side of the head and neck
- Left subclavian a.—to the left superior limb

Descending Part of Aorta (two parts):
- Thoracic part of descending aorta:
  - Bronchial branches—to the bronchi, lower trachea, respiratory bronchioles, adjacent lymph nodes, pulmonary vessels, pericardium, and part of the esophagus
  - Esophageal branches—to the esophagus
  - Pericardial branches—to the pericardial sac
  - Mediastinal branches—to the mediastinal areolar tissue, pericardium, adjacent lymph nodes, and thymus
  - Superior phrenic aa.—to the superior aspect of the diaphragm
  - Posterior intercostal aa.—to the thoracic wall
  - Subcostal aa.—below the last ribs
- Abdominal part of descending aorta:
  - Inferior phrenic aa.—to the inferior aspect of the diaphragm and adrenal glands
  - Lumbar aa.—to the posterior abdominal wall and renal capsule
  - Celiac trunk—to the stomach, spleen, esophagus, pancreas, duodenum, gallbladder, and liver
  - Superior mesenteric a.—to most of the small intestine and proximal portion of the colon
  - Renal aa.—to the kidneys, ureters, and adrenal glands
  - Inferior mesenteric a.—to the descending colon and rectum
  - Middle adrenal aa.—to the adrenal glands
  - Testicular/Ovarian aa.—to the testis, ureter, and epididymis/ovary, uterus, and uterine tube
  - Median sacral a.—to the bony sacrum, coccyx, and rectum
  - Common iliac aa.—to the pelvis, abdominal wall, and inferior limbs

The aortic arch supplies three large branches: brachiocephalic trunk, left common carotid artery, and left subclavian artery (Figure 15-18). The **brachiocephalic trunk** is the largest branch of the aortic arch. It divides into the **right subclavian artery** which is distributed to the right superior limb and the **right common carotid artery** which is the main vessel to the right side of the head. The other two branches of the aortic arch are the **left common carotid artery** and the **left subclavian artery**. They are symmetrical to their right counterparts except for having individual origins (*vs.* a truncal origin) from the aortic arch. Each common carotid artery courses superiorly toward the head and divides into two large branches near the level of the mandible: external carotid artery and internal carotid artery (Figure 15-19).

The **external carotid artery** supplies vessels to the thyroid gland, pharynx, face, occipital and posterior auricular regions and then terminates by dividing into the **maxillary** and **superficial temporal arteries**. Each **internal carotid artery** supplies several branches to the deep structures of the head and then passes through the carotid canal of the temporal bone to terminate as the major input to the **cerebral arterial circle**. The latter is a vascular ring around the infundibulum of the pituitary gland on the inferior aspect of the brain. It gives origin to several named vessels that supply the brain.

The left and right subclavian arteries course laterally just underneath the clavicles. They supply four branches to the shoulder region before they leave the thoracic cavity by passing through the thoracic inlet (Figure 15-21):

1. **Vertebral artery**—courses superiorly through the ipsilateral transverse foramina of the cervical vertebrae. It supplies tiny branches to cervical structures and then enters the skull through the

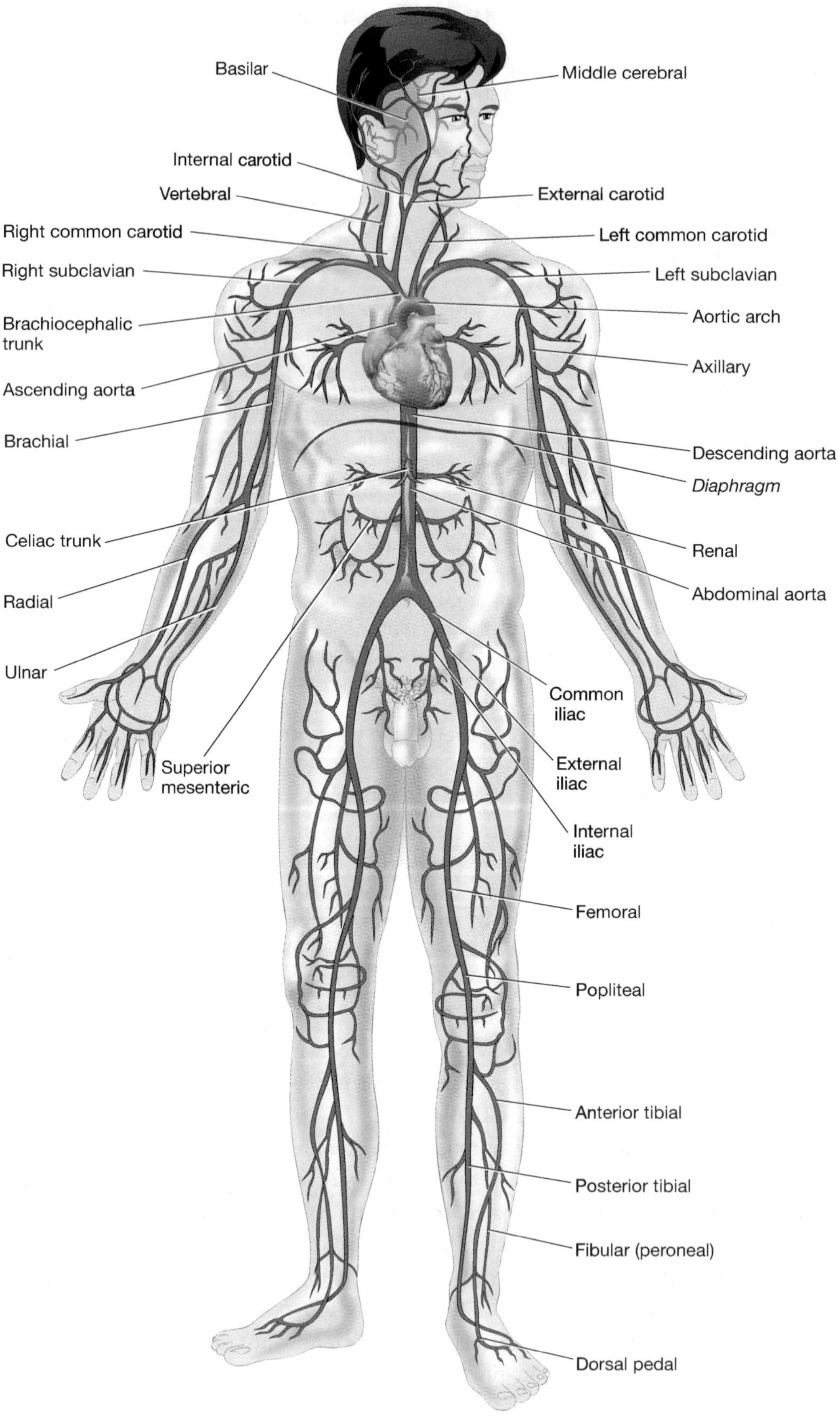

Figure 15-17
Major Systemic Arteries

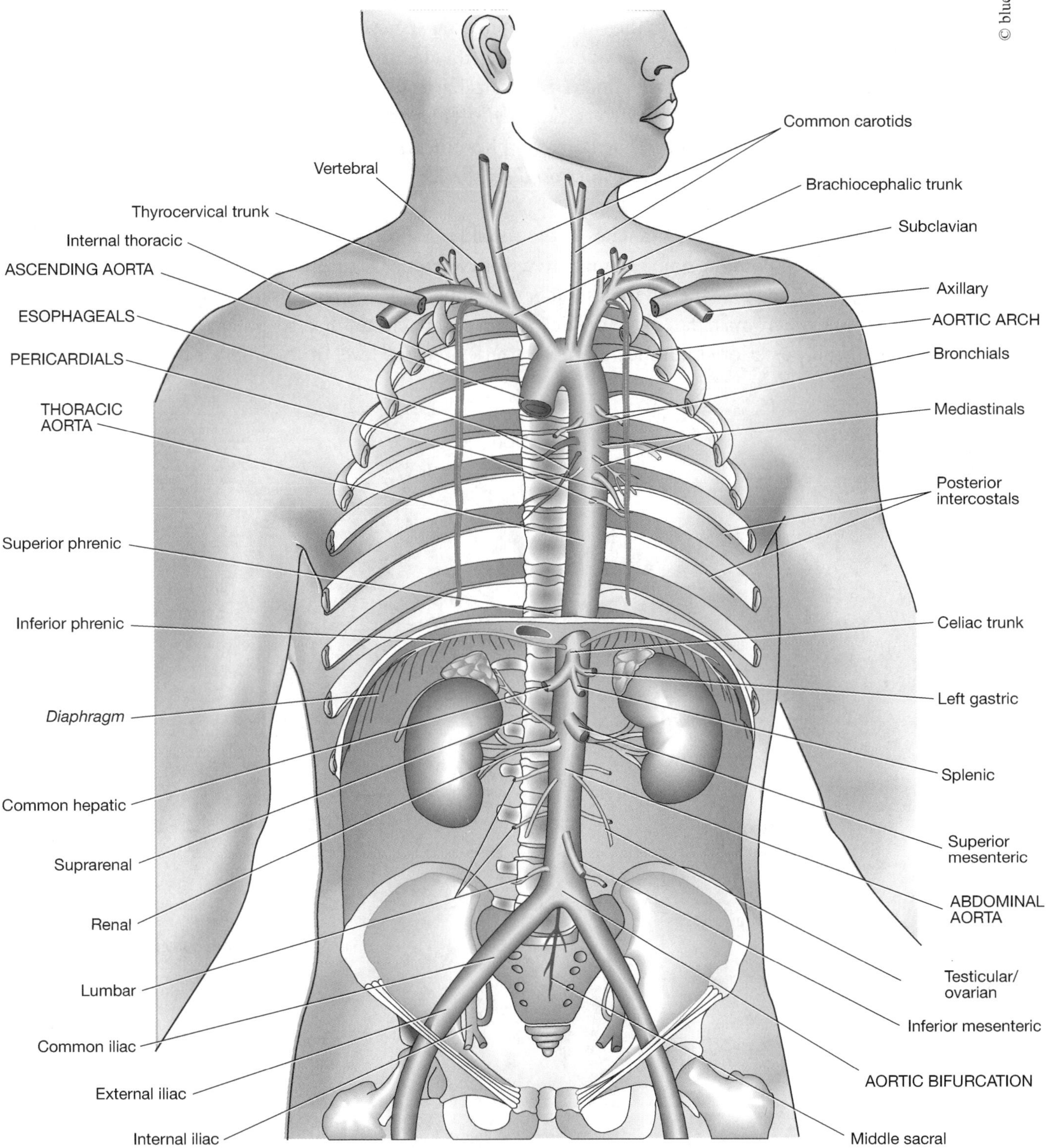

Figure 15-18
Branches of the Aorta

foramen magnum. The left and right vertebral arteries then unite to form the single **basilar artery** which is the major posterior input to the cerebral arterial circle (*see internal carotid artery*).

2. **Internal thoracic artery**—courses inferiorly along the posterior side of the anterior thoracic wall and supplies vessels to the ribs and intercostal structures.
3. **Thyrocervical trunk**—a short vessel which divides to form the inferior thyroid artery, the suprascapular artery and the transverse cervical artery.
4. **Costocervical trunk**—a short vessel which divides to form the deep cervical artery and the supreme intercostal artery. The latter supplies the posterior intercostal arteries in the first two intercostal spaces (*see posterior intercostal arteries*).

After supplying the four branches of the shoulder region, the subclavian artery courses over the first rib at which point its name changes to **axillary artery** (Figure 15-21). The axillary artery supplies several named branches to the shoulder and upper brachial regions including the superior thoracic, thoraco-acromial, lateral thoracic, subscapular, circumflex scapular, anterior circumflex humeral, and posterior circumflex humeral arteries. At the level of the inferior border of the teres

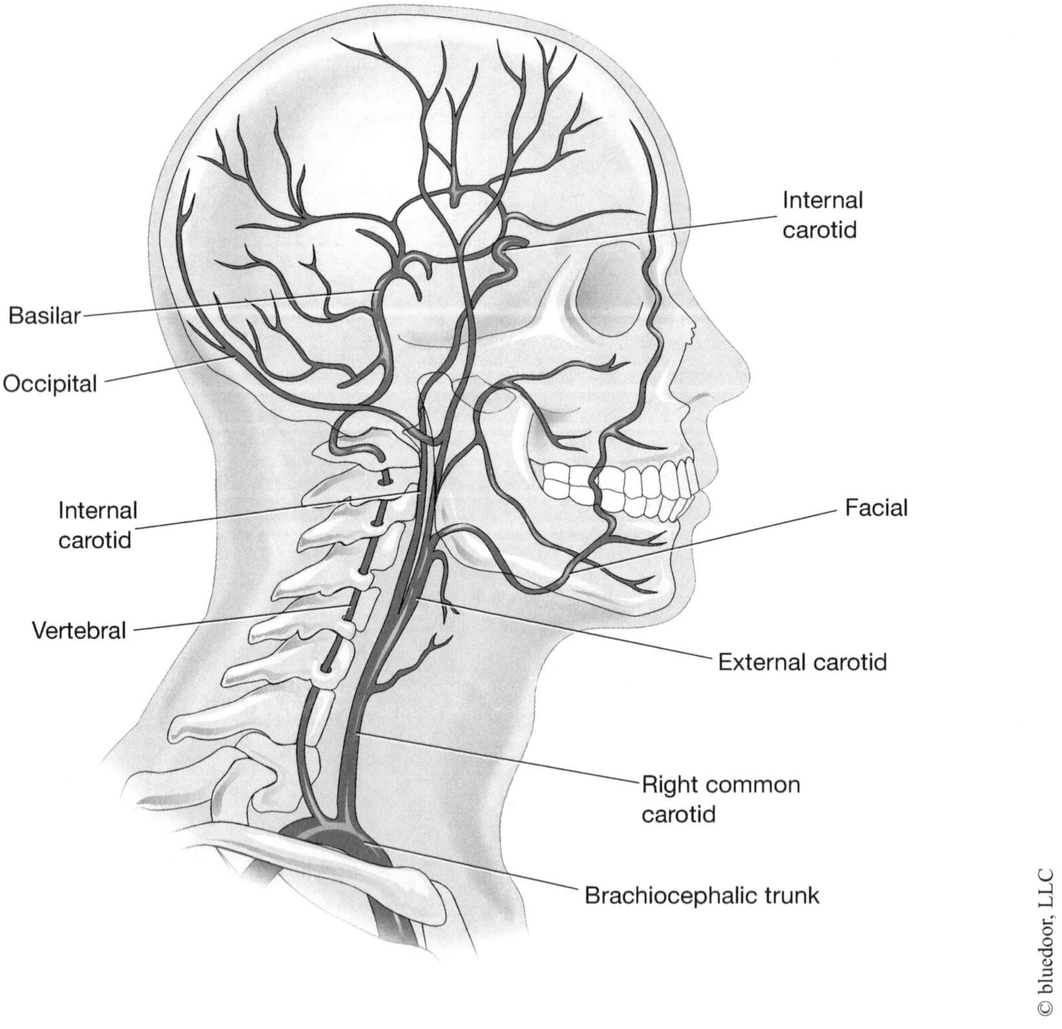

Figure 15-19
Arteries of the Head and Neck

major muscle, the axillary artery becomes the **brachial artery**. This vessel courses down the medial aspect of the superior limb and supplies several branches including the deep brachial, superior collateral ulnar, and inferior collateral ulnar arteries. The brachial artery terminates below the elbow by dividing into a **radial artery** (laterally) and an **ulnar artery** (medially). These supply several named branches to structures in the antebrachium and manus.

The thoracic part of the descending aorta supplies the last nine pairs of **posterior intercostal arteries** and a pair of **subcostal arteries** which parallel the intercostal vessels but are located below the last pair of ribs. The thoracic aorta also supplies bronchial, esophageal, pericardial, and mediastinal branches. These are small, variable in size and number, and are distributed to the structures implied by their names. The bronchial branches supply the lungs with arterial blood. Most individuals have two on the left side and a single, larger one on the right. Just above the diaphragm, the thoracic aorta supplies the left and right **superior phrenic arteries** to the diaphragm.

The abdominal part of the descending aorta supplies six sets of paired vessels (inferior phrenic, lumbar, middle adrenal, renal, testicular/ovarian, and common iliac arteries) and has four unpaired branches (celiac trunk, superior and inferior mesenteric arteries, and median sacral artery) (Figure 15-22). The small left and right **inferior phrenic arteries** to the diaphragm are the first vessels supplied by the abdominal aorta. They supplement the superior phrenic arteries from the thoracic aorta. There are four or five pairs of **lumbar arteries** that supply the vertebrae, musculature, and some of the skin in the lumbar region. These are analogous to the posterior intercostal and subcostal arteries supplied by the thoracic aorta. The first unpaired branch of the abdominal aorta is the large **celiac trunk**. It divides near its origin to form the left gastric artery, common hepatic artery, and splenic artery. The **left gastric artery** supplies parts of the stomach and sends branches to the lower

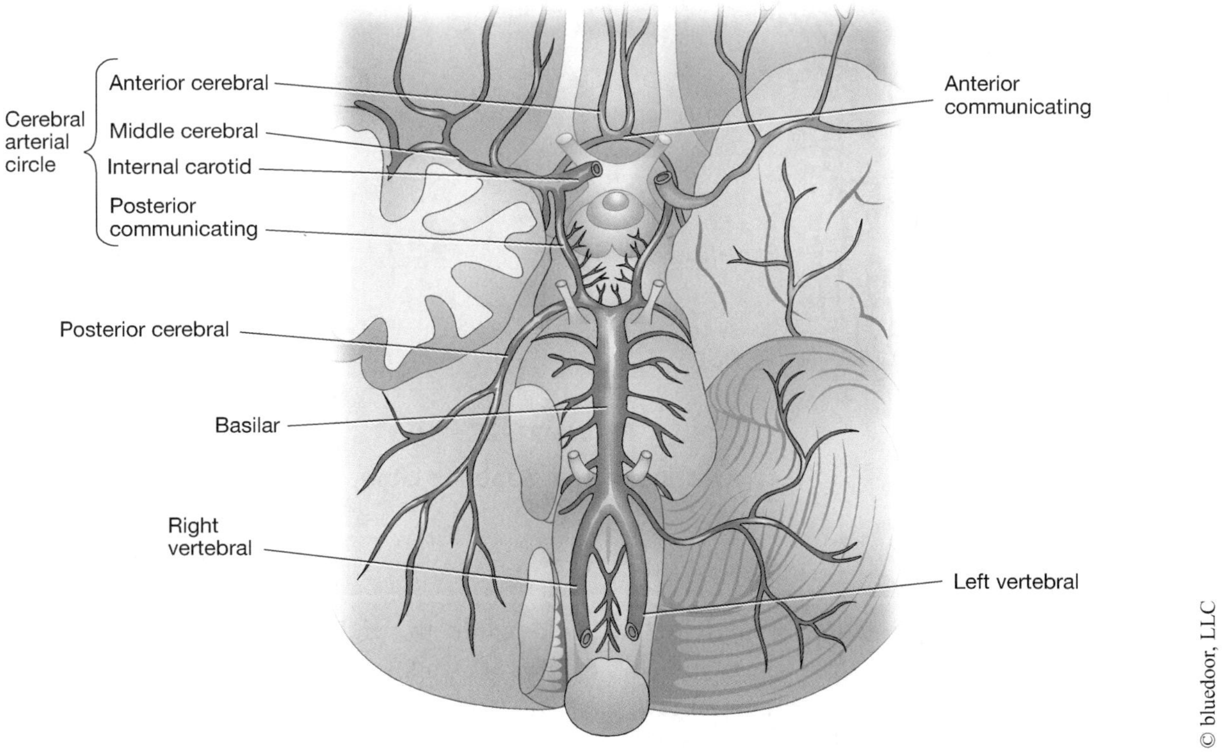

Figure 15-20
Arteries of Brain (Inferior Aspect)

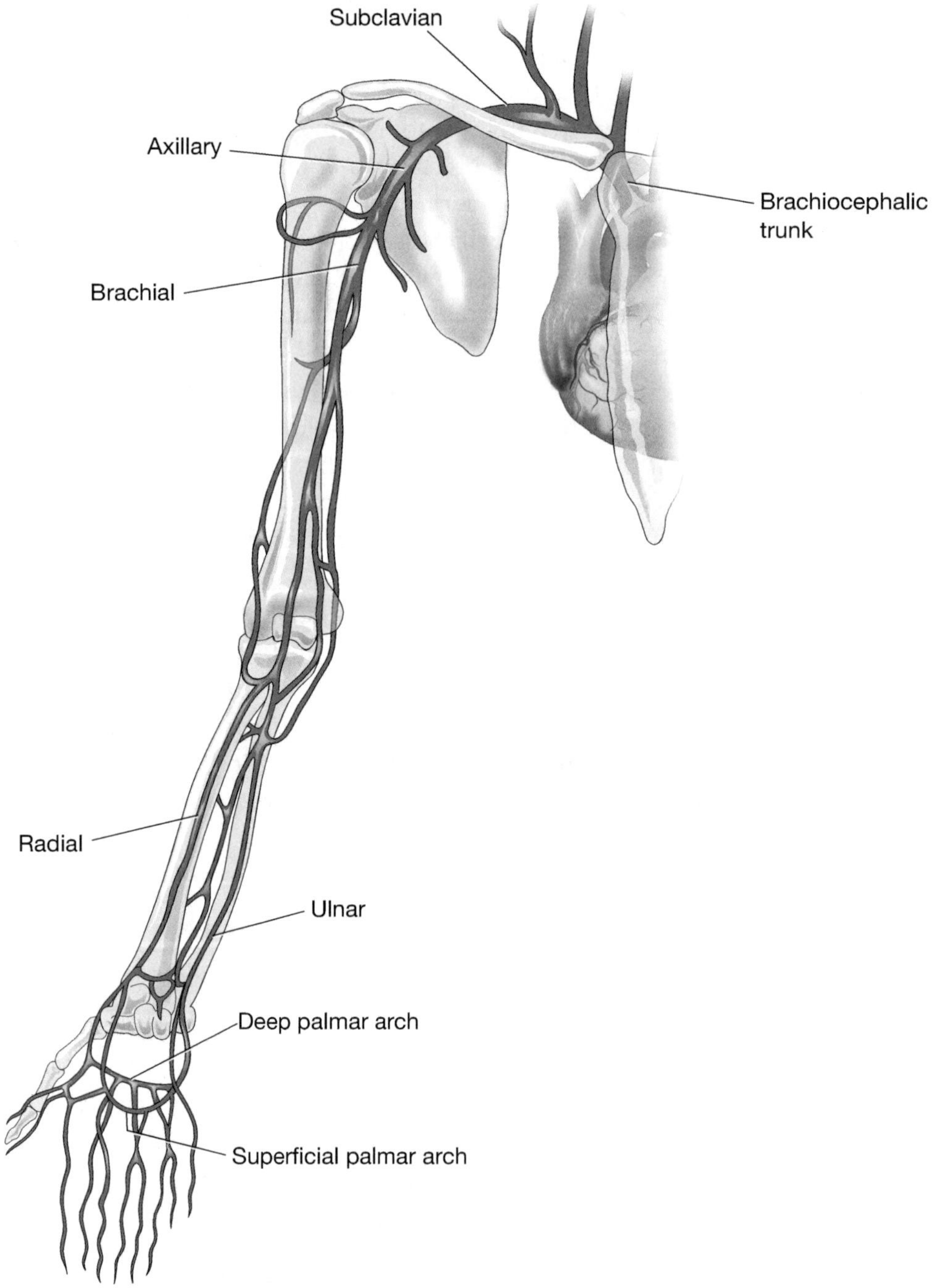

Figure 15-21
Arteries of the Superior Limb

esophagus. The **common hepatic artery** divides into the **right gastric artery** and the **proper hepatic artery**. The latter sends branches to the liver, gallbladder, stomach, duodenum, and pancreas. The **splenic artery** supplies branches to the spleen, pancreas, and stomach. After the celiac trunk arises, the abdominal aorta supplies the large, unpaired **superior mesenteric artery**. This vessel supplies branches to most of the small intestine (jejunal and ileal arteries) as well as to parts of the large intestine.

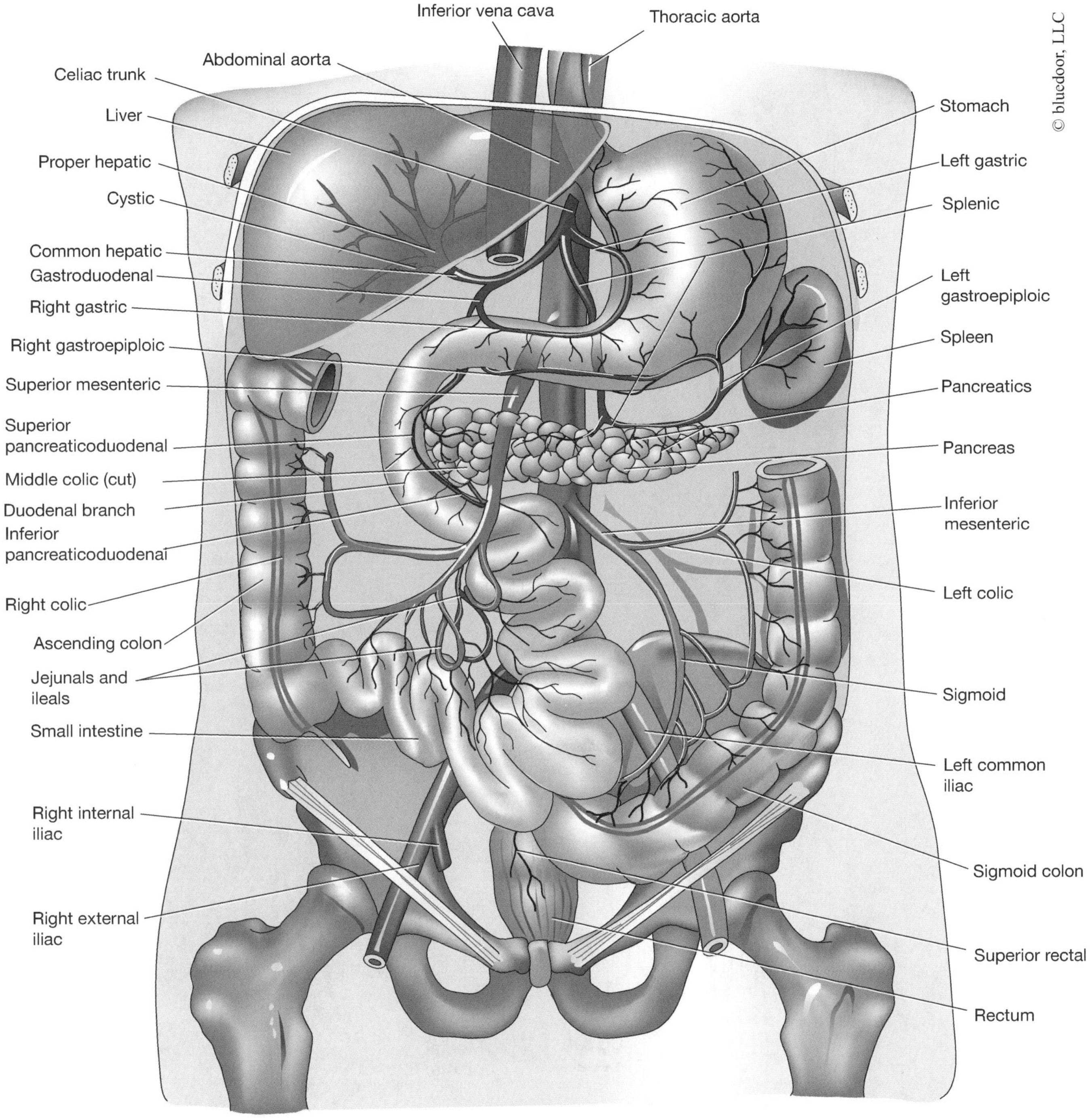

Figure 15-22
Arteries of the Abdomen

The left and right **middle adrenal arteries** arise from the aorta at about the same level as the superior mesenteric artery and are the largest vessels to the adrenal glands. They are supplemented by smaller superior adrenal arteries (branches of the inferior phrenic arteries) and the inferior adrenal arteries from the renal arteries. The large left and right **renal arteries** supply the kidneys. Each one receives approximately 10 percent of the cardiac output. The **testicular/ovarian arteries** supply the gonads. Their origin (from the area just below the kidneys) is related to the initial position of the

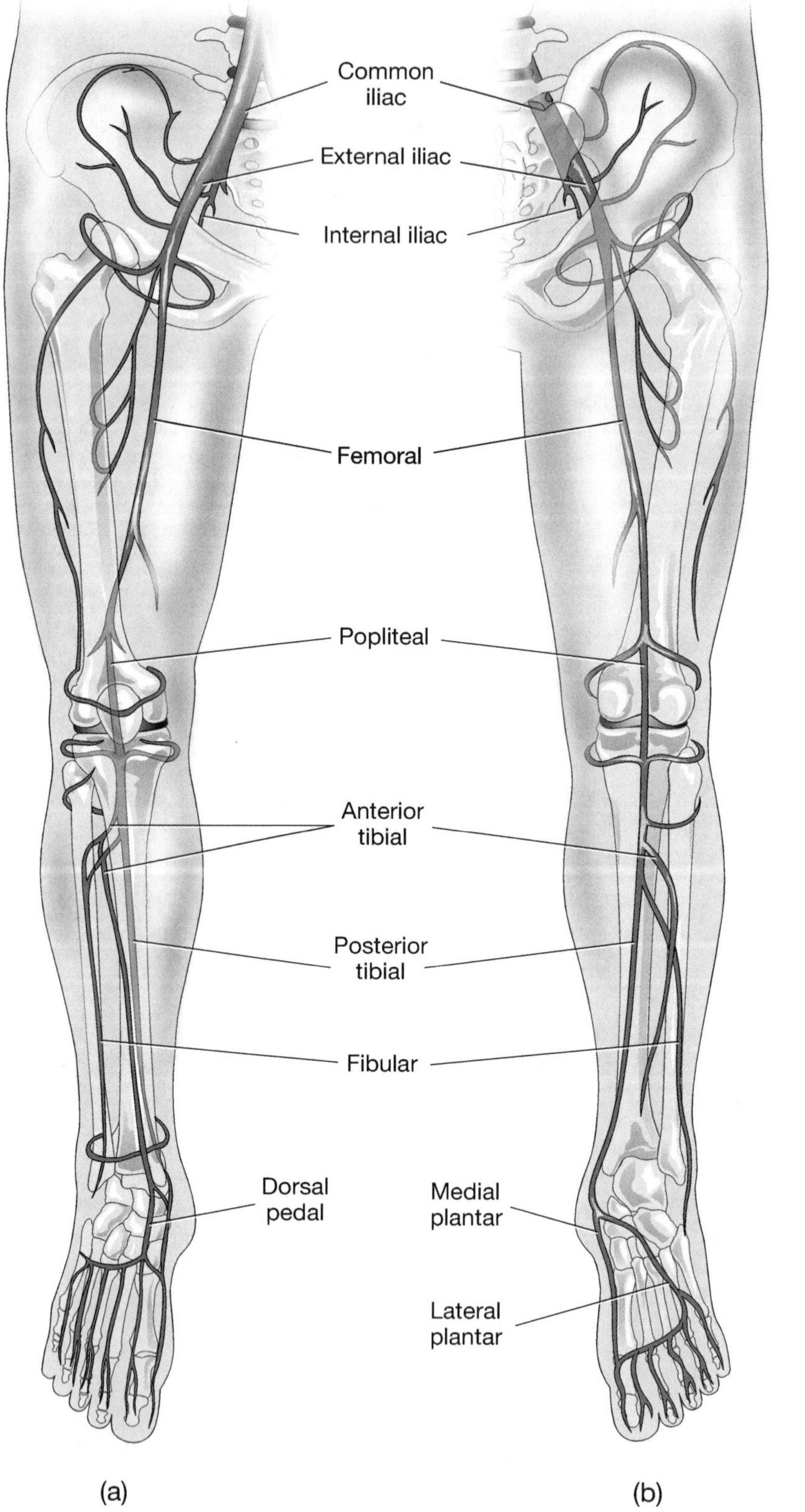

Figure 15-23
Arteries of the Inferior Limb (a) Anterior aspect (b) Posterior aspect

testes/ovaries during early development. The unpaired **inferior mesenteric artery** arises from the aorta below the testicular/ovarian arteries. It supplies several branches to the colon and rectum.

The last vessel to arise from the aorta before its termination is the small **median sacral artery** which is distributed to the sacral region. The aorta terminates by bifurcating into the left and right **common iliac arteries**. Each common iliac artery terminates after a course of several centimeters by dividing into an internal iliac artery which is distributed to the pelvic area and an external iliac artery to the inferior limb. The **internal iliac artery** supplies several named branches to musculoskeletal structures in the pelvic region as well as branches to the urinary bladder and reproductive viscera. The **external iliac artery** courses through the abdominal wall at the level of the inguinal ligament and, in passage, becomes the **femoral artery** (Figure 15-23). The femoral artery supplies five named branches (superficial epigastric, superficial circumflex iliac, deep femoral, external pudendal, and descending genicular arteries) and then becomes the **popliteal artery** when it enters the popliteal space on the posterior aspect of the knee. The popliteal artery is a short vessel that supplies several named branches to the genual region and then terminates by dividing into a larger **anterior tibial artery** and a smaller **posterior tibial artery**. These vessels supply several named branches in the crural region. As the anterior tibial artery crosses the talocrural joint, it becomes the **dorsal pedal artery** which is the largest arterial channel to the foot.

Objectives

17. Divide the aorta into its three major parts and list the branches that each one supplies.
18. Given the name of an artery, state its general distribution.

Major Systemic Veins

As mentioned earlier, most systemic veins follow arterial channels and are similarly named (Figure 15-24). However, the four largest (major) systemic veins do not parallel arterial channels: superior vena cava, inferior vena cava, azygos vein, and hepatic portal vein. The **superior vena cava** returns blood to the right atrium of the heart from the head, neck, thorax, and superior limbs. It is a short vessel which forms by the convergence of the left and right **brachiocephalic veins**.

Each brachiocephalic vein is a relatively short vessel formed by the convergence of the ipsilateral **internal jugular vein** carrying blood from the head, and the ipsilateral **subclavian vein** carrying blood from the superior limb. Much of the superficial venous drainage from the head is carried by the **external jugular vein** (Figure 15-25). It joins the subclavian vein before the latter converges with the internal jugular vein. Superficial venous channels in the superior limb which do not parallel arterial channels include the **cephalic vein** (on the lateral side of the limb), the **basilic vein** (on the medial side), and the **median cubital vein** (Figure 15-27). The latter is an anastomotic channel between the cephalic and basilic veins near the elbow. Superficial vessels on the back of the hand that drain into the cephalic and basilic veins are called **dorsal metacarpal veins**.

The **inferior vena cava** returns blood to the right atrium from the abdomen, pelvis, and inferior limbs. It forms within the abdominal cavity by the convergence of the left and right **common iliac veins**. Each of these is formed by the convergence of the ipsilateral **internal iliac vein** carrying blood from the pelvic region and the ipsilateral **external iliac vein** carrying blood from the inferior limb. Superficial veins in the inferior limbs that do not parallel arterial channels include the **dorsal metatarsal**

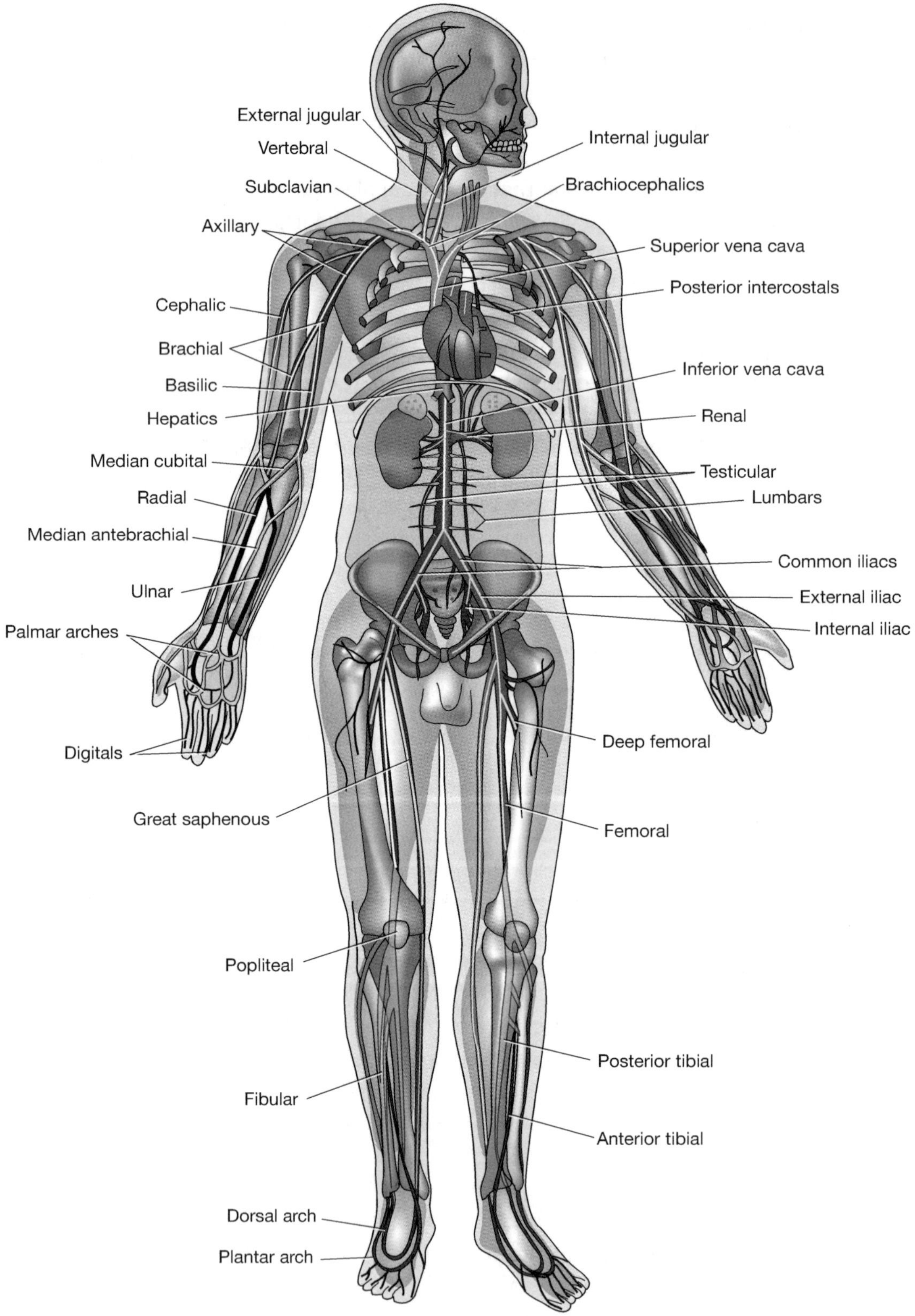

Figure 15-24

Major Systemic Veins

Most systemic veins parallel similarly named arterial channels. In females the veins labeled testicular in this diagram would be ovarian. Only the very largest veins are shown in this drawing.

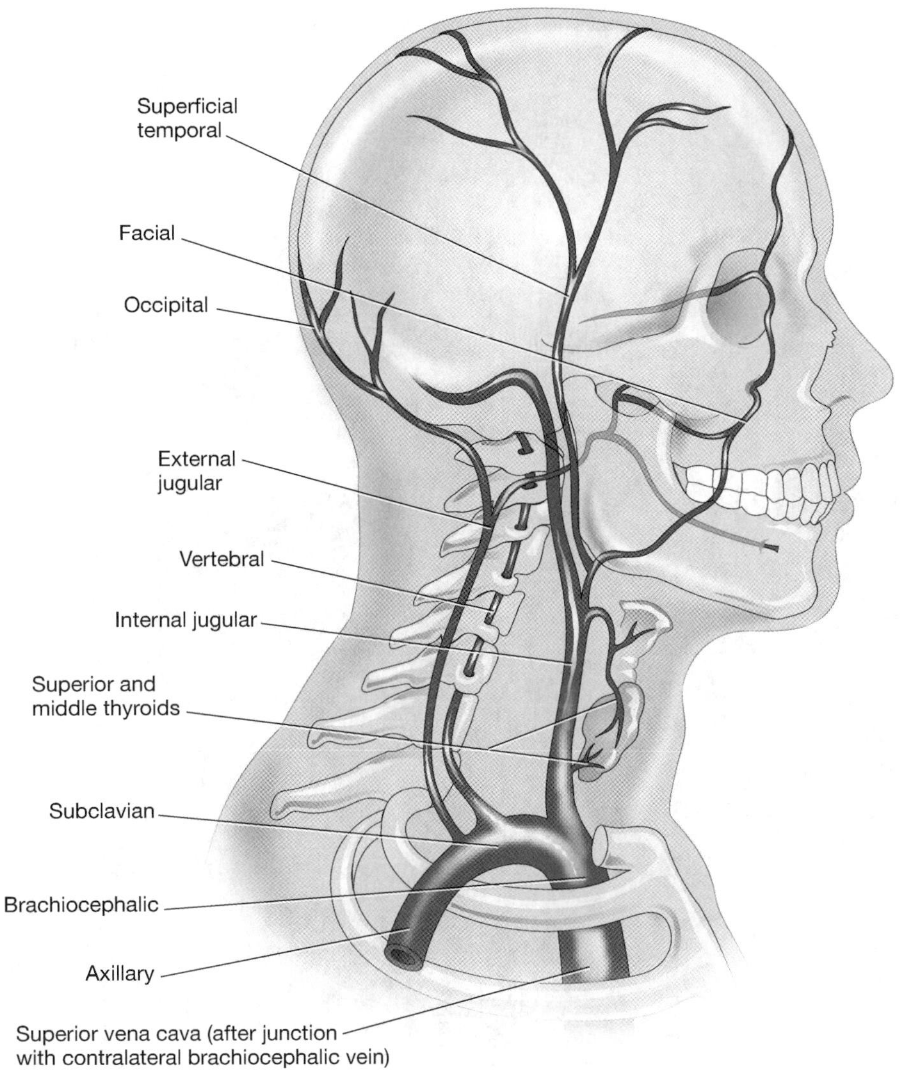

Figure 15-25
Veins of Head and Neck

veins on the superior aspect of the metatarsus (Figure 15-28). Some of these coalesce to form the **great saphenous vein** which ascends in front of the medial malleolus of the tibia. The great saphenous vein enters the femoral vein in the upper thigh. The **small saphenous vein** is a superficial vessel ascending in the posterior crural region. It enters the **popliteal vein** near the knee. As the inferior vena cava ascends along the posterior abdominal wall, it receives several tributaries including five pairs of **lumbar veins**, the left and right **renal veins**, three **hepatic veins**, and the left and right **inferior phrenic veins**. In addition to these, the **right testicular/ovarian vein** and the right adrenal vein usually join the inferior vena cava. Their contralateral counterparts usually drain into the left renal vein.

The **hepatic portal vein** is the large venous channel that receives most of the venous blood that has passed through capillary beds in the stomach, spleen, pancreas, and the small and large intestines (Figure 15-29). Nearly all of the blood which leaves the aorta through the celiac trunk, superior mesenteric, and inferior mesenteric arteries is involved in this pathway. It is called the **hepatic portal system** and its function is to allow the liver cells a chance to modify and detoxify materials

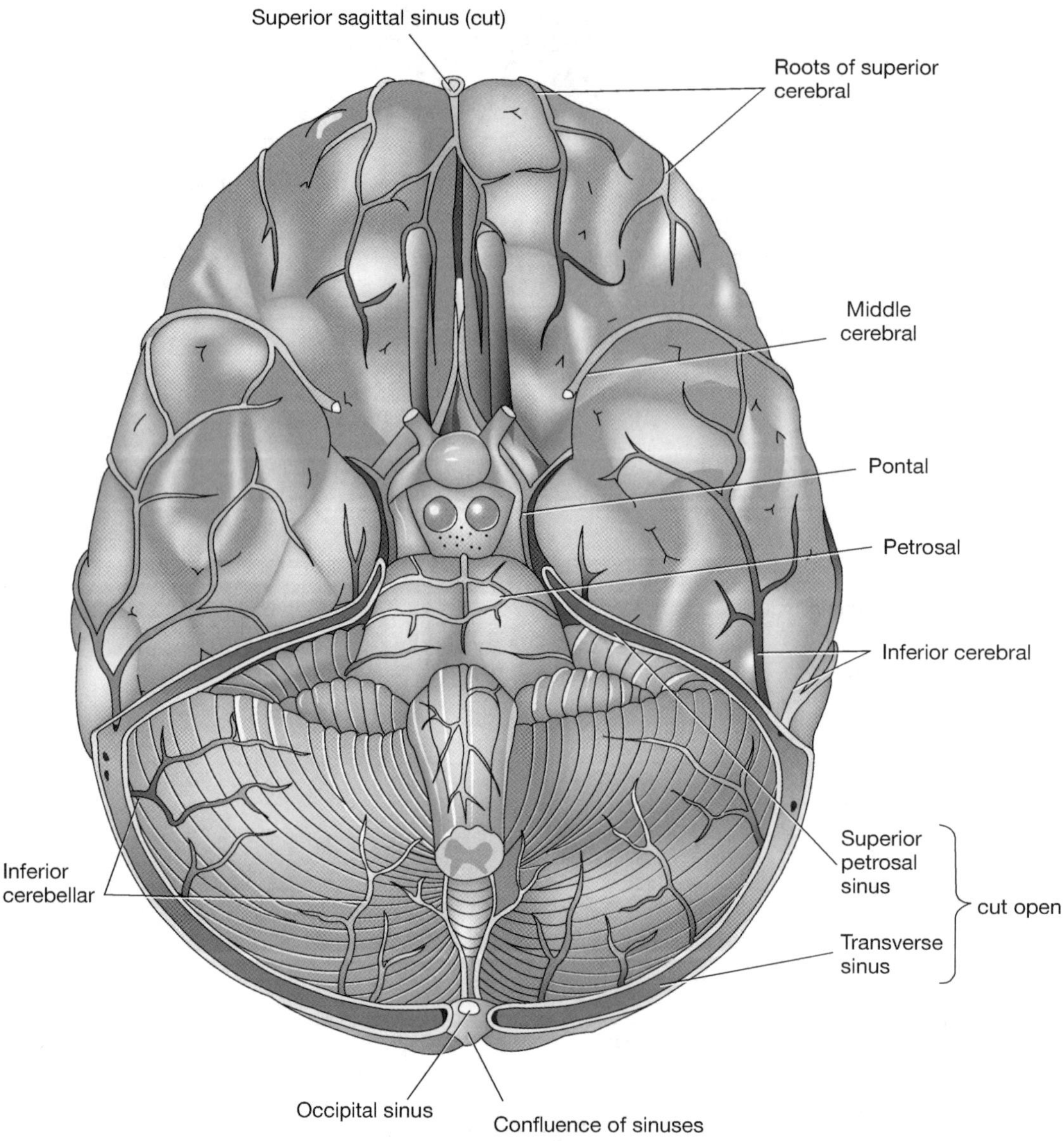

Figure 15-26
Veins of Brain

absorbed from the intestine before they circulate to the rest of the body. Two vessels unite to form the hepatic portal vein: **superior mesenteric vein** (draining primarily the small intestine) and the **splenic vein** (draining the spleen, stomach, pancreas, and large intestine). A number of other named vessels from abdominal digestive viscera drain into these two main tributaries of the portal vein. Within the liver, the hepatic portal vein divides to form many small branches that supply even smaller branches that drain into liver **sinusoids**. The latter are modified capillaries that allow close contact between blood and the liver cells (*see Chapter 17*). These sinusoids form the second set of capillaries that this blood passes through before returning to the heart. Blood in the sinusoids is joined by high oxygen (arterial) blood from branches of the proper hepatic artery. The latter supplies the oxygen needs of the liver cells. Venous blood leaves the liver through several **hepatic veins** (right, left, and middle) which join the inferior vena cava.

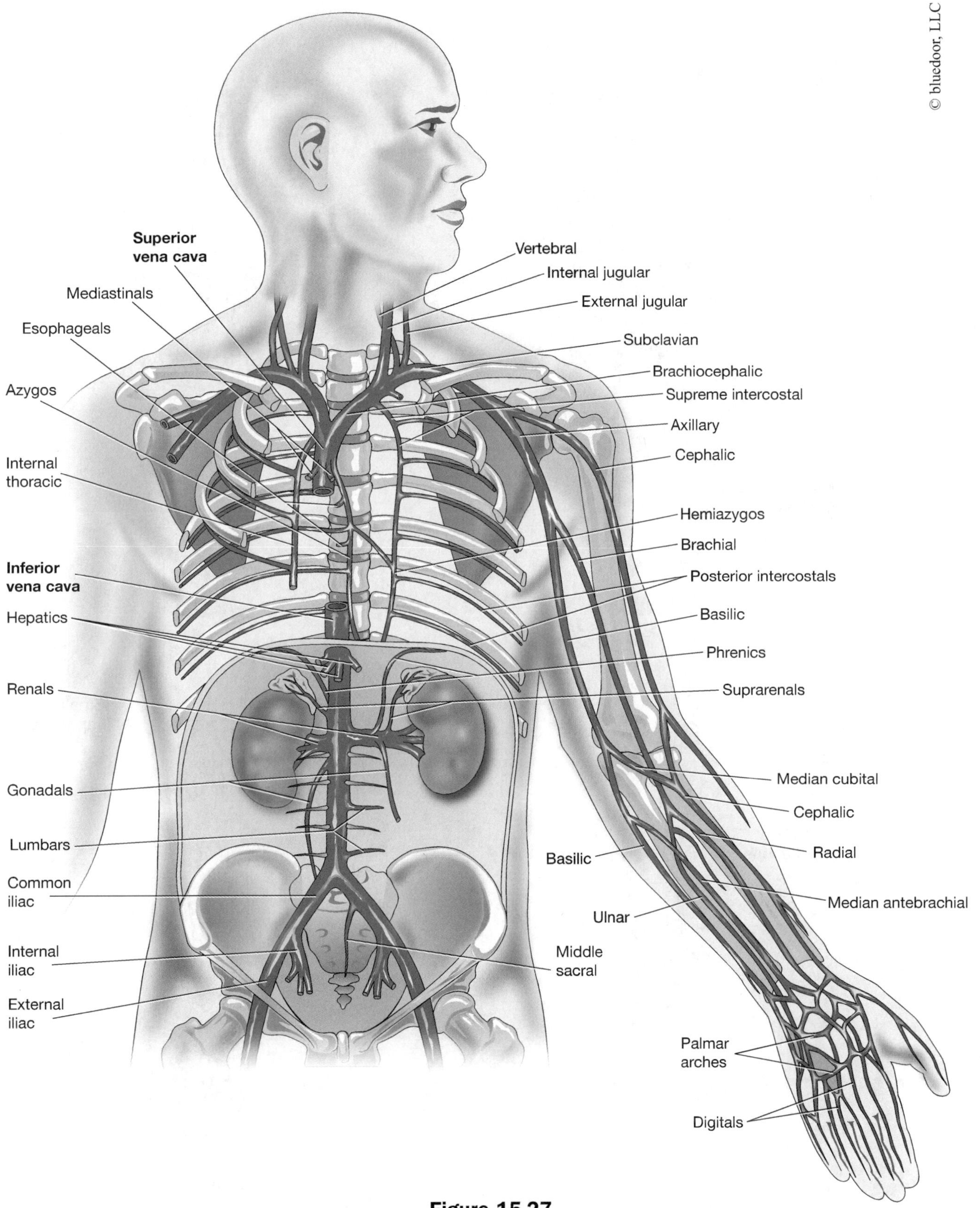

Figure 15-27

Veins of Superior Limb and Thorax

Note: "gonadal" vein (artery) is actually the testicular vein (artery) in males and the ovarian vein (artery) in females.

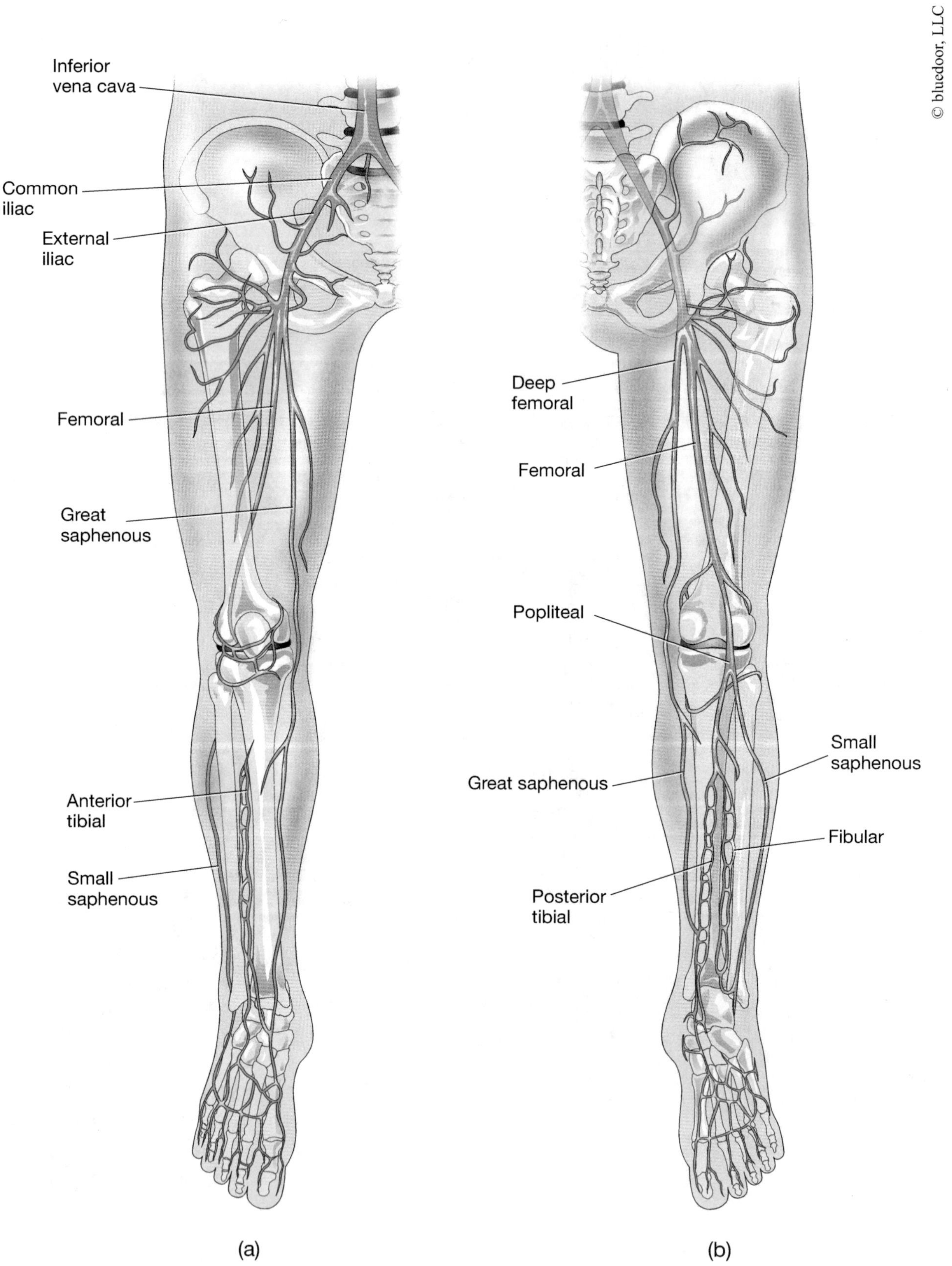

Figure 15-28

Veins of Inferior Limb (a) Anterior aspect (b) Posterior aspect

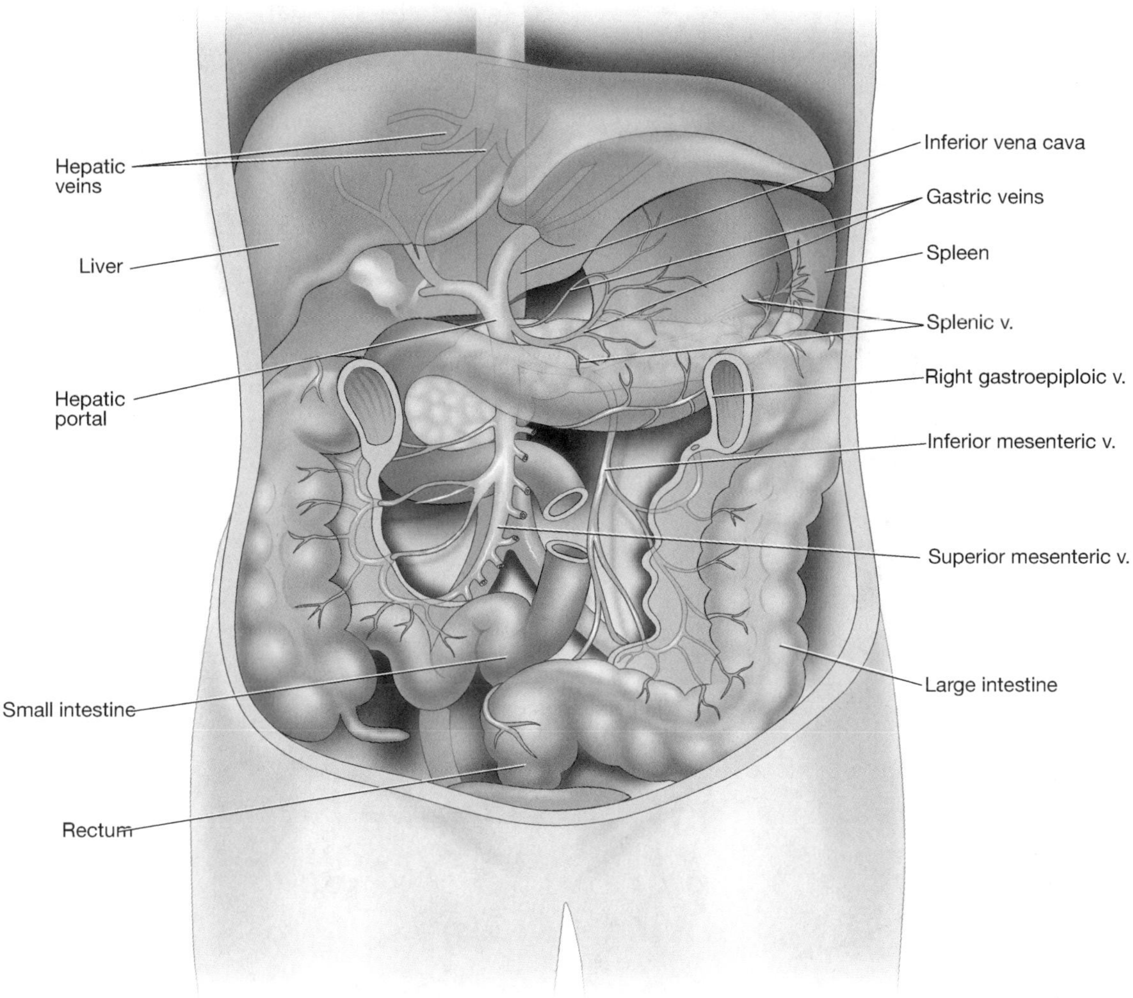

Figure 15-29
Hepatic Portal System

The arteries from whence this blood left the aorta are the celiac trunk, superior mesenteric artery, and inferior mesenteric artery.

The **azygos vein** is the major venous channel draining the thoracic wall (Figure 15-27). It empties into the superior vena cava just before the latter enters the right atrium. It courses along the posterior thoracic wall to the right of the median plane and receives blood from the right **posterior intercostal veins** as well as anastomotic channels from the **hemiazygos** and **accessory hemiazygos veins**. The latter are positioned parallel to the azygos vein but to the left of the median plane. The hemiazygos vein receives drainage from the last several left posterior intercostal veins (lower left thoracic wall) and the accessory hemiazygos vein drains the upper left posterior intercostal veins (upper left thoracic wall).

Objectives

19. Name the four major systemic veins, what coalesces to form each one, what parts of the body each drains, and where (into what) each one empties.

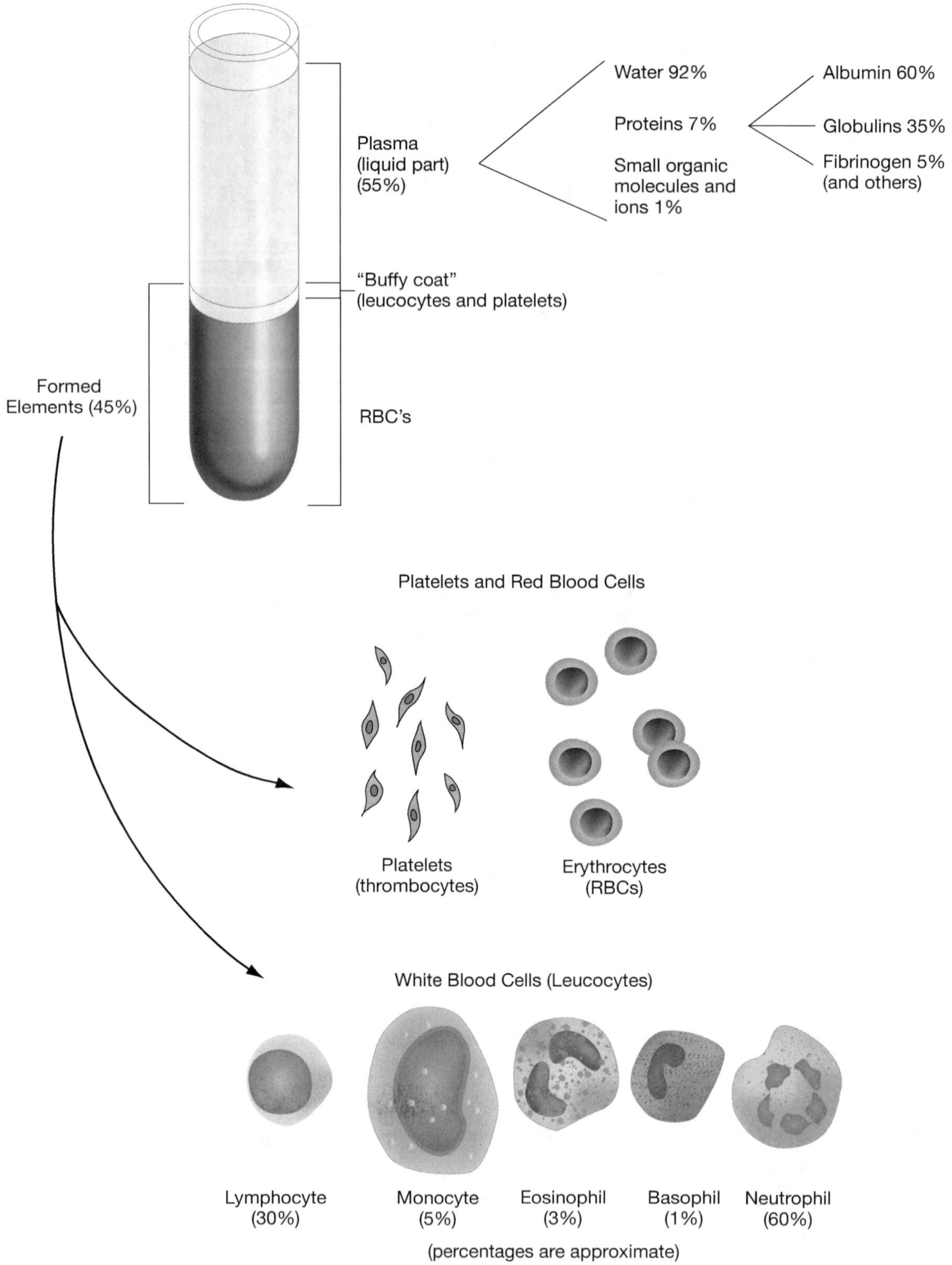

Figure 15-30

Composition of Blood

The formed elements of blood include erythrocytes (RBCs), leucocytes (WBCs) and platelets (thrombocytes). Plasma is about 92% water and most of the rest is proteins (albumin, globulins and fibrinogen).

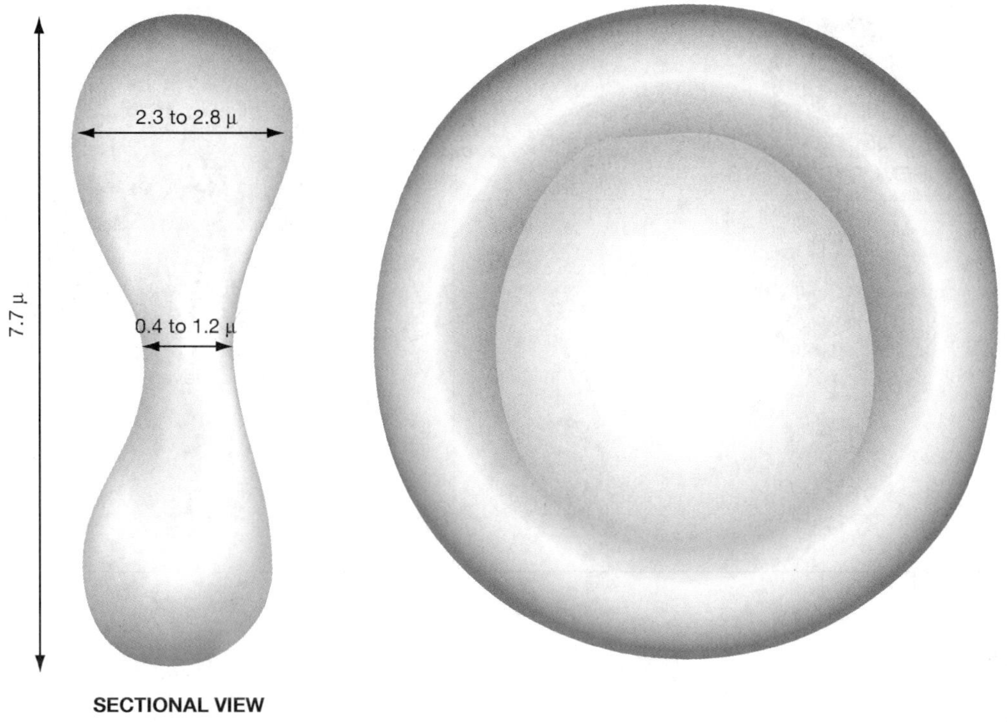

Figure 15-31

Erythrocytes (Red Blood Corpuscles)

By developmentally losing many organelles (including their nuclei), RBC's make more room for hemoglobin, the oxygen binding pigment. Their biconcave disc shape maximizes surface area to increase efficiency of oxygen absorption. There are about 5 million RBC's in each cubic millimeter of blood. That's 5 billion in each cc and five trillion in a liter. The average person has about 5 liters of blood—25 trillion RBC's. Each RBC contains over 250 million molecules of hemoglobin. Each hemoglobin can bind (carry) four molecules of oxygen.

Blood

Blood is the fluid connective tissue that circulates through the heart and vessels. An average-sized adult has a blood volume of about 5 liters which is, by coincidence, the approximate total volume of the average resting cardiac output each minute. Blood is about 55% **plasma** (fluid) and about 45% **formed elements** (Figure 15-30). Plasma is mostly water, is about 8% protein, and contains small amounts of electrolytes, carbohydrates, and lipids. Plasma proteins include **albumins** (which impart most of its osmotic pressure), globulins, and fibrinogen. **Globulins** are primarily immunoproteins and are subdivided into several groups. **Fibrinogen** is the soluble form of the clotting protein. It is converted to insoluble fibrin when the clotting mechanism is activated. **Blood serum** is the clear liquid that separates from blood as it clots (*i.e.*, blood plasma from which fibrinogen has been removed by the process of clotting).

The formed elements of blood include erythrocytes (red blood corpuscles or RBC's), leucocytes (white blood cells or WBC's), and thrombocytes (platelets). **Erythrocytes** are the most numerous and about 5 million are present in each cubic millimeter of blood (5 billion/milliliter) (Figure 15-30, 31).

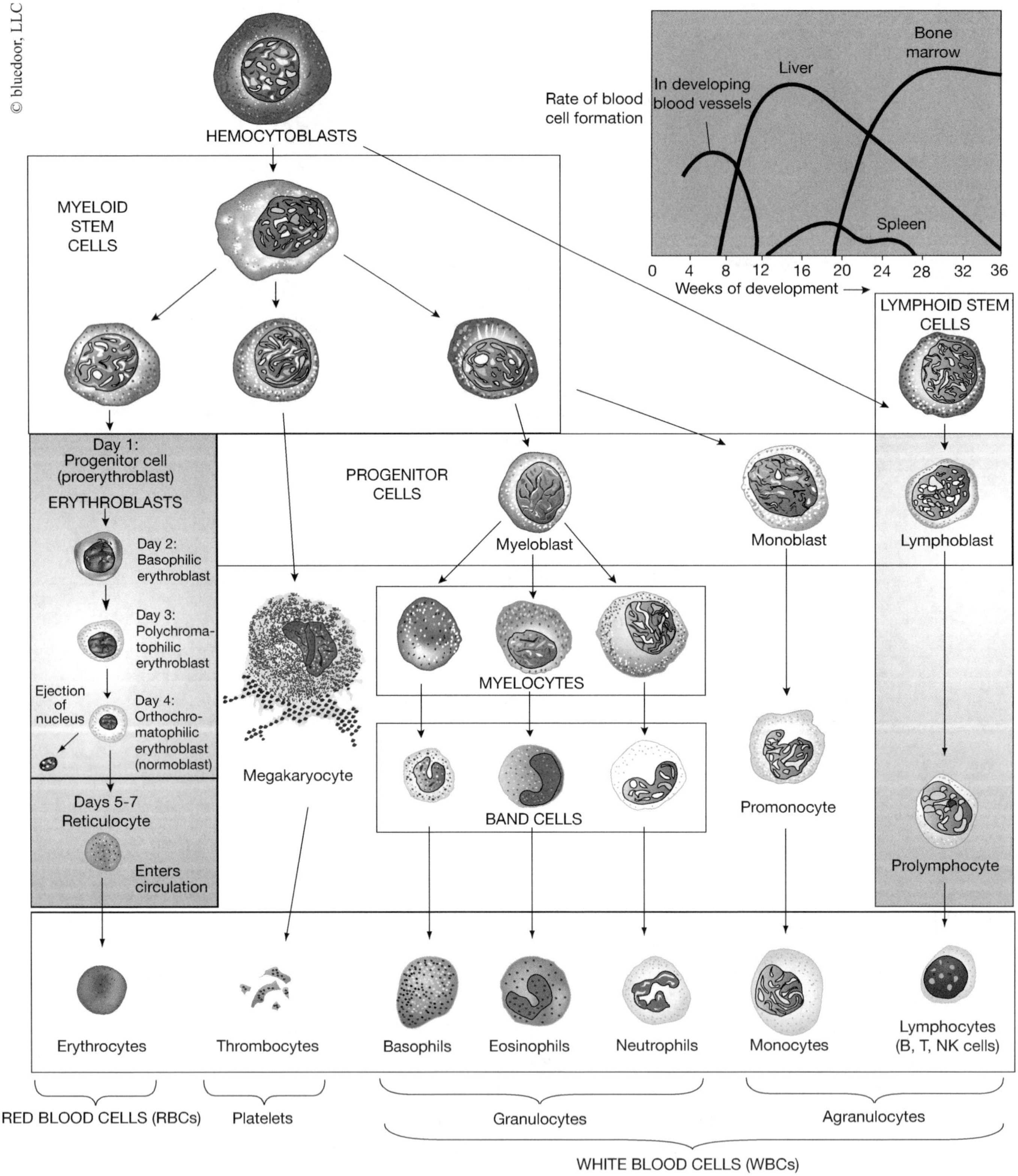

Figure 15-32

Origin and Differentiation of the Formed Elements of Blood

All formed elements of blood originate from a common stem cell, the hemocytoblast. Daughter cells of these precursors differentiate into erythroblasts, myeloblasts, monoblasts and lymphoblasts. Note that all granulocytes are derived from myeloblasts.

They are flattened, biconcave discs which are so specialized for oxygen transportation that they have lost their nuclei and mitochondria. The lack of a nucleus is the reason that they are often termed red blood *corpuscles vs.* red blood *cells.* Each one contains about 280 million molecules of **hemoglobin** which is the iron containing protein that transports oxygen. Each hemoglobin molecule can bind four molecules of oxygen (O_2). The O_2/hemoglobin (oxyhemoglobin complex) bond is passive, is concentration dependent, and is weakened by lower pH and higher temperature. In the lungs, the hemoglobin picks up oxygen (because the O_2 concentration is relatively high) and in the other areas of the body, O_2 is released and diffuses into a lower O_2 concentration area. Erythrocytes have a half-life of about 3 months after which they "wear out" and are phagocytized by cells in the liver, spleen, and bone marrow.

About 7000 leucocytes are present in each cubic millimeter of blood. **Leucocytes** are divided into two groups distinguished by the presence/absence of cytoplasmic granules. Those with granules are called **granulocytes** and include neutrophils, eosinophils, and basophils. **Neutrophils** are the most common white blood cells and account for about 60% of the total (4200/mm^3). Their name is derived from the fact that their cytoplasmic granules remain relatively colorless when stained with routine histologic stains. They are aggressive, phagocytic cells that attack invading microbes. **Eosinophils** are so named because their cytoplasmic granules stain red with eosin (one of the routine histological stains). They serve in certain detoxification schemes and secrete enzymes that dissolve blood clots. **Basophils** are the least numerous of all white blood cells (less than 1%). Their granules are blue with routine blood stains, and they contain heparin (an anticoagulant), histamine (a vasodilator), and serotonin (a vasoconstrictor).

The two types of **agranulocytes** (leucocytes which lack cytoplasmic granulations) are monocytes and lymphocytes. **Monocytes** are phagocytic and are the largest white blood cells. They pass through vessel walls and become **macrophages** (phagocytic cells within the body tissues). **Lymphocytes** play important roles in immune responses including the production of antibodies.

Thrombocytes (platelets) have several roles in the clotting mechanism. They are fragments of large bone marrow cells called **megakaryocytes**. They contain a chemical (serotonin) which serves as a vasoconstrictor, and they also activate the clotting mechanism which converts fibrinogen to fibrin. Blood cells are produced by a process called **hemopoiesis** (Figure 15-32). This includes **erythropoiesis**, which occurs in bone marrow, and **leucopoiesis** which also occurs primarily in the bone marrow (granulocytes and platelets) as well as in lymphatic tissue (some agranulocytes).

Objectives

20. Differentiate blood, plasma, and serum.
21. Name the formed elements of blood and state the function(s) of each one.
22. List the components of plasma.

Fetal Circulation

There are two major peculiarities of fetal biology which dictate anatomical differences in the fetal circulatory pattern compared to that of an adult: shrunken lungs (which preclude the passage of significant volumes of blood through the pulmonary circulation) and nutrient/waste exchange at the

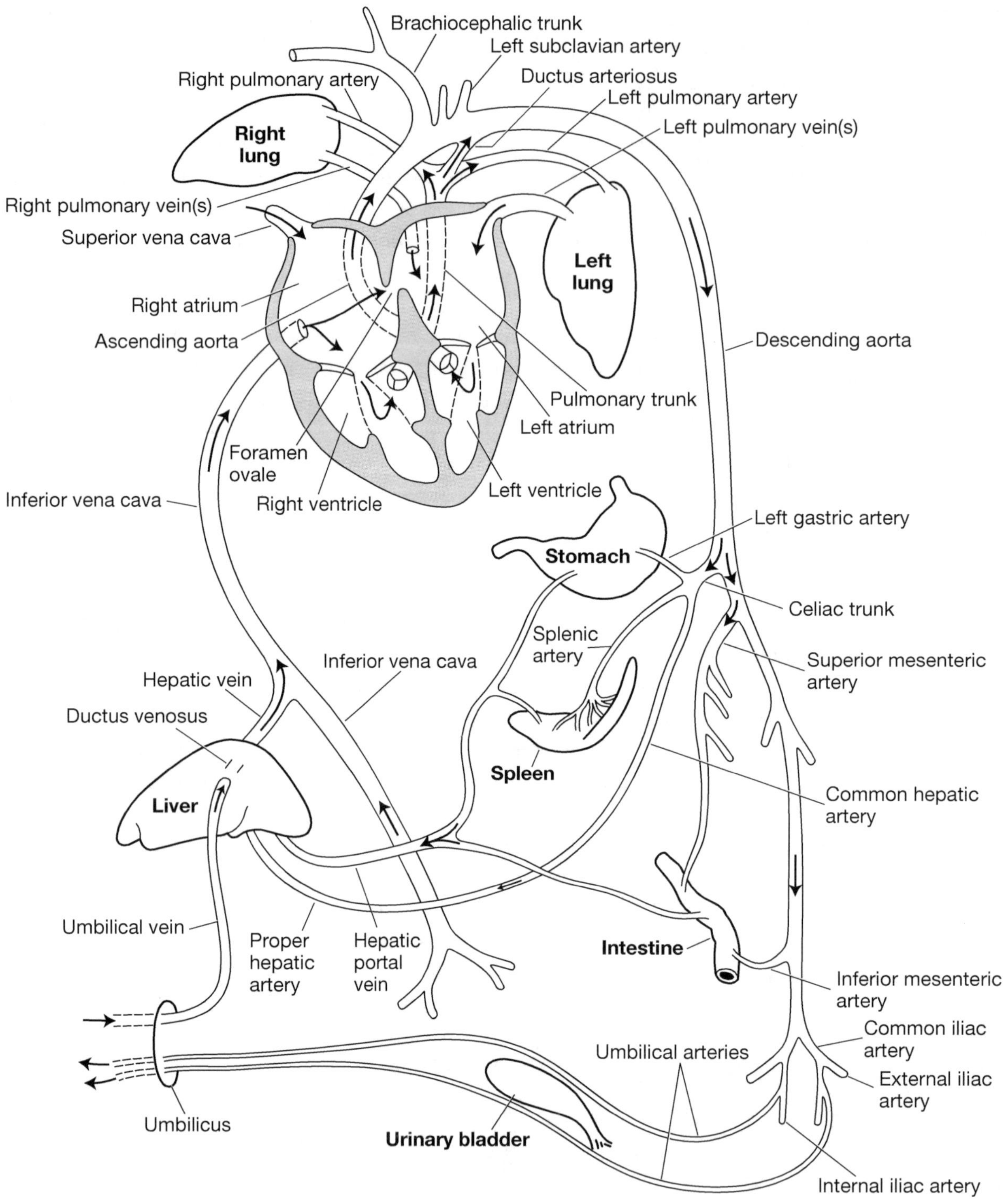

Figure 15-33

Circulatory Scheme in the Fetus

The fetal circulatory system includes two lung "bypasses" and umbilical vessels that transport blood to/from the placenta. The bypasses include the foramen ovale (an interatrial septal defect) and the ductus arteriosus (a vascular channel connecting the pulmonary trunk to the aorta). The umbilical vessels which carry blood to the placenta are the left and right umbilical arteries, which are the branches of the internal iliac arteries. The single umbilical vein returns highly oxygenated blood from the placenta to the fetus. The oxygen content of this blood is reduced in the liver, inferior vena cava and right atrium by mixing with blood of lesser oxygen content.

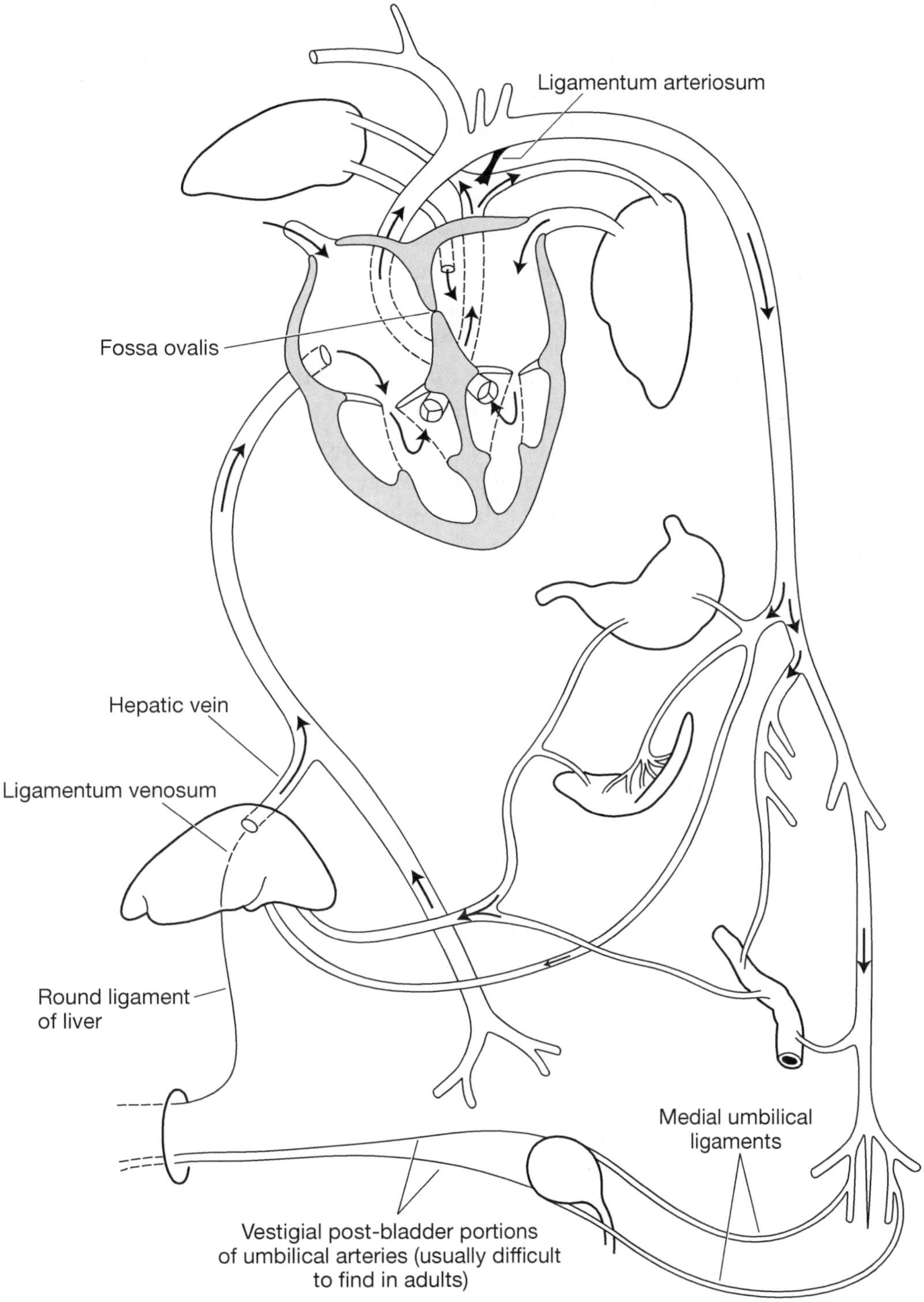

Figure 15-34

Circulatory Scheme in the Neonate and Adult

The foramen ovale closes to form the fossa ovalis as a result of greater left intra-atrial pressure due to more blood flowing to and returning from the expanded lungs. All other changes result from contraction of smooth muscle tissue in vessel walls related to increased oxygen tension (levels). (Structures are not drawn to scale, only those structures which undergo changes at birth are labeled; compare to Figure 15-33.)

placenta (which is physically distinct and remote from the fetus). Several fetal-specific anatomic structures are present because of these biological peculiarities including umbilical arteries, an umbilical vein, foramen ovale, and ductus arteriosus. The umbilical vessels carry blood to and from the placenta, and the foramen ovale and ductus arteriosus allow blood to bypass the pulmonary circulation (Figure 15-33). The left and right **umbilical arteries** are the pair of vessels which transport fetal blood to the placenta. They originate from the left and right internal iliac arteries, course to the umbilicus, and then travel to the placenta as part of the umbilical cord. After birth, the portions of the umbilical arteries within the abdomen regress to become fibrous cords termed **medial umbilical ligaments** which lie along the sides of the urinary bladder.

The **umbilical vein** is an unpaired vessel which returns oxygenated and nutrient laden blood from the placenta to the fetus. It courses from the umbilical cord through the umbilicus to the liver. Its continuation through the liver is called the **ductus venosus**. After birth, the portion of the umbilical vein between the umbilicus and liver fibroses to become the **round ligament of the liver**. The portion of the umbilical vein within the liver (ductus venosus) becomes the **ligamentum venosum**.

The **foramen ovale** is an interatrial septal passageway which allows some blood to bypass the lungs by flowing directly from the right atrium into the left atrium. After birth it normally closes by proliferation of fibrous connective tissues to form the **fossa ovalis**. In some cases the foramen ovale may remain sufficiently patent (open) to cause a circulatory disturbance. However, the pressures in the left and right atria are not significantly different postnatally, and so blood does not typically flow through a patent foramen ovale.

The **ductus arteriosus** is a vascular connection between the pulmonary trunk (usually at the base of the left pulmonary artery) and the aortic arch. It allows most of the blood in the pulmonary trunk to bypass the lungs by shunting it directly into the aorta. After birth, the ductus arteriosus fibroses to become a fibrous cord termed the **ligamentum arteriosum**. Occasionally it fails to regress and remains present as a **patent ductus arteriosus** (**PDA**). This condition causes a characteristic heart murmur which occurs continuously (throughout the cardiac cycle) and is commonly called a *machinery murmur*. PDA often requires surgical correction by ligation because of the circulatory disturbances that it causes.

The circulation of blood in the fetus is the same as that in the adult except for its flow to/from the placenta and the fact that most of it bypasses the non-functional fetal lungs. The maternal and fetal cardiovascular systems are completely separate, but their capillary beds are in close proximity within the placenta. Oxygen and other nutrients diffuse through the maternal capillaries of the placenta and are picked up by the red blood corpuscles flowing through the fetal placental capillaries. This highly oxygenated blood returns to the fetus through the umbilical vein and is shunted through the liver in the ductus venosus. As it leaves the liver through the hepatic veins, it is joined (and *diluted*) by the blood draining from the liver tissue. It then enters the inferior vena cava where it is further diluted by blood of low oxygen tension returning from the inferior limbs and lower abdomen. In the right atrium, the oxygen content of the blood is reduced once again by venous blood returning to the heart from the head, thorax, and superior limbs via the superior vena cava. Some of the blood in the right atrium flows directly into the left atrium through the foramen ovale (thereby bypassing the lungs) and the rest flows into the right ventricle (as it does in the neonatal/adult cardiovascular system). From the right ventricle, this latter blood enters the pulmonary trunk en route to the lungs. However, a large percentage of it bypasses the lungs by flowing directly into the aortic arch through the ductus arteriosus. The total volume continuing to the lungs is quite small. This latter blood returns from the lungs to the left atrium where it is joined by the blood entering through the foramen ovale. Left atrial blood is pumped into the left ventricle and then into the aorta in the

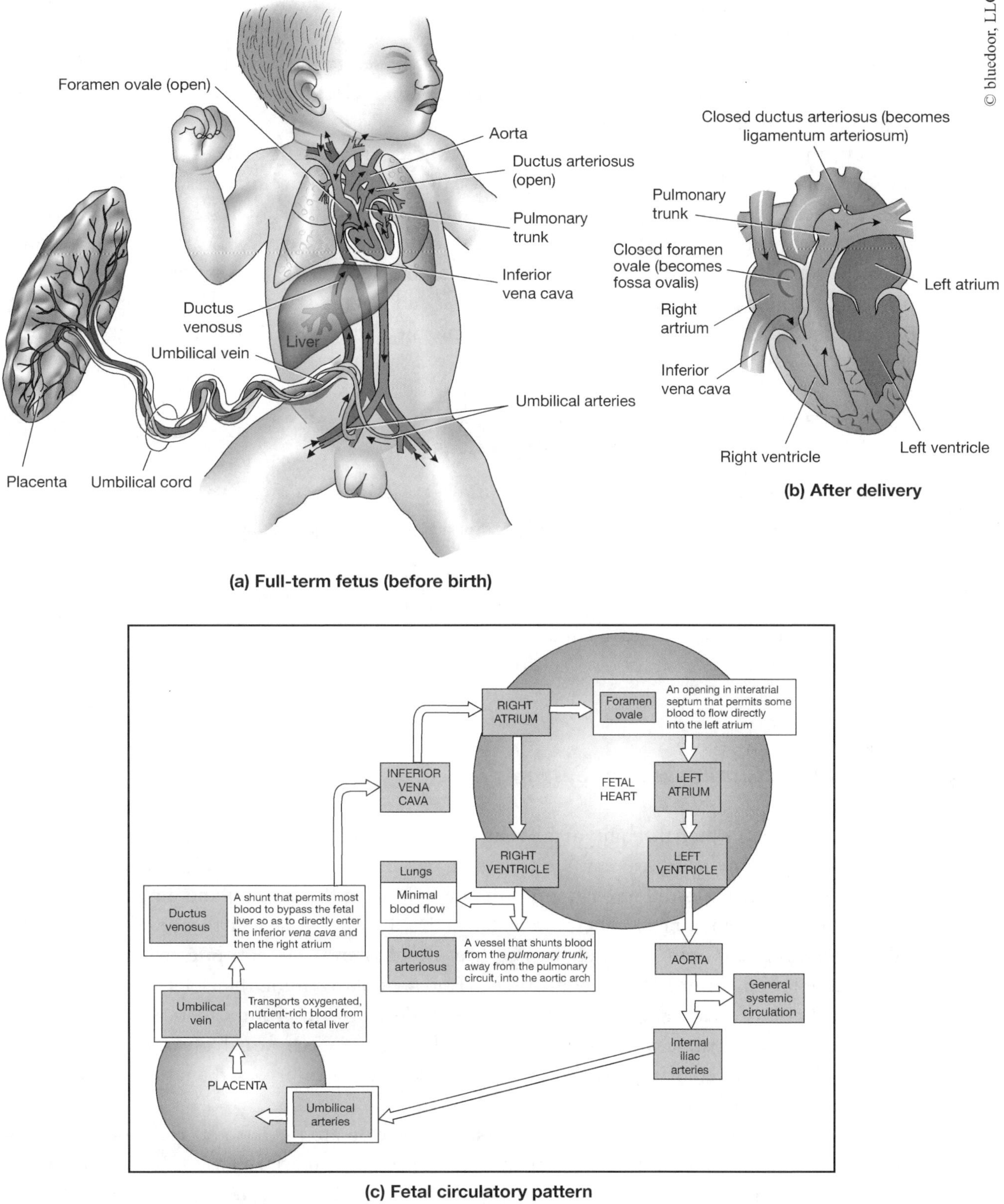

Figure 15-35

Changes in Circulation at Birth

(a) Full term fetus before birth showing the umbilical vessels carrying blood to/from the placenta and the two open pulmonary bypasses. (b) Neonate heart showing closure of the two pulmonary bypasses (foramen ovale of the heart and ductus arteriosus). (c) Schematic diagram of fetal circulation.

same manner as in the adult. The umbilical arteries originate from the internal iliac arteries and course along the sides of the urinary bladder en route to the umbilicus. They continue to the placenta within the umbilical cord. Note that the blood carried to the placenta in the umbilical arteries is not as low in oxygen as the blood in the fetal systemic veins (such as the superior vena cava and in the lower part of the inferior vena cava).

At birth, the first breath dilates the lungs and their expanded state reduces the flow resistance in the pulmonary circulation. The resulting increase in pulmonary flow increases the volume of blood entering the left atrium through the pulmonary veins. This functionally closes the foramen ovale by forcing a flap of tissue against it (termed the valve of the foramen ovale). As the neonate breathes, the increased oxygen concentration throughout the cardiovascular system causes smooth muscle in the walls of the umbilical vessels, ductus venosus, and ductus arteriosus to contract. This temporarily and functionally closes them and with time they fibrose (scar) to effect permanent closure (Figure 15-34, 35).

Objectives

23. List the two peculiarities of fetal biology that require fetal-specific cardiovascular structures.
24. Name the fetal-specific cardiovascular structures and state what each becomes after birth.
25. Follow blood through the fetal cardiovascular system and identify the three major places where the oxygen level of the blood is lowered due to mixing with blood of lower oxygen content.
26. State what happens at/shortly after birth to each fetal-specific cardiovascular structure.

Development of the Cardiovascular System

Blood vessels in human embryos first appear during the third week when the embryo is no longer able to satisfy its nutritional requirements by diffusion alone. Primitive connective tissue called mesenchymal cells differentiate from the mesoderm in the chorion and amnion (two of the extraembryonic membranes). These mesenchymal cells differentiate further into primitive cells called **angioblasts**. Groups of angioblasts called **blood islands** develop intercellular clefts which become the lumina of primitive blood vessels. The angioblasts lining the clefts become the lining endothelial cells of vessels and the central angioblasts develop into primitive blood cells. The blood islands form a plexiform network by proliferation of endothelial cells which grow toward each other and fuse. These extraembryonic vessels gradually penetrate the embryo and anastomose with intra-embryonic vessels which develop in a similar manner.

The first well defined intra-embryonic vessels to develop are the **left** and **right primitive aortae**. These curve around the primitive gut and course caudally (inferiorly) as the **left** and **right dorsal aortae**. Each one develops three major sets of branches: **intersegmental arteries** to the body wall, **vitelline arteries** to the yolk sac, and **umbilical arteries** to the placenta (Figure 15-37). The ventral portions of the primitive aortae unite to form the **aortic sac**. The aortic sac contributes a branch to each of the six pairs of pharyngeal arches as they form. These branches curve around the primitive gut, enter the dorsal aorta, and are called **aortic arches**. They are not all present simultaneously; the first pairs have already been obliterated by the time the last pair arises. Some of the arches and some parts of others contribute to definitive arteries (Figure 15-37; Table 15-3).

Three pairs of primitive venous channels develop: the cardinal veins which parallel the paired aortae, the vitelline veins which carry blood from the yolk sac toward the primitive heart, and the umbilical veins which originate in the chorion and carry oxygenated blood to the embryo. The **left** and **right cardinal veins** which drain the embryo proper are each divided into a **precardinal vein** (anterior to the heart) and a **postcardinal vein** (posterior to the heart). The postcardinals are later replaced by **subcardinal** and **supracardinal veins**. The changes which occur during venous development are more extensive than those which occur among developing arteries. Factors involved include shifts of position and flow direction, anastomoses, local transformations, loss by atrophy, and newly formed vessels which replace older ones already present (Figure 15-38).

The **vitelline veins** enter the embryo via the stalk of the yolk sac and form an anastomotic network around the duodenum. They then enter the liver, form the hepatic sinusoids, and continue to the sinus venosus of the primitive heart. The vascular network around the duodenum forms the portal vein and the vessel draining the intestinal loop (superior mesenteric vein) is derived from the right vitelline vein. The distal part of the left vitelline vein disappears. The umbilical veins returning blood from the placenta enter the fetus through the umbilicus, pass along the sides of the urinary bladder, and continue past the liver to the heart. They soon become connected to the hepatic sinusoids. The proximal parts of both and the remainder of the right one then disappear leaving only the left one to carry blood to the fetus. The intrahepatic portion of the left umbilical vein forms the ductus venosus.

The various derivatives of the cardinal veins form most of the intra-embryonic venous channels. At first they form a zygomorphic pattern. With further development, those on the right side enlarge and the left ones shunt blood to the opposite side via anastomoses. Ultimately, most of the ones on the left side diminish in size and are obliterated.

The heart begins developing at the end of the third week as a pair of mesodermally derived strands of cells near the head of the embryo. These strands become hollow and are known as **endocardial tubes**. When they first begin contracting, the left and right endocardial tubes fuse to form the single **cardiac tube**. Rapid elongation of this tube causes it to buckle and form various bulges which later develop into definitive heart chambers. By the end of the fourth week (when the embryo is about 5 mm long) the following parts can be recognized: **sinus venosus**, **atrial region**, **ventricular region**, and **bulbus cordis** (Figure 15-36). The sinus venosus is the most posterior (caudal) part of the primitive heart and consists of **left** and **right sinus horns**. Each horn receives the ipsilateral vitelline, umbilical, and common cardial veins. The sinus venosus joins the atrium just anterior (cranial) to it. The primitive atrium consists of a single chamber with left and right bulges destined to become the auricles of the definitive atria. The atrial lumen continues into primitive ventricle. A shallow groove (interventricular sulcus) separates it from the bulbus cordis. The latter is formed by the most anterior part of the primitive heart. The bulbus cordis is divided into three parts: proximal, middle, and distal. The **proximal part of the bulbus cordis** (next to the primitive ventricle) becomes the trabecular part of the right ventricle. The **middle part of the bulbus cordis** becomes the **conus cordis** which forms the outflow tracts of both ventricles. The **distal part of the bulbus cordis** is called the **truncus arteriosus**. It forms the initial portions of the aorta and pulmonary trunk (Figure 15-36).

The development of the definitive heart from the primitive, single-tubed, folded structure described above involves the formation of septae in the atrium and ventricles and the development of valves. The atrium is partitioned by ingrowth of two partitions of tissue termed the **septum primum** and **septum secundum**. These two septae do not completely separate the two sides of the atrium from each other and the remaining opening forms the **foramen ovale**. The ventricular area is divided by ingrowth of a ridge known as the **muscular part of the interventricular septum**. This septum

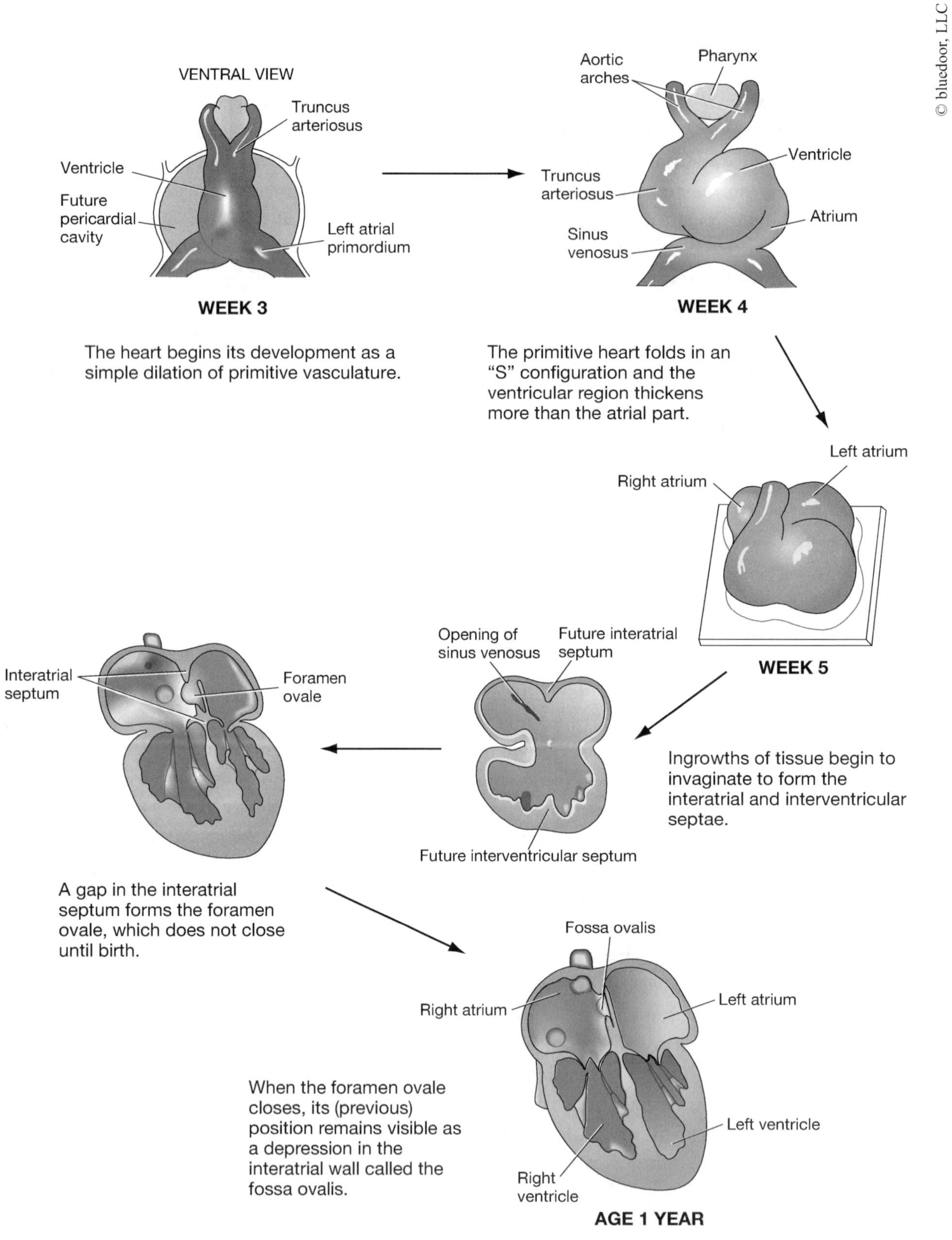

Figure 15-36
Development of the Heart

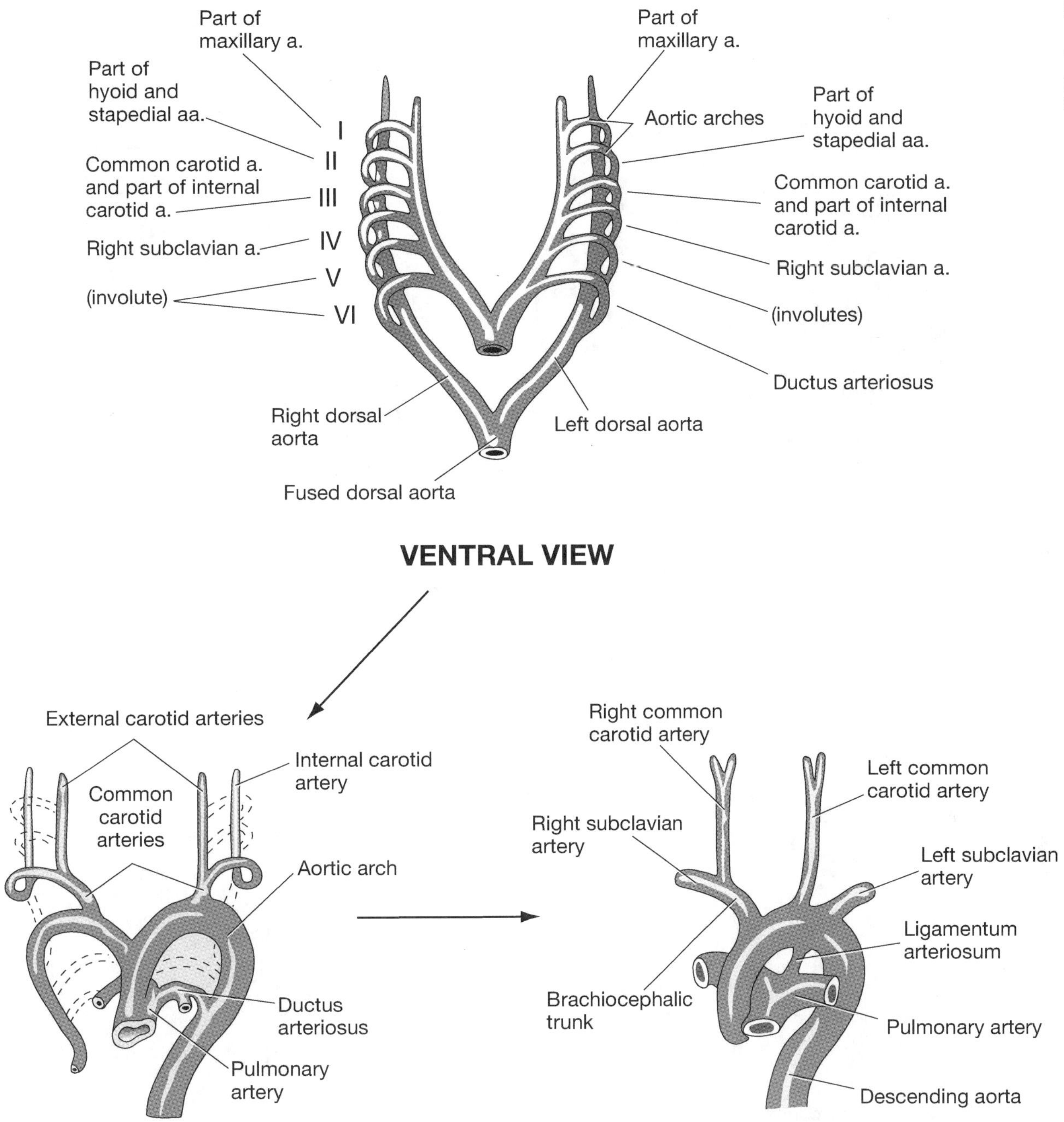

The ductus arteriosus forms a pulmonary bypass in the fetal circulatory system that allows blood to bypass the (nonfunctional) lungs.

After birth, the ductus arteriosus is (normally) closed (first by contraction of smooth muscle tissue and later by proliferation of fibrous connective tissue). If this closure fails, a patent (open) ductus arteriosus exists, causing a serious (and if uncorrected, possibly fatal) circulatory abnormality.

Figure 15-37

Fates of the Aortic Arches

Six pairs of aortic arches form. These are numbered I-VI to correspond to the pharyngeal arches through which they course. Although the fifth pair involutes without forming a definitive structure, the others contribute to definitive vasculature (*see Table 15-3*).

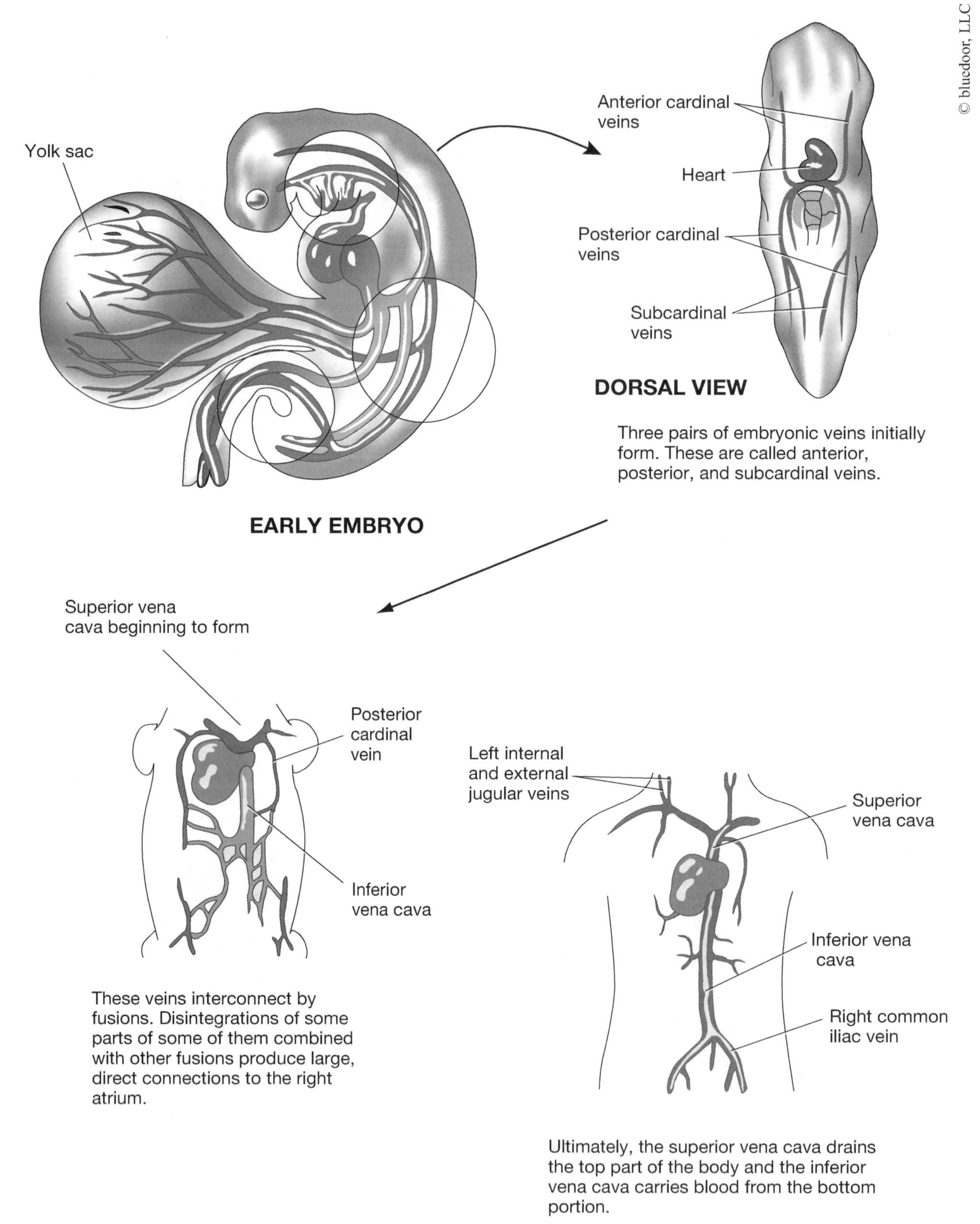

Figure 15-38

Development of the Vena Cavae

fails to completely divide the left and right ventricles but the division is soon completed by ingrowth of a pair of truncoconal ridges which also ingrow the truncus arteriosus and separate the lumina of the pulmonary trunk and aorta. These ridges spiral up through the truncus arteriosus such that the aorta originates from the left ventricle but lies initially to the right of the pulmonary trunk. Likewise, the pulmonary trunk originates from the right ventricle but lies initially to the left of the aorta.

Development of the two atrioventricular valves between the atria and ventricles and the two semilunar valves between the ventricles, aorta, and pulmonary trunk completes the development of the heart. With such a complex series of events contributing to the normal cardiac development, it is not surprising that so many developmental anomalies exist. If either septum (atrial or ventricular) fails to develop properly, septal defects may be present. Atrial septal defects are often benign unless they are large, but ventricular septal defects are quite serious due to the discrepancy in left/right pressures and the subsequent shunting of blood from left to right. **Tetralogy of Fallot** is a set of four simultaneously occurring cardiac anomalies consisting of (1) stenosis of the pulmonary valve; (2) ventricular septal defect; (3) overriding aorta; and (4) hypertrophy of the right ventricle. Failure of a valve to develop constitutes a **valvular atresia** and **valvular stenosis** often has a developmental cause. Failure of the truncoconal ridges to spiral as they grow through the truncus arteriosus causes the aorta to originate from the right ventricle and the pulmonary trunk from the left ventricle. This is a relatively common condition called **transposition** of the great vessels (Figure 15-39).

Table 15-3 The Six Pairs of Aortic Arches and Their Fate

Arch	*Fate*
First	Forms part of maxillary artery
Second	Forms part of hyoid and stapedial arteries
Third	Forms the common carotid artery and part of the internal carotid artery
Fourth	Left one forms the aortic arch, right one forms the right subclavian artery
Fifth	Disappears early without forming a definitive structure
Sixth	Right one disappears, left one forms the ductus arteriosus

Objectives

27. Name the embryonic precursor cell that forms the primitive blood cells and linings of the blood vessels.
28. List the three sets of arteries that the primitive aorta supplies.
29. Indicate the role of the two septae in dividing the developing atria and ventricles.

Clinical Considerations

Systemic blood pressure is clinically monitored by use of a device called a **sphygmomanometer**. Older versions of this instrument consist of an inflatable cuff which is placed around the brachium and a pressure gauge which is calibrated in millimeters of mercury (mm Hg). The cuff is inflated until it totally obliterates blood flow through the brachial artery. Then the cuff pressure is slowly released until blood first begins to flow in the artery again, as evidenced by the characteristic sounds (**Korotkoff sounds**) heard through a stethoscope placed at the cubital fossa (crook of the elbow). This pressure is called the **systolic arterial pressure** and averages about 120 mm Hg in normal indi-

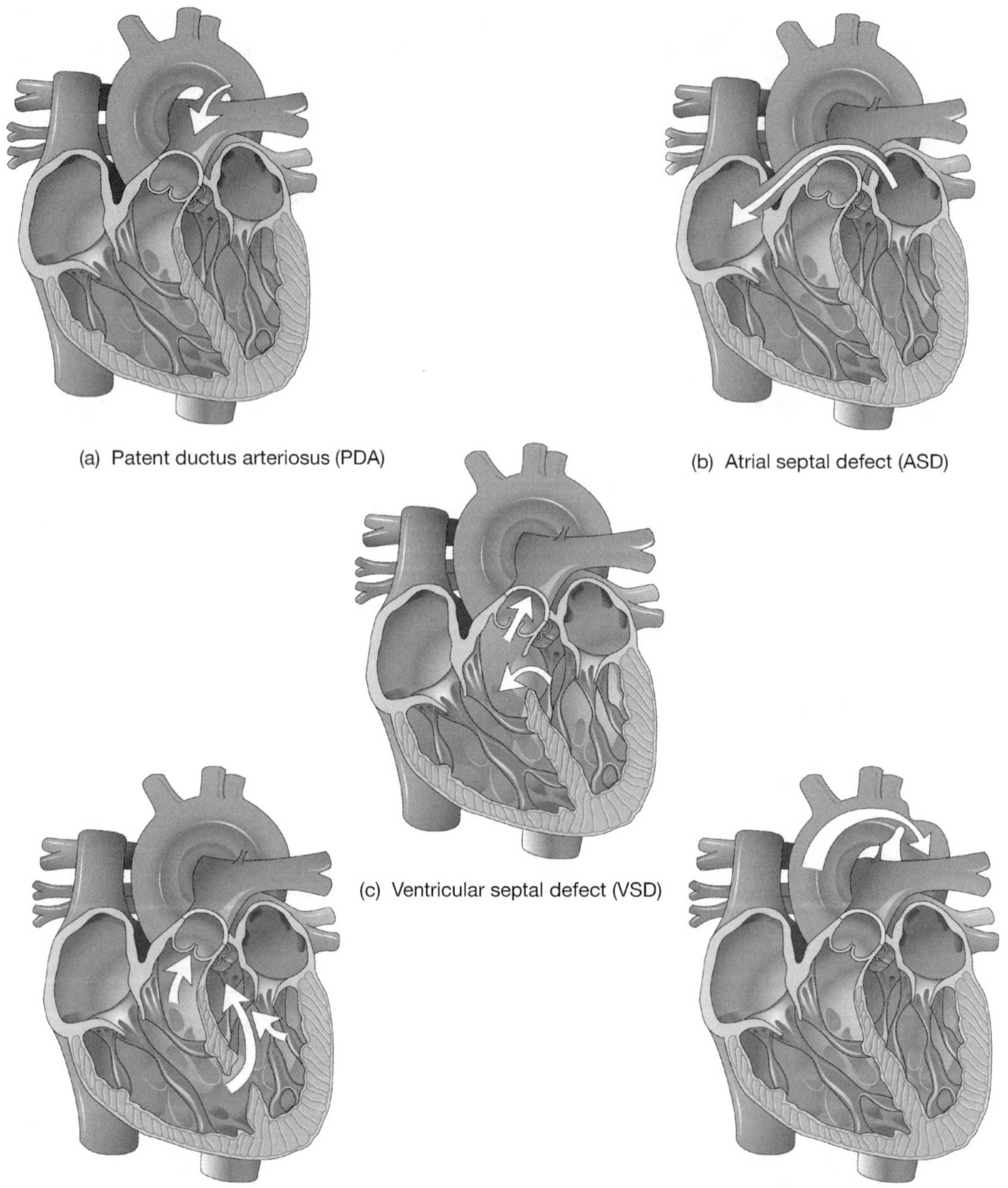

Figure 15-39

Congenital Defects of the Cardiovascular System

Patent ductus arteriosus (a) is the most common cause of the "blue baby" syndrome. Blood flows "backward" in a patent ductus from the aorta to the pulmonary trunk and causes pulmonary hypertension. Patent foramen ovale (b) produces an atrial septal defect. This structural abnormality is usually not serious since the pressures in the two atria are similar. Ventricular septal defect (c) allows blood to flow from the left ventricle (higher pressure) to the right ventricle. If large, it may dictate surgery right after birth. Tetralogy of Fallot (d) includes four structural abnormalities: pulmonary stenosis, overriding aorta, right ventricular hypertrophy, and a ventricular septal defect. Coarctation of the aorta (e) involves extreme narrowing of the aortic lumen.

viduals. Pressure in the cuff is then slowly released until no sounds are heard in the stethoscope. The pressure at which this occurs is the **diastolic arterial pressure** and typically measures about 80 mm Hg. The difference between the systolic and diastolic pressures is the **pulse pressure**. High blood pressure is called **hypertension** and is a health hazard because it puts an excessive load on the heart and can cause rupture of vessels. Modern sphygmomanometers still use the pressure cuff, but once applied, everything is monitored automatically and a stethoscope is not needed.

A precipitous drop in blood pressure is termed **circulatory shock**. It can result from significant blood loss (**hypovolemic shock**), extreme emotional disturbance (**neurogenic shock**), from paralysis of precapillary sphincters of arterioles by bacterial toxins (**endotoxic shock**), from a significant reduction in the heart's ability to pump (**cardiogenic shock**), and from a number of other causes. Shock can be life-threatening because it reduces cerebral arterial flow below critical levels. It is treated with intravenous fluid administration (to increase the blood pressure), corticosteroids (to restore vascular endothelial integrity), and antimicrobial agents to combat bacteria that may have crossed the mucous membranes (especially of the digestive system) while the pressure was reduced.

The electrical activity of the heart is measured by a specialized instrument called an **electrocardiograph**. This device measures the electrical potential difference between various points on the body surface which occur because of the electrical activity of the heart. It produces a graphed printout of this electrical activity called an **electrocardiogram** (**EKG** or **ECG**) (*see Figure 15-8*). A number of different cardiac diseases can be detected using EKGs including atrophy and hypertrophy of different parts of the heart and **heart block**. The latter refers to impairment of the normal impulse transmission within the heart. Over a dozen types are recognized. The best known forms involve reduced conduction between atria and ventricles (A-V blocks) and are classified as **first degree block** (prolongation of A-V conduction time), **second degree block** (some, but not all, atrial impulses reach the ventricles), and **complete (third degree) A-V block** (*no* atrial impulses reach the ventricles). Individuals with complete blocks and even some with second degree blocks may need a **cardiac pacemaker**. This device artificially initiates impulses that stimulate the heart.

A **heart attack** is the lay term for **myocardial infarction**. This is a localized insufficiency of blood supply to the myocardium resulting in damage or death of cardiac muscle tissue. It often occurs following reduced diameter of cardiac arteries due to **arteriosclerosis**, a condition of decreased resiliency ("hardening") of the vessels related to deposition of abnormal material in the tunica intima or tunica media. In severe cases, cardiac bypass surgery may be performed to install "detour" routes so that blood can flow past the constricted portions of the vessels.

Heart rate is usually monitored by manually checking the **pulse rate** in peripheral vessels. The most common method is to compress the radial artery against the radius in the distal antebrachium. However, compression of the common carotid, brachial, dorsal pedal arteries, and other vessels can also be used (Figure 15-17). Pulse rate is one of the three vital signs routinely checked by health professionals: temperature, pulse rate, and respiratory rate (commonly acronymed TPR). A typical resting heart rate is around 70 contractions/minute. An elevated rate is called **tachycardia** and a lowered rate is **bradycardia**.

The heart is auscultated with a stethoscope to monitor the sounds that it produces. The two **normal heart sounds** (first and second heart sounds or "lub-dub") should occur distinctly and in rapid succession followed by a somewhat longer period before they recur. Abnormal heart sounds (murmurs) are any deviations from those normally heard and are related to turbulent blood flow associated with valvular stenoses and insufficiencies, septal defects (abnormal passageways between the left and right chambers), and to patent ductus arteriosus. Cardiac auscultation is used to characterize two important parameters of the murmur: when it occurs in the cardiac cycle (systolic, dias-

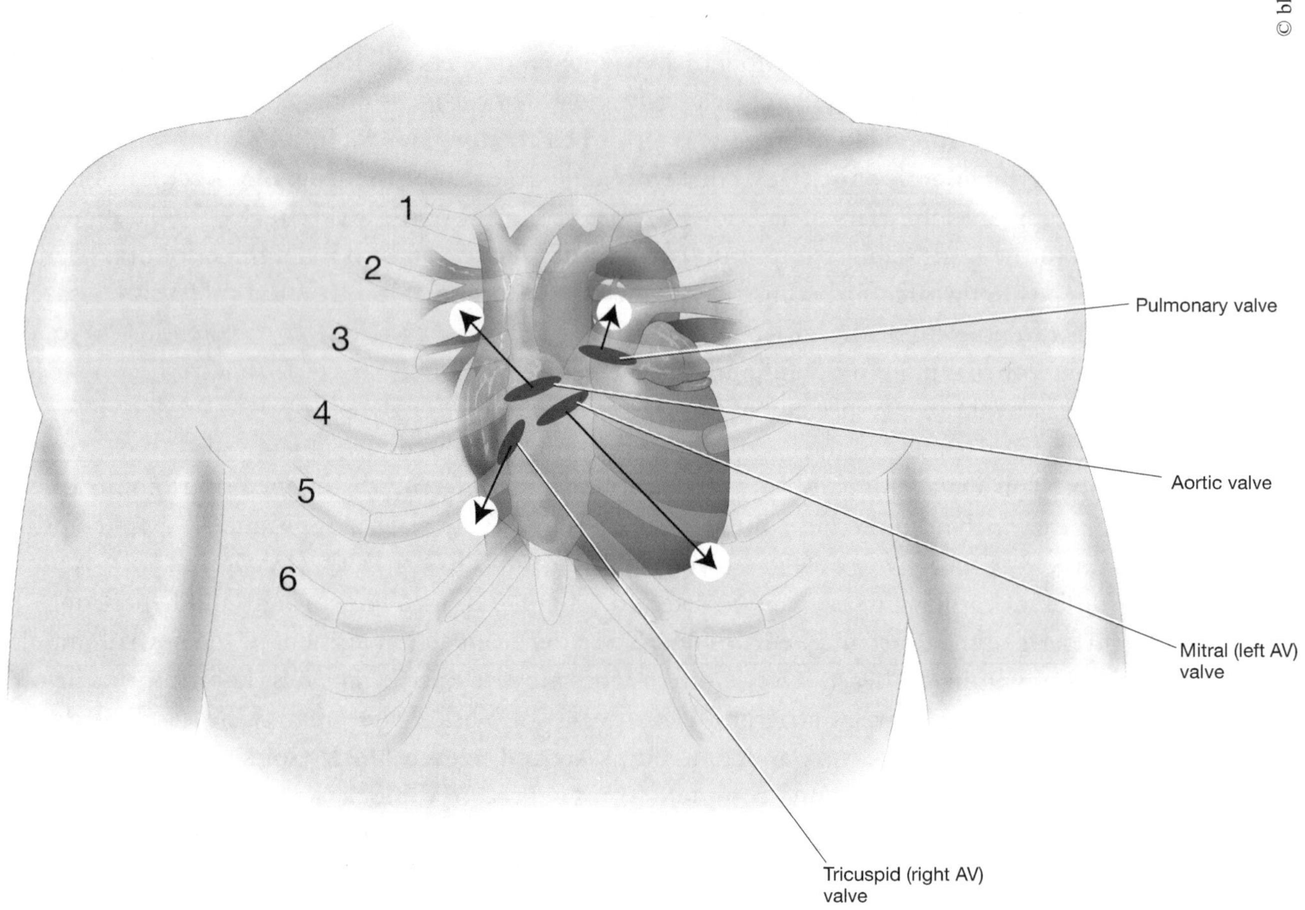

Figure 15-40

Points of Maximal Sound Intensity During Cardiac Auscultation

Note that the points of maximal sound intensity for various heart valves do not correspond precisely to the actual locations of the valves. The difference is caused by the structures through which the sounds are conducted to the thoracic wall:

Aortic valve—loudest just right of anterior midline at level of second intercostal space (just below the sternal angle).

Valve of the pulmonary trunk—loudest left of anterior midline just beyond sternum at the level of the second intercostal space.

Left atrioventricular (mitral) valve—loudest in the left fifth intercostal space just medial to a sagittal plane through the left nipple.

Right atrioventricular (tricuspid) valve—loudest in the right fifth intercostal space near the anterior midline.

tolic, continuous), and where (on the chest wall) it is heard the loudest. The four heart valves each have a point of maximal sound intensity which occurs at a location on the chest wall that is close to (but does not *exactly* correspond to) the anatomical location of the valve. These locations are (aortic valve: right side of sternum just below sternal angle; pulmonary valve: left side of sternum in the second intercostal space; tricuspid valve: apex of heart on the right side; mitral valve: apex of heart) illustrated in Figure 15-40. Using deductive reasoning, a systolic murmur heard loudest in the right third intercostal space would most likely be caused by stenosis of the aortic valve.

Blood transfusions are performed to restore blood volume in traumatized or surgical patients. There are many different blood types but the two of most concern in transfusion patients are the A-B-O blood groups and the Rh factor. Blood is classified as **type A**, **B**, **AB**, or **O** depending on the type(s) of antigen that the red blood corpuscles have in (on) their cell membranes. Type A blood has plasma antibodies against B, and type A individuals should not be given type B or AB blood because agglutination (clumping) of the transfused blood cells will occur (Table 15-4). Individuals with type B blood should not be given type A or AB blood for the same general reason. Type O blood does not have A or B antigens on the erythrocytes and these individuals are sometimes called **universal donors**. Type AB individuals have both A and B antigens on their RBC's but have no plasma antibodies and are called **universal recipients** since they can be given any other blood type (A, B, O) without serious consequence. In practice, blood transfusions are not performed until a cross match test confirms that no agglutination will occur.

The **Rh factor** is another group of antigens found on red blood corpuscles of most individuals. People with the antigens are said to be **Rh positive** and those lacking the factor are **Rh negative**. This becomes a critical factor in Rh negative women carrying Rh positive fetuses because the blood of the developing infant may sensitize the mother and cause her to develop antibodies to the factor. These will cross the placenta and cause hemolysis of the erythrocytes in the unborn. The condition is called **fetal erythroblastosis** and can be fatal to the baby. Usually the firstborn is not affected, but the mother's antibodies levels are often high enough to cause problems with subsequent pregnancies. This condition is routinely prevented by an immunosuppresent injection given to the mother during gestation.

Table 15-4 ABO System of Blood Types

Blood Type	*Genotype*	*Antigens on RBC's*	*Antibodies in Plasma*	*Can Donate to...*	*Can Receive...*
A	$I^A I^A$ or $I^A i$	A	anti-B	A, AB	A, O
B	$I^B I^B$ or $I^B i$	B	anti-A	B, AB	B, O
AB	$I^A I^B$	AB	none	AB	A, B, AB, O
O	ii	none	anti-A, anti-B	A, B, AB, O	O

Objectives

30. Define sphygmomanometer and explain how it and a stethoscope are used to monitor blood pressure.
31. Define and differentiate the types of circulatory shock.
32. Differentiate electrocardiograph from electrocardiogram and define the various degrees of heart block.
33. Define: heart attack, arteriosclerosis, tachycardia, bradycardia, and hypertension.
34. Differentiate the major ABO blood types and explain what is meant by the Rh factor.

Clinical Case Studies

Case 1—A teenager suffering chronic fatigue underwent a physical exam. The physician's assistant noted an obvious cardiac murmur heard loudest high on the anterior chest wall just to the right of the midline. The murmur occurred between the first and second heart sounds but not between the second and (next) first heart sounds. State a tentative diagnosis.

Case 2—Parents of a three-year-old boy had him examined because he would bleed excessively from even the smallest scratches. In several instances, it had taken more than an hour to control his hemorrhages. State a tentative diagnosis.

Case 3—A 63-year-old man suffered severe weakness and almost lost consciousness three times in a period of two weeks. A fourth time occurred a few days later while visiting some of his family members. The man's oldest son, fearing a heart attack, happened to check his father's pulse during the last episode, and found it to be exceptionally slow (35 beats/minute). State a tentative diagnosis.

Points to Ponder

Lub-dub. We take it for granted. Seventy times a minute, when we are at rest. That's 4200 times each hour, 100,800 times a day and 36,732,000 times each year. But we don't always rest. Sometimes the heart contracts two or three times as fast. Pumps two or three thousand gallons of blood a day—five or six thousand gallons in a football lineman (maybe more on game days). The only rest it gets is the short period between dub and the next lub. Called diastole (and memorized "dilate"), this brief respite is somewhat longer than systole (memorized "squeeze").

Lub-dub. If you haven't heard the normal heart sounds, find someone you know well (or would like to know better) and lay your ear on their chest. A stethoscope is helpful but less fun, and is not necessary. Lub-dub. (Even if you have a stethoscope you may want to pretend you don't!)

Located within the thoracic cavity and forming a major part of the thoracic partition known as the mediastinum, the heart symbolically represents the soul, the seat of emotion, even life itself. Four chambers, four valves, three layers, two ends, two sides, the heart is fed by two major arteries. When flow is reduced in these or their branches by atherosclerosis or lodged emboli, cardiac muscle tissue dies and the impending obituary will read heart attack. In a better but still serious scenario, a cardiac surgeon will delicately suture blood vessels in place (harvested from some less needed site on the same victim) to bypass the narrowed or blocked vessels. The obituary waits for another day in some future year.

In college I shamelessly sold my body at the rate of 25 dollars a pint to the local hospital laboratory. I never met any of those that my blood may have saved, but the 25 dollars (a lot of money in those days) fed me for a week. I never missed it—that tenth of my blood volume that I traded periodically in exchange for money. In fact, I impatiently watched the calendar as the mandatory three weeks passed until I could do it again... and again. Until my sophomore year in veterinary college when I came down with mononucleosis (compliments of Vicki). At least that was the tentative diagnosis. Unfortunately, the physician labeled me as a hepatitis suspect which ended my career as a professional blood donor and cost me $433.33 a year in donor's compensations. Years later, I'm back at it as a plasma prostitute. Twice a week I go to a plasma center with all of the college kids and other derelicts that are donating that day. We sit there and wonder why the others do it and then the movie comes on (that we have all seen seven times) and we just lay back and wait till our bottle fills.

Red blood corpuscles are amazing structures. To increase their capacity for hemoglobin, they lose their nuclei and most other organelles at maturity, making room for over a quarter of a billion molecules of the oxygen binding pigment called hemoglobin. To maximize their ability to quickly bind and release oxygen, RBC's assume a flattened, biconcave disc shape which increases their surface area to volume ratio. Relatively small for cells, there are 5 million per cubic millimeter of blood, 5 billion in each cubic centimeter, 5 trillion in each liter, 25 trillion in each average sized (70 kg.) individual. Slightly more in males than in females, more in mountain dwellers than in lowlanders, more in athletes than in couch potatoes. The presence/absence of two particular proteins in the RBC's allows hematologists and medical laboratories to define four blood types: A, B, AB (both proteins), and O (neither protein). The presence/ absence of another protein allows blood to be classified Rh positive or negative. Not content to let it go at that, hematologists (a group of confirmed malcontents) have several other typing systems as well. As a result, when you feel a quart low you can't just pull a bottle of 10W30 off the shelf. Instead, a careful cross-matching is done to prevent the possibility of a transfusion reaction. None of us want that obituary yet.

Slang and Obsolete Nomenclature

UNOFFICIAL TERM	OFFICIAL DESIGNATION
aortic semilunar valve	aortic valve/valve of the aorta *[valva aortae]*
pulmonary semilunar valve	pulmonary valve/valve of the pulmonary trunk *[valva trunci pulmonalis]*
bicuspid valve	left atrioventricular/mitral valve *[valva atrioventriculare sinistra/mitralis]*
left border of heart	pulmonary surface *[facies pulmonalis]* of heart
moderator band	trabecula septomarginalis *[trabecula septomarginalis]*
left/right auricle (as chamber)	left/right atrium *[atrium sinistrum/dextrum]*
left/right auricle	auricle of left/right atrium *[auricula atrii sinistra/dextra]*
bundle of His	atrioventricular bundle *[fasciculus atrioventricularis]*
portal vein	hepatic portal vein *[vena portae hepatis]*
brachiocephalic artery	brachiocephalic trunk *[truncus brachiocephalicus]*
pulmonary artery	right/left pulmonary artery *[arteria pulmonis dextra/sinistra]*
pulmonary vein	right/left, superior/inferior pulmonary vein *[vena pulmonis dextra/sinistra, superior/inferior]*
hepatic artery	common/proper hepatic artery *[arteria hepatica communis/ propria]*
carotid artery	common/external/internal carotid artery *[arteria carotis communis/externa/interna]*
jugular vein	internal/external jugular vein *[vena jugularis interna/externa]*
celiac artery	celiac trunk *[truncus coeliacus]*
thoracic aorta	thoracic part of aorta *[pars thoracica aortae]*
circle of Willis	cerebral arterial circle *[circulus arteriosus cerebri]*
gonadal arteries	testicular/ovarian arteries *[arteriae testiculares/ovaricae]*
spermatic artery	testicular artery *[arteria testicularis]*
platelet	thrombocyte *[thrombocytus]*
polymorphonuclear leucocyte	neutrophil *[granulocytus neutrophilicum]*

Review Questions

1. Which of the following is not an organ of the cardiovascular system?
   A. artery
   B. capillary
   C. vein
   D. blood
   E. heart

2. The first heart chamber encountered by blood in a pulmonary vein is the
   A. right atrium.
   B. right ventricle.
   C. left atrium.
   D. left ventricle.
   E. pericardial cavity.

3. Which layer of the heart wall consists of only one layer of serous membrane?
   A. epicardium
   B. myocardium
   C. endocardium
   D. parietal pericardium
   E. interventricular septum

4. Which heart valve is open during ventricular systole?
   A. mitral valve
   B. bicuspid valve
   C. aortic valve
   D. tricuspid valve
   E. left atrioventricular valve

5. Most of the blood leaving the aorta through the brachiocephalic trunk eventually flows back toward the heart in the...
   A. left subclavian vein.
   B. right common carotid vein.
   C. azygos vein.
   D. right brachiocephalic vein.
   E. right internal jugular vein.

6. Which vein is not correctly matched with the area that it drains?
   A. inferior vena cava—abdomen, pelvis, inferior limbs
   B. azygos vein—thoracic wall
   C. pulmonary veins—lungs
   D. superior vena cava—head, neck, superior limbs
   E. hepatic portal vein—stomach, intestine, spleen, pancreas, liver

7. Which branch of the abdominal part of the descending aorta is paired?
   A. superior mesenteric artery
   B. common carotid artery
   C. celiac trunk
   D. posterior intercostal artery
   E. common iliac artery

8. Find the false statement about blood:
   A. It is about 55% plasma and 45% formed elements.
   B. The formed elements include granulocytes, monocytes, platelets, RBC's, and lymphocytes.
   C. The protein fraction of plasma includes globulins, albumins, and fibrinogen.
   D. It can be classified into four major "ABO" types and two major "Rh" types.
   E. Removal of fibrinogen from blood leaves a fluid called serum.

9. Which vessel in a fetus should carry blood with the lowest oxygen (percentage)?
   A. umbilical vein
   B. femoral vein
   C. inferior vena cava (superior part)
   D. umbilical artery
   E. pulmonary trunk

10. Which fetal structure does not initially close due to the increased overall oxygen levels after birth?
    A. ductus venosus
    B. umbilical arteries
    C. umbilical vein
    D. foramen ovale
    E. ductus arteriosus

Thought Questions

1. Why can't cardiac murmurs be detected by electrocardiography (EKG)?

2. The standard treatment for circulatory shock is the administration of intravenous fluids, corticosteroids and antibiotics. What is the logic behind this regimen?

3. A systolic murmur is heard loudest just to the right of the manubrium of the sternum. State a tentative diagnosis.

4. Compare the overall diameter, wall thickness, volume of blood transported per unit time, and the relative flow speed (mm/sec) of blood within an artery and its satellite vein.

5. Why is it that type O blood can usually be transfused into recipients who have A, B, or AB blood without ill effects but type O individuals are likely to suffer a major transfusion reaction if type A, B, or AB blood is administered to them?

6. What causes the drop in systolic blood pressure from 120 mm Hg in a major systemic artery to about 35 mm Hg at the arteriole end of a capillary?

7. Why does blood in superficial vessels (*i.e.,* the metacarpal veins on the posterior metacarpal region) appear blue in color?

8. Since the lungs in a fetus are nonfunctional in O_2/CO_2 exchange, why does some blood travel to them in the pulmonary arteries? (*i.e.,* why aren't the lungs *completely* bypassed by the foramen ovale and ductus arteriosus)?

9. If the resting heart rate (about 70 contractions/minute) is doubled, the cardiac output (amount of blood pumped by the heart each minute) is more than doubled. Explain this apparent discrepancy.

10. What two peculiarities does blood have in relation to the other body components?

11. "Blood doping" is a term describing the unethical practice of an athlete who has some blood withdrawn, stored for a few weeks, and then infused back into his own circulatory system just prior to an endurance competition. What advantage would this procedure give?

12. Do the left and right ventricles pump the same volume of blood per unit of time? Is the volume of blood in the systemic circulation the same as that in the pulmonary circulation?

13. Why do arteries and veins have tiny vessels within their walls?

14. Why is it that a major arterial channel can often be ligated (tied off) without seriously disrupting the blood supply to its area of distribution?

15. Why is patent (open) foramen ovale usually inconsequential, but patent ductus arteriosus is usually quite serious (and often requires surgical intervention)?

16. What does the term *trunk* imply when used in the name of an artery?

17. Arteries are named on the basis of their course and distribution. What two kinds of anatomic features occur at the origin of arteries?

18. Four organs have a dual blood supply (receive blood of both high and low oxygen levels). At the tissue level, the organs differ in how that blood is distributed. Explain.

19. What purpose do arteriovenous shunts serve?

20. Why do the testicular arteries originate fairly high on the abdominal aorta instead of closer to the testes themselves?

21. Calculate (estimate) the total number of RBC's in an average-sized person.

Answers to Clinical Case Studies

Case 1—The location of the murmur implicates the aortic valve. Since the murmur occurs when the aortic valve is open, the logical tentative diagnosis is aortic stenosis. Stenotic valves cause murmurs (only) when they are in the open position and insufficient valves cause murmurs (only) when they are in the closed position.

Case 2—Excessive bleeding often indicates a problem with the blood clotting mechanism. In some individuals, this is a genetic (heritable) trait called hemophilia and is related to inadequate production of one or more of the clotting factors in blood or production of one or more defective clotting factors.

Case 3—The symptoms exhibited by this man are compatible with a complete heart block at the A-V node. When this occurs, the inherent rhythmicity of the ventricular myocardium (about 35 beats/minute) is often enough to sustain life, but may cause weakness and/or loss of consciousness. This patient underwent surgery to have a cardiac pacemaker installed.

Answers to Review Questions

1. D. Blood is a tissue.
2. C.
3. A. B, C, and E are not serous membrane and D is not part of the heart wall.
4. C. A=B=E and D are closed.
5. D. The brachiocephalic trunk supplies blood to the right side of the head and to the right superior limb.
6. E. The problem is the liver.
7. E. B and D are paired but are not branches of the abdominal part of the descending aorta.
8. E. Removal of fibrinogen from *plasma* leaves fluid called serum.
9. B. Systemic veins carry blood with the lowest oxygen level.
10. D. The foramen ovale closes due to increased pressure in the left atrium from increased pulmonary venous inflow.

Answers to Thought Questions

1. Cardiac murmurs are abnormal heart sounds. EKG's detect electrical activity.

2. Fluids elevate the blood pressure (which has dropped). Antibiotics combat bacterial invaders (which may have crossed mucous membranes during the low blood pressure). Steroids restore capillary wall integrity (which is often compromised).

3. Stenosis of the aortic valve. The location indicates the aortic valve and the fact that the aortic valve is open during systole implies that stenosis is the pathological feature. (Stenotic valves cause murmurs when they are in the open position and insufficient valves cause murmurs when they are closed.)

4. The artery is smaller in overall diameter than the vein. It also has a thicker wall than the vein, carries a slightly larger volume of blood per unit of time, and the blood in it is moving much faster than that in the vein.

5. Type O erythrocytes have no A or B antigens on them and so the anti-A and anti-B antibodies present in type A, B, or AB recipients do not cause them to agglutinate. (The anti-A and anti-B antibodies in the donor blood get so diluted going into the recipient that they do not cause agglutination either.) When type A, B, or AB blood enters a type O recipient, the recipient's anti-A and anti-B antibodies cause agglutination of the transfused RBC's. The critical factor in transfusion reactions is what occurs between the antibodies in the recipient's plasma and the antigens on the donor's RBC's. Potential reaction between the donor's antibodies and the recipient's antigens is of much less consequence due to dilution of the donor's antibodies related to slow administration of a relatively small quantity of blood. In practice, an *in vitro* cross-match is performed between a recipient's blood and that of a potential donor.

6. A small part of the drop is due to friction. A larger part is due to the fact that the total cross sectional area at the capillary level (of all capillaries) is larger than the cross sectional area of the main arterial channels supplying those capillaries. "Ballooning" of the thin-walled peripheral vessels also plays a role.

7. The blood in the superficial veins is dark red and the overlaying tissue translates this to a bluish color.

8. This is necessary to establish the circulatory channels that must take over at birth.

9. The cardiac output is a product of the heart rate (contractions/minute) and the stroke volume (amount of blood pumped/contraction). As the heart rate increases, so does the stroke volume.

10. It is the only liquid tissue and it is the only *tissue* that is considered to be a major component of a body system.

11. After "doping", an individual has a higher than normal red blood cell count which increases the oxygen carrying capacity of the blood.

12. There is a much larger volume of blood in the systemic circulation than in the pulmonary circulation at any given moment, but the ventricles do pump identical volumes of blood.

13. These tiny vessels (vasa vasorum) are necessary to nourish the tissues within their walls which are too thick for nutrients and waste products to diffuse through from the blood within their lumina.

14. Most regions of the body have multiple vessels that supply them. If one is ligated, the others typically enlarge to supply the same total flow to the area under consideration. This concept is called collateral circulation.

15. The pressures in the two atria are nearly identical and so there is little or no blood flow (right-left or left-right) through a patent foramen ovale. On the other hand, a patent ductus arteriosus allows significant left-right flow through the ductus. This blood "should" have gone through the aorta to the body.

16. Most "trunks" divide (branch) almost immediately into two or three arteries.

17. Arteries originate at branching points or at major landmarks (where the parent vessel passes a particular anatomic feature).

18. In the liver and in the pituitary gland, the high and low oxygen blood mixes within the tissue. In the heart the low oxygen blood is passing through the chambers (but not through the cardiac tissue). In the lungs, the low oxygen blood enters capillary beds where it becomes oxygenated. The small, high oxygen vessels associated with the lungs are the bronchial vessels which supply primarily the bronchial tree.

19. They allow variation in the amount of high oxygen blood delivered to particular loci and allow some thermoregulation.

20. The testes begin their development (as do the ovaries) fairly high in the abdominal cavity just below the kidneys. When the testes migrate through the lower anterior abdominal wall to enter the scrotum, their arteries (which originate near the renal arteries) migrate with them by "stretching." However, the origins of the testicular vessels do not move.

21. There are 5 million RBC's in each cubic millimeter of blood. Since there are 1,000 cubic millimeters in one cc (milliliter), there are 1,000 x 5 million RBC's therein (5 billion = 5×10^9). There are 1,000 ml (cc) in a liter and an average sized individual has 5 liters of blood. (5 billion x 1,000 = 5 trillion and 5 x 5 trillion = 25 trillion.)

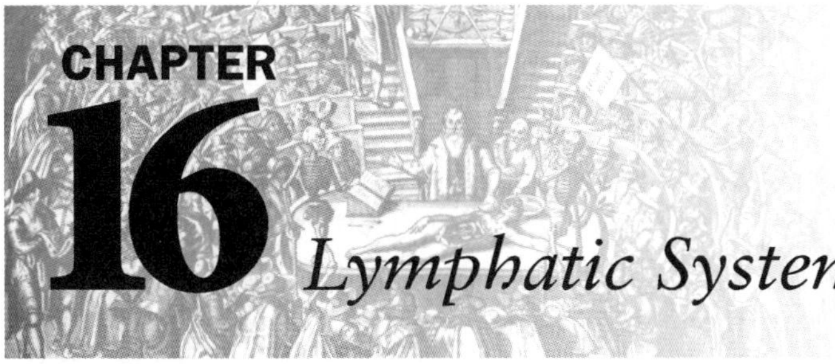

CHAPTER 16 *Lymphatic System*

Chapter Outline and Key Concepts

INTRODUCTION

The lymphatic system includes a group of organs that contain developing lymphocytes and a network of vessels that transport lymph.

FUNCTIONS

The lymphatic system returns excess tissue fluid to the blood, produces lymphocytes and antibodies, and absorbs lipids from the intestinal lumen.

FORMATION OF INTERSTITIAL FLUID AND LYMPH

Extracellular fluid (tissue fluid, interstitial fluid) that enters lymphatic capillaries is called lymph.

Interstitial fluid is formed continuously because capillary walls are very thin and the net "out" pressure through them exceeds the net "in" pressure.

LYMPHATIC VESSELS

Blind-ended lymphatic capillaries absorb excess interstitial fluid.

Lymphatic capillaries drain into larger lymphatic vessels.

Lymph eventually enters main lymphatic channels called trunks.

The right jugular, subclavian, and bronchomediastinal (lymphatic) trunks drain into the right lymphatic duct which joins the right brachiocephalic vein.

The thoracic duct is the largest lymphatic vessel, receiving lymph from both inferior limbs, the abdomen, and the left side of the upper body and transporting it to the left brachiocephalic vein.

LYMPHATIC ORGANS

Lymph nodes are positioned along the course of lymphatic vessels and lymph flows through them.

Groups of developing lymphocytes within various lymphatic organs produce antibodies.

The spleen is the largest lymphatic organ.

The thymus produces precursors of T lymphocytes and then involutes after puberty.

The tonsils are four paired groups of lymphatic nodules in the pharyngeal region.

Lymphatic nodules in the wall of the intestine are called aggregations of lymphatic nodules ("Peyer's patches").

DEVELOPMENT OF LYMPHATIC ORGANS

The thymus develops from mesodermal parts of the third pharyngeal pouches.

The spleen, lymphatic vessels, and lymph nodes develop from mesodermal condensations.

The tonsils develop from mesoderm in the area of the pharynx.

CLINICAL CONSIDERATIONS

Edema is the swelling that results from the collection of excess tissue fluid and has many causes.

Neoplastic lymphatic tissue is called a lymphoma.

Inflammation of lymph nodes (lymphadenitis) and lymphatic vessels (lymphangitis) occurs in some diseases.

Tonsillitis is the most common affliction of the lymphatic system.

Selected Definitions

Accessory spleen—a small parcel of splenic tissue separated from the main part of the spleen. Such developmental anomalies occur in about ten percent of the population and are clinically inconsequential.

B lymphocytes (**B cell**)—those lymphocytes primarily responsible for humeral (antibody) immunity. B-cell precursors in mammals originate in bone marrow tissue, migrate to other loci, and under the right conditions, differentiate into plasma cells and memory B cells.

Cisterna chyli—a small vesicular abdominal structure into which the intestinal trunks and lumbar trunks empty. The cisterna chyli is continued superiorly by the thoracic duct.

Edema—the accumulation of excess interstitial fluid – classically causing some localized or generalized swelling. It may occur in subcutaneous tissue or in various body cavities.

Germinal center (**of a lymphatic nodule**)—the lighter staining, central area of a lymphatic nodule within a lymph node. The stem cells for lymphocytogenesis are located therein and are actively dividing to form lymphocytes.

Lymph—interstitial fluid that has entered a lymphatic capillary. Lymph is the fluid in any lymphatic vessel and it re-enters the circulating bloodstream where the thoracic duct and the right lymphatic duct empty into the left and right brachiocephalic veins.

Lymphadenitis—inflammation of one or more lymph nodes – often those along the course of lymphatic drainage from a site of localized infection. Such lymph nodes enlarge and are often painful when gently pressured.

Lymphangitis—inflammation of lymphatic vessels. It sometimes results in red streaking on the skin surface.

Lymphatic nodule—a cluster of developing lymphocytes within a lymph node, tonsil, or within the intestinal wall. Developing lymphocytes produce antibodies.

Lymphatic trunk—any of the smallest named lymphatic vessels. Three of the lymphatic trunks drain into the right lymphatic duct and all of the others drain into the cisterna chyli or directly into the thoracic duct.

Lymph node—a small, spheroid organ occurring along the course of a lymphatic vessel. Lymph nodes contain developing lymphocytes in clusters called lymphatic nodules.

Lymphoma—neoplasia (cancer) of any lymphatic tissue. *Dorland's Medical Dictionary* has about 50 entries under lymphoma and most of the specific types are malignant.

Palatine tonsil—one of the four paired organs composed primarily of subepithelial lymphatic tissue located in the pharyngeal region (the others are lingual, pharyngeal, and tubal tonsils). Palatine tonsils are the only ones easily evaluated visually and they are removed during routine tonsillectomies.

Plasma hydrostatic pressure—the physical pressure exerted by blood pushing outward against the lining of a capillary. Systemic plasma hydrostatic pressure averages about 37 mm of Hg and tends to force water, electrolytes, and small organic molecules out through the capillary wall and into the interstitial space.

Plasma osmotic pressure—the pressure imparted by the "non-water" content of plasma (especially albumens) which tends to "draw" water into capillary lumina by osmosis. Plasma osmotic pressure averages about 25 mm Hg in systemic capillaries.

Red splenic pulp—the microscopic portion of the splenic parenchyma that has a reddish appearance due to blood within the splenic sinusoids. Red blood corpuscles forced through splenic sinusoids are often ruptured if they are already damaged or nearly worn out.

Right lymphatic duct—the smaller and shorter of the two lymphatic ducts. It is formed by the union of the right subclavian and right jugular trunks, and receives the right bronchomediastinal trunk before it empties into the right brachiocephalic vein.

Thoracic duct—the largest lymphatic vessel in the body. Coursing from the cisterna chyli to the left brachiocephalic vein, the thoracic duct is the termination for the left bronchomediastinal, left subclavian, and left jugular trunks, and (via the cisterna chyli) it also drains the intestinal and both lumbar trunks.

Tissue fluid—interstitial fluid, intercellular fluid. All extracellular fluid in the body (except for plasma, lymph, and secretory products) is tissue fluid.

T lymphocyte (**T cell**)—lymphocytes whose cytogenic ancestry includes the thymus. T cells are the cells primarily responsible for cell mediated immunity and are often subdivided into three groups: helper, killer, and suppressor T cells.

White splenic pulp—the microscopic part of the splenic parenchyma that consists of lymphatic nodules. It has a purple appearance with routine histological stains.

Etymology ***Persona non grata*** **—"An unwelcome guest."**

aden (G), *gland*—lymphadenitis
angi (G), *vessel*—lymphangitis
chylos (G), *juice*—cisterna chyli
cisterna (L), *box, chest*—cisterna chyli
ectomy (L), *surgical removal*—tonsillectomy
hydro (G), *water*—hydrostatic
itis (L), *inflammation*—tonsillitis
lympha (L), *water*—lymph
staticus (L), *static*—hydrostatic
thymus (G), *thymus gland*—thymus
tonsil (L), *tonsil*—tonsil

Introduction

The **lymphatic system** is a collection of organs containing groups of developing lymphocytes called lymphatic nodules and an extensive network of thin-walled lymphatic vessels that resemble veins in general structure. The lymphatic organs include lymph nodes, spleen, thymus, tonsils, and aggregations of lymphatic follicles (nodules) in the intestinal wall (Figure 16-1).

Functions

The lymphatic system **collects excess tissue fluid** (interstitial fluid, extracellular fluid) and returns it to the venous channels of the cardiovascular system. Because of this function, the lymphatic system is a functional subsidiary of the cardiovascular system and the two are often combined by those who prefer to "lump" systems together. When tissue fluid enters lymphatic vessels, it becomes lymph by definition. As the lymph is transported through the lymphatic channels, it filters through lymph nodes. These are aggregations of mature and developing lymphocytes (and monocytes), thus the lymphatic system **produces lymphocytes**. Lymphocytes **produce antibodies** (immunoglobulins) when exposed to antigens (foreign proteins) present in the lymph. These antibodies and the phagocytic monocytes produced in lymphatic organs are an important line of body defense. Another role of the lymphatic system is the **absorption of lipids** from the digestive system. Fats more readily enter the lymphatic capillaries within the intestinal villi than the capillaries of the cardiovascular system.

Objectives

1. List the components of the lymphatic system.
2. State the functions of the lymphatic system.

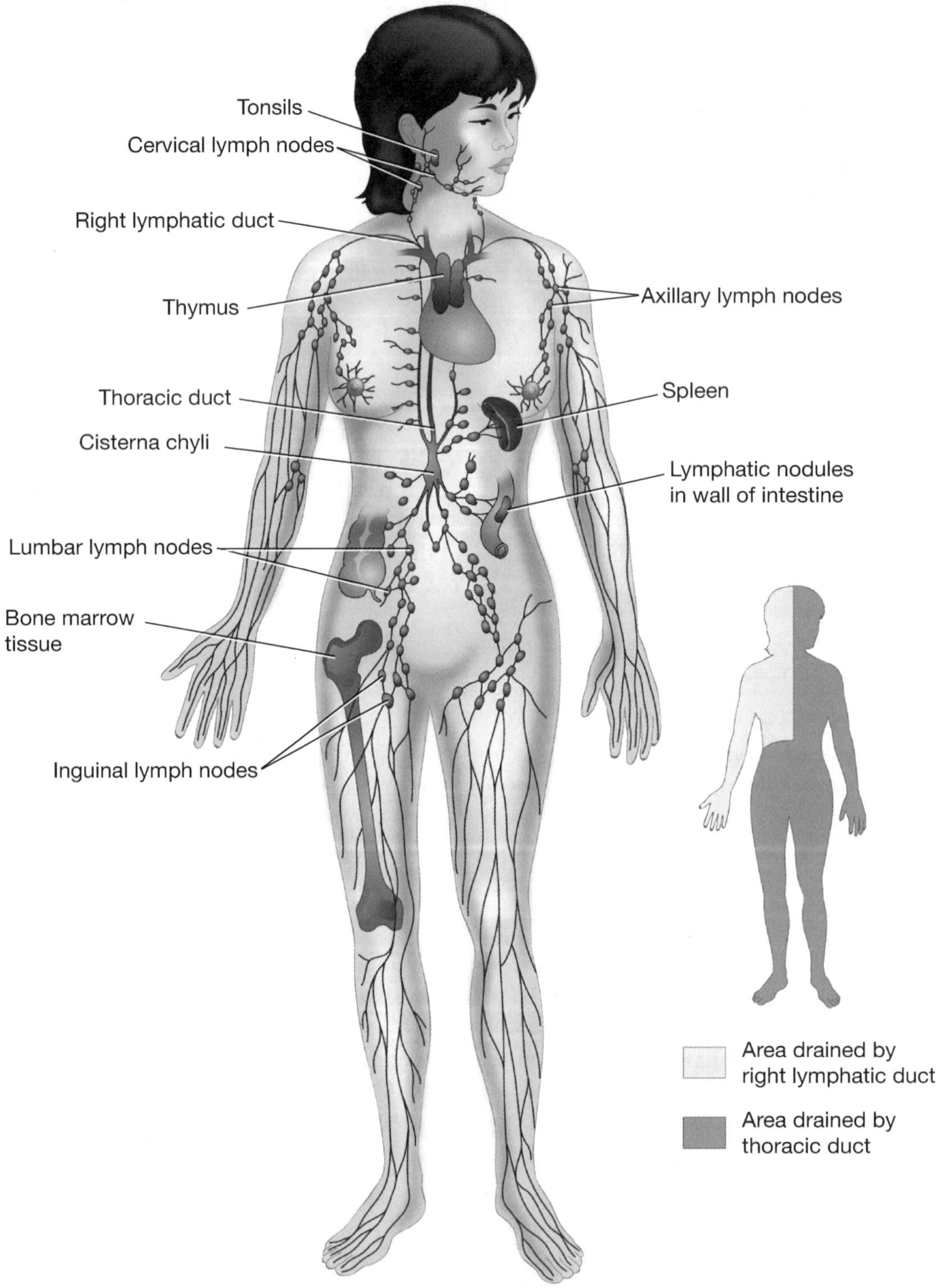

Figure 16-1

Components of the Lymphatic System

Lymphatic organs include lymph nodes, thymus, tonsils, spleen, subepithelial aggregations of lymphatic nodules in the intestinal wall, and a series of lymphatic vessels. Note that the lymphatic vessels draining the right half of the head, neck, and thorax, and those from the right superior limb drain into the right lymphatic duct. All other lymphatic drainage enters the thoracic duct.

Lymph Formation and Flow

Lymph and interstitial (tissue) fluid are two names for essentially the same substance. **Interstitial fluid** is the fluid within the intercellular (interstitial) matrix of the body. Because capillaries are porous they tend to "leak" a small percentage of the fluid portion of blood into the intercellular space. If this interstitial fluid is not drained away, an excess will build up and cause edema. The hemodynamics involved in the formation of interstitial fluid are illustrated in Figure 16-2. There are four pressures operating on blood within a capillary: plasma hydrostatic, plasma osmotic, interstitial fluid hydrostatic, and interstitial fluid osmotic pressure. **Plasma hydrostatic pressure** is the remaining physical pressure imparted to the blood by the contraction of the heart. At the capillary level it averages about 37 mm Hg and tends to force fluid through the capillary wall into the extracellular space. **Plasma osmotic pressure** is the pressure imparted by the blood albumins (primarily) which tends to "draw" water through the semi-permeable capillary wall into the lumen. It averages about 25 mm Hg in capillaries. The **interstitial fluid hydrostatic pressure** is a low (1-2 mm Hg) physical pressure which results from the presence of fluid already present in the extracellular space. It tends to move fluid back into the capillary lumen. **Interstitial fluid osmotic pressure** is a very weak (1 mm Hg) pressure due to the low concentration of solutes in the extracellular fluid. It tends to move fluid out of the capillaries. The net pressure which tends to move fluid out of capillaries is a simple summation of the two "out" pressures and the two "in" pressures. When any of these pressures are altered, circulatory disturbances such as edema (excessive accumulation of tissue fluid) may result. When excess tissue fluid enters lymphatic capillaries it is called **lymph** (Figure 16-3).

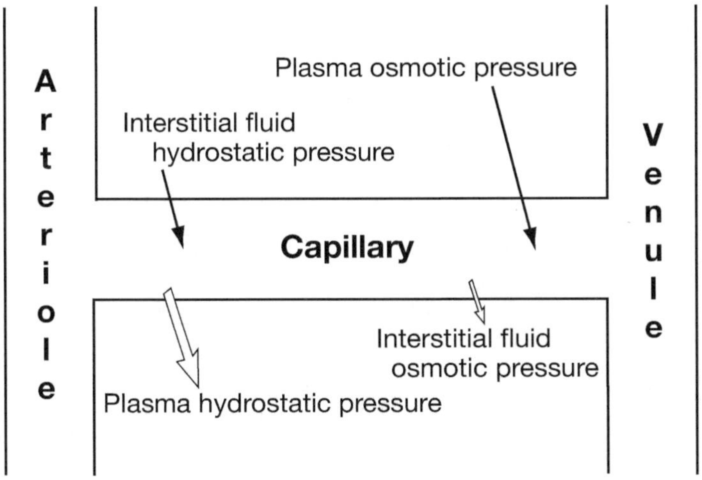

Plasma hydrostatic pressure	37 mm Hg (out)
Plasma osmotic pressure	25 mm Hg (in)
Interstitial fluid hydrostatic pressure	2 mm Hg (in)
Interstitial fluid osmotic pressure	1 mm Hg (out)
Net pressure	11 mm Hg (out)

Figure 16-2

Formation of Interstitial Fluid

There are four pressures acting on blood as it flows through a capillary. Plasma hydrostatic pressure and interstitial fluid osmotic pressure (white arrows) tend to move fluid out of a capillary into the intercellular space. Plasma osmotic pressure and interstitial fluid hydrostatic pressure (black arrows) tend to move fluid from the intercellular (interstitial) space back into a capillary. The net difference between the total of the two "in" pressures and the two "out" pressures (11 mm Hg out with the values shown here) explains why capillaries have a slight tendency to "leak" fluid into the intercellular space.

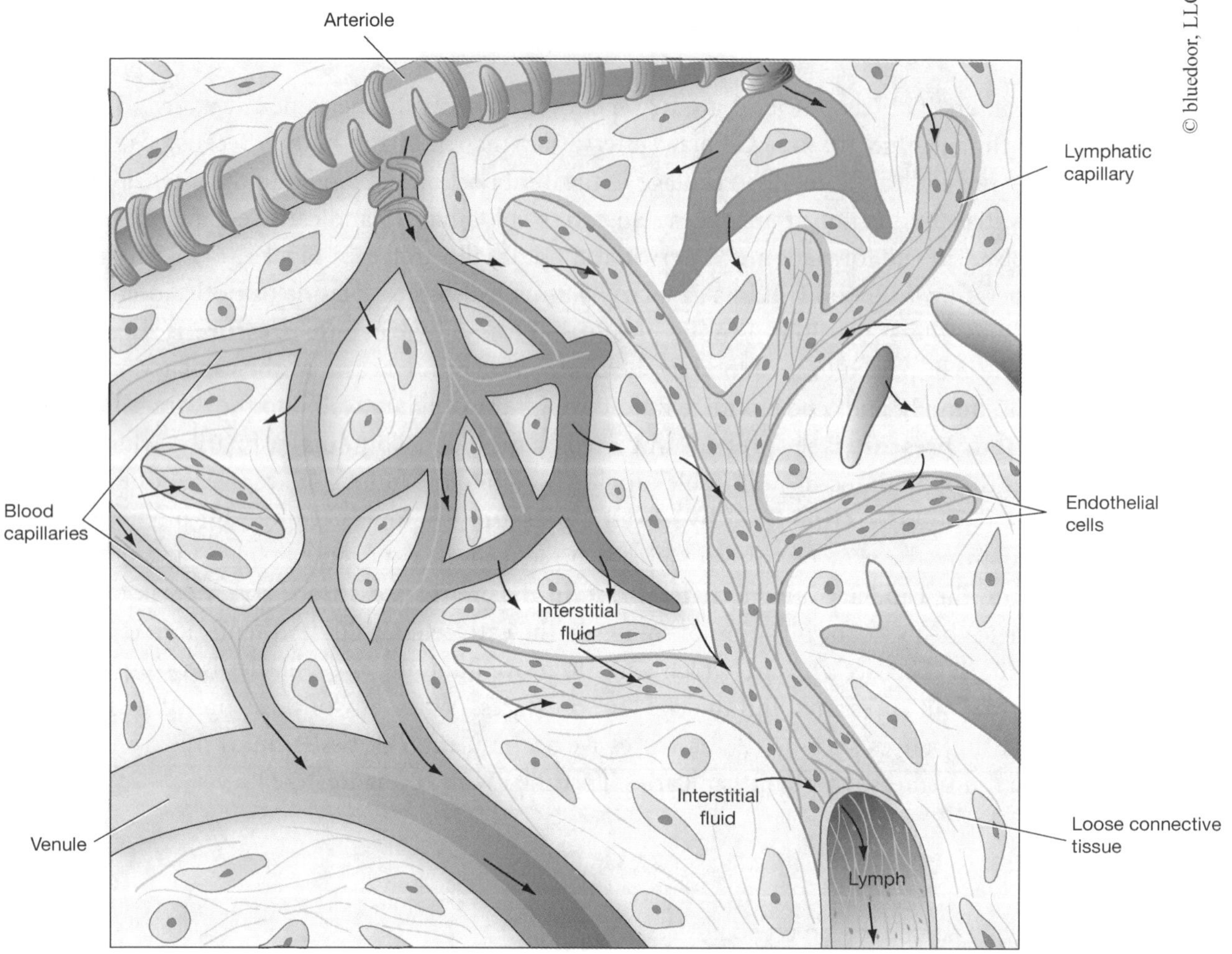

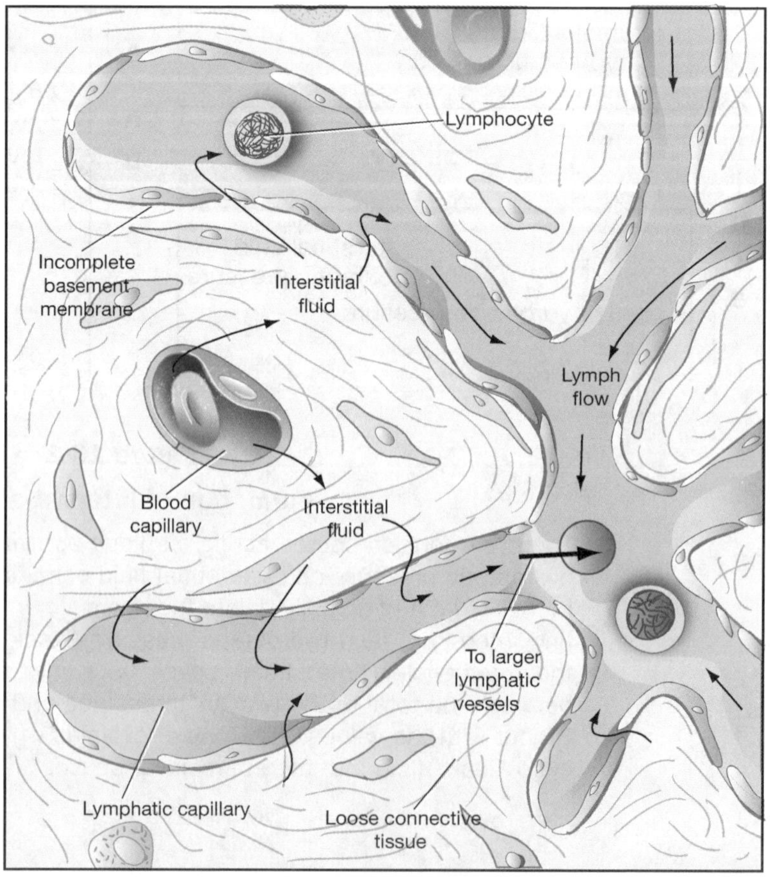

Figure 16-3

Absorption of Interstitial Fluid

Excess interstitial fluid formed by "leaking" through the blood capillary wall is absorbed into blind-ended lymphatic capillaries. After absorption, this fluid is called lymph and flows through a progressively larger series of lymphatic channels that ultimately enter either the right lymphatic duct or the thoracic duct. These ducts empty into the right and left brachiocephalic veins.

Objectives

3. Differentiate lymph from interstitial (extracellular) fluid.
4. Explain how lymph forms by discussing and quantifying the four pressures acting on fluid in and around capillaries.

Lymphatic Vessels

Lymphatic vessels include lymphatic capillaries and larger lymphatic vessels. **Lymphatic capillaries** are structurally similar to regular cardiovascular capillaries. However, they are blind-ended and drain into lymphatic vessels instead of venules (Figure 16-3). Essentially all vascularized tissues are permeated by lymphatic capillaries. As excess tissue fluid enters them by diffusing through their walls, it becomes **lymph**. Lymphatic capillaries within the intestinal villi called **central lymphatic vessels** ("lacteals") serve as absorption routes for lipids from the ingesta. The continued formation of lymph (passage of tissue fluid through the lymphatic capillary walls) forces that already present in vessels to flow centrally into larger lymphatic vessels. These resemble veins structurally, but have thinner walls, and they are not named. Some of those in the limbs have valves that prevent backflow. The lymphatic vessels drain into several named major lymphatic channels called **lymphatic trunks**. These include paired (left and right) lumbar trunks, bronchomediastinal trunks, subclavian trunks, jugular trunks, and a series of intestinal trunks. The left and right **lumbar trunks** receive lymphatic vessels draining the inferior limbs, pelvic walls and viscera, large intestine, kidneys, and adrenal glands. The **intestinal trunks** receive lymphatic vessels from the liver, stomach, spleen, pancreas, and small intestine. Lymphatic vessels draining the lungs empty into the left and right **bronchomediastinal trunks**. The major lymphatic channels draining the superior limbs are the left and right **subclavian trunks**. The head is drained by the left and right **jugular trunks**. The lymphatic trunks coalesce to form two main lymphatic vessels: thoracic duct and right lymphatic duct. The **thoracic duct** is the largest lymphatic vessel in the body. It begins in the abdomen as a vesicular enlargement called the **cisterna chyli** near the level of the second lumbar vertebra, into which the lumbar and intestinal lymphatic trunks open. The thoracic duct courses superiorly along the aorta through the aortic hiatus of the diaphragm and empties into the left brachiocephalic vein near the confluence of the internal jugular and subclavian veins. En route, it receives the left bronchomediastinal, left subclavian, and left jugular trunks. The **right lymphatic duct** is considerably smaller than the thoracic duct and is only 2–3 cm long. It is formed by the union of the right subclavian and right jugular lymphatic trunks and receives the right bronchomediastinal trunk before it empties into the right brachiocephalic vein (Figure 16-4).

Objectives

5. Compare a lymphatic capillary to a typical cardiovascular capillary.
6. Name the lymphatic trunks and indicate which ones drain into the thoracic duct and which three drain into the right lymphatic duct.

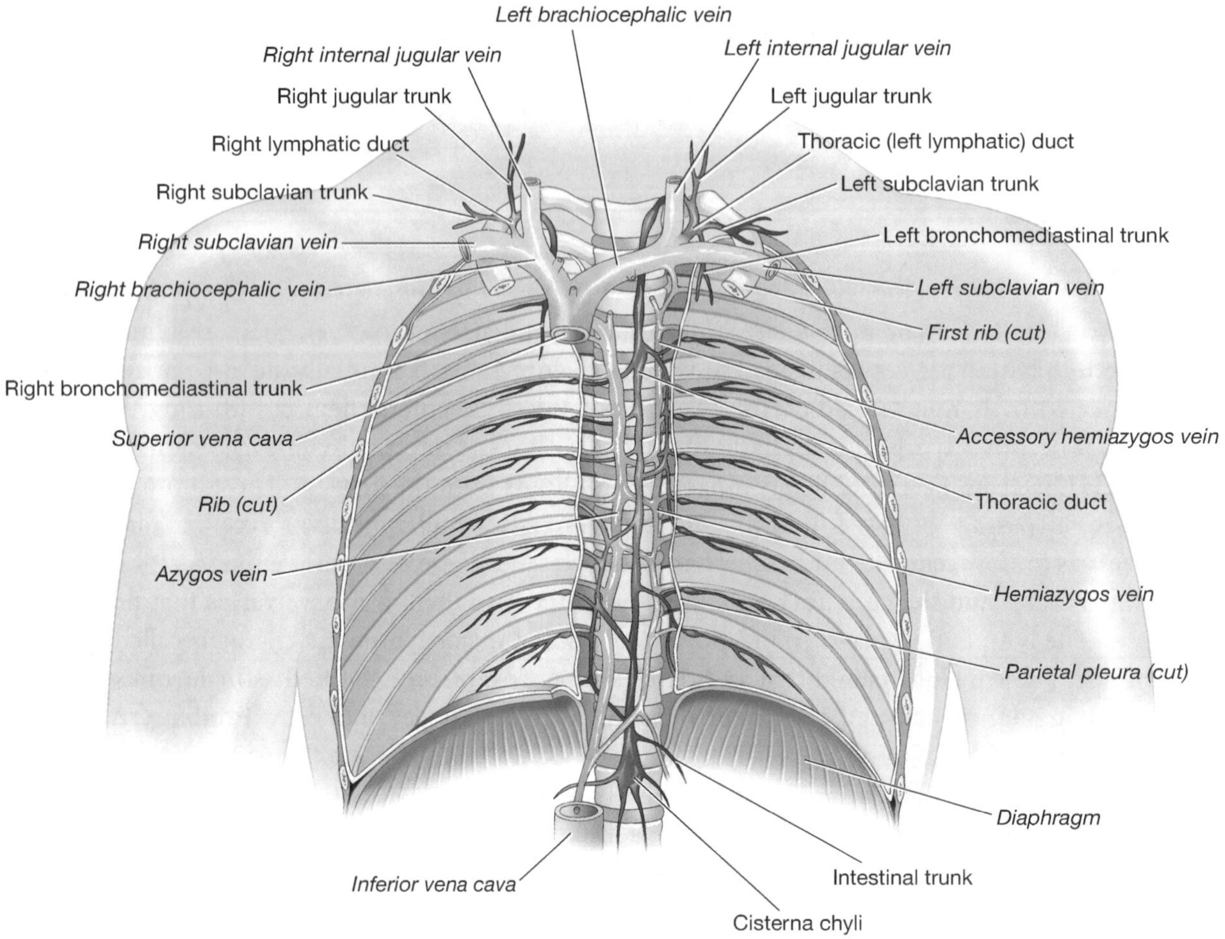

Figure 16-4

Thoracic Duct, Right Lymphatic Duct and Lymphatic Trunks

The thoracic duct is the largest lymphatic vessel in the body. It carries lymph from the inferior limbs, abdomen, left superior limb, and left half of the head, neck, and thorax. The right lymphatic duct carries lymph from the remainder of the body (right side of the head, neck, thorax, and right superior limb). Both of these lymphatic vessels drain into the systemic venous system via the left and right brachiocephalic veins formed by the convergence of the ipsilateral internal jugular and subclavian veins.

Lymphatic Organs

In addition to lymphatic vessels, the lymphatic system includes lymph nodes, spleen, thymus, tonsils, and subepithelial aggregations of lymphatic nodules. All of these latter organs contain groups of developing lymphocytes (Figure 16-6). When mature, these lymphocytes become circulating lymphocytes, but during development they produce large quantities of antibodies (gamma globulins).

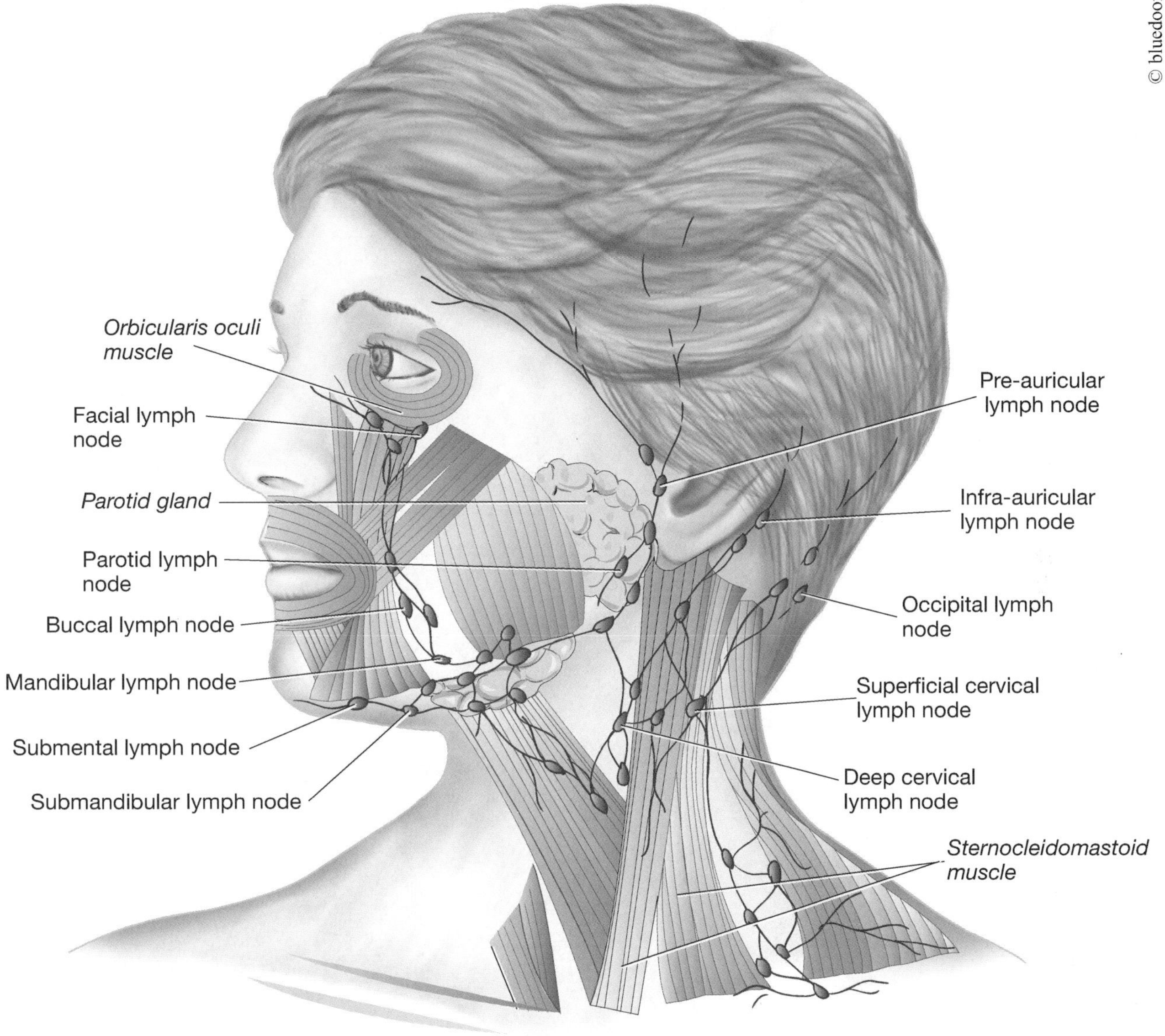

Figure 16-5
Lymph Nodes and Lymphatic Drainage

Lymph nodes are spheroid or bean-shaped structures which lie along the course of lymphatic vessels (Figure 16-1). They consist of a capsule of dense irregular connective tissue proper surrounding numerous groups of developing lymphocytes called **lymphatic nodules** (Figure 16-7). The younger (more recently formed) lymphocytes near the middle of each lymphatic nodule form a lighter staining area called the **germinal center**. More mature, terminally differentiated lymphocytes near the periphery of the nodule are called plasma cells and actively produce antibodies. The outermost of these cells eventually lose their connections to the reticular connective tissue framework of the lymph node. They flow with the lymph into the circulating bloodstream to become circulating lymphocytes. **Trabeculae** of connective tissue proper extend inward from the capsule and

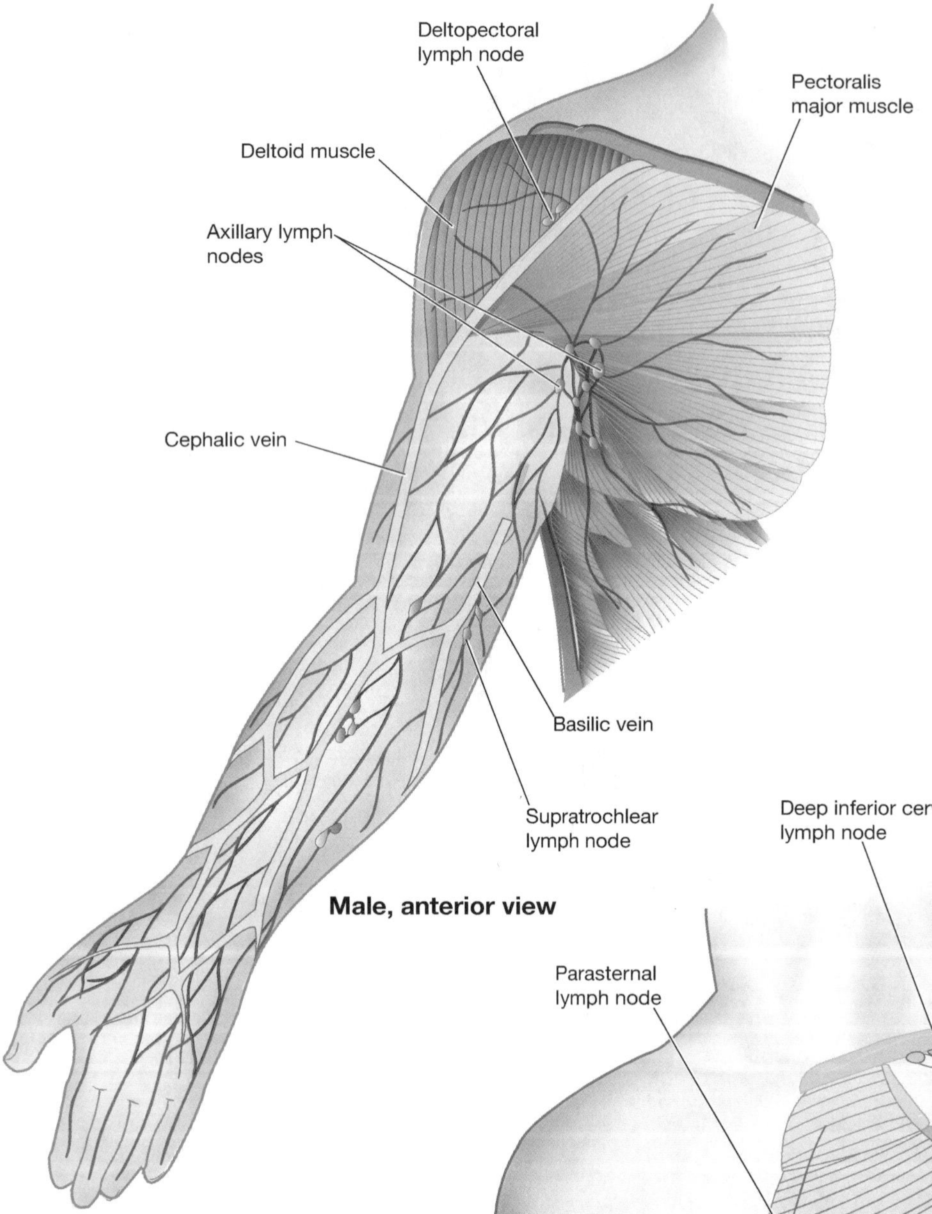

Male, anterior view

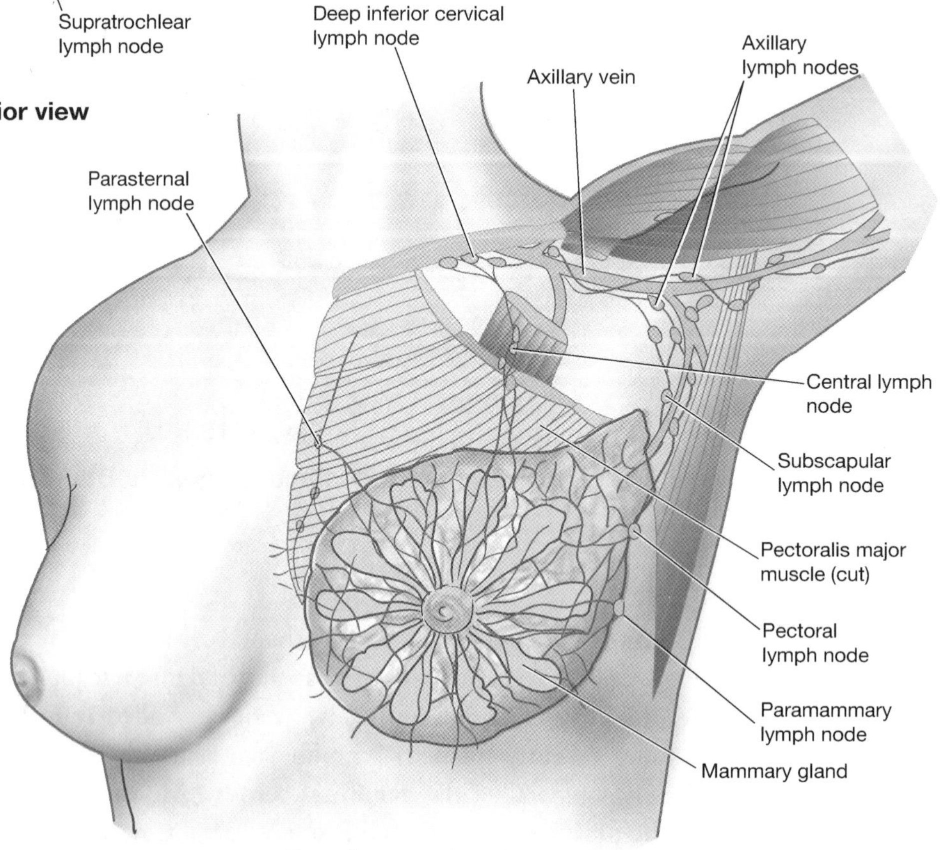

Female, anterior view

Figure 16-5 *(continued)*

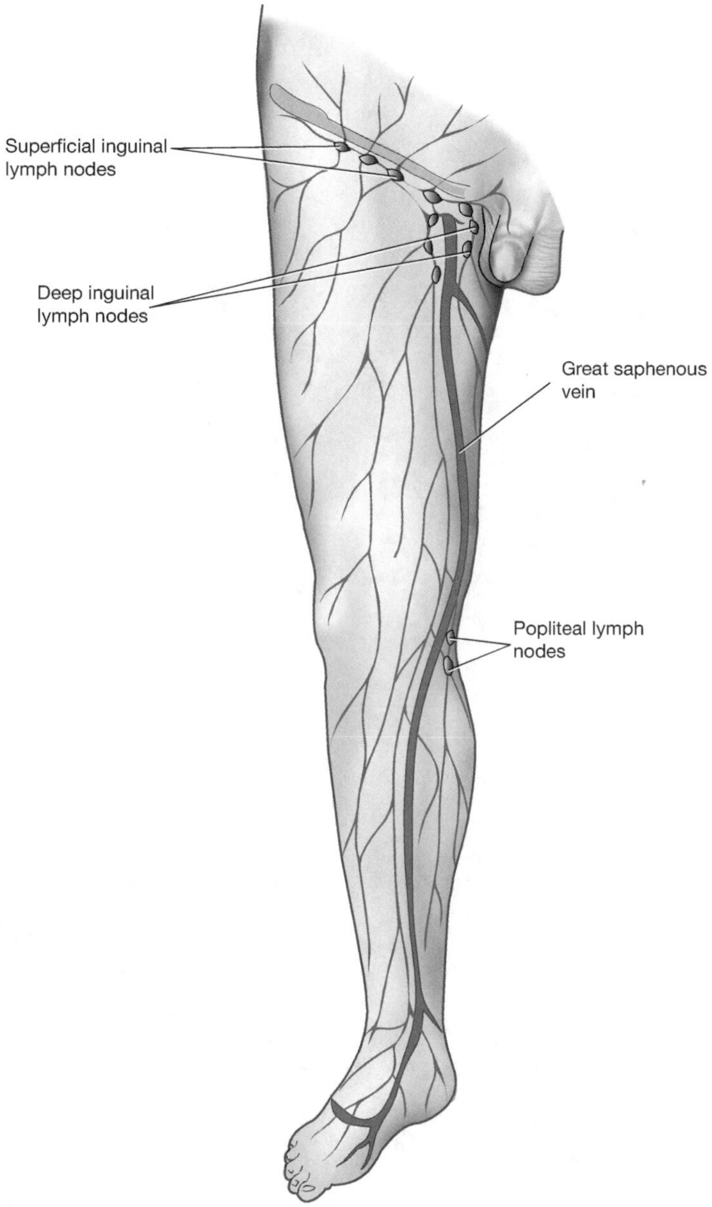

Figure 16-5 *(continued)*

separate some of the nodules from each other. Several **afferent** (incoming) **lymphatic vessels** pass through the convex surface of the lymph node and one or two **efferent** (outgoing) **lymphatic vessels** leave at a depression called the **hilum**. As lymph flows through a lymph node, it exposes the developing lymphocytes to foreign material (antigens) and induces the production of antibodies (immunoproteins, gamma globulins). Lymph typically encounters more than one lymph node as it flows back toward the venous system. These are named according to their location and about two hundred have been catalogued. Some of them are so small that they are essentially microscopic. Lymph nodes are important clinically for several reasons. Because of their significant enlargement in response to some pathogens, they are important indicators of infection. Judging the "normal size" of a lymph node, however, presents a difficult diagnostic problem because there is no absolute norm. There can be considerable size variation in specific lymph nodes between individuals and variations

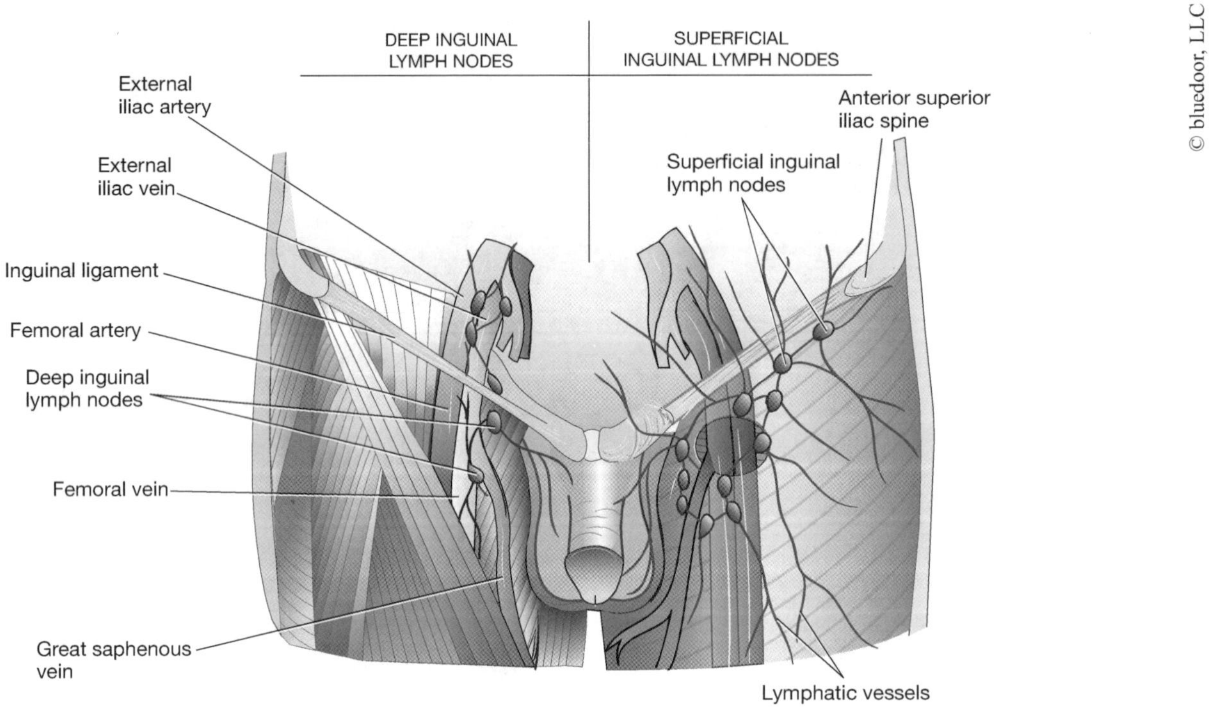

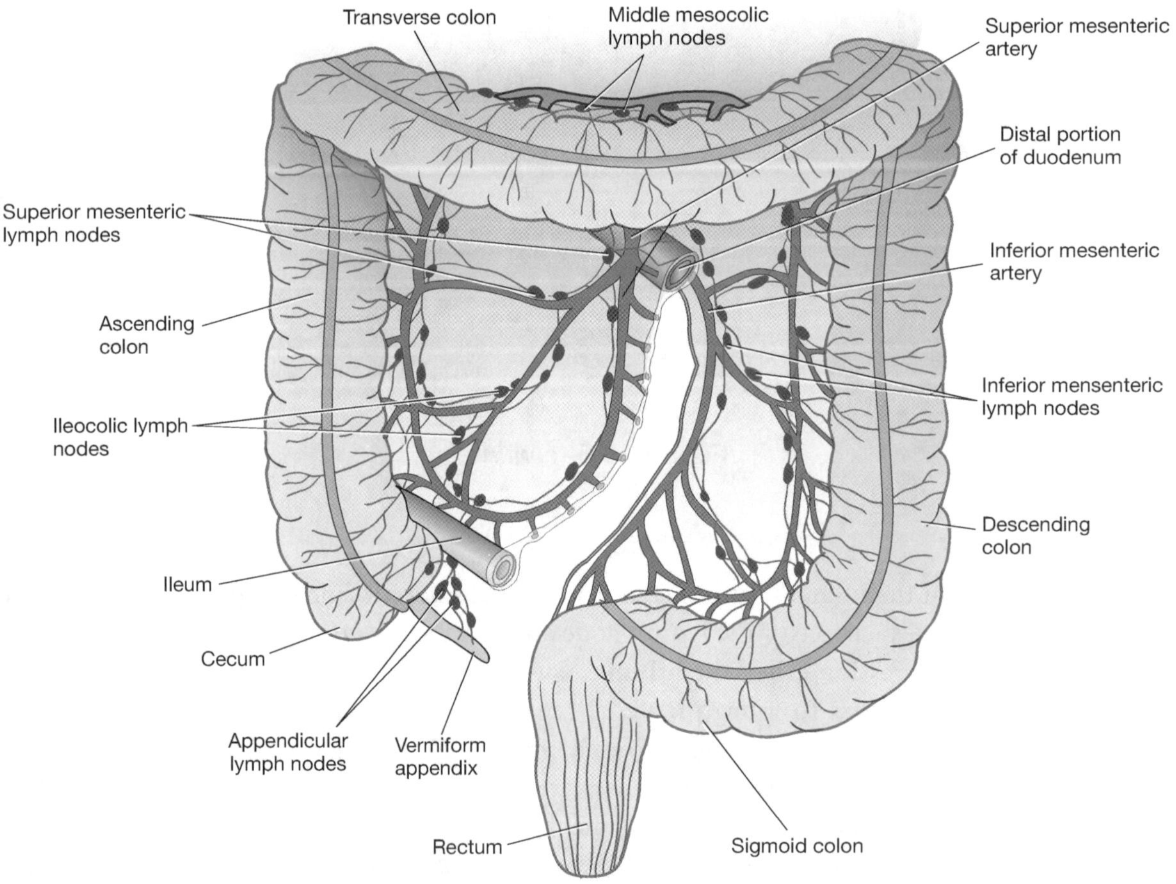

Figure 16-5 *(continued)*

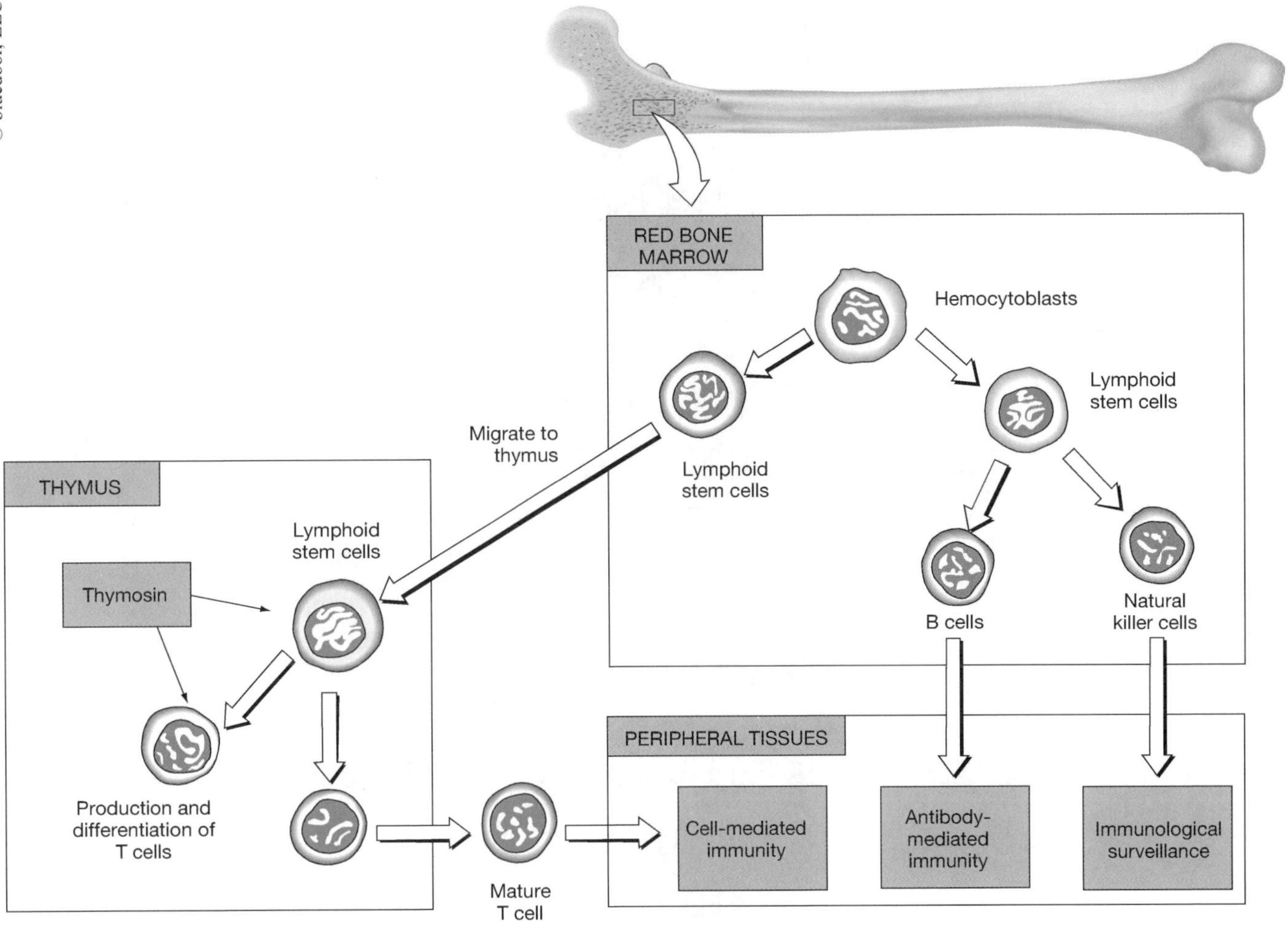

Figure 16-6
Derivation of Lymphocytes

Lymphocytes are derived from hemocytoblastic precursors in bone marrow tissue. Some of the lymphoid stem cells remain for a time in the bone marrow giving rise to cells that produce B lymphocytes and natural killer cells. Other lymphoid stem cells originate in the thymus and their derivatives become T lymphocytes.

even occur between left and right sides. Infectious organisms and neoplastic cells carried by lymph may be trapped in lymph nodes and initiate metastases. Lymph nodes that are so affected are often painful and undergo significant enlargement.

The **spleen** is the largest single lymphatic organ and is positioned in the left superior quadrant of the abdomen along the lateral aspect of the greater curvature of the stomach (Figure 16-8). The spleen is flattened and elongated with diaphragmatic and visceral surfaces, anterior and posterior extremities, and superior and inferior borders. Blood vessels, lymphatic vessels, and nerves attach to a linear hilum on the visceral surface. The spleen is surrounded by a fibrous connective tissue capsule containing smooth muscle tissue. The parenchyma of the spleen contains many lymphatic nodules and phagocytic cells interspersed within reticular connective tissue. Histologically, the areas occupied by lymphatic nodules are called white pulp and the remainder of the splenic parenchyma

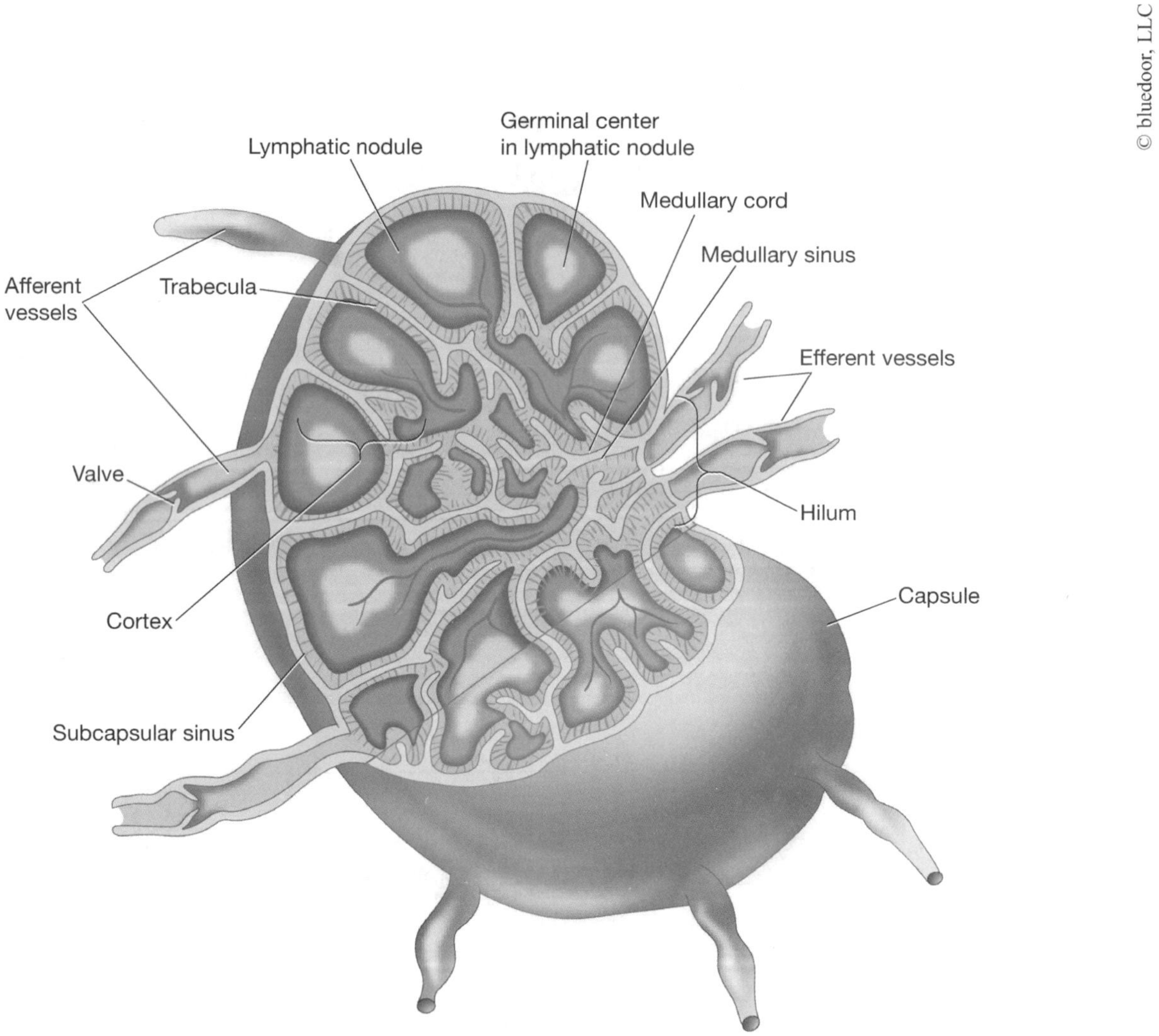

Figure 16-7

Structure of a Lymph Node

Lymph nodes occur along the course of lymphatic vessels. Several afferent (incoming) lymphatic vessels penetrate the capsule and one or two efferent (outgoing) lymphatic vessels leave a depressed area called the hilum. As lymph flows through the node, it percolates around the lymphatic nodules. This exposes the developing lymphocytes to antigens so that they can produce appropriate antibodies. As lymphocytes mature, they leave with the outgoing lymph to become circulating lymphocytes in the blood.

is called red pulp. Splenic phagocytes act as blood "filters" and are especially active in removing worn out erythrocytes from the circulation. Because of its high degree of vascularity, the spleen is said to "store" red blood corpuscles. The smooth muscle in the capsule enables it to contract in cases of hypovolemic shock, thus adding these erythrocytes to the general circulation. In about ten percent of the population, one or more separate splenic bodies called **accessory spleens** are located in the greater omentum near the spleen.

The **thymus** is a lymphoid organ located in the lower cervical and upper mediastinal regions

(Figure 16-9). It functions in early life to establish normal immunological competency. It reaches its largest size at puberty and rapidly involutes (regresses) thereafter. The thymus consists of left and right lobes within a connective tissue capsule. The cells within the thymus are called thymocytes. They are believed to be derived from bone marrow and fetal liver precursor cells. After spending time in the thymus they "seed" other lymphatic organs and their progeny become specialized circulating lymphocytes called T lymphocytes. The thymus produces a hormone called **thymosin** which is believed to activate these lymphocytes and/or their precursors. Histologically, the thymus contains localized spherical or ovoid bodies composed of concentric layers of epithelial cells containing keratohyalin and bundles of cytoplasmic filaments. These are called thymic corpuscles (Hassall's corpuscles) and their significance remains unknown.

Tonsils are subepithelial aggregations of lymphoid tissue in the pharyngeal region (Figure 16-10). They include palatine, pharyngeal, tubal, and lingual tonsils. The **palatine tonsils** are located in the lateral walls of the fauces (gullet) and can be easily observed using a mirror. They are the ones typically enlarged in "tonsillitis" and are removed during tonsillectomies. The **pharyngeal tonsils** are groups of lymphatic nodules embedded in the posterior wall of the nasopharynx. The term *adenoid* can variously mean a pharyngeal tonsil or hypertrophy thereof. The **tubal tonsils** are collections of lymphatic nodules near the pharyngeal openings of the auditory tubes. **Lingual tonsils** are similar aggregations under the dorsal surface of the posterior aspect of the tongue. Subepithelial lymphoid tissue is also found in the intestinal wall. These collections of lymphatic nodules are officially named **aggregations of lymphatic nodules** but they are also known as "Peyer's patches", "intestinal tonsils", and MALT (mucosa-associated lymphatic tissue) (Figure 16-11). These are more common in the large intestine than in the small, and within the latter, they are more common in the ileum than in the duodenum or jejunum.

Objectives

7. Sketch and label the components of a lymph node.
8. Structurally differentiate the spleen from a lymph node.
9. State the unusual features of the thymus and name the specialized cells of its parenchyma.
10. Name the four groups of tonsils. Which of these are easiest to detect using a mirror?

Development of Lymphatic Organs

The thymus initially develops during the fifth week of gestation from the ventral parts of the left and right third pharyngeal pouches (Figure 16-12). There is also a small contribution from the ventral parts of the fourth pharyngeal pouches. The two thymic primordia migrate medially and posteriorly into the thorax and fuse. A slender stalk of the thymic tissue left behind in this migration breaks up into small fragments which usually disappear. Sometimes they remain embedded in the thyroid gland or as isolated thymic nests.

The splenic primordium appears during the fifth week of gestation as a mesenchymal condensation between the doubled peritoneum supporting the stomach (mesogastrium). It bulges into the left part of the peritoneal cavity and remains close to the stomach as it develops further.

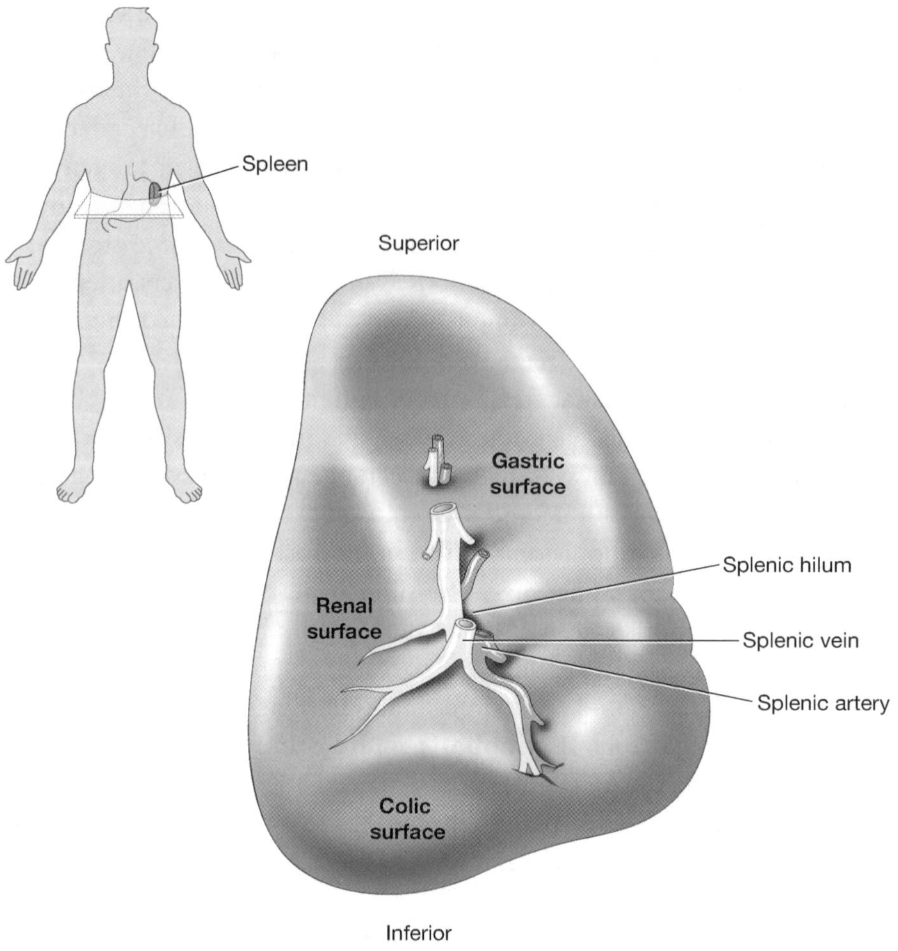

Figure 16-8
Spleen

The spleen varies in absolute dimensions but averages about 5 cm wide and 12 cm long. The visceral surface of the spleen is officially subdivided into renal, colic, and gastric surfaces corresponding to the organs that they contact. The splenic artery supplies numerous branches to the stomach as well as several branches which enter the splenic hilum. This arborization complicates splenectomies since several vessels must be separately ligated (tied off) and severed before the spleen can be removed.

The lymphatic vasculature was originally believed to be formed by venous branches. Later evidence has indicated that it develops from clefts in the mesenchyme (primitive connective tissue) which connect to the venous channels secondarily. The cells lining the clefts become flattened endothelial cells and the clefts fuse to form an arborizing system of lymphatic channels. Dilation of the abdominal portion of a retroperitoneal lymphatic channel forms the cisterna chyli. The thoracic duct and the right lymphatic duct form from two large lymphatic channels called the (embryonic) right and left thoracic ducts. Eventually, the adult thoracic duct develops from the inferior portion of the embryonic right thoracic duct, an anastomosis between the embryonic right and left thoracic ducts, and the superior portion of the embryonic left thoracic duct. The adult right lymphatic duct

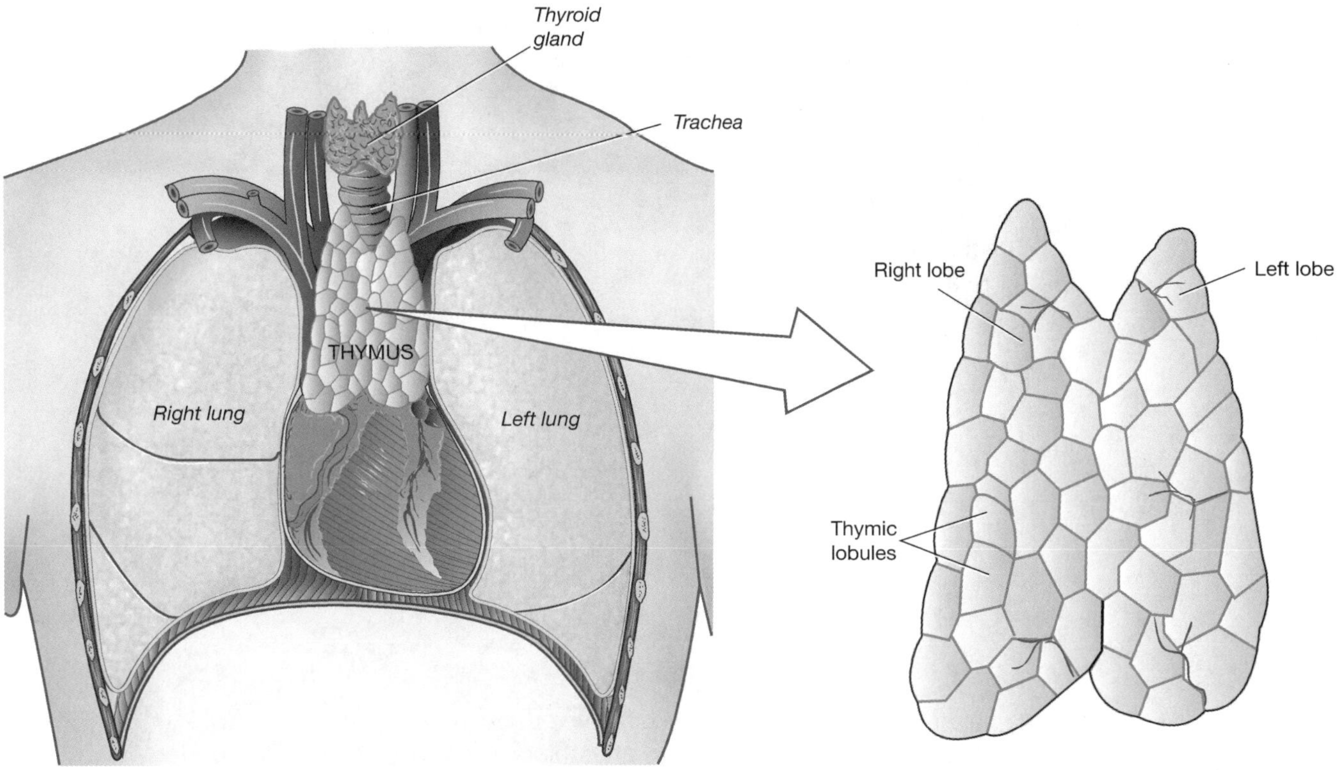

Figure 16-9

Thymus

The thymus reaches its largest size at puberty and decreases in size by an atrophic process called involution. The right and left lobes of the thymus eventually become indistinguishable and form a single mass located superior to the convergence of the left and right brachiocephalic veins.

is developed from the superior portion of the embryonic right thoracic duct. The lymph nodes appear during the third month of development along the course of the lymphatic vessels.

The palatine tonsils develop initially from the left and right second pharyngeal pouches. An invasion of mesoderm is followed by infiltration of lymphatic tissue during the third to fifth months of gestation. The tubal tonsils develop from aggregations of lymph nodules around the pharyngeal opening of the auditory tubes. The pharyngeal tonsils (adenoids) develop from an aggregation of lymph nodules in the wall of the nasopharynx. The lingual tonsils develop from lymphatic nodules embedded in the root of the tongue.

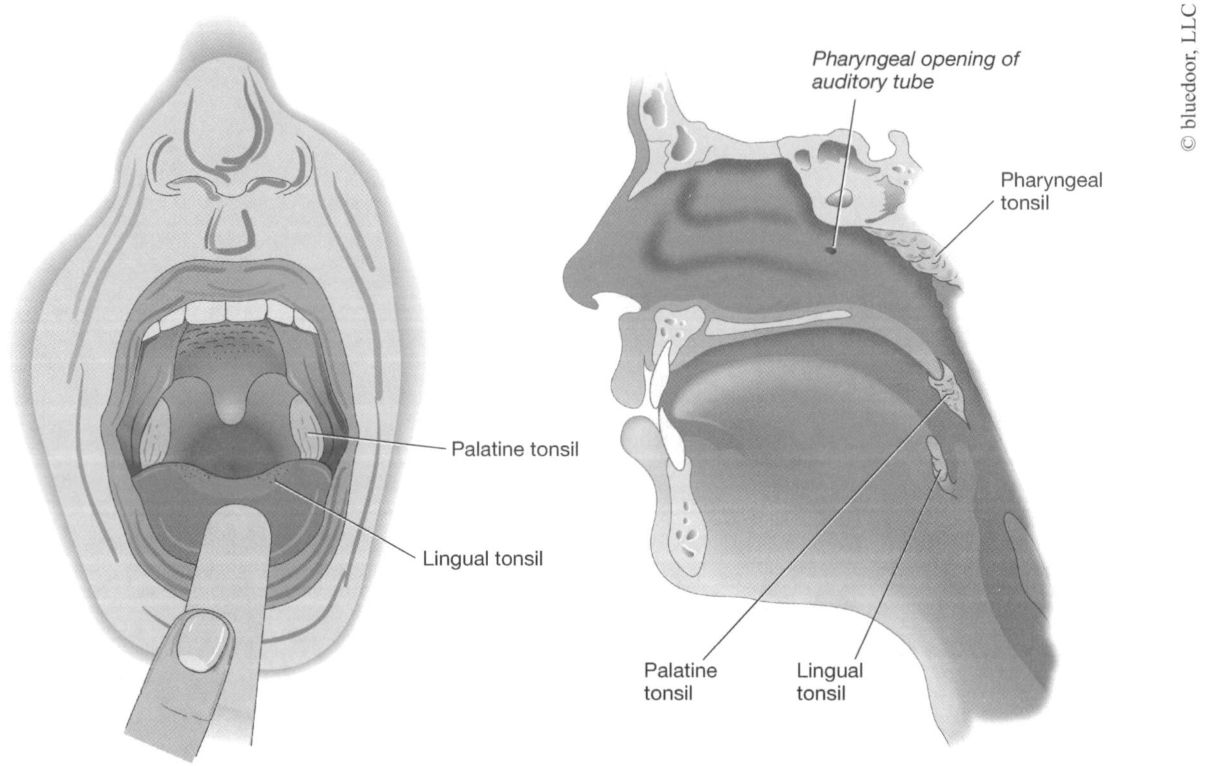

Figure 16-10

Tonsils

Only the palatine tonsils can be easily observed through the open mouth. They are removed during routine tonsillectomies and enlarged pharyngeal tonsils are often resected, as well. The lingual tonsils at the base of the tongue and the tubal tonsils (buried in the soft tissue around the openings of the auditory tubes) have little surgical significance.

Objectives

11. State the primary germ layer that gives rise to most lymphatic components.

Clinical Considerations

The normal flow of lymph can be disturbed by a number of conditions. When excess interstitial fluid collects in the tissues, localized or generalized swelling occurs and the condition is called **edema**. There are several general causes of edema and over thirty specific types have been recognized. In malnourished individuals or those with certain types of liver diseases, lowered levels of blood proteins (especially albumins) can result in reduced plasma osmotic pressure. This leads to excessive movement of plasma fluids outward through the capillary walls. Increased permeability of capillary walls from physical trauma can also lead to edema. Physical obstruction of lymphatic drainage causes edema and may involve conditions as innocuous as socks with elastic bands that are

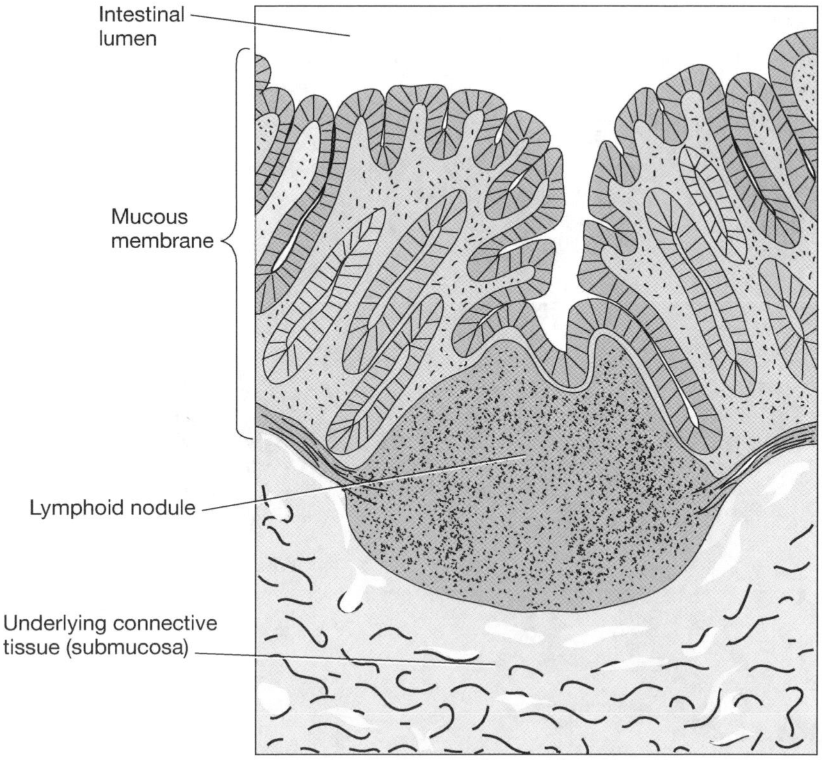

Figure 16-11

Subepithelial Aggregations of Lymphatic Nodules

Lymphatic nodules adjacent to the intestinal epithelium appear in the small intestinal wall and progressively increase in number in the lower part of the alimentary canal.

too tight to serious parasitic diseases such as gnathostomiasis or elephantiasis. Even heart failure can cause edema by changing the hydrostatic pressures in various parts of the cardiovascular system.

The fact that lymph nodes often trap neoplastic cells may temporarily halt or slow the spread of some cancerous conditions. Regional lymph nodes are often removed during cancer surgeries to ensure that any entrapped cancer cells are removed as well. Lymphatic tissue itself may become neoplastic. This condition is called **lymphoma** and includes several specific syndromes. Most of them are malignant.

Inflammation of lymph nodes is called **lymphadenitis**. Inflamed nodes enlarge and are often painful. Once enlarged, they often remain quite prominent for several months and may never return to their former size. Chronic inflammation may lead to abscess formation. If lymphatic vessels are inflamed, the condition is called **lymphangitis** and may result in red linear streaking visible on the surface of the skin. This is the classic "blood poisoning" syndrome.

The spleen is sometimes ruptured (severely traumatized) by sharp blows to the abdomen. In fact, the spleen is the abdominal organ most frequently injured from trauma. When ruptured, it bleeds profusely. Fortunately, the spleen is not a vital organ and may be removed without serious consequence because its functions are assumed by other reticuloendothelial organs. In children and adolescents, however, repair of a ruptured spleen is preferable to removal because of its role in anti-

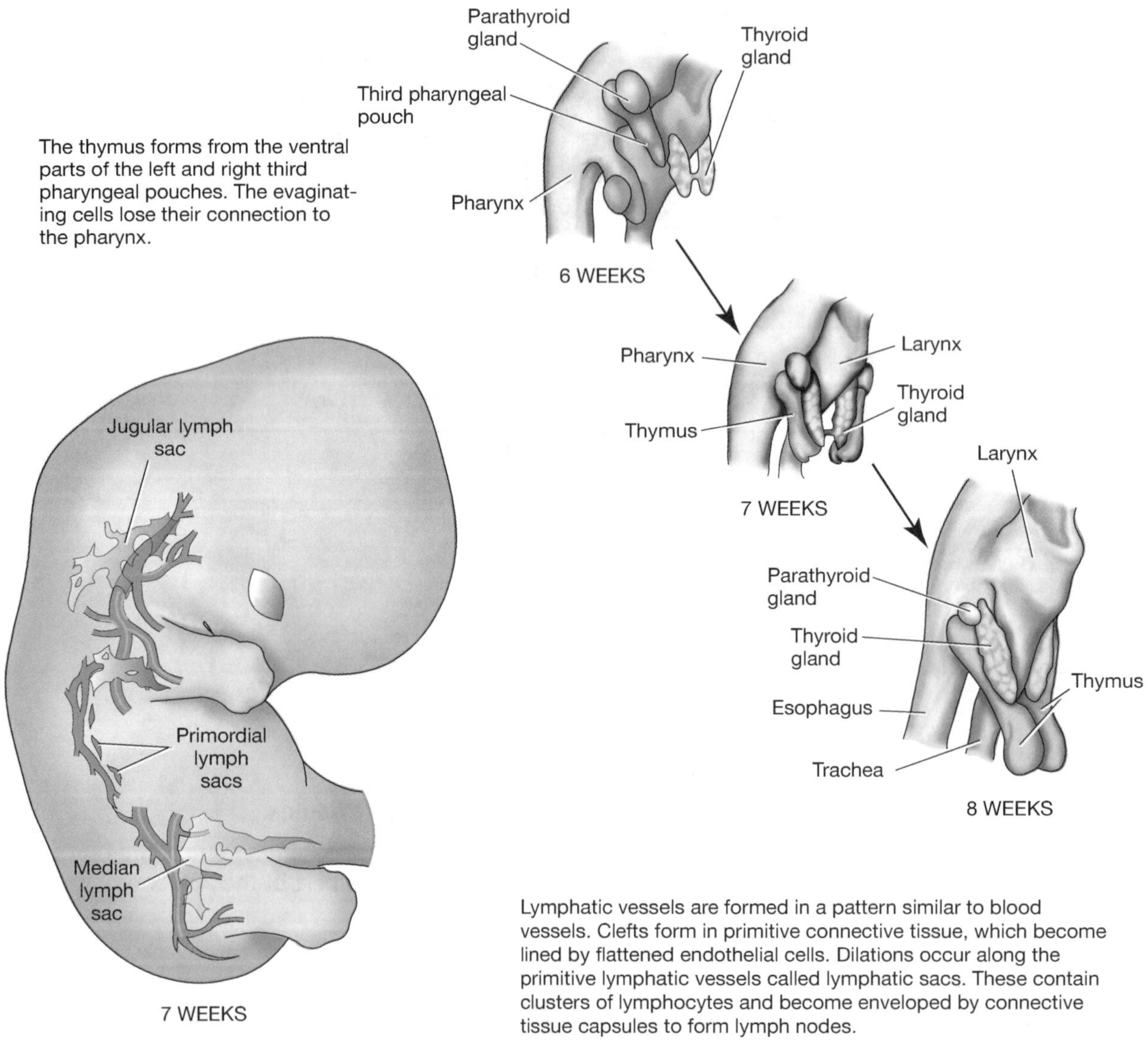

Figure 16-12
Development of the Lymphatic System

body production. When the spleen is diseased, it may enlarge to 10 times (or more) of its normal size. This enlargement is called **splenomegaly**.

Tumors of the thymus are rare, usually benign, and are called **thymomas**. They may compress the trachea and cause dyspnea or coughing. Compression of the superior vena cava may also occur causing blood to engorge the veins of the neck and head.

Recurring bouts of **tonsillitis** in a patient may cause the attending physician to recommend a **tonsillectomy**. Considerable hemorrhage often occurs during this surgery, especially in adults. Enlargement of the pharyngeal tonsils (adenoids) can obstruct the movement of air so severely that patients may be forced to breath through the mouth. If tubal tonsils become involved, the openings of the auditory tubes may be blocked by the swelling. **Otitis media** may result from this blockage.

When developing lymphocytes (plasma cells) are first exposed to a foreign protein (antigen) they begin producing gamma globulins (antibodies) that cross react with those proteins. This initial antibody output, called the **primary antibody response**, requires several days to develop and the total antibody output is relatively low. Thus, even though antibodies are produced, this response is typically "too little and too late" to prevent the progression of the disease. However, once exposed to a particular antigen in this manner, a subsequent exposure (weeks, months, years later) will result in a **secondary antibody response** which produces many more antibodies and only requires a few hours to occur. This quicker production and larger antibody output are usually sufficient to prevent the disease. Standard vaccination procedures use an injection of killed or attenuated microorganisms to produce a primary response. Subsequent exposure to virulent strains of the same organism do not result in development of the disease because a secondary immunological response occurs.

Immunity implies resistance to disease and there are many specific subtypes. **Innate immunity** occurs when one species simply is not susceptible to certain diseases of another species. Humans, for example, are innately immune to canine distemper (the disease just doesn't occur in humans). **Non–specific immunity** includes such factors as fever (elevated body temperature), phagocytosis, and interferon production. Interferons are proteins produced by the body during viral infections. They effectively prevent other kinds of viral infections from occurring simultaneously. **Passive immunity** results from the presence of antibodies in the bloodstream that the individuals did not produce themselves. Examples include the transfer of antibodies from mother to neonate through the colostrum (first milk) as well as the injection of gamma globulins into individuals who have recently been exposed to an infectious disease (like hepatitis C) to which they are not immune. **Natural immunity** results from exposure to or development of an infectious disease. **Active immunity** refers to the presence of circulating antibodies that individuals themselves produce in response to exposure to an antigen (either through a vaccination or clinical exposure). **Humoral immunity** implies that antibodies are present regardless of their original source. **Cell-mediated immunity** is that attributable to T lymphocytes which can occur through their release of lymphokines or through direct attack by the so-called "killer T cells".

Autoimmune diseases include several syndromes in which antibodies are produced that react with an individual's own proteins. These can occur when antibodies produced in response to foreign antigens occasionally cross-react with an individual's own proteins. It can also occur when one develops antibodies against one's own tissue that is not normally exposed to the bloodstream (lens of the eye, thyroglobulin, sperm). Autoimmune diseases can also occur when foreign antigens combine with one's own proteins and antibodies are produced that cross react with the "self" part of that combination. Finally, antibodies are sometimes produced in response to newly formed antibodies, themselves (which the body mistakenly considers to be "foreign").

Objectives

12. Define edema and state several causes.
13. Differentiate lymphadenitis from lymphangitis.
14. Define primary and secondary antibody response, and innate, active, and passive immunity.

Clinical Case Studies

Case 1—A teenager, failing to wear a seat-belt, was thrown up against the steering wheel during a car accident. In the emergency room, his blood pressure dipped precariously low and results of an abdominal puncture (paracentesis) demonstrated the presence of free blood in the peritoneal cavity. The emergency room physician sent him to surgery. Why?

Case 2—A few days after suffering a deep puncture wound to the instep of her foot, a young woman noticed some faint, linear red streaks extending up her leg. The original wound remained painful due to an infection. What caused the red streaks?

Case 3—A few days after the onset of a severe sore throat, a high school basketball player noticed firm, palpable lumps on the lateral aspects of his neck. They were moderately painful when digital pressure was applied. What could cause these enlargements?

Points to Ponder

Often dubbed the "immune" system, the lymphatic system is a better name because not all of its functions involve immunity, and also because some of the immune responses (like phagocytosis) may involve cells from other systems. Some of the misconceptions about lymphatic organs have an air of truth. The spleen is often said to store RBC's—probably because contraction of its smooth muscle capsule, brought on by epinephrine, will force its blood content back into the general circulation. In the process, some of these RBC's, relentlessly squeezed, will rupture as they are forced through the splenic pulp—just as a balloon will eventually burst when played with by kids. The weaker RBC's—those worn thin by previous weeks of rubbing shoulders with the endothelial cells lining the blood vessels—are most likely to break. A marvelous way to get rid of the old to make way for new ones.

When India ink (a suspension of microscopic carbon particles) is injected subcutaneously into an animal, the particles will enter the lymphatic vessels and color both them and the lymph nodes along their course a startling black color. Likewise, bacteria that worm their way into the lymphatic vessels are trapped in the next lymph node they encounter. There, phagocytes, the cellular "hit men" of the microbial world, engulf them in an untimely end, and developing lymphocytes and plasma cells manufacture antibodies that coat and identify them as well as any future cousins that may attempt an invasion. The alternative (sometimes happens) is that the invaders will get through all the lymph nodes and end up in the circulating blood. Blood, like the blood agar down in the microbiology lab, is a great nutritional medium for bacterial growth. The next few hours after a bacterial septicemia has been seeded will determine if the body defenses, led by phagocytes and antibodies, will react faster than the bacteria can reproduce themselves. Septicemias are scary.

Why does one typically suffer certain diseases, like chicken pox, only once? A child without immunity exposed to the virus will begin producing antibodies via lymphocytes and plasma cells within a few days. Unfortunately, this initial antibody output, called the primary response, takes too long to develop and results in too few antibodies to prevent the disease. However, weeks, months, or even years later, when re-exposed to the disease, antibodies in large quantities are produced within a few hours of exposure. This large number of antibodies occurring within hours of the subsequent exposure is called a secondary response and is usually sufficient to prevent the disease.

Of course one does not have to actually contract a disease to be immune to it. Humans have innate immunity to some diseases (canine distemper, for example). They can also be artificially "exposed" to microbial diseases via attenuated or killed vaccines that produce the antibody response but not the disease. Antibodies can also be orally passed to neonates via colostrum and antibodies themselves can be injected in the form of gamma globulins. These latter types of passive antibody transmissions result in temporary and relatively weak immunity as compared to the active forms (from vaccination or disease) where individuals manufacture their own antibodies.

Slang and Obsolete Nomenclature

UNOFFICIAL TERM	OFFICIAL DESIGNATION
Peyer's patches	aggregations of lymphatic nodules [*noduli lymphaticus aggregatus*]
intestinal tonsils	aggregations of lymphatic nodules [*noduli lymphaticus aggregatus*]
right thoracic duct	right lymphatic duct [*ductus lymphaticus dexter*]
left lymphatic duct	thoracic duct [*ductus thoracicus*]
thymus gland	thymus [*thymus*]
splenic hilus	splenic hilum [*hilum splenicum*]
Hassall's corpuscles	thymic corpuscles

Review Questions

1. The lymphatic organ most easily observed in a living individual is the...
   A. thymus.
   B. palatine tonsil.
   C. spleen.
   D. thoracic duct.
   E. pharyngeal tonsil.

2. Which lymphatic structure is mismatched with its location?
   A. spleen—adjacent to greater curvature of the stomach
   B. thymus—anterior part of base of neck and upper thoracic cavity
   C. lymph nodes—along the course of the thoracic duct
   D. subepithelial aggregations of lymphatic nodules—within wall of vermiform appendix
   E. tonsil—pharyngeal region

3. Which of the following is not a function of the lymphatic system?
   A. production of lymphocytes
   B. absorption of lipids
   C. production of antigens
   D. collection of excess tissue fluid
   E. return of lymph to the bloodstream

4. Which of the four pressures acting in/around cardiovascular capillaries should be most affected by severe starvation?

A. plasma (capillary) osmotic pressure
B. interstitial fluid osmotic pressure
C. interstitial fluid hydrostatic pressure
D. plasma (capillary) interstitial pressure
E. If severe starvation would not affect any of the above, choose this response.

5. How are lymphatic capillaries and cardiovascular capillaries alike?
A. both empty into venous channels
B. both carry blood
C. both connect to arterioles
D. both are open ended
E. If none of the above satisfy the premise, choose this response.

6. Which lymphatic trunks unite to form the right lymphatic duct?
A. right jugular, subclavian, and lumbar lymphatic trunks
B. left jugular, bronchomediastinal, and subclavian lymphatic trunks
C. right jugular, bronchomediastinal and lumbar lymphatic trunks
D. right subclavian, jugular, and bronchomediastinal trunks
E. left bronchomediastinal, subclavian, and jugular trunks

7. Which statement regarding the spleen is true?
A. It is the developmental source of T lymphocytes.
B. It regresses after puberty.
C. It is a vital organ.
D. Accessory spleens are present in about ten percent of the population.
E. The spleen dilates during hypovolemic shock as it attempts to increase the blood volume.

8. Which of the following is not one of the pairs of named tonsils?
A. palatine tonsils
B. tubal tonsils
C. laryngeal tonsils
D. pharyngeal tonsils
E. lingual tonsils

9. Which item is not associated with a lymph node?
A. capsule
B. white pulp
C. efferent lymphatic vessels
D. lymphatic nodules
E. germinal centers

10. Which statement best describes why interstitial fluid is continuously formed?
A. There are many kinds of cells that secrete it.
B. Lymphatic capillaries have thin walls.
C. The total "out" pressure at capillaries is greater than the total "in" pressure.
D. The blood capillaries are fenestrated.
E. The lymph nodes actively produce it.

Thought Questions

1. Explain why the first major organ to receive most lipid materials absorbed from the digestive system is the heart but the first major organ to receive other absorbed nutrients is the liver.

2. Discuss the hydrodynamics of fluid "leakage" through capillary walls.

3. Which lymphatic trunks are drained by the thoracic duct? Right lymphatic duct?

4. How do T lymphocyte producing cells (originally formed in the thymus) get scattered into several parts of the body?

5. Why can even a moderately tight constricting band around an extremity (or part thereof) cause soft tissue swelling?

6. Why are regional lymph nodes often removed (along with neoplastic tissue) during cancer surgeries?

7. Palatine tonsils that repeatedly become inflamed (tonsillitis) are sometimes surgically removed. This surgery used to be performed more frequently than it is today. Why?

8. In what ways does the spleen differ from a lymph node anatomically?

9. What is unusual about the thymus as a body organ?

10. Which lymphatic organ is most likely to be ruptured from an abdominal blow (as might occur from an impact with the steering wheel if one has a car accident while driving "seat-belt-less")?

11. Compare and contrast lymphatic and cardiovascular capillaries.

12. How does lymph vary from interstitial fluid (= "tissue fluid" = extracellular fluid)?

13. Which cells produce antibodies? Where are these cells found?

14. Of the four pressures acting within and around cardiovascular capillaries, which one is most likely affected by:
    A. starvation?
    B. high blood pressure?
    C. depositions of large quantities of abnormal protein in the extracellular space?

15. Why does a hand "swell" after a game of handball?

16. Why do microfilarial parasites that block lymphatic capillaries cause edema?

17. The same lymphatic vessel can be termed *afferent* and *efferent*. Explain.

18. Discuss the major functions of the lymphatic system.

19. Where does lymph re-enter the circulating blood?

20. A surgeon sometimes needs to visualize the abdominal lymphatic vessels during surgery. How can this be accomplished?

21. Differentiate several different usages of *trunk* in gross anatomy.

Answers to Clinical Case Studies

Case 1—Free blood in the peritoneal cavity is a grave sign that rupture of intra-abdominal vasculature has occurred. This patient went into hypovolemic shock and was literally bleeding to death internally. Infusion of sterile saline, plasma, and finally whole blood stabilized him sufficiently for surgery. When his abdomen was opened, the surgeon discovered a ruptured spleen which he removed. After rinsing the blood out of the peritoneal cavity with sterile, physiological saline solution, the surgeon examined the rest of the patient's abdominal viscera. Finding no other abnormalities, the surgeon closed the abdominal incision and the patient recovered. Since the spleen is a non-vital organ, it can be removed when it has been traumatized.

Case 2—Often called "blood poisoning" in folk medical circles, these red streaks are caused by inflammation of lymphatic channels that are carrying bacteria away from the site of the infection.

Case 3—Inflamed lymph nodes cause these painful enlargements. When lymph, carrying bacteria or their toxins, enters a lymph node, it causes an inflammatory response. Once enlarged in this manner, lymph nodes seldom return to their original size—although they do regress some when the inflammation subsides.

Answers to Review Questions

1. B.

2. C. Lymph nodes are found along the course of smaller lymphatic channels but not along the thoracic duct.

3. C. The lymphatic system produces antibodies.

4. A. Severe starvation impacts the liver's ability to synthesize albumins (the major blood component responsible for plasma osmotic pressure).

5. E. A, B, C, and D refer to cardiovascular capillaries only.

6. D. All of the other lymphatic trunks drain into the thoracic duct.

7. D. A and B are true for the thymus and E is false because of the word "dilates."

8. C.

9. B. White pulp is found in the spleen.

10. C.

Answers to Thought Questions

1. Lipids are absorbed primarily into the lymphatic channels within the small intestinal villi. These drain into the intestinal lymphatic trunks, which empty into the cisterna chyli. From there, lymph is transported via the thoracic duct and the latter drains into the left brachiocephalic vein. Therefore, the heart is the first major organ to receive absorbed lipids. Other nutrients absorbed through the small intestinal wall enter regular cardiovascular capillaries. From there, they are transported to the liver via the hepatic portal system.

2. When the four pressures acting in and around capillaries (two osmotic pressures and two hydrostatic pressures) are summated, the net "out" pressure is greater than the net "in". Consequently, fluid is forced out through the permeable walls of the capillaries and they are said to leak. The two "out" pressures are the capillary (plasma) hydrostatic pressure and the interstitial fluid osmotic pressure. The two "in" pressures are capillary (plasma) osmotic pressure and interstitial fluid hydrostatic pressure.

3. The thoracic duct receives all of the lymphatic trunks from the left side of the upper body, the whole abdomen, and both inferior limbs. These include the left and right lumbar trunks, all intestinal trunks, and the left jugular, left subclavian, and left bronchomediastinal trunks. The right lymphatic duct receives lymph from the right jugular, right subclavian, and right bronchomediastinal trunks.

4. They are distributed by the flow of blood and lymph.

5. Flow of lymph within superficial lymphatic vessels is easily disrupted.

6. The lymphatic channels often serve as conduits for metastasis of cancer cells and these cells often lodge in the regional lymph nodes.

7. Palatine tonsillectomies sometimes involve severe hemorrhage as a surgical complication. To eliminate this possibility, tonsillectomies are not routinely performed.

8. The spleen receives no afferent lymphatic vessels. Thus, it does not "filter" lymph as lymph nodes do. The spleen is much larger than lymph nodes and its capsule contains smooth muscle which can contract, forcing the blood within it back into the general circulation. The lymphatic nodules within the spleen are also organized differently than those within lymph nodes.

9. It is relatively large at birth, reaches its maximum size at puberty, and then it regresses (involutes) to the point where thymic tissue is difficult to find in most adults.

10. Spleen.

11. Lymphatic capillaries are blind-ended, transport lymph, and drain into larger lymphatic channels. Cardiovascular capillaries join arterioles to venules and transport blood.

12. Newly formed lymph is essentially identical to interstitial fluid. As it flows through lymph nodes, it picks up antibodies and lymphocytes.

13. Antibodies are produced primarily by plasma cells and lymphocytes. They are found in lymph nodes, tonsils, spleen, bone marrow tissue, and subepithelial aggregations of lymphatic nodules.

14. A. plasma (capillary) osmotic pressure
    B. plasma (capillary) hydrostatic pressure
    C. interstitial fluid osmotic pressure

15. Trauma due to hitting the ball increases the permeability of cardiovascular capillaries. Because of the increased permeability, excess tissue fluid is formed. As larger organic molecules leak into the interstitial space, they increase the interstitial fluid osmotic pressure which compounds the problem.

16. Blockage of the lymphatic capillaries prevents the tissue fluid from draining away. Since it is continuously formed, edema results.

17. After an efferent lymphatic vessel leaves a lymph node, it often encounters other lymph nodes along its course. Thus, what was "efferent" becomes "afferent" as it approaches the next lymph node.

18. The lymphatic system collects excess tissue fluid, produces lymphocytes and antibodies, and absorbs lipids from the intestinal lumen.

19. The two terminal lymphatic channels (thoracic duct and right lymphatic duct) enter the large systemic veins near the heart. In most individuals these vessels are the left and right brachiocephalic veins.

20. The patient is fed a high lipid drink prior to surgery (cream, for example). The lipid micelles are absorbed into the lymphatics and cause the lymph to assume an opaque white color that is easily visible through the lymphatic vessel walls.

21. When unmodified, *trunk* refers to the portion of the body to which the neck and limbs attach. It is divided into the thorax, abdomen, pelvis, and back. The sympathetic trunks (left/right) parallel the vertebral column. Some arteries are termed trunks (pulmonary trunk, brachiocephalic trunk) as are some of the larger lymphatic vessels. Trunk is also used as a regional part of some structures (trunk of the corpus callosum, trunk of the atrioventricular bundle, *etc.*).

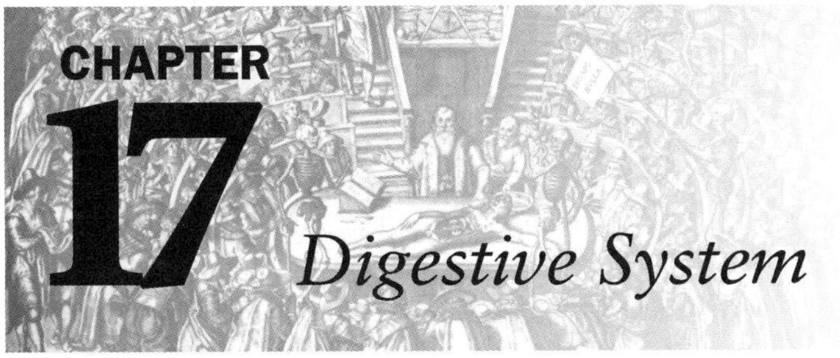

CHAPTER 17 *Digestive System*

Chapter Outline and Key Concepts

INTRODUCTION

The digestive system includes the organs that form the alimentary canal (digestive tube) as well as the salivary glands, liver, gallbladder, pancreas, and the associated ducts.

"GI tract" is a frequently used misnomer for the digestive system.

FUNCTIONS OF THE DIGESTIVE SYSTEM

The digestive system is involved in nutrient intake (prehension, mastication, deglutition, emulsification, hydrolysis, absorption) as well as in solid waste elimination (defecation).

LAYERS OF THE TUBULAR DIGESTIVE ORGANS

Most digestive organs have four identifiable layers in their walls: mucosa, submucosa, tunica muscularis, and tunica adventitia or serosa.

A mucosa (mucous membrane) has three layers: lining epithelium, lamina propria (c.t. proper), and muscularis mucosae.

ORAL CAVITY AND FAUCES

The oral cavity is the space behind the oral opening (mouth) which contains the teeth and the anterior portions of the tongue.

The fauces (gullet) is the short passageway that connects the oral cavity to the pharynx.

TONGUE

The tongue is the mucus covered skeletal muscle structure that is divided into an apex, body, and root.

The tiny projections on the surface of the tongue, called lingual papillae, are divided into 6 types by shape.

TEETH

Teeth cut and grind ingesta and are anchored to the maxillae and mandible by gomphoses.

A given tooth has a crown (exposed beyond the gum), neck (at the gum), and one or more roots (not visible) that surround a pulp cavity containing dental pulp.

Teeth are structurally formed by three substances: enamel, dentin, and cementum.

The thirty-two teeth of an adult consist of eight incisors, four canines ("cuspids"), eight premolars ("bicuspids"), and 12 molars.

A given tooth can be identified anatomically by using upper/lower, left/right, the tooth type, and a number to indicate its relative position within its grouping.

Dental professionals designate individual teeth by shorthand numerical or quadrant systems.

A tooth has several surfaces: lingual (palatal), vestibular (labial or buccal), masticatory (occlusal), and approximate (mesial or distal).

Neonates are usually edentulous at birth, erupt their first teeth at about six months, and have a full set of deciduous teeth at about two years.

Permanent teeth begin sequentially replacing deciduous teeth at about six years of age and most individuals have a full set of permanent teeth, except for third molars (wisdom teeth), by their teenage years.

The permanent dental formula is $2[I\frac{2}{2}C\frac{1}{1}P\frac{2}{2}M\frac{3}{3}]=32$ and the deciduous dental formula is $2[I\frac{2}{2}C\frac{1}{1}P\frac{2}{2}]=20$.

PHARYNX

The pharynx is a passageway that joins the fauces to the esophagus, and the nasal cavity to the larynx.

The pharynx is divided into three parts: nasal, oral, and laryngeal.

ESOPHAGUS

The esophagus joins the pharynx to the stomach and has three regional divisions: cervical, thoracic, and abdominal.

STOMACH

The stomach stores ingesta and begins the hydrolysis of proteins.

The stomach is "C"-shaped with greater and lesser curvatures and four named regions: cardiac part, fundus, body, and pyloric part.

Among the specialized cells in the gastric mucosa are parietal cells (hydrochloric acid), principal cells (pepsinogen), and mucus secreting cells.

The stomach is very distensible and its mucosa has distinct folds when the wall is not stretched.

SMALL INTESTINE

The small intestine is the major organ involved in the hydrolysis and absorption of ingesta.

The small intestine is divided into duodenum (12 inches), jejunum (8 feet), and ileum (12 feet).

The duodenum is divided into superior, descending, horizontal, and ascending parts and has three named flexures associated with it.

The descending part of the duodenum receives the hepatopancreatic ampulla and accessory pancreatic duct.

Absorption in the small intestine is enhanced by the increased surface area related to folds, villi, and microvilli.

LARGE INTESTINE

The large intestine is about 5-6 feet long and includes the cecum, colon, rectum, and anal canal.

The colon is the largest component of the large intestine and has three straight portions (ascending, transverse, descending colon) and three curved portions (right colic flexure, left colic flexure, sigmoid colon).

Most of the large intestine is sacculated due to the presence of taeniae coli (longitudinal bands of smooth muscle in the tunica muscularis).

SALIVARY GLANDS

There are three major pairs of salivary glands: parotid, submandibular, and sublingual glands.

The ducts of the major salivary glands open into the oral vestibule (parotid gland) or oral cavity proper (sublingual and submandibular glands).

Numerous small minor salivary glands are located in the cheeks, lips, palate, and tongue.

LIVER

The liver is the largest gland, largest internal organ, and is divided into four named lobes.

The liver cells (hepatocytes) are arranged in functional groups that form microscopic subunits called liver (hepatic) lobules.

Portal triads containing tiny branches of the hepatic portal vein, proper hepatic artery, and biliary duct system surround each liver lobule.

Blood from portal triads flows centrally in the sinusoidal spaces of each lobule and enters the central vein therein.

Bile, manufactured by hepatocytes, flows peripherally in bile canaliculi to enter the biliary ductules within the portal triads.

Blood from the central veins of the liver lobules leaves the liver via the 3–4 hepatic veins.

Bile in the biliary ductules flows into larger channels which coalesce to form two large (left and right) hepatic ducts leaving the liver.

The hepatic ducts unite to form the common hepatic duct which continues toward the descending duodenum as the bile duct after the origin of the cystic duct.

The bile duct joins the pancreatic duct to form the hepatopancreatic ampulla which enters the descending duodenum at the major duodenal papilla.

GALLBLADDER

The gallbladder is a distensible storage reservoir for bile that is positioned between the quadrate and right lobes of the liver.

Bile enters/leaves the gallbladder through the cystic duct which joins the common hepatic duct to form the bile duct.

PANCREAS

The pancreas has a head, body, tail, and two ducts.

The pancreatic duct joins the bile duct to form the hepatopancreatic ampulla which enters the descending duodenum at the major duodenal papilla.

The accessory pancreatic duct enters the descending duodenum at the minor duodenal papilla.

Most pancreatic cells produce pancreatic juice which leaves the pancreas through its ducts.

The alpha and beta cells in the pancreatic islets produce glucagon and insulin, respectively.

ABDOMEN, ABDOMINAL CAVITY; PERITONEUM, PERITONEAL CAVITY

The space within the abdomen is called the abdominal cavity and is continuous with the pelvic cavity.

The serous membrane lining the abdominal and pelvic cavities and covering all organs therein is called peritoneum.

The potential space "inside" the peritoneum is called the peritoneal cavity.

Parietal peritoneum (lining the walls of the abdominal and pelvic cavities) is distinguished from visceral peritoneum on the surface of organs.

Parietal peritoneum passing from one organ to the abdominal wall or from organ-to-organ is double layered and given specific names.

DEVELOPMENT OF THE DIGESTIVE SYSTEM

The primitive alimentary canal, derived primarily from endoderm and mesoderm, is divided into foregut, midgut, and hindgut.

The liver, gallbladder, and pancreas all develop from the terminal part of the foregut.

CLINICAL CONSIDERATIONS

Harelip and cleft palate are developmental conditions of the "top" end of the alimentary canal.

Teeth are subject to decay and improper positioning (malocclusion).

Ulceration commonly occurs in the stomach or small intestine.

Intestinal obstructions can occur due to ingestion of foreign bodies or constipation.

Appendicitis requires surgical removal of the vermiform appendix.

Selected Definitions

Absorption—the process wherein water, electrolytes, small organic molecules, and lipids pass through the lining epithelium of the alimentary canal and enter the vasculature. Most biological macromolecules must be hydrolyzed before they can be absorbed.

Alimentary canal—the digestive tube beginning at the mouth and ending at the anus. It has seven major regional subdivisions: mouth/oral cavity, gullet (fauces), pharynx, esophagus, stomach, small intestine, and large intestine.

Anal canal—the very last part of the large intestine. It opens at the anus and is about two centimeters long.

Bile canaliculi—the smallest biliary channels. Bile canaliculi course between the hepatocyte-lined walls of adjacent hepatic sinusoids and they empty into the biliary ductules that form one of the three components of each hepatic triad.

Connecting peritoneum—peritoneum that is neither on the body wall or diaphragm (parietal peritoneum) nor on a particular organ (visceral peritoneum). Parietal and visceral peritonea are both single-layered, but the variously named connecting peritonea are all double-layered.

Crown of a tooth—the portion of a tooth that can be visualized (above the gumline). It is composed of enamel (superficially) and dentin (deeply) around the pulp cavity.

Deglutition—the physical act of swallowing. It is initiated by voluntarily moving a bolus of ingesta into the oral part of the pharynx and forcing it into the esophagus by movements of the lingual and pharyngeal muscles.

Hepatic (portal) triad—a tight grouping of biliary ductule, a branch of the proper hepatic artery, and a branch of the hepatic portal vein which occurs at several loci around each hepatic lobule. Blood from the artery and vein flows centrally through the hepatic sinusoids, and bile produced by the hepatocytes flows peripherally through the bile canaliculi to enter the biliary ductule.

Hepatic sinusoids—the large diameter, modified capillaries through which blood flows within a hepatic lobule. Sinusoids receive blood from the peripherally located portal triads and empty it into the central veins of the lobules.

Hepatopancreatic ampulla—the passageway formed by the convergence of the bile duct with the pancreatic duct. It courses through the duodenal wall and opens at the tip of a mucosal projection termed the *major duodenal papilla.*

Minor duodenal papilla—the conical mucosal projection from the luminal wall of the duodenum whereon the accessory pancreatic duct opens. It is located superior to the major duodenal papilla.

Muscularis mucosae—a layer of muscle tissue found in some mucous membranes. The muscularis mucosae of the intestinal wall is not involved in peristalsis but causes folds and rugae which, in turn, increase the surface area through which absorption can occur.

Numerical tooth designation—the most common way of designating individual teeth in the dental profession. The permanent teeth are numbered 1-32 beginning with the upper right posterior molar, and the deciduous teeth are lettered A-T in a similar pattern.

Peristalsis—rhythmic involuntary contractions of muscle tissue that move material through tubular structures. In the digestive system, peristalsis moves ingesta through the alimentary canal.

Pharynx—that portion of the alimentary canal common to the respiratory and digestive systems. It has three named regional subdivisions (nasal, oral, laryngeal) and is connected to other structures by a total of seven openings.

Pylorus—the junction of the stomach and duodenum. The pylorus is differentiated from the pyloric canal (luminal passageway), pyloric sphincter muscle (thickened tunica muscularis), pyloric opening (stomach end of the pyloric canal), and the pyloric part of the stomach.

Small intestine—that portion of the alimentary canal beyond the stomach that is longer and smaller in diameter than the large intestine. Divided into duodenum, ileum, and jejunum, the small intestine is the major organ of hydrolysis and absorption.

Submucosa (tunica submucosa)—a layer of connective tissue proper located adjacent to the mucosa of mucous membranes. Submucosa is highly vascularized.

Taeniae coli—the three thickened bands within the longitudinal layer of the tunica muscularis that are easily visualized on the outer surface of the cecum and colon. Contractual tone within them causes the sacculations (haustra) that characterize most of the large intestine.

Tunica muscularis—a layer of muscle tissue primarily involved in peristalsis which is located in the wall of a visceral organ. In the intestine, the tunica muscularis has only two layers (inner circular and outer longitudinal), but in the stomach there are three.

Vermiform appendix—the finger-like projection from the cecum of the large intestine. Its length, small diameter, and single opening predispose it to the inflammatory syndrome called appendicitis.

Etymology ***Quod cibus est aliis, aliis est venenum*—"What is food to some is poison to others."**

adventicius (L), *outside*—tunica adventitia
alimentum (L), *nourish*—alimentary
anus (L), *ring*—anus
caecus (L), *blind*—cecum
caries (L), *decay*—dental caries
caruncula (L), *a little piece of flesh*—caruncle
commissura (L), *a joining together*—commissure
deciduus (L), *to fall off*—deciduous
dent (L), *tooth*—dental
digerere (L), *to divide*—digest
duodeni (L), *twelve each*—duodenum
emulgere (L), *to milk out*—emulsification
falx (L), *sickle*—falciform
filiform (L), *having the shape of a thread*—filiform
flextere (L), *to bend*—flexure
folium (L), *leaf*—foliate
frenum (L), *small bridle*—frenulum
fungi (L), *mushroom*—fungiform
halitus (L), *breath*—halitosis
haustrum (L), *machine for drawing water*—haustra
hernia (L), *rupture*—hernia
ileum (L), *groin, viscera*—ileum
jejunum (L), *"empty after death"*—jejunum
kreas (G), *flesh*—pancreas
kystis (G), *bladder, pouch*—cystic
lentil (L), *shaped like lentil seeds*—lentiform
metrium (L), *layer of uterus*—mesometrium
pan (G), *all*—pancreas
pertonos (G), *stretched over*—peritoneum
pharynx (L), *throat*—pharynx
philtron (G), *dimple in upper lip*—philtrum
proprius (L), *own, particular*—lamina propria
pyloros (G), *gate keeper*—pylorus
rectus (L), *straight*—rectum
salivarius (L), *slimy*—salivary
salping (L), *uterine tube*—mesosalpinx
sigma (G), *Greek letter sigma*—sigmoid
taeniae (L), *a band of muscle*—taeniae coli
uva (L), *grape, bunch of grapes*—palatine uvula
vallare (L), *to wall off*—vallate
villus (L), *shaggy hair*—villi

Introduction

The **digestive system** includes the organs which collectively form the so-called "alimentary canal", the gallbladder, and a number of associated glands and duct systems. The tubular design, mucous membrane lining, and openings at the body surface qualify the digestive system as one of the visceral body systems (*see Chapter 1*). It is the only visceral system with two widely separated openings (mouth and anus). The digestive system is often called the "gastro-intestinal" ("GI") tract—a misnomer that ignores all of its organs above the stomach. The alimentary canal is the tubular portion of the digestive system that transports ingesta. It includes the oral cavity, fauces (gullet), pharynx, esophagus, stomach, small intestine, and large intestine. Other digestive organs located in or opening into the alimentary canal via a duct are teeth, tongue, salivary glands, pancreas, liver, and gallbladder. The major glands include salivary glands, liver, and pancreas (Figure 17-1). In addition to these, there are many microscopic glands within the mucosal lining of the tubular organs.

Objectives

1. List the organs, in order, that make up the alimentary canal and list the other organs of the digestive system.

Functions of the Digestive System

The digestive system functions in nutrient intake as well as in solid waste elimination. **Nutrient intake** is a complex, multi-step phenomenon that includes prehension, mastication, deglutition, emulsification and hydrolysis, and absorption. **Prehension** is the process of getting food materials into the oral cavity and is delegated primarily to the superior limbs. **Mastication** is the physical degradation of ingesta within the oral cavity. It primarily involves grinding and mashing of solid food materials with the teeth. **Deglutition** is the physical process of swallowing. This involves the voluntary act of forcing ingested material posteriorly with the tongue until it enters the esophagus where involuntary peristalsis moves it on into the stomach. **Emulsification** is the initial breakdown of lipids in which they are dispersed as tiny droplets within the ingesta. **Hydrolysis** is the chemical "de-polymerization" of proteins, carbohydrates, and fats which releases their basic organic building blocks. **Absorption** is the physical passage of nutrients through the mucosal lining of the intestinal wall and into its cardiovascular capillaries (most nutrients) and lymphatic capillaries (fat micelles). **Solid waste elimination** involves the dehydration of non-absorbed ingesta to form feces which are periodically removed from the body by **defecation**.

Objectives

2. State the two major functions of the digestive system and subdivide the concept of nutrient intake into its separate processes.

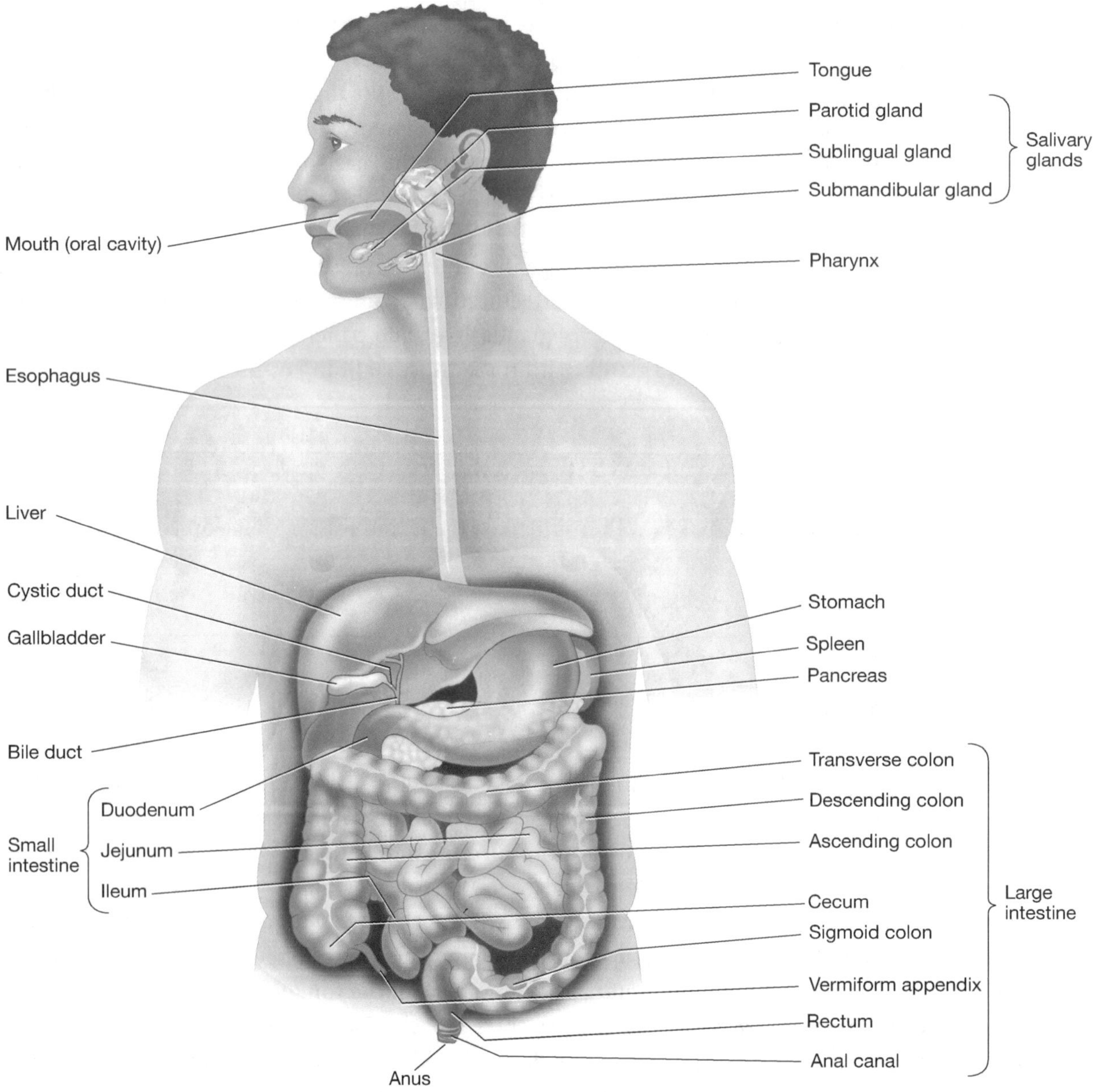

Figure 17-1

Major Components of the Digestive System

In addition to the components of the 9 meter-long alimentary canal with which ingesta makes direct contact, the digestive system includes a number of accessory digestive organs (salivary glands, pancreas, liver, and gallbladder).

Layers of the Tubular Digestive Organs

Most tubular organs of the digestive system have four identifiable layers in their walls: mucosa, submucosa, tunica muscularis, and tunica adventitia/serosa (Figure 17-2). The **mucosa** (**mucous membrane**) is the innermost layer and it surrounds the lumen. It is composed of three named layers: epithelium, lamina propria, and muscularis mucosae. The **epithelium** lines the lumen. It varies in type from stratified squamous epithelium in the oral cavity, fauces, pharynx, and esophagus to simple columnar epithelium from the stomach on down. The stratified squamous epithelium is primarily a protective lining whereas the simple columnar epithelium has secretory and absorptive roles. Unicellular mucous glands (goblet cells) within the simple columnar epithelium secrete a lubricative and protective layer of mucus. The **lamina propria** is a layer of connective tissue proper which surrounds the epithelium. It supports the epithelium physically, is highly vascularized, and serves as a pathway for nerve fibers within the mucosa. The lamina propria in many regions contains lymphatic nodules which react to bacterial invaders by producing antibodies against them. The **muscularis mucosae** is smooth muscle tissue which surrounds the lamina propria. It causes the mucosa in the stomach and small intestine to have numerous folds which greatly increase their surface area. The **submucosa** is a relatively thick and highly vascularized layer of connective tissue proper that surrounds the muscularis layer of the mucosa. It, in turn, is surrounded by the **tunica muscularis** which is a relatively thick layer of smooth muscle tissue that is primarily responsible for the peristaltic and other movements of the esophagus, stomach, and intestine. It is innervated by both sympathetic and parasympathetic (VE) neurons. The outermost layer of most parts of the alimentary canal is connective tissue proper which in some places is covered by simple squamous epithelium called **mesothelium** to form a **serous membrane** (**tunica serosa**). In places where the organs are not covered by serous membrane, the mesothelium is not present and the connective tissue proper, by itself, is called the **tunica adventitia**.

Objectives

3. Name and state the composition of the four major layers of the walls of the tubular digestive organs and similarly identify the layers of the mucosa.

Oral Cavity and Fauces

The **oral cavity** is the part of the digestive system that houses the teeth and the anterior part of the tongue. Anteriorly, it is enclosed by the upper and lower **lips** which surround and form the boundaries of the **mouth**. Technically, the mouth is only the opening and the space inside is the oral cavity (Figure 17-3). However, in common usage, mouth often includes the oral cavity, as well. The upper lip has a median groove on its anterior surface termed the **philtrum** and a tiny median projection along its margin termed the **tubercle**. The junctions of the lips at the **angles** ("corners") of the mouth are called **labial commissures.** On the posterior side of each lip is a delicate, median fold of mucosa called the **labial frenulum** which attaches to the base of the gums on the midline. Laterally, the oral cavity is bounded by the cheeks. The superior aspect of the oral cavity is formed by the palate. The latter is divided into the (anterior) **hard palate** which is supported by the maxil-

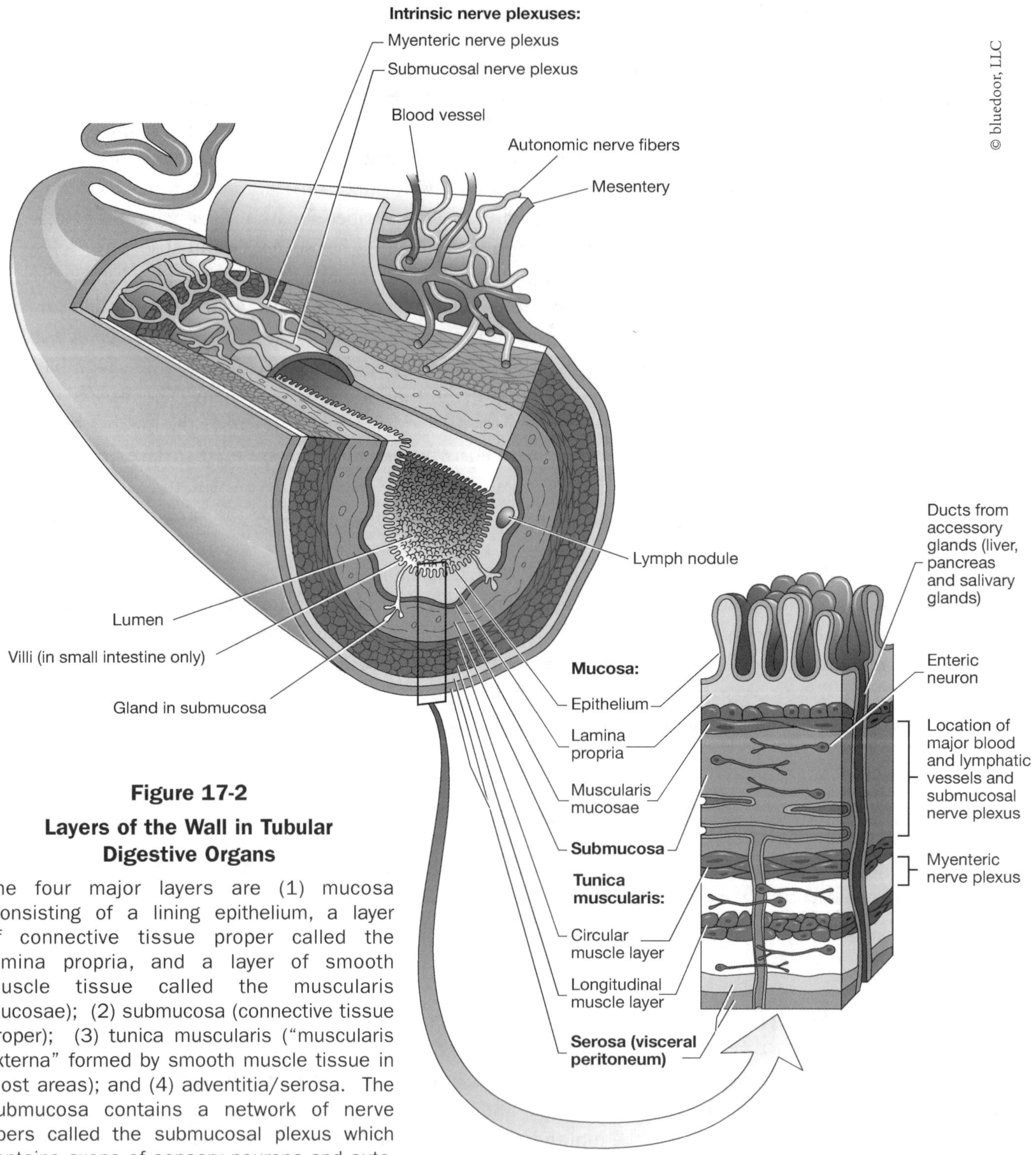

Figure 17-2

Layers of the Wall in Tubular Digestive Organs

The four major layers are (1) mucosa (consisting of a lining epithelium, a layer of connective tissue proper called the lamina propria, and a layer of smooth muscle tissue called the muscularis mucosae); (2) submucosa (connective tissue proper); (3) tunica muscularis ("muscularis externa" formed by smooth muscle tissue in most areas); and (4) adventitia/serosa. The submucosa contains a network of nerve fibers called the submucosal plexus which contains axons of sensory neurons and autonomic neurons as well as parasympathetic (terminal) ganglia. The tunica muscularis contains a similar plexus called the myenteric plexus. Parasympathetic stimulation increases muscular tone and activity and sympathetic stimulation inhibits or relaxes muscular tone and activity.

lae and palatine bones and the **soft palate** (posteriorly) which has no skeletal support. The hard palate is crossed anteriorly by a number of ridges termed **transverse palatine folds**. A subtle median projection just behind the front teeth is called the **incisive papilla**. The tongue occupies most of the floor of the oral cavity. The teeth divide the oral cavity into the **oral cavity proper** (bounded by the teeth) and the **oral vestibule** (between the lips or cheeks and the teeth).

Posteriorly, the oral cavity is connected to the pharynx by a short tubular passageway termed the **fauces** (**gullet**). The superior wall of this passageway is formed by the anterior portion of the soft palate. A median projection from the posterior border of the soft palate hangs inferiorly and is termed the **palatine uvula**. The posterior borders of the palate on each side of the uvula are called **palatopharyngeal arches**. Folds of the soft palate anterior to these extend inferiorly to join the tongue as the **palatoglossal arches**. The **palatine tonsils** are located in depressions (formed by the arches) in the lateral walls of the fauces. During deglutition, the soft palate is forced superiorly by ingesta elevated by the base of the tongue. This closes the opening into the nasal cavity and forces ingesta down into the oral and laryngeal parts of the pharynx.

Objectives

4. Identify the boundaries of the oral cavity and its two major subdivisions.
5. Define fauces and discuss its landmarks.

Tongue

The **tongue** is a mobile digestive organ that has several functional roles in the digestive system. It assists mastication by positioning ingesta where the teeth can macerate it. The tongue also has numerous **gustatory organs** (taste buds) (*see Chapter 10*) embedded in its surface and plays a major role in deglutition by moving ingesta posteriorly and then acting as a plunger to force it into the esophagus during deglutition. The tongue is a flattened organ consisting of a root, body, and apex (Figure 17-4). The **root** of the tongue is attached to the hyoid bone and forms the anterior wall of the inferior part of the pharynx. The **body** and **apex** of the tongue are located in the oral cavity. The parenchyma of the tongue includes four **intrinsic muscles**: superior longitudinal, inferior longitudinal, transverse, and vertical lingual muscles. These skeletal muscles are assisted in lingual movements by **extrinsic muscles** attaching the tongue to the mandible (genioglossus m.), to the styloid process of the temporal bone (styloglossus m.), to the greater horn of the hyoid bone (hyoglossus m.), and to the lesser horn of the hyoid bone (chondroglossus m.).

The mucosa on the dorsum and margin of the tongue forms small projections termed **lingual papillae**. Six types have been identified based on their shapes: filiform, conical, fungiform, vallate, foliate, and lentiform. **Filiform papillae** are the most numerous and form the light colored, hair-like projections over most of the dorsum of the tongue. **Conical papillae** resemble filiforms but are larger and located primarily on the posterior aspect of the tongue. **Fungiform papillae** are mushroom-shaped and interspersed among the filiform papillae. They are the second most numerous type of papilla and form tiny pink "dots" which can be observed over the tongue's surface. **Lentiform papillae** resemble fungiforms but are less elevated. **Vallate papillae** resemble large fungiforms and are located near the posterior aspect of the oral cavity. Only a few are present. **Foliate papillae** are found on the edges of the tongue near the palatoglossal arches. **Taste buds** (gus-

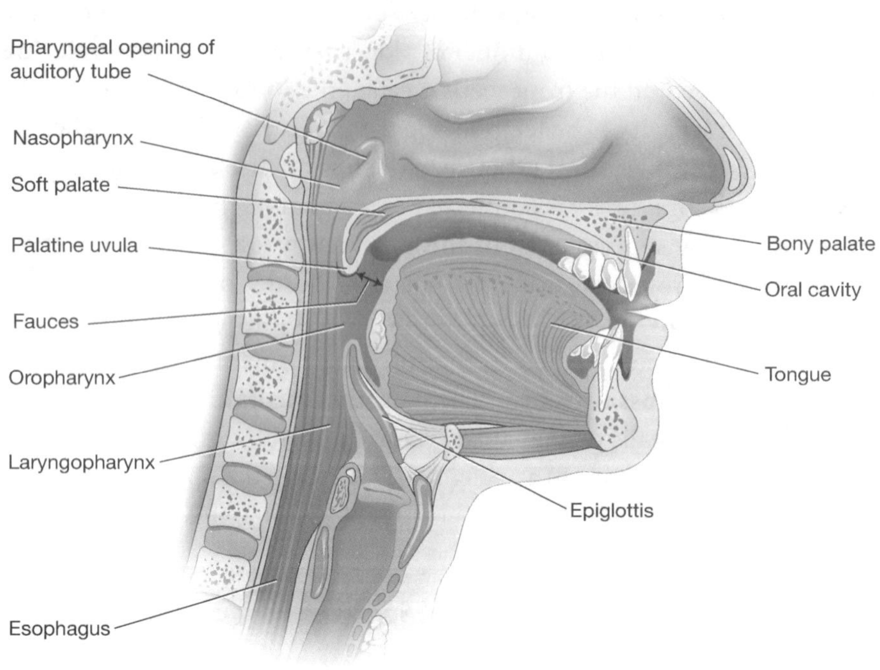

Sagittal section of head

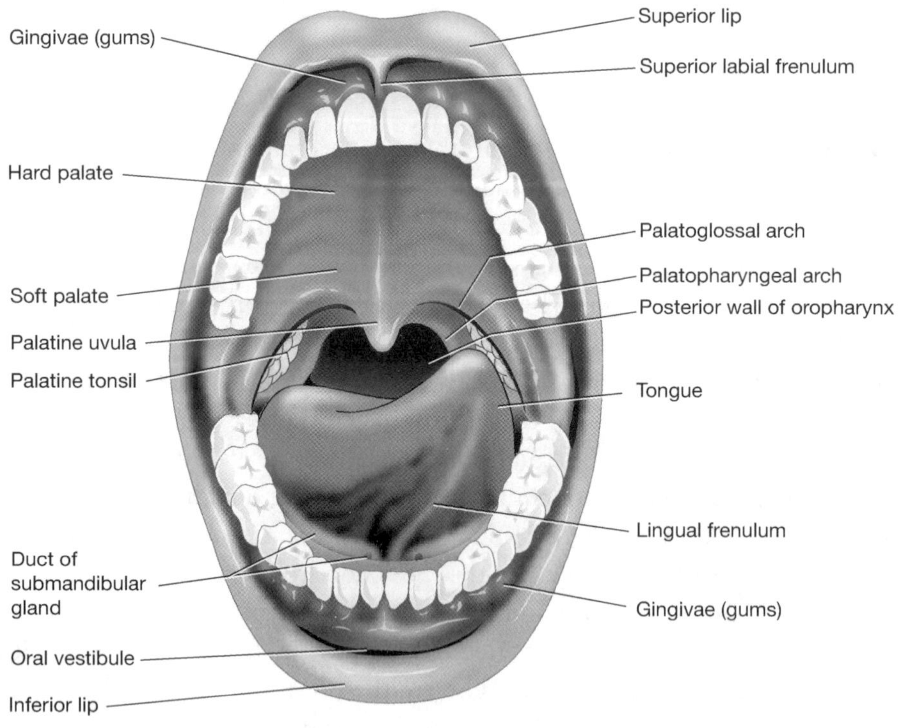

Oral cavity, Anterior aspect

Figure 17-3
Oral Cavity and Associated Structures

The hard palate and soft palate separate the nasal cavity (above) from the oral cavity and fauces (below). The nasal cavity opens posteriorly into the nasopharynx and the oral cavity is continued through the fauces into the oropharynx.

tatory organs) are collections of gustatory and supporting cells within the epithelium of fungiform and vallate papillae. They are chemoreceptors and are discussed in Chapter 10.

The dorsum of the tongue is divided by a **median groove** which continues anteriorly from the blind foramen (see below) to its apex. The **terminal groove** is an indentation which extends laterally from the blind foramen and divides the dorsum of the tongue from the root of the tongue. The vallate papillae are located at the terminal groove. Only the anterior half of the tongue can be easily observed. It is divided from the posterior half by a median indentation termed the **blind foramen** of the tongue (Figure 17-4). This marks the original site of origin of the tissue that forms the thyroid gland. The inferior aspect of the tongue is attached to the floor of the oral cavity by a median fold of oral mucosa termed the **lingual frenulum**. On each side of this frenulum is a ridge of mucosa termed the **sublingual fold.** Each sublingual fold ends anteriorly in a projection termed the **sublingual caruncle**. The combined ducts of the sublingual and submandibular (salivary) glands open on these caruncles.

Objectives

6. Sketch the superior (dorsal) surface of the body and apex of the tongue and label its major landmarks.
7. Differentiate the six types of lingual papillae.

Teeth

Teeth are the major organs of mastication and are anchored into the maxillae and mandible by dentoalveolar joints (gomphoses). A tooth has three major external parts: crown, neck, and root (Figure 17-5). The **crown** of a tooth is the visible portion that projects beyond the gingiva (gums). Elevations or mounds on the crown are termed cusps or tubercles. The **root** of a tooth is the embedded portion which occupies a dental alveolus in the maxilla (superior teeth), or in the mandible (inferior teeth). Some teeth have single roots. Others have two or more. The connective tissue proper which anchors each tooth in its socket is called the **periodontium** or **periodontal ligament**. The **neck** of a tooth is the portion at the junction of the crown and root(s). In many teeth it is visibly constricted.

There are three major mineralized substances forming a tooth. The crown is covered by **enamel** which is composed of calcium salts and is the hardest substance in the body (harder than bone). The root of a tooth is enveloped by **cementum** which is a bone-like connective tissue to which the periodontium attaches. Deep to the enamel and cementum is **dentin** which is harder and denser than bone but softer than enamel. The dentin surrounds a hollow space termed the **pulp cavity** which is filled with soft tissue (vessels, nerves, etc.) termed the **dental pulp**. These enter and leave through passageways at the tips of the roots termed **canals of the roots**.

A typical adult has 32 teeth with 16 in the **upper** (**superior**) **dental arch** and 16 in the **lower** (**inferior**) **dental arch** (Figure 17-5). These are divided into four groups: incisors, canines, premolars, and molars. The four teeth adjacent to the median plane as well as the teeth just lateral to them are **incisor teeth** (eight total in the mouth). These teeth are sharp-edged and specialized for nipping and cutting. **Canine teeth** are the teeth posterolateral to the incisor teeth and are used for tearing fibrous tissues. These are commonly called "eye" teeth or "cuspids" (four total). The two teeth pos-

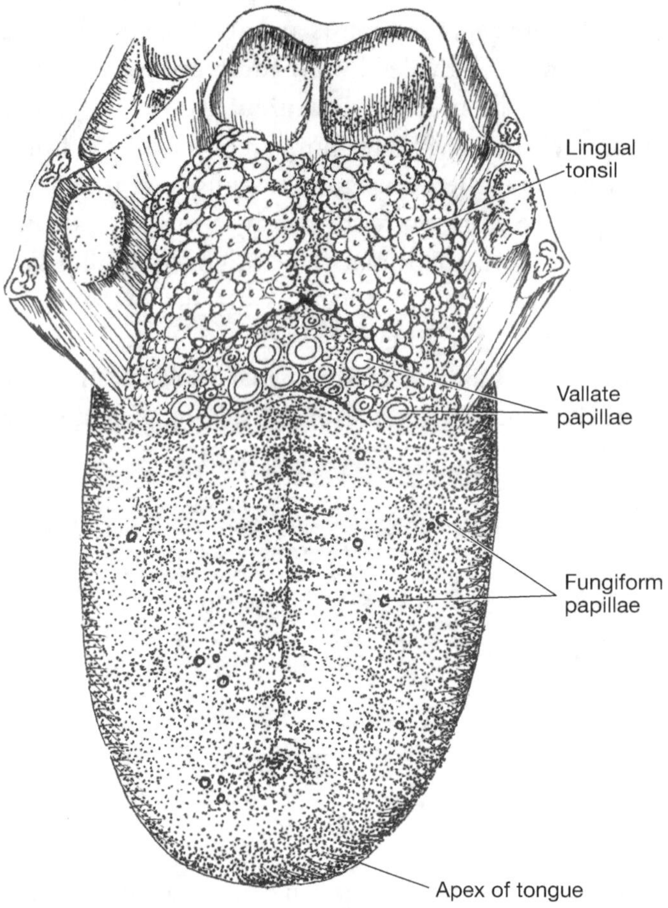

Figure 17-4

Tongue

The tongue occupies three different parts of the alimentary canal: oral cavity, fauces, and oropharynx. It functions in mastication, deglutition, and in the special sense of taste. The gustatory chemoreceptors (taste buds) are microscopic structures associated with some of the lingual papillae.

terior to each canine tooth are **premolar teeth** (eight total). These are often called "bicuspids" because they have two major cusps. **Molar teeth** are the last three teeth on each side of each dental arch (12 total). The last one on each side of each arch is often called the **wisdom tooth**. Molars are primarily used for grinding and crushing ingesta.

A given tooth has several defined surfaces: masticatory (occlusal), lingual, vestibular, and approximate. The **masticatory (occlusal) surface** is the surface that faces the opposite dental arch. The **lingual surface** is the surface of a tooth adjacent to the tongue. Notice that this is posterior on the incisor teeth, but it is medial on the premolars and molars. On superior teeth, the lingual surface is sometimes called the **palatal surface**. The **vestibular surface** is the surface oriented toward the oral vestibule. On the incisors and canines this is a **labial surface**. On the premolars and molars the vestibular surface is a **buccal surface**. The **approximate surface** is the surface that faces adjacent teeth in the same dental arch (*i.e.,* the surface "between" adjacent teeth). This is the "dental

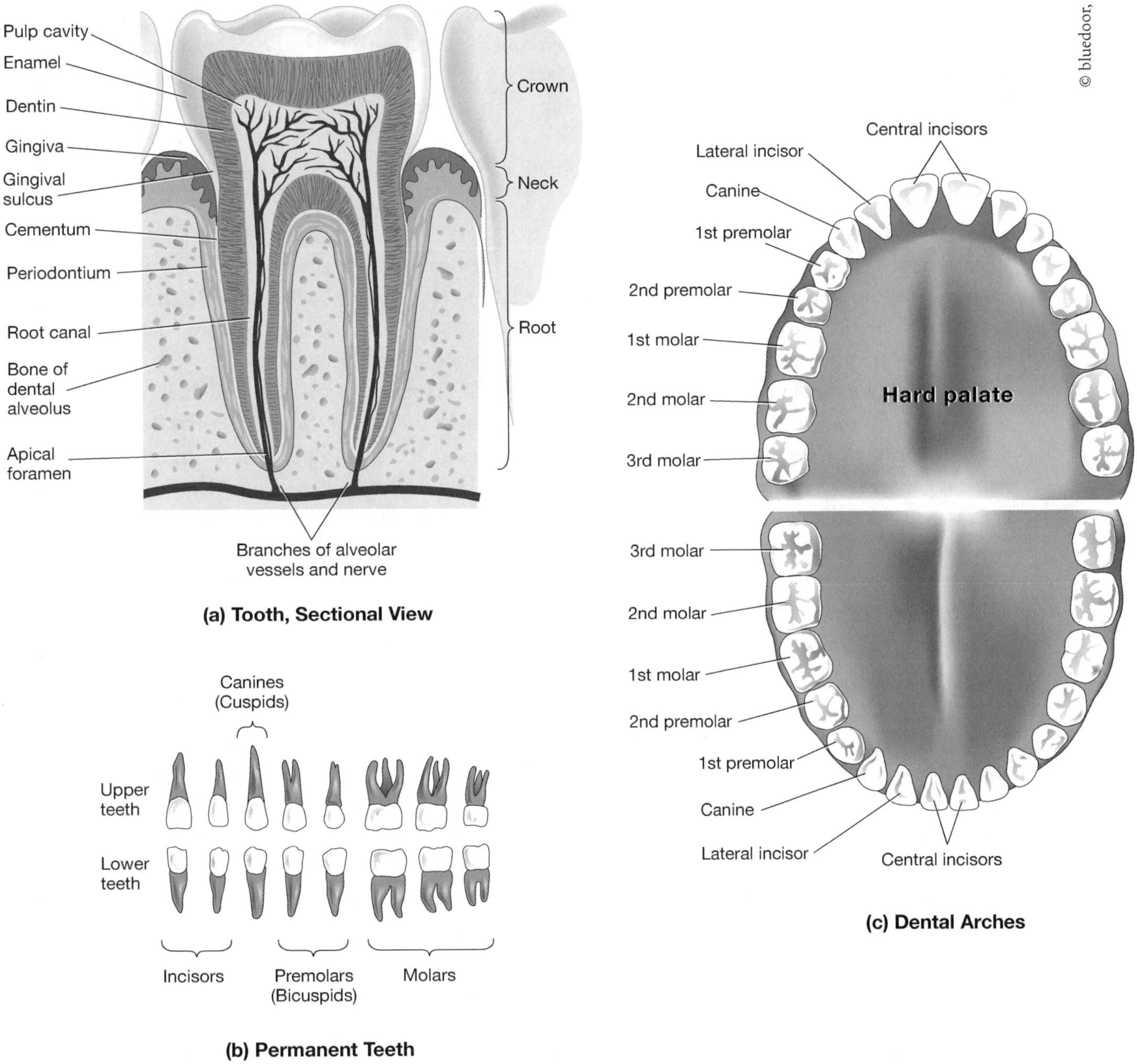

Figure 17-5
Teeth

The structure of an individual tooth is shown in sagittal section (a). Some teeth have single roots and some are multi-rooted (b). The connective tissue proper that "glues" the roots into the dental alveoli is called periodontium (= periodontal ligament or "membrane"). A full set of permanent teeth is illustrated in (c). Deciduous teeth are smaller and do not include any molars. Individual teeth can be named anatomically (superior, inferior, left, right, tooth type and number) or they can be designated numerically by 1-8 or 1-32 numerical systems as explained in the text and in Table 17-1.

floss" surface. Teeth have two of these and the terms **mesial** and **distal** are applied to distinguish them. The mesial surface of a tooth is the approximate surface that is oriented toward the median plane as one moves forward (and then medial) along the dental arch. The distal surface is the opposite approximate surface. Note that the distal surface of a wisdom tooth is not adjacent to another tooth. A region where the mesial surface of one tooth actually touches the distal surface of an adjacent tooth is called the **contact area**.

Infants are edentulous (without teeth) at birth and their first teeth usually erupt (break through the gums) at about six months of age. This is followed by a sequential eruption of other teeth until a full set of **deciduous teeth** is present at about two years of age. These are sequentially replaced by **permanent teeth** beginning at about six years of age. By age 13 all permanent teeth except the third molars (wisdom teeth) should have erupted. The latter erupt after 17 years of age (sometimes they fail to erupt at all). Deciduous teeth resemble permanent teeth except that they are smaller and no true molars are present (the deciduous premolars are often called "molars").

Dental formulae are used as a shorthand method of designating the particular dental complement of a given mammalian species. Letters are used to symbolize each tooth type and fractions indicate the number of each type present with the numerator designating the superior arch and the denominator representing the inferior arch. Because of bilateral symmetry, only one side (left or right) of the arch is symbolized and the whole expression is bracketed and multiplied by two to arrive at the correct total number of teeth. Using I (incisor), C (canine), P (premolar), and M (molar), the permanent dental formula is $\mathbf{2[I\frac{2}{2}\,C\frac{1}{1}\,P\frac{2}{2}\,M\frac{3}{3}] = 32}$. The deciduous dental formula is $\mathbf{2[I\frac{2}{2}\,C\frac{1}{1}\,P\frac{2}{2}] = 20}$.

Teeth are individually identified using tooth type, left/right, and inferior/superior. In addition, teeth within a given type are numbered (from the median plane) except canine teeth. Thus, there are first (central) and second (lateral) incisors; first and second premolars; and first, second and third molars on each side of each arch. Specific identification of a given tooth requires all of this information (*i.e., second upper left premolar*). Some dentists use a shorthand system that uses numbers, and letters. The 32 adult teeth are numbered 1-32 with the upper right third molar being number 1 and the upper left third molar numbered 16. The lower left third molar is 17 and the lower right third molar is tooth number 32. In this system the twenty deciduous teeth are lettered A–T (also beginning at the posterior aspect of the upper right dental arch). Another system numbers the teeth in each quadrant 1-8 beginning with the central incisor and working posteriorly (Table 17-1). Right, left, upper, and lower are acronymed R, L, U, and L, respectively. Note that the permanent molars have no deciduous predecessors. Dentists often refer to the deciduous premolars as "molars".

Objectives

8. State the permanent and deciduous human dental formulae.
9. Sketch a tooth in sagittal section and label its crown, neck , root, pulp cavity, enamel, dentin, cementum, periodontium, and dental alveolus.
10. Name and differentiate the several surfaces of a given tooth.
11. Properly designate any tooth using anatomic nomenclature and the numerical (1-32) system.
12. State the ages by which: a) the first deciduous teeth erupt, b) a full set of deciduous teeth is present, c) the first permanent teeth erupt, and d) all permanent teeth except the third molars have erupted.
13. State the official name for each of the following: front teeth, eye teeth, cuspids, bicuspids, wisdom teeth.

Table 17-1 Comparison of Ways to Designate Teeth

Numerical (Permanent)	(Deciduous)	Quadrant	Anatomic Name
1		UR8	right superior third molar tooth[1]
2		UR7	right superior second molar tooth
3		UR6	right superior first molar tooth
4	A	UR5	right superior second premolar tooth
5	B	UR4	right superior first premolar tooth
6	C	UR3	right superior canine tooth
7	D	UR2	right superior second/lateral incisor tooth
8	E	UR1	right superior first/central incisor tooth
9	F	UL1	left superior first/central incisor tooth
10	G	UL2	left superior second/lateral incisor tooth
11	H	UL3	left superior canine tooth
12	I	UL4	left superior first premolar tooth
13	J	UL5	left superior second premolar tooth
14		UL6	left superior first molar tooth
15		UL7	left superior second molar tooth
16		UL8	left superior third molar tooth[2]
17		LL8	left inferior third molar tooth[3]
18		LL7	left inferior second molar tooth
19		LL6	left inferior first molar tooth
20	K	LL5	left inferior second premolar tooth
21	L	LL4	left inferior first premolar tooth
22	M	LL3	left inferior canine tooth
23	N	LL2	left inferior second/lateral incisor tooth
24	O	LL1	left inferior first/central incisor tooth
25	P	LR1	right inferior first/central incisor tooth
26	Q	LR2	right inferior second/lateral incisor tooth
27	R	LR3	right inferior canine tooth
28	S	LR4	right inferior first premolar tooth
29	T	LR5	right inferior second premolar tooth
30		LR6	right inferior first molar tooth
31		LR7	right inferior second molar tooth
32		LR8	right inferior third molar tooth[4]

1. Upper right wisdom tooth 3. Lower left wisdom tooth 2. Upper left wisdom tooth 4. Lower right wisdom tooth

Pharynx

The **pharynx** is the organ which joins the fauces (gullet) to the esophagus, and the nasal cavity to the larynx (Figure 17-3). It is divided into three parts: nasal, oral, and laryngeal. These are commonly (unofficially) called the nasopharynx, oropharynx, and laryngopharynx. The **nasal part of the pharynx** is the uppermost portion and is located above the level of the soft palate. It is continuous anteriorly with the nasal cavity and the left and right auditory tubes open into it (there are actually seven openings into/out of the pharynx). The **oral part of the pharynx** lies below the level of the soft palate. It is continuous anteriorly with the fauces (gullet) and the line of demarcation between them is formed by the left and right palatopharyngeal folds. Inferiorly, the oral part of the pharynx is continuous with the **laryngeal part of the pharynx**. The latter is positioned around and behind the opening into the larynx. Its laryngeal opening is called the **aditus laryngis**. The laryngeal pharynx continues inferiorly into the esophagus. Functionally, the pharynx separates ingesta from inspired air and (usually) sends each down its appropriate passageway. Some of its mechanics have already been addressed (see *soft palate* in the *Oral Cavity* discussion) and more discussion is present in the next chapter (*Respiratory System*).

Objectives

14. Define pharynx and differentiate its three parts.

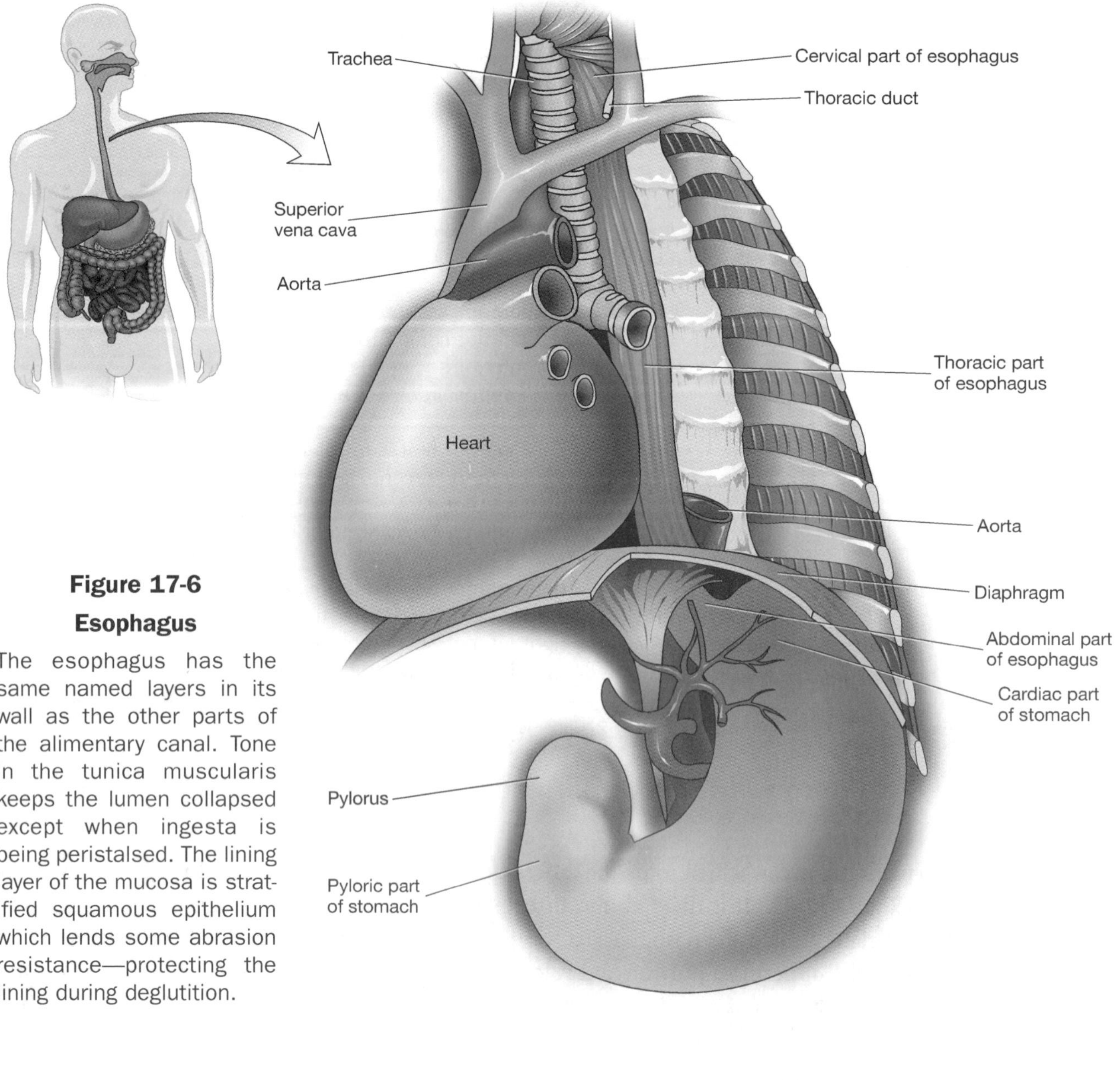

Figure 17-6
Esophagus

The esophagus has the same named layers in its wall as the other parts of the alimentary canal. Tone in the tunica muscularis keeps the lumen collapsed except when ingesta is being peristalsed. The lining layer of the mucosa is stratified squamous epithelium which lends some abrasion resistance—protecting the lining during deglutition.

Esophagus

The **esophagus** is a tubular organ connecting the pharynx to the stomach (Figure 17-1, 6). It is about 25 cm long and is positioned posterior to the trachea. The esophagus is divided into three parts: cervical, thoracic, and abdominal. The **cervical part** of the esophagus is the portion within the neck. It joins the laryngeal part of the pharynx. The **thoracic part** courses inferiorly through the central portion of the thorax within the partition (mediastinum) that separates the right lung from the left one. At the diaphragm, the thoracic esophagus courses through the esophageal hiatus to become the short **abdominal part** which joins the cardiac part of the stomach.

Functionally, the esophagus transports ingesta from the pharynx to the stomach by peristaltic contractions of the tunica muscularis within its wall (Figure 17-7). In the upper part of the esophagus, this muscular layer is skeletal muscle tissue and in the lower part it is smooth muscle tissue. The muscularis in the central portion is a mixture of skeletal and smooth muscle tissue. **Esophageal glands** within the mucosa produce **mucus** which lubricates the lining to facilitate the passage of ingesta. The esophagus is lined with stratified squamous epithelium to protect it from abrasion.

Objectives

15. Name the three parts of the esophagus and indicate the composition of the tunica muscularis in the top, middle, and bottom thirds.

Stomach

The **stomach** is a C-shaped distensible organ located primarily in the left superior quadrant of the abdomen. It stores ingesta and mixes it with acid and proteolytic enzymes to begin the digestion of proteins. The stomach has four major parts: cardiac part, fundus, body, and pyloric part (Figure 17-8, 9, 10). The **cardiac part** ("cardia") is the portion where the esophagus attaches and its opening from the esophagus is termed the **cardiac ostium**. The **fundus** is the portion which bulges to the left and above the attachment of the esophagus. It directly contacts the diaphragm. The **body** is the large central portion of the stomach and the **pyloric part** is the funnel-shaped terminal portion including the narrow passageway (pyloric canal) into the duodenum. The portion of the stomach leading down to the canal is called the pyloric antrum. The junction of the stomach with the duodenum is termed the **pylorus**. *Pylorus* is an abused anatomic term that has been variously used to mean the pyloric part of the stomach, pyloric antrum, pyloric canal, pyloric opening, and pyloric sphincter muscle. Here a **pyloric opening** (ostium) leads into a short **pyloric canal**. The pyloric opening can be closed by contraction of the **pyloric sphincter muscle** which is a thickened part of the tunica muscularis. It controls the entry of stomach contents into the duodenum. Exteriorly the stomach has anterior and posterior surfaces, and lesser and greater curvatures. The **lesser curvature** extends along the superior aspect of the cardiac part, body, and pyloric part, and the **greater curvature** is located along the opposite (inferior) border. The mucosa of the stomach has numerous longitudinal **gastric folds** which allow distensibility. The epithelial surface is marked with depressions called **gastric pits**. These mark the openings of simple tubular glands called **gastric glands**. The two major types of cells within these glands are parietal cells and principal (chief) cells. The **parietal cells** secrete hydrochloric acid and the **principal cells** secrete pepsinogen. The hydrochloric

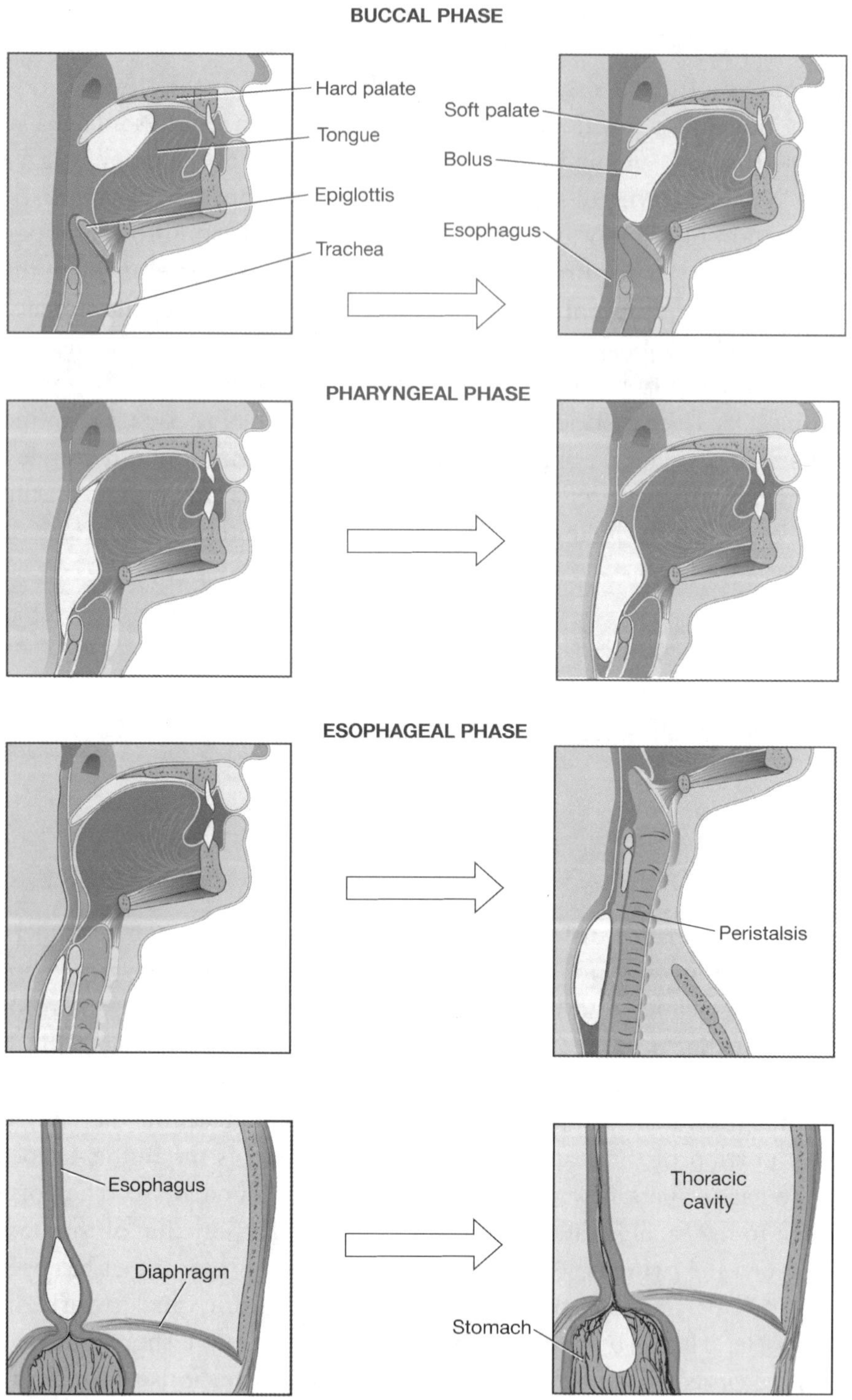

Figure 17-7

Deglutition

The tongue initiates deglutition by forcing ingesta back into the gullet and pharynx. The base of the tongue continues the process by pushing the ingesta into the cervical (upper) part of the esophagus. Peristalsis then moves the bolus (moistened, masticated ball of ingesta) down through the thoracic and abdominal parts of the esophagus and into the stomach.

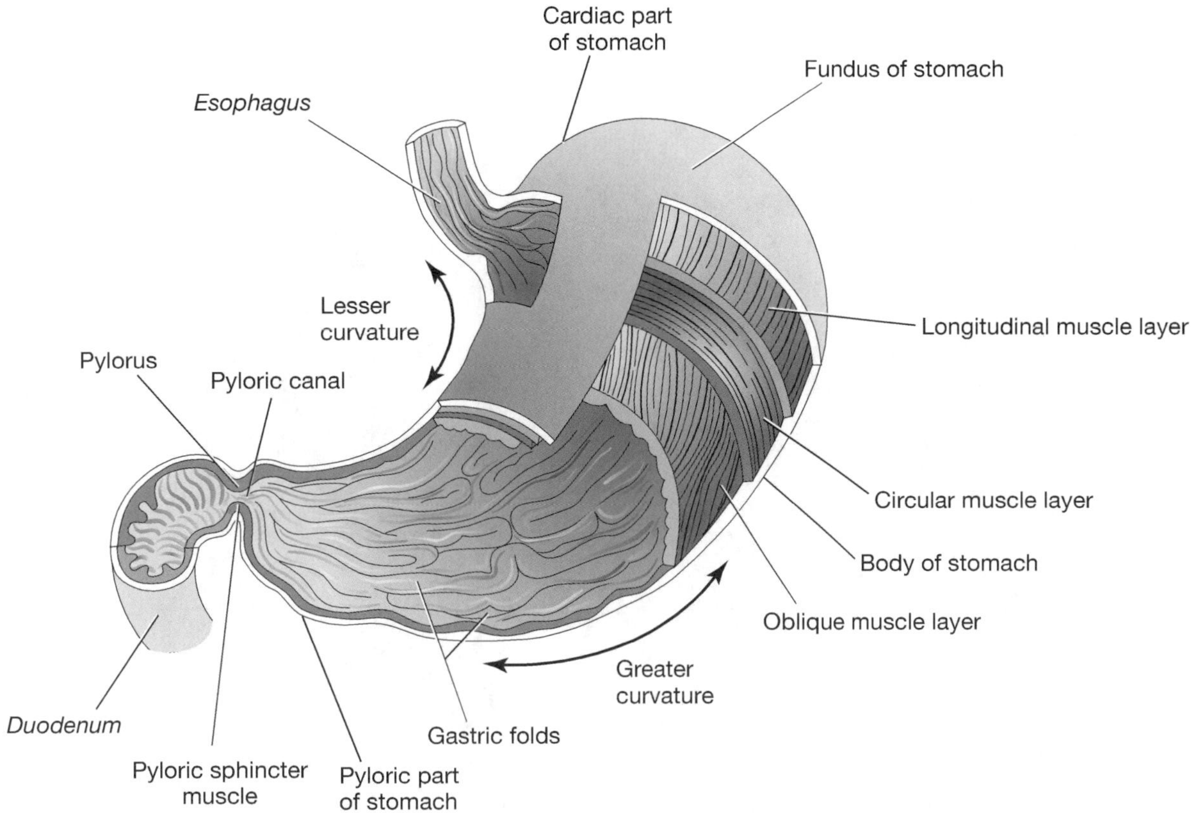

Figure 17-8

Stomach

The stomach has four major regions: cardiac part, fundus, body, and the pyloric part. The cardiac part is the portion where the esophagus enters. The fundus bulges to the left. The body is the main part of the stomach and the pyloric part is that portion which narrows down to join the duodenum at the pylorus.

acid and pepsin already present convert the pepsinogen to pepsin (a proteolytic enzyme which begins the breakdown of proteins). **Mucus producing cells** within the glands and on the lining surface secrete the mucus that protects the stomach wall from autodigestion. The tunica muscularis of the stomach is especially well-developed with three identifiable layers: longitudinal, circular, and oblique. As these muscles contract, ingesta is mixed, moistened with gastric juice, and then moved into the small intestine. The stomach absorbs some water (and alcohol, if present) from its contents, but very little else. It is primarily a receiving and holding reservoir.

Objectives

16. Diagram and label the stomach.
17. Differentiate pylorus, pyloric ostium, pyloric sphincter muscle, pyloric canal, and pyloric part of the stomach.
18. Name the three major cell types in the lining epithelium of the stomach and state the function of each.

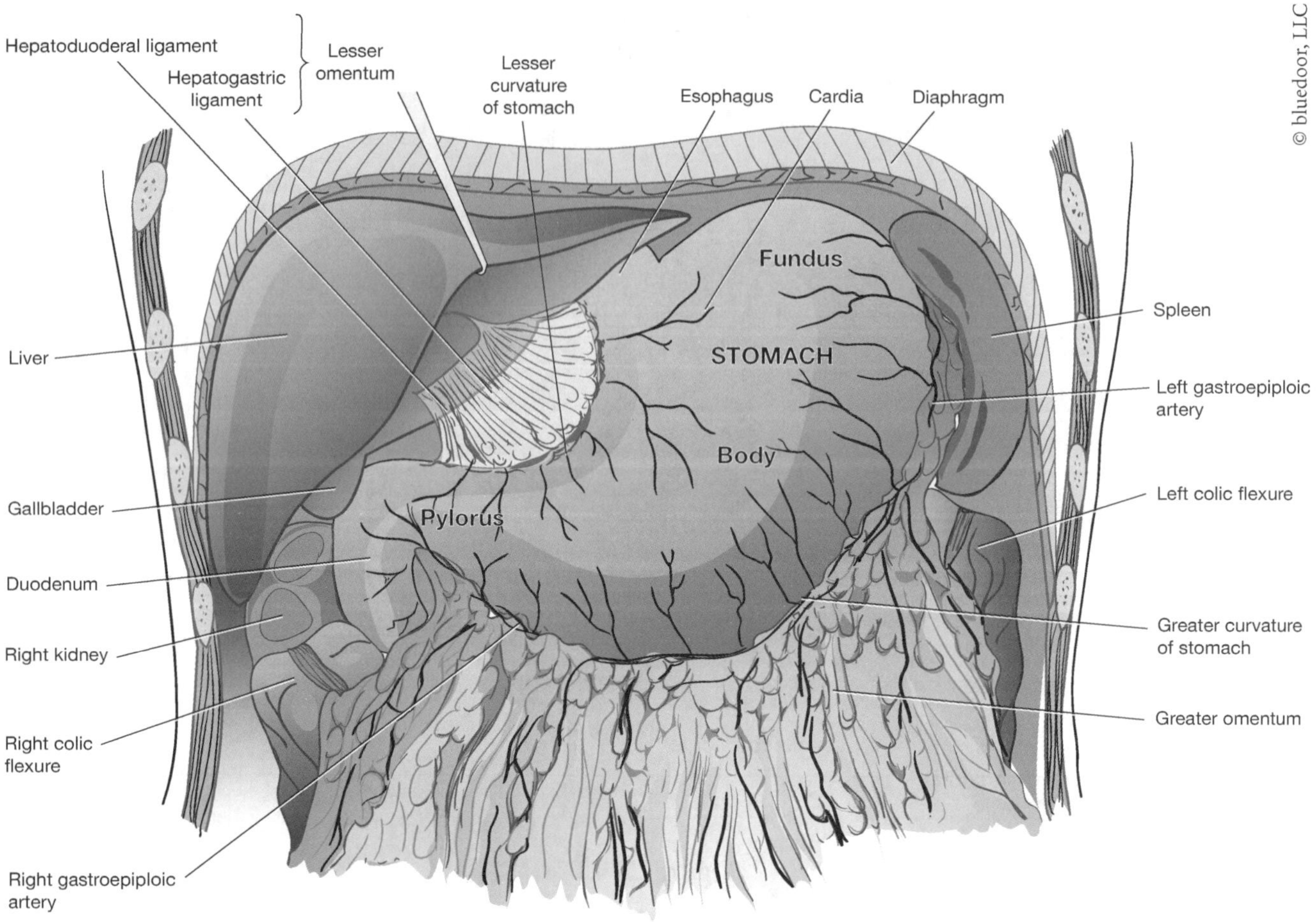

Figure 17-9

Relationship of the Stomach to Other Structures

The stomach lies below the diaphragm adjacent to the liver (above), the spleen (to the left), and the pancreas and intestine (below). The serous membrane reflecting off the greater curvature (greater omentum) covers the pancreas and intestine in this illustration. A similar reflection of peritoneum from the lesser curvature (lesser omentum) connects to the liver.

Small Intestine

The **small intestine** joins the stomach to the large intestine. It receives liquified ingesta (called **chyme**) from the stomach; mixes it with bile, pancreatic juice, and intestinal secretions; and serves as the major organ of hydrolysis and absorption (Table 17-2; Figure 17-12, 13, 14). The small intestine is about 21 feet (6-7 m) long and about an inch (2.5 cm) in diameter in an average individual. It is divided into three named segments: duodenum, jejunum, and ileum. The **duodenum** leaves the stomach at the pylorus, is the shortest segment (measuring about 12 inches (30 cm) in length), and has several named parts. The initial portion is directed superiorly and is called the **superior part** of the duodenum. It bends to the right and downward at the **superior duodenal flexure** to continue as the **descending part** of the duodenum. The descending duodenum courses inferiorly along the right abdominal wall and bends to the left at the **inferior duodenal flexure** to continue as the **hor-**

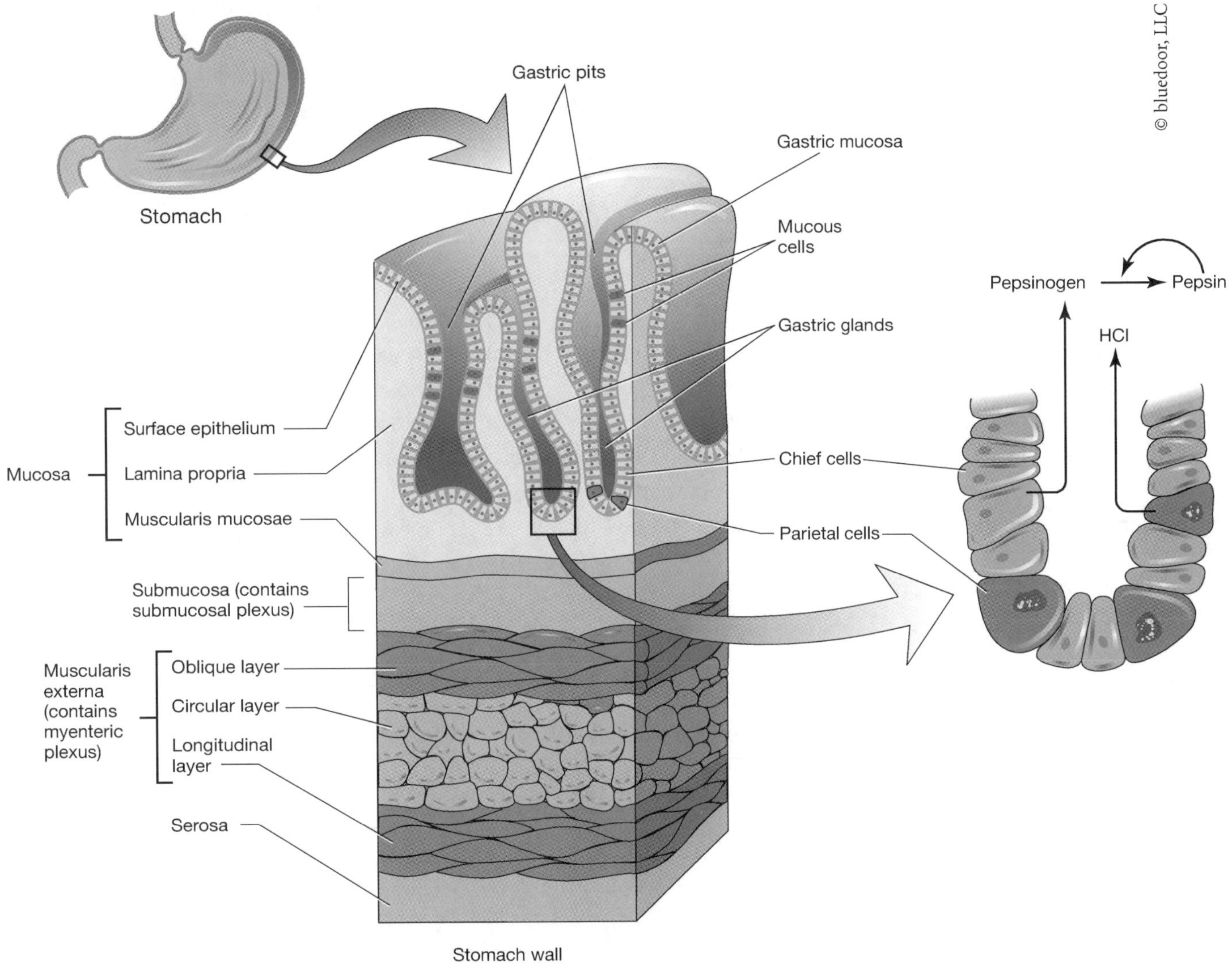

Figure 17-10

The Stomach Wall

The stomach is lined with simple columnar epithelium. It forms evaginations called gastric glands (simple tubular glands), the openings of which are called gastric pits. Three major types of cells are associated with the gastric glands: parietal cells (secrete HCl), principal (chief) cells (secrete pepsinogen), and mucous cells (secrete mucus).

izontal (**inferior**) **part** of the duodenum. The horizontal part turns upward to form the **ascending part** of the duodenum which joins the jejunum at a bend termed the **duodenojejunal flexure**. The descending duodenum receives the hepatopancreatic ampulla and accessory pancreatic duct. They open on mucosal projections termed the **major** and **minor duodenal papillae** (*see Figure 17-17*). The smaller minor duodenal papilla is located about 2 cm above the major one. The **jejunum** is about eight feet (2.5 m) long and the **ileum** is approximately twelve feet (4 m) in length. These two parts of the small intestine are essentially devoid of named landmarks. The ileum joins the large intestine by projecting into it at the **ileal papilla**. A thickened portion of the tunica muscularis at this point is called the **ileocecal** (**ileal**) **valve**. In contrast to the duodenum, which has several named subdivisions, the only landmark on the jejunum is the duodenojejunal flexure and the only one on the ileum is the ileocecal (ileal) valve (Table 17-3). A comparison of the three parts of the small intestine is shown in Table 17-3 and some of the differences are illustrated in Figure 17-14.

Table 17-2 A Comparison of the Small and Large Intestine

	Small Intestine	*Large Intestine*
Total length	21± feet	5–6 feet
Named parts	3 (duodenum, jejunum, ileum)	4 (cecum, colon, rectum, anal canal)
Villi	present	absent
Taeniae coli/sacculations	absent	present
Major functions	hydrolysis and absorption of most nutrients	absorption of water and electrolytes
Significant clinical conditions	ulceration and obstruction	diverticulosis and neoplasia

Table 17-3 A Comparison of the Three Parts of the Small Intestine

	Duodenum	*Jejunum*	*Ileum*
Length	1 foot	8 feet	12 feet
Relative length of villi	short	longer	longest
Submucosal glands	+	—	—
Relative number of goblet cells	+	++	+++
Number of aggregates of lymphatic nodules	+	++	+++
Named landmarks	several	duodenojejunal flexure	ileal (ileocecal) valve
Suspending peritoneum	mesoduodenum	mesentery (mesojejunum)	mesentery (mesoileum)
Primary digestive role	hydrolysis	hydrolysis and absorption	absorption

The mucosa of the small intestine forms **circular** (transversely oriented) **folds** due to contractions of the muscularis mucosae. These allow distensibility and increase the surface area available for absorption. Microscopic, finger-like projections of the intestinal mucosa called **intestinal villi** increase the surface area to maximize absorption. The simple columnar epithelial cells comprising the lining epithelium have **microvilli** projecting from their surface membranes to further increase the absorptive surface area. Simple tubular **intestinal glands** invaginate the mucosa at the bases of the villi. The secretory cells of these glands produce some enzymes that aid those present in pancreatic juice in the digestion of proteins, carbohydrates, and lipids. In the duodenum, submucosal glands ("Brunner's glands") are also present which produce additional mucus to protect the duodenal lining from the acidity of the chyme from the stomach. Lymphatic nodules are present within the mucosa of all parts of the small intestine but are especially numerous in the ileum.

Objectives

19. List, in order, the three main parts of the small intestine and schematically draw and label the landmarks of the duodenum.
20. List the structural modifications found in the small intestine that increase its absorptive capacity.

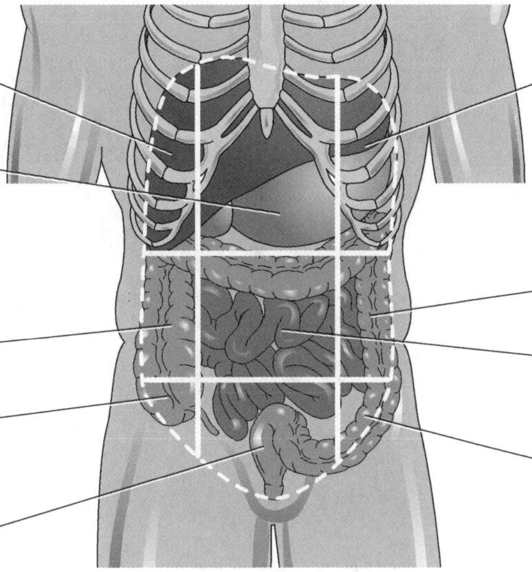

Figure 17-11
Abdominal Regions

The nine official regions illustrated here are used less often by medical practitioners than the four quadrants delineated by the median plane and a transverse plane through the umbilicus.

Large Intestine

The **large intestine** forms the terminal portion of the digestive system. It is only about five feet (1.5 m) long but is much larger in diameter (5 cm) than the small intestine. The large intestine functions primarily in the absorption of water and electrolytes. This dehydrates unabsorbed chyme (ingesta) to form feces which are temporarily stored and subsequently expelled from the body by defecation. The large intestine has four named segments: cecum, colon, rectum, and anal canal. The **cecum** forms a pouch-like diverticulum below the ileal papilla (Figure 17-15). It has a finger-like projection termed the **vermiform appendix** which is prone to infection and abscessation (appendicitis). The cecum is continuous above the ileal papilla with the **colon**. The latter forms the major portion of the large intestine and is divided into three straight segments (ascending, transverse, and descending colons), each of which is followed by a curved segment (right colic flexure, left colic flexure, and sigmoid colon).

The **ascending colon** courses superiorly from the cecum near the right side of the abdomen. It bends 90 degrees to the left near the liver as the **right colic flexure** and continues horizontally to the

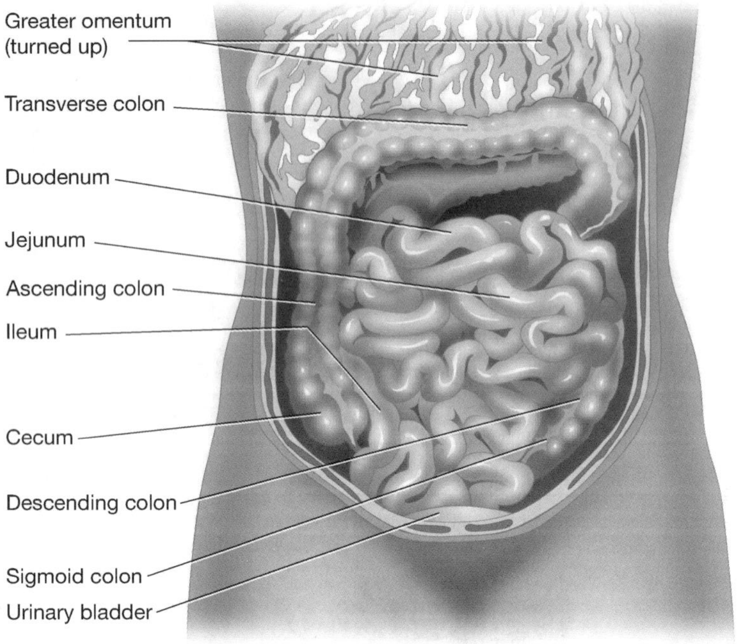

Figure 17-12
Intestine

The small intestine includes the duodenum, jejunum, and ileum and the large intestine is divided into four parts (*see Figure 17-15*). Most of the duodenum is hidden in this perspective and only parts of the large intestine are visible.

left as the **transverse colon**. Near the left abdominal wall, the transverse colon bends inferiorly 90 degrees as the **left colic flexure**. The latter continues inferiorly as the **descending colon** along the left abdominal wall to the pelvis. There, it angles medially and forms an S-shaped portion termed the **sigmoid colon**.

The remaining few inches of the large intestine are located on the median plane. They include the **rectum** (approximately 6 inches long) and the **anal canal** (about one inch long). Distention of the rectum by feces causes the sensation relating to the need to defecate. The anal canal serves as the terminal passageway and it opens at the **anus**. A thickened region of the outer layer of smooth muscle in the tunica muscularis of the anal canal forms the involuntary **internal anal sphincter muscle**. The **external anal sphincter muscle** is a skeletal muscle that encircles the anus.

The tunica muscularis of the large intestine has three distinct longitudinal bands called **taeniae coli**. These parallel the intestinal axis and are approximately equally spaced around the wall. They cause the formation of segmental **sacculations** (**haustra**) along its length. Small fat-filled pouches called **epiploic appendices** are present in the serosa. The mucosal lining of the large intestine lacks villi but does have simple tubular glands. These contain an especially large number of goblet cells interspersed among simple columnar epithelial cells.

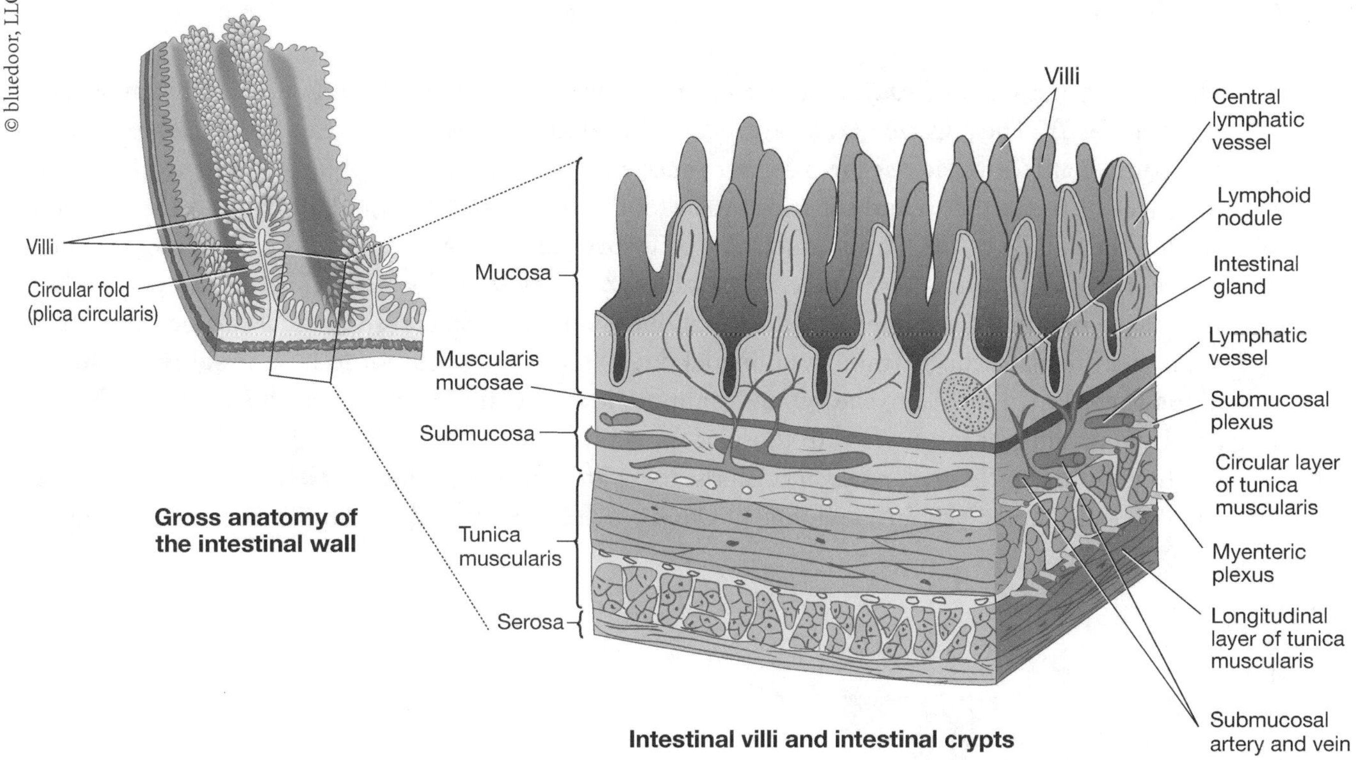

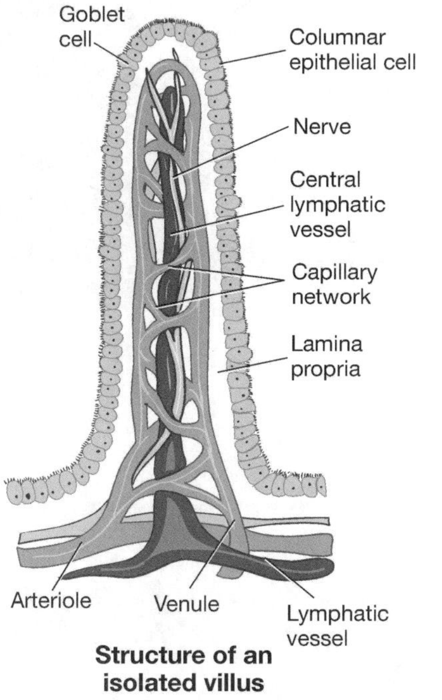

Figure 17-13
Structure of the Small Intestine Wall

The small intestinal mucosa increases its total surface area by circular folds, villi, and microvilli. The simple tubular glands (crypts) at the bases of the villi produce small intestinal juice which contains several hydrolytic enzymes. When nutrients are absorbed through the intestinal wall, they enter the capillaries therein. Most of them are absorbed directly into the bloodstream via regular cardiovascular capillaries. Lipids, however, are absorbed into specialized lymphatic capillaries (central lymphatic vessels = lacteals).

Objectives

21. Diagram and label the large intestine including its four major components and their various landmarks.
22. Differentiate the functional roles of the stomach, small intestine, and large intestine.
23. State the approximate lengths of the various parts of the alimentary canal.

Salivary Glands

There are three pairs of **major salivary glands**: parotid, sublingual, and submandibular glands (Figure 17-16). The **parotid glands** are located below and anterior to the ears. The duct from each one courses anteriorly across the masseter muscle to enter the oral vestibule on the medial side of the cheek opposite the second superior molar tooth. It opens at the tip of a tiny mucosal elevation termed the papilla of the parotid duct. An accessory parotid gland may be present along the duct where it crosses the masseter muscle. The **sublingual glands** are located below the tongue on each side of the midline. Each one has a duct that opens on the ipsilateral sublingual caruncle as well as a number of smaller ducts (minor sublingual ducts) that open posterior to it. The **submandibular glands** are located medial to the left and right bodies of the mandible. Their ducts open at the left and right sublingual caruncles with those of the sublingual glands.

In addition to the major salivary glands, there are numerous **minor salivary glands** including labial, buccal, molar, palatine, and lingual glands. These are located within the mucosa in the posi-

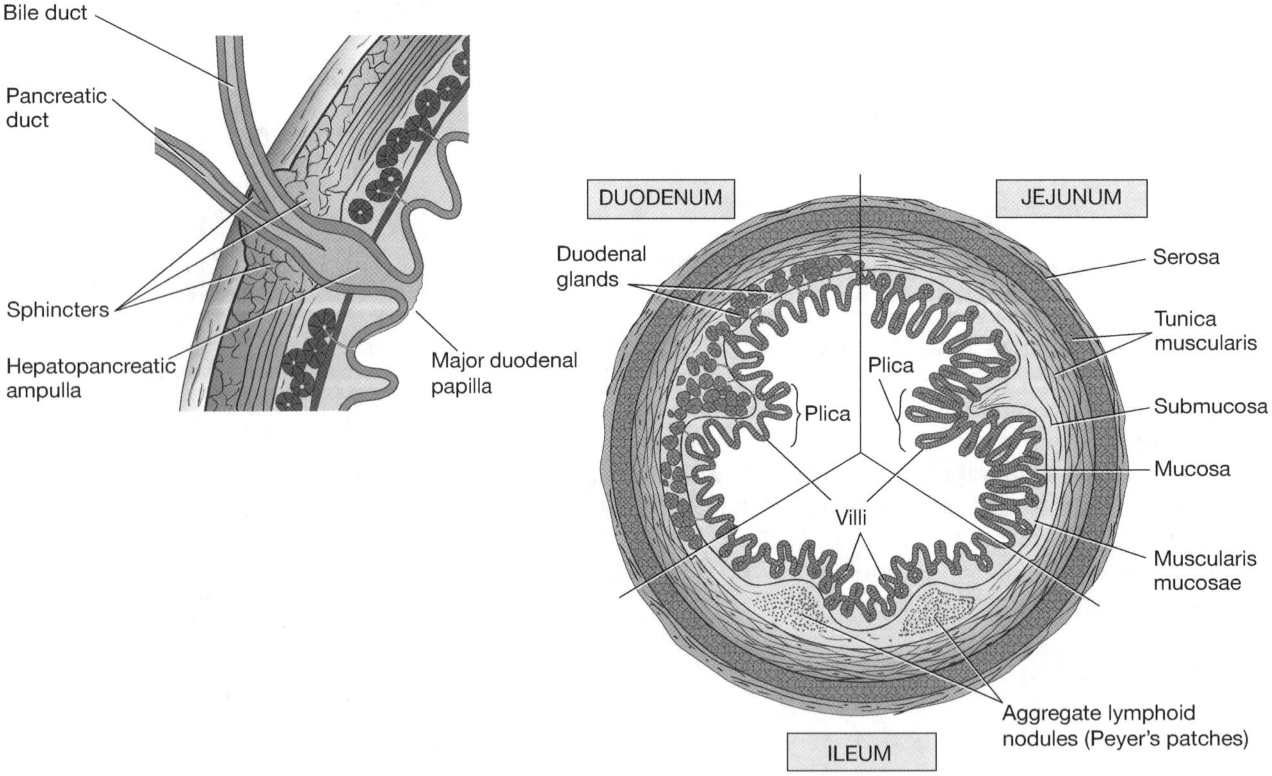

Figure 17-14

Structural Differences in the Small Intestinal Segments

The duodenum has well-developed glands in the submucosa and the ileum has numerous aggregations of lymphatic nodules in the same location. This drawing fails to emphasize that the villi in the lower (ileal) part of the small intestine are significantly longer than those in the duodenum or jejunum.

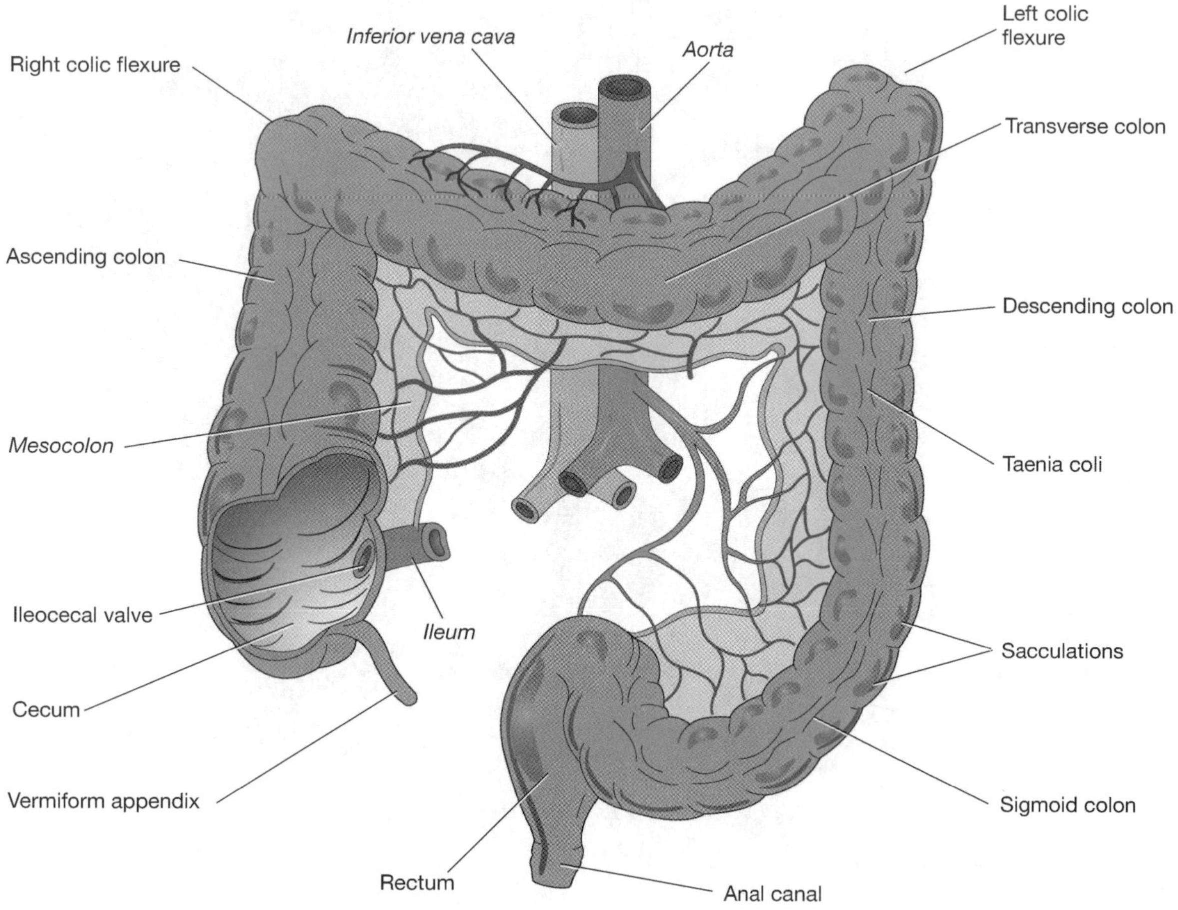

Figure 17-15
Large Intestine

The four regions of the large intestine are the cecum, colon, rectum, and anal canal ("anorectal" canal). The colon is divided into three straight regions and three curved regions.

tions implied by their names. The molar glands are several well-developed buccal glands located near the last molar teeth. The salivary glands produce a total of 1-2 liters of saliva each day. Saliva serves primarily as a lubricant but some of it also contains an **amylase** which hydrolyzes starch. Like the other glands of the digestive system, the salivary glands are controlled by both parts of the ANS. Parasympathetic impulses cause the secretion of large volumes of watery saliva. This occurs at the sight, smell, or even thought of desirable food. Sympathetic impulses result in a smaller quantity of thicker (more viscous) saliva.

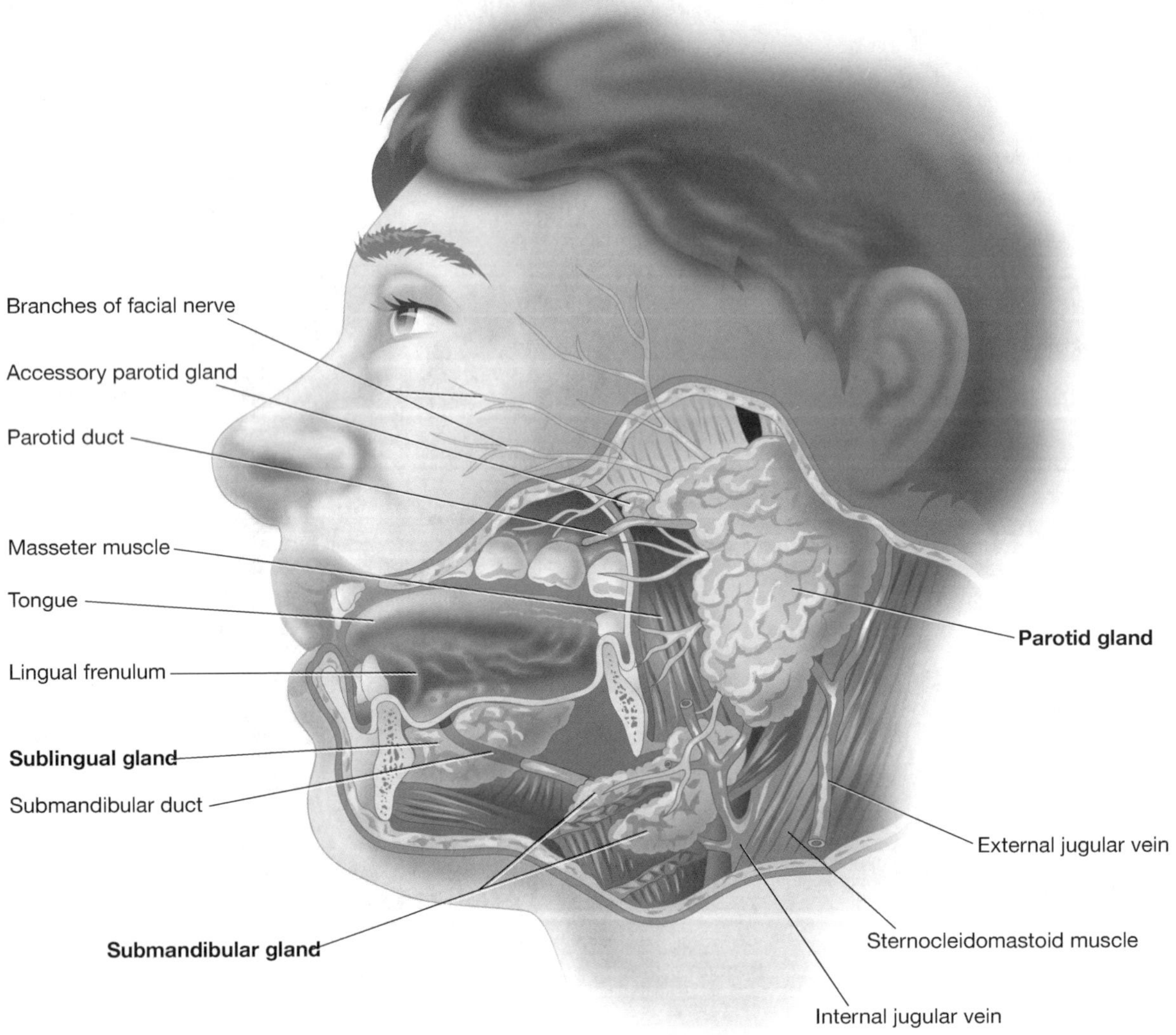

Figure 17-16

Salivary Glands

The three major pairs of salivary glands are the parotid, submandibular, and sublingual glands. The saliva that they produce contains a weak amylase but functions primarily as a lubricant for mastication and deglutition. The parotid duct opens into the oral vestibule near the second superior molar tooth. The ducts of the sublingual and submandibular glands open on the sublingual caruncles under the tongue. In some individuals, pressure on the sublingual and submandibular glands (especially when yawning) will cause a small stream of saliva to involuntarily squirt out of the oral cavity. This is sometimes termed "gleeking".

Objectives

24. Name the three major pairs of salivary glands, state where each pair is located, and indicate where the ducts from each open into the oral cavity.

Liver

The **liver** is the largest internal organ (3-4 lbs) and the largest gland in the body. It is located immediately inferior to the diaphragm and is structurally divided into four lobes: right, left, quadrate, and caudate. These surround a hilar area on the inferior aspect termed the **hepatic porta** where the hepatic portal vein, proper hepatic artery, and common hepatic duct are located. The **right lobe** is the largest one and is separated from the small, anteroinferiorly located **quadrate lobe** by the gallbladder. The **caudate lobe** is a small lobe located above and behind the hepatic porta. The **left lobe** is second in size only to the right lobe (Figure 17-17, 18).

The **liver cells** (**hepatocytes**) are arranged around central veins to form functional units called **liver lobules** (Figure 17-19). **Hepatic** ("portal") **triads** are located at several loci around the periphery of each lobule. Each of these consists of a tiny branch of the hepatic portal vein, a branch of the proper hepatic artery and a biliary ductule. Blood flows from the artery and vein into spaces between the hepatocytes called **sinusoidal capillaries** (sinusoids). Phagocytes called stellate macrophages ("Kupffer cells") line these vessels. They are the second capillaries in the hepatic portal system (*see Chapter 15*) and allow the hepatocytes access to absorbed metabolites and toxins. Blood from the arterial and venous channels mixes in the sinusoids and flows centrally to the **central vein**. The central veins from adjacent lobules coalesce to form venous channels which empty into three or four hepatic veins. These leave the liver and drain into the inferior vena cava near the diaphragm. Hepatocytes produce **bile** as an exocrine product. Bile aides in the emulsification, digestion, and absorption of lipids. It is secreted directly into tiny biliary channels called **bile canaliculi** which are located between adjacent hepatocytes. These channels are entirely separate from the sinusoids and bile flows peripherally in them to empty into the **biliary ductules** within the hepatic triads. These ductules empty into larger biliary channels which coalesce to form the **left** and **right hepatic ducts**. The latter join to form the **common hepatic duct** which receives the **cystic duct** and then continues toward the descending duodenum as the **bile duct**. The latter is usually joined by the pancreatic duct to form the **hepatopancreatic ampulla** and this combined passageway opens at the tip of the major duodenal papilla. Note that bile which is temporarily stored in the gallbladder must traverse the cystic duct twice—once to enter the gallbladder and once again when leaving it.

Objectives

25. Name the lobes of the liver and state where the gallbladder is located relative to them.
26. Diagram and label a hepatic lobule and discuss the flow of blood and bile through it.

Gallbladder

The **gallbladder** is a storage reservoir for bile secreted by the liver (Figure 17-17, 18). It is located in the **fossa for the gallbladder** which is a depression positioned on the visceral (inferior) surface

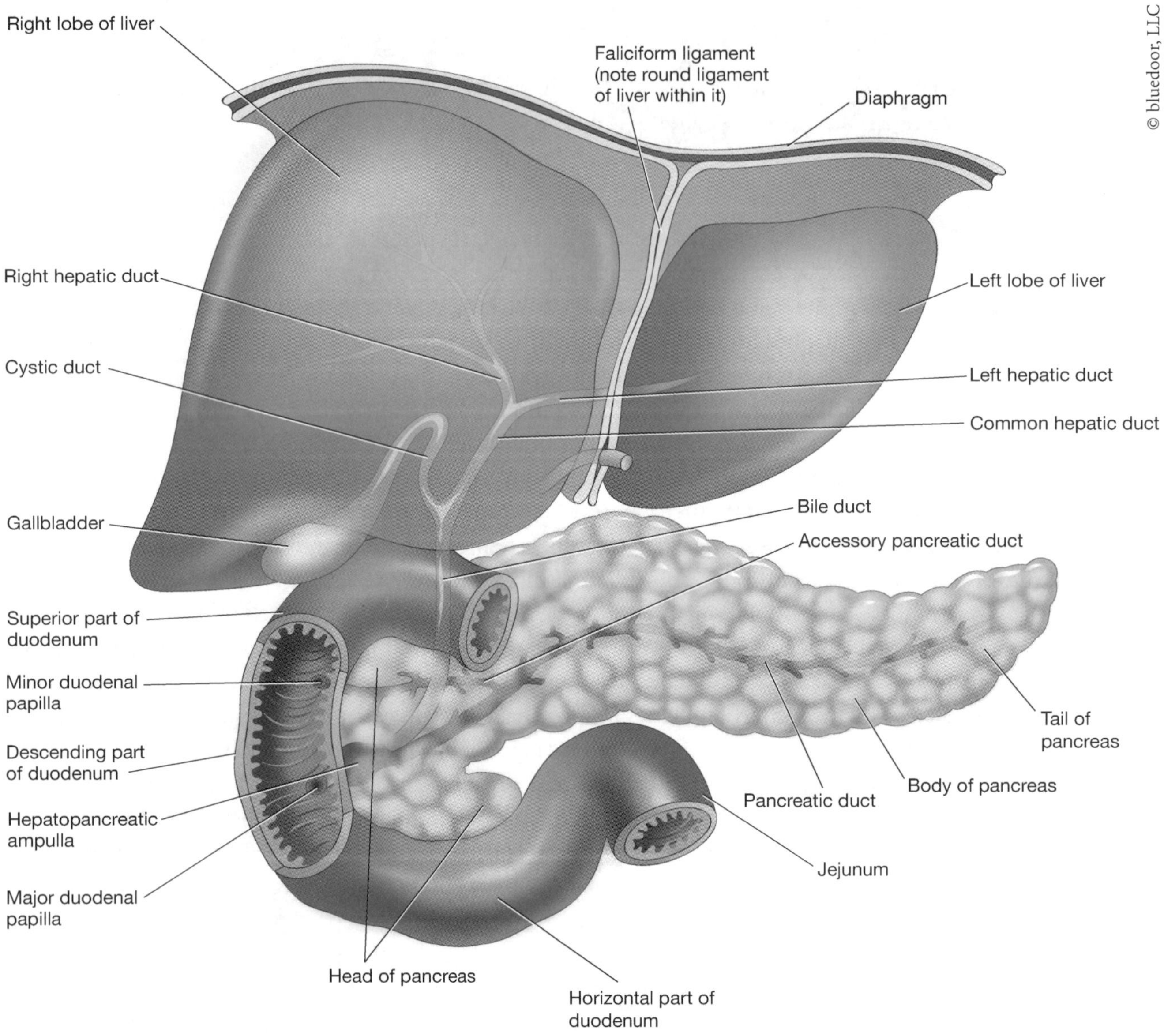

Figure 17-17

Liver, Gallbladder, Pancreas, and Duodenum

The descending duodenum has been sectioned to show the terminations of the accessory pancreatic duct at the minor duodenal papilla and the hepatopancreatic ampulla at the major duodenal papilla.

of the liver at the junction of the right and quadrate lobes. The gallbladder consists of a **fundus** (inferiorly), **body**, and **neck** which connects to the cystic duct. It distends as it fills with bile and contracts via smooth muscle in its tunica muscularis to force bile back into the cystic duct and thence on into the bile duct and descending duodenum. As bile is secreted by the liver it may continue directly into the duodenum if the **sphincter muscle of the hepatopancreatic ampulla** within the wall of the duodenum is relaxed. If the sphincter muscle is contracted, bile will be forced into the cystic duct and (temporarily) stored in the gallbladder.

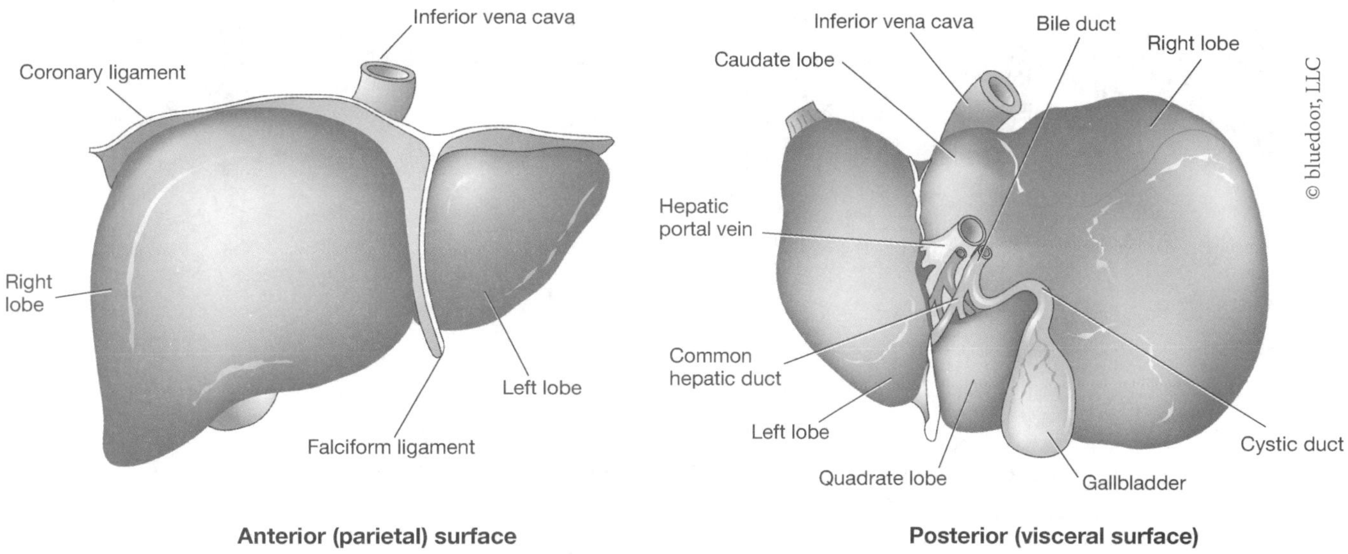

Figure 17-18

Gross Features of the Liver

The liver lies just below the diaphragm within the abdominal cavity. It has four lobes, two surfaces, and a hilum (porta hepatis) where vessels and biliary channels enter/leave.

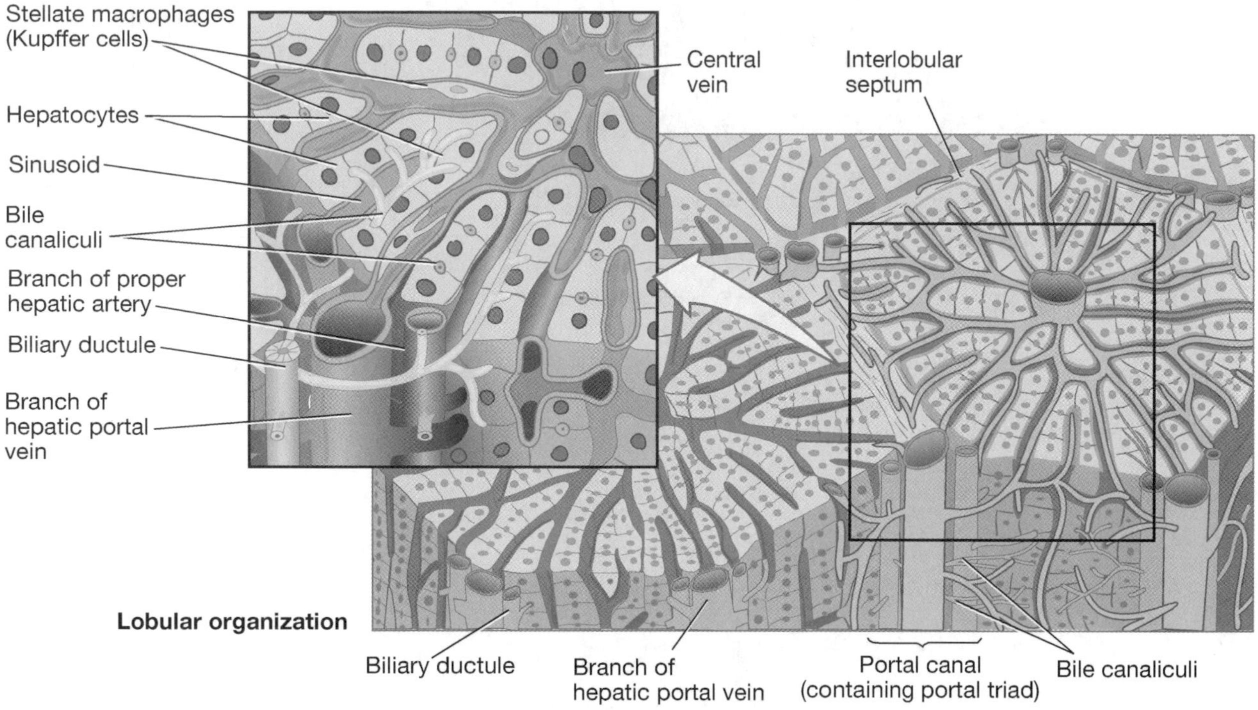

Figure 17-19

Microstructures of the Liver

The hepatic parenchyma is divided into groups of hepatocytes that are surrounded by connective tissue proper. Each group constitutes a liver lobule. Within a liver lobule, blood flows centrally (centripetally) through the modified capillaries called liver sinusoids. Blood from the branches of the portal vein mixes with the arterial blood from the branches of the proper hepatic artery. Bile, a secretory product of the hepatocytes, flows peripherally (centrifugally) through the bile canaliculi and empties into a biliary ductule within a hepatic triad. Note that blood and bile are located in completely separate passageways.

Objectives

27. Diagram and label the biliary duct system.

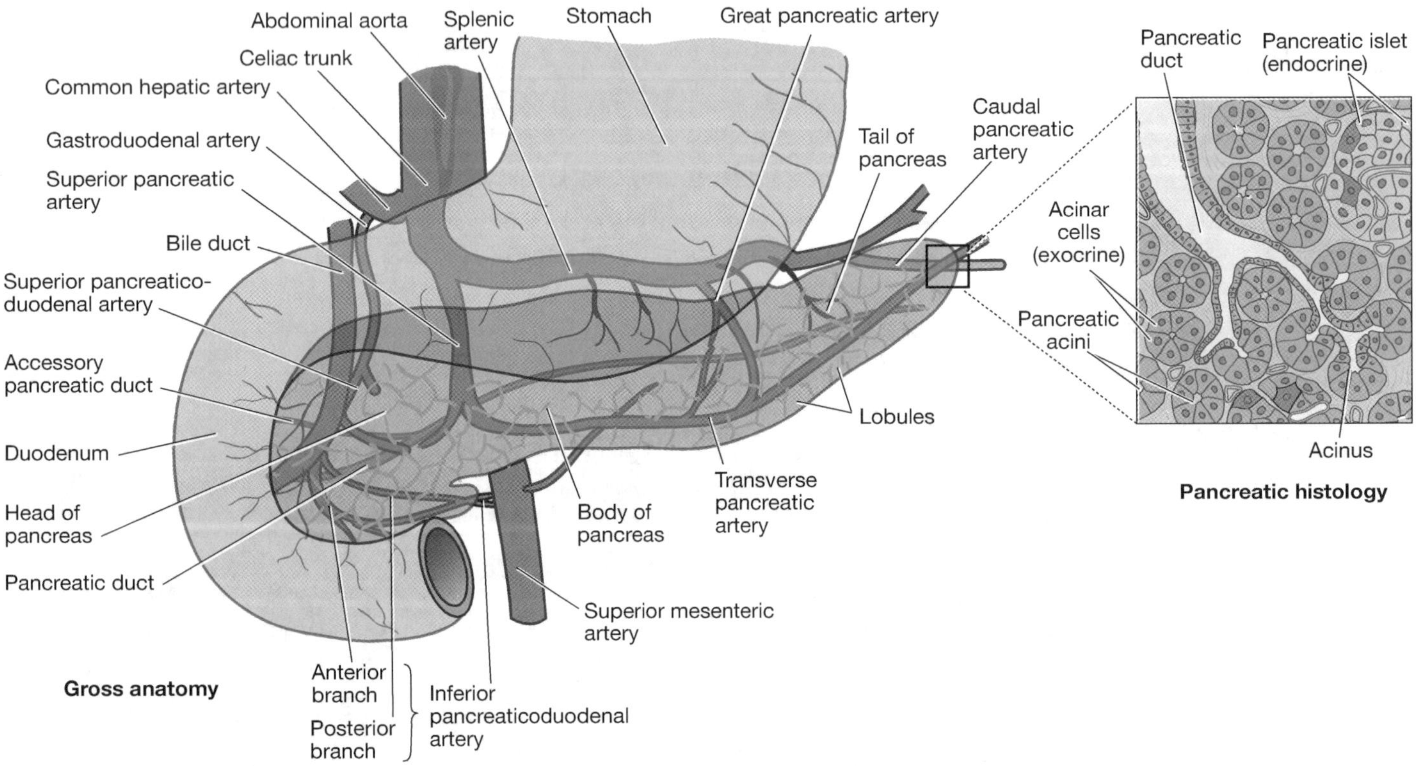

Figure 17-20

Pancreas

Grossly, the pancreas has three main parts: head (against the duodenum), body, and tail. Pancreatic juice is transported toward the descending duodenum by the pancreatic duct and the accessory pancreatic duct. The pancreatic duct joins the bile duct to form the hepatopancreatic ampulla. This combined passageway opens at the major (greater) duodenal papilla. The accessory pancreatic duct opens at the minor duodenal papilla. Insulin and glucagon are produced by the cells of the pancreatic islets.

Pancreas

The **pancreas** is located adjacent to the duodenum within the abdominal cavity. It consists of a head, body, and tail (Figure 17-17, 20). The **head of the pancreas** is the widest part and is positioned against the descending duodenum at the inferior duodenal flexure. The **body of the pancreas** extends to the left along the horizontal part of the duodenum and continues toward the spleen. The **tail of the pancreas** is the tapered left extremity. The pancreas produces **pancreatic juice** as an exocrine product and two hormones: insulin and glucagon. Pancreatic juice is the most important digestive fluid in the body. It contains a number of different enzymes that hydrolyze proteins, carbohydrates, and fats. It is secreted by **pancreatic acinar cells** and drains into a series of channels that coalesce to form the **pancreatic duct**. The pancreatic duct joins the bile duct to form the hepatopancreatic ampulla and this combined passageway empties into the descending duodenum at the major duodenal papilla. A smaller **accessory pancreatic duct** branches from the pancreatic duct and typically enters the duodenum independently at the minor duodenal papilla. There is a considerable individual variation in the two pancreatic ducts. The most common ones are failure of the accessory pancreatic duct to join the duodenum, and failure of the two pancreatic ducts to communicate with each other. Scattered among the pancreatic acinar cells are groups of endocrine cells known as **pancreatic islets**. These contain **alpha cells** which produce glucagon and **beta cells** which secrete insulin (*see Chapter 14*).

Objectives

28. List the three gross parts of the pancreas, name its two ducts, and indicate where each one terminates.
29. List the three main cell types present in the pancreas, state what each produces, and indicate which two are found in the pancreatic islets.

Abdomen, Abdominal Cavity; Peritoneum, Peritoneal Cavity

The **abdomen** is the region of the body below the thorax and above the pelvis. The space within it is called the **abdominal cavity** and is continuous below with the space inside the pelvis. Some anatomists prefer to combine the two as the abdominopelvic cavity. The abdominal portion is larger than the pelvic part and it contains many of the digestive, urinary, and reproductive organs, as well as a few vessels, nerves, and endocrine organs. The **peritoneum** is a serous membrane that lines the abdominal and pelvic cavities and adheres to all organs therein (Figure 17-21). The peritoneum on the abdominal wall, pelvic wall, and on the underside of the diaphragm is called the **parietal peritoneum**. That which is adherent to the surfaces of the organs is called **visceral peritoneum**.

Organs such as the kidneys, adrenal glands, and the abdominal portions of the aorta and inferior vena cava which have peritoneum only on their anterior surfaces are said to be **retroperitoneal** ("behind the peritoneum"). The potential space between the parietal and visceral peritoneum is the **peritoneal cavity**. It is a closed cavity (except for the openings of the left and right ovarian bursae in females) that contains nothing except a small amount of serous fluid. The fused, double layers of connecting peritoneum which extend between the parietal peritoneum and various organs are given special names. There are many more of these than the ones described in Table 17-4. Diverticula from the main part of the peritoneal cavity between and around various organs form the paravesicular fossae (both sexes), the rectovesicular excavation (males) and the recto-uterine and vesico-uterine excavations (females).

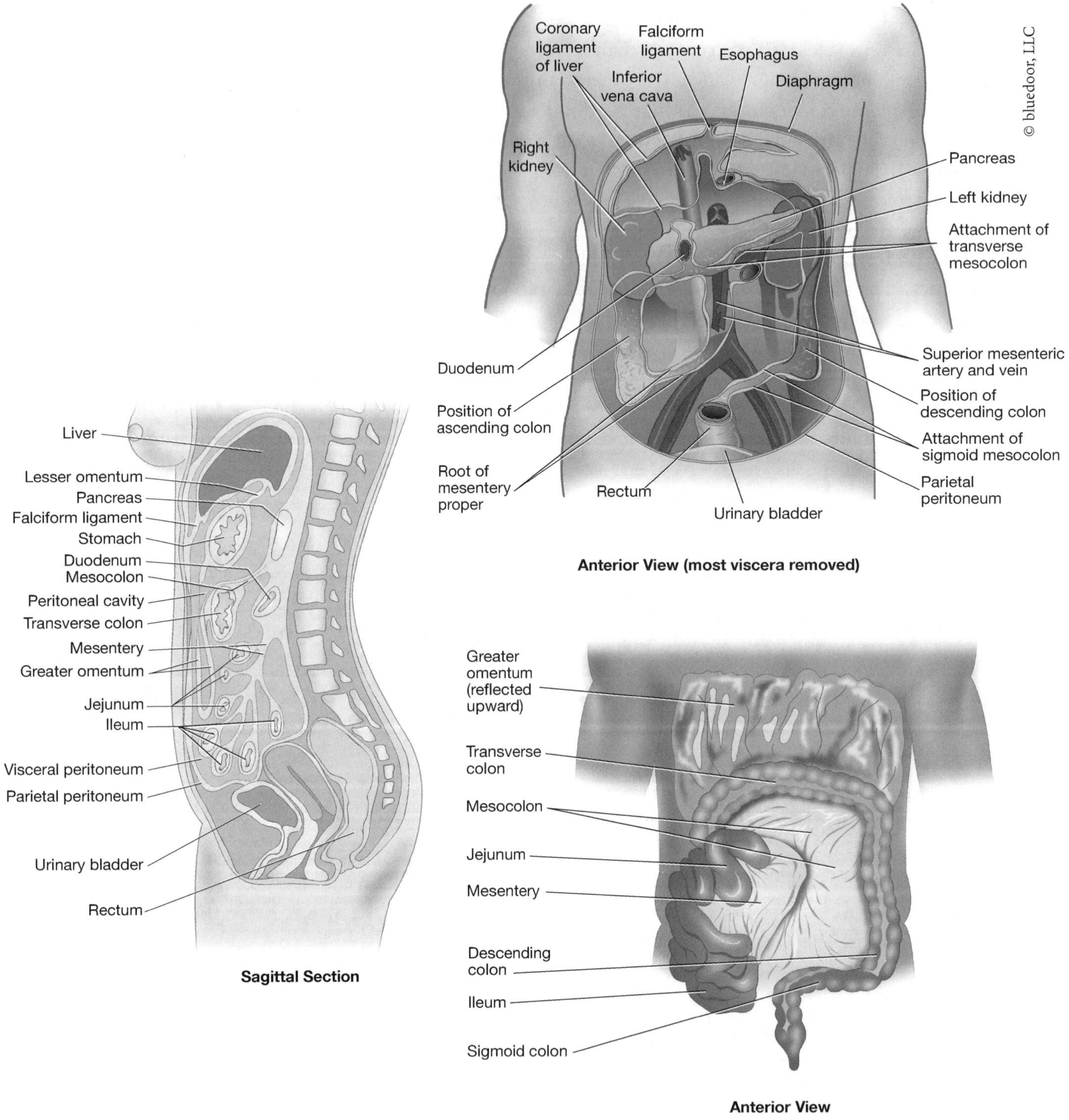

Figure 17-21

Peritoneum and the Peritoneal Cavity

The serous membrane lining the abdominal cavity is called peritoneum. On the body wall, it is designated parietal peritoneum and on the surfaces of organs it is called visceral peritoneum. The doubled layers of parietal peritoneum between the body wall and various organs are given specific names (*see Table 17-4*).

Table 17-4 Examples of Connecting Peritoneum

These are all double-layered sheets of peritoneum (two layers fused together) in contrast to the single layers that cover organs (visceral peritoneum) or line the walls of the abdominal cavity (parietal peritoneum). This is only a partial listing.

Greater omentum—the redundant peritoneum that extends from the greater curvature of the stomach to the transverse colon and thence to the posterior abdominal wall. It has five named subdivisions: gastrophrenic, gastrosplenic, gastrocolic, phrenicocolic, and splenorenal ligaments.

Lesser omentum—the peritoneum extending from the liver to the lesser curvature of the stomach and upper portion of the duodenum. It has two major subdivisions: hepatogastric and hepatoduodenal ligaments.

Falciform ligament—the peritoneum extending to the liver from the diaphragm and anterior body wall. The round ligament of the liver lies within it.

Coronary ligament of the liver—the peritoneum that reflects from the inferior surface of the diaphragm to the liver.

Triangular ligaments of the liver (right and left)—the peritoneum that extends from the right or left lobe of the liver to the diaphragm. It is continuous with the coronary ligament.

Hepatorenal ligament—the peritoneal fold that passes from the posterior aspect of the visceral surface of the liver to the anterior aspect of the right kidney to form the right margin of the epiploic foramen.

Mesentery—the peritoneum that extends from the posterior abdominal wall to support the jejunum and ileum.

Mesocolon—the peritoneum that extends from the posterior abdominal wall to support the colon. It is divided into the ascending, transverse, descending, and sigmoid mesocolons, and the meso-appendix.

Broad ligament of the uterus—the peritoneum that supports the female reproductive viscera. It is divided into the mesosalpinx, mesovarium, and mesometrium.

- **Mesosalpinx**—the part of the broad ligament of the uterus above the mesovarium that encloses the uterine tube.
- **Mesovarium**—the part of the broad ligament of the uterus between the mesosalpinx and mesometrium that holds the ovary in place.
- **Mesometrium**—the part of the broad ligament of the uterus below the mesovarium that encloses the uterus.

Objectives

30. Differentiate abdomen, abdominal cavity, peritoneum, and peritoneal cavity.
31. Define retroperitoneal and list several structures to which the term applies.

Development of the Digestive System

The primitive intestinal tube from which the membranous and glandular epithelium lining the alimentary canal is derived from endoderm is called the **gut**, and is divided into three segments: **foregut**, **midgut**, and **hindgut** (Figure 17-22). These give rise to the linings of specific digestive organs as well as the linings of the organs of the lower respiratory system (Table 17-5). The muscular and connective tissue components of the various digestive organs are derived from the mesoderm which lies adjacent to the primitive gut.

The primitive gut is initially formed by the **head** (cranial) and **tail** (caudal) **folds** which enclose part of the endoderm within the embryo. The midgut remains connected to the extraembryonic yolk sac by the vitelline duct and the hindgut is joined to the allantois, another extra-embryonic structure (Figure 17-18). At the cranial end of the developing gut, a depression in the surface ectoderm termed the **stomodeum** contacts the endoderm to form a thin partition termed the **buccopharyngeal membrane**. This ruptures soon after its formation to form an open connection between the **foregut** and the external environment (Figure 17-19). A similar membrane, the **cloacal membrane**, initially separates the caudal part of the **hindgut** from an ectodermal depression termed the **proctodeum** (Figure 17-20). This cloacal membrane is divided into an anterior **urogenital membrane** and a posterior **anal membrane** by a septum of tissue termed the **urorectal ridge** (Figure 17-20).

The **midgut** is initially a very short segment of the alimentary canal extending from the anterior intestinal portal to the posterior one and connected to the yolk sac by the **vitelline duct** (Figure 17-20). It undergoes rapid elongation during development to form a **primary intestinal loop** which twists 270 degrees (counterclockwise when viewed from the ventral aspect) on itself and continues to elongate (Figure 17-21). The various parts of this loop form the intestinal tube. Sometimes a vestige of vitelline duct can be found on the ileum (Meckel's diverticulum). Vitelline fistulae or cysts can also occur.

The liver, gallbladder, and pancreas all develop as evaginations from the terminal part of the foregut (Figure 17-22). The pancreas initially develops as separate dorsal and ventral primordia which fuse to form the definitive pancreas. Separate ducts (pancreatic and accessory pancreatic) remain in the adult.

Table 17-5 Derivatives of the Primitive Gut

Foregut—pharynx and its derivatives, distal portion of transverse colon, larynx, trachea, bronchial tree, lungs, esophagus, stomach, proximal part of duodenum, liver, gallbladder, biliary ducts,

Midgut—distal part of duodenum, jejunum, ileum, cecum, vermiform appendix, ascending colon, and initial part of transverse colon

Hindgut—distal portion of transverse colon, descending colon, sigmoid colon, rectum, superior part of anal canal, lining of urinary bladder and most of urethra

Objectives

32. State the major derivatives of the foregut, midgut, and hindgut.

Clinical Considerations

The digestive system is subject to so many acquired diseases and developmental anomalies that any discussion of them would either be either quite lengthy or woefully inadequate. Only a few examples will be given. In the oral cavity, failure of left and right primordia to fuse properly during gestation can produce a **harelip** (split lip) or **cleft palate**. The latter may be so severe that it negates the newborn's ability to suckle and interferes with deglutition. Viral infections of the oral mucosa can produce localized ulcerations called **canker sores** that can be quite painful. Localized thermal damage from ingesting food that is too hot is also common.

Figure 17-22
Development of the Digestive System

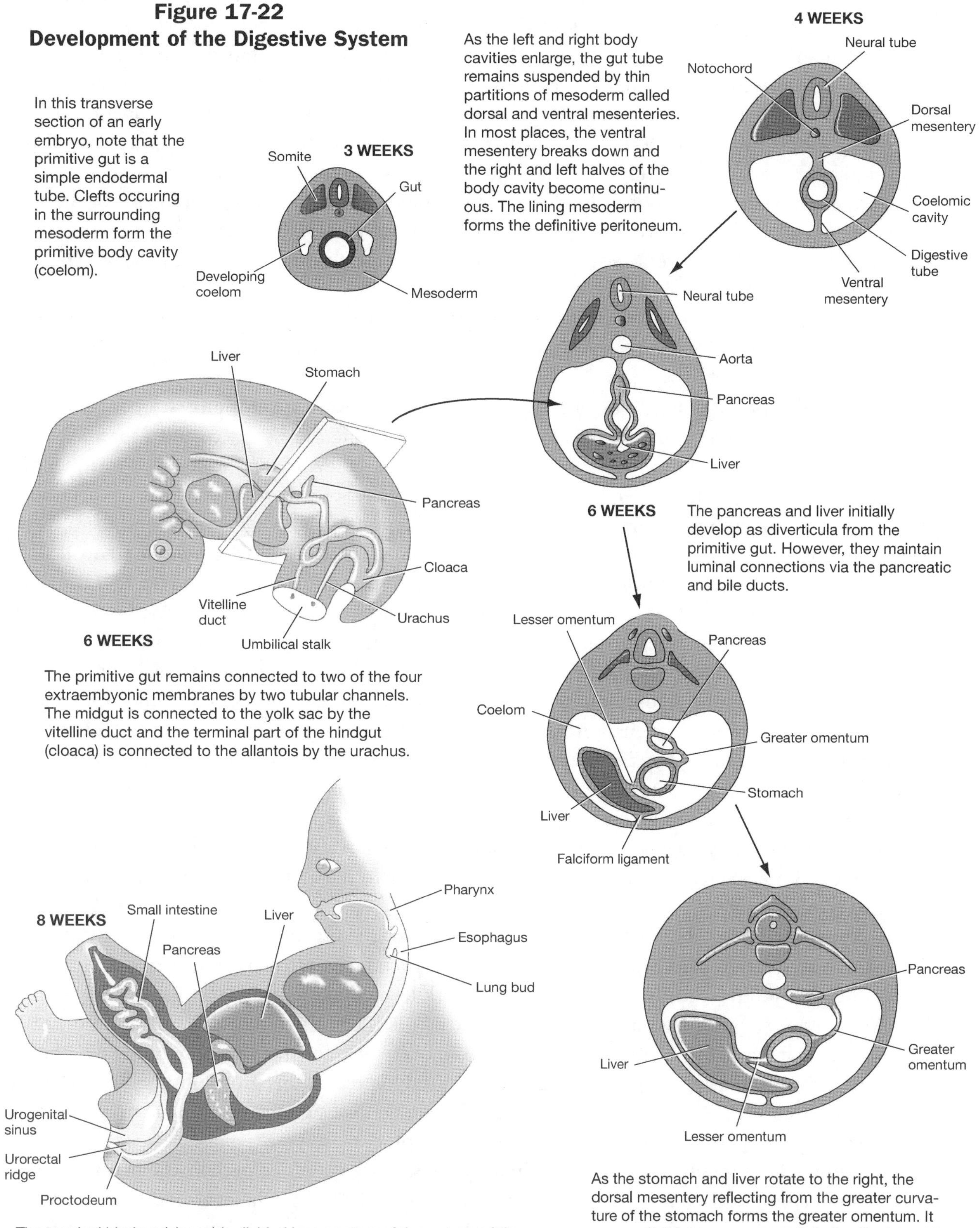

In this transverse section of an early embryo, note that the primitive gut is a simple endodermal tube. Clefts occuring in the surrounding mesoderm form the primitive body cavity (coelom).

As the left and right body cavities enlarge, the gut tube remains suspended by thin partitions of mesoderm called dorsal and ventral mesenteries. In most places, the ventral mesentery breaks down and the right and left halves of the body cavity become continuous. The lining mesoderm forms the definitive peritoneum.

The pancreas and liver initially develop as diverticula from the primitive gut. However, they maintain luminal connections via the pancreatic and bile ducts.

The primitive gut remains connected to two of the four extraembyonic membranes by two tubular channels. The midgut is connected to the yolk sac by the vitelline duct and the terminal part of the hindgut (cloaca) is connected to the allantois by the urachus.

The terminal hindgut (cloaca) is divided by a septum of tissue termed the urorectal ridge. The space anterior to this septum becomes the urogenital sinus (which forms urinary structures) and the posterior space becomes the proctodeum, which develops into the rectum and anal canal.

As the stomach and liver rotate to the right, the dorsal mesentery reflecting from the greater curvature of the stomach forms the greater omentum. It surrounds the pancreas enroute to its attachment to the posterior body wall. The ventral mesentery reflecting from the lesser curvature of the stomach to the liver becomes the lesser omentum. That portion of it between the liver and anterior body wall becomes the falciform ligament.

The majority of the problems in the oral cavity relate to the teeth and involve decay, malocclusion, or periodontal disease. **Tooth decay** (dental caries) is caused by acids produced by bacteria and is partially related to poor oral hygiene. Decayed portions may be abraded with dental drills and replaced with restorations ("fillings") of gold or silver alloys or enamel colored polymers. Severely damaged teeth may require especially large restorations called caps or crowns. Improper tooth positioning is called **malocclusion**. It is usually related to crowding of the oral cavity but can also be caused by habits including thumb sucking and tongue thrusting. Orthodontic treatment can significantly improve most cases of malocclusion. **Periodontal disease** includes problems of the gums and dental alveoli. These are often related to poor oral hygiene. **Gingivitis** (inflammation of the gums), for example, can be caused by the build up of plaque near the necks of the teeth. **Halitosis** is a foul odor from the mouth.

Inflammation of the pharynx (**pharyngitis**) due to bacterial or viral infections is commonly called a "sore throat". It and the esophagus may be severely damaged by ingestion of strong acids or bases such as *Draino®*.

The lining of the stomach sometimes ulcerates. **Peptic ulcers** are erosions of the mucosa of the stomach or duodenum due to hydrochloric acid. These are often stress related and a specific bacterium seems to be involved in most cases as well. Sometimes they respond to medical treatment but severe cases may require surgery. Surgical severance of the vagal nerve trunks (or of their gastric branches) is sometimes performed to reduce the production of hydrochloric acid, and the ulcerated segment of the stomach wall may be removed. The stomach is also subject to **pyloric stenosis** which involves a narrowing of the pylorus. Affected individuals have difficulty moving ingesta through this opening and surgery may be required to enlarge the passageway. It is usually detected in infants and a classic sign is an abnormal frequency of spitting up. Partial gastrectomy (removal of part of the stomach) is occasionally done because of cancer or to help obese patients control their body weight.

The small intestine is subject to physical obstruction, traumatic perforation, and strangulation due to torsion (twisting on its long axis) or volvulus (twisting a loop or knotting). **Intestinal obstruction** from foreign bodies is a relatively common problem in toddlers who try to ingest most anything that they put into their oral cavities. Obstruction may require surgical intervention (**enterotomy**) to remove the offending object. Obstruction may also occur due to severe **constipation**. In mature individuals, colonic cancer may require removal of a significant segment of the large intestine. Surgical creation of an artificial anal opening in the abdominal wall in these patients is called a **colostomy**.

Appendicitis is inflammation and/or abscessation of the vermiform appendix. The classic sign is severe abdominal pain. Individuals with acute appendicitis often have discomfort localized at **McBurney's point** which is an imaginary landmark located at one-third the distance between the right anterior superior iliac spine and the umbilicus. This condition may prove fatal if not treated because the infected organ may burst and release an overwhelming quantity of toxins and pathogenic bacteria. Infected appendices are surgically removed to prevent this probability. Since the appendix is apparently a vestigial organ with no remaining digestive significance, it is often removed any time a surgeon happens to open an abdomen for any other reason (*see Points to Ponder 2*).

Mumps is a viral disease affecting primarily the salivary glands (especially the parotid glands). It is an uncomfortable but not serious condition unless it also affects the pancreas or testes where it can cause serious consequences. **Viral hepatitis** is a contagious disease involving the liver. It is a serious disease that can be fatal.

The liver is a critical organ that is closely monitored with laboratory tests and biopsies in the living and histopathic evaluation in those deceased. An interesting observation reported by pathologists performing autopsies is that toxic conditions of the liver (poisoning, alcoholism, *etc.*) typically produce their first changes near the periphery of hepatic lobules. This logically follows the pattern of blood flow within the lobule (peripheral to central). Chronic heart failure, on the other hand, causes central lobular degeneration due to the back pressure related to poor pumping by the heart.

The gallbladder occasionally becomes filled with **gallstones** which form by the precipitation of insoluble materials. These may cause essentially no problem within the gallbladder but one may block the cystic duct or bile duct with serious consequences. Some individuals have their gallbladders removed because of this problem. Such individuals still produce bile and still transport it from the liver to the duodenum in their bile duct, but they do not have any ability to store bile. They often have more problems with fatty (greasy) meals than do individuals with intact gallbladders because they cannot store significant quantities of bile.

A **hernia** is an abnormal passageway through which various organs may protrude and possibly become strangulated. Typical hernias involve weakened areas in the abdominal wall through which loops of intestine or other abdominal organs may pass. Diaphragmatic hernias involve abnormal openings in the diaphragm or enlargements of the normal ones. Surgical intervention is usually required for permanent closure.

Radiographic evaluation of the alimentary canal often includes ingestion of a radiopaque positive contrast medium (barium sulfate) that coats the luminal walls of the digestive tube and makes the various portions of it radiographically obvious. Radiographic visualization of the large intestine may involve administration of the contrast medium in enema form.

Peritonitis is inflammation of the peritoneal membrane which lines the abdominal cavity. It is nearly always caused by bacterial infection and is usually related to a penetrating abdominal wound that releases bacteria from the intestinal lumen. Rupture of an inflamed appendix (*see appendicitis above*) can also cause severe peritonitis.

Objectives

33. Define: harelip, cleft palate, malocclusion, gingivitis, periodontal disease, peptic ulcers, enterotomy, appendicitis, hernia, peritonitis.

Clinical Case Studies

Case 1—A frantic mother rushed her four-year-old boy to the emergency room after he admitted that he had swallowed a rubber pencil eraser. Standard radiography did not demonstrate the eraser's presence and the youngster was asked to swallow some barium sulfate (Esophatrast®). Several minutes later, radiography was performed again and a radiolucent (dark) area the size and shape of the alleged eraser was observed within the white (radiodense) shadow caused by the barium sulfate. Why did the eraser show up after the barium sulfate but not before?

Case 2—A nineteen-year-old college sophomore entered the emergency room with a complaint of bleeding and ulcerated gums that had steadily worsened over the past two weeks. The patient also complained of severe fatigue and had bruises over several areas of his body where he could not remember any traumatic incidents. The emergency room physician questioned the young man closely about his diet. What condition might the physician suspect?

Case 3—A new mother, anxious to begin breast feeding her firstborn, was unable to tolerate the experience because she found it too painful. Since her nipples were not exceptionally sensitive, what could explain the pain she felt?

Points to Ponder

The 24-hour, thirty foot trip of a salt and vinegar chip changes it from something profitable for Lays® to that most vile and shunned but perfectly normal waste product called feces (and several other, less socially acceptable aliases). Along the way it will be crushed, moistened with saliva (and perhaps soda pop), mixed with hamburger (or whatever else was on the menu at the time), acidified down to pH 2, peristalsed and emulsified to form a nondescript muck known to physiologists as chyme, alkalized back up to a neutral pH, and assaulted with a myriad of hydrolytic enzymes — some of which will ignore it and others will, indeed, hydrolyze. Many of the resulting monomeric subunits will cross the small intestinal mucosa into blood capillaries or lacteals and will be swept to various destinations where they will be burned for energy or reassembled into polymers and perhaps stored in places where we don't need any more but get it anyway. The non-absorbed remainder is moved on to the last few feet of the tube where a lot of water and some ions are routinely removed leaving the unwanted, the unmentionable, to gain sufficient mass to get the owner's attention and temporarily interrupt the daily routine. Deposited unceremoniously in one of the receptacles designed for that very purpose (if handy) or discreetly near a log or tree in some forest, it fulfills the saying... "from dust to dust" — just as the rest of our bodies eventually do after death.

Physiologists talk a lot about some juices: saliva, gastric juice, pancreatic juice, bile. Less fuss is made about intestinal juice or the secretions of the microscopic glands lining the esophagus. Saliva is primarily a lubricant to facilitate deglutition. Swallowing is a talent we've had since before birth. Before mom's milk, we swallowed amniotic fluid, practicing for the future. Swallowing is easy when stuff is fluid—less so when it is dry or when one sits across from someone incredibly attractive. The act begins voluntarily when a bolus (that's a fancy word for glob of stuff) is forced by the tongue into the gullet and on into the oropharynx. At that point an involuntary reflex occurs involving several of the pharyngeal muscles and movements of the base of the tongue which propel the bolus (glob) on its merry way down the esophagus. Sometimes when we sit across from that person, we forget to chew something enough (potato chips are bad about this) and it pains us all the way down to the stomach— as we try desperately to soften the edges with swallows of whatever liquid is available.

Vomiting is a temporary reversal in the travel direction of the early digestive process. It's the stomach's way to "just say no!" In grade school, vomiting is a faddish social event which can be triggered by anybody's reaction to spinach. We are simultaneously fascinated by the process and repulsed by the result — because the spinach is even uglier when mixed up with unidentifiable chunks of other stuff. The major propulsion force comes from a violent abdominal press which squeezes the stomach. With its pyloric sphincter tightly contracted and everything above relaxed, the contents are ejected forcefully and unceremoniously— ready or not. Sometimes, as if to punish us further, the spasmodic contractions occur a few times after everything seems to be emptied— an unpleasant event known in vomiting circles as the "dry heaves." Historically, the Romans are said to have glutenously overeaten and then induced vomiting— a practice continued today by individuals with certain psychological eating disorders.

The intestine's way to "just say no" is diarrhea— but there's not room to run on about that here.

Points to Ponder 2

In the fall of 2001, I came to work one Friday morning feeling a bit out of sorts (even before I taught any classes). Within a couple of hours I was vomiting violently and my pulse had slowed to the low fifties. Negotiating a stair was a major obstacle. I drove myself home (and apologize to any and all who may have been on the road at the time). I tried to lay down but frequent bouts of animated vomition caused me to beat a frequent path between the bed and bath. Nausea, more severe than any I had ever had, was my only real symptom on Friday. That night marked a new record for personal misery as I was up and down all night with severe dry heaves. Attempts to combat my growing dehydration were negated when ingested liquid was ejected from my stomach as soon as I swallowed it. By the next morning, McBurney's point became severely tender and I diagnosed myself as having acute appendicitis. My wife drove me down to the emergency room of the local hospital. Rumors of my arrival spread like wildfire and my former students, now nurses, orderlies, and med-techs, cast lots and drew straws for phlebotomy rights and other invasions of my personal space. A CAT-scan confirmed the appendicitis and I was whisked into surgery within the hour.

When I awakened, the nausea was gone and I felt great. The surgeon had removed my vermiform appendix via fiberoptic technology utilizing three small "puncture" type incisions through my abdominal wall. I was discharged the next morning, did yard work that afternoon, and went on a four day-long canoe trip three days later.

The appendix is a funny vestige. We could care less about it until it becomes inflamed, and then we hate it—with a passion.

Slang and Obsolete Nomenclature

UNOFFICIAL TERM	OFFICIAL DESIGNATION
GI system	digestive system (apparatus) [*digestive apparatus*]
muscularis externa	tunica muscularis [*tunica muscularis*]
common bile duct	bile duct [*ductus biliaris*]
bicuspid tooth	premolar tooth [*dens premolaris*]
eye tooth	canine tooth [*dens caninum*]
cuspid tooth	canine tooth [*dens caninum*]
wisdom tooth	third molar tooth [*dens molaris tertius*]
deciduous molars*	deciduous [*dentes decidui premolares*] premolar teeth
hepatic flexure of colon	right colic flexure [*flexura coli dextra*]
splenic flexure of colon	left colic flexure [*flexura coli sinistra*]
duodenal papilla	major/minor duodenal papilla [*papilla duodeni major/minor*]
appendix	vermiform appendix [*appendix vermiformis*]
anorectal canal	anal canal [*canalis analis*]
buccal cavity	oral cavity [*cavitas oris*]
uvula	palatine uvula [*uvula palatina*]
gastric rugae	gastric plicae (folds) [*plica gastricae*]
chief cells	principal cells [*exocrinocytus principalis*]
large bowel	large intestine [*intestinum crassum*]
anterior/parietal surface of liver	diaphragmatic surface [*facies diaphragmatica*] of liver

* The molar teeth have no deciduous predecessors.

posterior surface of liver	visceral surface [*facies visceralis*] of liver
sphincter of Oddi	sphincter muscle of the hepatopancreatic ampulla [*m. sphincter ampullae hepatopancreatica*]
parotid (mandibular, sublingual) salivary gland	parotid (mandibular, sublingual) gland [*glandula parotidea/submandibularis/sublingualis*]
Kupffer cell	stellate macrophage [*macrophagocytus stellatus*]
Crypts of Lieberkuhn	intestinal glands [*glandulae intestinales*]
Brunner's glands	duodenal glands [*glandulae duodenales*]
Meissner's plexus	submucosal plexus [*plexus submucosus*]
Auerbach's plexus	myenteric plexus [*plexus myentericus*]
Stensen's duct	parotid duct [*ductus parotideus*]
Wharton's duct	submandibular duct [*ductus submandibularis*]
Rivini's ducts	minor sublingual ducts [*ductus sublinguales minores*]

Review Questions

1. Which digestive organ is not part of the alimentary canal?
   A. vermiform appendix
   B. spleen
   C. fauces
   D. pharynx
   E. gallbladder

2. The intestinal wall has___ named layer(s) of membranous epithelium, ___ named layer(s) of smooth muscle tissue, and ____ named layer(s) of c.t. proper (in addition to the thin layer that is part of the parietal peritoneum).
   A. 2—1—2
   B. 2—2—2
   C. 1—2—2
   D. 2—2—1
   E. 3—3—2

3. Which item is located in the oral vestibule?
   A. opening of submandibular gland
   B. sublingual caruncle
   C. lingual frenulum
   D. incisive papilla
   E. opening of the duct of the parotid gland

4. Which statement about teeth is false?
   A. Most infants are edentulous at birth and their first deciduous teeth begin to erupt after a few months of age.
   B. The dental formula of a typical 5 year-old is $2\,[\mathrm{I}\tfrac{2}{2}\ \mathrm{C}\tfrac{1}{1}\ \mathrm{P}\tfrac{3}{3}] = 20$.
   C. A typical tooth has two approximate ("contact") surfaces, and one occlusal surface.
   D. The full adult dental formula is $2[\mathrm{I}\tfrac{2}{2}\ \mathrm{C}\tfrac{1}{1}\ \mathrm{P}\tfrac{2}{2}\ \mathrm{M}\tfrac{3}{3}] = 32$.
   E. The canine teeth are tooth numbers 6, 11, 22, and 27 in the 1-32 numbering system.

5. Which "pyloric" structure is largest?
   A. pyloric sphincter muscle
   B. pylorus
   C. pyloric canal
   D. pyloric part of stomach
   E. pyloric opening

6. Which statement about the intestine is false?
   A. The small intestine is about four times as long as the large intestine.
   B. Complex nutrients are hydrolyzed in the small intestine and absorbed in the large intestine.
   C. Villi are present only in the small intestine and sacculations are present only in the large intestine.
   D. The large intestine has four major named parts and the small intestine has three.
   E. The ileum is the longest part of the small intestine and the colon is the longest part of the large intestine.

7. Which item is false?
   A. Bile can be transported to the duodenum without entering the cystic duct or the gallbladder.
   B. Both bile and pancreatic juice enter the duodenum at the major duodenal papilla.
   C. The gallbladder is positioned between the right lobe and caudate lobe of the liver.
   D. Within a liver lobule, bile is transported peripherally in bile canaliculi and blood is transported centrally in sinusoids.
   E. A hepatic (portal) triad within the liver consists of a branch of the hepatic portal vein, a branch of the proper hepatic artery and a biliary ductule.

8. Which cell of the digestive system is correctly matched with an exocrine product?
   A. beta cell of pancreatic islet—insulin.
   B. parietal cell of stomach—pepsinogen.
   C. goblet cell—mucus.
   D. hepatocyte—pancreatic juice.
   E. If more than one of the above satisfy the premise, choose this response.

9. A bullet passed through the abdomen from front to back. En route, it passed through the alimentary canal three times and the left kidney once. Based on this information one should assume that it passed through visceral peritoneum at least____ time(s), parietal peritoneum at least ____ time(s), and it must have entered the peritoneal cavity at least____ time(s).
   A. 4—2—1
   B. 7—1—4
   C. 4—3—2
   D. 7—3—2
   E. 4—2—4

10. Which organ is matched incorrectly with the general direction that ingesta would move within it?
    A. stomach—right
    B. transverse colon—left
    C. horizontal part of duodenum—left
    D. oral cavity—inferior
    E. right colic flexure—turn from superior to medial

Thought Questions

1. Many individuals have their wisdom teeth surgically removed. On the 1-32 arabic numbering system, which teeth are they missing (after the surgery)?

2. Differentiate pylorus, pyloric sphincter, pyloric part of the stomach, pyloric opening, pyloric canal.

3. What criteria could be used to determine that an isolated segment of intestine is colon *vs.* small intestine?

4. *Large intestine* and *colon* are often (incorrectly) used interchangeably. Since they are not synonymous, what do you think is the reason for this common error?

5. Is the digestive system synonymous with alimentary canal? GI system? Explain.

6. Why can some (very) toxic substances be ingested with no ill effects?

7. What purpose does muscularis mucosae serve? What does tunica muscularis do?

8. Which of the lingual papillae have associated taste buds and how are the four principal taste modalities distributed on the tongue?

9. Discuss the distribution of smooth and skeletal muscle tissue within the wall of the esophagus and relate the distribution to the voluntary and involuntary aspects of deglutition and vomiting.

10. The duct of the parotid gland can be translocated to moisten the eyeball in individuals suffering from xerophthalmia. How can this be successful (since there are digestive enzymes in saliva) and why is the parotid gland chosen?

11. Do individuals that have had their gallbladders removed still produce bile? Explain.

12. Discuss the relationship of the abdominal organs to the peritoneum and peritoneal cavity.

13. What feature of "connecting" peritoneum distinguishes it from the rest of the parietal peritoneum and from visceral peritoneum?

14. Discuss the flow of blood and the flow of bile through a hepatic lobule. Use this to explain why chronic alcoholics have damaged hepatocytes near the periphery of liver lobules whereas heart failure patients have central lobular pathology.

15. Which part of the pharynx does not transport ingesta? The pharynx is considered to be a digestive organ but some anatomists prefer to place it in the respiratory system. What might their logic be?

16. Some individuals do not have an accessory pancreatic duct. What else will these individuals lack?

17. The lingual surface of some teeth is on their medial aspect but on other teeth it is on the posterior aspect. Explain.

18. Dento-alveolar joints (gomphoses) are very strong fibrous joints that allow very little motion. How do they stretch (violate) the definition of joints?

19. Gastric juice has a very low pH due to its hydrochloric acid content. Chyme in most of the intestine, however, has a near neutral pH. How does this pH change occur?

20. A surgeon performed an enterotomy to remove a quarter lodged in the ileum of a small child. Would he incise the mesenteric border (where the mesentery attaches) or the opposite (antimesenteric) border? Why?

21. Why is the small intestine much more actively involved in hydrolysis/absorption than the stomach or large intestine?

Answers to Clinical Case Studies

Case 1—Erasers are close to the same radiographic density as the body's soft tissue. Consequently they are often not visible in a standard radiograph. By putting the radiodense material around it, the eraser becomes visible as a blacker (radiolucent) image within a whiter (radiodense) background. After determining that the size of the eraser was unlikely to block the alimentary canal, the patient was released and the mother was advised to monitor the boy's bowel movements over the next few days to insure that he did not show signs of constipation.

Case 2—With signs of classic scurvy in this patient (vitamin C deficiency) the physician became suspicious that the young man suffered malnutrition. When his diet was found to consist exclusively of junk food, the physician prescribed vitamin C and the young man's symptoms disappeared within a few days. Among other things vitamin C is necessary for the integrity of capillary walls. That is why individuals with vitamin C deficiency bruise easily and often bleed from their gums.

Case 3—Although most neonates are edentulous (toothless), some babies are born with erupted teeth. These individuals are often weaned early!

Answers to Review Questions

1. E. B is not a digestive organ and so it doesn't satisfy that part of the premise.

2. B. The membranous epithelia are simple columnar epithelium (lining) and mesothelium (simple squamous epithelium of the visceral peritoneum). The layers of smooth muscle tissue are muscularis mucosae and tunica muscularis. The layers of connective tissue proper are the lamina propria and the submucosa.

3. E. The other structures are in the oral cavity proper.

4. B. There are only two premolars in each position in the deciduous dental formula.

5. D.

6. B. Absorption of most nutrients occurs in the small intestine, too.

7. C. The gallbladder lies between the right and quadrate lobes of the liver.

8. C. A is matched with an endocrine product and B and D are incorrectly matched with products.

9. B.

10. D. Ingesta moves posteriorly within the oral cavity.

Answers to Thought Questions

1. The wisdom teeth are 1, 16, 17, and 32. Therefore, individuals who have had these teeth extracted are missing those numbers.

2. The pylorus is the name of the junction of the stomach and small intestine (duodenum). Its luminal passageway is the pyloric canal and the gastric end of the pyloric canal is the pyloric opening (ostium). The pyloric sphincter is the well developed smooth muscle sphincter in the wall of the pyloric part of the stomach. The pyloric part of the stomach is the portion of the stomach adjacent to the pylorus.

3. The large intestine is larger in diameter than the small intestine, but this would be difficult to ascertain on a single, isolated specimen. Of more value might be the presence/absence of taeniae coli, sacculations, and epiploic appendages— all characteristics of the colon.

4. Most of the large intestine is colon— which probably accounts for the common error.

5. Digestive system and alimentary canal are often used interchangeably, but technically, the alimentary canal includes only the tubular digestive organs that ingesta encounters. Left out of the alimentary canal concept are the salivary glands, pancreas, liver, gallbladder and their associated ducts. "GI (gastrointestinal) system" is often used as a synonym for digestive system but it is a misnomer since it only implicates the stomach and intestines.

6. Sometimes toxic substances are altered by the digestive system into harmless substances. The proteins in ingested rattlesnake venom, for example, are rendered harmless because they are hydrolyzed down to their component amino acids. Other toxic substances cause no harm because they remain in the intestinal lumen and are not absorbed. Barium sulfate, a contrast agent used to render the alimentary canal visible in radiographs is harmless when ingested (because it is not absorbed).

7. Muscularis mucosae alters the configuration of the mucous membrane lining—forming folds and spirals. The tunica muscularis is primarily involved in peristalsis.

8. Fungiform and vallate papillae are the only ones with taste buds. The sweet receptors are concentrated at the apex of the tongue, the bitter receptors at the posterior aspects, sour receptors on the sides of the tongue, and those responding to salt overlap the sweet and sour areas.

9. At the upper end of the esophagus, the tunica muscularis is skeletal muscle tissue. This assists deglutition since the initiation of the swallowing process is voluntary. In its middle section, the tunica muscularis gradually changes to smooth muscle tissue and is entirely smooth muscle tissue adjacent to the stomach. The latter part of swallowing (as ingesta nears the stomach) is involuntarily controlled by this smooth muscle tissue. Vomiting is involuntary and is effected primarily by inhibition of the esophageal musculature as well as by spasmodic, forceful contractions of the stomach and abdominal muscles.

10. The parotid gland is chosen for this procedure because its duct is superficially accessible and is long enough to easily reach the eye. The only digestive enzyme in saliva, a weak amylase which hydrolyzes starch, is harmless to the eye.

11. Yes— but without the gallbladder, they have no place to store it. The bile that they produce passes directly down the biliary duct system into the duodenum.

12. The abdominal organs are covered by the peritoneum that lines the abdominal cavity. Consequently they are invaginated into the peritoneal cavity, but are not inside of it. This is akin to shoving one's fist into the side of a large soft balloon. The fist is pushed into (invaginated into) the side of the balloon, but is not inside of the balloon.

13. "Connecting" peritoneum is always two layers of peritoneum adherent to each other. These double layers are not on the body wall and are not on the organs. Instead, they attach (connect) organs to the body wall or to each other. Unlike the visceral peritoneum and regular parts of the parietal peritoneum, each segment of connecting peritoneum is given a specific name depending on its attachments.

14. Blood flows centrally from the arterial and venous components of the hepatic triads through the hepatic sinusoids (modified capillaries) into the central vein. Bile, which is manufactured by the hepatocytes, enters the bile canaliculi and flows peripherally through the lobule to enter the biliary ductules of the portal triads. In essence, blood and bile flow in different directions through different structures within the liver lobules. Because blood flows centrally through hepatic lobules, blood-borne toxins (like alcohol) will damage the peripheral hepatocytes more severely than the central ones. In chronic heart failure patients, the venous back pressure damages the centrally located hepatocytes more severely than the peripheral ones.

15. Nasopharynx. All parts of the pharynx transport air during respiration, but only the oral and laryngeal parts of the pharynx are normally involved in transporting ingesta. Since respiration can involve all parts of the pharynx, but digestion usually only involves two, an argument could be that the pharynx "belongs" to the respiratory system.

16. Such individuals do not have a minor duodenal papilla.

17. On the front teeth (incisors) the lingual surface (tongue side) is posterior. On the premolars and molars (located lateral to the tongue) the lingual surface is medial. On canine teeth (located at the front "corners" of the oral cavity) the lingual surface is posteromedial because the teeth are angled relative to the tongue.

18. Most joints are junctions of bones and/or cartilages. Teeth are not bones nor are they cartilages.

19. Pancreatic juice has a basic pH. When it mixes with acidic ingesta from the stomach, the pH of the chyme brought back to a near neutral pH.

20. A surgeon will incise the antimesenteric border because the nerve and blood supply enters the mesenteric side. An incision on the antimesenteric side should disrupt less of the nerve and blood supply which will promote better post-surgical healing and function.

21. The small intestine produces a few hydrolytic enzymes in its lining epithelial cells, but more importantly, it receives several powerful ones from the pancreas. The stomach has only one proteolytic enzyme (pepsin) but nothing that will break down carbohydrates, lipids, or nucleic acids. The small intestine also has a huge absorptive surface area due to its circular folds, villi, and microvilli. By the time ingesta reaches the large intestine, most of the major nutrients have been absorbed.

CHAPTER 18 Respiratory System

Chapter Outline and Key Concepts

INTRODUCTION

The respiratory system includes the nose, nasal cavity, paranasal sinuses, larynx, trachea, bronchial tree, and lungs.

Functionally, the respiratory system includes conducting passageways and the pulmonary alveoli which exchange O_2/CO_2.

The conducting passageways thermoregulate inspired air to body temperature, moisturize it to 100% relative humidity, and remove most particulate matter from it.

FUNCTIONS OF THE RESPIRATORY SYSTEM

Functions of the respiratory system include O_2/CO_2 exchange, acid/base balance, vocalization, participation in the abdominal press maneuver, protective reflexes, and olfaction.

NOSE, NASAL CAVITY, AND PARANASAL SINUSES

The nose has a root, bridge, apex, and wings that surround the nasal openings.

The nasal cavity is divided in half by the nasal septum which includes membranous, cartilaginous, and bony portions.

Four pairs of paranasal sinuses invaginate bones of the head: frontal, maxillary, sphenoid, and ethmoid sinuses.

Most of the nasal cavity and paranasal sinuses are lined by ciliated pseudostratified columnar epithelium (containing goblet cells).

PHARYNX

Officially part of the digestive system, the pharynx is used as an air conducting passageway, as well.

LARYNX

The larynx joins the laryngeal part of the pharynx to the trachea and serves as the vocal organ.

The larynx is stiffened by three paired and three unpaired cartilages.

The vocal folds are mucosal folds lining the larynx that can be adducted, abducted, and tensed by skeletal muscles to close and open the glottis, and to change the pitch of the voice during vocalization.

TRACHEA AND BRONCHIAL TREE

The trachea is a tubular structure about 5 inches long and an inch in diameter extending inferiorly from the larynx.

Sixteen to 20 "C"-shaped hyaline cartilages stiffen the tracheal wall to prevent its collapse during inspiration.

Inferiorly, the trachea bifurcates to form the left and right principal bronchi.

Each principal bronchus divides to form lobar bronchi which, in turn divide to form segmental bronchi.

Tiny passageways called bronchioles conduct air beyond the bronchi and are distinguished from the latter by the lack of cartilage in their walls.

The smallest (respiratory) bronchioles open into pulmonary alveoli.

Mucus produced by cells in the trachea and bronchial tree entraps dirt particles, and ciliated cells in these loci help "sweep" the dirt-laden mucus up and out of the respiratory passageways.

LUNGS

The right and left lungs occupy the thoracic cavity and are separated from each other by a partition termed the mediastinum (formed by the heart, esophagus, trachea, vessels, and the mediastinal pleura on each of its sides).

Each lung has a narrow (superior) apex, a base, and four surfaces: costal, diaphragmatic, mediastinal, and interlobar.

Pulmonary alveoli exchange O_2/CO_2 through three layers that form the so-called air/blood barrier: lining (simple squamous) epithelial cells, a thin layer of c.t. proper, and the lining endothelium of the surrounding capillaries.

THORAX, THORACIC CAVITY; PLEURAE, PLEURAL CAVITY

The thorax is the superior, anterior part of the trunk and the organ-containing space within it is the thoracic cavity.

The thoracic cavity is divided by the mediastinum into two lung-containing spaces that are lined by serous membranes termed pleura(e).

Pleura on the inside of the thoracic wall, on top of the diaphragm, and on each side of the mediastinum is collectively termed parietal pleura and regionally distinguished as costal, diaphragmatic, and mediastinal, respectively.

Pleura on the surface of each lung is termed visceral (pulmonary) pleura.

The potential space between the visceral and parietal pleura on each side forms the left and right pleural cavities.

DIAPHRAGM

The diaphragm is a skeletal muscle forming a dividing partition between the thoracic and abdominal cavities.

The contractile parts of the diaphragm surround a central tendon.

Three passageways transmit structures through the diaphragm: (vena) caval foramen (inferior vena cava), esophageal hiatus (esophagus and vagal nerve trunks), and aortic hiatus (aorta, thoracic duct, and azygos vein).

MECHANICS OF RESPIRATION

Movement of air into the lungs (inspiration) occurs when the intrapleural pressure drops below atmospheric pressure.

The intrapleural pressure can be reduced by contracting the diaphragm (which makes the thoracic cavity longer) or by increasing the diameter of the thoracic cavity by rib movements (or both).

Expiration occurs naturally if the diaphragm is relaxed (due to the natural tendency of the lungs to contract via elastic fibers and surface tension of the fluid lining the alveoli).

Expiration can be forced by an abdominal press.

Four non-overlapping pulmonary volumes are identified: residual, expiratory reserve, tidal, and inspiratory reserve volumes.

Combinations of two, three, or four of the pulmonary volumes form four pulmonary capacities: inspiratory, functional reserve, vital and total lung capacities.

DEVELOPMENT OF THE RESPIRATORY SYSTEM

The nasal passageways develop as thickened ectoderm (nasal placodes) which invaginates.

The palate forms from horizontally growing mesoderm plates (palatine shelves).

The laryngotracheal bud evaginates from the anterior part of the pharynx to form the larynx, trachea, and bronchial tree.

CLINICAL CONSIDERATIONS

The abdominal thrust ("Heimlich") maneuver is used to dislodge objects blocking the lower air conducting passageways (especially larynx/trachea).

Foreign material sometimes found in the thoracic (pleural) cavity includes blood (hemothorax), lymph (chylothorax), air (pneumothorax), and pus (pyothorax).

Carbon monoxide poisoning is insidious since CO is a colorless, odorless gas.

Pneumonia (pneumonitis) is inflammation of the lungs—usually caused by an infectious agent.

Bronchitis (inflammation of the bronchial tree) is a common respiratory ailment.

Selected Definitions

Air-blood-barrier—a physiological term referring to the thin layers that separate air in the pulmonary alveoli from blood in the capillaries surrounding the alveoli. These layers include the respiratory epitheliocytes lining the alveoli and the endothelial cells of the capillaries.

Anatomic dead space—the air-filled volume of the nasal cavity and air conducting passageways. Air within it enters the respiratory system during inspiration but does not reach the pulmonary alveoli.

Bronchial tree—a collective name for the two principal bronchi, the five lobar bronchi, and the 19-20 segmental bronchi. The segmental bronchi give rise to bronchioles.

Bronchioles—small, air conducting tubules within the lungs. The largest bronchioles arise from segmental bronchi and are distinguished from them by the lack of cartilage in their walls.

Bronchus—any of a number of air conducting passageways between the trachea and bronchioles. Bifurcation of the trachea gives rise to the two principal bronchi, and divisions of the latter form the lobar and segmental bronchi.

Dyspnea—difficult breathing. Causes of dyspnea include asthma, chronic obstructive pulmonary disease, pneumonia, and anaphylactic shock.

Larynx—the "voicebox". The larynx is stiffened by several cartilages and has a number of small skeletal muscles whose contractions abduct, adduct, or tense the vocal folds.

Mediastinum—the partition that lies between the lungs and separates the left and right pleural cavities. It consists of the left and right mediastinal pleurae and all of the structures which lie between them.

Nasal cavity—the air-filled space beginning at the nares and terminating at the choanae. The nasal cavity is separated from the oral cavity by the palate and is divided into left and right halves by the nasal septum.

Pleura—either one of the two (left/right) serous membranes that are associated with the lungs within the thoracic cavity. The pleura on each lung is called visceral pleura and the parietal pleura which reflects onto surrounding structures is called costal, mediastinal, or diaphragmatic according to its location.

Pleural cavity—either of the two serous body cavities into which the lungs are invaginated. Both pleural cavities and the intervening pericardial cavity are located within the thoracic cavity.

Pneumothorax—the presence of air in one or both pleural cavities. It may enter the cavity via a ruptured lung or from a hole in the thoracic wall.

Pulmonary alveoli—the microscopic "air sacs" in the lungs. The thin walls of pulmonary alveoli and surrounding capillaries allow exchange of oxygen and carbon dioxide between the air of the alveoli and the circulating blood.

Respiratory epitheliocytes—the simple squamous epithelial cells that line pulmonary alveoli. These should not be confused with the homonymous respiratory epithelium.

"**Respiratory epithelium**"—the unofficial name sometimes applied to the epithelium lining the air conducting passageways of the respiratory system. It is composed of ciliated pseudostratified columnar epithelium.

Superior thoracic aperture ("**thoracic inlet**")—the opening at the top of the thoracic cavity. It is bounded skeletally by the first pair of ribs, the first thoracic vertebra, and the top of the sternum.

Surfactant—the lipoprotein secreted by the granular epitheliocytes found in pulmonary alveoli. It reduces the surface tension of the fluid lining the pulmonary alveoli (which would otherwise prevent inspiration).

Tidal volume—the quantity of air inhaled or exhaled at any given time. The average resting tidal volume is about 500 cc.

Thorax (**chest, pectus**)—the anterior, superior portion of the trunk. It contains the thoracic cavity, pleural cavities, pericardial cavity, and a number of organs.

Total lung capacity—the total quantity of air that both lungs can hold. It can be subdivided into four volumes: residual, expiratory reserve, tidal, and inspiratory reserve.

Trachea—the "windpipe". The trachea is a cartilage-stiffened, mucosa-lined tube, about twelve centimeters long, that conducts air from the larynx to the bronchial tree.

Etymology ***Dum spiro spero***—"**While I breathe, I hope.**"

arytaenoid (L), *ladle shaped*—arytenoid
asthma (G), *to blow*—asthma
bronchos (G), *throat, trachea*—bronchus
chonae (G), *funnel*—choana
chylos (G), *juice*—chylothorax
concha (L), *conch, shell shaped*—conchae
emphysema (G), *inflation, swelling*—emphysema
glottis (G), *tongue*—glottis
krikos (G), *ring*—cricoid
pleura (L), *side, rib*—pleura
pnea (G), *breathing ,breath*—dyspnea
pneu (G), *air*—pneumothorax
pneumon (G), *lung*—pneumonia
pyon (G), *pus*—pyothorax
respirare (L), *to breath*—respiration
rima (L), *slit, fissure*—rima glottidis
thyroydes (L), *shield-shaped*—thyroid
trachea (L), *windpipe*—trachea

Introduction

The **respiratory system** is the visceral body system that is involved with the exchange of carbon dioxide in the blood for atmospheric oxygen. It includes the nose, nasal cavity, paranasal sinuses, larynx, trachea, bronchial tree, and lungs (Figure 18-1). In addition to these, the pharynx (officially listed as an organ of the digestive system) is often included because air must pass through it to move from the nasal (or oral) cavity to the larynx (and vice-versa). The respiratory organs from the nose down to and including the larynx are often grouped as the "upper" respiratory system, and the trachea, bronchial tree, and lungs comprise the "lower" respiratory system. Conceptually, most respiratory organs can be considered to be air conducting passageways. The microscopic pulmonary alveoli ("air sacs") in the lungs serve as the only structures directly involved with oxygen/carbon dioxide exchange. The conducting passageways affect inspired air in three ways before it reaches the alveoli: they moisten it (to 100% relative humidity), raise (or lower) it to body temperature, and clean it by entrapping dust and other particulate matter in mucus. These changes are important to protect the delicate lining cells of the pulmonary alveoli.

Objectives

1. Name the major parts of the respiratory system in the order that inspired air encounters them.
2. Differentiate the "upper" and "lower" parts of the respiratory system.

Table 18-1 Modified Respiratory Movements

Protective Reflexes:

Cough—a reflex characterized by a sudden explosive forcing of air through the rima glottidis. This includes a deep inspiration followed by the complete closure of the rima glottidis. This is followed by a strong expiration that pushes the rima glottidis open and sends a blast of air through the upper respiratory tract. This reflex can be stimulated by foreign objects in the larynx, trachea or against the epiglottis.

Sneeze—a reflex characterized by spasmodic contraction of the expiratory muscles that forcefully expels air through the nose and mouth. Irritation of the nasal mucosa is the inciting stimulus.

Non-protective Reflexes:

Laugh—the expression of mirth, pleasure, derision, or nervousness by explosive, interrupted expiratory efforts similar to those which occur during crying.

Cry—an expression of unhappiness (or sometimes elation) with inspirations followed by numerous, short expirations, during which the rima glottidis is open and the vocal folds vibrate. Lacrimal secretions flood the conjunctival sac and characteristic facial expressions accompany the respiratory movement.

Sigh—a long, deep inspiration immediately followed by a shorter but forceful expiration.

Yawn—a deep inspiration through the open mouth. It may be stimulated by fatigue, drowsiness, or another's yawn.

Hiccup (hiccough)—a spasmodic diaphragmatic contraction followed by spasmodic closure of the rima glottidis which produces a sharp inspiratory sound. Stimuli may include irritation of the sensory nerve endings of the alimentary canal.

Valsalva maneuver—forced expiratory effort with closed mouth and nose. This can be used by scuba divers to pressurize the tympanic cavities through the auditory tubes.

Functions of the Respiratory System

The most obvious function of the respiratory system is the exchange of carbon dioxide in the blood (a waste product) for atmospheric oxygen (a nutrient). This is a cooperative venture of the respiratory and cardiovascular systems and occurs by gaseous diffusion through the alveolar and capillary walls. In addition to **O_2/CO_2 exchange**, the respiratory organs are also involved in acid/base balance, protective reflexes, vocalization, and some of them are also involved in the abdominal press and olfaction. **Acid/base balance** is the control of body pH within the relatively narrow range compatible with life (7.35-7.45). This function is shared with the cardiovascular and urinary systems. The role of the respiratory system is to rid the body of CO_2, thereby reducing its H_2CO_3 (carbonic acid) content. This riddance elevates the pH and decreases the acidity of body fluids. **Protective reflexes** of the respiratory system include coughing and sneezing. These are modified respiratory movements that help expel foreign matter from the upper respiratory system. Other (non-protective) reflexes and movements in which the respiratory system plays a role include laughing, sobbing, sighing, yawning, hiccuping, and the Valsalva maneuver (Table 18-1).

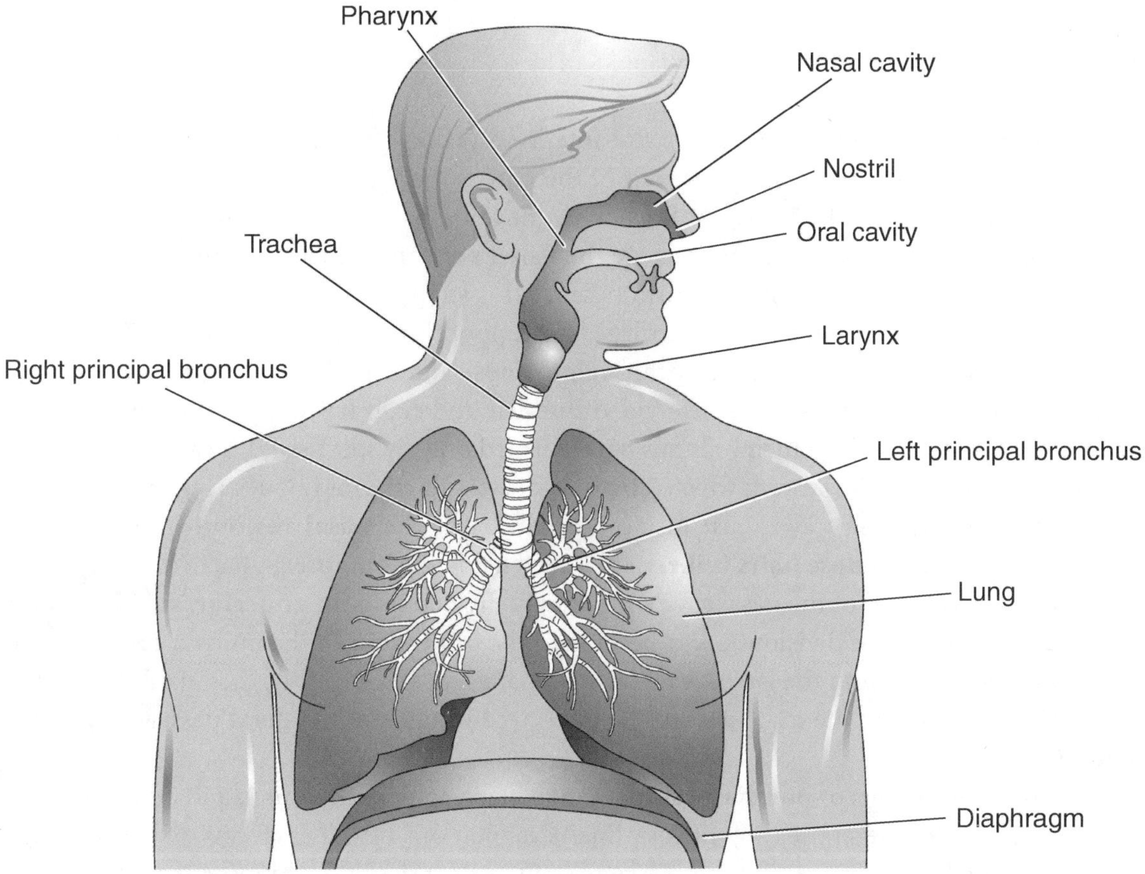

Figure 18-1

Organs of the Respiratory System

The respiratory system is a visceral body system that includes seven major components: nose, nasal cavity, paranasal sinuses, larynx, trachea, bronchial tree, and lungs. The respiratory system also uses the pharynx (a digestive organ) as an air conducting passageway.

Vocalization (phonation) is the production of the sounds involved in verbal communication. Most vocal sounds are initiated by forcing air up the trachea and between the vocal folds causing them to vibrate. The production of intelligible language requires the coordinated contraction of laryngeal muscles, varying degrees of abdominal compression, and coordinated movements of the mandible, tongue, and lips. **Abdominal compression** is mainly produced by contraction of the muscles forming the abdominal wall. Maximal compression can be obtained only when the lungs are expanded by inspiration and the laryngeal passageway is blocked by fully adducting the vocal folds. **Olfaction** is the sense of smell. The olfactory cells are located in the respiratory epithelium lining the nasal cavity (*see Chapter 10*).

Objectives

3. List the functions of the respiratory system and note which two are also functions of the cardiovascular system.
4. Describe the various modified (protective and non-protective) respiratory movements.

Nose, Nasal Cavity, and Paranasal Sinuses

The **nose** occupies a central position on the anterior aspect of the face. Its external features include the root, bridge, apex, and wings. The **root** of the nose is the superior portion that joins the inferior aspect of the forehead. The **bridge** of the nose is the anterior aspect along the midline. The **apex** is the tip at the inferior end and the **wings** are the flared portions which surround the nasal openings. The superior half of the nose is quite firm because it is supported by the left and right nasal bones. The inferior portion contains several cartilages for support but is relatively flexible (Figure 18-2).

The **nasal cavity** is the passageway through the nose and superior to the palate. It begins at the left and right **nostrils** (**nares**) and is divided into left and right halves by the **nasal septum**. This median partition includes a membranous part (formed only by soft tissue), a cartilaginous part, and an osseous portion. The latter is formed by the vomer and ethmoid bones (Figure 18-2). The initial portion of the nasal cavity just inside each nostril is the **nasal vestibule**. Its passageway is screened by numerous **nose hairs** (**vibrissae**) which help filter out foreign particulate matter. Above the vestibule, each half of the nasal cavity is partially divided into the **superior**, **middle**, and **inferior nasal meatus**. These divisions occur because of the projections of the mucosa covered nasal conchae (*see Chapter 6*) from the lateral wall of the nasal cavity. Posteriorly, each half of the nasal cavity communicates with the nasal part of the pharynx through an ipsilateral passageway termed the **choana**.

There are four pairs of **paranasal sinuses**: maxillary, sphenoid, frontal, and ethmoid (*see Figure 6-6*; *Figure 18-2*). The sinuses are mucosa-lined evaginations of the nasal cavity that invaginate the bones indicated by their names. They serve to lighten the skull and add resonant intonation to the voice but have no other known functions. They cannot serve as warming, moistening, or "cleaning" passageways because their narrow, single connections to the nasal cavity do not allow significant movement of air.

The nasal cavity and paranasal sinuses (as well as the larynx, trachea, and bronchial tree) are lined by **ciliated pseudostratified columnar epithelium**, also unofficially called "**respiratory epithelium**" (not to be confused with *respiratory epitheliocytes* which form the lining epithelium of

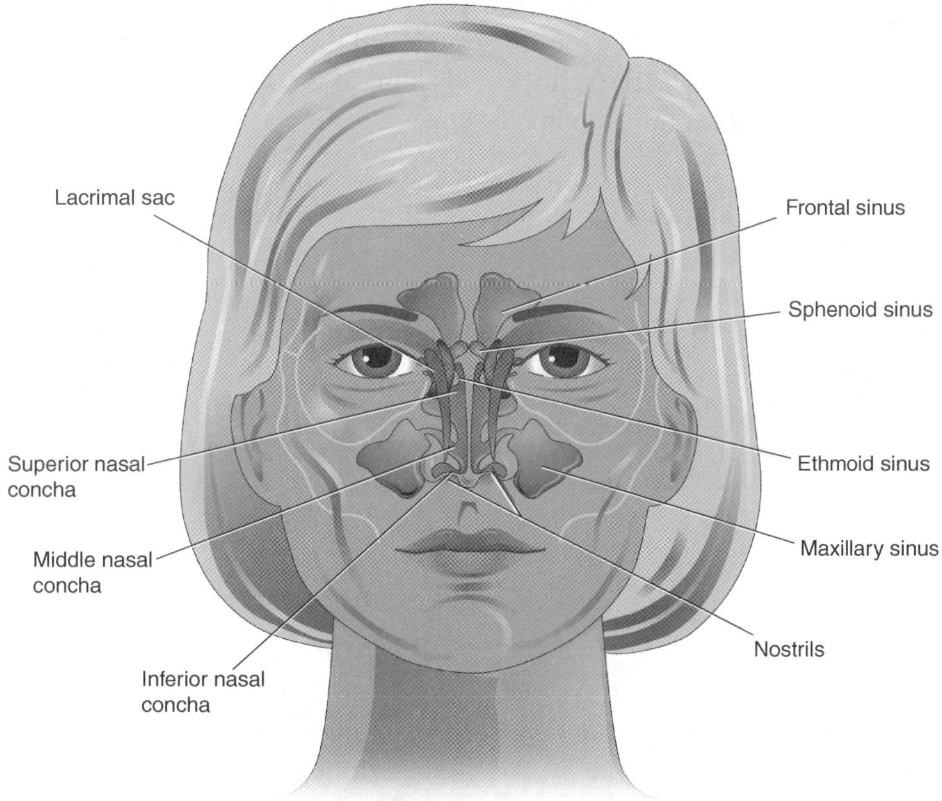

Figure 18-2

Components of the Upper Respiratory System

The paranasal sinuses are air-filled diverticulae from the nasal cavity that invade the frontal, ethmoid, and sphenoid bones as well as the maxillae. In the midsagittal section of the head, the close relationship of the digestive and respiratory systems at the pharynx is evident. Initially, they are separated by the palate (hard palate anteriorly and soft palate posteriorly), but they join at the bottom, posterior edge of the soft palate where the oropharynx begins. The mucosa covered nasal conchae (superior, middle, and inferior) partially divide each half of the nasal cavity into a superior, middle, and inferior meatus. Note that the superior and middle nasal conchae are parts of the ethmoid bone but the inferior nasal concha is a separate bone.

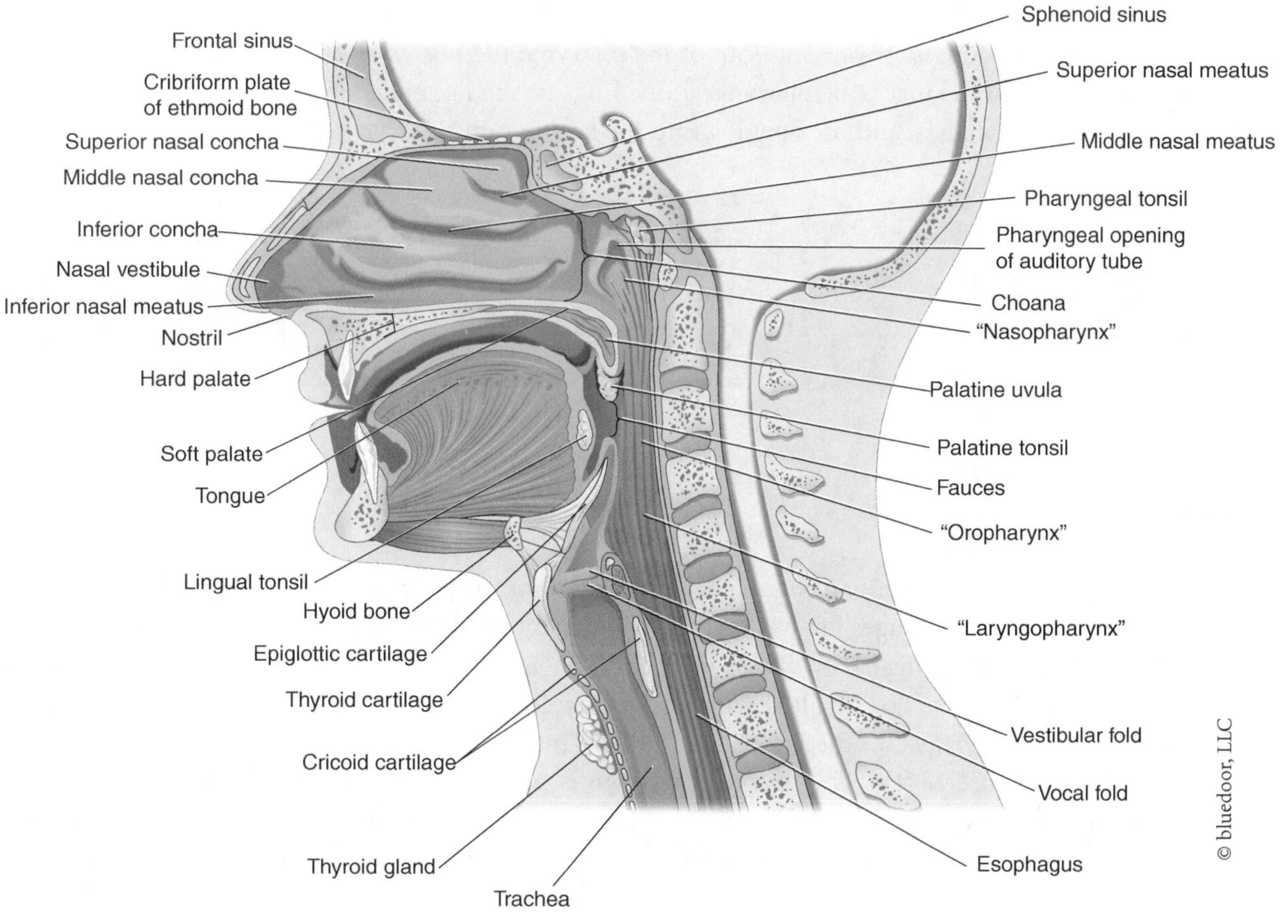

the alveoli of the lungs). **Goblet cells** interspersed among the columnar epithelial cells produce mucus which helps to moisturize inspired air, and prevent desiccation of the passageway linings. This mucus also entraps particulate matter which the wave-like motion of the ciliated cells moves up and out of the bronchial tree and trachea. The respiratory epithelium in the superior part of the nasal cavity contains the olfactory cells which function in olfaction.

Objectives

5. Differentiate nose and nasal cavity.
6. Explain how the nasal septum and nasal conchae divide the nasal cavity into six meatus.
7. Name the four pairs of paranasal sinuses.
8. State the four word histological classification of respiratory epithelium.

Pharynx

The pharynx is officially listed as part of the digestive system (*see Chapter 17*). However, air must pass through it during inspiration and expiration. Consequently, many anatomists consider it to be an organ shared by the respiratory and digestive systems. Air inspired through the nose/nasal cavity enters the nasal part of the pharynx, then passes down through the oral and laryngeal parts to enter the larynx. Air inspired through the oral cavity passes through only the oral and laryngeal parts. There are 7 passageways into/out of the pharynx: the posterior openings of the two halves of the nasal cavity (choanae), the pharyngeal openings of the left and right auditory tubes, the fauces (gullet), the esophagus, and the opening into the larynx (aditus laryngis).

Objectives

9. List the seven openings into/out of the pharynx and indicate which ones are normally traversed by ingesta or inspired air.

Larynx

The **larynx** is a complex organ about 5 cm long that joins the pharynx to the trachea. It is composed of a framework of cartilages joined together by ligaments and lined by a mucous membrane (Figure 18-3). The nine laryngeal cartilages include three unpaired cartilages (thyroid, epiglottic, and cricoid) and three pairs of smaller cartilages (arytenoid, corniculate, and cuneiform). Several small laryngeal muscles attach to these cartilages and are involved in tensing, adducting or abducting the vocal folds (Figure 18-4). The **thyroid cartilage** is the largest one and is trough-shaped with an open posterior aspect. Its anterosuperior midline projection forms the **laryngeal prominence** ("Adam's apple"). Superior and inferior horns project from each side of its posterior aspect. The

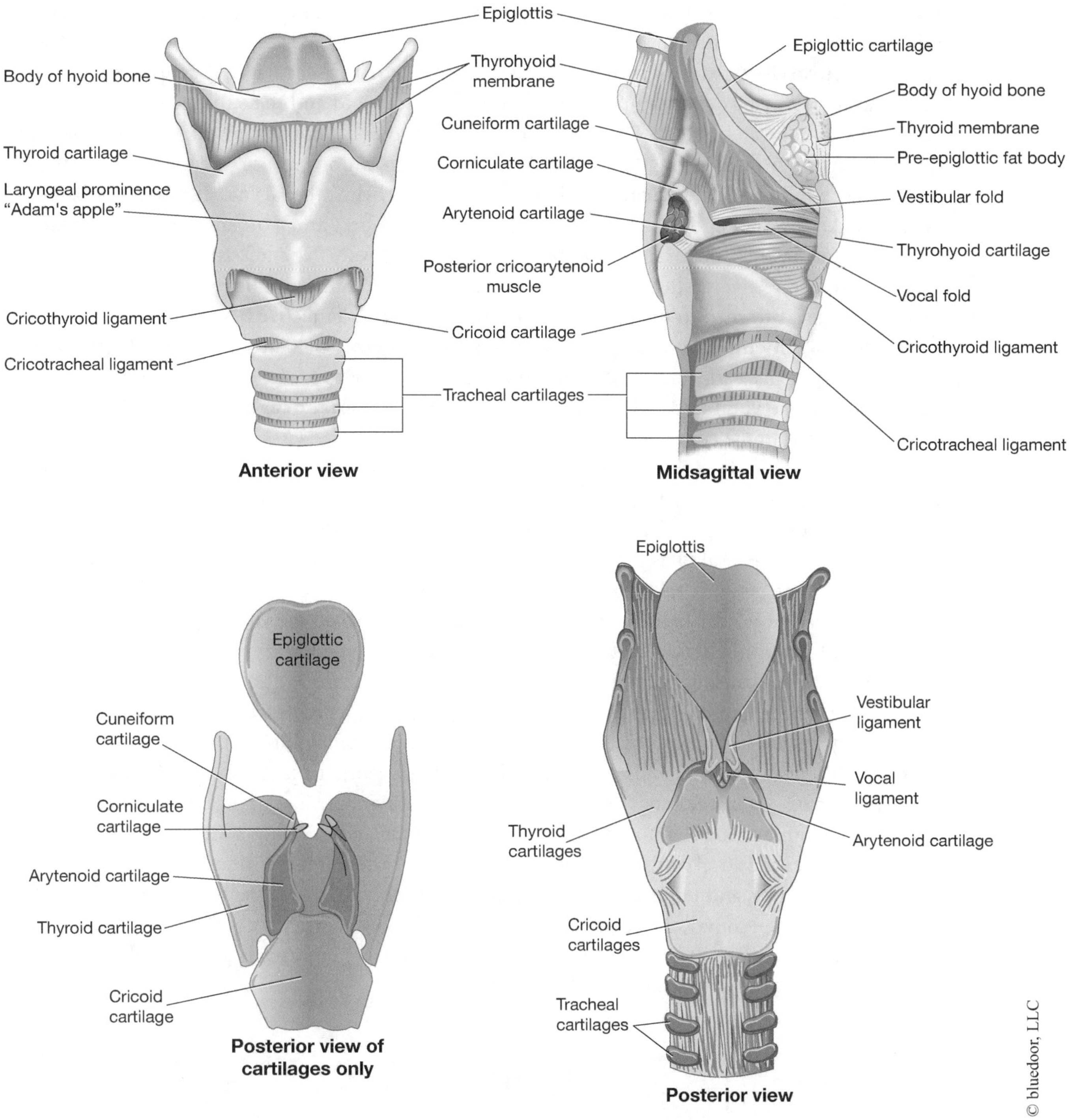

Figure 18-3

Cartilages and Ligaments of the Larynx

The larynx is stiffened by three unpaired cartilages (thyroid, cricoid, and epiglottic cartilages) and three pairs of smaller cartilages (arytenoid, corniculate, and cuneiform cartilages). The mucosa which lines the larynx (not illustrated here) forms soft tissue folds around the left and right vocal ligaments called vocal folds. These folds can be adducted/abducted and tensed/relaxed by a number of small laryngeal muscles (also not shown here). Air forced between partially abducted vocal folds produces the vibrations that allow us to talk.

thyroid cartilage is joined to the hyoid bone above it by connective tissue proper termed the **thyrohyoid membrane**. The inferior horns form synovial joints with the sides of the cricoid cartilage. The **epiglottic cartilage** extends posterosuperiorly from the thyroid cartilage. It guards the opening into the larynx. During deglutition, contraction of the infrahyoid and the suprahyoid muscles elevates the hyoid bone and larynx. The base of the tongue forces the epiglottis back over the opening to prevent ingesta from entering the larynx. With its investment of mucosa, the epiglottic cartilage is termed the **epiglottis**. The **cricoid cartilage** is positioned below the larynx. It resembles a signet ring (looks like a class ring) in shape with a narrow anterior aspect and a broader posterior portion. The cricoid cartilage is anchored to the thyroid cartilage above by the left and right cricothyroid joints and by connective tissue proper termed the median cricothyroid ligament. Inferiorly, the cricoid cartilage is attached to the first tracheal cartilage by the connective tissue proper termed the **cricotracheal ligament**. The small, paired **arytenoid cartilages** articulate with the posterior aspect of the cricoid cartilage at the cricoarytenoid joints. These cartilages provide attachment for the posterior aspects of the vocal folds. The paired **corniculate** and **cuneiform cartilages** are very small and are embedded in the edges of the aryepiglottic fold.

The **laryngeal cavity** is the passageway through the larynx. Its superior opening is called the **aditus laryngis** and is bounded anteriorly by the epiglottis and laterally by the **aryepiglottic folds**. The latter are folds of mucosa that extend from the arytenoid cartilages to the epiglottis. The **vocal folds** ("cords") are mucosal folds that project from the lateral walls of the laryngeal cavity. The vocal folds and the space between them (**rima glottidis**) are collectively termed the **glottis**. Each vocal fold surrounds a fibroelastic band of connective tissue proper termed the **vocal ligament**. These ligaments extend from the thyroid cartilage (anteriorly) to the arytenoid cartilages (posteriorly). To inspire and expire air during normal respiration, the vocal folds are abducted by contracting some of the small laryngeal muscles that attach to (and rotate) the arytenoid cartilages. Abduction of the vocal folds opens the rima glottidis and allows free movement of air through the larynx. To affect an abdominal press, the vocal folds are fully adducted to close the rima glottidis. This prevents air from being forced out of the lungs as the abdominal viscera are pushed up against the diaphragm. Vocalization is initiated by slightly abducting the vocal folds and expiring a stream of air between them. This causes the vocal folds to vibrate. The sounds of these initial vibrations are modified by the tongue, teeth, lips, and paranasal sinuses to form the individually characteristic voice. To produce a higher pitched sound, the vocal folds are stretched more tightly by contracting the cricothyroideus muscle to change the angle of the cricothyroid joints. This stretches the vocal folds more tautly and causes them to vibrate with a higher frequency.

Objectives

10. Name the cartilages of the larynx and indicate which are paired.
11. Explain how and why the vocal folds are tensed, abducted, and/or adducted.

Trachea and Bronchial Tree

The **trachea** is a tubular structure about 12 cm long and 2.5 cm in diameter. It extends from the larynx at the level of C6 to its terminal bifurcation at the level of T5. The patency of the tracheal lumen is maintained by the presence of 16-20 **tracheal cartilages** embedded in its wall. These hyaline car-

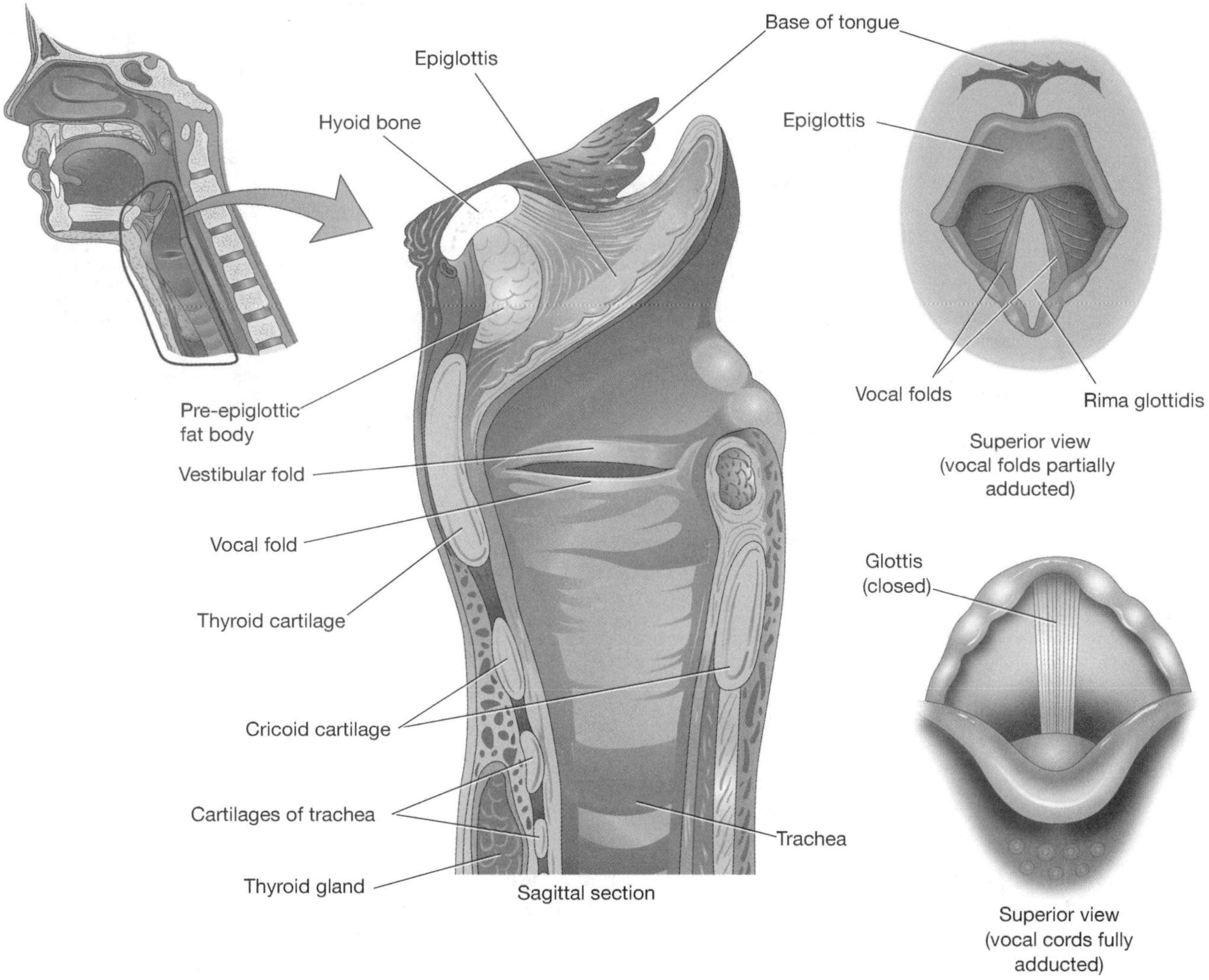

Figure 18-4

Vocal Folds

The left and right vocal folds extend from the thyroid cartilage (anteriorly) to the left and right arytenoid cartilages (posteriorly). By rotating the arytenoid cartilages toward/away from each other (with small muscles), the vocal folds can be fully abducted (separated) for free breathing. For vocalization, the vocal folds are only partially abducted and vibrate in the exhaled air to produce sound. Total adduction of the vocal folds (completely blocking the airway) is necessary during an abdominal press.

tilages are "C-shaped" with the "open" part of the "C" facing posteriorly. Smooth muscle and elastic tissue fill in this gap. Each cartilage is joined to its counterparts above and below by **tracheal anular ligaments**. The lining mucosa resembles that of the larynx and bronchial tree. Inferiorly, the trachea terminates by dividing at the **tracheal bifurcation** into the left and right **principal bronchi**.

The **bronchial tree** is the group of passageways that channels air into and out of the lungs. It consists of three size categories of bronchi: principal, lobar, and segmental. The **left** and **right principal** ("primary") **bronchi** are the largest and attach to the tracheal bifurcation. Each one conducts

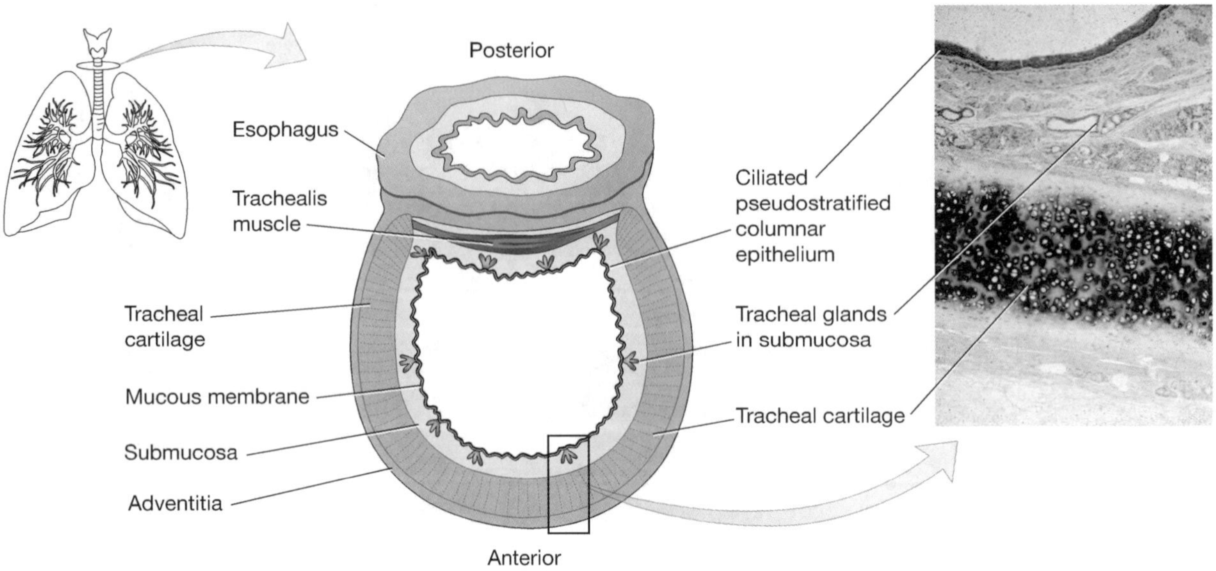

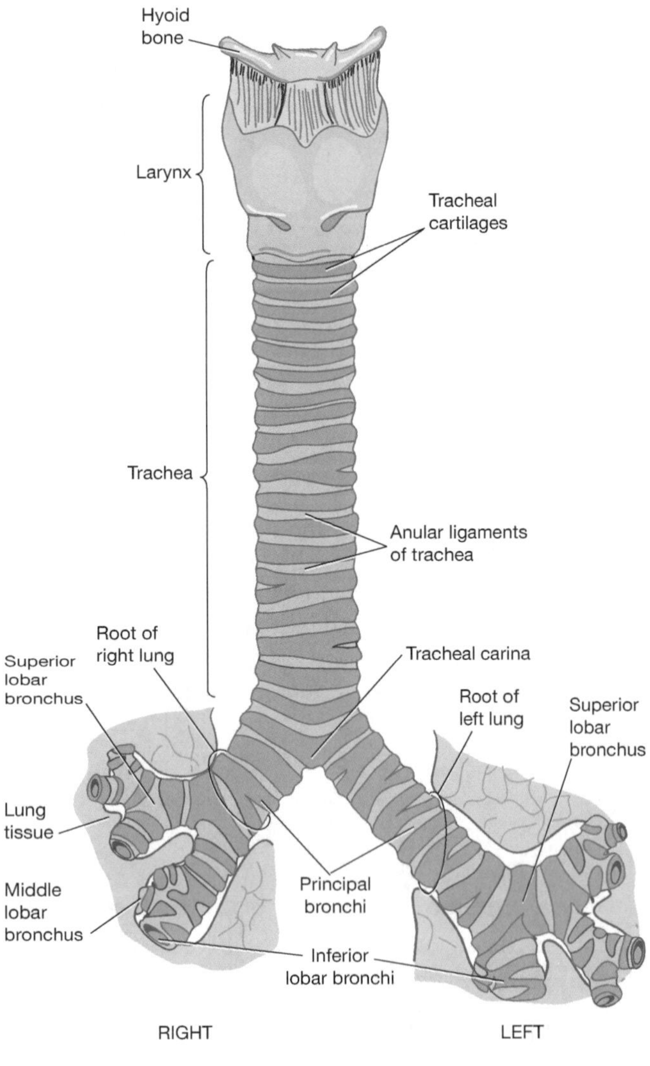

Figure 18-5

Trachea and Bronchial Tree

The trachea courses only 4–5 inches inferiorly from the larynx before it bifurcates to form the left and right principal bronchi. The two main divisions of the left principal bronchus and three main divisions of the right one are termed lobar bronchi because they conduct air to a particular pulmonary lobe. The respiratory mucosa has goblet cells in its lining epithelium which secrete mucus that entraps dirt particles and ciliated pseudostratified columnar epithelial cells to "sweep" the dirt-laden mucus up and out of the air conducting passageways.

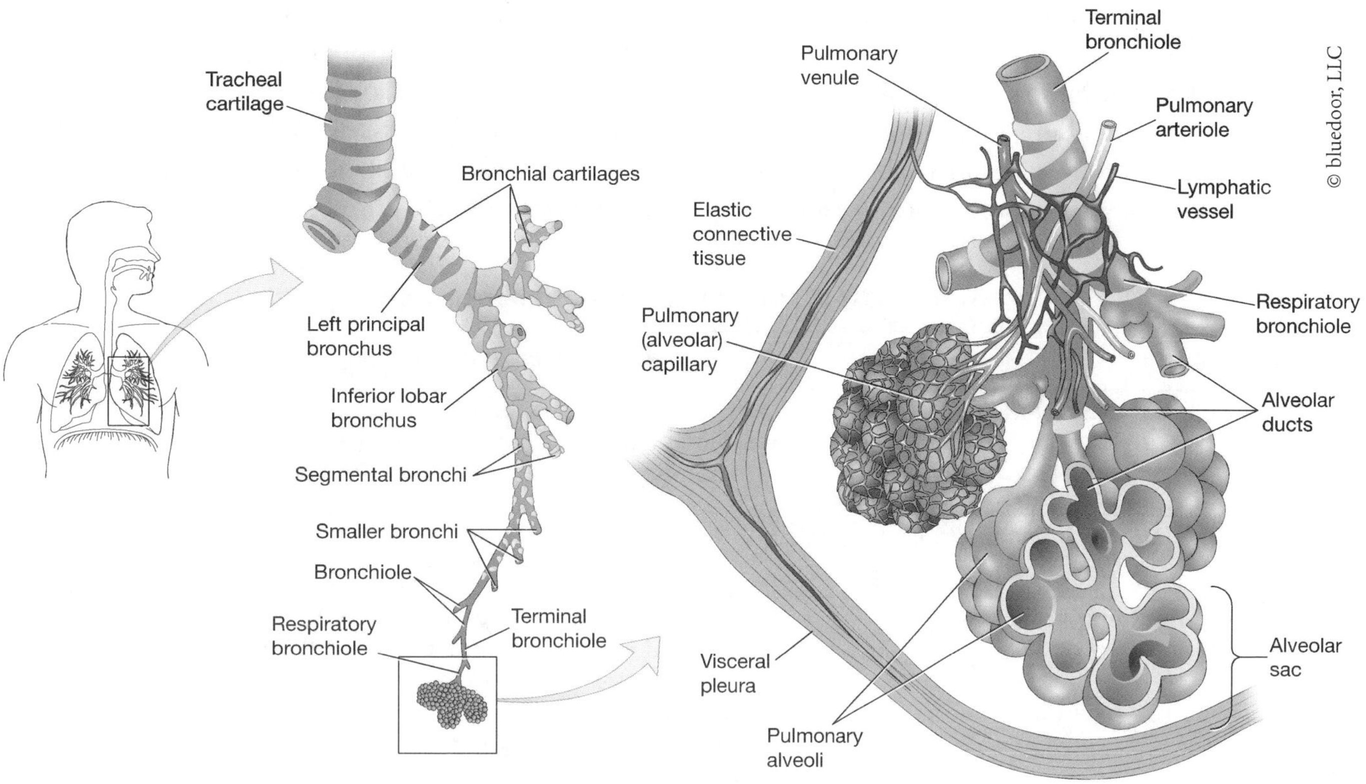

Figure 18-6

Lobar and Segmental Bronchi and Bronchioles

As the air conducting passageways branch and become smaller in diameter, the amount of cartilaginous "stiffener" that they contain is reduced. When cartilage disappears completely, the passageways are called bronchioles. For clarity, the degree of branching has been underrepresented. Most conducting tubes branch over 20 times before reaching the pulmonary alveoli within the pulmonary lobules.

air to/from the ipsilateral lung. The **left principal bronchus** is about 5 cm long and courses laterally from the trachea at about a 45 degree angle. The aortic arch loops over it from anterior to posterior. The **right principal bronchus** is shorter (2.5 cm) and larger in diameter than the left one. It angles laterally from the axis of the trachea at only about 25 degrees and thus is more vertically oriented than the left one. The principal bronchi divide to form the **lobar bronchi** that enter and supply the individual lobes of the lungs. There are three lobar bronchi on the right side (right superior, middle, and inferior lobar bronchi). The left principal bronchus divides into only two lobar bronchi (left superior and inferior lobar bronchi) because the left lung has only two lobes. Within the lungs, the lobar bronchi divide to form **segmental bronchi**. There are typically 10 segmental bronchi on the right side and nine on the left (the first left one, however, divides almost immediately to form two—*see Table 18-2*). Each segmental bronchus conducts air to/from a specific portion of a lung termed a **bronchopulmonary segment** (Figure 18-8).

Structurally the bronchi resemble the trachea. In the larger bronchi, the cartilages are single, "C-shaped" entities that resemble the tracheal cartilages. In the smaller bronchi, the cartilages exist in multiple pieces instead of single structures. At the level where cartilage is no longer present, the passageways are called **bronchioles**. The largest of these are about one millimeter in diameter. They terminate by forming **alveolar ducts** which supply the pulmonary alveoli (*see Lung*). The respiratory epithelium lining of the bronchioles loses its mucus producing goblet cells and then its ciliated cells as it nears the pulmonary alveoli. Loss of the goblet cells "above" the ciliated cells insures that mucus will not be produced in areas that lack means (cilia) of moving it.

Table 18-2 Divisions of the Bronchial Tree

Lobar bronchi	*Segmental bronchi (abbreviation)*
Right superior lobar bronchus	apical segmental bronchus (BI) posterior segmental bronchus (BII) anterior segmental bronchus (BIII)
Right middle lobar bronchus	lateral segmental bronchus (BIV) medial segmental bronchus (BV)
Right inferior lobar bronchus	superior segmental bronchus (BVI) medial basal segmental bronchus (BVII) anterior basal segmental bronchus (BVIII) lateral basal segmental bronchus (BIX) posterior basal segmental bronchus (BX)
Left superior lobar bronchus	apicoposterior segmental bronchus (BI + BII) anterior segmental bronchus (BIII) superior lingular bronchus (BIV) inferior lingular bronchus (BV)
Left inferior lobar bronchus	superior segmental bronchus (BVI) medial basal segmental bronchus (BVII) anterior basal segmental bronchus (BVIII) lateral basal segmental bronchus (BIX) posterior basal segmental bronchus (BX)

Objectives

12. Explain the role of cartilage in the wall of the trachea and bronchi.
13. Discuss the anatomy of the bronchial tree including principal, lobar, and segmental bronchi.
14. Structurally differentiate bronchi and bronchioles.
15. Explain why it is advantageous to have ciliated cells extend "deeper" into the bronchial passageways than goblet cells.

Lungs

The right and left **lungs** occupy a significant portion of the thoracic cavity and are separated from each other by a thoracic partition termed the mediastinum (*see Thorax/Thoracic Cavity*). The narrow, superior end of each lung is the **apex** and the broad inferior end is the **base** (Figure 18-7). Vessels, nerves, and branches of the bronchial tree enter each lung on its medial aspect at a locus

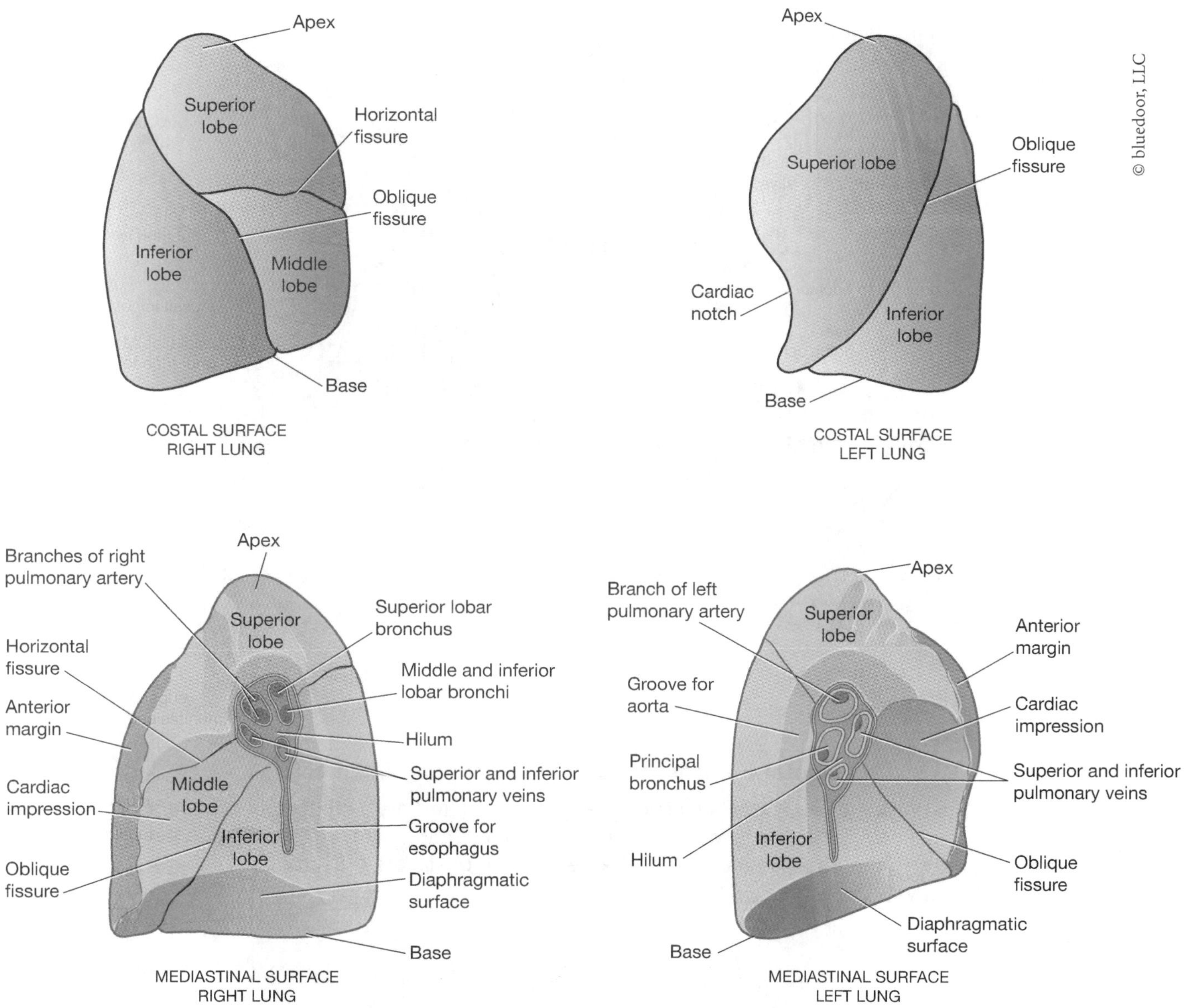

Figure 18-7

Lungs

Each lung has an apex, base, hilum, and four named surfaces. The right lung has three lobes (superior, middle, and inferior) but the left one has only two (superior and inferior).

termed the **hilum**. The lungs are divided into lobes by clefts called **fissures**. The left lung has a single cleft termed the **oblique fissure** which divides it into the **inferior** and **superior lobes**. The right lung has two fissures (**horizontal** and **oblique**) which divide it into three lobes: **superior**, **middle**, and **inferior**. Each lung has four surfaces: diaphragmatic, costal, interlobar, and mediastinal. The **diaphragmatic surface** is the inferior aspect which is adjacent to the diaphragm. The **costal surface** encompasses the anterior, lateral, and posterior aspects which face the ribs. The **interlobar surfaces** are the surfaces between adjacent lobes that face each other. The **mediastinal surface** is the medial aspect of the lung which lies adjacent to the mediastinum. The hilum is located on this sur-

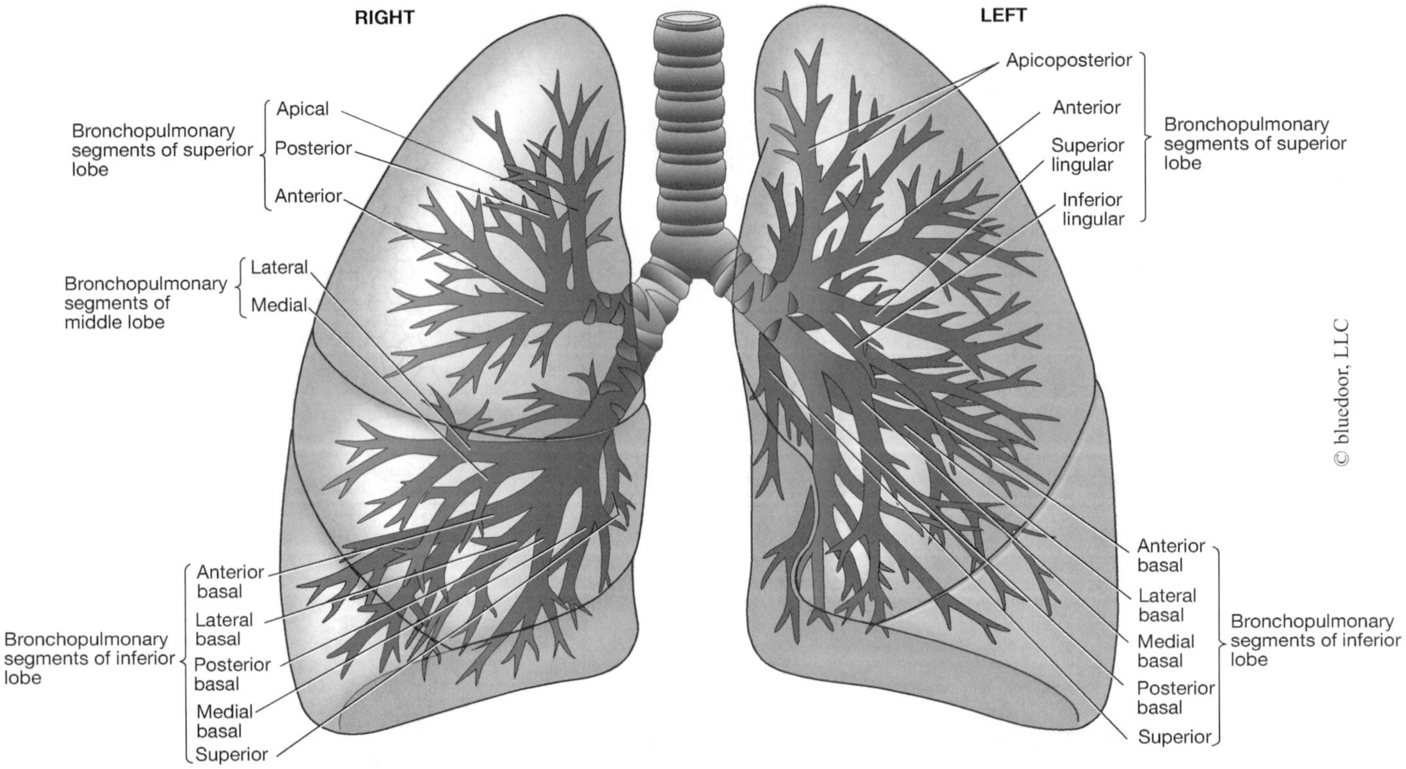

Figure 18-8

Segmental Bronchi and Bronchopulmonary Segments

The portion of each lung supplied by a segmental ("tertiary") bronchus is called a bronchopulmonary segment. These are named the same as the segmental bronchi that supply them and they are also designated by roman numeral acronyms (*see Table 18-2*).

face and the heart causes an indentation (concavity) called the **cardiac impression**. On the anterior border of the left lung this impression forms a concavity termed the **cardiac notch**.

The functional subunits of the lungs are microscopic structures called **pulmonary alveoli** (Figure 18-9, 10). Each alveolus is a sac-like dilation and some occur as evaginations from the walls of the smallest bronchioles (respiratory bronchioles). Most of them, however, occur as clusters supplied by **alveolar ducts**. Each lung contains 75-175 million alveoli and they provide a large surface area (70 m^2) for the exchange of pulmonary gases. The alveoli are lined by simple squamous epithelium and two different cell types can be identified. Most of the cells are **respiratory epitheliocytes** ("type I alveolar cells") with some **granular epitheliocytes** ("type II alveolar cells") interspersed among them. Respiratory epitheliocytes form part of the so-called "**air-blood-barrier**" (**respiratory membrane**). This consists of the three layers that gases must pass through from the alveolus to the blood (and vice versa): respiratory epitheliocytes of the alveolar wall, a thin layer of connective tissue proper, and the endothelium (simple squamous epithelium) forming the capillary wall. The granular epitheliocytes produce a surface tension reducing agent called **surfactant**. This lessens the tendency of the lungs to collapse from the surface tension of the thin layer of fluid (water plus a tiny amount of surfactant) lining the alveoli.

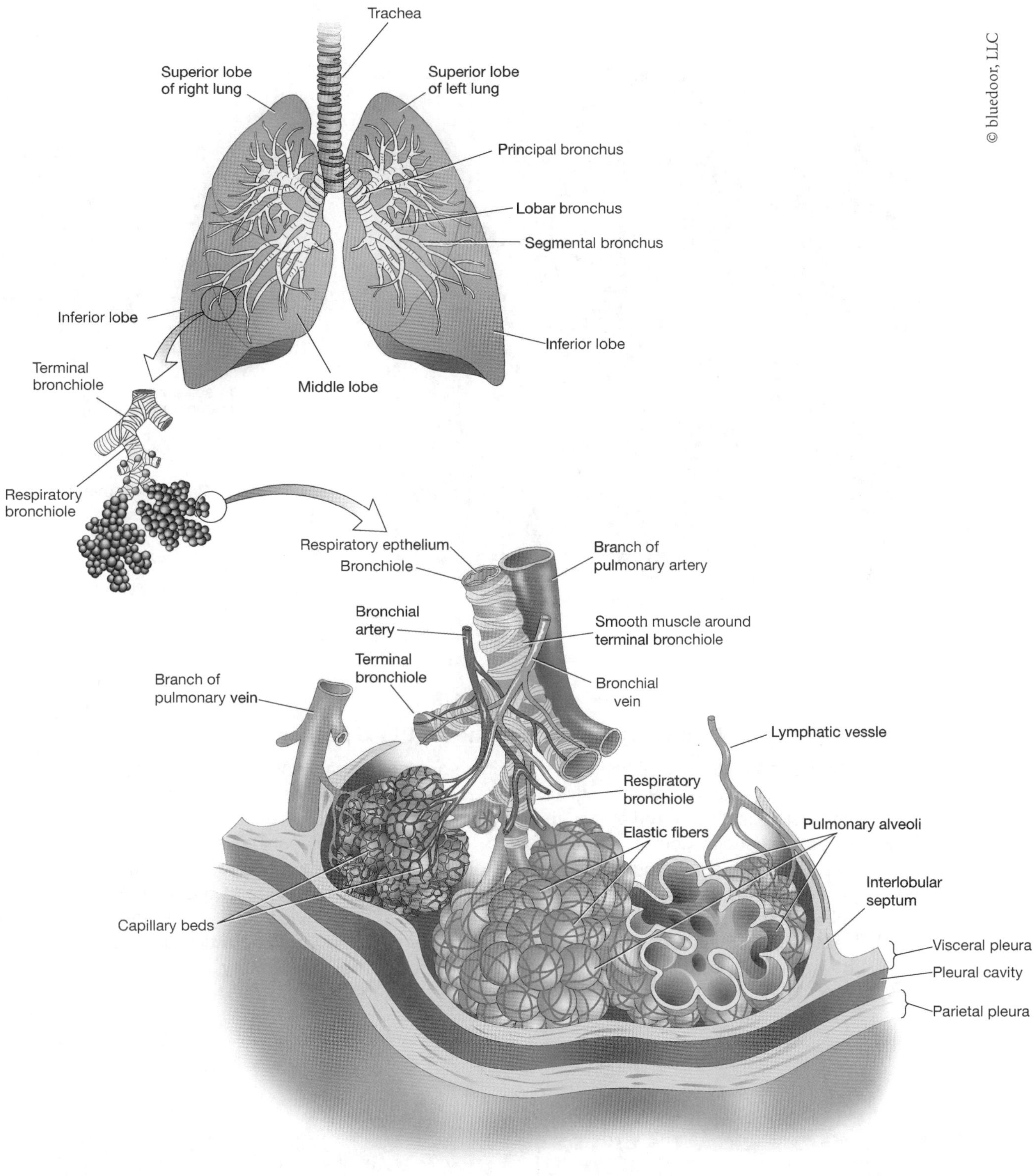

Figure 18-9

Organization of Pulmonary Lobules

A pulmonary lobule consists of the group of alveoli supplied by a respiratory bronchiole. A dense capillary bed surrounds each alveolus to facilitate O_2/CO_2 exchange through the alveolar wall.

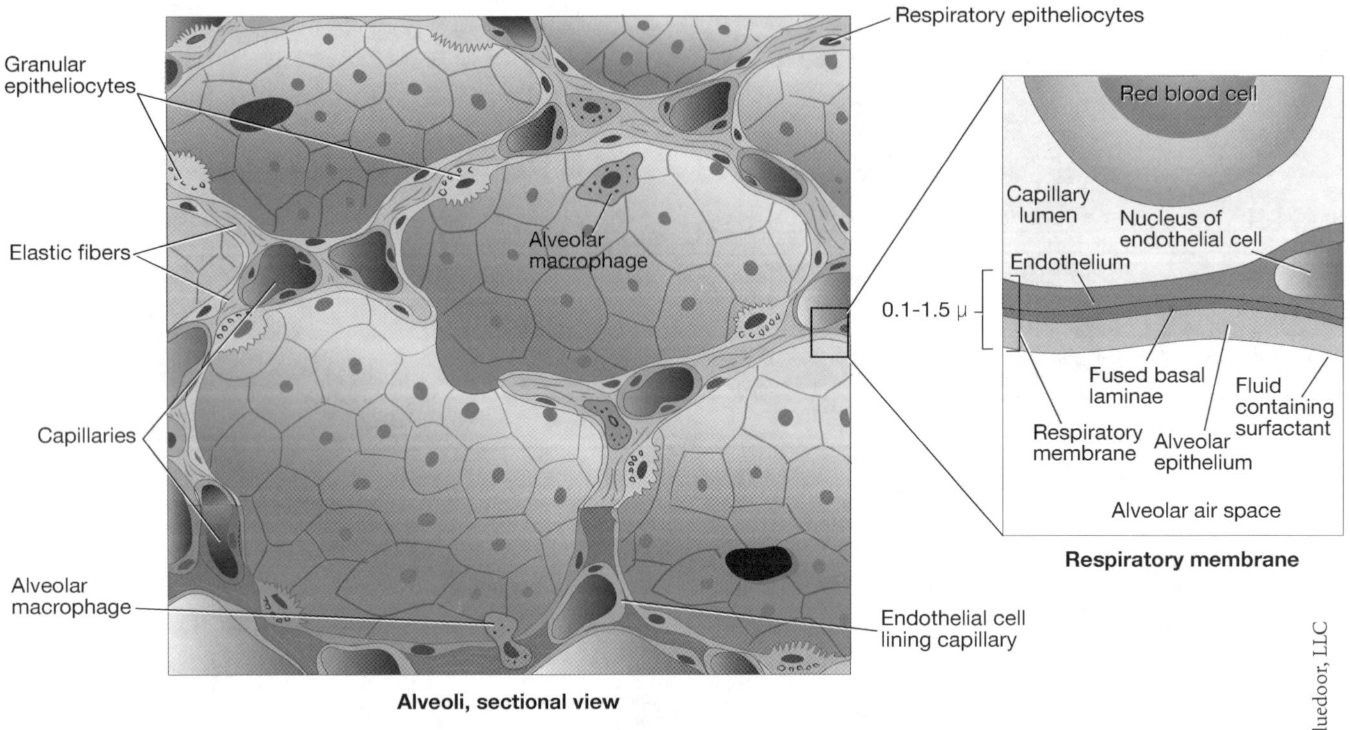

Figure 18-10

Pulmonary Alveoli and the Air-Blood-Barrier

Most of an alveolar wall consists of simple squamous epithelial cells called respiratory epitheliocytes. Physiology texts often designate these as "type I pulmonary alveolar cells." Scattered among the respiratory epitheliocytes are smaller numbers of granular epitheliocytes ("surfactant cells," "type II pulmonary alveolar cells.") These secrete a lipoprotein called surfactant that lowers the surface tension of the thin layer of fluid lining the alveolus. Phagocytic macrophages perform a defensive role in the alveoli by engulfing bacteria. The pulmonary capillaries lie between adjacent alveoli. Their endothelial wall, the respiratory epitheliocytes and a tiny amount of intervening tissue forms the so-called air-blood-barrier (respiratory membrane) which separates the air in the alveoli from the blood in the capillaries.

Objectives

16. Name and define the four surfaces of a lung and state where the hilum is located.
17. Discuss the anatomy of a pulmonary alveolus including the three layers that O_2 and CO_2 must diffuse through (*i.e.*, the components of the "air-blood-barrier").
18. Name (be very specific) the structures which must be ligated (tied off) and transected (severed) to perform a pulmonectomy and a pulmonary lobectomy.

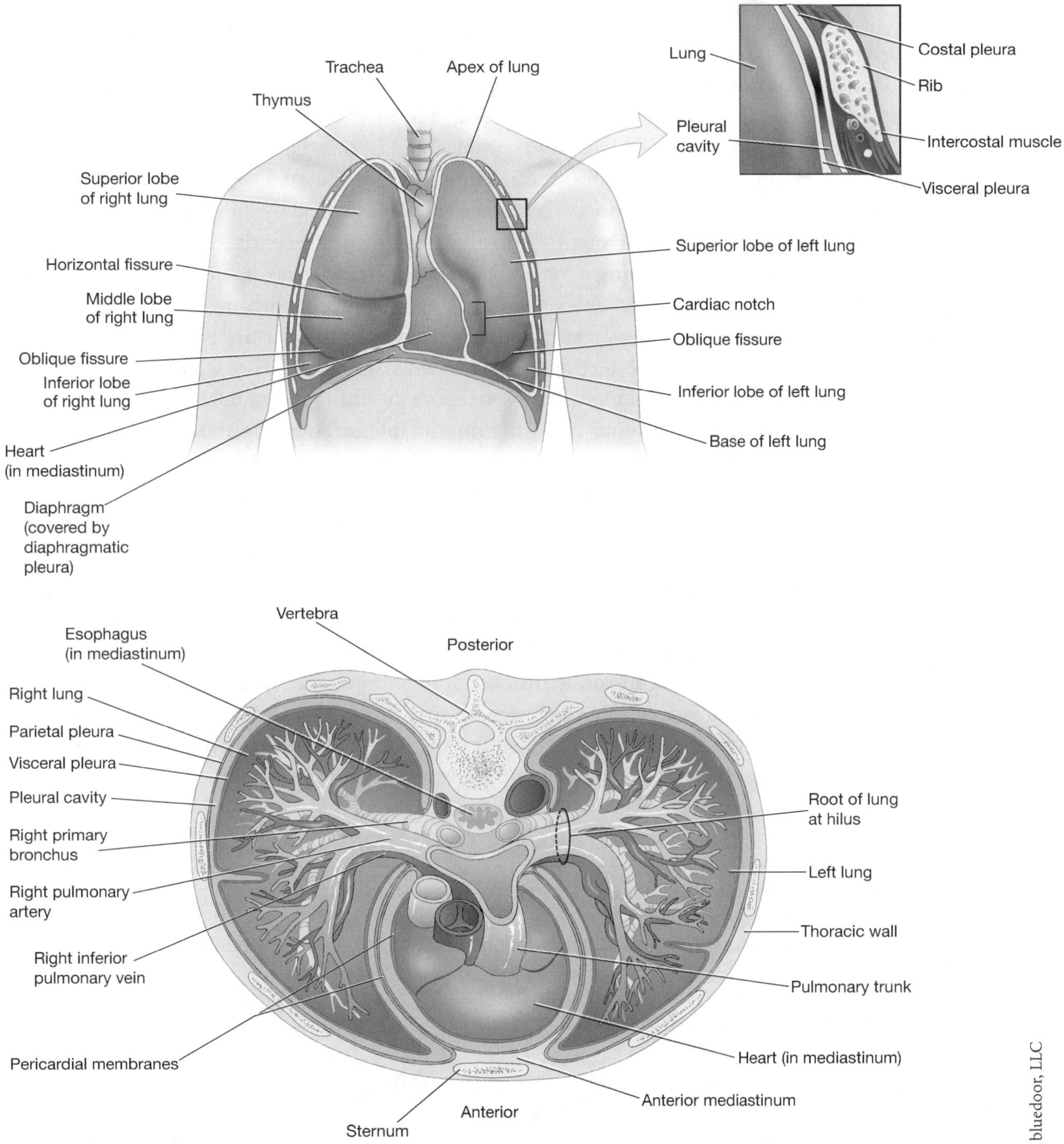

Figure 18-11

Sections of Thorax

The thoracic cavity is the space within the thorax that contains the thoracic organs. These organs invaginate (but are not inside of) three serous body cavities contained within the thoracic cavity: left and right pleural cavities and the pericardial cavity.

Thorax, Thoracic Cavity; Pleurae, Pleural Cavity

The **thorax** is the regional segment of the trunk inferior to the neck, anterior to the back, and superior to the abdomen. The **thoracic cavity** is the organ-filled space within the thorax (Table 18-3). It has three boundaries: superior thoracic opening, thoracic wall, and inferior thoracic opening. The **superior thoracic opening** is commonly called the "thoracic inlet" and is enclosed by the manubrium sterni, first pair of ribs, and the first thoracic vertebra. It transmits the esophagus, trachea, vagal nerve trunks, and a number of vessels and other structures. The **thoracic wall** is formed by the thoracic vertebrae, ribs, sternum, and the soft tissues that surround them. It forms a protective enclosure around the thoracic organs. The **inferior thoracic opening** is formed by the twelfth thoracic vertebra as well as by the lower aspects of the rib cage and sternum. This opening is closed by the diaphragm. The thoracic cavity is completely divided by a median partition termed the **mediastinum**. It is formed by the heart, esophagus, trachea, aorta, some vessels, thoracic duct, and vagal nerves as well as the pleura which covers them. The mediastinum is divided into a superior mediastinum (above the heart) and an inferior mediastinum. The latter is further subdivided into an anterior mediastinum (anterior to the heart), middle mediastinum (containing the heart) and posterior mediastinum (behind the heart). Most of the neurovascular structures in the inferior mediastinum occupy the middle and posterior mediastina.

The two halves of the thoracic cavity are lined by a serous membrane termed pleura. **Pleura** covers the walls of the thoracic cavity and invests the surfaces of the thoracic organs. Pleura on the lungs is termed **visceral pleura**. That lining the walls of the thoracic cavity is termed **parietal pleura** and is regionally subdivided into the **diaphragmatic pleura** (covering the superior aspect of the diaphragm), **costal pleura** (lining the thoracic wall), and **mediastinal pleura**. The latter covers the lateral aspects of the organs that form the mediastinum and in some areas the left and right layers fuse to each other due to a lack of other intervening structures. The very small spaces between the visceral and parietal pleurae on each side constitute the left and right **pleural cavities** (Figure 18-11). They contain essentially nothing except a minute amount of serous fluid.

Table 18-3 Location of Thoracic Organs

Structures Located Totally Within the Thoracic Cavity: heart, pericardial cavity, lungs, pleural cavities, lymph nodes, and superior vena cava.

Structures That Pass Through the Thoracic Cavity: esophagus, thoracic duct, sympathetic trunks, and vagal nerve trunks.

Structures that Pass Into or Out of the Thoracic Cavity: trachea, inferior vena cava, right lymphatic duct, azygos vein, aorta, and other vessels.

Objectives

19. Differentiate the thorax/thoracic cavity and the pleura/pleural cavity.
20. Define the two major subtypes of pleurae and the three regional subdivisions of the parietal pleura.
21. Schematically represent the thorax, trachea, principal bronchi, lungs, diaphragm, and heart in a frontal section. Draw in the pleural membranes and pericardium. Be able to use this drawing to answer penetration questions (arrows, bullets) regarding serous membranes and serous body cavities.
22. List those structures located totally within the thoracic cavity, those that pass through it, and those that enter/leave it.
23. Define mediastinum and indicate the structures which are included in it.

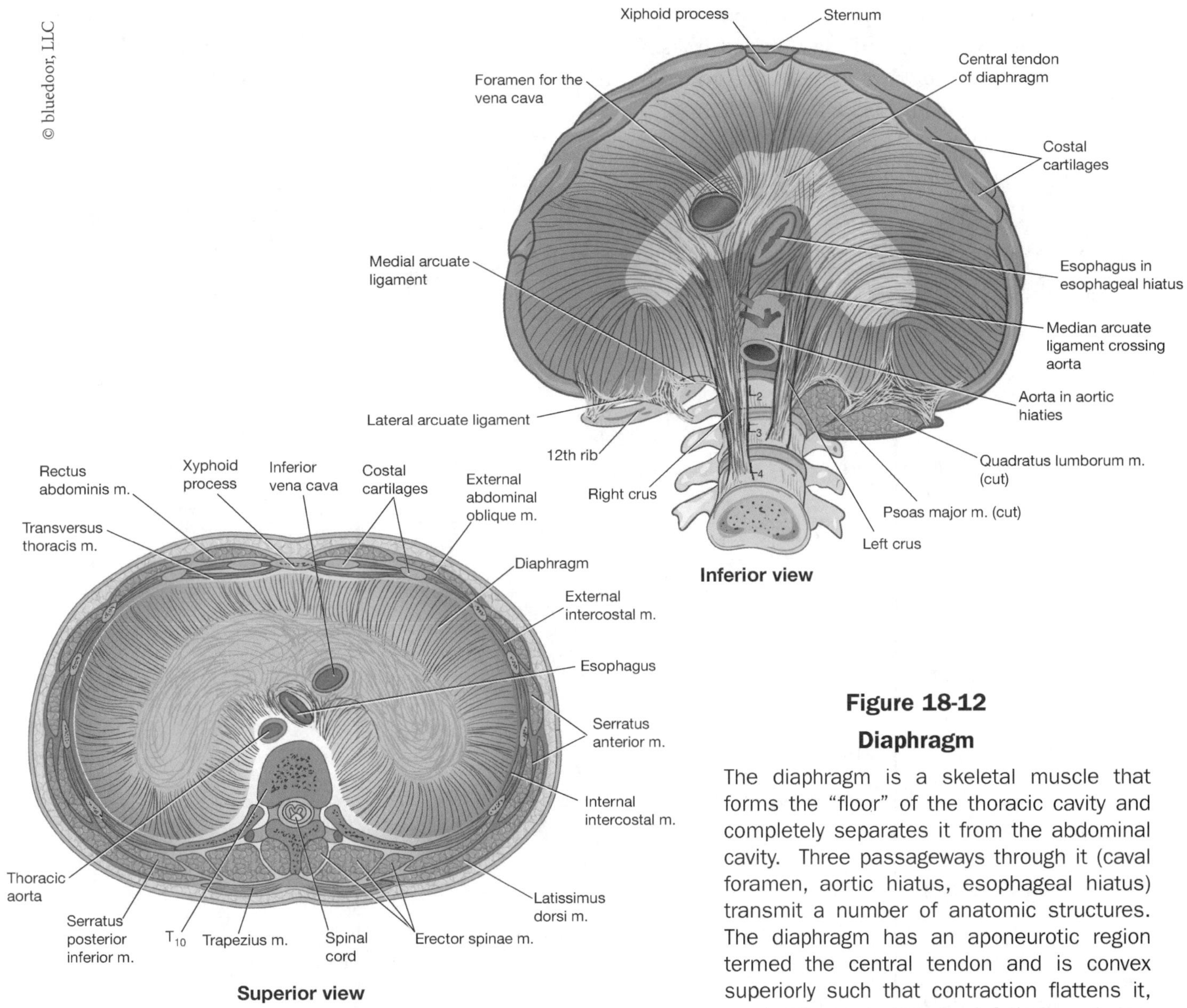

Figure 18-12

Diaphragm

The diaphragm is a skeletal muscle that forms the "floor" of the thoracic cavity and completely separates it from the abdominal cavity. Three passageways through it (caval foramen, aortic hiatus, esophageal hiatus) transmit a number of anatomic structures. The diaphragm has an aponeurotic region termed the central tendon and is convex superiorly such that contraction flattens it, moving the central tendon inferiorly, and elongating the thoracic cavity (top to bottom).

Diaphragm

The **diaphragm** (thoracoabdominal diaphragm) is a skeletal muscle that forms a partition between the thoracic and abdominal cavities (Figure 18-12). The contractile portion of the diaphragm consists of three named parts (sternal, costal, and lumbar) that surround a **central tendon**. The **sternal part** is the anterior portion which attaches to the sternum. The **costal part** attaches to the inner surfaces of the ribs, and the **lumbar part** attaches to the lumbar vertebrae. The latter portion is divided into right and left **crura**. The diaphragm has three named openings which transmit other anatomic structures: aortic hiatus, esophageal hiatus, and vena caval foramen. The **aortic hiatus** is located in the posterior portion between the crura. It transmits the descending aorta, azygos vein, and thoracic duct. The **esophageal hiatus** is located in the fleshy part of the left crus and transmits the esophagus and vagal nerve trunks. The **vena caval foramen** is the opening through which the inferior vena cava passes. It is located in the central tendon to the right of the median plane and is often called the *caval foramen*.

Objectives

24. Name the three openings in the diaphragm and state what each one transmits.

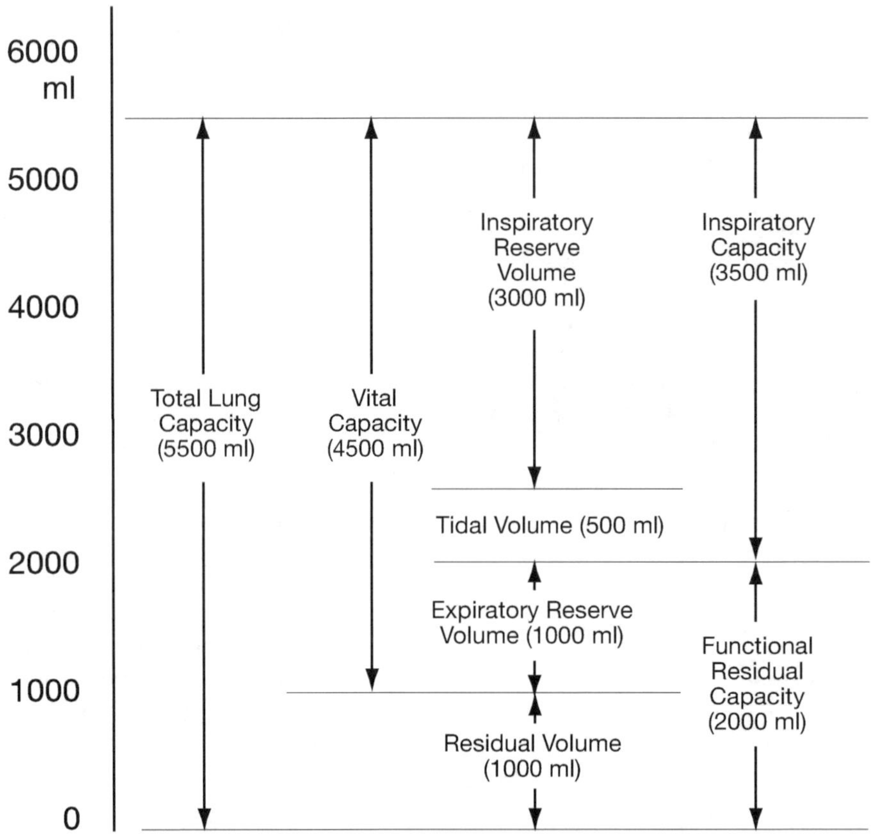

Figure 18-13

Respiratory Volumes and Capacities

Total lung capacity is the total amount of air that the lungs can hold and represents the sum of four non-overlapping volumes. These volumes include residual volume (which cannot be exhaled), expiratory reserve volume (*can* be exhaled but currently is not), tidal volume (the amount of air inhaled and exhaled), and inspiratory reserve volume (which *can* be inhaled but currently is not). The sum of the "top three" volumes is called the vital capacity. The sum of the "top two" volumes constitutes inspiratory capacity and the sum of the "bottom two" volumes is the functional residual capacity.

Mechanics of Respiration

The physical movement of air into the lungs is called **inspiration**. This is effected primarily by contraction of the diaphragm with some assistance from the muscles of the thoracic wall. In its relaxed state, the diaphragm assumes a dome-like configuration with the abdominal aspect markedly concave. Contraction of the diaphragm flattens this cavity, forcing the liver and other abdominal viscera inferiorly. This lengthens the thoracic cavity and reduces the intrapleural pressure. Elevation

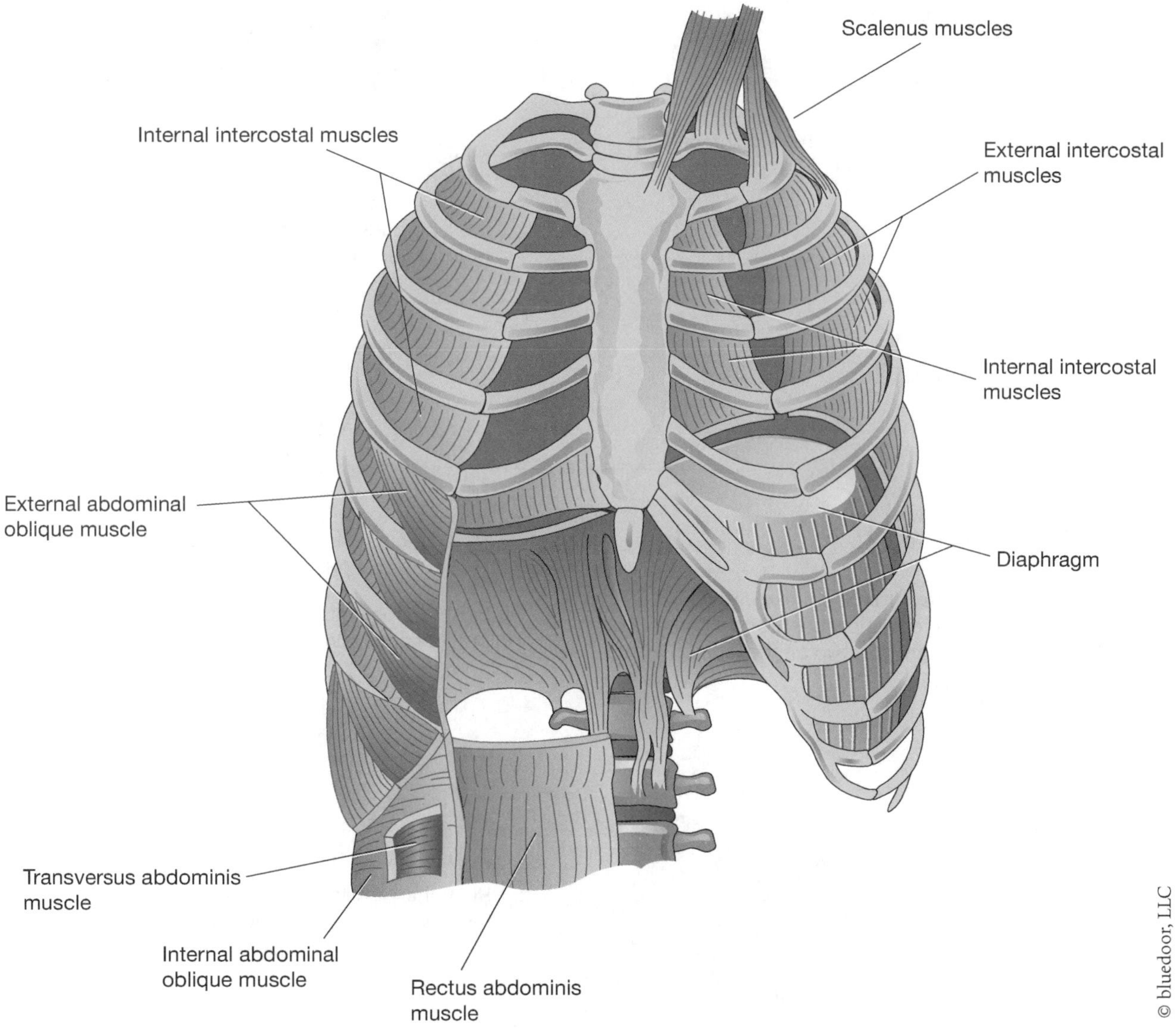

Figure 18-14

Respiratory Muscles

Passive respiration involves mostly diaphragmatic movements to elongate and shorten the thoracic cavity. Forced respiration recruits a number of other muscles that elevate and depress the ribs. Elevation of the ribs increases the diameter of the thoracic cavity and depression of the ribs narrows it.

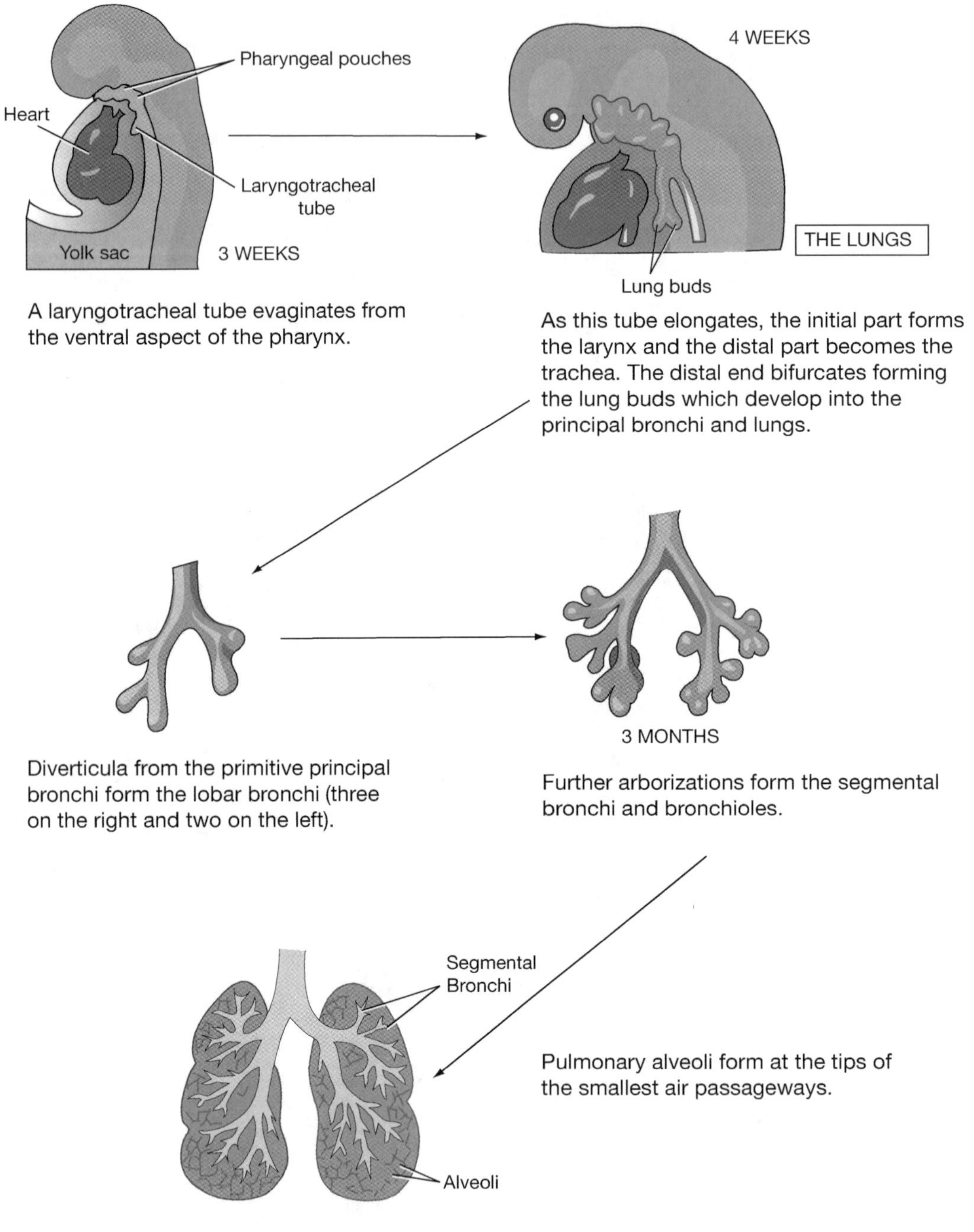

Figure 18-15

Development of Respiratory Organs

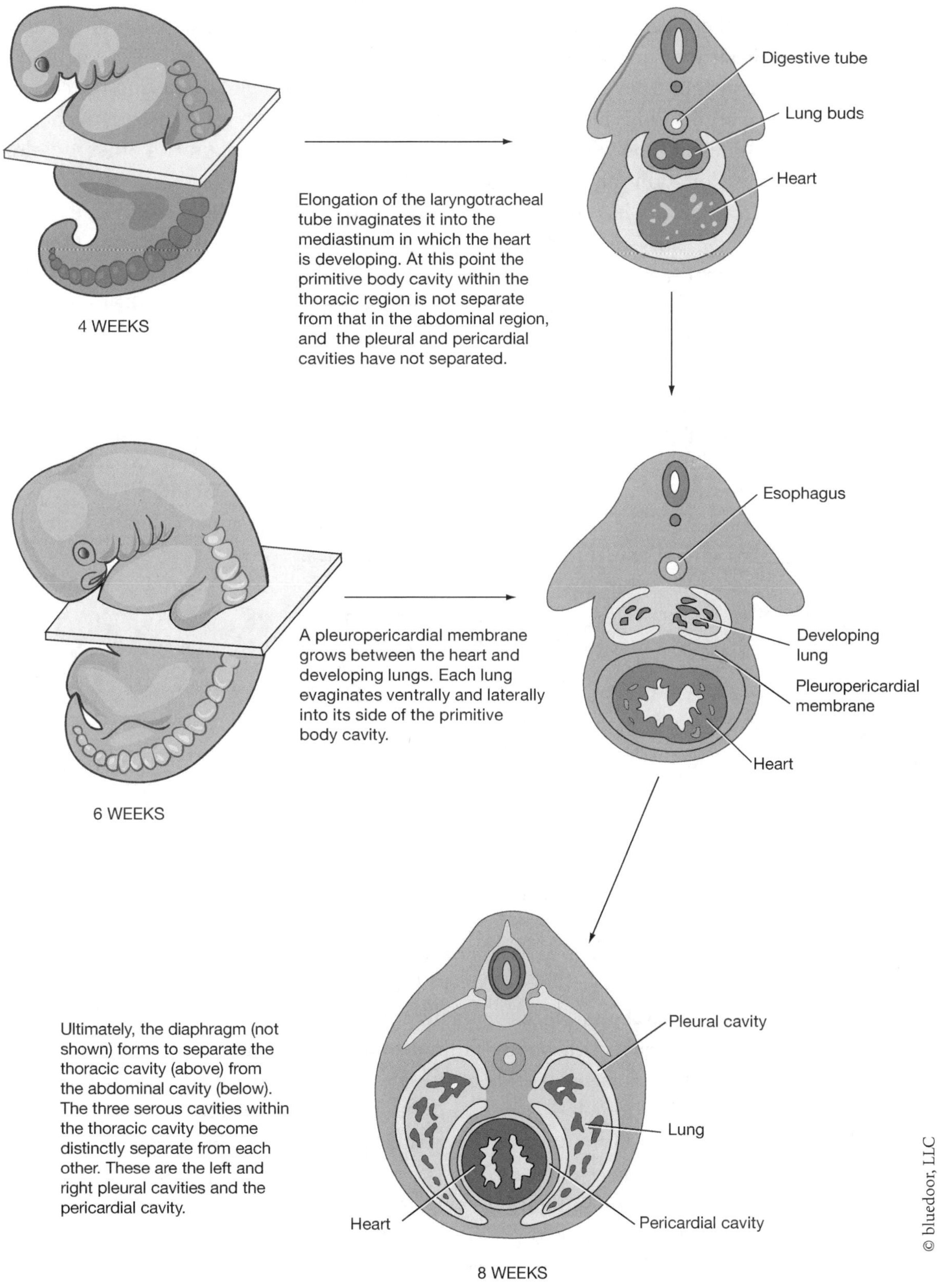

Figure 18-16

Development of the Pleural and Pericardial Cavities

of the rib cage by the scalenus and other muscles slightly increases the diameter of the thoracic cavity which further decreases the intrapleural pressure. This results in inflation of the lungs from atmospheric air pressure. **Expiration** is largely a passive process caused by the natural tendency of the lungs to shrink. They have considerable elastic tissue in their stroma and the surface tension of the thin layer of fluid lining each alveolus also contributes to their tendency to collapse. Consequently, expiration will occur simply by relaxing the diaphragm and other muscles of inspiration. Forced expiration can be effected by an abdominal press.

The volume of air which is inspired and expired is termed the **tidal volume**. In an average-sized individual at rest, this is only about 500 ml but it is markedly increased during exercise. The total amount of air that can be forcefully inhaled and exhaled is called the **vital capacity**. It consists of the tidal volume plus the inspiratory and expiratory reserve volumes. The **inspiratory reserve volume** is the volume that can be forcefully inspired (3000 ml) after a tidal inspiration. The **expiratory reserve volume** is the volume that can be forcefully exhaled (1000 ml) after a tidal expiration. Even after forcing out all air possible, about 1000 ml remains in the lungs. This is called the **residual volume**. The **total lung capacity** includes all four lung volumes (Figure 18-13). Two other lung capacities are defined by physiologists: **inspiratory capacity** and **functional residual capacity.** The inspiratory capacity is the sum of the tidal volume and inspiratory reserve volume. The functional residual capacity is the sum of the expiratory reserve volume and the residual volume. Note that each lung "capacity" is a sum of two, three or all four lung "volumes."

Objectives

25. Explain the mechanics of respiration.
26. Name two things that cause the lungs to have a tendency to collapse.
27. Define the four lung volumes and the four lung capacities and state their inter-relationships.

Development of the Respiratory System

The upper part of the respiratory system begins its development at about four weeks of gestation as paired, thickened areas of ectoderm called **olfactory** (**nasal**) **placodes** (*see Figure 12-13*). These invaginate to form **nasal pits** which eventually connect to the nasal cavity. The latter is separated for a time from the oral cavity below it by a thin **oronasal membrane**. When this membrane ruptures during the seventh week, a single large **oronasal cavity** is formed. Mesodermal plates called **palatine shelves** grow horizontally across this cavity to form the palate which separates the definitive oral and nasal cavities. At the same time, a vertical plate develops on the median plane which forms the nasal septum and separates the nasal cavity into right and left halves.

The lower part of the respiratory system begins its development at four weeks as a diverticulum called the **laryngotracheal bud** that evaginates anteriorly from the lower pharynx (Figures 18-15, 18-16). As this bud elongates, the upper portion forms the larynx, the middle part forms trachea, and the lower part bifurcates to form the left and right principal bronchi. These divide and elongate to complete the development of the bronchial tree. At their ends, the branches of the bronchial tree form bronchioles and ultimately pulmonary alveoli. This is finally complete at about 26 weeks of gestation.

Objectives

28. Name the structures that grow horizontally to divide the nasal cavity from the oral cavity and name the structure that branches off the pharynx to form the lower respiratory system.

Clinical Considerations

Aspirated objects, swollen mucous membranes, and traumatic injuries to the trachea can all block the respiratory passageways. If the blockage occurs in the upper part of the respiratory system, a skin incision can be made over the cricoid cartilage followed by an incision into the trachea. A plastic or metal tube is then inserted to restore an open airway below the obstruction. This procedure is called a **tracheostomy**. Another method of insuring a patent airway is tracheal **intubation**, which is the insertion of a tube through the oral cavity and larynx and on into the trachea. Foreign objects can be suctioned out of the lower respiratory passageways. Those that lodge in the lower bronchial tree generally become wedged in the right principal bronchus or one of its branches because the left principal bronchus diverges from the trachea at a sharper angle. The **abdominal thrust maneuver** (also called the "Heimlich" maneuver) can sometimes be used to "pop" an obstruction out of place. This maneuver, which usually must be applied by a second party, uses the remaining air in the lungs to dislodge the object. The would-be rescuer approaches the choking individual from behind, reaches around the victim's trunk, and positions a fist on the anterior abdomen just below the sternum. Then, using the other arm in a "bear hug" squeeze, the fist is suddenly and very powerfully forced into the abdomen resulting in air being squeezed out of the lungs, and (hopefully) dislodging the obstruction.

Laryngitis is inflammation of the larynx. Sore throat, hoarseness, cough, and dysphagia (difficulty in swallowing) can all accompany laryngitis. It is usually caused by respiratory infections or by irritants such as cigarette smoke. In severe cases, the swelling of the vocal folds is so marked that they will not vibrate properly and "loss of voice" occurs.

Stab and gunshot wounds (open thoracic wall), as well as lung damage from cancer or a broken rib, can introduce air into the pleural cavities and result in **pneumothorax**. Blood can enter the pleural cavities in a like manner and result in **hemothorax**. Severe infectious processes within the thorax can result in pus accumulation (**pyothorax**) and a rupture of the thoracic duct or other large lymphatic channels can cause **chylothorax** (lymph in the pleural cavity). A **diaphragmatic hernia** (ruptured diaphragm) allows the liver, stomach, and/or intestines to enter the thoracic cavity. Hernias require surgical intervention. All of these conditions can prevent the lung(s) from inflating (**atelectasis**). Fluid or gas in the pleural cavities can be drawn out with a large syringe by inserting a needle through the thoracic wall. Any condition that results in the incomplete expansion of the lungs may cause difficulty in breathing (**dyspnea**).

Pleurisy or **pleuritis** is the inflammation of the pleural membranes. Friction of the pleurae can cause pain during the early stages, and fluid accumulation. In severe cases, the visceral and parietal pleurae may permanently fuse together.

Carbon monoxide poisoning results from the remarkably strong tendency of carbon monoxide to bind with hemoglobin to form carboxyhemoglobin (the bond is much stronger than that between oxygen and hemoglobin). This prevents hemoglobin from binding with oxygen and causes hypoxia. **Hypoxia** is a condition where there is low oxygen supply to the tissues despite adequate blood flow. Carbon monoxide poisoning can result from exhaust fumes of gas engines and from tobacco smoke. The condition is treated by administering pure oxygen and can be fatal if not immediately corrected.

Asthma is a chronic, inflammatory disorder that causes narrowing of the airways. Spasms of smooth muscles in the walls of the smaller bronchi and bronchioles causes bronchoconstriction. The patient may have the most difficulty during exhalation. **Emphysema** is a condition characterized by abnormally large pulmonary air spaces due to the destruction of alveolar walls. This reduces the surface area for gaseous exchange and thus, blood oxygen levels are lowered. Any physical exertion can cause breathlessness. Over time, the thorax of an affected individual enlarges, forming a "barrel chest", to compensate for the added exertion of breathing.

Pneumonia is the acute infection or inflammation of the pulmonary alveoli. Affected alveoli have a reduced ability to function in O_2/CO_2 exchange. This reduces the blood oxygen levels while blood carbon dioxide levels remain the same (carbon dioxide more readily diffuses across the alveoli than oxygen). A bacterium called *Streptococcus pneumoniae* is the most common cause of pneumonia. Another bacterium (*Mycobacterium tuberculosis*) produces the infectious disease called **tuberculosis** (**TB**). Lung tissue is destroyed by the tuberculosis organism and is replaced by fibrous connective tissue. The fibrous tissue reduces the elasticity of the lungs.

Cystic fibrosis is an inherited disease of the secretory epithelia. It affects the respiratory passageways, salivary glands, pancreas, and sweat glands. Patients with cystic fibrosis have an inability to transport chloride ions across plasma membranes of some epithelial cells. The production of thick secretions in the passageways causes difficult breathing. The excessive secretions inflame the mucous membranes and result in replacement of normal tissue with fibrous connective tissue. Cystic fibrosis is the most common lethal genetic disease among Caucasians. It is believed that 5% of the population are genetic carriers.

Scuba divers get excess nitrogen dissolved into their blood because they are breathing compressed air at higher than atmospheric pressures (air is 80% nitrogen). Depending on how deep they dive and how long they remain at depth, they need to ascend slowly and often need to stop at certain depths for a short time on the way back to the surface to allow the excess nitrogen to leave their bloodstream in their exhaled air. Otherwise, the nitrogen tends to form bubbles within the bloodstream (akin to the CO_2 bubbles that form when a carbonated drink is suddenly depressurized by opening it). A diver with this affliction is said to have the "**bends**" (**decompression sickness**). The latter may be simply painful, or if too many bubbles form and cerebral vessels are blocked, may be fatal. Divers who descend to extreme depths while breathing compressed air may get so much nitrogen in their bloodstream that they suffer **nitrogen narcosis** (**rapture of the deep**). This is caused by the effect that high concentrations of nitrogen have on the brain. A euphoric state is produced similar to intoxication with alcohol. Affected individuals have been known to remove their diving equipment and perish.

Objectives

29. Explain how to perform the abdominal thrust (Heimlich) maneuver.
30. Explain how pneumothorax, hemothorax, or a diaphragmatic hernia can result in dyspnea.

Clinical Case Studies

Case 1—A 28-year-old man, dining at a restaurant with his wife, suddenly grabbed at his throat and tumbled out of his chair onto the floor. An alert diner at a nearby table came to the man's rescue by administering a "bear hug" maneuver from behind—forcing a fist into the victim's abdomen. The choking man recovered immediately. Explain what happened.

Case 2—A 58-year-old housewife who had smoked cigarettes heavily for many years became noticeably short of breath after climbing a stair or walking out to her mailbox. Her labored breathing became progressively worse and she was finally put on supplemental oxygen 24 hours a day. Even though she had not smoked for the last several years, her ability to intake oxygen steadily decreased and she died three years later. Suggest a diagnosis.

Case 3—A high school senior involved in a car accident suffered a crushing injury to his thoracic region. In the emergency room his labored breathing worsened and the attending physician quickly installed a chest tube and began withdrawing air to relieve his dyspnea. Radiography confirmed a complete collapse of his left lung and partial collapse of his right one. No abdominal viscera were observed in the thoracic cavity. What could have caused his pulmonary collapse?

Points to Ponder

Respiration. It's a voluntary but subconscious vital act that we take for granted until it is compromised by the dyspnea associated with anaphylactic shock, pneumothorax, or severe pneumonia. In the broad sense of the term, respiration encompasses the mechanics of ventilation (moving air into and out of the lungs), oxygen/carbon dioxide exchange in the lungs and body tissues, and oxygen utilization by the cells.

Open the chest wall with a scalpel or tear a lung with the end of a broken rib and the lung on that side collapses. Its innate tendency to shrink is due to elastic fibers within its stroma, and the surface tension of the fluid lining its alveoli. Close up the wound and the collapsed lung gradually re-inflates over the next few days as the air (that ought not to be there in the first place) is slowly reabsorbed from the pleural cavity. Pneumothorax can also occur from a spontaneously ruptured lung. Same bottom line. Collapse of a lung doesn't have to be due to air in there. It can also occur from anything else that's not supposed to be in the pleural cavity: blood (intrathoracic hemorrhage), lymph (ruptured thoracic duct), liver, intestines (diaphragmatic hernia), *etc., etc.*

The "gee whiz" facts regarding the respiratory system are impressive. The total length of all the capillaries in the two lungs is said to be one thousand miles. The total surface area of the pulmonary alveoli is about one thousand square feet. A red blood corpuscle carries about 280 million molecules of hemoglobin and each of those can bind to four molecules of oxygen. Thus, an RBC can carry about a billion molecules of oxygen and routinely picks up over 90% of that number in the split second that it takes to pass through a pulmonary capillary bed. The resting tidal volume of an average-sized individual is about 500 ml and we intake that about 14 times a minute. That's seven liters each minute, 420 liters each hour, and 10,080 liters each day (at rest). On its way in to the delicate alveoli, inspired air is thermoregulated to body temperature, brought to 100% relative humidity and cleaned of a significant amount of its particulate matter.

Surface tension explains why a wasp can land on a mud puddle—it also explains why carefully placed razor blades can float on water, and as noted above, is a major reason why lungs, left to their own devices, collapse. In the lungs, this surface tension is produced by the thin layer of fluid lining the pulmonary alveoli. It is so powerful that were it not for surfactant, that famous lipoprotein that reduces surface tension, we couldn't inhale. A premature infant struggles to do just that because surfactant is not produced until the last part of gestation. Thus, babies arriving early may not have enough. They labor every time for what you and I don't even think about 12-14 times a minute, 800 times an hour, and 20,000 times a day.

Anaphylactic shock is a hypersensitive (allergic) reaction which causes such severe bronchial constriction that it may be fatal. I've been there twice—once was just a close call that I was able to fight off myself after a bunch of Texas fire ants (37) decided to sting me more or less simultaneously. A number of welts, severe dyspnea, and I was fine two hours later. The other time would have been fatal had I not received multiple injections of epinephrine at the point where I passed out due to anoxia. This particular episode was induced by injection of a tetanus antitoxin injection which contained horse serum—a material I had developed a hypersensitivity to several years earlier from a similar injection of the same material.

Severe dyspnea is a scary affliction. I have felt the terror personally and have seen it twice on the face of my wife who is severely hypersensitive to bee stings. Both times she came close to death and both times I was thankful for my veterinary medical training and background which averted otherwise fatal consequences.

My mother died in 1983 from complications related to chronic emphysema. Brought on by years of smoking cigarettes, emphysema slowly reduced her ability to exchange O_2/CO_2 in her lungs as the walls between adjacent pulmonary alveoli collapsed and her individual alveoli coalesced and enlarged. For the last few years of her life, she had to inhale supplemental oxygen and was tethered to an oxygen tank in the middle of the house by clear plastic tubing that followed her everywhere and forced her to retrace her steps when she rounded a table, chair, or other object. A small, portable oxygen tank gave her a larger degree of mobility—allowing her to go shopping with the rest of us.

Slang and Obsolete Nomenclature

UNOFFICIAL TERM	**OFFICIAL DESIGNATION**
primary bronchus	principal bronchus *[bronchus principalis]*
secondary bronchus	lobar bronchus *[bronchus lobaris]*
tertiary bronchus	segmental bronchus *[bronchus segmentalis]*
vocal cord, true vocal cord	vocal fold *[plica vocalis]*
false vocal cord	vestibular fold *[plica vestibularis]*
respiratory epithelium	ciliated pseudostratified columnar epithelium *[epitheliopseudostratificatum columnare ciliatum]*
nasopharynx	nasal part *[pars nasalis]* of the pharynx
oropharynx	oral part *[pars oralis]* of the pharynx
laryngopharynx	laryngeal part *[pars laryngis]* of the pharynx
alveolar epithelial cell	respiratory epitheliocyte *[epitheliocytus respiratorius]*
type I alveolar cell	respiratory epitheliocyte *[epitheliocytus respiratorius]*
surfactant cell	granular epitheliocyte *[epitheliocytus granularis]*
type II alveolar cell	granular epitheliocyte *[epitheliocytus granularis]*

Review Questions

1. Inspired air does not have to pass through which of the following to reach the pulmonary alveoli?
   A. nose
   B. bronchioles
   C. bronchi
   D. pharynx
   E. larynx

2. Which directional aspect of a lung is mismatched with the name of the surface?
   A. inferior—diaphragmatic surface
   B. anterior—costal surface
   C. posterior—posterior surface
   D. lateral—costal surface
   E. medial—mediastinal surface

3. The right lung has_____ fissures, _______ lobes, and ____ segmental bronchi.
   A. 2—2—9
   B. 2—3—10
   C. 1—2—9
   D. 1—2—10
   E. 2—3—3

4. Which structure is found totally within the thoracic cavity?
   A. aorta
   B. esophagus
   C. superior vena cava
   D. trachea
   E. inferior vena cava

5. Which structure is mismatched with the diaphragmatic passageway that transmits it?
   A. aorta—aortic hiatus
   B. azygos vein—aortic hiatus
   C. vagal nerve trunks—esophageal hiatus
   D. superior vena cava—caval foramen
   E. esophagus—esophageal hiatus

6. Which statement about the mediastinum is false?
   A. It includes most structures within the thoracic cavity except the lungs, and parts of the bronchial tree.
   B. It consists of the left and right mediastinal pleurae and all structures between them.
   C. It is the partition between the lungs formed by several body structures.
   D. It is the partition between the left and right pleural cavities formed by several body structures.
   E. If all of the above are true, choose this response.

7. Find the incorrect statement.
   A. The larynx contains three unpaired and three paired cartilages.
   B. The vocal ligaments, surrounded by vocal folds, attach to the thyroid cartilage (anteriorly) and to the arytenoid cartilages (posteriorly).
   C. To vocalize, breathe normally, and effect an abdominal press, the vocal folds must be partially abducted, fully abducted, and fully adducted, respectively.
   D. To raise the pitch of the voice, the vocal folds must be abducted.
   E. The vocal folds and the space between them are collectively called the glottis.

8. Many of the functions of the respiratory system depend partially on interactions with the muscular system. Which one of the following depends least on the muscular system?
   A. air movement into/out of the lungs
   B. vocalization
   C. protective reflexes (coughing/sneezing)
   D. acid/base balance
   E. abdominal compression

9. Paranasal sinuses invade all of the following bones except the...
   A. sphenoid bone.
   B. temporal bone.
   C. ethmoid bone.
   D. maxillae.
   E. frontal bone.

10. The total lung capacity of an individual is 6000 ml, the residual volume is 1500 ml and the tidal volume is 500 ml. Calculate the vital capacity.
    A. 1000 ml
    B. 4500 ml
    C. 2500 ml
    D. 55000 ml
    E. If the vital capacity cannot be calculated from the data given, choose this response.

Thought Questions

1. Why are cartilages necessary to prevent collapse of bronchial walls during inspiration, but are not necessary (or present) to prevent bronchiolar collapse?

2. How can an abdominal press force expiration?

3. Discuss the physical relationship of the lungs and the pleural membranes (pleurae).

4. Sometimes a lung spontaneously collapses and then over the next few days, spontaneously re-inflates. Suggest a logical explanation.

5. The bony limits of the thoracic cavity are formed by components of the axial skeleton collectively

termed the thoracic cage. What bones form the thoracic cage and which of these form the skeletal limits of the thoracic inlet?

6. The portion of the inferior vena cava that passes through the caval foramen of the diaphragm is physically adherent to the diaphragm that surrounds it. What effect would this and the change in intrapleural pressure during respiration have on the diameter of the inferior vena cava?

7. Why do lungs appear black radiographically?

8. Discuss the functional role of respiratory epithelium.

9. Respiratory therapists refer to the "anatomical dead space" in the respiratory system. What is meant?

10. What causes the faint whistling sounds that occur when an individual with severe bronchitis forcefully exhales?

11. A healthy lung will collapse if it is torn (by a penetrating wound), if the integrity of the thoracic cavity is compromised by a hole in the chest wall, or by a large diaphragmatic hernia. Explain why.

12. A healthy lung, surgically removed from an individual, will collapse. If this lung is placed in a vacuum jar and air in the jar is evacuated with a vacuum pump, what will happen?

13. What are the positions of the vocal folds during an abdominal press, during vocalization, and during normal respiration? How are these positions achieved?

14. Once mucus collects in paranasal sinuses (during sinusitis) how does it get out?

15. Why do most individuals inspire through their oral cavities (*vs.* nasal cavities) during heavy exercise?

16. Which parts of the pharynx are traversed by inspired air?

17. Why are (significantly) premature neonates often dyspneic?

18. A bullet passing through the thoracic cavity may enter pleural cavities several times enroute but it can only pass through a total of two different pleural cavities. Explain the several/two discordance.

19. In birds, some of the bones are connected to the conducting parts of the respiratory system with the net result that the medullary cavities are full of air instead of bone marrow tissue. What advantage does this pose?

20. The conducting passageways of the respiratory system thermoregulate inspired air to body temperature, clean it, and adjust its relative humidity to 100% before it reaches the pulmonary

alveoli. Since forced inspiration can occur in a fraction of a second, how are all of these functions completed in such a short time?

21. When the thoracic cavity is opened surgically, the patient must be put on "positive pressure ventilation". Why?

Answers to Clinical Case Studies

Case 1—This man's airway became blocked with ingesta. The first aid administered, called a "Heimlich maneuver" after its discoverer, unblocked the airway by forcing residual air in the lungs up the trachea and literally blowing the airway clear. Note: If you're ever in a situation where this needs to be done, make sure that you are *very* forceful. If you do not use *sufficient* and *sudden* force the first time, you may compound the problem by forcing air around the obstruction without dislodging it. Then, insufficient air may remain in the lungs to do the procedure a second time.

Case 2—The signs in this patient indicate chronic emphysema—a disease often related to heavy smoking wherein the walls between adjacent pulmonary alveoli break down, resulting in fewer, larger alveoli. These enlarged alveoli fail to exchange O_2/CO_2 as efficiently as small ones (due to their relatively reduced surface area) and can, as in this patient, lead to a dependency on supplemental oxygen, and subsequent death.

Case 3—Since the patient had no external holes in his thoracic wall, and no abdominal viscera within the thorax (indicating a diaphragmatic hernia), the pulmonary collapse likely occurred from a ruptured lung due to the impact or one torn by the jagged end of a broken rib. The presence of free air in the pleural cavity (pneumothorax) in the absence of chest wall perforations is diagnostic for a ruptured lung.

Answers to Review Questions

1. A. It can pass through the oral cavity, instead.

2. C. The anterior, lateral, and posterior aspects of a lung constitute the costal surface.

3. B.

4. C.

5. D. The inferior vena cava passes through this opening.

6. E.

7. D. The vocal folds must be stretched (tensed) to raise the pitch of the voice.

8. D.

9. B. There are some air filled spaces within the temporal bone (epitympanic recesses), but they are diverticula from the tympanic (*vs.* nasal cavity). These diverticula are sometimes called mastoid cells or "mastoid sinuses."

10. B. Total lung capacity minus residual volume = vital capacity.

Answers to Thought Questions

1. Bronchi are more susceptible to collapse because their walls are relatively weaker when compared to their overall diameter than those of bronchioles. This comparison can be likened to the strength of a (soda) paper straw—if expanded to a few feet in diameter, its walls would be relatively weak.

2. An abdominal press forces abdominal viscera against the underside of the diaphragm—forcing it up against the lungs above it and ejecting the air within the lungs by direct pressure on them.

3. The pleurae are serous membranes that cover the lungs. At the hilar region of each lung, pleura reflects onto the mediastinum and forms a continuous lining that also covers the superior aspect of the diaphragm below and the inside of the thoracic wall around the lung. The potential space between the visceral pleura on the lung and the rest of the (parietal) pleura is called the pleural cavity. The lungs are invaginated into the pleural cavity but are not inside of it.

4. Occasionally a lung will spontaneously rupture (develop a hole). Air then passes out of the hole and fills the pleural cavity. Lacking the partial vacuum around it, the lung then collapses. Small tears in lungs often heal on their own. Reabsorption of the air in the pleural cavity occurs spontaneously and allows (causes) the lung to re-inflate.

5. The thoracic cage is formed by the sternum, ribs, and the thoracic vertebrae. The bony limits of the thoracic inlet are formed by the superior aspect of the sternum, the first pair of ribs, and the first thoracic vertebra.

6. As the diaphragm contracts for inspiration, it moves inferiorly and this would tend to stretch the inferior vena cava (like a rubber band). However, the intrapleural pressure drops during inspiration and this would tend to enlarge the inferior vena cava by allowing it to "balloon". When the diaphragm relaxes for expiration the opposite effects occur.

7. They contain a lot of air which doesn't absorb x-rays and so the x-ray beam easily passes through them and exposes the film. When developed, exposed x-ray film is black.

8. Respiratory epithelium, also known as ciliated pseudostratified columnar epithelium lines most of the tubular parts of the respiratory system down through the bronchiole level. Goblet cells within it secret mucus to entrap particulate matter and produce moisture that helps humidify inspired air. The ciliated cells help move the dirt-laden mucus up and out of the air passageways.

9. The anatomical dead space is the total volume of the air conducting passageways. At the end of an expiration, air within these passageways is not expelled from the body. Instead, this air is the first to re-enter the pulmonary alveoli during the next inspiration.

10. These noises, known to medical practitioners as *rales*, are caused by air squeezing through bronchiolar passageways which are partially blocked by excessive mucus and its entrapped debris.

11. The first two of these situations allow air to enter the ipsilateral pleural cavity. The third allows abdominal viscera to enter the cavity. The presence of anything in a pleural cavity prevents or reduces the ability of a lung to inflate.

12. Nothing. The lung can't inflate because there is no air available in the vacuum jar.

13. During an abdominal press the vocal folds are fully and forcefully adducted. During normal inspiration, they are fully abducted. For vocalization the vocal folds are partially abducted with a narrow space between them. A number of small skeletal muscles associated with the larynx are involved in changing the positions and tensions of the vocal folds.

14. Mucus leaves the paranasal sinuses by the tiny passageways which connect them to the nasal cavity. When these passageways become inflamed and the surrounding tissues swell, they are sometimes blocked.

15. There is less resistance to the movement of large volumes of air through the oral cavity.

16. When breathing through the nose, all three parts of the pharynx are traversed by air. During mouth breathing, only the oral and laryngeal parts of the pharynx serve as air passageways.

17. Surfactant is not produced in significant quantities until very late in gestation. Without it, the surface tension in the thin fluid layer lining the alveoli is so high that inspiration is difficult or impossible (without assistance).

18. There are only two pleural cavities but the bullet can enter each several times by alternately passing through lung tissue of different pulmonary lobes.

19. Air in some of the medullary cavities (*vs.* bone marrow tissue) reduces the total body weight. The dry weight of the skeleton of an eagle is less than the total weight of its feathers.

20. As the bronchial tree branches into the bronchiolar network, the total number of passageways increases exponentially. The surface area to volume ratio of these microscopic tubes is so high that essentially all inspired air makes direct contact with their walls.

21. When a pleural cavity is surgically invaded, that lung collapses because the relative vacuum created by the closed cavity is lost. Air must be forced into the lungs with positive pressure.

CHAPTER 19 Urinary System

Chapter Outline and Key Concepts

INTRODUCTION

The urinary system contains only four types of organs: kidneys, ureters, urinary bladder, and urethra.

The urinary organs form, transport, store, and excrete urine.

FUNCTIONS OF THE URINARY SYSTEM

As urine is formed by the kidneys, wastes are eliminated, blood pressure and pH are regulated, and water and electrolyte levels are controlled.

Low oxygen levels stimulate the kidneys to produce a hormone (erythropoietin) that increases the rate of RBC production.

KIDNEYS

The kidneys are located in the posterior abdominal cavity, just below the ribs.

Gross renal landmarks include superior/inferior extremities, medial/lateral borders, and anterior/posterior surfaces.

The medial indentation along the medial border is termed the renal hilum.

Five structures enter/leave the renal hilum: artery, vein, nerve plexus, lymphatics, and the ureter.

Internally, the renal parenchyma is divided into cortex and medulla, and the renal medulla is divided into renal pyramids which drain into minor renal calices.

Minor renal calices unite to form major calices which unite to form the renal pelvis which is continuous with the ipsilateral ureter.

Functional renal subunits (nephrons) have three parts: glomerulus, glomerular capsule, and renal tubule.

Renal tubules are divided into four main segments: proximal convoluted tubule, nephron loop, distal convoluted tubule, and collecting tubule.

RENAL CIRCULATION AND URINE FORMATION

The renal artery divides to form anterior and posterior branches near the renal hilum and these supply several segmental arteries.

Branches of the segmental arteries called interlobar arteries course peripherally between renal pyramids to form arcuate arteries at the corticomedullary junction.

Branches of the arcuate arteries called interlobular arteries branch to form the microscopic afferent arterioles that supply blood to glomeruli.

After passing through glomeruli, blood enters the peritubular capillaries around renal tubules and then drains through a series of venous channels that parallel the arterial ones.

Urine is formed by filtration, secretion, and selective reabsorption.

About 20% of the cardiac output flows into the renal arteries.

Ten percent of the renal blood flow becomes filtrate and 99% of the filtrate volume is reabsorbed.

URETERS

The left and right ureters connect the renal pelvis of each kidney to the urinary bladder.

Urine is transported through the ureters by peristalsis resulting from contractions of smooth muscle tissue within the ureteral walls.

Vesicoureteral reflux is prevented largely by the angle at which the ureters pass through the urinary bladder wall.

URINARY BLADDER

The urinary bladder has an apex, body, fundus, neck, and trigone.

Like the ureters and urethra, the urinary bladder is lined with transitional epithelium.

Both smooth and skeletal muscle sphincters must relax to facilitate urine flow into the urethra.

URETHRA

The urethra is longer in males (18-20 cm) than in females (2.5-3.0 cm).

In males the urethra is divided into prostatic, membranous, and spongy parts.

The urethra of males functions in the reproductive system (to transport semen) but in females the urethra serves the urinary system only.

DEVELOPMENT OF THE URINARY SYSTEM

Three successive stages of kidneys develop embryologically: pronephros, mesonephros, and metanephros.

The definitive kidneys (metanephros) and ureters arise from mesoderm along the urogenital ridges.

The urinary bladder and urethra arise from a primitive gut diverticulum called the urogenital sinus.

CLINICAL CONSIDERATIONS

Urinary calculi (precipitated deposits) may block portions of the urinary system.

Urinary dialysis cleanses the blood by periodically filtering it through external devices.

Urinary incontinence is the inability to urinate voluntarily and is classified as neurogenic, non-neurogenic, or paradoxical (depending on its cause).

Selected Definitions

Erythropoietin—a hormone produced by the kidney that stimulates bone tissue to produce erythrocytes. Reduced blood oxygen levels stimulate the kidneys to produce more erythropoietin.

Filtrate—the fluid composed of water, electrolytes, and small organic molecules which passes through the glomerular walls and enters the lumen of the glomerular capsule. The composition of filtrate is modified by secretion and selective reabsorption as it flows through the renal tubule.

Glomerular ("Bowman's") capsule—the portion of a nephron into which the glomerulus is invaginated. The internal wall of the glomerulus is composed of specialized cells called podocytes which coat the glomerular vessels.

Glomerulus—the tuft of small vessels that form the vascular component of a nephron. These vessels are fenestrated and are coated with podocytes.

Kidney —the paired urinary organ that forms urine by filtration, secretion, and selective reabsorption. In doing so, it helps regulate body water and electrolyte levels, blood pressure, and prevents the accumulation of certain metabolic wastes such as urea.

Micturition (urination)—the movement of urine from the urinary bladder through the urethra from which it is excreted. This involves relaxation of the sphincters of the urinary bladder and contraction of the muscle tissue within the bladder wall.

Minor renal calyx (calix)—the small, funnel-shaped structure into which the urine produced by one renal pyramid drains. These coalesce to form two or three larger collecting channels (major renal calyces) that converge, in turn, to form the renal pelvis.

Nephron—a functional subunit of the kidney consisting of a glomerulus, glomerular capsule, and renal tubule. Each kidney contains an estimated one million nephrons.

Nephron ("Henle's") loop—the second portion of the renal tubule. It is divided into three named parts: proximal straight tubule, attenuated tubule, and distal straight tubule.

Podocytes—the specialized cells that coat the glomerular vessels. Gaps between the "foot processes" (pedicels) of adjacent podocytes form the "filtration slits" (cytotrabeculae) which determine the maximum size of filtered molecules.

Renal collecting tubule—the terminal segment of a renal tubule. It has three named subcomponents: renal arcuate tubule, straight collecting tubule, and papillary duct.

Renal cortex—the outer part of the renal parenchyma (opposite of the renal hilum). Most of the glomeruli and glomerular capsules are located therein.

Renal medulla—the inner portion of the renal parenchyma (near the hilum). It is divided into segments called renal pyramids which drain newly formed urine into funnel-like collecting structures called minor renal calyces.

Renal tubule—the portion of a renal tubule that adds substances to filtrate by secretion and removes material by selective reabsorption. It is divided into four major segments: proximal convoluted tubule, nephron loop, distal convoluted tubule, and renal collecting tubule.

Renin—a hormone produced by the kidney that converts the circulating protein, angiotensinogen, to angiotensin I. In the lungs, the latter is converted to angiotensin II which is a powerful vasoconstrictor that elevates the blood pressure.

Uremia—the presence of high levels of urea $[CO(NH_2)^2]$ in the blood. Urea is an end product of protein metabolism and high levels in the blood are toxic.

Ureters—the left and right organs that transport urine from the kidneys to the urinary bladder. Their small diameter predisposes them to blockage from urinary calculi.

Urethra—the tubular channel through which urine is excreted from the urinary bladder. The short urethra of females makes them more susceptible to ascending bladder infections than males where the urethra courses down the whole length of the penis.

Urinary bladder—the expansible organ that receives urine from the left and right ureters. It temporarily stores the urine and then empties it through the urethra.

Urinary calculus—a concretion formed by precipitation within some part of the urinary system. Variously named renal, ureteral, cystic or urethral calculi according to the organ they occupy, urinary calculi can be composed of phosphates or oxalates (which are usually radiopaque) or they can be formed of urates or cystine (which are usually radiolucent).

Urinary incontinence—the loss of control over urination. Urinary incontinence is divided into three etiological categories: neurogenic, non-neurogenic, and paradoxical.

Etymology *Aqua vitae*—**"Water of life."**

arcus (L), *bow*—arcuate artery
calculatus (L), *pebble*—urinary calculi
calyx (L), *chalice*—minor renal calyx
cortex (L), *bark*—renal cortex
cystis (L), *bladder, pouch*—cystitis
detrusus (L), *to push down*—detrusor muscle
diabetes (G), *siphon*—juvenile diabetes
dipsa (G), *thirst*—dipsomania
fistula (L), *pipe*—fistulize
glomus (L), *ball*—glomerular capsule
glyc (G), *sweet*—glycosuria
hilum (L), *trifle*—renal hilum
hydr (L), *water*—hydrocele
incontinentia (L), *inability to retain a bodily discharge voluntarily*—neurogenic incontinence
insipidus (L), *lacking taste*—diabetes insipidus
medulla (L), *deep part*—renal medulla
melleus (L), *resembling honey*—diabetes mellitus
nephr (G), *kidney*—nephrectomy
noct (L), *night*—nocturia
olig (G), *few*—oliguria
patere (L), *to be open*—patent urachus
posis (G), *drinking*—hydroposia
ptosis (G), *fall*—nephroptosis
pyel (G), *trough*—pyelectasis
ren (L), *kidney*—renal papilla
strictus (L), *to draw tight*—urethral stricture
topos (G), *place*—ectopic ureter
trigonus (L), *triangular*—urinary bladder trigone
urachus (L), *to hold urine*—urachus
ureter (L), *urinary duct*—ureterolithotomy
urethra (L), *urinary canal*—urethra
uria (L), *within the urine*—albuminuria
urina (L), *urine*—urinology
vesica (L), *bladder*—vesicoureteral reflux

Introduction

The **urinary system** is the simplest of the visceral body systems and is composed of only four major organs: kidneys, ureters, urinary bladder, and urethra (Figure 19-1). The kidneys form urine and the ureters, urinary bladder, and urethra transport, store, and excrete it. Because of the intimate physical relationships of some organs of the urinary and reproductive systems (especially in males), the two systems are sometimes combined as the **urogenital system**.

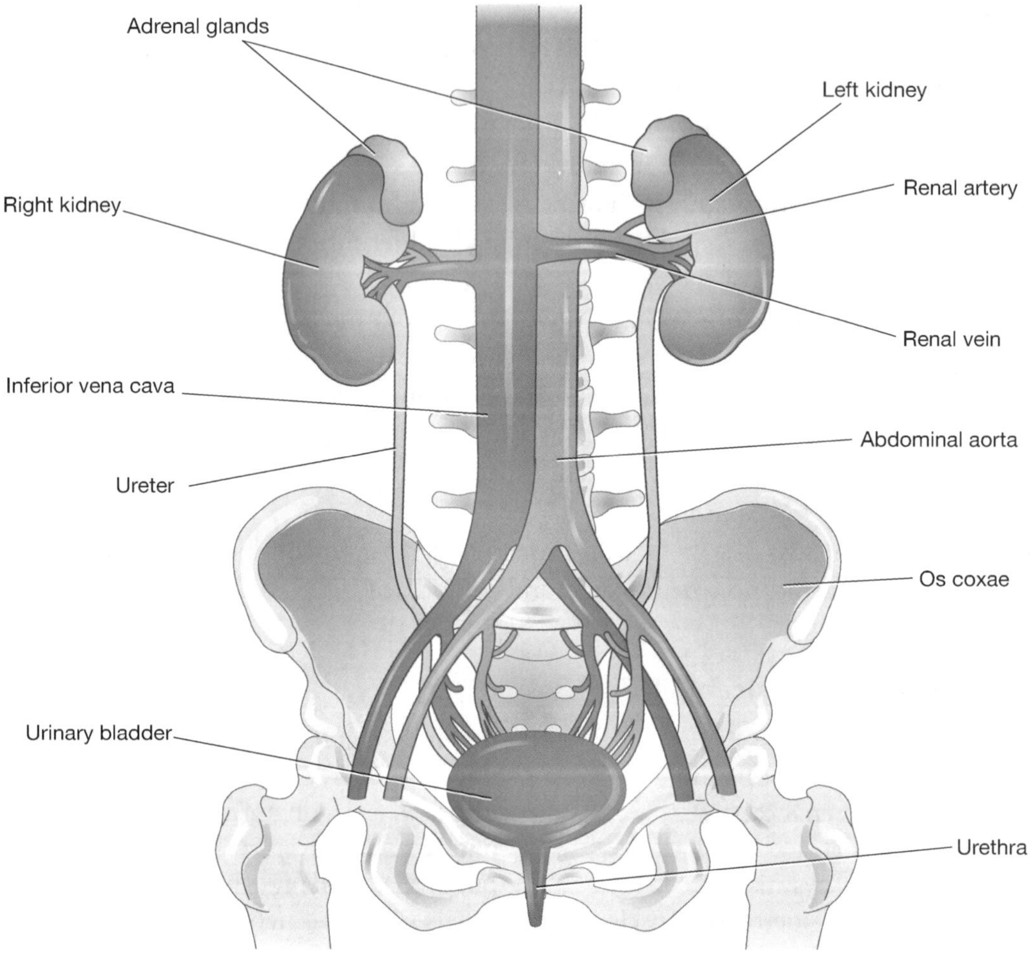

Figure 19-1

Urinary System

Only four major kinds of organs make up the urinary system: kidneys, ureters, urinary bladder, and urethra. Of these, only the urethra is sexually dimorphic. The urethra of males is several centimeters longer than that of females since it extends through the penis.

Objectives

1. List the four major urinary organs and their functions regarding urine.
2. Explain why the urinary system is often conceptually combined with the reproductive system (urogenital system).

Functions of the Urinary Organs

The overall functions of the kidneys, ureters, urinary bladder, and urethra can be summarized as the **formation**, **transportation**, **storage**, and **excretion of urine**, respectively. By forming and excreting urine, the urinary system partially regulates the contents of the extracellular fluid. The exact composition of the urine can be varied in regard to pH, sodium (Na^+) content, and selected other components as needed to help keep the internal body environment within the narrow limits compatible with life. Several specific functions of the urinary system are related to its role in urine formation and excretion:

1. **Waste product elimination**. The urinary system rids the body of urea and a number of other metabolic wastes. Urea is the principal end product of nitrogen metabolism and about one ounce is eliminated in the urine each day.
2. **Blood pressure regulation**. The kidneys regulate body fluid content directly by forming urine which reduces the fluid content of the body. They also manufacture a hormone (**renin**) which increases blood pressure by converting circulating angiotensinogen (inactive) to angiotensin I. This is, in turn, converted to angiotensin II (a powerful vasopressor) as blood flows through the lungs.
3. **Acid/base balance**. The kidneys help the lungs and cardiovascular system regulate body pH by excreting hydrogen (acid) ions and reabsorbing bicarbonate ions from the filtrate.
4. **Electrolyte balance**. When the blood content of potassium (K^+) ions increases, aldosterone (a mineralocorticoid) is released from the adrenal cortex. This hormone stimulates the reabsorption of sodium (Na^+) from renal filtrate in exchange for potassium.
5. **Production of erythropoietin**. This hormone is produced and released by the kidneys in response to lowered blood oxygen concentrations. It stimulates the formation of new erythrocytes (erythropoiesis) by the bone marrow.
6. **Hydroregulation**. By regulating the water loss in the urine, the kidneys help control the total body water content. Antidiuretic hormone (ADH) interacts with the renal tubules to effect the reabsorption of water as urine is formed.

Objectives

3. State the functions of the urinary system and indicate which one is shared with the cardiovascular and respiratory systems.
4. List the two hormones produced by the kidneys and indicate their functions.

Kidneys

The **kidneys** are the most important and complex organs of the urinary system. By forming urine and producing two hormones (renin and erythropoietin), they are responsible for all urinary system functions except the physical aspects of urine transport, storage, and excretion. The kidneys are located in the posterior abdominal cavity at the level of the last thoracic to the third lumbar vertebrae. The right

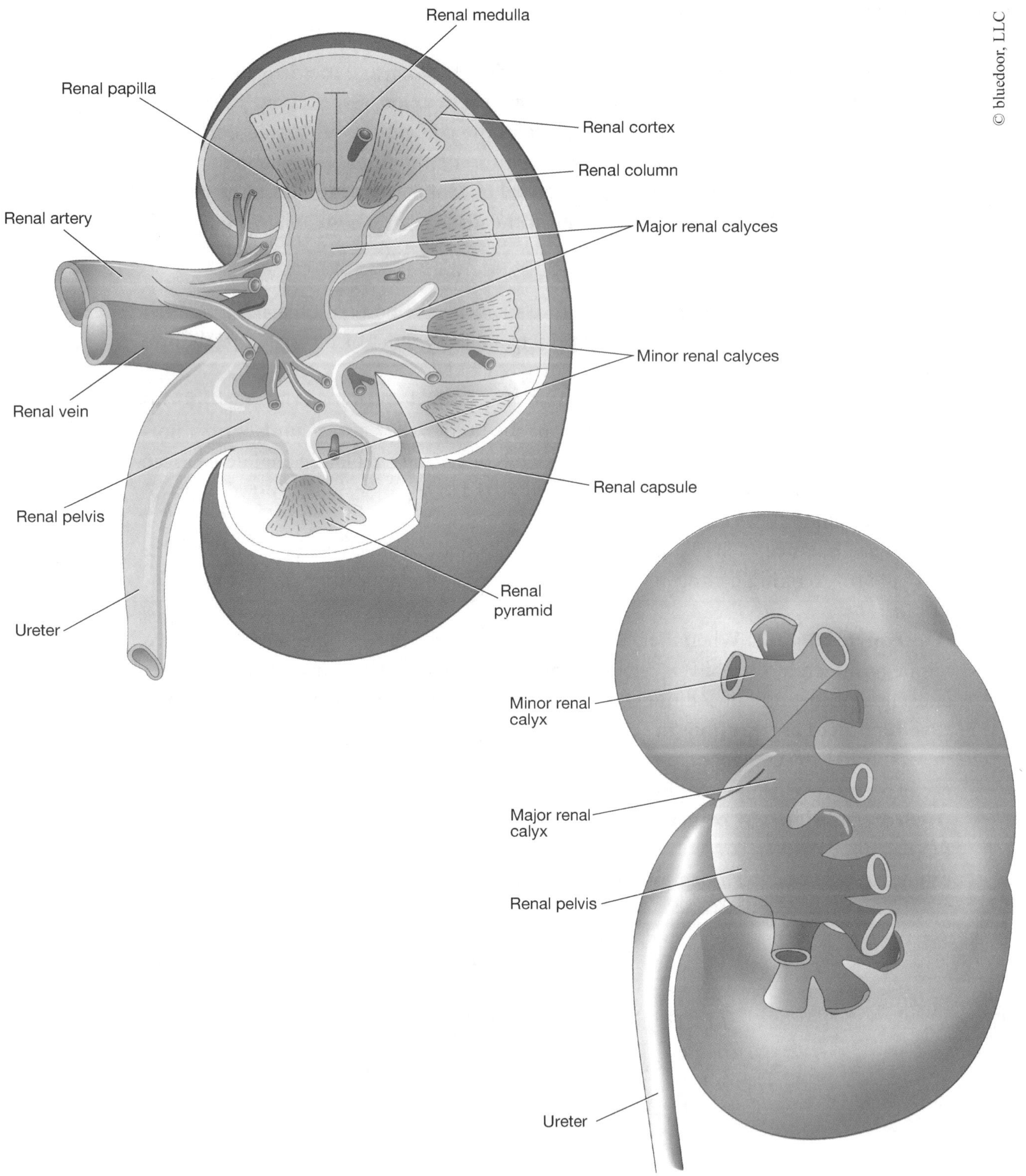

Figure 19-2

Anatomy of the Kidney

Each kidney has two extremities, two surfaces, two borders, and a medially located hilum. In frontal section the cortical/medullary arrangement of renal tissue can be seen as can the division of the renal medulla into pyramids. Each renal pyramid drains into a minor renal calyx and the latter coalesce to form the major renal calyces which, in turn, join to form the renal pelvis. Calyx can be spelled with either a "y" or an "i."

kidney is usually forced into a position somewhat lower than the left one by the large right lobe of the liver. Each kidney is bean-shaped and measures about 10 cm long, 6 cm wide, and 2.5 cm thick (Figure 19-2). The **superior extremity** is capped by the ipsilateral adrenal (suprarenal) gland. The **inferior extremity** is free. The **lateral border** of the kidney is convex and the **medial border** is concave. The central part of the indentation along the medial border where the renal artery, vein, nerve plexus, lymphatic vessels, and ureter attach is called the **renal hilum**. The **posterior surface** of each kidney lies adjacent to the diaphragm, transversus abdominis, quadratus lumborum, and psoas major muscles. The **anterior surface** is covered by peritoneum, and a significant quantity of adipose tissue called the **pararenal fat body** is deposited around each kidney. Because they have peritoneum only on their anterior surfaces, the kidneys (like the adrenal gland, abdominal part of the descending aorta, and inferior vena cava) are said to be retroperitoneal in location.

Objectives

5. Roughly sketch a kidney and label its extremities, borders, and hilum.
6. List five structures that attach at the renal hilum.

Structurally, each kidney is covered by a **fibrous capsule** of connective tissue proper (Figure 19-2). When sectioned, the outer **renal cortex** can be distinguished from the inner **renal medulla**. The medulla is composed of 8-15 conically shaped segments termed **renal pyramids** separated by partitions of tissue extending inward from the cortex termed **renal columns**. The hilar tip of each renal pyramid is termed a **renal papilla** and projects into a small, funnel-shaped structure termed a **minor renal calix**. These, in turn, coalesce to form two or more **major renal calices**. The major calices unite to form the **renal pelvis**. The pelvis is continuous at the renal hilum with the ureter.

Objectives

7. Roughly sketch a coronally sectioned kidney and label the renal cortex, medulla, columns, pyramids, minor renal calices, major renal calices, and renal pelvis.

The urine forming subunits of the urinary system are called **nephrons**. These perform the filtration, secretion, and selective reabsorption involved in urine formation. About one million nephrons are present in each kidney. Each nephron consists of a glomerulus, glomerular capsule, and an elongated portion termed the renal tubule (Figure 19-3). The **glomerulus** is a convoluted tuft of modified (fenestrated) vessels that receives blood from an afferent glomerular arteriole and is drained by an efferent glomerular arteriole. Most glomeruli are located in the renal cortex and their respective renal tubules extend down into the renal medulla. The **glomerular capsule** is the initial portion of the nephron into which the glomerulus is invaginated. The side of the glomerular capsule into which the glomerular vasculature is invaginated is called the **vascular pole** and the opposite side, which attaches to the renal tubule is the **tubular pole**. The glomerular capsule consists of an outer, relatively impervious **external wall** formed by simple cuboidal epithelial cells and an **internal wall** which is formed by specialized cells called **podocytes** (Figure 19-4).

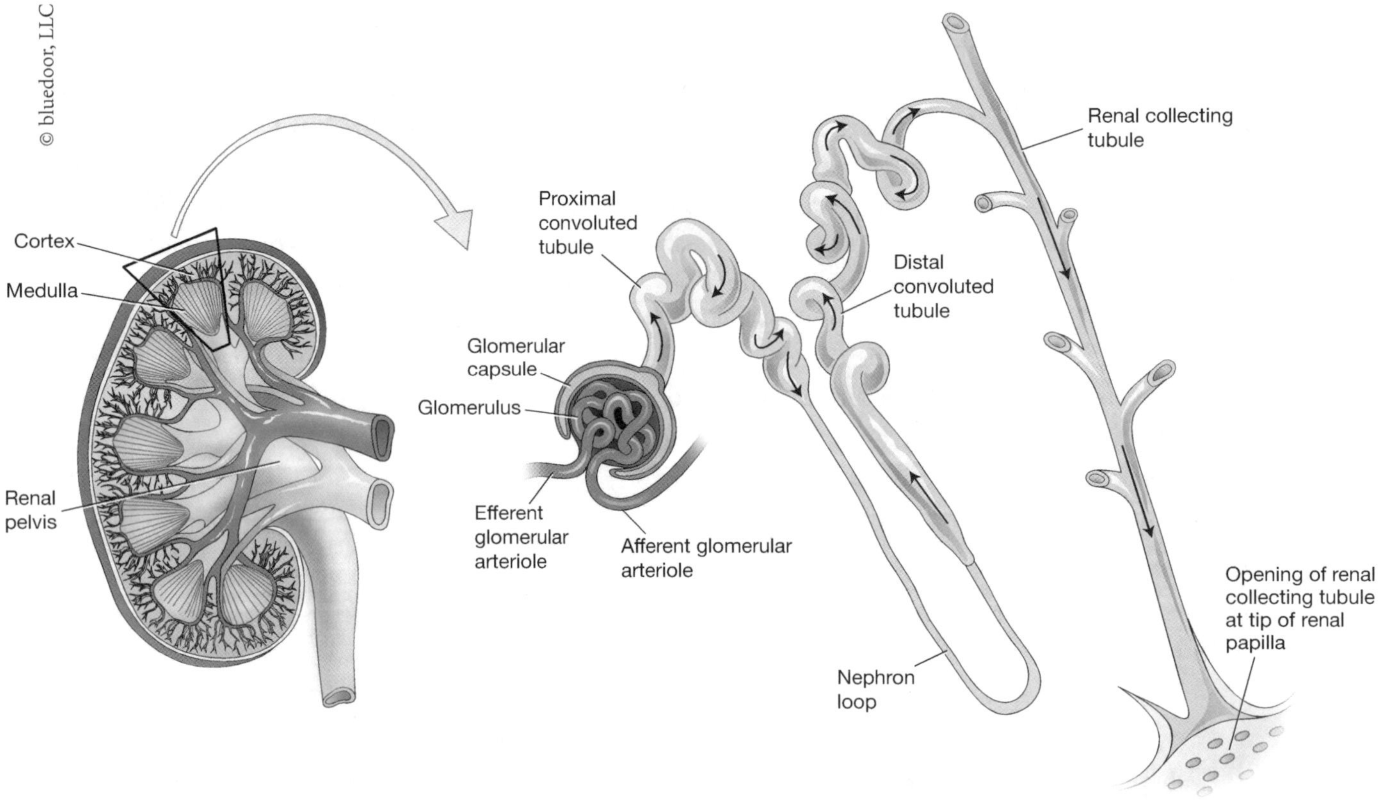

Figure 19-3

Schematic Structure of a Nephron

Each nephron has three major components: glomerulus, glomerular capsule, and renal tubule. The glomerulus and glomerular capsule (taken together) comprise the renal corpuscle which is involved in filtration. The renal tubule is divided into four major parts that are involved in secretion and selective reabsorption. Note that the nephron loop ("loop of Henle") and the renal collecting tubule are subdivided into three parts each (*see Table 19-1*).

The podocytes are adherent to the external surface of the glomerular vessels. Finger-like projections called **pedicels** (**cytopodia**) from adjacent podocytes interdigitate with each other but leave tiny intervening spaces called **filtration slits** (**cytotrabeculae**). These slits are so narrow that they only allow the passage of water and small molecules (blood cells and large organic molecules cannot pass through them). As blood flows through each glomerulus, part of its fluid portion passes through the vessel walls and filtration slits, and then enters the glomerular capsule as **filtrate**. This fluid is modified during its passage down the renal tubule by secretion and selective reabsorption to form **urine**.

The **renal tubule** is the portion of the nephron involved in secretion and selective reabsorption. These processes modify filtrate by adding additional things to it and reabsorbing other entities from it to form definitive urine. The tubule is an elongated passageway composed of simple cuboidal epithelium and consisting of four major segments: proximal convoluted tubule, nephron loop, distal convoluted tubule, and renal collecting tubule. The **proximal convoluted tubule** is the initial tortuous portion of the renal tubule (Figure 19-3). The **nephron loop** is a long hairpin-shaped segment, divided into three named subparts (Table 19-1), that extends toward the renal hilum where it turns sharply and returns toward the glomerulus. The nephron loop has been popularly called the

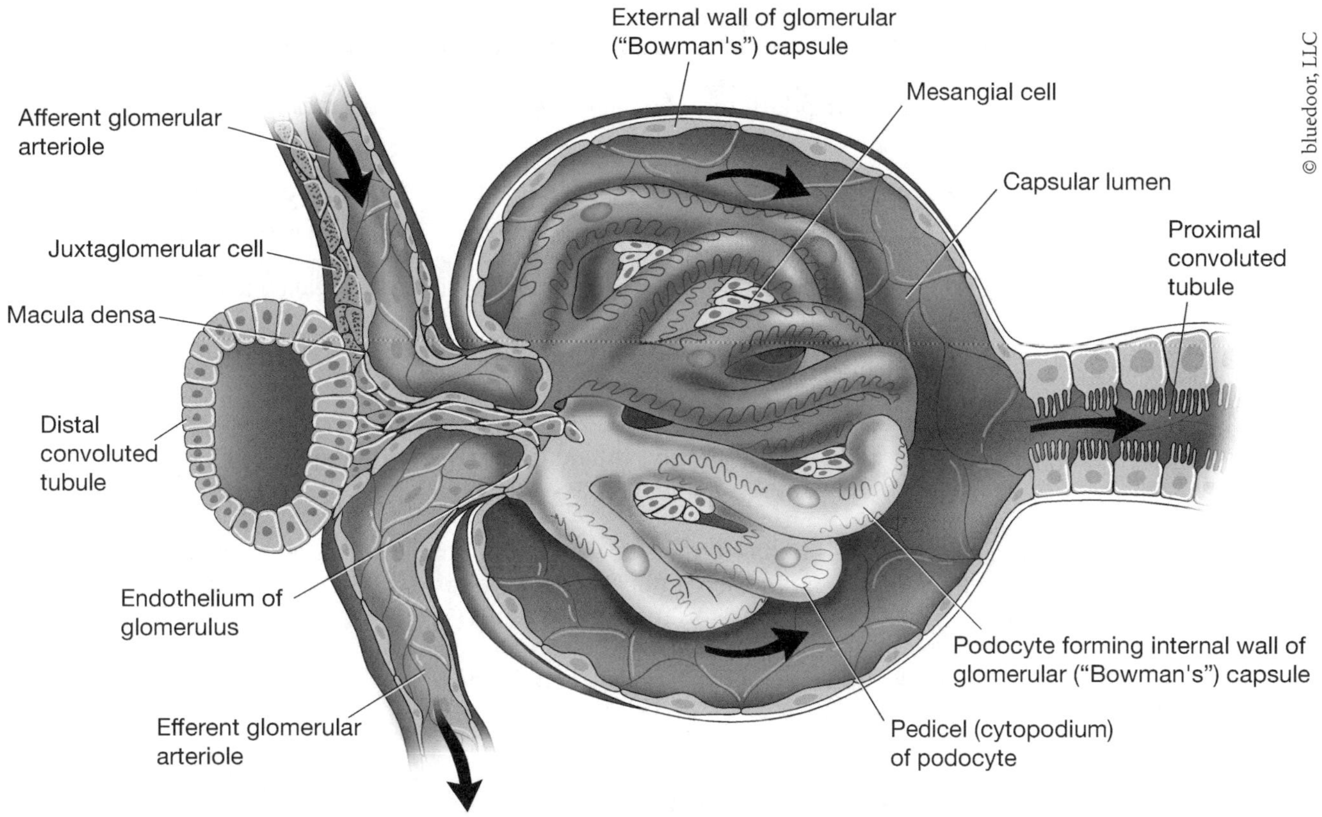

Figure 19-4

Microstructure of the Glomerulus and Glomerular Capsule

The glomerulus is a tuft of blood vessels supplied by an afferent glomerular arteriole and drained by an efferent glomerular arteriole. These vascular loops are physically tied together and supported by mesangial cells. Although the glomerular vessels are fenestrated (perforated), the size limiting factor in determining what can/cannot pass through the internal wall of the glomerular capsule to become filtrate is the width of the filtration slits between the podocytes. These cells coat the glomerular vessels and interlock their cytoplasmic processes called pedicels (cytopodia) leaving the narrow gaps called filtration slits (cytotrabeculae) through which water, electrolytes, and small organic molecules can easily pass.

"loop of Henle". Much of it consists of a very thin-walled portion called the **attenuated tubule**. The portion of the latter extending toward the renal hilum is the **descending part** of the attenuated tubule and that returning toward the glomerulus is the **ascending part**. Near the glomerulus, the renal tubule again becomes tortuous as it forms the **distal convoluted tubule**. At one point the distal convoluted tubule is in direct contact with the afferent arterioles of the glomerulus. Cells in this portion of the distal tubule form a dark area called the **macula densa** (Figure 19-4). They interact with the **juxtaglomerular cells** of the afferent arterioles that produce renin (*see Chapter 14*). The distal convoluted tubule then empties into the **renal collecting tubule** which has three named components (Table 19-1). Each renal collecting tubule courses toward and empties into a minor renal calix by opening at the tip of a renal papilla. Each renal collecting tubule consists of several **arcuate tubules** (from different nephrons), a **straight tubule** (into which the arcuate tubules empty), and a portion near the tip of a renal papilla called the **papillary duct** (Table 19-1).

Table 19-1 Definitions of Some Subparts of the Renal Tubule

Nephron Loop ("loop of Henle")	The elongated hairpin turn that dips into the renal medulla. It is divided into three parts: **Proximal straight tubule**—the initial thick part of the nephron loop which leaves the proximal convoluted tubule and descends into the renal medulla. **Attenuated tubule**—the thin part of the nephron loop. **Distal straight tubule**—the terminal part of the nephron loop which joins the distal convoluted tubule.
Renal collecting tubule	A term that encompasses all parts of the renal tubule after the distal convoluted tubule. Renal collecting tubule is a collective name for the following three items: **Renal arcuate tubule ("connecting tubule," "junctional tubule")**—the short segment of the renal tubule between the distal convoluted tubule and the straight collecting tubule. **Straight collecting tubule**—the portion of a renal tubule which receives renal arcuate tubules from several adjacent nephrons and, after receiving the last arcuate tubule, becomes (is continuous with) the papillary duct. **Papillary duct**—the terminal part of a nephron which continues down to the tip of a renal papilla and opens into a minor renal calyx.

Objectives

8. List the three major components of a nephron and the four sequential subparts of a renal tubule.
9. List the three processes involved in urine formation and indicate which of the three major parts of a nephron are involved in each.
10. Explain how filtration occurs using the terms glomerulus, internal wall of glomerular capsule, podocyte, pedicel, and filtration slit.
11. Indicate the name and location of the cells that produce renin.

Renal Blood Flow and Urine Formation

Each **renal artery** is a large vessel that carries about 10 percent of the cardiac output. As it approaches the renal hilum, the artery divides into two major branches (anterior and posterior). The anterior branch divides to form four segmental branches that supply the anterior half of the kidney (including the renal extremities). The posterior branch supplies the main portion of the posterior part of the kidney (Figure 19-5). These segmental branches divide to form **interlobar arteries** which ascend in the renal columns between renal pyramids (Figure 19-5). At the corticomedullary junctions, these form loops called **arcuate arteries** which supply tiny **interlobular arteries** to the cortex and medulla. The **afferent arteriole** which supplies each glomerulus arises as a branch of one of these interlobular arteries. The **efferent arteriole** which drains each glomerulus feeds a network of **peritubular capillaries** (Figure 19-5) around the renal tubule. Blood in these drains into the interlobular veins and subsequently leaves the kidney through the **renal vein**.

The kidneys form urine by **filtration**, **secretion**, and **selective reabsorption**. About twenty percent of the total cardiac output (5.0 liters/minute) flows into the left and right renal arteries (Table

19-2). This renal blood flow (about 1.0 liter/minute) enters progressively smaller vessels within the kidneys (as outlined above) and eventually flows through the glomeruli. At the glomeruli, about ten percent of its volume is filtered through the glomerular walls and filtration slits into the lumina of the glomerular capsules. This fluid, called filtrate, is mostly water but it also includes electrolytes and small organic molecules (including some albumin). Filtrate (averaging 100 ml/minute) then flows through the renal tubules where secretion and selective reabsorption modify it to form urine. About 99% of the initial filtrate volume is reabsorbed in the renal tubule (especially in the proximal convoluted tubules and papillary ducts). The principal substance reabsorbed is water, but amino acids, albumin, acetoacetic acid, and even some urea is reabsorbed. The remaining filtrate (about 1 ml/minute) passes out of the papillary ducts and into the minor renal calices as urine. The volume of urine formation (one tenth of one percent of the renal blood flow) can be significantly altered by fluid and electrolyte levels.

Objectives

12. Name, in order, the vessels through which blood flows in a kidney.
13. Outline the volumetrics of urine formation beginning with an average resting cardiac output of 5.0 liters/minute.

Ureters

The **ureters** transport urine from the renal pelvis to the neck of the urinary bladder (Figure 19-6). Each one is divided into an upper abdominal part and a lower pelvic part. The ureter has three major layers in its wall: a mucous membrane lining, a tunica muscularis layer, and a serosal layer. The **mucosa** has only two layers (in contrast to the three found in most other mucous membranes): a lining of transitional epithelium (4-5 cells thick) surrounded by **lamina propria** (c.t. proper). The **tunica muscularis** consists of layers of smooth muscle tissue. The inner layer (adjacent to the mucosa) is longitudinally oriented. This is surrounded by a circular layer. The lower third of the ureter has a third (external longitudinal) layer of smooth muscle tissue. The outer part of the ureteral wall consists in most areas of a **serosa** composed of visceral peritoneum. To move urine toward the urinary bladder, the muscularis layer contracts in peristaltic waves. The ureters penetrate the wall of the urinary bladder at oblique angles which increases the length of their passageway through the bladder wall. This allows increasing pressure of urine in the bladder to act as a passive "valve" to keep the terminal portion of the ureteral lumen squeezed "shut" except when peristaltic waves force more urine into the bladder. Closure of the terminal parts of the ureters prevents backflow of urine from the urinary bladder into the ureters (vesicoureteral reflux) which can cause pressure at the kidneys leading to renal degeneration.

Objectives

14. Discuss how the oblique passage of each ureter through the urinary bladder wall forms a functional valve to help prevent vesicoureteral reflux.

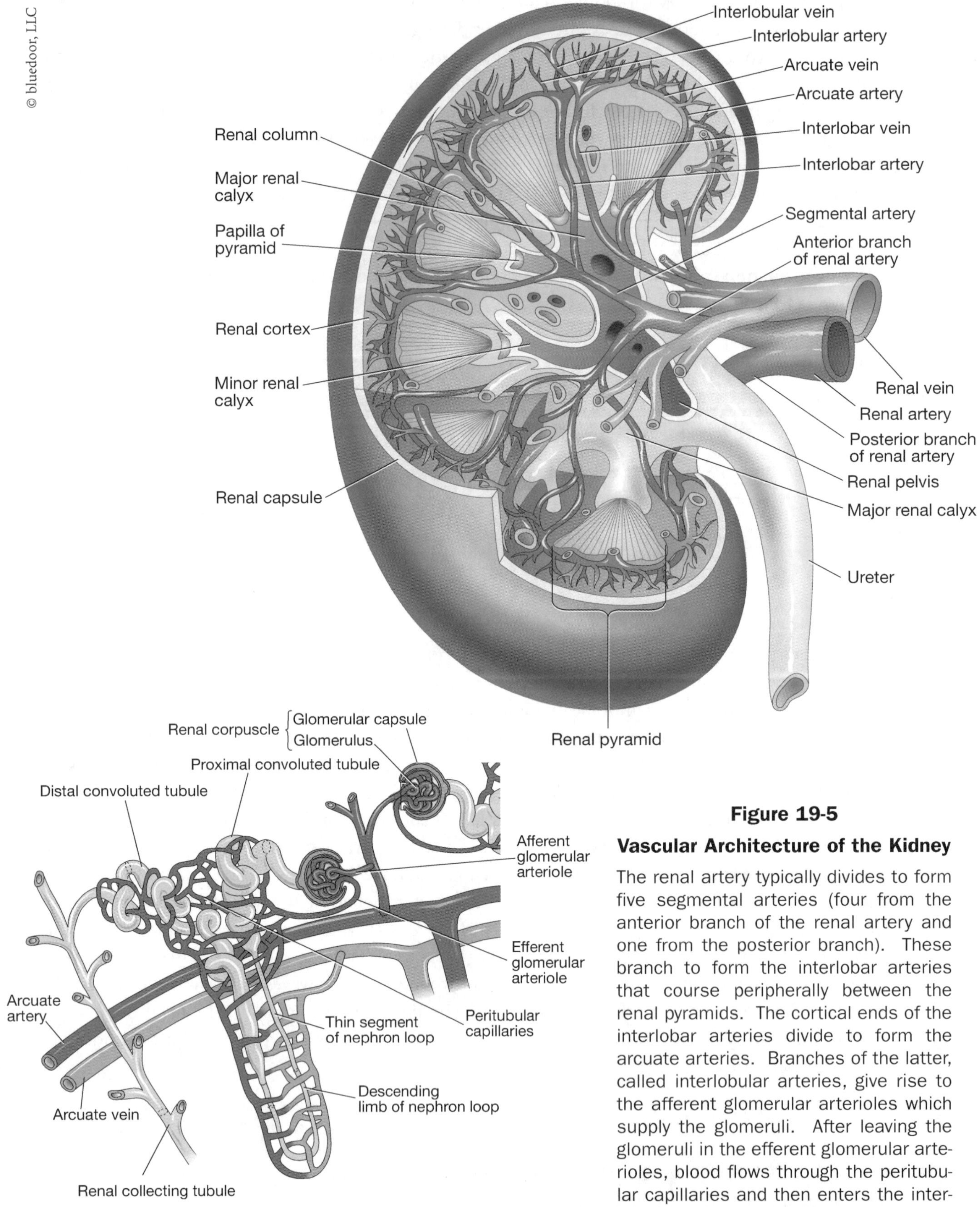

Figure 19-5

Vascular Architecture of the Kidney

The renal artery typically divides to form five segmental arteries (four from the anterior branch of the renal artery and one from the posterior branch). These branch to form the interlobar arteries that course peripherally between the renal pyramids. The cortical ends of the interlobar arteries divide to form the arcuate arteries. Branches of the latter, called interlobular arteries, give rise to the afferent glomerular arterioles which supply the glomeruli. After leaving the glomeruli in the efferent glomerular arterioles, blood flows through the peritubular capillaries and then enters the interlobular veins and then a series of larger veins that parallel the arterial supply.

Table 19-2 Volumetrics of Urine Formation

The figures given are approximate values for an average-sized (70 kg) individual in a typical state of hydration. Note that the volume of urine formed each minute represents 0.02% of the cardiac output, 0.1% of the renal blood flow, and 1% of the filtrate volume.

	Volume (ml/minute)
Cardiac output (C.O.)	5000
Renal blood flow (20 % of C.O.)	1000
Filtrate formed (10 % of renal flow)	100
Filtrate volume reabsorbed (99 %)	99
Remaining filtrate volume (urine)	1

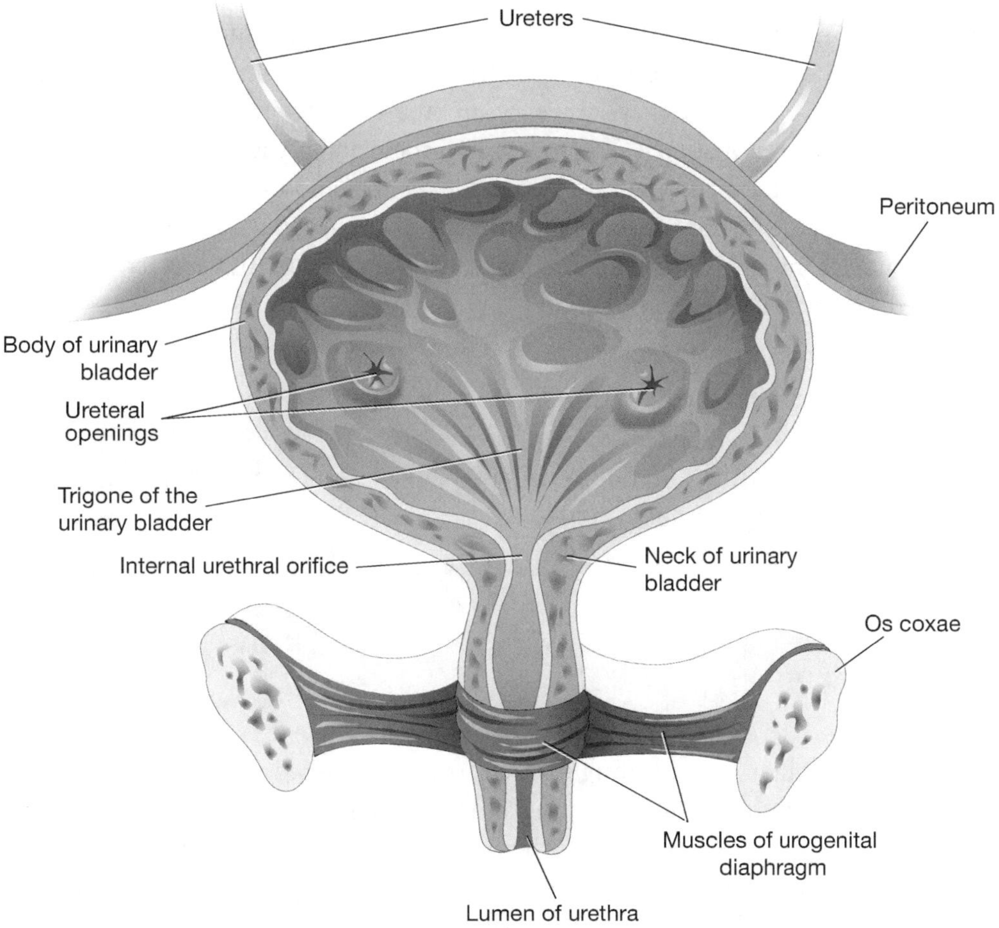

Figure 19-6

Urinary Bladder and Urethra (Frontal Section)

The trigone of the urinary bladder is a triangular area formed by the internal urethral orifice and the two ureteral openings. Tiny flaps of mucosa across the latter and the oblique passage of the ureters through the urinary bladder wall help form the functional valves which prevent vesicoureteral reflux as the bladder fills. The detrusor muscle in the urinary bladder wall is the outer of the three thin layers of smooth muscle tissue which form the tunica muscularis.

Urinary Bladder

The **urinary bladder** stores urine until it can be eliminated (Figure 19-6). It consists of an apex, body, fundus, and neck. The **apex of the urinary bladder** is located superoanteriorly. The **body of the urinary bladder** is the expanded portion and the **neck** is the narrowed part which joins the urethra. The **fundus** is the base of the urinary bladder formed by the convex posterior bladder wall. On its interior wall is a triangular area termed the **trigone of the urinary bladder** which is formed by the left and right ureteral openings and the internal opening of the urethra. The bladder wall has four layers: mucosa (epithelium, lamina propria, and muscularis mucosae), submucosa, tunica muscularis, and serosa. The lining tissue of the **mucosa** is **transitional epithelium** which is 6-8 cells thick in an empty bladder. These cells are globular (rounded) when the bladder is empty but they flatten as they become stretched when the bladder fills. The **tunica muscularis** of the urinary bladder consists of three layers of smooth muscle tissue. The outer one is named the **detrusor muscle**. These contract to empty the bladder during urination. The tunica muscularis is modified at the neck of the bladder to form a thickened portion surrounding the urethra. This acts as an involuntary sphincter muscle which is controlled by the ANS and is called the sphincter muscle of the urinary bladder ("internal sphincter muscle"). Skeletal muscle fibers surrounding the initial portion of the urethra called the urethral sphincter muscle ("external sphincter muscle") serve as a voluntary control of urination (micturition). The process of urination is initiated by the stimulation of stretch receptors within the bladder wall. Afferent impulses from these receptors result in reflex motor impulses which stimulate the smooth muscle in the bladder wall and inhibit the smooth muscle forming the sphincter muscle of the urinary bladder. Voluntary relaxation of the urethral sphincter muscle is then required for urination to occur. In effect, both sphincter muscles must be relaxed for normal urination to occur.

Objectives

15. Schematically represent a sagittally sectioned urinary bladder and label the apex, body, neck, fundus, and the internal and external urethral sphincters.

Urethra

The **urethra** is the tubular organ through which urine is excreted from the urinary bladder to the exterior. In males the urethra is 18-20 cm long and is divided into three segments (Figure 19-7). The proximal portion (3 cm) is surrounded by the prostate and is termed the prostatic part. The next centimeter (membranous part) penetrates the urogenital diaphragm. The remainder courses through the penis as the spongy part. The terminal, enlarged portion of the spongy part is called the navicular fossa. Transitional epithelium lines the prostatic part and changes to pseudostratified columnar epithelium in the membranous and spongy portions. This changes to stratified columnar and near its termination, the urethra is lined with stratified squamous epithelium. The lamina propria which surrounds the epithelium is invaginated by numerous urethral lacunae into which mucus secreting urethral glands open.

In females the urethra is only 2.5-3.0 cm long (Figure 19-7). Its mucous membrane lining is similar to that of males but has deep longitudinal folds.

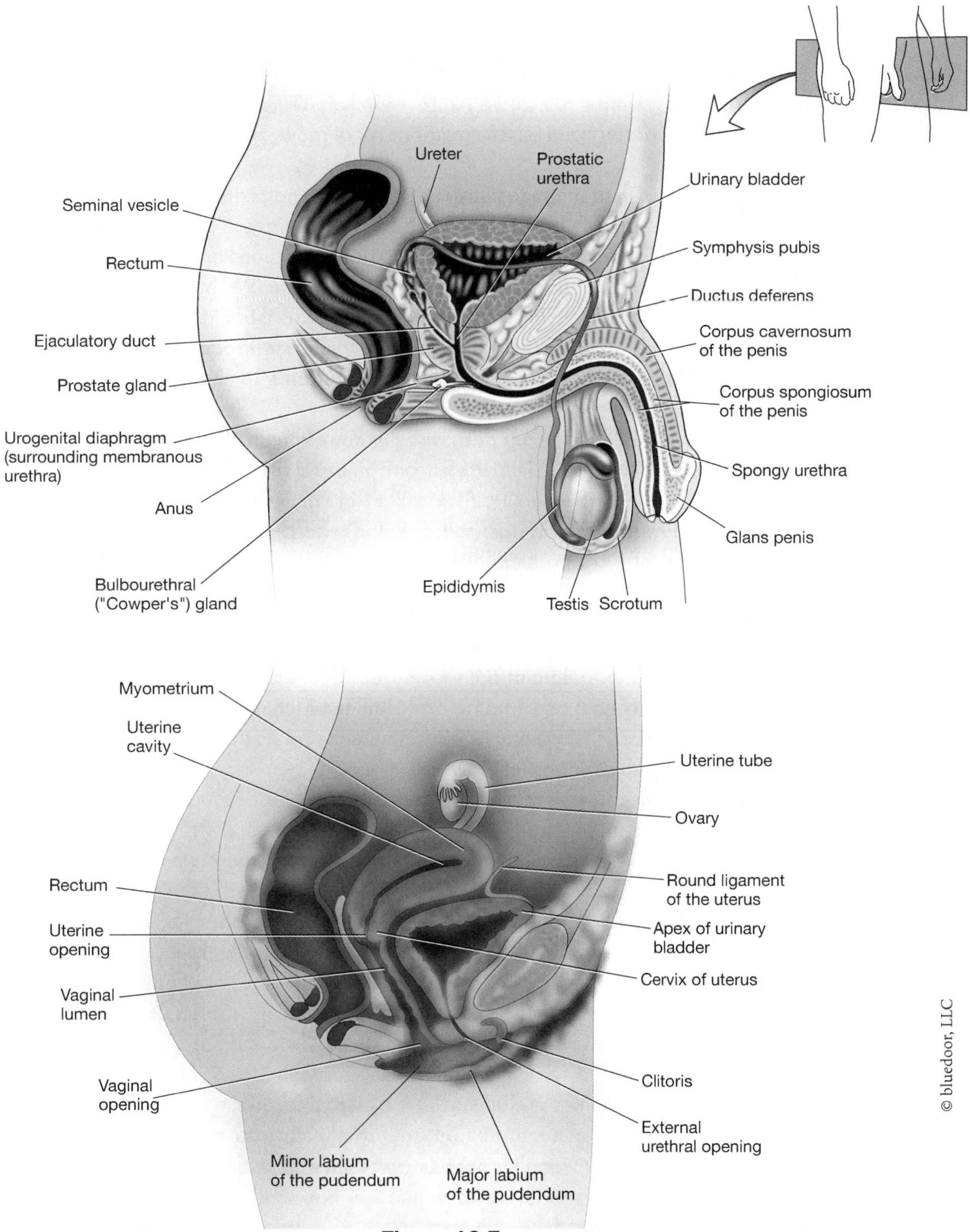

Figure 19-7

Urethra in a Male *vs.* a Female

In males the urethra extends the full length of the penis. The initial portion (within the prostate gland) is the prostatic urethra. The short portion passing through the urogenital diaphragm is called the membranous urethra. The remainder, within the penis, is the spongy urethra. In females the urethra is significantly shorter and is not divided into regional segments. The short overall length of the urethra in females predisposes them to ascending infections of the urinary bladder.

Objectives

16. Explain why men suffer cystitis (urinary bladder inflammation) from ascending urethral infections less often than women.

Development of the Urinary System

The urinary and reproductive systems both develop from folds of mesoderm called the left and right **urogenital ridges**. Development begins in the fourth week of gestation and the kidneys first begin to function at about three months. The definitive kidney develops as the third of three successive types of kidneys in mammalian embryos. The first primordium is called the **pronephros** (Figure 19-8). It appears during the fourth week, lasts only until week six, and never becomes functional in human embryos. The pronephros consists of 7-10 rudimentary tubules which form along the superior aspect of the urogenital ridge. These empty into a **pronephric duct** which courses posteriorly to empty into a terminal portion of the primitive hindgut termed the cloaca. The cranial part of the pronephric duct and the primitive pronephric tubules disappear (regress) during the sixth week, but the remaining part of the duct persists and becomes the drainage channel for the second primitive kidney, the **mesonephros**. The latter ("middle kidney") develops during the sixth week from the middle part of the urogenital ridge and takes over the terminal pronephric duct (it becomes the **mesonephric duct**). In the middle of the second month the mesonephros forms a large mass on each side of the midline consisting of numerous tubules which connect to the duct. By the end of the second month, however, the mesonephros degenerates and its duct becomes the ductus deferens in males. In females the duct almost entirely disappears.

The third renal primordium is termed the **metanephros**. It becomes the definitive kidney and becomes functional as the mesonephros degenerates. The main part of the renal parenchyma develops from a specialized part of the lower urogenital ridge called the **metanephrogenic mass**. The tubular part of the urinary system develops as a diverticulum of the mesonephric duct near the cloaca. This diverticulum, called the **ureteric bud**, expands and invades the metanephrogenic mass (Figure 19-8). The lower part of the bud becomes the ureter and the upper portion which contacts the metanephrogenic mass becomes the renal pelvis, calices, and papillary ducts ("collecting tubules"). As these ducts penetrate the metanephric tissue, small clusters of cells along the sides of the papillary ducts form **renal vesicles** which form the nephrons (Figure 19-8). The terminal end of each nephron invaginates to form the glomerular capsule and the other end joins the papillary duct. Each renal tubule continues to elongate after its initial formation resulting in the formation of the proximal convoluted tubule, nephron loop, and distal convoluted tubule. Even though the kidneys initially develop in the lower abdominal region, they migrate superiorly (anteriorly) during development.

The urinary bladder develops as a diverticulum of the **urogenital sinus**, which is, in turn, derived from the primitive **cloaca** (Figure 19-8). It is connected exteriorly to the **allantois** (one of the four extraembryonic membranes—*see Chapter 22*) by a stalk known as the **urachus**, which courses through the umbilical cord. Failure of this passageway to become totally obliterated at birth may result in a condition called patent urachus, which is characterized by urine dribbling from the umbilicus.

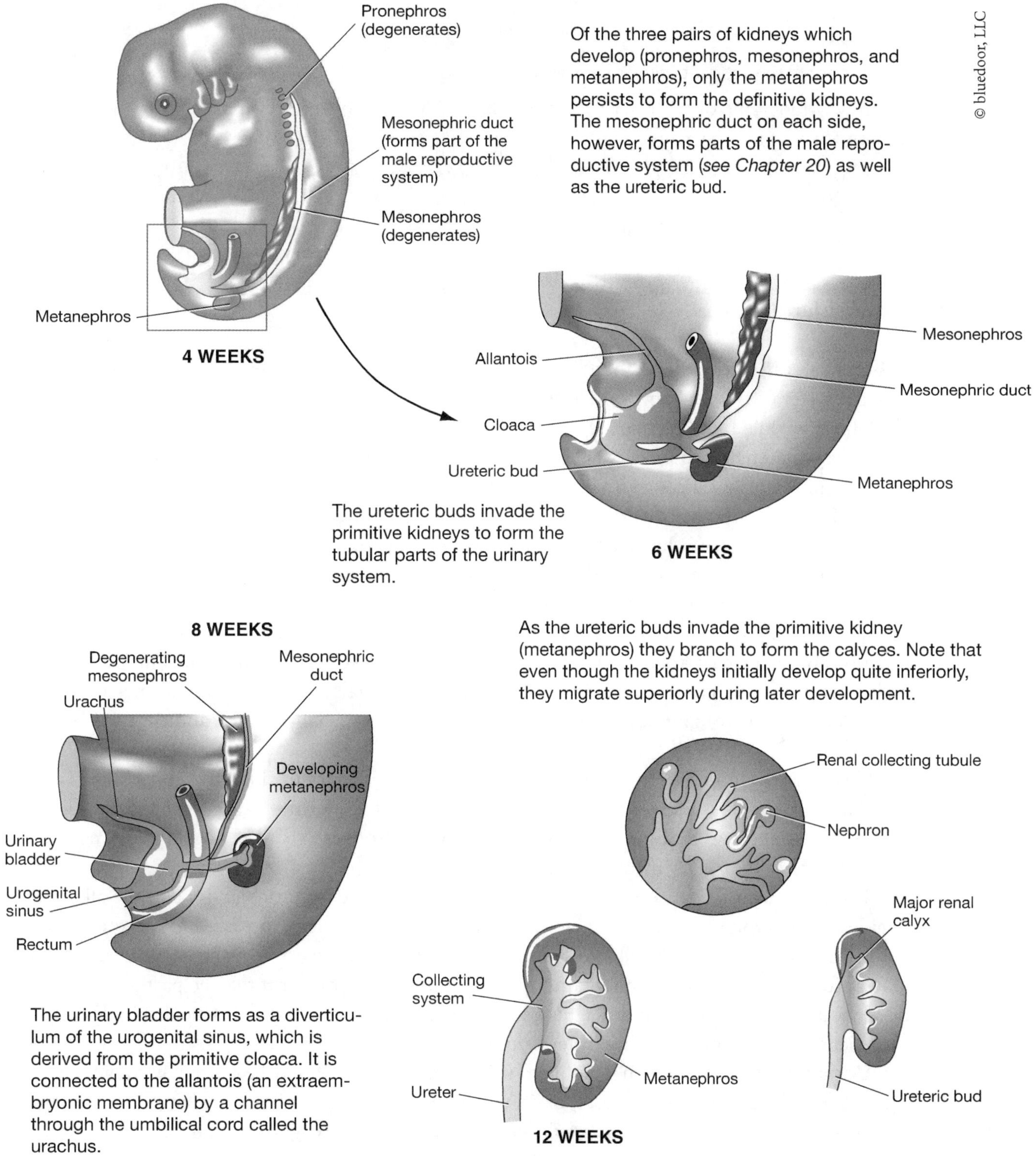

Figure 19-8
Development of the Urinary System

Objectives

17. Name the three sequential types of kidneys that develop in mammals.
18. Explain why the lining of the urinary bladder and urethra are considered to develop from the same endoderm as that of the terminal intestine.
19. Indicate what structure fails to close properly in those neonates that have urine dribbling from the umbilicus.

Clinical Considerations

Urinary calculi, often called "stones", are precipitated deposits that sometimes block portions of the urinary system. Those composed primarily of phosphates or oxalates are usually visible radiographically while those composed of urates or cystine are radiolucent. If these lodge in the renal pelvis they may enlarge to form "staghorn" calculi, named for their numerous branches which extend into the minor renal calices. These may require surgical removal. Calculi may also pass down the ureters often accompanied by extreme pain. Urinary calculi are classified as renal, ureteral, cystic, or urethral calculi based on the organ in which they are located.

Removal of a kidney is termed **nephrectomy** and may be necessary due to injury, cancer, or other disease. The retroperitoneal location of the kidneys makes it possible to remove them without actually invading the peritoneal cavity. At least one functional kidney is necessary to perform the functions of the urinary system. If both are diseased, an excessive build-up of urea may occur in the blood. This is called **uremia** and, if excessively high, can be fatal. Such individuals may require frequent (and expensive) **urinary dialysis** in which blood is artificially filtered and cleansed by external devices.

Ureters may fail to develop proper connections to the urinary bladder and end blindly causing **hydronephrosis**. The latter is a degenerative condition of the kidney caused by the back-pressure of blocked urine flow. **Ectopic** (abnormally positioned) **ureters** can also end in the uterus, vagina, or urethra causing urinary incontinence.

The **urachus** is a fetal connection between the apex of the urinary bladder and the allantois (a fetal, extraembryonic membrane). During gestation it allows urine to pass through the umbilical cord to be absorbed from the allantois by the maternal circulation at the placenta. It usually degenerates after birth. Sometimes it remains open as a **patent urachus** or it may be partially patent and develop cysts. This condition is diagnosed in neonates by the presence of urine dribbling from the umbilicus. It may require surgical intervention.

Urinary incontinence is an inability to urinate voluntarily. It may be caused by congenital malformations, urinary bladder diseases, or by trauma to the bladder and/or urethra. Incontinence is classified as neurogenic, non-neurogenic, and paradoxical. **Neurogenic incontinence** involves the nerve supply to the urinary bladder. This may result from direct damage to the sacral nerves or portions of the spinal cord which supply the bladder, or it may result from a lesion of the CNS between the brain and the sacral part of the spinal cord. **Paradoxical incontinence** typically results from partial obstruction of the urethra. In this case, the urinary bladder is typically distended. This is the only type of incontinence that is associated with difficulty in passing a catheter up the urethra into the urinary bladder (Table 19-3). **Non-neurogenic incontinence** encompasses all types which are not neurogenic and paradoxical. These include some types of ectopic ureters, congenital problems of the urethra, patent urachus, and some types of endocrine imbalances.

Cystitis is inflammation of the urinary bladder. It is usually caused by bacterial infections and is more common in females. The relatively short urethra of females (compared to those in males—3 cm *vs.* 20 cm) predisposes them to ascending bacterial infections of the urethra and urinary bladder.

Radiographic visualization of parts of the urinary system may be indicated in some disease syndromes. This may be accomplished by injecting air or other contrast medium into the urethra or urinary bladder. Intravenous injection of certain radiopaque dyes which are eliminated in the urine can also be performed. When the individual is subsequently radiographed, these cause the kidneys, ureters, and urinary bladder to be radiographically visible.

Urinalysis is a laboratory analysis of urine to help evaluate the health of the urinary system. Urine has normal levels of a number of components and these are altered in characteristic ways in various urinary diseases.

A number of developmental anomalies occur in the urinary system. One kidney fails to develop at a rate of 1:2500 births. This is usually inconsequential. Fusion of the left and right kidneys to form a single "horseshoe" kidney occurs in 1:6000 births. Double ureters from one kidney and failure of a ureter to make proper connections (noted earlier) also occur. In males, failure of left and right primordia to fuse properly may cause the urethra to open on top (dorsal surface) of the penile body (**epispadias**) or underneath the penile body (**hypospadias**) rather than at the tip of the glans penis.

Table 19-3 Types and Differentiation of Urinary Incontinence

Type	*Normal Urination*	*Distended Bladder*	*Easily Catheterized*
Neurogenic	–	+	+
Non-neurogenic	+	–	+
Paradoxical	–	+	–

Objectives

20. Define: urinary calculi, uremia, ectopic ureter, patent urachus, cystitis, epispadias, and hypospadias.
21. Differentiate the three types of urinary incontinence.

Clinical Case Studies

Case 1—A 49-year-old man suffered lower abdominal pain of sudden onset. The pain was so severe that he laid down on the floor and was unable to move. Later in the day, the pain subsided and he noticed that his urine had a pink tint. Alarmed, he drove himself to a 24-hour clinic where a urinalysis was positive for blood. Suggest a likely cause of his condition.

Case 2—A 29-year-old woman with chronic back pain had some symptoms of kidney disease. She was admitted to the radiology unit of a regional hospital for a special diagnostic procedure called an IVP (intravenous pyelogram). In this procedure, a radiopaque organic iodine solution was administered intravenously and then the renal area of her abdomen was radiographed as the contrast medium was eliminated through her urine. Only her left kidney was observed on the subsequent x-ray films. It appeared normal in size, shape, and location. Is it possible to have only one kidney?

Case 3—A 32-year-old man suffered swelling of his ankles, feet, abdomen, and the areas around his eyes. Urinalysis revealed the presence of a significant amount of protein in his urine and blood tests showed a lower than normal level of plasma albumin. How could these facts be related to the swelling this patient suffered?

Points to Ponder

"To be or not to be..." a mere 14 letters further down the alphabet and Shakespeare's famous quote would have been more urinary than legendary. Second only to blood as the body's most famous liquid, urine is a reviled waste product—aromatic as it is formed and ammoniacal from bacterial degradation soon thereafter. Beyond the mostly water composition, its specific content varies—hour to hour, day to day. Sometimes clear, sometimes turbid. We learn when young not to eat the yellow snow.

For every milliliter of urine formed, about 1000 ml of blood pass through the kidneys. This happens each minute in an averaged sized individual. Ten percent of this 1000 ml becomes filtrate (100 ml) and 99% of the filtrate volume is reabsorbed in each kidney's one million renal subunits called nephrons. The reabsorption figures are impressive. To make about 1.5 liters of urine each day, about 1500 liters of blood flow through the kidneys, 150 liters of filtrate are formed, and 148.5 liters of water are reabsorbed along with 225 grams of glucose and 3 pounds of sodium chloride.

One kidney can be lost (donated, surgically removed) without seriously impacting renal function. In fact, about 0.04% of the population is born unirenal. Since they are hung on the posterior body wall and extend below the lower ribs, the kidneys are vulnerable to contusions from sharp blows to the lower back. This is the anatomic basis for the "kidney punch" of boxing. The fibrous attachment to the posterior body wall dictates that a kidney has peritoneum only on its anterior surface. For this reason the kidneys are said to occupy a retroperitoneal position (literally behind the peritoneum). This is a distinction that they share with only a few other organs (adrenal glands and the abdominal parts of the aorta and inferior vena cava). By forming urine, the kidneys play important roles in a number of homeostatic mechanisms including hydro-regulation, acid/base balance, waste product elimination, blood pressure regulation, and electrolyte balance.

Day to day, our occupation with urine is a re-occurring but fleeting scuttle to a socially acceptable depository. When illness strikes, however, biomedical personnel become obsessed with ours. We are requested to fill a cup (doesn't have to be clear to the top, but if some is good, more is better! Right?). They analyze for color, specific gravity, pH, check for sugar, protein, *etc. etc.* (It's amazing what can be learned by going through a person's trash.).

Once formed by its kidney bean namesake, urine is quietly transported to the urinary bladder by the left and right ureters. These tiny tubes peristalse their cargo as it is formed—sometimes faster, sometimes slower. About the only time most people have solid testimony that ureters exist is when they see them in the anatomy laboratory or when a urinary calculus lodges in or passes down a ureter. Then we know—sometimes on our hands and knees and curled in the fetal position in pain.

How much can a urinary bladder hold? There's a lot of individual variation. High school boys have contests using a quart jar measuring device. Harry Pierce beat us all—something over a quart. It's more impressive now—looking back—knowing that Harry processed 100 liters of filtrate, filtered 1000 liters of blood, and pumped 5000 liters—just to fill the jar. What a man!

In the anatomical battles of the sexes, men win the average body size and length of the urethra contests. The male urethra is 6-7 times as long as that of females. This makes men much less susceptible to ascending urinary tract infections, but much more susceptible to perineal traumatic incidents.

Slang and Obsolete Nomenclature

UNOFFICIAL TERM	OFFICIAL DESIGNATION
Bowman's capsule	glomerular capsule *[capsula glomerularis]*
slit pores	filtration slits *[cytotrabeculae]*
trigone	trigone of urinary bladder *[trigonum vesicae]*
loop of Henle	nephron loop *[ansa nephrica]*
bladder	urinary bladder *[vesica urinaria]*
Malpighian corpuscle	renal corpuscle *[corpusculum renale]*

Review Questions

1. Using a cardiac output of 5.0 liters/minute and an average state of hydration, one would expect...
   A. 100 ml of filtrate formed each second.
   B. 1.0 ml of urine formed each hour.
   C. 99 ml of filtrate reabsorbed/minute.
   D. 1000 liters of blood to flow to the kidneys each minute.
   E. If one should expect more than one of the above, choose this response.

2. To remove a kidney, the structures which will be severed (and ligated) do not include the (ipsilateral)...
   A. renal lymphatic vessels.
   B. renal vein.
   C. renal artery.
   D. urethra.
   E. plexus of nerves.

3. The size limiting factor in determining what filtrate contains is...
   A. fenestra.
   B. pedicel.
   C. podocytes.
   D. spaces between adjacent podocytes.
   E. the RBC's.

4. The three major components of a nephron are...
   A. glomerular capsule, renal tubule, and nephron loop.
   B. proximal convoluted tubule, nephron loop, and distal convoluted tubule.
   C. glomerulus, glomerular capsule, and papillary duct.
   D. glomerulus, renal capsule, and renal tubule.
   E. If none of the above list the three main parts of a nephron, choose this response.

5. Consider:
   a. interlobular artery b. glomerulus c. interlobar artery
   d. renal artery e. renal vein f. peritubular capillaries
   g. arcuate artery
   Which lists these in the order that systemic arterial blood will encounter them?
   A. a, b, c, d, e, f, g
   B. d, c, g, a, b, f, e
   C. d, a, c, g, b, e, f
   D. d, c, a, g, b, f, b
   E. c, g, a, b, f, e, d

6. Which part of the kidney is most heavily involved with secretion?
   A. glomerulus
   B. renal pelvis
   C. proximal convoluted tubule
   D. minor renal calix
   E. ureter

7. Which organ is not retroperitoneal?
   A. kidney
   B. abdominal portion of the descending aorta
   C. abdominal portion of the inferior vena cava
   D. spleen
   E. adrenal gland

8. Women suffer more from ascending cystitis than men because women...
   A. have shorter ureters than men.
   B. are not as clean as men.
   C. have more bacteria in their urinary bladder (than men).
   D. are more delicate (than men).
   E. If none of the above satisfy the premise, choose this response.

9. Urinary calculi are never found in the ________________.
   A. renal pelvis
   B. urethra
   C. urinary bladder
   D. glomeruli
   E. toilet

10. Which word is properly defined?
    A. filtrate—the fluid that enters a minor renal pelvis
    B. nephrotomy—removal of a kidney
    C. urinalysis—production of excessive quantities of urine
    D. ectopic urethra—condition in which a ureter is improperly positioned
    E. micturition—urination

Thought Questions

1. Because the kidneys are positioned against the posterior abdominal wall, they are covered only on one side by peritoneum and are said to be retroperitoneal. Name some other retroperitoneal structures.

2. How do the kidneys variously influence the number of erythrocytes in Pacific Islanders vs. the Indians of the Andean highlands?

3. State the relationship of podocytes, pedicels, and filtration slits.

4. Follow a drop of filtrate through a renal tubule naming the subparts in order.

5. At what point does filtrate become urine?

6. Which part(s) of a nephron are actively involved in secretion and reabsorption?

7. How much filtrate is formed in an average individual in one day (24 hours)?

8. As the urinary bladder fills and the resulting pressure "closes" the terminal ends of the ureters, how does additional urine continue to enter the bladder?

9. To remove a kidney, what five structures must be transected at the renal hilum? A surgeon is most concerned about ligating (tying off) which three of these?

10. Follow a drop of urine from the point of its formation to the point of its excretion and name all of the structures (in order) that it encounters.

11. Which components of blood become filtrate?

12. As various components of filtrate (especially water) are reabsorbed from the renal tubule, what vessels do they enter?

13. If a kidney has approximately one million nephrons, why does it have considerably fewer straight collecting tubules and papillary ducts?

14. Which organs of the urinary system are lined by transitional epithelium?

15. In addition to the difference in overall body size, what other factor may contribute to the observation that women seem to have "smaller" urinary bladders than men?

16. A small boy going into a public men's room for the first time may find it difficult or impossible to urinate. Why?

17. What is the difference between a renal calculus, a ureteral calculus, a cystic calculus, and a urethral calculus?

18. Which type of urinary incontinence is characterized by a distended urinary bladder, lack of ability to urinate normally, and a urinary bladder that cannot be catheterized?

19. What condition is characterized by urine leaking from the umbilicus?

20. How can an individual with an ectopic ureter exhibit both normal bladder filling/emptying as well as continuous, uncontrolled dribbling of urine?

21. What is the source of the excess "amine" groups that are combined to form the urea that is subsequently eliminated through the urine?

Answers to Clinical Case Studies

Case 1—Severe pain of this type coupled with blood in the urine is pathognomonic for urinary calculi—usually indicating passage of a stone down the ureter. Some individuals have recurring episodes involving calculi. Apparently, they are more likely to form in some individuals' body chemistries than in others'. Those afflicted are advised to drink lots of water. "Flushing" the urinary passageways is a reasonable but not foolproof preventative procedure.

Case 2—Yes. Some individuals are born with only one. In this case, the radiology technician filmed her lower abdomen and "found" the other kidney in an abnormal position near her urinary bladder. "Pelvic kidneys" as these are called sometimes cause clinical difficulties because the ureter gets kinked. This causes back pressure and can result in degeneration of the involved kidney. Pelvic kidneys may result from traumatic incidents that tear the kidneys away from their normal position and allow them to drop into the pelvic cavity. They may also occur when kidneys fail to "ascend" in the abdominal cavity during development or when the supporting pararenal fat which holds them in position is reabsorbed during extreme weight loss.

Case 3—Since urine should be essentially free of albumin, this patient has a renal function problem. The loss of albumin into the urine is causing the low blood albumin level. This in turn reduces the plasma osmotic pressure within the capillaries which is the largest pressure preventing fluid loss through the capillary wall. With this reduced, the capillaries become exceptionally "leaky" and this explains the edema suffered by this patient.

Answers to Review Questions

1. C. The errors in the other choices are: A, second should be minute; B, hour should be minute; D, liters should be ml (or 1000 should be 1.0).

2. D. The ipsilateral ureter would be severed but not the urethra.

3. D. The material passes between the pedicels of podocytes. The fenestrations in the arteriolar walls of the glomerulus are larger.

4. E. The three components are: glomerulus, glomerular capsule, and renal tubule.

5. B.

6. C. The glomerulus (A) is involved in filtration, the renal pelvis (C), the minor renal calix (D) and ureter (E) have nothing to do with urine formation.

7. D.

8. E. B and D are nonsense. A would be the answer if ureters were changed to urethra. The urinary bladders in both sexes are normally bacteria free.

9. D. Urinary calculi ("stones") can be found everywhere that urine occurs. Those that are passed can even be found in the toilet!

10. E. The definition in choice A describes urine. In B, note that nephrotomy refers to an incision into a kidney. Urinalysis (C) refers to a laboratory analysis of urine. D confuses urethra and ureter.

Answers to Thought Questions

1. Adrenal glands, and the abdominal parts of the aorta and inferior vena cava.

2. Kidneys of Pacific Islanders produce less erythropoietin because the oxygen content of the air they breathe is higher. (This hormone stimulates bone marrow to produce RBC's.) Consequently, islanders have a lower concentration of RBC's in their blood than highland people.

3. Podocytes are cells forming the internal walls of the glomerular capsules. Their finger-like processes, called pedicels, interdigitate. The intervening spaces between pedicels are called filtration slits.

4. Proximal convoluted tubule, nephron loop, distal convoluted tubule, renal collecting tubule.

5. Filtrate becomes urine when it leaves the papillary duct and enters a minor renal calix at the tip of a renal papilla.

6. Renal tubule (all of its subparts).

7. 100 ml of filtrate are formed each minute x 60 minutes/hour x 24 hours/day = 144000 ml/day = 144 liters/day.

8. Peristaltic contractions of the ureteral walls overcome the pressure produced by the functional "valves."

9. Ureter, renal artery, renal vein, renal lymphatic vessels and renal nerve plexus. Surgeons are more concerned about the first three than the last two.

10. Minor renal calix, major renal calix, renal pelvis, ureter, urinary bladder, urethra.

11. Water, electrolytes, and small organic molecules. In some disease states, other (larger) molecules may enter filtrate as well.

12. Peritubular capillaries (these are supplied by the efferent arterioles).

13. Each straight collecting tubule receives the renal arcuate tubules of several nephrons and then drains into a single papillary duct (*see Table 19-1*).

14. Urethra, urinary bladder, ureters, (as well as the renal pelvis and calices).

15. The female pelvic cavity is more crowded with reproductive organs than that of males.

16. Even though he voluntarily relaxes his urethral sphincter muscle (skeletal muscle tissue), anxiety may prevent him from being able to relax the sphincter muscle of his urinary bladder (smooth muscle tissue).

17. Location.

18. Paradoxical incontinence (caused by urethral obstruction).

19. Patent urachus.

20. As the kidney connected to the normal ureter produces urine, the urinary bladder fills normally and can be emptied normally. Urine produced by the kidney connected to the ectopic ureter, bypasses the bladder and enters the urethra directly as it is produced. This causes continuous dribbling of urine from the urethra.

21. These amines are derived from transamination/oxidative deamination reactions that are performed on amino acids to make the latter into non-amine containing hydrocarbons. An individual on a high protein diet will produce more free amines (than most individuals) as amino acids are modified into citric acid (Kreb's) cycle intermediates and used for energy. Compounds with amine groups are unacceptable to energy cycle enzymes.

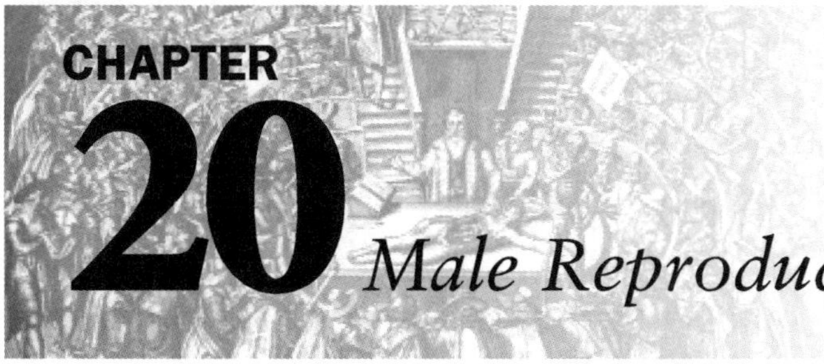

CHAPTER 20 Male Reproductive System

Chapter Outline and Key Concepts

INTRODUCTION

The male reproductive system includes the testes, epididymides, deferential ducts, penis, and three kinds of accessory sex glands. The urethra, which is part of the urinary system, also functions in the male reproductive system.

FUNCTIONS

The male reproductive system produces testosterone, sperm, the other components of semen, and participates in sexual intercourse.

TESTIS

The paired testes are located in the perineal region within a cutaneous pouch termed the scrotum.

Testicular lobules contain microscopic seminiferous tubules in which developing sperm are found.

Sustentacular cells within the seminiferous tubules support developing sperm, and interstitial cells between the tubules produce testosterone.

EPIDIDYMIS

The epididymis consists of a head, body, and tail and is located on the posterior surface of the ipsilateral testis.

Efferential ducts conduct sperm from the testis into the duct of the epididymis within the head of the epididymis.

The duct of the epididymis is a tortuous tube (about 20 feet long) that serves as a maturation site for recently formed sperm.

SPERMATOGENESIS

Primitive male sex cells called spermatogonia (2N) divide mitotically to form primary spermatocytes (2N).

Each primary spermatocyte divides (first meiotic division) to form two secondary spermatocytes (N) and each of these divides (second meiotic division) to form two spermatids (N).

Spermatids undergo metamorphic changes to become spermatozoa, a process called spermiogenesis.

All cells in the spermatogenic series are invaginated into sustentacular cells which metabolically support them.

The major parts of a sperm are the head, neck, and flagellum (tail).

DUCTUS DEFERENS

Continuous with the tail of the epididymis and terminating in the urethra, the ductus deferens is primarily a sperm transport tube.

En route to the urethra, the ductus deferens penetrates the abdominal wall and the prostate.

MALE URETHRA

The urethra in males is 18-20 cm long, belongs to the urinary system but serves the reproductive system as well. It is divided into prostatic, membranous, and spongy parts.

The spongy part of the urethra extends through the penis and opens terminally at the end of the glans penis.

PENIS

Regionally the penis is divided into a root (formed by left and right crura), body, and glans penis.

Redundant skin covering the glans penis is termed the prepuce and is partly removed if circumcision is performed.

Within the penis are three erectile bodies: two corpora cavernosa (dorsally) and a corpus spongiosum (ventrally) which surrounds the urethra.

ERECTION, COPULATION, AND EJACULATION

Erection is produced by increased arterial flow into the erectile bodies and decreased venous drainage from those bodies.

Copulation (sexual intercourse, coitus) involves insertion of a male's erect penis into a female's vagina.

Ejaculation occurs when pleasurable sensory impulses initiate a reflex causing semen to be forcefully expelled through the urethra.

ACCESSORY SEX GLANDS

The paired seminal vesicles secrete fructose, prostaglandins, and fibrinogen through a duct that joins the ejaculatory duct of the ductus deferens.

The unpaired prostate surrounds the urethra and contributes acid phosphatase, citric acid, clotting enzyme, profibrinolysin, and calcium ions to semen.

The paired bulbourethral glands secrete a lubricating fluid into the urethra that cleanses it and lubricates the glans penis for intromission.

INGUINAL CANAL AND SPERMATIC CORD

The inguinal canal is a passageway through the anteroinferior abdominal wall and its openings are the superficial and deep inguinal rings.

The spermatic cord is the extra-abdominal ductus deferens and the structures associated with it (testicular artery, vein, nerve, lymphatic and the tiny deferential vessels).

A slip of the internal abdominal oblique muscle called the cremaster muscle follows the spermatic cord down into the scrotum.

The peritoneum that follows the spermatic cord through the inguinal canal is called the vaginal tunic and the similar extension of the peritoneal cavity is called the vaginal cavity.

SCROTUM

The scrotum is a cutaneous pouch divided by a septum that houses the testes.

The wall of the scrotum is composed of skin (externally), parietal vaginal tunic (internally) and a middle layer termed the tunica dartos.

The tunica dartos contains smooth muscle tissue and is thermoregulatory.

DESCENT OF THE TESTIS AND FORMATION OF THE VAGINAL CAVITY

The testes originate in the abdomen just below the kidneys and developmentally follow the gubernaculum through the inguinal canal.

The peritoneal investment on the surface of each testis, epididymis, and ductus deferens becomes visceral vaginal tunic as the testes descend.

DEVELOPMENT OF THE MALE REPRODUCTIVE SYSTEM

Primordia for most of the reproductive organs are similar in males and females and will be considered together in Chapter 21.

CLINICAL CONSIDERATIONS

Paraphimosis and phimosis are mechanical disorders of the prepuce which can occur in uncircumcised males only.

Cryptorchidism is usually inconsequential if unilateral but often causes sterility if bilateral.

Prostate cancer and prostatic hyperplasia are relatively common disorders and can mechanically interfere with urination.

Impotence (inability to achieve or maintain an erection) should be distinguished from sterility (inability to produce viable sperm).

Selected Definitions

Cremaster muscle—the fascicle of skeletal muscle tissue that follows the spermatic cord into the scrotum. It arises from the internal abdominal oblique muscle and allows a male to voluntarily elevate his testes.

Cryptorchid—a male with one testis (unilateral) or both (bilateral) testes undescended. Such an individual is typically sterile but not impotent.

Dartos muscle—the smooth muscle tissue present in the middle layer of the scrotal wall. It has a thermoregulatory function and contracts when a male is cold (drawing the testes up closer to the trunk).

Duct of the epididymis—the tortuous passageway within the epididymis. Efferential ducts from the testis transport sperm to it, and it is continued as the ductus deferens at the tail of the epididymis.

Ductus ("vas") deferens—the tubular organ that transports sperm from the tail of the epididymis to the urethra. Because sperm may spend some time therein, the ductus deferens is said to "store" sperm.

Efferential ducts—the tiny channels that transport sperm from the rete testis to the duct of the epididymis. They penetrate the superior extremity of the testis and then penetrate the head of the epididymis to reach the duct.

Erection—engorgement of the erectile bodies of the penis with blood, causing it to lengthen and stiffen. Erection occurs during sexual excitement in adult males and with little or no provocation in younger ones.

Ejaculatory duct—the last part of each ductus deferens into which the duct of the ipsilateral seminal vesicle opens. The ejaculatory duct passes through the prostate to join the urethra.

Gubernaculum testis—the paired connective tissue proper structure that guides each testis through the inguinal canal and down into the scrotum. Its vestige forms the ligament of the tail of the epididymis.

Impotent—adjective applied to a male who cannot maintain the erection necessary for sexual intercourse. Impotence is often psychological and is unrelated to sperm production.

Inguinal canal—the paired passageway through the lower anterior wall of the trunk that transmits the ipsilateral spermatic cord (in males). Its outer opening (superficial inguinal ring) is a slit in the aponeurosis of the external abdominal oblique muscle and its inner opening (deep inguinal ring) is formed by the internal abdominal oblique muscle, the tendon of the rectus abdominis muscle, and the inguinal ligament.

Interstitial ("Leydig") cells of the testis—the cells located between the seminiferous tubules of the testis that produce testosterone. These cells are not as sensitive to elevated temperatures as the spermatogenic cells in the seminiferous tubules.

Pampiniform plexus—the name applied to the redundancy of the testicular vein in the spermatic cord. Its multiple channels allow more efficient heat transfer wherein the cooler venous blood absorbs some of the core body heat carried toward the testis by the arterial blood.

Prepuce—the redundant skin covering the glans penis. Its removal (circumcision) is sometimes done for religious and/or hygienic reasons.

Rete testis—the dilated passageway in the middle of the testis from which the seminiferous tubules emanate (and then return). Several efferential ducts transport sperm from the rete testis to the head of the epididymis.

Semen—the fluid released when a male ejaculates. It includes sperm, prostatic secretions, and secretions from the seminal vesicles.

Spermatic cord—the (left or right) ductus deferens and the other structures that accompany it through the ipsilateral inguinal canal and down into the scrotum. These structures include the tiny deferential vessels as well as the testicular artery, vein, nerve, and lymphatic vessel.

Spermatogenesis—the formation of spermatozoa (sperm) from their stem cell precursors (spermatogonia). This involves the processes of mitosis, meiosis, and metamorphosis, and includes intermediate cell types called primary spermatocytes, secondary spermatocytes, and spermatids.

Spongy part of the (male) urethra—that part of the urethra that is surrounded by corpus spongiosum. It has been called the "penile" urethra.

Sustentacular cells of testes—large cells in the seminiferous tubules into which the spermatogenic cells are physically invaginated. They support the spermatogenic cells physically and metabolically.

Vaginal tunic—the name applied to peritoneum that accompanies each testis, epididymis, and spermatic cord through the inguinal canals into the scrotum. The visceral vaginal tunic (adherent to the testis, epididymis, and ductus deferens) is separated from the parietal vaginal tunic (lining the inguinal canal and scrotum) by the vaginal cavity.

Etymology ***Vae soli*—"Woe to the solitary man."**

albugineus (L), *white*—albuginea
balan (L), *acorn*—balanitis
caverna (L), *cavern*—corpus cavernosa
dartos (G), *flayed*—dartos
de (L), *down, away*—detumescence
detumescere (L), *to cease swelling*—detumescence
didymos (G), *twin, testicle*—epididymis
fertilis (L), *to bear, produce*—infertility
glans (L), *acorn*—glans
gubernaculum (L), *to steer*—gubernaculum
gubernare (L), *rudder*—gubernaculum
impotentia (L), *lack of self-control*—impotence
inguin (L), *groin*—inguinal
kremaster (G), *to hang*—cremaster
kryptos (G), *hidden*—cryptorchidism
nocturnus (L), *of night*—nocturnal

orchis (G), *testicle*—orchitis
pampinus (L), *tendril*—pampiniform
phimosis (G), *muzzling, stopping up of an orifice* – paraphimosis
priapismos (G), *to be lewd*—priapism
rete (L), *net*—rete
seminiferous (L), *semen producing*—seminiferous
serere (L), *to sow*—semen
sperm (G), *seed*—sperm
sustentaculm (L), *prop, support*—sustentacular
tumescere (L), *to swell up*—detumescence

Introduction

The male reproductive system is one of the visceral body systems and includes the testes, epididymides, deferential ducts, and penis as well as several accessory sex glands: seminal vesicles, prostate gland, and bulbourethral glands (Figure 20-1, 2). The male and female reproductive systems are necessary for procreation but they are not vital to sustain the life of an individual. Testosterone, a hormone produced by the testes, plays a minor role in functions other than procreation: maintenance of muscle, nervous, and bone tissue and it assists in the retention of certain elements including nitrogen, calcium, phosphorus, and potassium.

Objectives

1. List the organs of the male reproductive system.

Functions

There are four major functions of the male reproductive system:

1. **Production of male sex hormones**, mainly testosterone. This powerful hormone controls the development and function of some of the male reproductive organs, promotes the production of male secondary sex characteristics (including increased muscle and bone mass, deepening of voice, and increased facial hair), and is responsible for libido.
2. **Production of male sex cells** (spermatozoa = sperm). Sperm are produced in the testes through a process of mitotic and meiotic cell division called spermatogenesis. Meiosis reduces the chromosome number of the sperm to 23 (from 23 pairs). Meiotic cell division halves the chromosome number in ova as well. During fertilization the chromosome number is restored to the proper total of 46 (23 pairs of chromosomes).
3. **Production of semen**. Semen is the mixture of sperm and fluid expelled during ejaculation. The majority of this fluid is from the seminal vesicles (60%), followed by prostate secretions (20% to 40%), and mucus from both the bulbourethral glands and the glands of the urethra. The typical volume of ejaculum is 3.5 ml. Each milliliter contains approximately 120 million sperm.
4. **Copulation** is the sexual union of a male and female. The erect penis of the male is inserted into the vaginal lumen of the female. Penile erection is a circulatory phenomenon controlled by nervous impulses. Continued stimulation of the penis during copulation results in a summation of sensory impulses leading to ejaculation.

Objectives

2. State the functions of the male reproductive system.

Testis

The left and right testes are located in the perineal region within a cutaneous pouch termed the scrotum. Each one measures about 5 cm long and 2.5 cm thick. The testes produce male sex cells (spermatozoa) and male sex hormone (testosterone). Each testis (plural = testes) is encapsulated by dense connective tissue proper called the **tunica albuginea** of the testis (Figure 20-3). This capsule continues superoinferiorly along the axis of the testis and forms a fibrous cord within the testis termed the **testicular mediastinum**. **Testicular septula** (small septa) extend from the mediastinum to divide the testicular parenchyma into approximately 250 segments called **testicular lobules**.

Within each testicular lobule are several microscopic, tortuous passageways called **seminiferous tubules**. The total length of these tubules in each testis exceeds 700 meters. The seminiferous

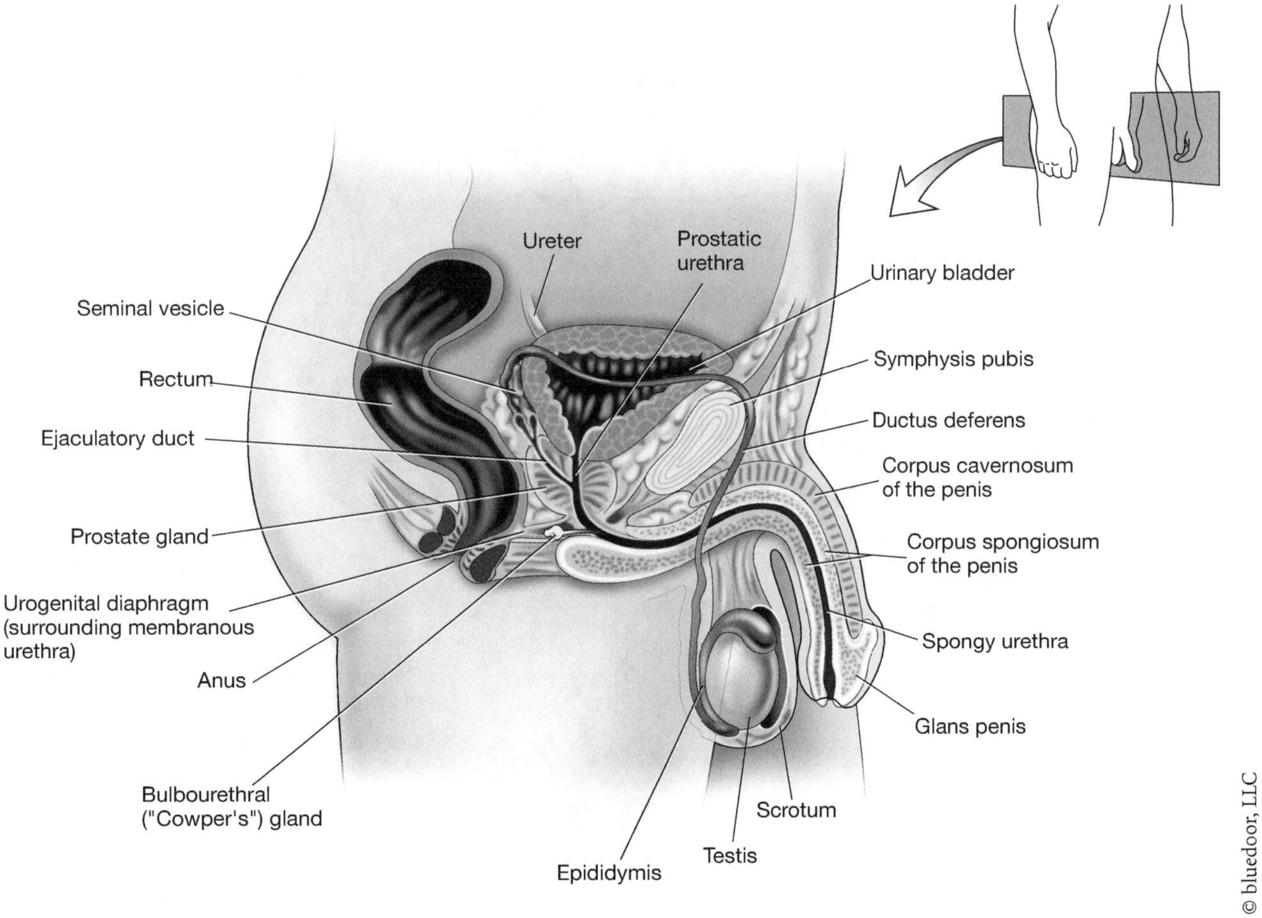

Figure 20-1
Sagittal Section of Male Reproductive System

tubules include loop-like, contorted seminiferous tubules which join straight seminiferous tubules. The latter enter a common collecting area within the mediastinum testis called the **rete testis**. Sperm leave the rete testis via 15 to 20 **testicular efferent ductules** that penetrate the tunica albuginea and enter the head of the epididymis. In addition to sperm producing cells (spermatogenic cells), the seminiferous tubules also contain **sustentacular cells** ("Sertoli" cells) which provide developing sperm with support, protection, and nutrition. **Interstitial cells** ("cells of Leydig") are located between the seminiferous tubules. They produce testosterone.

Objectives

3. Draw a coronal section of a testis and label the following: testicular septula, testicular lobules, seminiferous tubules, and interstitial cells.
4. List the function(s) of the following testicular cells: interstitial cells, sustentacular cells, and spermatogenic cells.

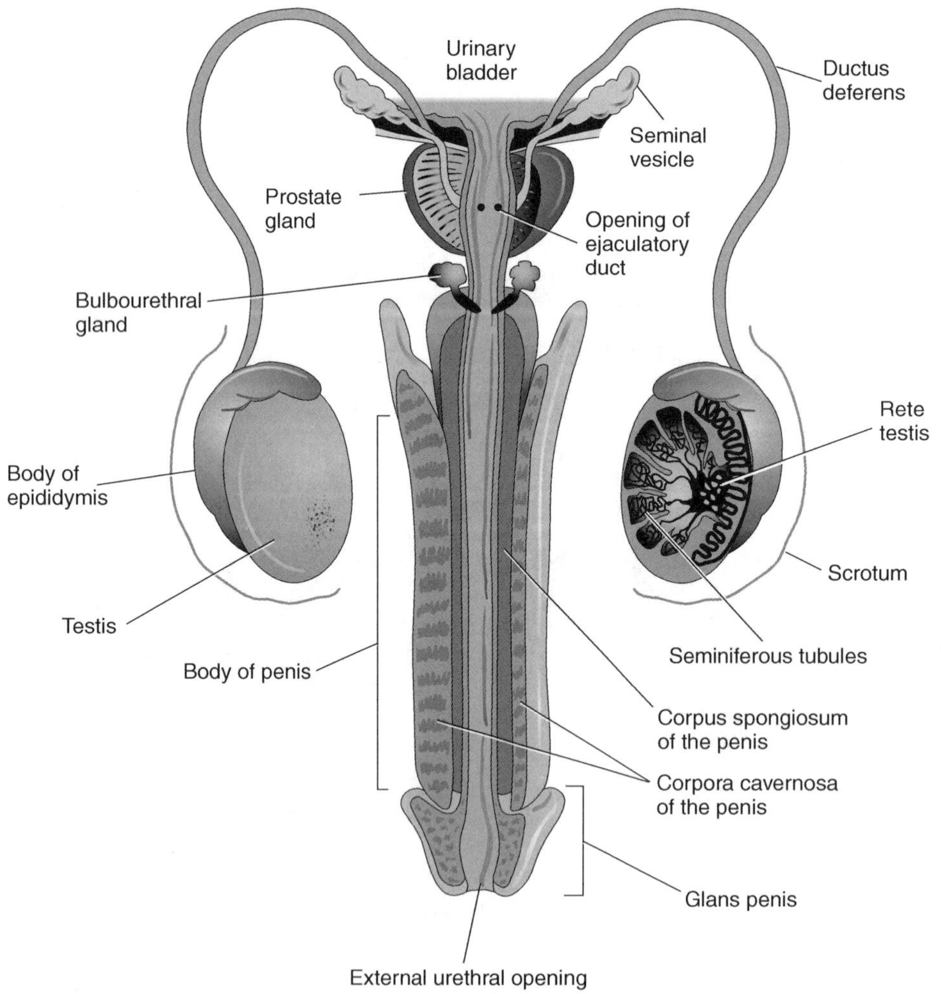

Figure 20-2
Anterior View of Male Reproductive System

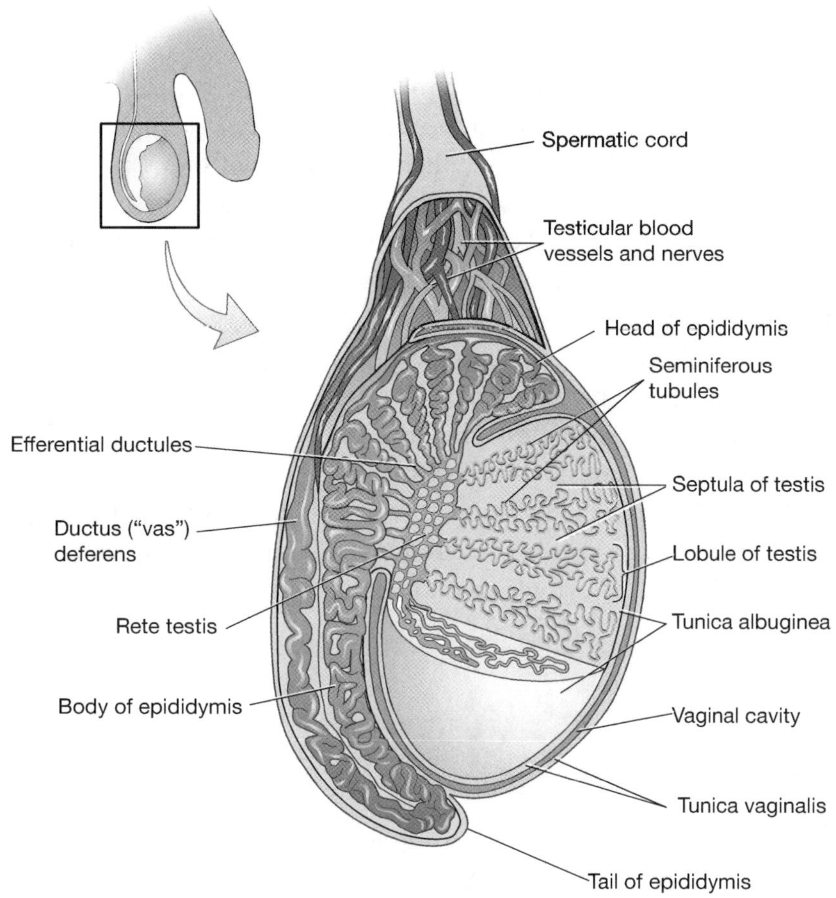

Figure 20-3

Testis and Epididymis

Sperm produced in the seminiferous tubules of the testis collect in the rete testis and are then transported to the duct of the epididymis via the efferential ductules. In the tortuous duct of the epididymis they complete their development by manufacturing an enzyme necessary to penetrate the zona pellucida of an ovum (*see Chapter 21*).

Epididymis

The **epididymis** (plural = epididymides) is a vertically oriented, elongated structure located on the posterior surface of each testis (Figure 20-3). It is divided into three parts: head, body, and tail. The superiorly oriented **head of the epididymis** receives sperm from the testis through the efferential ductules. The **body of the epididymis** is located along the posterior aspect of the testis and is continuous with the tail at the inferior pole of the testis. The **tail of the epididymis** turns 180 degrees and is connected to the ductus deferens. The single, tortuous passageway within the epididymis measures 5-6 meters in total length and is called the **duct of the epididymis**. Sperm complete their maturation within this duct (*see spermatogenesis below*).

Objectives

5. Explain the phenomenal difference in the length of the epididymis *vs.* the length of its duct.

Spermatogenesis

Spermatogenesis is the process of formation of spermatozoa (singular = spermatozoon) which begins at puberty and continues throughout the male's lifetime. Development of sperm occurs within the seminiferous tubules of the testes at a phenomenal rate of thousands per second. Four functional, mature sex cells (spermatozoa) are developed from a single primary spermatocyte in contrast to oogenesis where only one functional cell (ovum) is produced from each precursor cell (Figure 20-4, 5). The basement membrane of each seminiferous tubule is lined with primitive sex cells called **spermatogonia**. Spermatogonia are diploid (46 chromosomes) germ cells that undergo continuous mitotic division. Some of them migrate away from the basement membrane and become **primary spermatocytes**. Each primary spermatocyte undergoes a first meiotic division to form two secondary spermatocytes. **Secondary spermatocytes** are haploid (23 chromosomes) because the first meiotic division reduces the chromosome number by half. Each secondary spermatocyte undergoes a second meiotic division to become two immature sperm called **spermatids**. Spermatids attach to large, specialized nurturing cells called **sustentacular** ("Sertoli") **cells** and undergo metamorphic changes that include the loss of cytoplasm and changes in shape. This series of changes is called

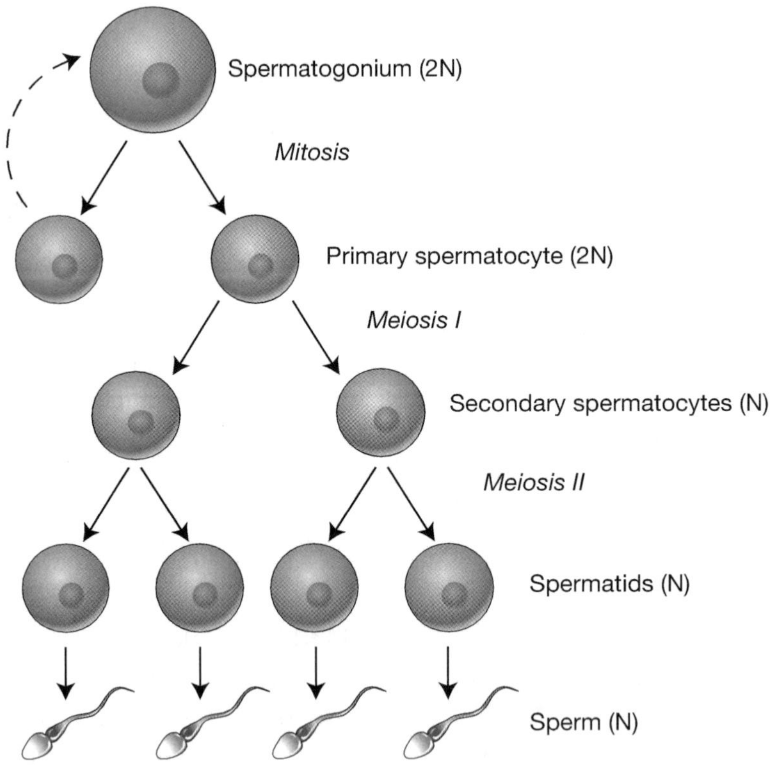

Figure 20-4
Spermatogenesis

The primitive stem cells from which sperm are derived are called spermatogonia. When they divide by mitosis, some of the daughter cells differentiate into primary spermatocytes. The two divisions of meiosis produced four spermatids from each primary spermatocyte. The latter undergo metamorphic change (without nuclear division) to become sperm. This last step of spermatogenesis, wherein spermatids differentiate into sperm, is called spermiogenesis.

spermiogenesis and includes developing a flagellum (tail) (Figure 20-5). At the end of spermiogenesis, the cells are called **spermatozoa** (**sperm**). They are released from the sustentacular cells, leave the testis, and enter the duct of the epididymis. After several days in the epididymis, the sperm are capable of motility and fertilizing ova. Some sperm can be stored in the epididymis, but most

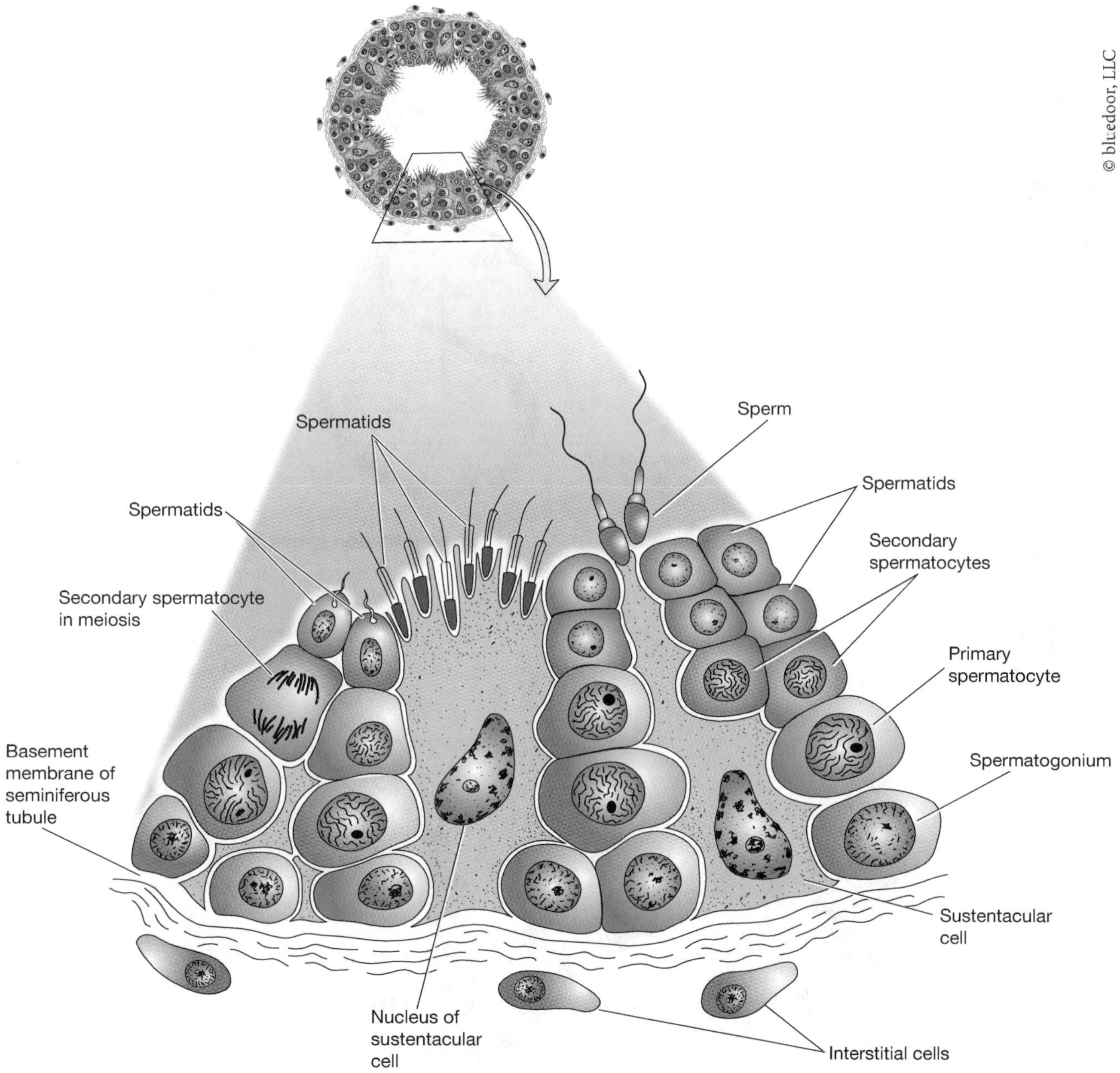

Figure 20-5

Section of a Seminiferous Tubule

The spermatogenic cells form several layers in each seminiferous tubule with the primitive stem cells (spermatogonia) adjacent to the wall (basement membrane). Spermatogenesis produces primary and secondary spermatocytes and finally spermatids which undergo metamorphic changes to become sperm. The huge sustentacular cells serve as physical and metabolic support for the spermatogenic cells. The interstitial cells located between seminiferous tubules produce testosterone.

are stored in the ductus deferens where they await emission and ejaculation. Sperm can survive in the male reproductive tract for several months before being reabsorbed (if not ejaculated first). However, sperm can only survive in the female reproductive tract for about 24-48 hours. The process of spermatogenesis, from mitotic division of a spermatogonium to the end of maturation of

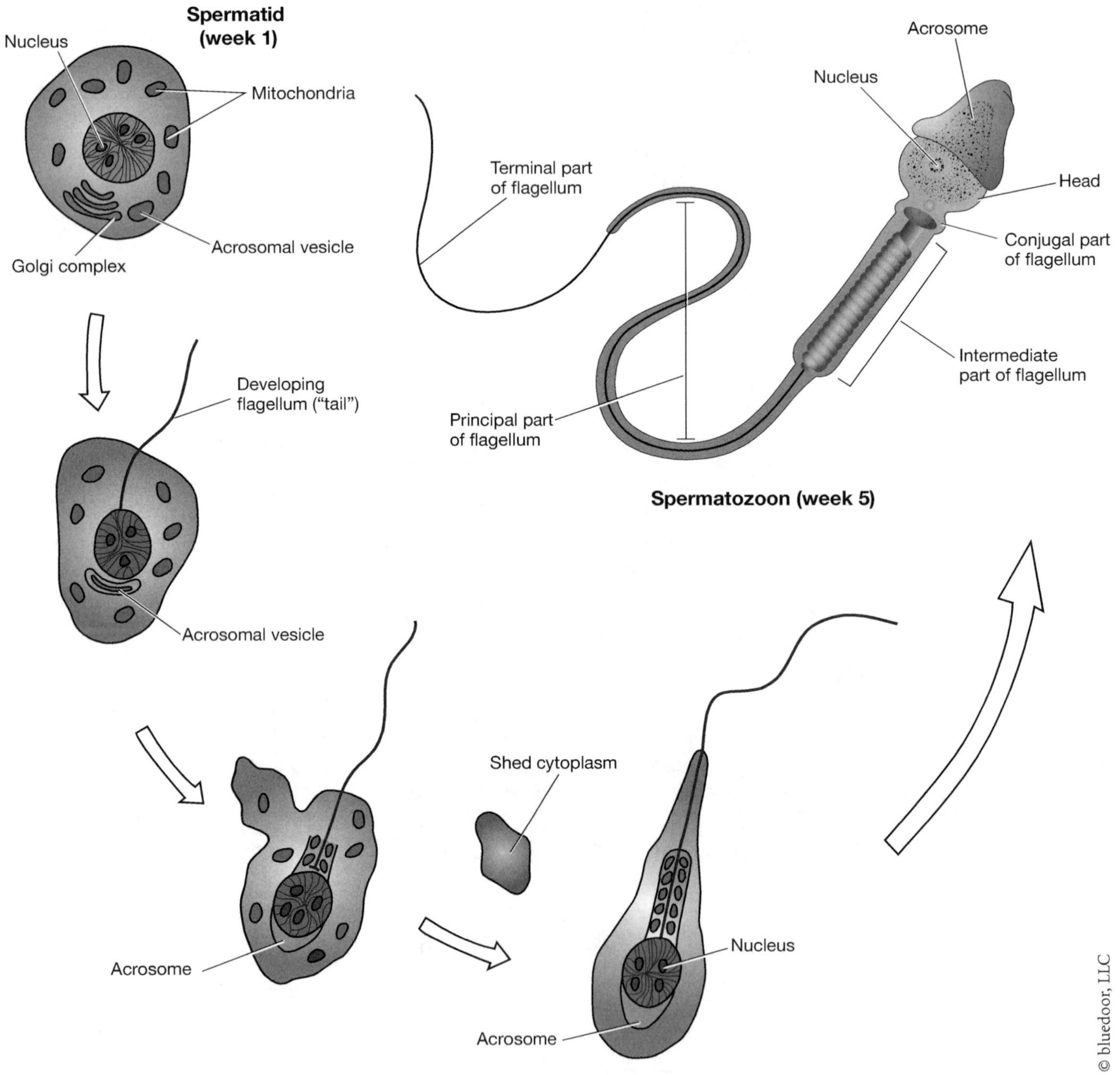

Figure 20-6

Spermiogenesis and Spermatozoon Structure

Spermiogenesis is the metamorphic process by which spermatids are converted to sperm. Sperm are streamlined male sex cells that have a relatively small quantity of cytoplasm. The genetic material is contained within 23 chromosomes in the head. The remainder of the cell is the flagellum with several identifiable regions. The flagellum is often called the "tail" and some authors call its initial parts "neck" and/or "midpiece."

a spermatid is about 72 days. In a mature male that is not sexually active, seminal fluid is periodically "ejaculated" during sleep as **nocturnal emissions** ("wet dreams").

Sperm constitute less than one percent of semen. The typical sperm count in an ejaculum is between 40 to 250 million per milliliter. A sperm count below 10 million per milliliter constitutes **oligospermia**. Men with oligospermia are likely to have fertility problems. Typical sperm motility is 50 percent and less than 40 percent is considered abnormal.

The parts of a developed spermatozoon are the head and flagellum (tail) (Figure 20-6). The majority of the **head** consists of the nucleus (most of the cytoplasm was removed during its metamorphosis from a spermatid. The head of a sperm is tipped by an acrosome which contains powerful hydrolytic and proteolytic enzymes that can literally destroy the male reproductive tract if prematurely released. Cholesterol in the seminal fluids coats the acrosome and prevents the enzyme release. After ejaculation, the sperm become mobile, move away from the cholesterol, and become capacitated (have the ability to release the enzymes and penetrate an ovum). The **flagellum** of a sperm is divided into four segments: conjugal part, intermediate part, principal part, and terminal part. The conjugal part, which joins the head has often been called the "neck" and the intermediate part has sometimes been called the "midpiece." This segment contains numerous mitochondria which provide energy (ATP) to move the rest of the flagellum. Sperm can "swim" at a rate of 1 to 4 mm per minute, but have no sense of direction until they are very close to an ovum. At that point chemotaxis directs them toward their objective.

Objectives

6. Diagram and label the process of spermatogenesis.
7. Schematically represent and label a transverse section of a seminiferous tubule.
8. Diagram and label a spermatozoon and differentiate sperm from semen.

Ductus Deferens

The **ductus deferens** is a muscular tube which is a continuation of the duct of the epididymis (Figure 20-1, 6). It is about 45 cm long and courses from the tail of the epididymis at the inferior pole of the testis to the urethra. The ductus deferens passes through the anteroinferior abdominal wall accompanied by several structures to collectively form the spermatic cord. Within the abdominal cavity the ductus deferens loops around the ipsilateral ureter on the posterior aspect of the urinary bladder, passes through the prostate, and then enters the urethra. Near its termination, each ductus deferens enlarges to form the **ampulla of the ductus deferens**. The urethral end of each ductus deferens is called the **ejaculatory duct** (Figure 20-7) and is joined by the excretory duct of the ipsilateral seminal vesicle. The terminal end of each ejaculatory duct connects to the prostatic part of the urethra. As sperm are transported through the ductus deferens, fluid is added to suspend them. Bilateral surgical interruption of the ductus deferens (vasectomy) renders a male sterile.

Objectives

9. List and define the subparts of the ductus deferens.

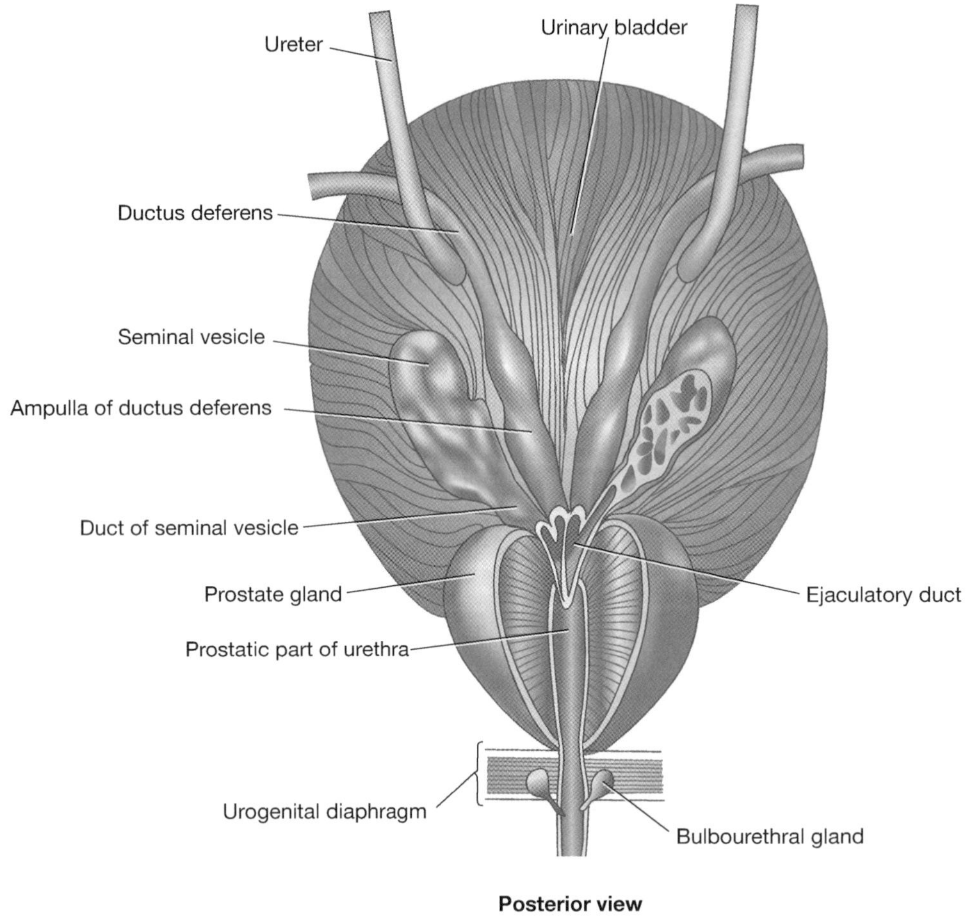

Figure 20-7

Ductus Deferens and Accessory Sex Glands

The terminal part of each ductus deferens (after the duct of the ipsilateral seminal vesicle joins it) is called the ejaculatory duct. Prostatic secretions enter the urethra through numerous microscopic channels called prostatic ductules.

Male Urethra

The male urethra belongs to the urinary system but also functions in the reproductive system. (*see Chapter 19*). It is 18-20 cm long and is divided into three parts: prostatic, membranous, and spongy. The initial portion within the prostate gland is called the **prostatic part of the urethra** (Figure 20-7, 8) and receives the openings of the left and right ejaculatory ducts. A ridge called the **urethral crest** projects from the posterior wall of the prostatic part of the urethra. Numerous **prostatic ducts** open into the urethra on either side of this crest. Prostatic secretions pass through these ducts to mix with sperm and vesicular fluids to form semen. The **membranous part of the urethra** is the section within the urogenital diaphragm. It is the shortest (1-2 cm) part of the male urethra and is less distensible than the other parts, partially due to the surrounding urethral sphincter muscle. The **spongy part of the urethra** is the portion within the penis (some authors call it the "penile urethra"). It is surrounded by erectile tissue called corpus spongiosum penis and terminates at the **external urethral ostium** at the tip of the glans penis. The ducts of the left and right bulbourethral glands enter the spongy part of the urethra just inferior to the urogenital diaphragm. **Urethral glands** located in the spongy part of the urethra secrete a mucus-like substance that is similar to the secretion of the bulbourethral glands.

Objectives

10. List and define the subparts of the urethra.

Penis

The male copulatory organ is called the penis and it includes the root, body, and glans (Figure 20-8). The **root of the penis** is divided into left and right crura, each of which attach to the ipsilateral pubis. The **body of the penis** includes most of its length, and the distal penile extremity is called the glans penis. The **glans penis** flares proximally to form the **corona of the glans penis**. The redundant skin extending over the glans penis is called the **prepuce** (**foreskin**) **of the penis**. This skin is attached to the ventral aspect of the penis by the **frenulum** of the prepuce. In circumcised males, the foreskin has been partially removed by surgery.

The penis contains three tubes of erectile tissue: a left and a right corpus cavernosum penis and the corpus spongiosum penis. The **corpora cavernosa penis** form the main portion of the body of the penis (Figure 20-8). They diverge proximally into the left and right crura which attach the root of the penis to the pubes. The **corpus spongiosum penis** surrounds the spongy part of the urethra and is located inferior to the corpora cavernosum penis. Its proximal end is slightly enlarged to form the **bulb of the penis** and the distal end of the corpus spongiosum penis forms the erectile tissue within the glans penis. The three erectile bodies consist of cavernous spaces which can fill with blood to effect erection. They are each surrounded by dense fibrous non-expansible connective tissue termed the **tunica albuginea** of the penis.

Objectives

11. Explain what is surgically removed during circumcision of a male.
12. Diagram and label a transverse section through the body of a penis.

Erection, Copulation, and Ejaculation

Penile erection is a circulatory phenomenon controlled by nervous impulses. Parasympathetic impulses initiate increased blood flow to penile arteries and cause partial occlusion of penile veins. This causes engorgement of the erectile bodies of the penis (corpora cavernosa penis and corpus spongiosum penis). The engorgement results in the enlargement and stiffening of the penis called **erection**. **Detumescence** (decrease in penile size associated with loss of erection) is caused by reduced arterial blood flow to the penis and increased venous drainage from the erectile bodies.

Copulation (also known as sexual intercourse, sexual union, or coitus) is the procreative act whereby a man's erect penis is inserted into a woman's vagina. Lubrication of the glans penis and vagi-

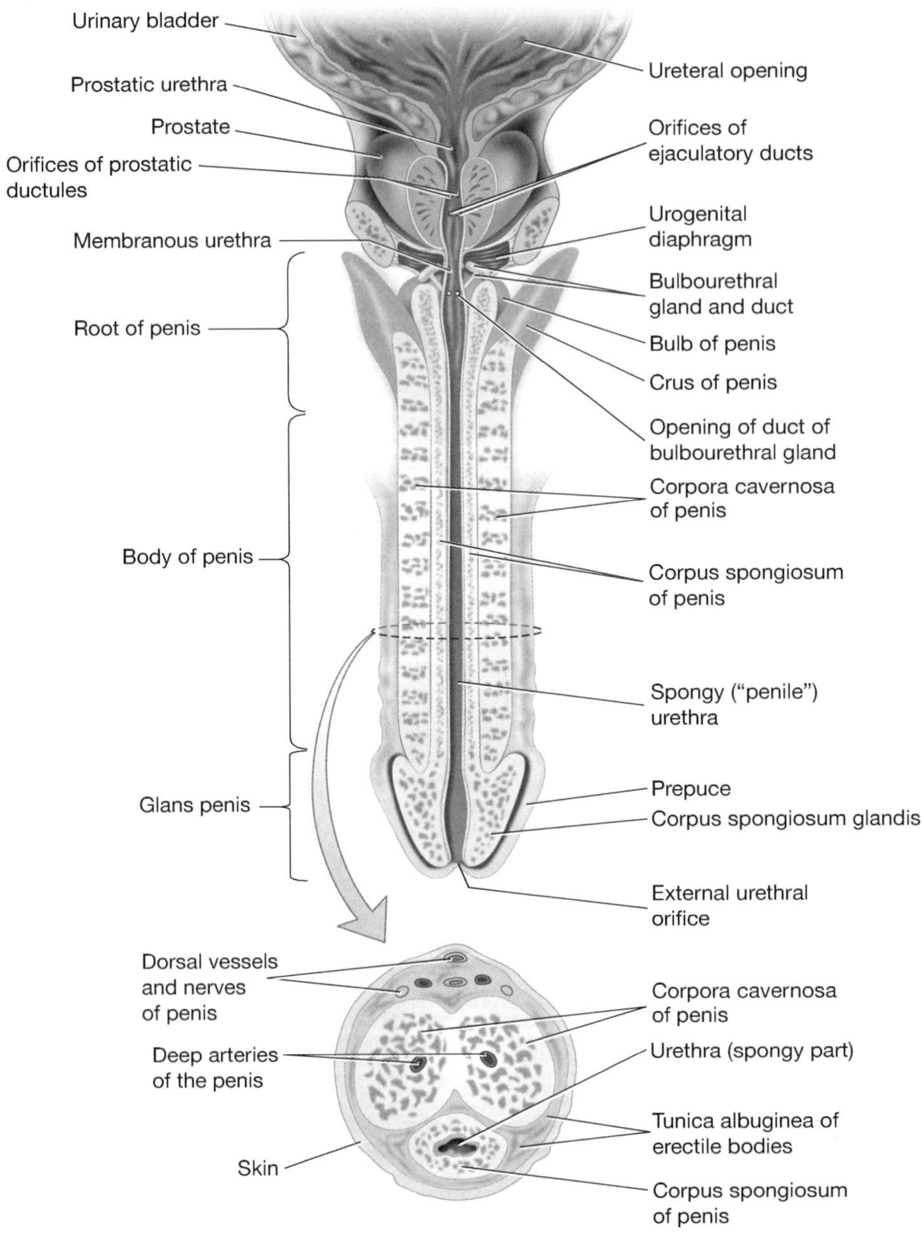

Figure 20-8
Penis

The three erectile bodies of the penis become engorged with blood during sexual arousal. The left and right corpora cavernosa do not extend the full length of the penis but stop at the glans. The unpaired corpus spongiosum expands distally to form the erectile tissue within the glans. Proximally the corpus spongiosum expands to form the bulb of the penis.

na are necessary for this process and natural lubricant is provided by the bulbourethral glands of males and the major vestibular glands of females. Stimulation of the penis causes **emission** (movement of sperm from the epididymides to the ejaculatory ducts and the release of secretions from the accessory sex glands). Continued stimulation of the penis and clitoris during intercourse may result in a summation of pleasurable sensory impulses termed **orgasm** ("climax"). In males, orgasm is typically accompanied by **ejaculation** of semen. This occurs through rhythmic contractions of the bulbospongiosus and urethral muscles which results in peristaltic waves within the corpus spongiosum penis surrounding the urethra. The force of these contractions may cause the semen to spurt from the urethral orifice. Orgasm in females involves spasmodic contractions of the uterus and uterine tubes which may help propel sperm through the female reproductive tract.

Objectives

13. Explain the phenomenon of penile erection.
14. Differentiate emission, orgasm, and ejaculation.

Accessory Sex Glands

The three major male accessory sex glands are the seminal vesicles, prostate, and bulbourethral glands. The **seminal vesicles** are a pair of elongated structures which extend about 5 cm along the lateral aspects of the ampulla of each ductus deferens on the posterior aspect of the urinary bladder (*see Figure 20-6*). Each one has an excretory duct that empties into the ejaculatory duct of the ipsilateral ductus deferens. The seminal vesicles secrete a mucoid substance which contains fructose, prostaglandins, and fibrinogen. *Fructose* is a nutrient for sperm and the *prostaglandins* cause the cervical mucus of the female to be more receptive to sperm. They may also be responsible for reverse peristaltic contractions in the uterus and uterine tubes. *Fibrinogen* creates a weak coagulum that immobilizes sperm for the first 15 to 20 minutes after ejaculation. The **prostate gland** (**prostate**) is a spheroid structure about 4 cm in diameter which surrounds the initial part of the male urethra (Figure 20-7). It secretes a milky, thin, alkaline fluid that contains calcium ions, acid phosphatase, citric acid, clotting enzyme, and profibrinolysin. The alkalinity of the prostate secretions neutralizes acidic fluids within the vagina and vulva. Profibrinolysin breaks down the weak coagulum formed after ejaculation. The paired **bulbourethral glands** ("Cowper's" gland) are less than a centimeter in diameter. They secrete a *lubricating fluid* during sexual arousal that assists intromission (insertion of the penis into the vaginal lumen). It also cleanses the urethra and neutralizes any residual acidity from urine. The ducts of the bulbourethral glands empty into the initial portion of the spongy part of the urethra.

Objectives

15. Name the male accessory sex glands, state their location, and state what each secretes.

Inguinal Canal and Spermatic Cord

The oblique passageways through the anteroinferior abdominal wall that transmit each ductus deferens and several other structures are called the **inguinal canals**. The external opening of each canal is a "hole" in the aponeurosis of the external abdominal oblique muscle called the **superficial inguinal ring**. The internal opening is bounded by the internal abdominal oblique muscle, the tendon of the rectus abdominis muscle, and the inguinal ligament. It is called the **deep inguinal ring**.

The portion of the ductus deferens that courses through the ipsilateral inguinal canal and the neurovascular structures that accompany it constitute the **spermatic cord**. The accompanying structures include the tiny deferential vessels, as well as the testicular artery, veins, nerves, and lymphatic vessels. The testicular veins anastomose around the testicular artery forming a network called the **pampiniform plexus**. This plexus serves as a countercurrent heat exchanger that cools the arterial flow before it reaches the testis. The spermatic cord components are enveloped by peritoneum called the vaginal tunic. That which is adherent to the ductus deferens itself (and continues distally to cover the testis and epididymis) is called the **visceral vaginal tunic** and the remainder which lines the inside of the scrotum is the **parietal vaginal tunic**. The serous space between the parietal and visceral vaginal tunics is continuous with the peritoneal cavity and is called the **vaginal cavity** (cavity of the vaginal tunic—not to be confused with the vaginal lumen of a female). A slip of skeletal muscle from each internal abdominal oblique called the **cremaster muscle** attaches to the parietal vaginal tunic and follows the ipsilateral spermatic cord down into the scrotum. Contraction of this muscle elevates the testis.

Objectives

16. Define the inguinal canal and its openings.
17. Define spermatic cord and schematically represent and label a transverse section through it.

Scrotum

The testes are suspended from the perineum below the root of the penis within an expansible cutaneous pouch termed the **scrotum** (Figure 20-2). The scrotal wall has three layers: skin, tunica dartos, and parietal vaginal tunic. The **tunica dartos** is a thin layer of tissue deep to the **skin** composed mainly of smooth muscle tissue. The **parietal vaginal tunic** is formed by peritoneum that courses through the inguinal canal to line the ipsilateral scrotal cavity (Figure 20-9). The scrotum is divided into left and right chambers by a dividing wall of tissue termed the **scrotal septum**. The scrotum assists in the thermoregulation of the testes. Smooth muscle tissue within the tunica dartos (**dartos muscle**) contracts and relaxes in response to changing environmental temperatures. Relaxation of the muscle allows the testes to be suspended further from the perineum and helps cool them. Cold temperatures will cause reflex contraction of the dartos muscle which draws the testes closer to the perineum (a warmer location). The core body temperature is 37.0 degrees C but the temperature within the scrotum is normally maintained at less than 34.0 degrees C. This lower temperature is necessary for spermatogenesis in most mammals. In some mammals (bats, whales, elephants) the testes always remain in the abdominal cavity. Such animals are said to be *testicond*. In other mammals (such as members of the deer family) the testes move into the scrotum only during breeding season.

Objectives

18. Sketch and label a transverse section through the scrotum.
19. Explain how the tunica dartos functions in thermoregulation of the testis.

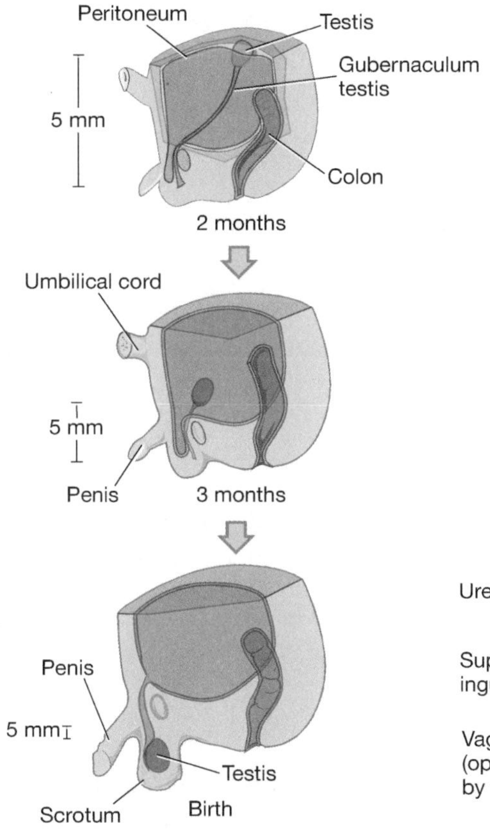

Descent of testis, lateral view

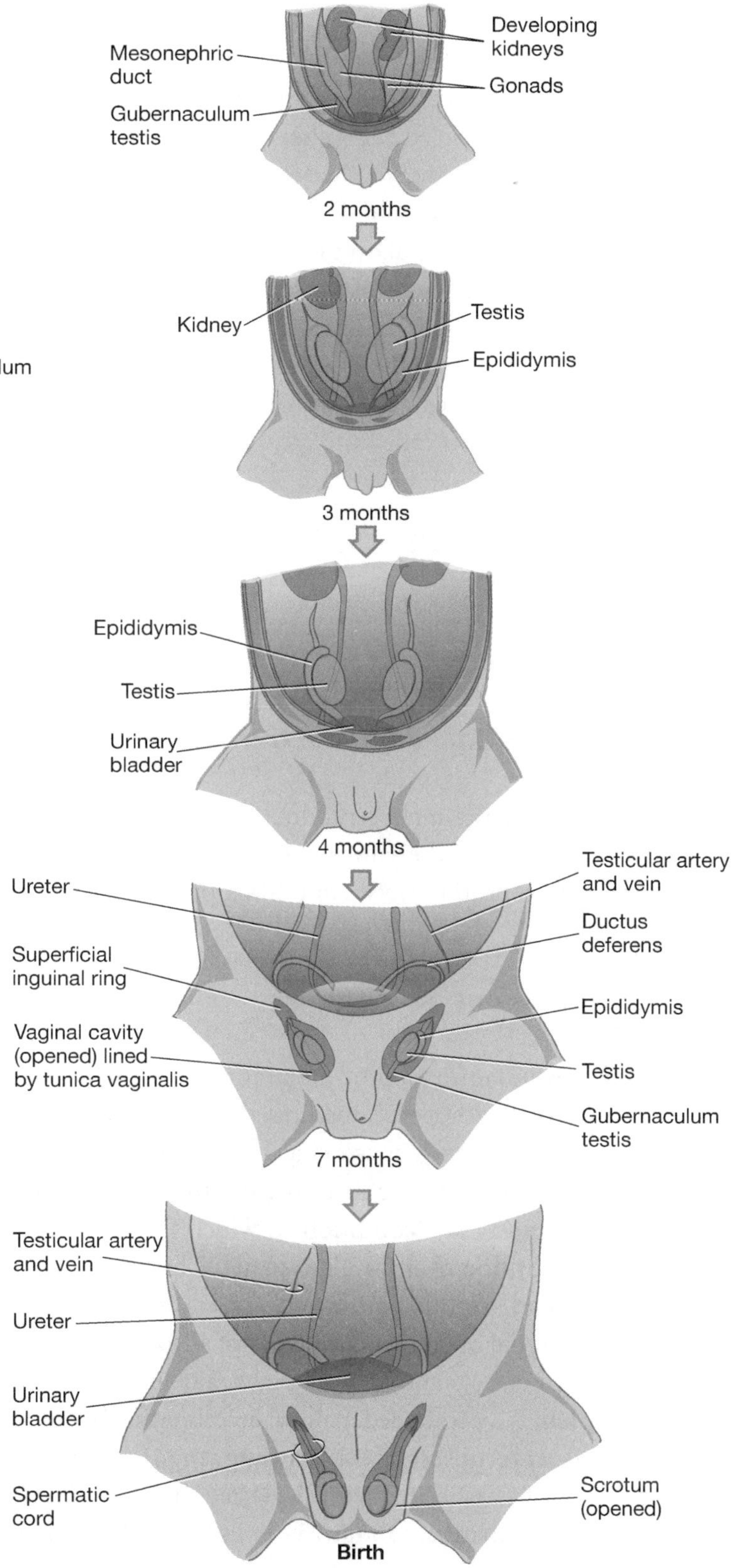

Descent of testis, anterior view

Figure 20-9
Descent of the Testes

During development, the testis and epididymis migrate through the lower anterior abdominal wall into the scrotum.They follow a connective tissue cord through the inguinal canal called the gubernaculum testis. Failure of one or both testes to complete this migration results in cryptorchidism (*see Clinical Considerations*).

Descent of the Testis and Formation of the Vaginal Cavity

What induces the testes to migrate down into the scrotum from the comparatively "safe" intra-abdominal site of early development is not fully understood. The descending testis follows a connective tissue cord called the **gubernaculum testis** (Figure 20-9). During their early development just inferior to the kidneys, the testes are enveloped by a surface covering of visceral peritoneum which they "take" with them during their descent into the scrotum. The peritoneum extending out through the inguinal canal on the surface of the ductus deferens, epididymis, and testis is termed the **visceral layer of the vaginal tunic**. This reflects off the inferior extremity of the testis to line the wall of the scrotum and inguinal canal as the **parietal layer of the vaginal tunic**. The **vaginal cavity** is the space between the visceral and parietal layers of the vaginal tunic. As noted previously, a fascicle from the internal abdominal oblique muscle adherent to the outer side of the parietal layer of the vaginal tunic is called the cremaster muscle.

Objectives

20. Differentiate the two regional parts of the vaginal tunic.

Development of the Male Reproductive System

Development of the male reproductive system is summarized in Figure 20-10. Most of the male organs develop from the same primordia as their female counterparts. See Chapter 21 for a general discussion of reproductive system development.

Clinical Considerations

Urethritis is inflammation of the urethra that can result from bacterial infections (including sexually transmitted pathogens), manipulation of urologic instruments, and trauma. It can be caused by ingestion of toxins such as wood alcohol or turpentine. Urethritis causes dysuria, a burning sensation during urination (micturition), and frequent, urgent urination.

Paraphimosis is a condition in which the prepuce is retracted and cannot be returned to its anatomical position over the glans penis. This may constrict blood flow and damage the glans penis if left untreated. Another abnormal condition of the prepuce is phimosis. **Phimosis** is caused by a stenotic preputial opening which will not allow the prepuce to be retracted over the glans penis. This prevents proper hygienic cleansing and may increase the risk of penile cancer.

Priapism is a prolonged, painful erection that is not related to sexual arousal. It generally affects the corpus cavernosum penis causing engorgement with blood that will not properly drain. Priapism can be associated with sickle cell disease, pelvic tumors, leukemia, spinal cord trauma, and can also be idiopathic. **Balanitis** is inflammation of the glans penis resulting from inadequate cleansing under the prepuce, skin diseases, priapism, or pathogens such as *Candida albicans.*

Varicocele can occur in the spermatic cord when there is an abnormal dilation of a vein due to congenital absence of valves or from acquired valvular incompetence. **Hydrocele** is a collection of fluid between the parietal and visceral layers of the vaginal tunic.

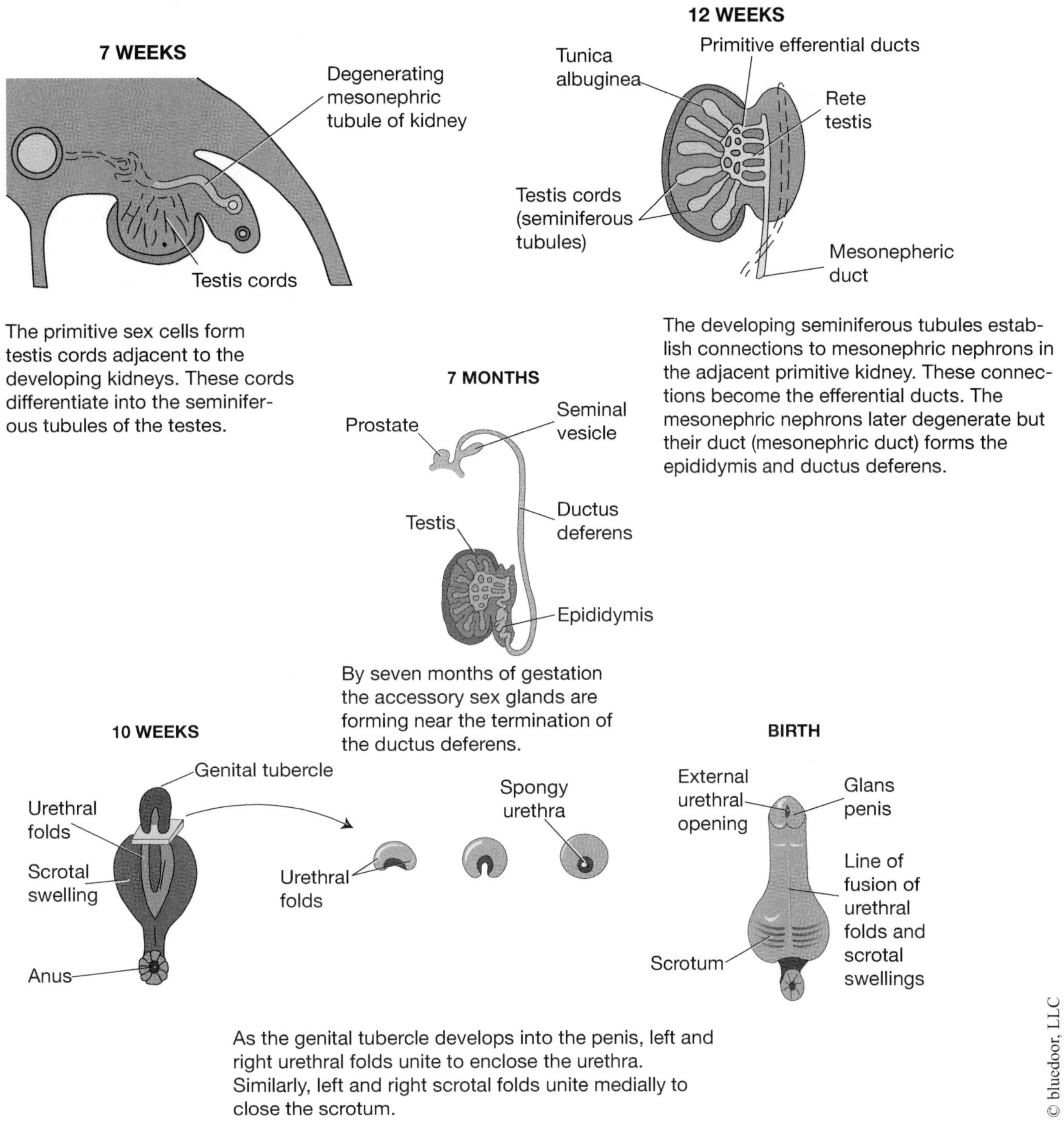

Figure 20-10

Development of Male Reproductive System

An **inguinal hernia** is an evagination of abdominal viscera (usually intestine) into the inguinal canal. This can compromise the blood supply of the herniated structure and compress the vasculature within the spermatic cord. Surgical intervention is usually indicated.

Cryptorchidism is the failure of one or both testes to descend into the scrotum. Undescended testes present an increased risk of testicular cancer and usually do not produce viable sperm. Their testosterone output, however, is undiminished. **Testicular torsion** is an abnormal rotation of a testis. Blood vessels become twisted and blood flow is arrested. The impeded blood flow can cause edema which may result in necrosis and atrophy of testicular parenchyma within a few hours. **Orchitis** is testicular inflammation which may be caused by pathogens or trauma.

Testicular cancer is the most common malignancy in males between the ages of 25 to 35. Some types are quite malignant. **Benign prostatic hyperplasia** (or hypertrophy) is the enlargement of the prostate gland. This condition causes compression of the prostatic urethra which can affect the urinary bladder and urine flow. Infection of the prostate can also cause the gland to enlarge. **Prostate cancer** is the third leading cause of cancer deaths in men (lung cancer is the first followed by colorectal cancer).

Infertility in males is the reduced or absent capacity to produce offspring. **Sterility** is the complete inability to induce conception (due to the lack of live or normal spermatozoa). **Impotence** is the inability of a male to maintain an erection.

Objectives

21. Differentiate phimosis *vs.* paraphimosis.
22. Explain why bilateral cryptorchids are usually sterile but not impotent.

Clinical Case Studies

Case 1—After participating in a wrestling meet, a high school junior had severe pain and swelling in his scrotal area. There was no history of perineal trauma during his match and no evidence that he had an inguinal hernia. Suggest a cause for the swelling.

Case 2—A sixth grade boy complained of moderate pain in his right inguinal region that seemed to worsen after hard play. After spending one afternoon rolling up large snowballs to build a snow fort with some friends, the pain became almost unbearable. Offer a tentative diagnosis.

Case 3—A 70-year-old retiree noted a gradual and significant reduction in the size of his urine stream and concurrent increase in the total time required to empty his urinary bladder. What is the most likely explanation?

Points to Ponder

The reproductive system has no vital organs. Convince a bunch of high school seniors of that fact and you'll land a position on the gold medal debate team! It has been observed that males of most higher species are naturally promiscuous. Even in mankind, monogamy exists largely because of social pressures related to cultural and/or religious taboos.

Most males seem to be glad that they are male—until the gears on their 10-speed bike slip when they are cranking up a hill. Sooner or later every male has an altercation of this type that makes him question nature's design. Males of most mammalian species carry their testes around (almost externally) in the scrotum. Sperm like to be cool, we are told. ("Look at me, I'm a sperm. I'm cool!") A fever kills them in high numbers. Anyway, that's the why on the scrotum. (Keep's 'em cool.) Some species get special dispensation to keep their testes in the abdomen. That's why you won't see an elephant or bat scrotum when you visit the zoo. Whales don't have scrota (that's plural) either. Maybe they did at one time, but in the cold ocean water... The most infamous scrotum in the animal kingdom is that of the mythical Onno bird of central Africa. The Onno has four inch legs, a six inch scrotum, and gets its name from the frantic call it emits every time it comes in for a landing ("Oh No!").

Sometimes one or both testes refuse to enter the scrotum, preferring instead, to remain in the relatively safer confines of the abdominal cavity. (Maybe they heard about the bicycle thing or read the autobiographies of abused cousins). Spermatogenesis is hampered by the higher temperature of the abdominal cavity and individuals with both testes undescended are likely to be sterile. That's bad news and it gets worse because undescended testes are also more susceptible to neoplasia. The good news is that the interstitial cells which produce testosterone are just as comfortable at higher temperatures. Nature sometimes plays cruel tricks and more than one bilateral cryptorchid, making the best of his theoretically sterile situation, has joined the ranks of fatherhood.

After sexual maturity, men produce sperm at an alarming rate and usually stop only because of death. The numbers are staggering—making you wonder how they have time for anything else. ("Yeah, I would have been taller but..."). Sperm are pathetic little cells. Smallest in the body. All head and tail. A nucleated flagellum with half a set of DNA. When conditions are right, they are enthusiastic swimmers with no sense of direction, and they wander aimlessly about whether on a microscope slide or vaginal mucosa. One has to observe the meanderings for only a few moments to realize that we would have become extinct long ago if they had to get someplace on their own.

Enter the penis. A marvel of vascularity, its erections are the result of engorgement of three erectile bodies with blood. Increase the arterial input into these while reducing the venous drainage and "voila"! This mechanism seems to have a mind of its own in junior high school. In some mammals, the penis even contains a real bone (os penis) for added rigidly. The tip of the penis, called the glans penis (no "d", please), is covered by some redundant integument called prepuce. One can easily understand its importance to a dairy bull walking through tall weeds, but it really isn't necessary in a pair of Jockeys® or Fruit-of-the-Looms® . Its surgical removal, called circumcision, is sometimes recommended for hygienic reasons but has been more commonly practiced as a religious rite.

Slang and Obsolete Nomenclature

UNOFFICIAL TERM	OFFICIAL DESIGNATION
penile urethra	spongy part *[pars spongiosa]* of urethra
vas deferens	ductus deferens *[ductus deferens]*
Cowper's gland	bulbourethral gland *[glandula bulbo-urethralis]*
vesicular gland	seminal vesicle *[vesicula seminalis]*
shaft of penis	body *[corpus]* of penis
corpus cavernosum/spongiosum	corpus cavernosum/spongiosum penis *[corpus cavernosum/spongiosum penis]*
glans	glans penis *[glans penis]*
cell of Leydig	interstitial cell (endocrinocyte) *[endocrinocytus interstitialis]*
Sertoli (nurse) cell	sustentacular cell *[epitheliocytus sustenans]*
scrotal cavity	vaginal cavity *[cavitas vaginalis]*
external inguinal ring	superficial *[superficialis]* inguinal ring
internal inguinal ring	deep *[profundus]* inguinal ring

Review Questions

1. Sperm are not present within the....
   A. ductus deferens.
   B. urethra.
   C. seminal vesicles.
   D. efferential ducts.
   E. epididymis.

2. During spermatogenesis, each_________________________results in the formation of _________sperm.
   A. primary spermatocyte—6
   B. secondary spermatocyte—2
   C. tertiary spermatocyte—8
   D. spermatid—2
   E. If none of the above fill the blanks correctly, choose this response.

3. Which structure does not pass all the way through the inguinal canal?
   A. ductus deferens
   B. testicular artery
   C. testicular nerve
   D. cremaster muscle
   E. vaginal tunic

4. Which of the following has no thermoregulatory function?
   A. scrotum
   B. cremaster muscle
   C. tunica dartos
   D. pampiniform plexus
   E. testicular artery and vein

5. A bilateral cryptorchid would probably be...
   A. sterile.
   B. impotent.
   C. impotent and sterile.
   D. neither impotent nor sterile.
   E. unable to maintain an erection.

6. Which of the following is not part of the scrotal wall?
   A. skin
   B. visceral vaginal tunic
   C. tunica dartos
   D. dermis
   E. dartos muscle

7. Which male reproductive structure is mismatched with a secretory product?
   A. prostate—clotting enzyme, acid phosphate
   B. testis—testosterone
   C. bulbourethral gland—lubricating fluid
   D. seminal vesicle—fructose
   E. seminal vesicle—prostaglandin

8. Which cell is not found within a testis?
   A. sustentacular cell
   B. interstitial cell
   C. spermatid
   D. leucocyte
   E. If all of the above are found within a testis, choose this response.

9. Which statement is true regarding seminiferous tubules?
   A. They contain sustentacular cells, interstitial cells, and the spermatogenic cells of the testis.
   B. They terminate in the rete testis.
   C. They serve as the site of sperm maturation.
   D. They are divided into groups within the testicular lobules that have different functions.
   E. They are found within the seminal vesicles.

10. Which part of the male reproductive system is shared with the urinary system?
    A. seminal vesicles
    B. prostate
    C. ureter
    D. bulbourethral gland
    E. If none of the above satisfy the premise, choose this response.

Thought Questions

1. What is the relationship between sterility and impotence?

2. Compare the functions of the dartos muscle and the cremaster muscle.

3. Explain the mechanics of penile erection.

4. Which part of the male reproductive tract is shared functionally with another system? Give other examples of shared organs.

5. Do vasectomized males ejaculate? Explain.

6. Are any of the organs of the male reproductive system vital to the life of the individual? Explain.

7. Why are so many sperm produced?

8. Explain why the testicular vessels originate relatively high in the abdomen.

9. Discuss the mechanics of ejaculation.

10. Why does prostatic hyperplasia interfere with urination?

11. Explain why men with bilateral cryptorchidism are usually sterile but not impotent.

12. What happens to sperm that are not ejaculated?

13. Explain why boys who reach puberty relatively early are often shorter as adults than those who mature later.

14. Discuss castrati singers.

15. How do the testes descend into the scrotum?

16. Why are the testes located in the scrotum?

17. If sperm can swim 3 millimeters per minute, how long will it take for them to swim 20 centimeters through the vagina, cervix, uterus, and uterine tube?

18. Explain the functional purpose of the secretions of each of the male accessory glands.

19. At what general age do men become dysfunctional sexually?

20. Discuss the different roles of the three populations of cells found in the testes.

21. Can a successfully vasectomized male father children?

Answers to Clinical Case Studies

Case 1—Testicular torsion, wherein a testicle is twisted relative to the spermatic cord coursing down to it, can reduce venous return from the involved testicle while allowing free flow within the testicular artery. The net result is swelling and pain. These cases are surgical emergencies because the testicular tissue quickly dies due to hypoxia.

Case 2—The symptoms are classic for an inguinal hernia. In many cases, a loop of intestine protrudes into/through the inguinal canal where it becomes partially strangulated and causes pain. Surgical repair involves reduction of the diameter of the inguinal canal such that abdominal viscera cannot invade it.

Case 3—These symptoms indicate that the urethra is becoming obstructed and the usual cause is prostatic enlargement due to hyperplasia or cancer. Since the prostate completely surrounds the initial part of the urethra, its enlargement can constrict the urethra and reduce urine flow.

Answers to Review Questions

1. C.

2. B.

3. D.

4. B. This muscle contracts in hostile situations.

5. A. Spermatogenesis would be inhibited by the higher body temperature.

6. B.

7. A. The prostate secretes acid phosphatase—an enzyme that hydrolyzes acid phosphates.

8. E.

9. B.

10. E.

Answers to Thought Questions

1. There is no direct relationship. Sterility implies the inability to produce viable sex cells and impotence is an inability to get or maintain an erection. A male can have either syndrome, both, or (best case scenario) neither.

2. The dartos muscle is smooth muscle tissue within the tunica dartos of the scrotal wall. It is involuntary and thermoregulatory, contracting when cold to position the testes closer to the trunk and relaxing when hot. The left and right cremaster muscles are slips of voluntary (skeletal) muscle off the internal abdominal oblique muscles. They can be contracted voluntarily in hostile situations to elevate the testes. (Hostile situations include jumping fences where clearance is critical and large dogs snapping at one's crotch!)

3. Blood flow to the penis increases. In addition, contraction of the ischiocavernosus muscle causes a "kinking" in the main venous drainage from the three erectile bodies of the penis. The increase in blood flow to these areas and decreased venous drainages causes them to engorge with blood and imparts the size increase and rigidity termed erection.

4. Urethra (urinary system). The pharynx is shared by the digestive and respiratory systems. In a slightly different sense the endocrine system shares organs with numerous other systems.

5. Yes, but their ejaculations contain no sperm. They consist of secretions of the accessory sex glands only.

6. No. The reproductive system (male and female) is the only body system that has no vital organs. The urethra of males technically "belongs" to the urinary system.

7. They get lost easily (and refuse to ask for directions). They are delicate, easily killed cells. They leave home with little survival gear and the attrition rate en route to the objective (ovum) is high.

8. The testes begin their development in the abdominal cavity just inferior to the kidneys. The testicular arteries originate there and then elongate as the testes descend into the scrotum.

9. Contractions of the bulbospongiosus muscle create hydrostatic compression waves in the blood within an erectile body called the bulb of the penis which is continuous with the corpus spongiosum penis. These compression waves cause peristaltic constrictions of the urethral lumen which propel semen through the urethra.

10. The prostate gland surrounds the urethra. Hyperplastic prostatic glands cause urethral constriction.

11. The higher temperature to which undescended testes are subjected interferes with spermatogenesis but not with production of testosterone by the interstitial cells. Sterility implies inability to produce viable sperm and this is the usual case with bilateral cryptorchids. Such individuals are, however, sexually competent and so they are not impotent.

12. They are forced out during nocturnal emissions ("wet dreams") in intact males. In vasectomized males they degenerate and are reabsorbed.

13. Testosterone inhibits growth at the epiphyseal cartilages. Consequently, boys who begin producing testosterone earlier in life than others are often shorter.

14. Members of boys choirs in Europe during recent centuries were subjected to castration to preserve their high voices. This barbaric practice is no longer continued.

15. During development, each testes "follows" a connective tissue proper cord termed the gubernaculum. The reason is not clear. However, it does appear to involve more than a simple traction mechanism.

16. A scrotal location allows them to remain a few degrees cooler than the core body temperature. The lowered temperature is necessary for spermatogenesis.

17. They will never make it on their own because they change directions frequently. Considerable peristaltic assistance from female viscera is necessary.

18. The bulbourethral gland secretion cleanses the urethra and lubricates the glans penis prior to intromission. The prostate secretions are alkaline and contain buffers to neutralize the acid environment of the vagina. Citric acid and phosphates serve as nutritional sources. The major nutritional source, however, appears to be fructose secreted by the seminal vesicles. Other substances secreted by the prostate and bulbourethral glands like prostaglandins, fibrinolysin, fibrinogen, clotting enzyme, *etc.* have specific roles as well.

19. They don't. Most men are fertile until death. However, impotence is often a nuisance in older men.

20. Interstitial cells produce testosterone (responsible for libido and male secondary sex characteristics). The spermatogenic series of cells include spermatogonia, primary and secondary spermatocytes, spermatids and sperm which represent various stages in the formation of male sex cells. The sustentacular cells are support cells for the spermatogenic cells.

21. Yes, but only for a few days because few sperm are "stored" in the ductus deferens distal to the transection site. Vasectomies can sometimes be surgically reversed.

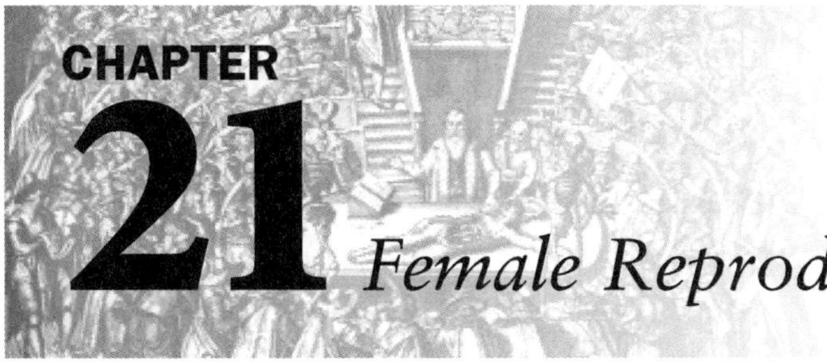

CHAPTER 21 Female Reproductive System

Chapter Outline and Key Concepts

INTRODUCTION

The female reproductive system includes the ovaries, uterine tubes, uterus, vagina, and the vulva (pudendum femininum).

FUNCTIONS

Functions of the female reproductive system involve oogenesis and ovulation, production of female sex hormones, copulation and fertilization, protection and nourishment of the developing conceptus, and parturition.

OVARY

The ovaries are located below the kidneys in the posterior part of the abdominal cavity.

Within the ovarian parenchyma, developing ova surrounded by other cells are called ovarian follicles.

At ovulation, an ovum and some of the surrounding follicular cells break through the tunica albuginea and visceral peritoneum on the ovarian surface and enter the ovarian bursa (a subdivision of the peritoneal cavity).

OOGENESIS

Cell divisions leading to the formation of female sex cells called ova is termed oogenesis.

In the first meiotic division, a primary oocyte (2N) divides unequally to form a secondary oocyte (N) and a vestigial first polar body (N).

The second meiotic division of the secondary oocyte is arrested at metaphase pending fertilization.

OVARIAN CYCLE

As the most mature follicle prepares for ovulation, its estrogen output inhibits other maturing follicles and causes them to degenerate.

At ovulation, a tiny amount of hemorrhage occurs and the blood laden empty follicle is called the corpus hemorrhagicum.

Follicular cells that remain in situ after ovulation begin producing progesterone, assume a yellow color, and are collectively termed the corpus luteum.

If fertilization does not occur, the corpus luteum regresses after a few days, and the falling progesterone level causes sloughing of the endometrium termed menstruation.

Scar tissue deposited in a degenerating corpus luteum forms a corpus albicans.

Within a few days of mensis, another follicle matures and the ovarian cycle repeats.

The ovarian cycle is hormonally interrupted by pregnancy, age, and sometimes periodically during times of severe emotional or physical stress.

UTERINE TUBES

The 2.5 inch long uterine tubes transport ovulated ova from the ovary to the uterus and serve as the usual site of fertilization.

The expandable, open end of the uterine tube almost completely surrounds the ovary and (usually) captures ova released from it.

Ova are transported toward the uterus by ciliary action in 1–2 days.

UTERUS

The uterus houses the conceptus during gestation and forces it out of the body at term.

Divided into a cervix, body, fundus, and two horns, the non-pregnant uterus is quite small.

The uterine wall has three layers from without inward: perimetrium (visceral peritoneum), myometrium, and a mucosal lining called endometrium.

Physiologically, the endometrium cycles through three

phases: menstrual phase (first 3-5 days), proliferative phase (up to ovulation at day 14) and secretory phase (the two weeks prior to the next menstruation).

BROAD LIGAMENT AND VESSELS OF THE FEMALE REPRODUCTIVE SYSTEM

The double-layered, connecting peritoneum that suspends the uterus, uterine tubes, and ovaries is called the broad ligament of the uterus and is divided into mesometrium, mesosalpinx, and mesovarium.

Three pairs of arteries (ovarian, uterine, vaginal) supply the female reproductive viscera.

VAGINA

The vagina receives the penis during sexual intercourse and serves as part of the birth canal at parturition.

Folds in the lining of the wall, called vaginal rugae, allow linear expansion during coitus and parturition.

PUDENDUM FEMININUM (VULVA)

Vulva encompasses all female external (or nearly external) genitalia including the mons pubis, labia, vaginal vestibule, vestibular bulbs, vestibular glands, and clitoris.

The clitoris resembles a small penis complete with glans and two erectile bodies but the urethra does not pass through it.

The labia majora pudendi are folds of skin on either side of the genital opening (rima pudendi).

DEVELOPMENT OF REPRODUCTIVE SYSTEMS

The gonads of both sexes develop from tissue called urogenital ridges.

In males, primitive mesonephric ducts become the efferential ducts, epididymis, and ductus deferens on each side.

In females, primitive paramesonephric ducts form the uterine tubes, uterus, and vagina.

The external genitalia in both sexes develop from mesodermal (cloacal) folds which fuse anteriorly to eventually form the genital tubercle.

The genital tubercle becomes penis (male) or clitoris (female) and the folds behind it become the labia majora pudendi (female) or fuse to form the scrotum in males.

CLINICAL CONSIDERATIONS

Permanent sterilization can be effected by tubal ligation.

Ovarian cysts develop when follicles mature but don't ovulate.

PMS (pre-menstrual syndrome) encompasses behavioral/emotional changes that are associated with the ovarian cycle.

Hysterectomy is surgical removal of the uterus.

Selected Definitions

Amenorrhea—absence of menstrual periods. This can be caused by prepubescence, pregnancy, menopause, stress, low body weight, hormonal imbalances, and certain traumatic injuries.

Broad ligament—the double layer of peritoneum that suspends the female reproductive viscera within the abdominal cavity. Its subdivisions, (mesovarium, mesosalpinx, mesometrium) support the ovary, uterine tube, and uterus, respectively.

Cervix of the uterus—the narrow, constricted portion of the uterus at its inferior aspect. The cervical canal within it joins the uterine lumen to the vaginal lumen and markedly dilates at parturition.

Corpus luteum—a yellow-colored mass of cells in an ovary representing follicular cells left behind after a recent ovulation. These produce progesterone for a few months if fertilization occurs, but only for a few days if it does not.

Corpus albicans—the small scar formed by proliferation of connective tissue proper at the site of an involuting corpus luteum. Accumulation of corpora albicantes after years of ovarian cycling is a factor in menopause.

Cystic ovary (polycystic ovary)—an ovary containing multiple cysts. These typically result from follicles which mature but do not ovulate and often cause hormonal imbalances which interfere with normal ovarian cycling.

Endometriosis—aberrant proliferation of endometrial-like tissue. When it occurs within the uterus it is called *endometriosis interna* or *adenomycosis*. Elsewhere it is sometimes termed *endometriosis externa*.

First polar body—the smaller cell resulting from uneven cytokinesis at the end of the first meiotic division of oogenesis. It serves as a repository for 23 chromosomes and its scant allotment of cytoplasm dictates that it has no further biological future.

Hymen—the fold of mucous membrane which commonly narrows the opening of the vagina in virginal females. Sometimes it completely occludes the vaginal opening (imperforate hymen).

Hysterectomy—surgical removal of the uterus. This is typically indicated by neoplasia or intractable endometriosis interna.

Menarche—the first menstrual period in a young female. This signals puberty and marks the onset of adolescence.

Myometrium—the middle and thickest of the three layers of the uterine wall. Smooth muscle tissue within it contracts to expel the fetus at (or sometimes before) the end of gestation.

Oogenesis—the process of sex cell formation in females. It begins with stem cells called oogonia and progresses through primary and secondary oocytes, but does not reach its final stage (definitive ovum) unless fertilization occurs.

Ovulation—the process wherein a mature ovum (secondary oocyte) and a few accompanying follicular cells (corona radiata) leave the ovary. They must penetrate the tunica albuginea of the ovary and the visceral peritoneum coating the ovary.

Salpingitis—inflammation of the uterine tubes. It is usually caused by infectious organisms and often results in temporary or permanent sterility.

Tubal ligation—the common form of permanent sterilization in females. It may be accomplished by constricting, severing, or crushing the uterine tubes, which renders them ineffective in transporting sperm and ova.

Uterine tube ("fallopian tube," "oviduct")—the small tubular channel, a few centimeters long, that joins the ovarian bursa (surrounding the ovary) to the uterine horn. It transports ova toward the uterus, sperm toward the ovary, and serves as the usual site of fertilization.

Vesicular ovarian follicle—a maturing ovarian follicle containing a fluid-filled cavity (antrum). These have also been called "graafian", "secondary", and "tertiary" follicles.

Vestibular bulbs—the erectile bodies in the wall of the vaginal vestibule. These develop from the same primordia as the corpus spongiosum of the penis in males.

Vulva (pudendum femininum)—a term encompassing all of the external (or nearly external) female reproductive structures. These include the major and minor labia pudendi, clitoris, vestibular bulbs, mons pubis, vestibular glands, and the vaginal vestibule.

Zona pellucida—the thick, halo-like layer of protein/polysaccharide that encases a secondary oocyte at ovulation. Penetration of this layer by a sperm requires enzymes contained in its acrosome.

Etymology ***Dex femina facti*—"A woman was the leader in the deed."**

antrum (L), *cave*—antrum
bursa (L), *bag, purse*—bursa
cervix (L), *neck*—cervix
corona (L), *garland, crown*—corona radiata
cumulus (L), *heap*—cumulus
ektopos (G), *away from a place*—ectopic
fimbria (L), *fringe*—fimbriae
heme (G), *blood*—corpus hemorrhagicum
hymen (G), *membrane*—hymen
hystera (G), *womb*—hysterectomy
luteus (L), *yellow*—corpus luteum
oophoron (L), *ovary*—oophrons
ovum (L), *egg*—ovum
primo (L), *first*—primordial
pudere (L), *to be ashamed*—pudendum
radiare (L), *to emit rays*—corona radiata
rrhagia (G), *to break, burst*—corpus hemorrhagicum
uterus (L), *womb*—uterus
vagina (L), *sheath, vagina*—vagina
vulva (L), *covering*—vulva

Introduction

The female reproductive system is one of the five visceral body systems. It includes the ovaries, uterine tubes, uterus, vagina, and the vulva—a collective term (equivalent to pudendum femininum) that encompasses all of the external (or nearly external) female genitalia (Figure 21-1). Like its male counterpart, the female reproductive system is not vital to sustain the life of an individual but it is necessary for the continuation of the species.

Objectives

1. List the major components of the female reproductive system in the order that they are encountered by an ovum.

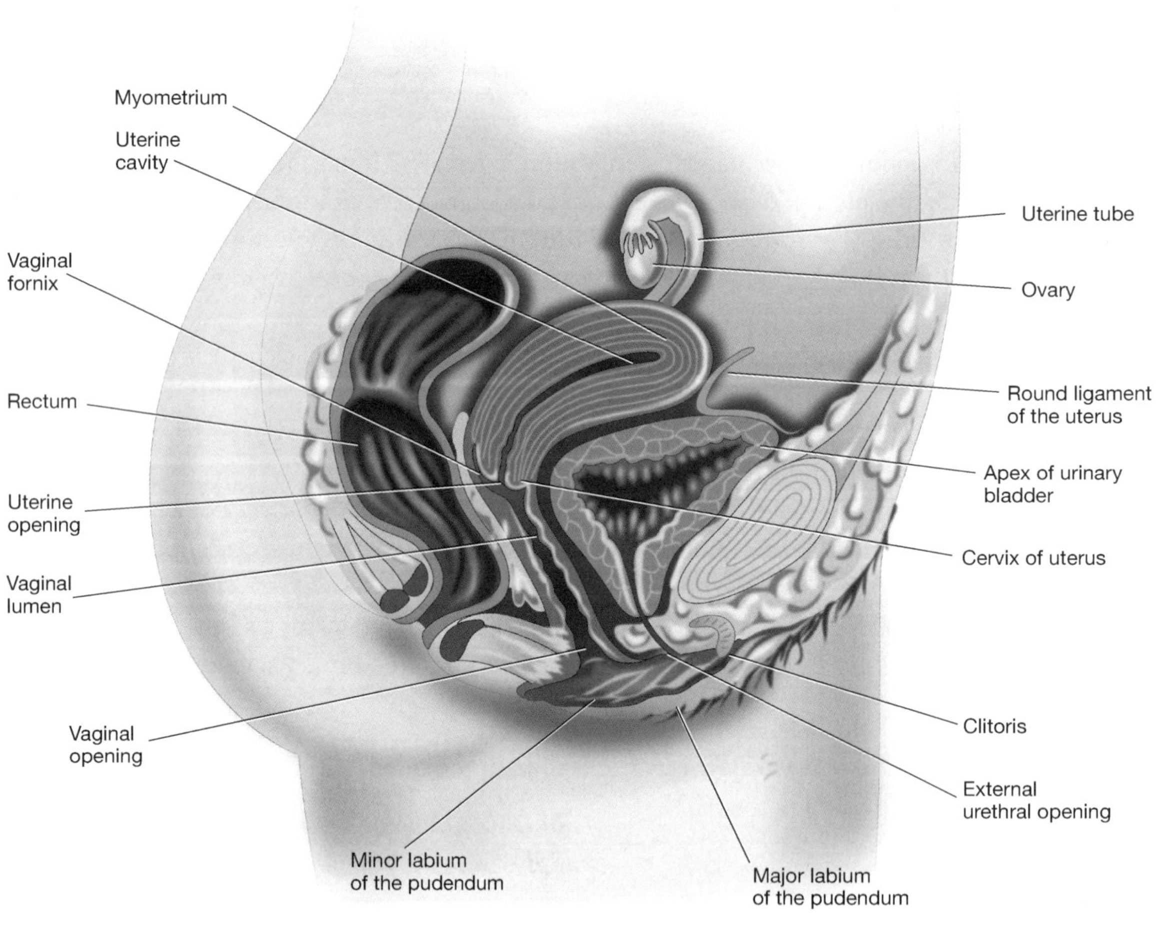

Figure 21-1

Female Reproductive Organs (Midsagittal Section)

The major components of the female reproductive system are the ovaries, uterine tubes, uterus, vagina, and several structures grouped collectively as the vulva (pudendum femininum). Included in the latter are the vaginal vestibule, vestibular bulbs, vestibular glands, clitoris, minor and major labia of the pudendum, and the mons pubis.

Functions

There are five major functions of the female reproductive system:

1. **Production of female sex cells** (ova) through meiotic cell division called oogenesis. Only a few hundred (400±) ova are ovulated during a female's lifetime (even fewer in individuals with large numbers of children).
2. **Production of female sex hormones**, especially estrogen and progesterone. Estrogen is the female counterpart of testosterone and is produced by the granulosa cells of developing follicles. It is responsible for the development of female secondary sex characteristics (thinner skin, different distribution of body fat and hair, *etc.*). Progesterone is the hormone produced by the corpus luteum of the ovary. It is often called the "hormone of pregnancy" since it keeps the uterine lining in a state conducive to pregnancy.
3. **Copulation and fertilization**. The vagina receives the penis of the male during sexual intercourse and serves as a depository for semen during ejaculation. The sperm are then transported through the uterus to the uterine tube(s) wherein they normally contact the ovum (ova).
4. **Protection and nutrition of the developing conceptus**. After fertilization in the uterine tube, the zygote continues to the uterus wherein it resides and develops until the termination of pregnancy.
5. **Transmission of the fetus**. At parturition, the fetus normally passes through the "birth canal" formed by the cervical canal and the vagina, and then emerges from the female reproductive system at the vulva.

Objectives

2. List five general functions of the female reproductive system.

Ovary

The left and right **ovaries** are located below the kidneys in the posterior part of the abdominal cavity. The lateral end of the ovary is oriented toward the uterine tube and is termed the **tubal extremity**. The medial end is adjacent to the uterus and is called the **uterine extremity**. This end of each ovary is attached to the lateral margin of the uterus by a cord in the broad ligament of the uterus called the **proper ligament of the ovary.** The tubal extremity of the ovary is suspended by a part of the broad ligament of the uterus termed the **suspensory ligament of the ovary.** Each ovary is an ovoid structure about 3.5 cm long and is covered with a layer of visceral peritoneum. Deep to the peritoneum is a dense layer of connective tissue proper termed the **tunica albuginea**. The parenchyma of the ovary is indistinctly divided into an **ovarian cortex** and **medulla**. Concentrated near the cortex are numerous developing **follicles** in various stages of maturity (Figure 21-2). Each ovarian follicle consists of a **developing ovum** surrounded by numerous cells termed **follicular epithelium (granulosa cells)**. These cells produce estrogen. Four major stages of follicular development are recognized: primordial, primary, secondary, and vesicular (tertiary). **Primordial ovarian follicles** consist of a developing ovum surrounded by a single layer of flattened follicular cells. With time, some of these progress to become **primary ovarian follicles**. These consist of a developing ovum surrounded by one or more layers of cuboidal (or even columnar) follicular cells. These are surrounded by a sheath of stromal cells termed the theca. As the primary follicles mature and become **secondary ovary follicles**, they develop a fluid-filled space called the **follicular antrum** (Figure 21-3). The developing ovum surrounded by several layers of follicular cells termed the **cumulus oophorus** projects into this antrum. As the secondary follicles mature into tertiary ovarian follicles, the layers of follicular cells immediately surrounding the ovum are termed the **corona radiata** and they are separated from it by a homogeneous membrane-like structure termed the **zona pellucida**. The latter is formed by microvilli of the oocyte, cellular processes of the follicular cells and an intervening basement membrane-like substance formed of glycoprotein. When ovulation occurs, the ovum, zona pel-

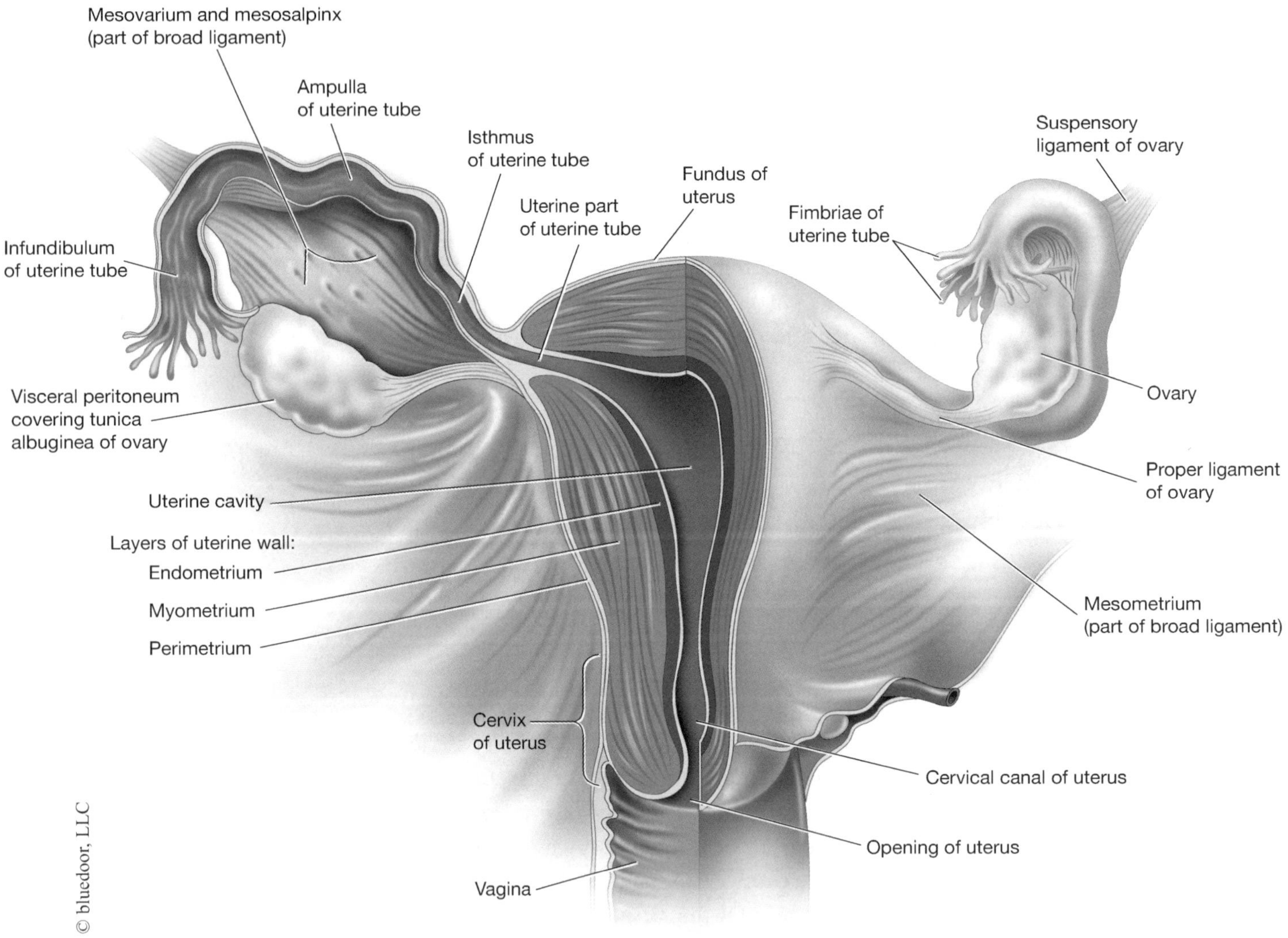

Figure 21-2

Ovaries, Uterine Tubes, and Uterus

Unlike their male homologues, the ovaries remain in the abdominal cavity and are covered by visceral peritoneum. The uterine tubes are each divided into four segments: infundibulum (which partially surrounds the ovary), ampulla, isthmus, and uterine part (buried within the ipsilateral horn of the uterus). The uterus is divided into a main part (body), two horns, a fundus, and the cervix (neck). The uterine wall has three named layers with the myometrium (middle layer) being the thickest. Part of the lining layer is sloughed in a cycling female to form menstrual flow.

lucida, and corona radiata break through the tunica albuginea and visceral peritoneum on the ovarian surface and enter a subdivision of the peritoneal cavity called the **ovarian bursa**.

Objectives

3. Diagram and label a vesicular (mature) ovarian follicle.

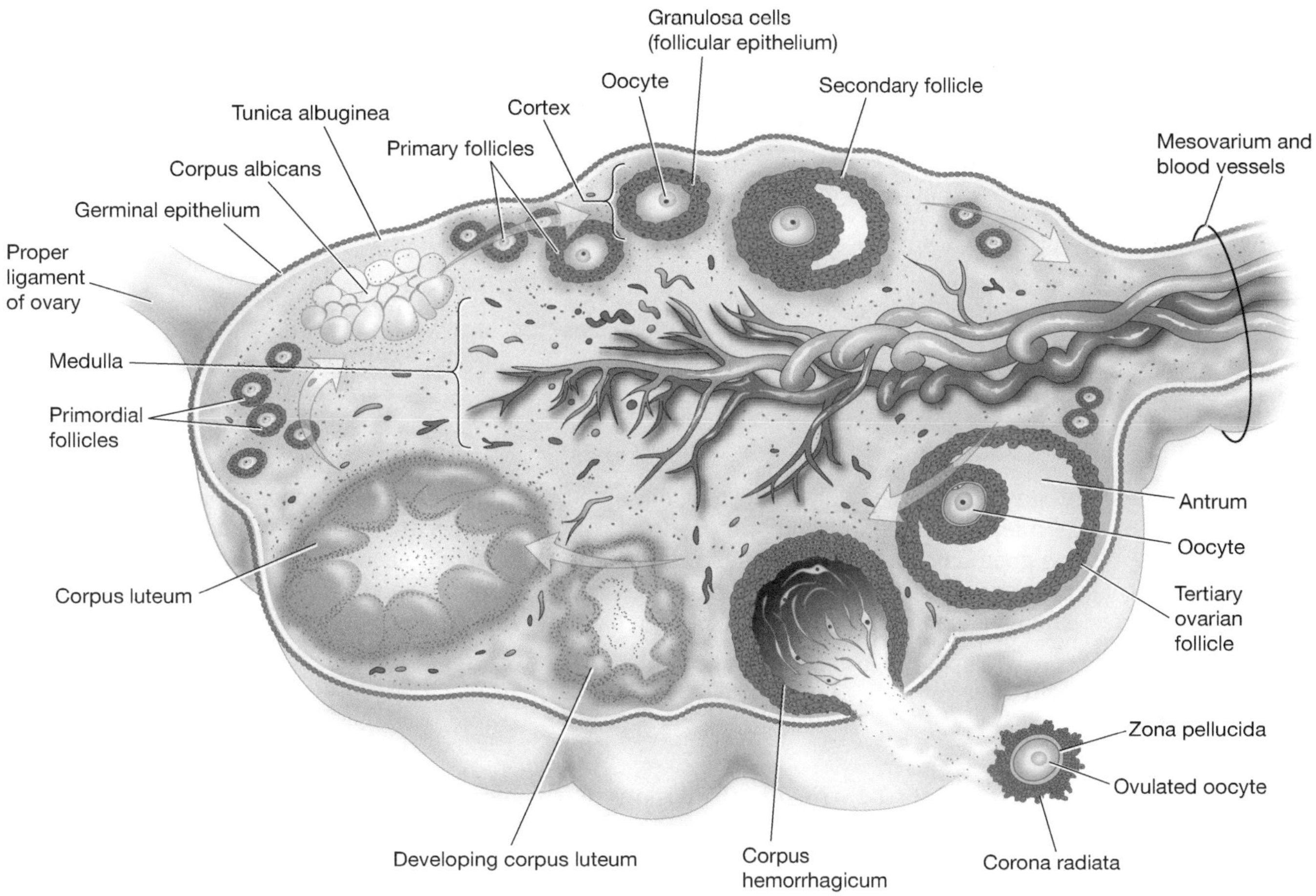

Figure 21-3

The Ovarian Cycle

Developing ova and the surrounding follicular (granulosa) cells are called ovarian follicles. Four stages of follicular development are recognized: primordial, primary, secondary, and tertiary. The follicular cells in tertiary follicles (often called "Graffian" or "mature" follicles) produce high levels of estrogen which facilitates ovulation. When ovulation occurs, the ovum and some surrounding follicular cells (collectively called the corona radiata) penetrate through the surface of the ovary into the peritoneal cavity where they are "captured" by the expanded, open end of the uterine tube. Hemorrhage in the follicular antrum from which ovulation just occurred forms the corpus hemorrhagicum. Follicular cells left behind turn yellow under the influence of luteinizing hormone from the hypophysis and form the progesterone producing corpus luteum. The corpus luteum eventually involutes to form a corpus albicans. Note: the various stages of follicular development do not migrate (move) around in the ovary. The arrows indicate various stages of development rather than changing locations.

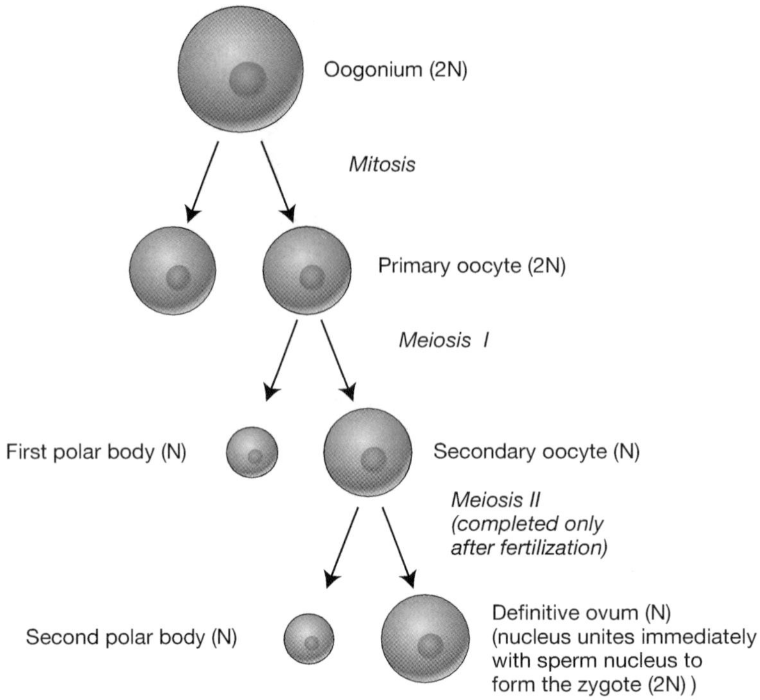

Figure 21-4
Oogenesis

Oogonia are formed only during the early months of gestational development. Mitosis of a few hundred thousand of these form primary oocytes. This is as far as oogenesis goes until puberty when these continue to develop into secondary oocytes (typically one at a time) within the tertiary (vesicular) follicles. Secondary oocytes are ovulated and complete their second meiotic division when (and only if) fertilized.

Oogenesis

Oogenesis encompasses the series of cell divisions in which the female primitive germ cells are converted to viable female sex cells capable of being fertilized by a sperm. The primitive sex cells are derived from endoderm which migrates into the ovaries during early embryonic development. These divide mitotically for a few months to form several million cells called **oogonia**. When this division stops, no new oogonia are produced. Near the end of gestation, the oogonia in the fetal ovaries begin meiosis and are called **primary oocytes** (Figure 21-4). Their division is arrested at prophase of the first meiotic division and newborn baby girls have about 350,000 of these in their ovaries contained within primordial follicles. At puberty some primordial follicles are hormonally stimulated to enlarge by gonadotropins to become primary follicles by the addition of several layers of follicular cells. A few of the primary follicles become vesicular follicles. The primary oocyte in a vesicular follicle completes its first meiotic division to form two dimorphic cells: a large **secondary oocyte** and a smaller **first polar body** which subsequently degenerates. The secondary oocyte then enters its second meiotic division and is arrested at metaphase until (unless) fertilization occurs (*see Chapter 22*).

Objectives

4. Schematically diagram and label oogenesis.

Ovarian Cycle

For reasons not totally understood but hormonally induced, only one ovarian follicle normally completes its development each month. This occurs 10-14 days after the onset of menstruation. Other follicles that are near maturation at that point regress and become atretic (degenerative). When the secondary oocyte and corona radiata cells break through the ovarian surface at **ovulation**, a small amount of hemorrhage occurs and the "empty" follicle at this stage is called a **corpus hemorrhagicum**. The follicular and thecal cells left behind soon form a yellow-colored **corpus luteum** which is 10-15 mm in diameter. The latter produces some estrogen and especially high levels of progesterone. Progesterone is known as the "hormone of pregnancy." If fertilization does not occur, the corpus luteum regresses after a few days to eventually form a white connective tissue proper structure termed the **corpus albicans**. The latter produces no hormones and is essentially a "scar." If fertilization does occur, chorionic gonadotropin produced by the developing placenta causes the corpus luteum to persist for 5-6 months, after which it regresses to the corpus albicans stage. When a woman reaches middle age, she ceases to ovulate and the loss of the monthly estrogen and progesterone peaks causes a cessation of menstruation. This is termed **menopause**.

Objectives

5. Discuss the ovarian cycle including ovulation; the sequential appearance of corpus hemorrhagicum, corpus luteum, and corpus albicans; and the hormonal changes that lead to menstruation.

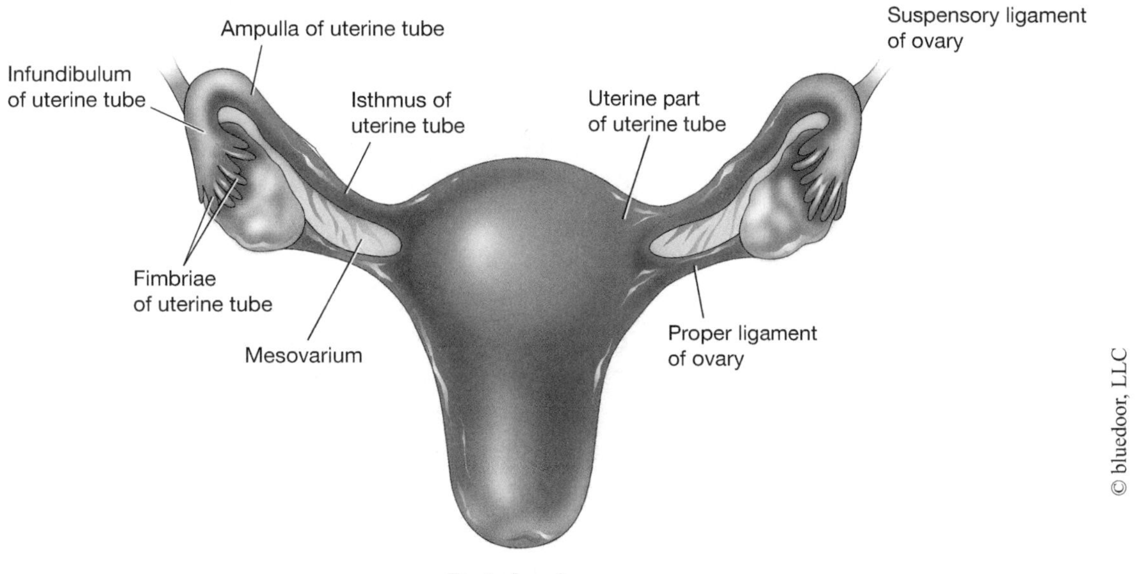

Figure 21-5

Parts of the Uterine Tube

The four parts of a uterine tube are labeled. Ciliated cells within its lining mucosa "sweep" ova toward the uterus. It takes about two days for this to occur even though the total distance is only about 7 cm. Since ova degenerate beyond fertilization in about 48 hours, fertilization nearly always occurs in the uterine tube rather than in the uterus. Sperm are small enough that peristalsis moves them up the uterine tube (between the cilia) at the same time that ova are being "ciliated" in the opposite direction.

Uterine Tubes

The **uterine tubes** (once called "Fallopian" tubes or "oviducts") form a tubular passageway from the ovaries to the uterus (Figure 21-1, 5). Each is about 7 cm long and 0.7 cm in diameter. The ovarian end of the uterine tube is enlarged and almost completely surrounds the ovary. This portion of the uterine tube is called the **infundibulum** and its opening is fringed with tiny finger-like projections termed the **fimbriae of the uterine tube**. At ovulation, the ovum (secondary oocyte) breaks free from the ovary and enters the space between the ovary and the surrounding infundibulum. This small space is a subdivision of the peritoneal cavity called the **ovarian bursa**. The ciliated lining of the infundibulum guides the ovum into the rest of the uterine tube where it is slowly transported to the uterus. The initial portion of the uterine tube beyond the infundibulum is called the **ampulla** of the uterine tube, the portion near the uterus is called the **isthmus** of the uterine tube and the part "buried" in the uterine wall is the **uterine part** of the uterine tube. In addition to transporting ova to the uterus, the uterine tubes transport sperm toward the ovary by peristaltic action and serve as the usual site of fertilization.

Objectives

6. State two unofficial names for the uterine tube and indicate its functions in reproduction.

Uterus

The **uterus** is the organ which houses the conceptus during gestation and plays an important functional role in expelling the fetus from the reproductive system at birth. It is located within the pelvis above the vagina and is positioned between the urinary bladder (anteriorly) and the terminal part of the large intestine (posteriorly). The non-pregnant ("**non-gravid**") uterus is surprisingly small with a length of about 7 cm, a thickness of about 2.5 cm, and a greatest width of about 5 cm. It is subdivided into body, fundus, left and right horns, and cervix (Figure 21-6, 7).

The **body of the uterus** is the main portion with the left and right **uterine horns** located superolaterally where the uterine tubes attach. The **fundus of the uterus** is the dome-like superior portion above the uterine tubes. The **cervix of the uterus** is the inferior constricted portion which joins the vagina. The **uterine cavity** narrows significantly at the **cervical canal** and opens into the vagina at the **uterine ostium**. Cervical glands within the wall of the cervical canal secrete a mucous plug during pregnancy which forms a barrier to protect the conceptus from ascending infections from the vagina.

The uterine wall has three layers: perimetrium, myometrium, and endometrium. The **perimetrium** is the serous membrane (visceral peritoneum) which invests the outer surface of the uterus. It reflects off each side of the uterus to become the doubled-layered **mesometrium** (part of the broad ligament). The **myometrium** is composed of several poorly defined layers of smooth muscle tissue. Some of this muscle tissue extends posteriorly from the uterus to join the rectum and form the recto-uterine muscle. The **endometrium** is the mucosal lining of the uterus. It is the only layer of the uterine wall that is involved in the menstrual cycle. If an egg is not fertilized after ovulation, the menstrual cycle begins in approximately two weeks. It is initiated by the falling levels of progesterone which occur as the corpus luteum regresses. The cycle has three parts: menstrual, proliferative, and secretory phases. The **menstrual phase** encompasses the first 3-5 days and is characterized by a bloody discharge caused by the sloughing endometrium. During the **proliferative phase** which continues to the time of ovulation (up to day 14±), the endometrial tissue regrows. The **secretory phase** occurs from ovulation until the next menstrual phase. During this period, the endometrium increases its vascularity and glandular secretions in preparation for a (potential) pregnancy. The first menstrual cycle is called **menarche**.

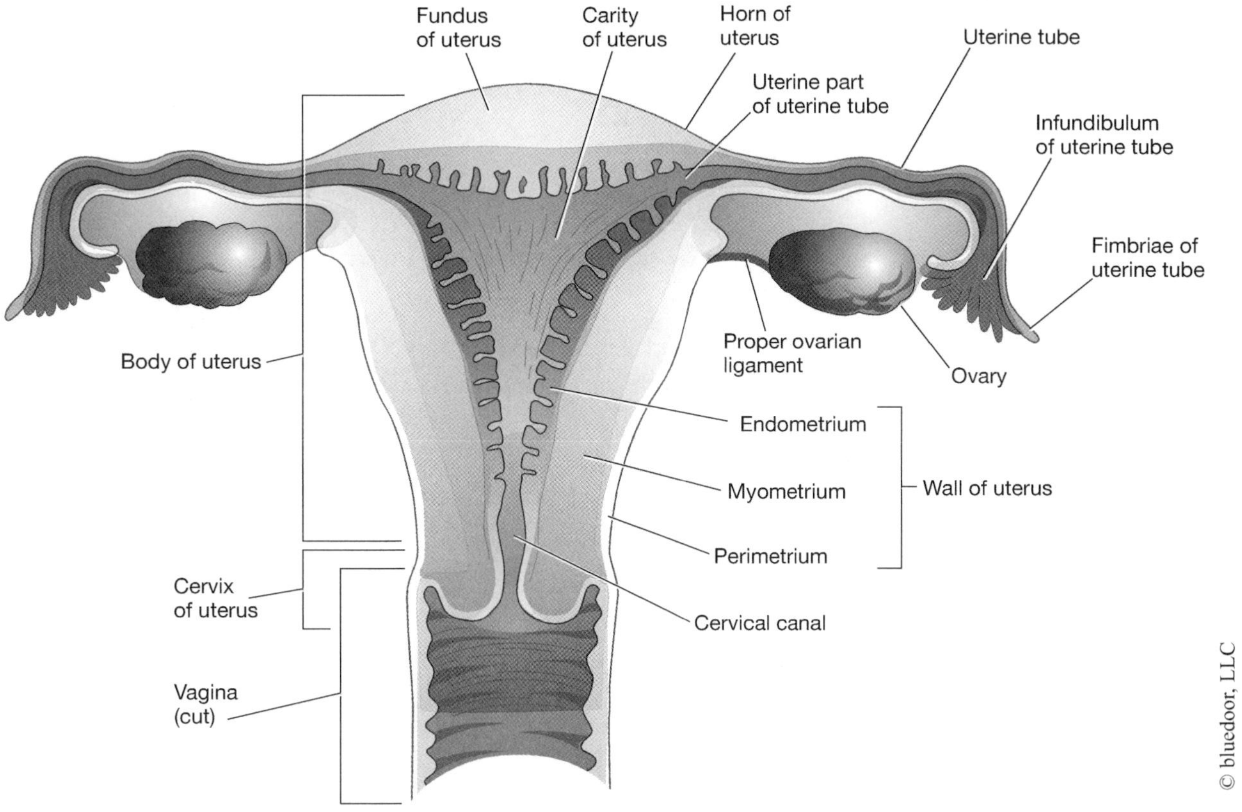

Figure 21-6
Uterus

The uterus is divided regionally into a body, fundus, cervix, and two horns. The uterine wall consists of three named layers which surround the uterine cavity.

Objectives

7. Define the three layers of the uterine wall and diagram the major landmarks of the uterus.

Broad Ligament and Vessels of the Female Reproductive System

The **broad ligament of the uterus** is the double-layered connecting peritoneum that supports the female reproductive system. It is regionally divided into mesometrium, mesosalpinx, and mesovarium. The **mesometrium** attaches to each side of the uterus and contains vestigial remnants of the

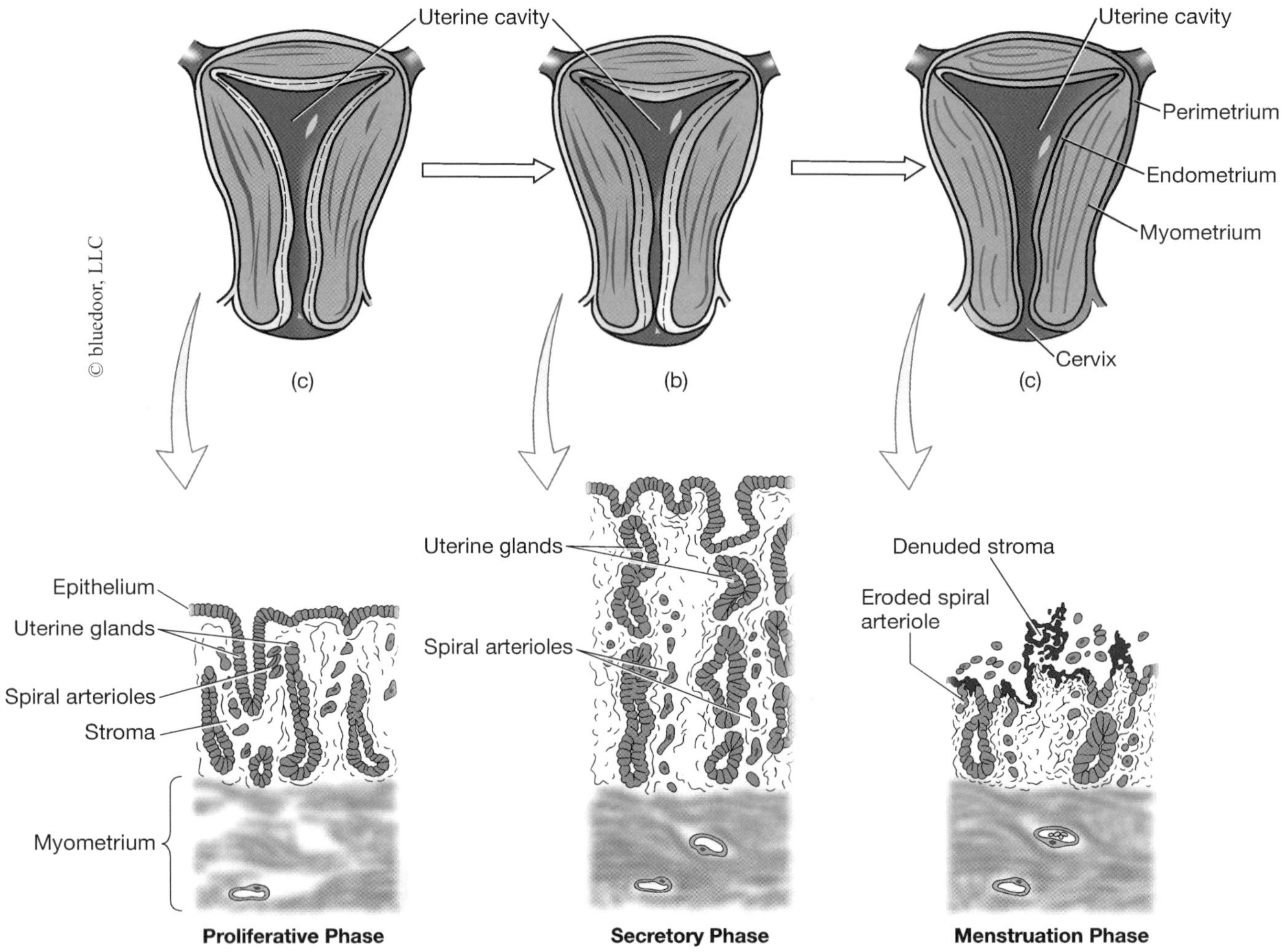

Figure 21-7

Changes in the Endometrium of a Cycling Female

Note that the endometrium is tremendously thickened in the secretory phase compared to the menstrual phase (c) or the proliferative phase (a).

left and right fetal **gubernacula** called **round ligaments** of the uterus. The **mesosalpinx** is the paired portion of the broad ligament that attaches to and supports the uterine tubes. It blends into the **mesovarium** which suspends the ovaries.

Three pairs of arteries supply the internal organs of the female reproductive system. The left and right **ovarian arteries** are direct branches of the aorta which course through the broad ligament to the ovaries. The left and right **uterine** and **vaginal arteries** originate from the internal iliac arteries and course through the broad ligament to the uterus and vagina. The uterine tubes are supplied by tiny anastomotic branches joining the ovarian and uterine arteries. Venous channels parallel all of these arteries.

Objectives

8. Differentiate the peritoneal structures that suspend the internal female reproductive organs.

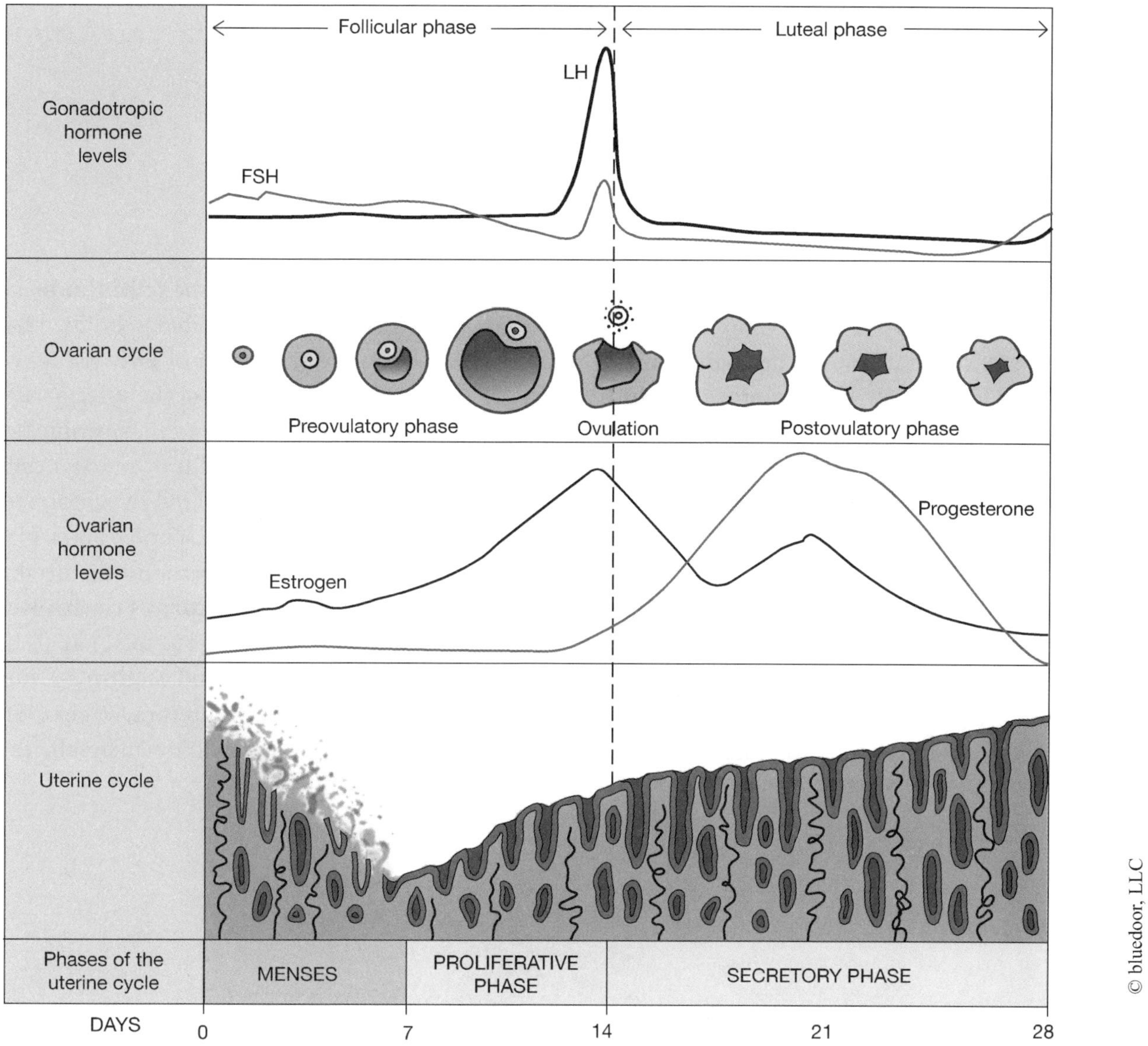

Figure 21-8

Cycling Hormone Levels, Follicles, and Uterine Endometrium

The bottom part of the diagram shows the histology of the uterine lining in different phases of the monthly cycle.

Vagina

The **vagina** receives the penis during sexual intercourse and serves as part of the birth canal at parturition. It is a tubular organ about 10 cm in length. The lining mucosa of the vaginal lumen has transverse folds termed **vaginal rugae** which allow linear expansion during coitus and parturition. The cervix of the uterus protrudes slightly into the lumen of the vagina forming a blind recessed area called the **vaginal fornix** (*see Figure 21-1*). Externally, the vaginal lumen opens into the vaginal vestibule at the **vaginal opening**. The **hymen** is a membrane which extends over much of the vaginal opening. In rare cases, the hymen forms a complete seal and surgical intervention may be required to allow drainage of menstrual fluids. During the first coitus, the hymen is stretched and sometimes torn.

Objectives

9. Differentiate vaginal lumen and vaginal cavity.

Pudendum Femininum (Vulva)

The external genitalia of the female are collectively called the **pudendum femininum** (**vulva**) (Figure 21-9). Included are the mons pubis, labia, vaginal vestibule, vestibular bulbs, vestibular glands, and clitoris. The **mons pubis** is the prominence caused by the pad of fatty tissue over the pubic crest. The **labia majora pudendi** are the left and right folds of skin on the inferior aspect of the trunk. They are joined at the anterior and posterior labial commissures and the opening between them is called the **rima pudendi**. Within this opening are left and right folds of mucosa called the **labia minora pudendi**. The anterior aspects of the labia minora extend around the clitoris to form its prepuce. The **clitoris** is the female homologue of the penis. It has crura, a body, and a glans clitoridis homologous to its male counterparts (Figure 21-9) but does not surround the urethra and has no corpus spongiosum. The erectile body within each crus is called the **corpus cavernosum clitoridis**. Physical stimulation of the clitoris leads to the pleasurable sensations termed female orgasm or climax. In some cultures the clitoris is (barbarically) removed. The **vaginal vestibule** is the space posterior to the clitoris and between the labia minora into which the urethra, vagina, and the vestibular glands open. The major and minor **vestibular glands** produce fluid which lubricates the

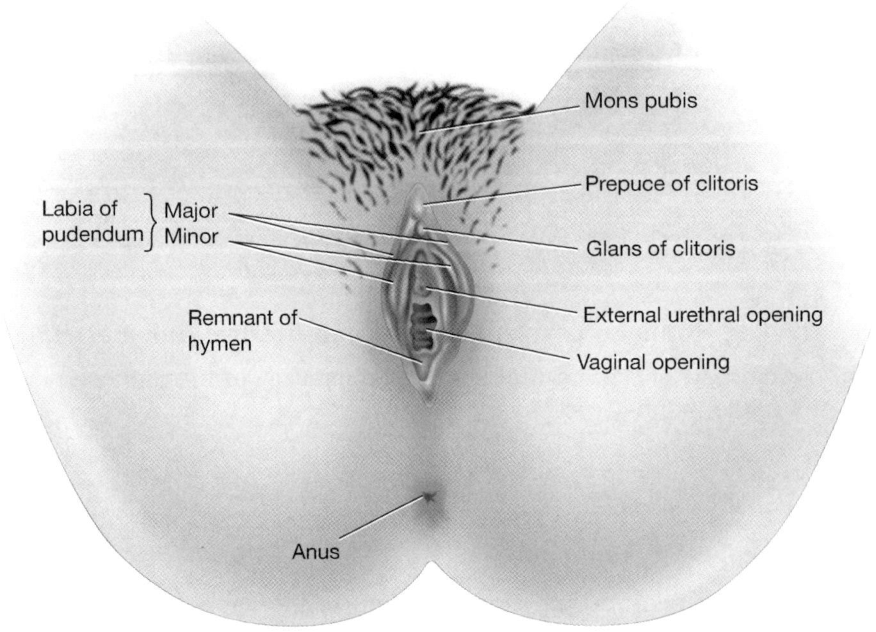

Figure 21-9

External Female Genitalia

The major labia of the pudendum are skin folds and the space between them is called the rima pudendi. The minor labia are folds of mucous membrane and the space between them forms the vaginal vestibule into which the vagina, urethra, and vestibular glands open.

vulva prior to intromission. The **vestibular bulbs** are left and right bodies of erectile tissue which are embedded in the walls of the vestibule. They engorge with blood during sexual intercourse.

Objectives

10. List the structures included in the vulva (pudendum femininum).

Development of the Reproductive Systems

Although the sex of an individual is determined at the time of fertilization (due to the gametes, one from each parent), the gonads are not distinguishable as male or female until the seventh week. They develop from the same (left and right) **urogenital ridges** that give rise to the kidneys (*see Chapter 19*). The **primordial germ cells** appear at about 21 days within the wall of the yolk sac (one of the extra-embryonic membranes). They then migrate into the mesoderm of the urogenital ridges where they are surrounded by groups of cells called **primitive sex cords**. The resulting structure (primordial sex cells surrounded by primitive sex cords within the urogenital ridge) is called an **indifferent gonad** because it cannot be distinguished as testis or ovary (Figure 21-10).

If the embryo is male, the indifferent gonad undergoes metamorphosis to become a testis. This involves a number of changes in which the primordial sex cells become **spermatogonia** and some of the surrounding cells become **sustentacular cells**. The cord-like structures made up of these two cell types become the seminiferous tubules of the definitive testis, but no lumen is present in the center of the tubule and no spermatogenesis occurs until sexual maturity. The mesodermal cells surrounding the developing seminiferous tubules become the **interstitial** (testosterone producing) **cells**.

If the embryo is female, the primordial sex cells break up into clusters which eventually form the **ovarian medulla**. The surface epithelium of the female gonad continues to proliferate (not so in males) and these cells invade the underlying mesoderm to form the **ovarian cortex**. These latter cells subsequently form the **oogonia** and the cells that surround them become **follicular cells**.

Male and female embryos develop two pairs of genital ducts: the **mesonephric** ("Wolffian") **duct** which extends from the mesonephros to the cloaca (*see Chapter 19*); and the **paramesonephric** ("Müllerian") **duct** which parallels the latter and also extends to the cloaca. In males, the mesonephric duct becomes the main genital duct (Figure 21-10). The paramesonephric duct degenerates except for vestiges which form the inconsequential appendix testis and the prostatic utricle. The most superior portion of the genital duct degenerates. However, the next portion forms the efferential ducts and the part immediately below becomes the epididymis. The remainder of the mesonephric duct becomes the ductus deferens which joins the urethra. In females, the paramesonephric duct forms the main genital duct. Its initial portion opens into the peritoneal cavity and forms the infundibulum and the rest of the uterine tube. The lower parts of the paramesonephric ducts unite to form the uterus and vagina.

The external genitalia in both sexes develop from a pair of mesodermal folds called **cloacal folds** (Figure 21-10). These fuse anteriorly to form a protuberance known initially as the **cloacal eminence** and later as the **genital tubercle**. Swellings occur on each side of the cloacal (genital) folds called **genital swellings**. With further development, the genital tubercle becomes the penis in males and the clitoris in females. In males the genital folds become known as **urethral folds** and they fuse

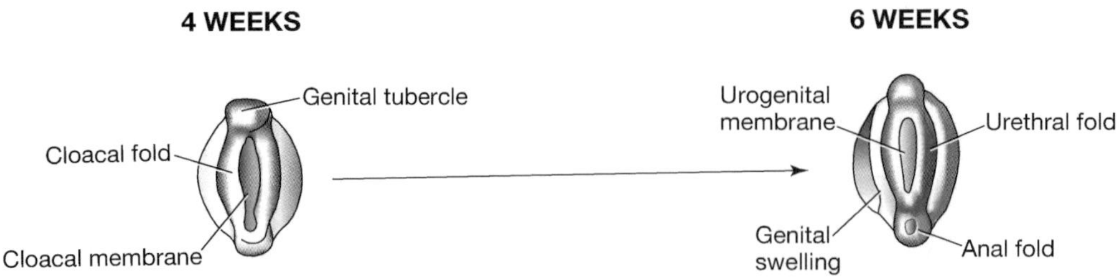

The genital tubercle, which forms the penis in the male, forms the clitoris in the female. The genital swellings on each side of the urethral folds differentiate into the major labia.

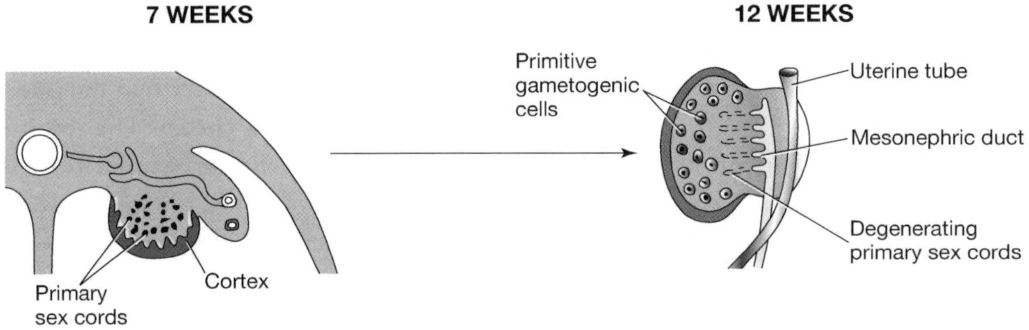

In females the primitive sex cords, which form the seminiferous tubules of males, degenerate. The primitive gametogenic cells migrate into the outer part of the urogenital ridge.

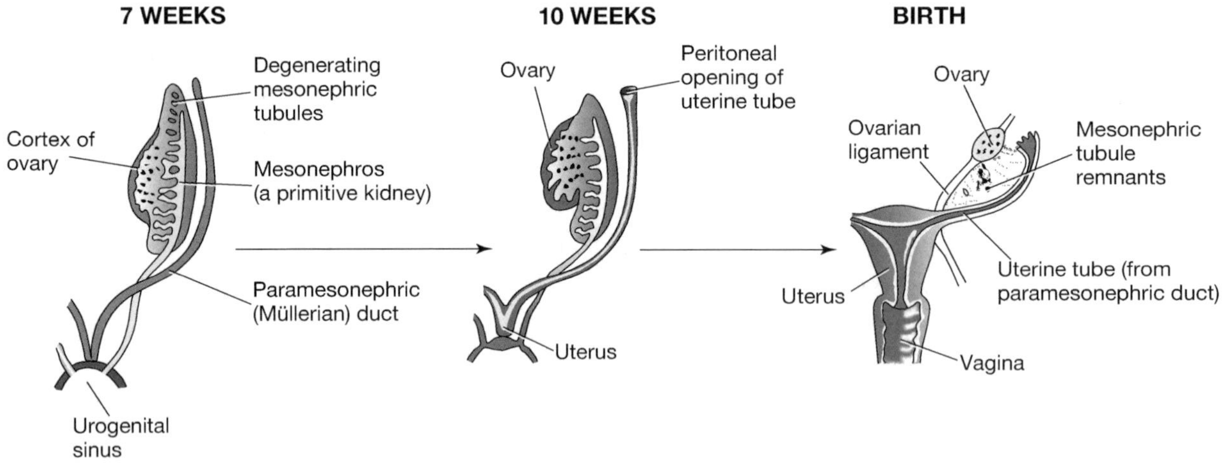

The paramesonephric ("Müllerian") ducts which develop near the mesonephric ducts, form the definitive uterine tubes. Where these unite, the uterus and vagina develop.

Figure 21-10

Development of the Female Reproductive System

on the underside of the penis to surround and enclose the urethral lumen. The genital swellings (just lateral to the genital folds) form the scrotum (*see Chapter 20*).

In females the genital tubercle elongates (less than in males) to form the clitoris. Instead of uniting to surround an extra-abdominal urethra, the genital folds remain separate as the labia minora. The open groove between them forms the vaginal vestibule. The genital swellings (located further laterally) enlarge to become the labia majora (Figure 21-10).

A summary of the developmental homologies between the male and female reproductive systems is presented in Table 21-1.

Table 21-1 Homologies of Male and Female Urogenital Organs

Because they both develop from the same primordia, male and female reproductive organs exhibit a large degree of homology. Some of these are obvious and some are more cryptic.

Male	***Female***
Testis	Ovary
Mesorchium	Mesovarium, mesosalpinx
Gubernaculum testis	Round ligament of the uterus
Prostatic urethra	Urethra
Membranous urethra	Vaginal vestibule
Penis	Clitoris
Prepuce of the penis	Prepuce of the clitoris
Corpus cavernosum penis	Corpus cavernosum clitoridis
Scrotum	Labium majus pudendi
Spongy urethra	Labium minus pudendi

Objectives

11. Indicate the homologies that exist between various components of the male and female reproductive systems.

Clinical Considerations

Ovarian tumors are not common in young women but **ovarian cysts** (enlarged follicles that fail to ovulate) occur relatively frequently. These usually spontaneously resolve, but in some cases they are surgically treated as a precautionary measure since they cannot be distinguished from neoplasms without histopathological examination. Permanent sterilization in women can be accomplished by ligating (tying off) the uterine tubes (**tubal ligation**). This procedure does not interfere with the ovarian cycle or menstruation. It simply blocks the uterine tubes and prevents fertilization. **Ectopic pregnancy** results from implantation of the blastocyst (*see Chapter 22*) in some location other than the uterus. The usual site is in a uterine tube (called a **tubal pregnancy**) where enlargement of the conceptus causes pain and its continued growth leads to rupture and hemorrhage. Surgical removal is usually performed to protect the individual. Abnormal menstrual cycles are relatively common problems involving the female reproductive system. Lack of cycles is termed **amenorrhea**. This is normal before puberty, during pregnancy, and after menopause, and it may also occur during periods of severe physical or emotional stress. Some women do not cycle while they are lactating (however, this has been repeatedly shown to be an unreliable method of birth control). **Dysmenorrhea** is painful menstruation characterized by severe menstrual cramps. Sometimes hormonal changes prior to menstruation cause physical and emotional changes and are collectively termed **pre-menstrual syndrome** (**PMS**). Excessive uterine bleeding is termed **menorrhagia**. Periodic hemorrhage between regular periods is called **metrorrhagia**. Removal of the uterus is called **hysterectomy** and is often indicated by uterine cancer. The ovaries are typically left in place to insure adequate natural levels of hormones. If the ovaries must be removed because of cancer or other disease, hormone replacement therapy is usually instituted. Proper positioning of the uterus in the pelvic cavity is necessary to prevent problems with fertility or parturition. Marked tilting (anterior/posterior) or prolapse (movement into the vagina) can also cause dysmenorrhea. Termination of pregnancy before seven months of gestation is termed abortion. **Spontaneous abortion** (**miscarriage**) often occurs when the mother or fetus is diseased. **Induced abortions** are intentional terminations of pregnancy. These raise significant issues of rights and morality. Inflammation of the vagina (**vaginitis**) or urinary bladder (cystitis) can occur from the trauma associated with frequent intercourse ("honeymoon disease") or from infectious organisms. The acidity of vaginal secretions prevents growth of most bacteria. Fungal infections from *Candida albicans* and protozoal infections from *Trichomonas vaginalis* are relatively common.

Endometriosis is a condition where endometrial-like tissue occurs in a non-uterine locus. Also called **endometriosis externa** or **adenomycosis externa**, this condition should not be confused with excessive proliferation of the uterine endometrium (*in situ*) which is called **endometriosis interna** or **adenomycosis**.

Objectives

12. Explain how an ectopic pregnancy can occur in a uterine tube and in the peritoneal cavity.
13. Differentiate amenorrhea, dysmenorrhea, PMS, menorrhagia, and metrorrhagia.

Clinical Case Studies

Case 1—A college sophomore complained of pelvic pain in association with unexplained cessation of menstrual cycles. Her last period had occurred six months earlier and she was not pregnant. Her physician monitored the woman's estrogen levels and found them to be quite high. Suggest a likely explanation for her symptoms.

Case 2—A young couple, married for five years, had been trying to conceive for the past 36 months. Frustrated, they sought medical advice. What are some of the general factors in infertility cases?

Case 3—A sexually active female body-builder, working out heavily for an upcoming competition, became concerned that she might be pregnant after missing two successive menses. A home pregnancy test kit failed to confirm pregnancy and she visited her physician for his advice. What might he have told her?

Points to Ponder

In most females, ovulation occurs once each lunar month. (Odd coincidence, that!) The ovaries taking alternating turns appear to be polite but in reality are controlled by estrogen concentrations. Estrogen is produced in very high levels by a mature follicle just prior to its ovulation and this same estrogen inhibits other follicles from entering the final throes of development. Due to higher concentrations of estrogen, this inhibitory effect is greater in the ovary of impending ovulation than in the contralateral one—hence the other ovary goes next. Some women can tell when they ovulate. They feel a twinge of pain when the ovarian surface ruptures and the ovum sallies forth, accompanied by a bunch of non-gametic friends that collectively make up the corona radiata. Body temperature elevations occur in association with ovulation, too. Couples experiencing conceptional difficulties are advised to chart her temperature rise and act accordingly—as though young people need encouragement!

The ovum is a large cell—big enough to see with the naked eye. It is the largest cell (in diameter) in the body. Unfertilized, it degenerates in a few days and is forgotten. Fertilized, it completes its second meiotic division, and after unceremoniously discarding unwanted genetic material in a second polar body, combines with the waiting sperm nucleus to form a zygote. (Males are taught to wait early on). Are zygotes alive? Certainly, but so are sperm, (although not for long once they leave home). To many biologists, the debate about when life begins is nonsensical—the self-righteous, uninformed arguing with the ignorant know-nots.

Wandering about in the peritoneal space around the ovary, the newly liberated (rejected?) ovum is induced, seduced, (fimbriated) into the enlarged, open end of Gabriele Fallopio's infamous tube. If this tube is bilaterally ligated ("tied"), the female is sterilized. Certain kinds of infections can cause scarring with the same end result. In the usual scenario, the ovum is slowly swept down the tube toward the uterus. It is here that it may meet those alien haploids that were recently deposited in the vagina. Peristalsed through the uterus and "up" the uterine tube, many of them will pass right by their objective, out the open end of the infundibulum and spend the next day exploring the peritoneal cavity without a flashlight. Like the boy digging through a pile of horse manure in search of the pony that surely must be there, they are ultimately disappointed.

Just as a balloon can only be pricked by one pin, the ovum can only be penetrated by one sperm. Chemical changes occur immediately that effectively block out additional suitors. ("Sorry boys, the position has been filled"). After her 23 chromosomes are pooled with his 23, the diploid honeymooner(s) spend(s) the next few blissful days becoming two, four, eight (you do the math) cells. Nutrition during this time is largely from that stored in her cytoplasm. That's one of the reasons why polar bodies are such pathetic little cells. Preparing for a several day fast, the developing ovum adopts a stingy, she-who-ends-up-with-the-most-cytoplasm-and-organelles-wins philosophy. One can criticize the morality here but it's hard to argue success!

Ova that are not fertilized degenerate and fail to implant in the uterus. When implantation does not occur, no placenta develops. With no placenta, there is no chorionic gonadotropin (CG). This hormone spills over in the urine causing the color change in the over-the-counter (do-it-yourself) home pregnancy test kits. The biological purpose of CG, however, is to encourage the cells of the corpus luteum to continue their production of progesterone. This is something they start to do right after ovulation but continue for only a few days unless they get the CG message to keep it up. Progesterone is necessary to keep the uterine lining compatible with pregnancy. Without sufficient quantities of progesterone, a spontaneous abortion will occur (in gravid uteri) or (if pregnancy has not occurred) the uterine lining will slough out to form the menstrual flow. In the procreative race of life, the false starts vastly outnumber the real ones.

Slang and Obsolete Nomenclature

UNOFFICIAL TERM	OFFICIAL DESIGNATION
cervix*	cervix of uterus *[cervix uteri]*
minor labium	minor labium of the pudendum *[labium minus pudendi]*
major labium	major labium of the pudendum *[labium majus pudendi]*
fallopian tube/oviduct	uterine tube *[tuba uterina]*
Bartholin's glands	major vestibular glands *[glandulae vestibulares majora]*
Graafian (secondary) follicle	vesicular follicle *[folliculi ovarici vesiculosi]*
vestibule	vaginal vestibule *[vestibulum vaginae]*
vaginal entrance	vaginal vestibule *[vestibulum vaginae]*
external orifice of cervix	opening of the uterus *[ostium uteri]*

* *Cervix* used alone refers to the anterior aspect of the neck.

Review Questions

1. Which of the following does not represent a part of the female reproductive system that a sperm might encounter?
   A. cervix
   B. vagina
   C. uterus
   D. uterine tube
   E. ovum

2. Which cell in the oogenic series is the first one with only 23 chromosomes in its nucleus?
   A. oogonia
   B. secondary oocyte
   C. second polar body
   D. primary oocyte
   E. definitive ovum

3. To reach the uterine tube, a secondary oocyte must pass through ...
   A. the tunica albuginea of the ovary and the uterine tube.
   B. visceral peritoneum and a synovial bursa.
   C. some connective tissue proper, a serous membrane, and a serous body cavity.
   D. the tunica albuginea of the ovary and a mucous membrane.
   E. the tunica albuginea of the ovary and the pleural cavity.

4. Which of the following would not affect the ovarian cycle?
   A. age
   B. pregnancy
   C. oral contraceptives
   D. sexual intercourse
   E. severe stress

5. Which statement is false concerning the uterine tubes?
   A. They are not part of the uterus.
   B. They serve as the usual site of fertilization.
   C. They are the most common site of ectopic pregnancies.
   D. They transport sperm "upstream" by ciliary action.
   E. They transport secondary oocytes toward the uterus and are sometimes called "fallopian" tubes.

6. The term vulva (pudendum femininum) does not include the ____________________.
   A. clitoris
   B. vagina
   C. vestibular bulb
   D. labia
   E. vestibular glands

7. Which set of male and female reproductive structures are not derived from the same primordia?
   A. penis—clitoris
   B. scrotum—labia majora pudendi
   C. gubernaculum testis—mesovarium
   D. spongy urethra—labia minora pudendi
   E. corpus spongiosum penis—vestibular bulbs

8. The clitoris resembles the penis structurally except that it ...
   A. has no prepuce.
   B. has no glans.
   C. does not surround the urethra.
   D. has no body.
   E. has no crura.

9. Which part of the uterus consists of serous membrane?
   A. endometrium
   B. broad ligament of the uterus
   C. myometrium
   D. perimetrium
   E. If more than one of the above satisfy the premise, choose this response.

10. Which part of the female reproductive system is mismatched with a function?
   A. ovary—oogenesis
   B. vagina—physical protection of developing conceptus
   C. uterus—parturition
   D. corpus albicans—production of progesterone
   E. If more than one of the above satisfy the premise, choose this response.

Thought Questions

1. What are the major differences in the processes of oogenesis *vs.* spermatogenesis?

2. Explain the statement... "sperm can be present in the vaginal lumen but not in the vaginal cavity."

3. At ovulation, usually only one secondary oocyte is released and the ovaries usually alternate (left-right-left-right) from month to month. What controls this?

4. What happens to sperm in the uterine tubes that don't fertilize ova?

5. Why is it necessary to add "of the uterus" when speaking of the female reproductive structure called the cervix?

6. Why does the uterine lining degenerate and slough each month in a cycling female (causing the menstrual flow)?

7. What roles do the uterine tubes play in the reproductive process?

8. In what ways is the clitoris similar to and different from the penis?

9. What female reproductive organ is homologous to the bulbourethral gland(s) of males?

10. In female sterilization via tubal ligation, why are the ovaries left in situ?

11. At ovulation, some of the follicular cells accompany the ovum as the corona radiata, but most of them remain behind in the ovary. What do these latter cells do next?

12. What differences should occur between normal ovaries from a 20 year-old woman *vs.* a 40 year-old?

13. Can ovulation be detected externally?

14. What is female circumcision?

15. What is the fate of the hymen?

16. Why aren't the mammary glands considered to be part of the female reproductive system?

17. What happens to unfertilized ova?

18. How does the uterine tube accomplish the remarkable feat of simultaneously transporting ova "downstream" and sperm "upstream"?

19. Fertility in females can be diminished by numerous problems including the fibrous proliferations called endometriosis, salpingitis, cystic ovaries, *etc.* How do each of these reduce fertility?

20. Compare and contrast the male and female reproductive systems in regard to their overall roles in the process of reproduction.

21. What can cause amenorrhea besides pregnancy, menopause, and prepubescence?

Answers to Clinical Case Studies

Case 1—High estrogen levels occur just prior to ovulation. Since this woman was not menstruating, it is likely that she suffered cystic ovaries. In this condition, follicles mature but fail to ovulate. This would explain both the high estrogen levels and the failure of menses.

Case 2—Infertility is usually related to no viable gametes or to a failure of these gametes to make physical contact. Fertility is easily evaluated in males by analysis of a semen sample where numbers, morphology, and motility of sperm can be evaluated. In females that are cycling normally, infertility is often related to previous infections which have caused scarring in the uterine tubes or to an abnormal positional relationship of the uterus relative to the vagina. If the uterus is tipped forward and down, for example, the passage of sperm into/through the uterine cervix may be hampered sufficiently to cause infertility.

Case 3—Females who are physically stressed and have very low body fat (as do body-builders) often have a temporary or extended cessation of ovulation. With more food intake and less stress after the competition, this individual began cycling normally again.

Answers to Review Questions

1. A. When used alone, cervix refers to the anterior aspect of the neck. The part of the female reproductive system using this term is the cervix of the uterus.

2. B. Each primary oocyte (2N) divides to form a secondary oocyte (N) and a first polar body (N).

3. C. A secondary oocyte must pass through the tunica albuginea of the ovary, the visceral peritoneum, and the ovarian bursa before it enters the infundibulum of the uterine tube.

4. D. Females of some mammalian species (but not humans) are induced ovulators. Ovulation does not occur in them unless sexual intercourse occurs.

5. D. The uterine tubes do transport sperm "upstream". However, this occurs by peristalsis rather than by ciliary action. On the other hand, ova are "swept" down the uterine tubes by ciliary action.

6. B. The vaginal vestibule is part of the vulva but the vagina, itself, is not.

7. C.

8. C.

9. D. The broad ligament is serous membrane, too. However, it attaches to but is not part of the uterus. Thus, it does not satisfy the premise ("which part of the uterus...").

10. E. Both B and D are mismatched with functions.

Answers to Thought Questions

1. Oogenesis and spermatogenesis both result in the formation of haploid sex cells. In oogenesis, only one sex cell is formed from each primary oocyte, but in spermatogenesis, four are formed from each primary spermatocyte. Spermatogenesis is a rapid, continual process with millions of definitive sperm produced each day. Oogenesis is halted in the second meiotic division (until fertilization) and a fertile female produces only a few hundred mature sex cells in her lifetime.

2. During sexual intercourse, sperm are deposited in the vaginal lumen of the female. The vaginal cavity is an extension of the peritoneal cavity in males and sperm are not present therein.

3. As a given follicle matures, the high estrogen levels produced by its follicular cells inhibit other follicles from completing the maturation process. Since the estrogen levels should be highest in the ovary of impending ovulation, the inhibition should be highest there. Consequently, the next ovulation will typically occur in the contralateral ovary.

4. They wander around in the female reproductive tract about 48 hours and then degenerate and die.

5. *Cervix* used alone denotes the anterior aspect of the neck.

6. The uterine lining proliferates under the influence of progesterone which is produced by the corpus luteum of the ovary following ovulation. In a cycling female, the corpus luteum regresses a few days after ovulation. As it does, the progesterone output falls. Without the progesterone to maintain it, the hypertrophied endometrium degenerates, sloughs, and menstrual flow results.

7. The uterine tubes transport sperm, ova, and serve as the normal site of fertilization.

8. The clitoris has two crura, a body, a glans clitoridis, and a prepuce similar to those of the penis. It also contains two corpora cavernosa (erectile bodies) similar to those of the penis. However, the clitoris does not surround the urethra, has no corpus spongiosum, and is much smaller than the penis.

9. Major vestibular gland(s).

10. They are left in place to produce female sex hormones.

11. They undergo luteinization under the influence of pituitary hormones to form the corpus luteum and then produce progesterone (for a few days if fertilization has not occurred or several weeks if it has).

12. The ovary of the 40 year-old woman contains more scar tissue (corpora albicantia) and fewer follicles than that of the 20 year-old.

13. Usually there is a rise in body temperature associated with ovulation and some women feel a twinge of pain when ovulation occurs.

14. Female circumcision is the term applied to the surgical removal of part or most of the clitoris. This barbaric practice is the norm in a few cultures.

15. The hymen is stretched and sometimes torn by sexual intercourse.

16. Some authors do include the mammary glands in the reproductive system due to their important nutritional role for the newborn. More often (and officially), mammary glands are considered to be part of the integumentary system.

17. Unfertilized ova degenerate and die (usually within a day of ovulation).

18. The ciliated cells lining the uterine tubes "sweep" the ova toward the uterus. Peristaltic waves transport sperm toward the ovary. The sperm are so small that they "sneak" between the downward beating cilia.

19. Endometriosis interna (= adenomycosis) reduces fertility because the thickened endometrium is less conducive to implantation. Salpingitis interferes with the transport of ova (down) and sperm (up) the uterine tubes. Cystic ovaries result when ovulation fails to occur and several follicles are trapped at (near) maturity. Without ovulation, fertilization cannot occur.

20. Both male and female reproductive systems produce gametes and participate in the sexual union that leads to fertilization. The female reproductive system, however, provides the fertilization site, houses and nourishes the conceptus, and delivers the offspring at birth.

21. Extreme stress (physical or emotional) can alter the release of pituitary gonadatropins (LH, FSH) such that ovarian cycles (temporarily) cease. Female athletes under a heavy training regimen and extremely thin individuals often cease cycling as well as individuals under extreme and/or continuous emotional stress.

CHAPTER 22 Human Development

Chapter Outline and Key Concepts

INTRODUCTION

The human body develops from a single cell into a complex structure of about one quadrillion ($1x10^{15}$) cells.

STAGES OF ONTOGENY

The developmental history of an individual is called *ontogeny* and the common biological history of a group of animals is *phylogeny.*

Ontogeny includes the following stages: gametogenesis, ovulation, copulation, fertilization, cleavage, gastrulation, organogenesis, growth, birth, maturation, senescence, and death.

Early developmental stages are often grouped as pre-embryonic period (encompassing everything through early organogenesis), embryonic period, and (when the fetus is recognizably human) the fetal period.

COPULATION

Copulation (coitus, sexual intercourse) is the procreative act wherein a man's erect penis is inserted into a woman's vagina.

During a male's orgasm (climax), semen is ejaculated from the penis, and (providing "barrier" type birth control is not in use) is moved through the uterus and uterine tubes by muscular contractions.

FERTILIZATION

Most sperm deposited in the vagina fail to enter the uterus and even fewer reach the uterine tubes.

Penetration of the zona pellucida of the ovum by a sperm is assisted by hydrolytic enzymes within an organelle called the acrosome.

After a sperm penetrates, the ovum undergoes a chemical change to prevent other sperm from entering.

Penetration by a sperm stimulates the ovum to complete its second meiotic division, eject the second polar body, and combine its nucleus with the sperm nucleus to form a zygote.

Multiple births can occur from complete division of the conceptus during early cleavage (identical or monozygotic siblings) or from fertilization of multiple ova (fraternal or multizygotic siblings).

Birth control techniques are designed to prevent ovulation, fertilization, or implantation.

CLEAVAGE AND IMPLANTATION

Initial cell divisions to form 2, 4, 8, *etc.*, cells occur synchronously, but the synchrony is lost after several generations of cells.

The solid ball of cells (morula) formed during cleavage hollows to create a fluid-filled blastocyst.

The blastocyst secretes chorionic gonadotropin to maintain the corpus luteum of the ovary and attaches to the lining of the uterine wall 5–7 days after fertilization.

GASTRULATION AND FORMATION OF THE BASIC TISSUES AND EXTRAEMBRYONIC MEMBRANES

The embryoblast within the blastocyst forms three primary germ layers: ectoderm, mesoderm, and endoderm.

Connective tissue and muscle tissue are derived from mesoderm, nervous tissue from ectoderm, and epithelium is derived from all three germ layers.

Four extraembryonic membranes form during and after gastrulation: amnion, chorion, yolk sac, and allantois.

The chorion and allantois form most of the fetal part of the placenta.

Within the placenta, fetal blood and maternal blood occupy separate but intimate capillary beds to facilitate nutrient/waste exchange.

ORGANOGENESIS AND GROWTH

Most organ rudiments are formed during the early part of the embryonic period (weeks 3-8 after fertilization).

The heart becomes functional during week 4-5 and the embryo is recognizably human by week 7-8.

PARTURITION

The typical gestational period is 266 days ± 2 weeks and the projected delivery date is calculated at 280 days from the onset of the last menstrual period.

Labor is divided into three stages: dilation, expulsion, and placental stages.

POSTNATAL DEVELOPMENT

There are six periods of postnatal development: neonatal period, infancy, childhood, adolescence, adulthood, and senescence.

The neonatal period lasts one month, infancy continues until the end of year two, and childhood blends into adolescence at puberty.

Adulthood and senescence are not clearly separated, but death is definite.

Selected Definitions

Adolescence—the developmental period, indefinite in time, between puberty and adulthood. For many individuals it is an emotionally unsettled period often characterized by an inflated or devalued self-image.

Blastocyst—the post-morula stage of development which implants in the endometrium. It consists of an inner cell mass (embryoblast) and a trophoblast surrounding a fluid-filled cavity.

Childhood—the developmental period, several years in length, between infancy and puberty. It has an arbitrarily assigned beginning (two years of age) and a variable termination.

Cleavage—the first several cell divisions of the zygote. These include the various named "cellular" stages of development (two cell, four cell, eight cell, *etc.*) as well as the morula, blastocyst, and blastula.

Embryoblast (inner cell mass)—the eccentric group of cells within a blastula that will develop into the definitive individual. After gastrulation, the descendants of these cells differentiate to form the four basic tissues and initiate organogenesis.

Embryonic period—the developmental period beginning two weeks after fertilization and lasting a total of six weeks. The first two weeks of development are called the pre-embryonic period.

Extraembryonic membranes—those membranous parts of a conceptus which do not ultimately form parts of the definitive individual. They include the chorion, amnion, allantois, and yolk sac.

Fetal period—that part of prenatal development wherein the conceptus is recognizably human. It begins at the end of the embryonic period (when the conceptus is eight weeks old) and lasts until birth.

Gametogenesis—the divisional process by which sex cells are developed. In males it is called spermatogenesis and in females it is termed oogenesis.

Gastrulation—the development of three primary germ cell layers. By this process, a blastula becomes a gastrula.

Infancy—the postnatal developmental period from thirty days of age to two years (when childhood formally commences). The first thirty days after birth constitute the neonatal period.

Intrauterine device (IUD)—a mechanical form of birth control, variable in design, that physically prevents nidation (implantation). IUD's are placed (and removed) through the cervical canal by gynecologists and are considered by some to be a passive form of abortion.

Monozygotic (identical) twins—twins that develop from a single zygote. An early stage of cleavage (two cell, four cell, eight cell) splits and each of the resulting cell masses develop into a complete individual (natural biological cloning).

Morula—a solid mass of cells (blastomeres) formed by cleavage of a zygote. When it develops a fluid-filled cavity with further divisions of its cells, it becomes a blastocyst.

Ontogeny—the biological development (history) of an individual. It follows the general pattern of ("recapitulates") the development of the group of animals to which that individual belongs.

Organogenesis—the stage of ontogeny in which primary and secondary organ rudiments differentiate. It occurs after gastrulation.

Phylogeny—the biological development of a group of related animal species. Mammals, for example, share most general developmental patterns (regardless of species).

Senility—old age or the physical and mental deterioration that occurs in old age. Premature senility is called senilism.

Trophoblast—the outer part of a blastula that does not contribute directly to the definitive individual. Trophoblastic cells embed in the endometrium and contribute to the formation of the chorion and amnion.

Urachus—a tubular channel through the umbilical cord in a fetus that connects the urinary bladder to the allantois. It involutes after birth to form the median ligament of the urinary bladder.

Zygote—the fertilized ovum. Its chromosome number is restored to 46 by the addition of the twenty-three chromosomes from the sperm, and it divides after about twenty-four hours to form the two cell stage.

Etymology ***Dil posse creari de nilo*—"Nothing can be created out of nothing."**

allantoeides (G), *sausage-shaped*—allantois
akme (G), *point*—acrosome
amnos (G), *lamb*—amnion
chorion (G), *leather*—chorion
cleven (ME), *to split*—cleavage
coire (L), *to come together*—coitus
echein (G), *to hold*—urachus
gaster (G), *belly*—gastrulation
geron (G), *old man*—gerontology
merum (L), *mulberry*—morula
nidus (L), *nest*—nidation
ont (G), *to be*—ontogeny
ouron (G), *urine*—urachus
phyl (L), *tribe, clan*—phylogeny
senescere (L), *to be old*—senescence
teras (G), *monster*—teratology
trephein (G), *to nourish*—trophoblast
zygotos (G), *yoked together* —zygote

Introduction

The human body develops from a single initial cell into a complex structure containing several hundred trillion (about one quadrillion) cells. This is remarkable in itself, but even more amazing is the fact that even though every cell has the same genetic material, some develop into kidneys, while others form lungs, heart, skin, *etc.* Most individuals have the same number of limbs, fingers, toes, and ears. What determines how and when certain cells and cell groups in the developing embryo form an evagination that will become a superior limb? How do cells "decide" how long a bone should be? How are all of the axonal connections within the central nervous system made? These are questions that embryologists, molecular biologists, and developmental biologists are attempting to answer. We know much more about *what* happens developmentally than we do about *why* and *how* it happens.

Stages of Ontogeny

The developmental history of an individual is termed **ontogeny**. Ontogeny can be contrasted to the evolutionary development of groups of related animals which is termed **phylogeny**. The often stated phrase, "...ontogeny recapitulates phylogeny..." refers to the fact that individual development often follows an evolutionary pattern. Parallel developmental patterns among the higher animals are obvious embryologically. All chordates have a notochord, a neural tube, and pharyngeal pouches. Renal development in more primitive phylogenetic lines involved a primitive urinary organ termed the

Table 22-1 Twelve Major Stages of Ontogeny

Gametogenesis—the formation of sex cells by meiosis (spermatogenesis in males and oogenesis in females). Its purpose is to reduce the chromosome number from 46 (2N) to 23 (N) prior to fertilization.

Ovulation—the release of a secondary oocyte and its accompanying corona radiata cells through the surface of the ovary. This occurs once each month in a sexually mature, non-pregnant female.

Copulation—sexual intercourse wherein a man's erect penis is inserted into the lumen of a woman's vagina. At male orgasm, sperm are ejaculated into the vagina and then permeate the uterus and uterine tubes.

Fertilization—the penetration of a secondary oocyte by a spermatozoon. This triggers completion of the second meiotic division and the newly formed definitive ovum (N) immediately combines with the sperm nucleus (N) to form a zygote (2N).

Cleavage—the initial mitotic divisions of the zygote which result in two cells, then four, eight, sixteen, *etc.*, to form a solid ball of cells termed a morula. Continued mitosis soon forms a fluid-filled hollow ball of cells termed a blastula (and, with further development, a blastocyst).

Gastrulation—the formation of the three primary germ layers. This occurs step-wise with the cells of the blastula termed the inner cell mass first separating into two layers (ectoderm and endoderm), followed by a third layer (mesoderm) between them. These three germ layers form the various tissues of the body.

Organogenesis—the differentiation of various tissue subtypes and their combinations to form specific body organs.

Growth—the continued development, enlargement, and refinement of body organs and their combinations to form organ systems.

Birth—the pivotal event in which a fetus is expelled from its mother's reproductive system and begins to sustain life partially independent of its maternal parent.

Maturation—the biological stages and changes from birth to sexual maturity. This can be subdivided into several post-natal phases including the neonatal period, infancy, childhood, adolescence, and adulthood. Once sexual maturity is reached, gametogenesis commences to initiate ontogeny in potential progeny.

Senescence—biological aging accompanied by gradual physical and functional deterioration. There is no single, distinct event separating maturation and senescence.

Death—the termination of an individual's life that occurs whenever organs in one or more systems are no longer able to maintain required (vital) body functions.

pronephric kidney. More advanced animals developed a more sophisticated organ termed the mesonephric kidney and higher mammals (including humans) have attained a third level of renal modification called the metanephric kidney. Intriguingly, however, kidney development in the higher mammals still involves pronephric and mesonephric stages. Another example of definitive development retracing evolutionary phases is the arterial pattern of mammals. It involves a series of aortic arches that prevail in fish as the arteries within the gills. The list of these sorts of developmental "mini-evolutions" is quite lengthy. Ontogeny does, indeed, replay many stages of evolutionary development and modification.

The 12 major sequential stages of ontogeny are gametogenesis, ovulation, copulation, fertilization, cleavage, gastrulation, organogenesis, growth, birth, maturation, senescence, and death. These are defined and briefly summarized in Table 22-1. They can be subgrouped in various ways. The eight stages which occur before birth constitute the prenatal period and the three which occur after birth collectively form the postnatal period. Embryologists often divide the prenatal period into four parts: gametogenesis, pre-embryonic period, embryonic period, and fetal period. **Gametogenesis** is the for-

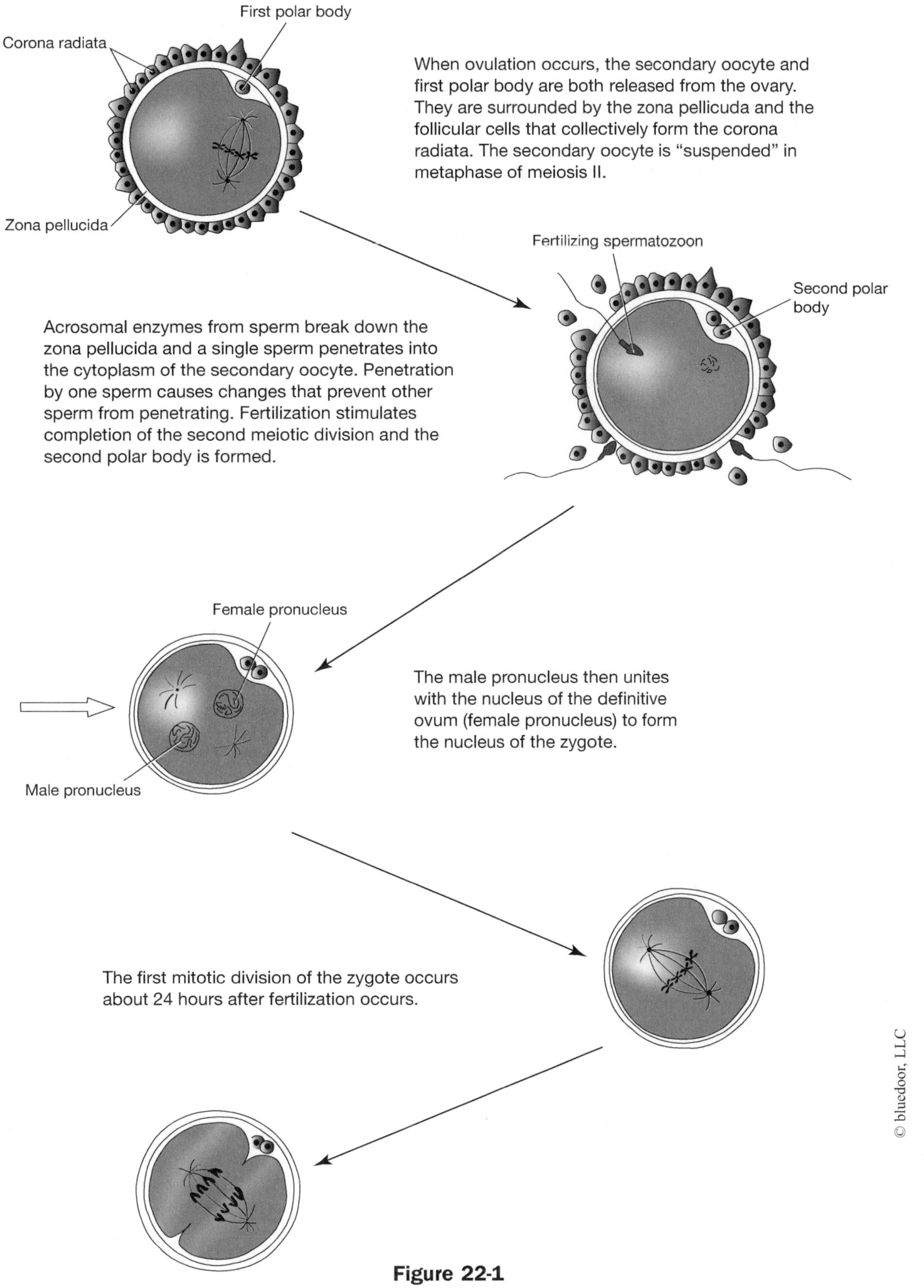

Figure 22-1

Fertilization and the Initiation of Cleavage

mation of sex cells by meiosis and is termed spermatogenesis in males and oogenesis in females. Its purpose is to reduce the chromosome number and form functional spermatozoa and ova. The **pre-embryonic period** lasts two weeks and encompasses ovulation, copulation, fertilization, cleavage, gastrulation, and the initial part of organogenesis. The **embryonic period** lasts six weeks and includes the remainder of organogenesis and the initial stages of growth. This is the most critical period of development in regard to teratogens (agents that cause physical defects). At the end of this period, the embryo is about 3.5 cm long and is recognizable as human. The remainder of intra-uterine life (from eight weeks after fertilization until birth) constitutes the **fetal period**.

Objectives

1. List the 12 major stages of ontogeny, the approximate length of time involved in each, and the major events that each one includes.
2. Group the appropriate ontogenic stages into the pre-embryonic, embryonic, and fetal periods.

Copulation

Copulation, also known as **coitus** or **sexual intercourse**, is the procreative act wherein a man's erect penis is inserted into a woman's vagina. Erection in the man is initiated by autonomic impulses which cause increased blood flow to and decreased venous drainage from erectile tissues of the penis. Similar mechanisms cause engorgement of the clitoris, vestibular bulbs, and areolas in females. The bulbourethral glands in the male and the vestibular glands of the female secrete lubricating fluids which facilitate intromission. Pressure and frictional forces from movement during intercourse act on sensory receptors in the glans penis and glans clitoridis. These may summate to effect a release of pleasurable sensations termed **orgasm** or **climax**. In males, climax includes spasmodic contractions of the bulbospongiosus muscle which create peristaltic waves in the corpus spongiosum penis and propel semen forcefully out of the urethra, a process called **ejaculation**. In females, orgasm causes rhythmic contraction of the perineal muscles as well as the smooth muscle tissue in the uterus and uterine tubes. These contractions assist movement of semen through the female organs to the upper parts of the uterine tubes where fertilization normally occurs.

Objectives

3. State several synonyms for sexual intercourse.
4. Explain the logic behind each of the major forms of birth control.

Fertilization

During ejaculation, several hundred million sperm are deposited in the vaginal lumen. Most of these fail to pass through the cervical canal of the uterus and simply drain out of the vaginal opening. Those that enter the uterus undergo a poorly understood change called **capacitation** which is neces-

Table 22-2 Methods of Birth Control*

Withdrawal—removal of the penis from the vaginal lumen prior to ejaculation. This is the least reliable method of birth control.
Rhythm—limitation of sexual intercourse to the non-fertile portion of the ovarian cycle.
Condom—a disposable sheath worn over the penis. It prevents impregnation or infection. A female version has been developed.
Diaphragm—a physical barrier placed in the vagina over the cervical opening of the uterus to deny sperm access to the uterus. It should be used with a spermicide.
Spermicide—a gel or foam that is toxic to sperm. It is placed in the vagina. Some forms are combined with a diaphragm-like device called a contraceptive sponge.
Vasectomy—surgical ligation/resection of the left and right ductus deferens to render a male permanently sterile by denying sperm their pathway of exit from the body.
Tubal ligation—ligation of the left and right uterine tubes to render a female permanently sterile by blocking the pathway between the ovary and the uterus.
Oral contraceptives—progesterone derivatives taken by females. These prevent ovulation in the same manner as the natural progesterone produced by the corpus luteum in a pregnant female.
Intrauterine device (IUD)—a small indwelling structure placed in the uterus by a physician. It prevents implantation and causes the conceptus to be sloughed (prevents nidation).
Subcutaneous implants—progesterone derivatives surgically implanted beneath the skin. These are slowly released and can prevent pregnancy for several years before they lose potency.
Abstinence—lack of sexual union is the only 100 percent guarantee against pregnancy. (It's fool proof!)
Vaginal ring—time-release, progesterone containing ring-shaped structure that can be self-inserted into the vagina and left *in situ* for three weeks. It is then removed for a week and another one inserted. In effect, it is similar to oral contraception but the hormones are absorbed vaginally.
Dermal patch—time release progesterone in a "band-aid" device. The progestins are absorbed transdermally.
"Morning-after pill" (levonelle)—a single dose oral contraceptive that prevents ovulation or implantation. It is considered to be an emergency contraceptive.

** A number of other methods have been researched, but have had side-effects or problems that have prevented their commercialization.*

sary to complete their ability to fertilize. Sperm are transported up the uterine tubes by peristalsis, and they normally meet the ovum (secondary oocyte) therein (only a few dozen normally contact an ovum). When a sperm contacts the egg, it must pass through the granulosa cells forming the corona radiata and then penetrate the zona pellucida (a thin transparent layer of protein/polysaccharide). Penetration is facilitated by digestive enzymes contained in a special organelle called the **acrosome** which caps the sperm's head (Figure 22-1). After one sperm penetrates the zona pellucida, a chemical change occurs which blocks others from entering. Penetration by the sperm stimulates the secondary oocyte to complete its second meiotic division into a definitive ovum and a diminutive second polar body (Figure 22-1). The sperm nucleus (23 chromosomes) then unites with the nucleus of the ovum (23 chromosomes) to form a single diploid (2N) cell termed the **zygote** which has 46 chromosomes (23 pairs). The diminutive second polar body degenerates and disappears.

As noted in the previous chapter, a secondary oocyte that is not fertilized does not complete its second meiotic division. In fact, it degenerates 12-24 hours after ovulation. Thus, fertilization cannot occur if copulation occurs more than 24 hours after ovulation. However, sperm can survive for 48 hours in the female reproductive tract and so fertilization can result from coitus occurring 1-2 days *before* ovulation. Most techniques of birth control prevent fertilization by preventing ovulation, by keeping sperm and ova separated, or by killing the sperm. Intrauterine devices, however, allow fertilization to occur but prevent implantation (adhesion of the blastocyst to the uterine wall). This mechanism is considered by some to be a form of abortion (Table 22-2).

Twins occur in slightly more than 1% of pregnancies. They can result from fertilization of two ova (**dizygotic twins**) or from division of the conceptus during early cleavage (**monozygotic twins**).

Dizygotic twins are commonly called fraternal twins and do not resemble each other any more than regular brothers and sisters. Monozygotic twins are identical twins. If they fail to completely separate, conjoined ("Siamese") twins may result. Triplets and other multiple births are quite rare. They may be identical, fraternal, or contain some identical siblings.

Objectives

5. Define a woman's fertile period relative to when ovulation and sexual intercourse occur.
6. Discuss the process of fertilization.
7. Differentiate monozygotic and fraternal twins.

Cleavage and Implantation

The initial divisions of the zygote occur synchronously and double the number of cells (two cells, four cells, eight cells, 16 cells, *etc.*). However, the individual cells decrease in size because implantation has not yet occurred and the only nutrients available are those which were present in the original cytoplasm of the zygote. The first division to form two cells usually occurs about a day after fertilization with two or three subsequent divisions forming a total mass of eight or 16 cells during the next 24 hours (Figure 22-2). By the third day, the conceptus consists of a solid mass of cells called a **morula**. It has also completed its slow journey down the uterine tube and has entered the uterus. By the fourth day, the center of the morula is filled with fluid and the resulting "hollow" ball of cells is called a **blastocyst**.

The inner cells on one side of the blastocyst form the **inner cell mass** (**embryoblast**) which forms the definitive embryo. The outer cells, collectively called the **trophoblast**, interact with the lining cells of the uterus during days 5-7 to effect **implantation** (**nidation**). This attachment usually occurs on the posterior wall of the body of the uterus. Enzymes secreted by the trophoblast digest an area of the endometrium and the blastocyst sinks into the resulting depression and fuses to the uterine wall. The anatomic stages through implantation are schematically illustrated in Figure 22-3. After implantation, some cells of the blastocyst secrete a hormone called chorionic gonadotropin that helps maintain the corpus luteum of the ovary. Progesterone from the corpus luteum prevents sloughing of the uterine lining (menstruation). For this reason it is often called the "hormone of pregnancy".

Objectives

8. Discuss cleavage using the terms morula, blastocyst, embryoblast, trophoblast, and implantation.

Gastrulation and Formation of the Basic Tissues and Extraembryonic Membranes

After implantation occurs, the embryoblast undergoes significant differentiation resulting in two distinct layers: ectoderm and endoderm. This is followed by formation of a third layer (mesoderm) between them. Ectoderm is the outer layer, mesoderm is the middle, and endoderm forms the inner

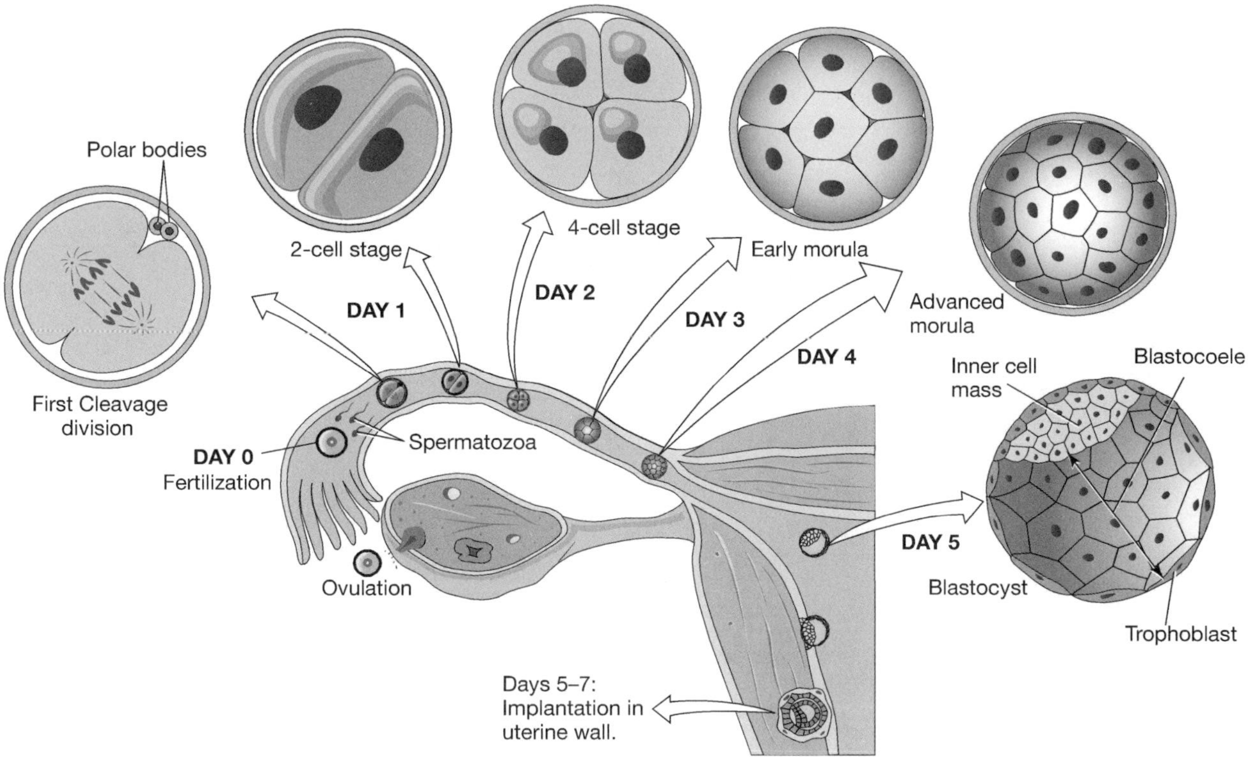

Figure 22-2

Cleavage and Formation of the Blastocyst

For the first few days of its existence, the conceptus is moving down the uterine tube toward the uterus.

layer. These three constitute the primary germ layers and from them all tissues in the body are derived. **Ectoderm** forms the nervous tissue and the epithelium covering the outer body surface. **Mesoderm** forms all of the muscle tissue and the connective tissue of the body as well as the kidneys and the epithelium of the serous membranes and blood vessels. **Endoderm** forms the lining epithelium and glands of the visceral body systems. More specific derivatives are listed in Table 22-3.

As the embryoblast undergoes gastrulation and organogenesis, the **extraembryonic membranes** develop. These include the amnion, chorion, yolk sac, and allantois. The **amnion** is derived from ectoderm and mesoderm. It forms a fluid-filled, balloon-like sac which envelopes the embryo. This cushions and protects the embryo during development. Because it contains cells that slough off the surface of the fetus or amniotic lining, amniotic fluid can be aspirated by needle biopsy (**amniocentesis**) and the cells can be examined for genetic defects such as Down syndrome. Biochemical analysis can also be performed to detect Tay-Sachs disease and other genetic disorders. Just before or during birth the amnion is naturally or iatrically (*i.e.*, caused by a physician) ruptured and the amniotic fluid is released. When this happens naturally to an expectant mother, she is said to have "broken her water."

The **chorion** is derived from ectoderm and mesoderm and is the major fetal contribution to the placenta (Figure 22-4). It is the outermost of the extraembryonic membranes and forms numerous finger-like extensions called chorionic villi which penetrate deeply into the uterine wall. Within these, the fetal blood passes through fetal capillaries in close proximity to maternal blood in maternal capillaries. This allows an exchange of nutrients and wastes (but not blood) between the fetus and mother.

The **yolk sac** forms from endoderm and mesoderm (Figure 22-4). It is an out-pouching of the

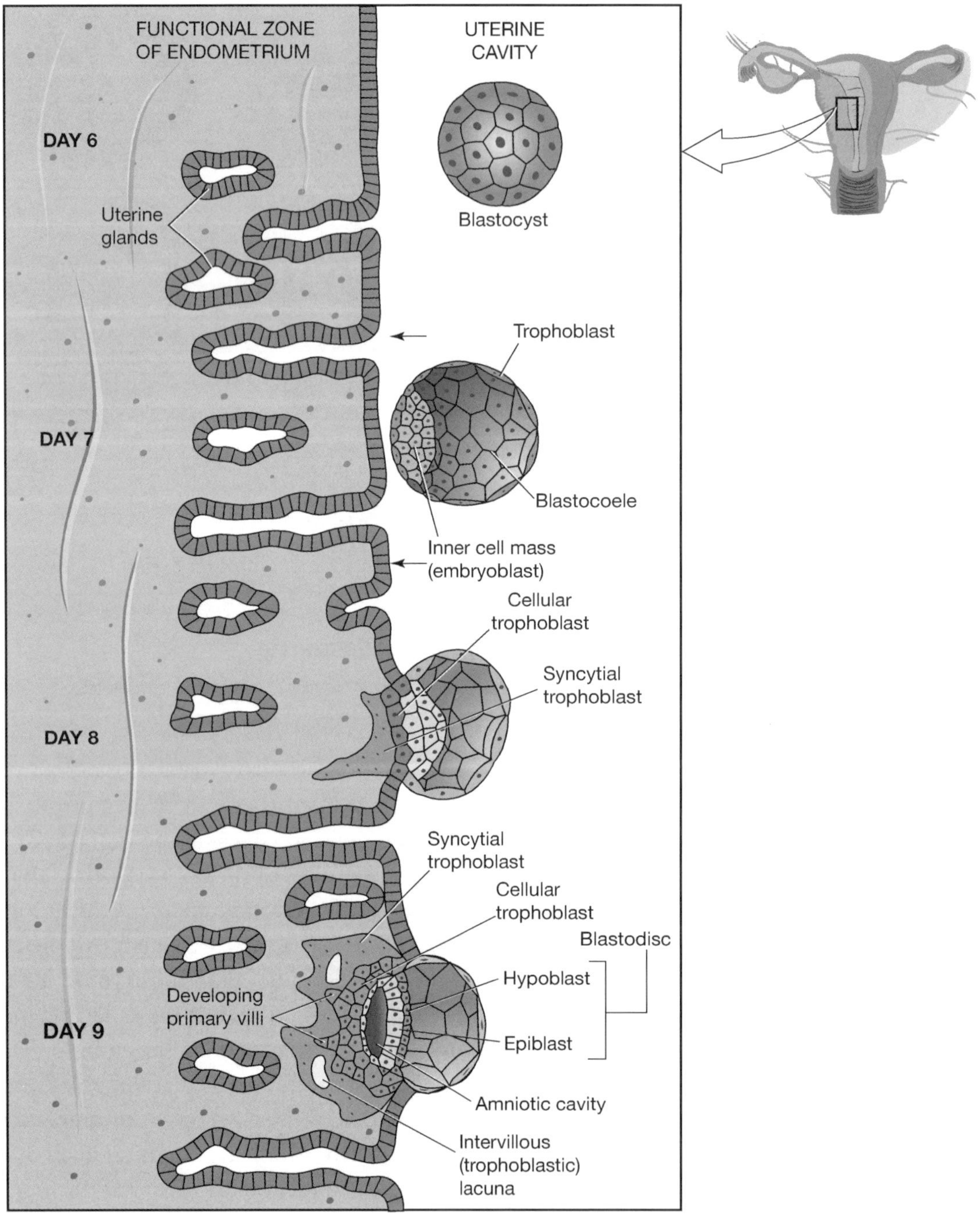

Figure 22-3

Nidation

As implantation proceeds, the cells of the embryoblast (inner cell mass, blastodisc) form an upper (epiblast) and a lower (hypoblast) layer. When a third layer forms between them, the process of gastrulation is underway and the three layers are identified as ectoderm, mesoderm, and endoderm.

Table 22-3 Derivatives of the Three Primary Germ Layers

Ectoderm:	
	Epidermis of skin including hair and nails
	Glands of skin
	Linings of oral cavity, nasal cavity, anal canal, and vagina
	Brain, spinal cord, sensory organs
	Lens of eye and epithelium of conjunctiva
	Pituitary gland
	Adrenal medulla
	Enamel of teeth
Mesoderm:	
	All muscle tissue (skeletal, smooth, cardiac)
	All connective tissue (fibrous c.t., bone, blood, cartilage, *etc.*)
	Dentin of teeth
	Adrenal cortex
	Kidneys and ureters
	Internal reproductive viscera
	Epithelium lining vessels, joint cavities, and the serous body cavities
Endoderm:	
	Lining epithelium and glands of digestive, respiratory, and (parts of) urogenital systems
	Thyroid and parathyroid glands
	Thymus

primitive gut which produces blood cells for the early embryo and some of its cells migrate into the developing gonads to become the spermatogonia or oogonia. After a few weeks, the yolk sac normally degenerates in mammals. If it remains, it may form an evagination from the ileum (near the cecum) called **Meckel's diverticulum**.

The **allantois** forms from mesoderm and endoderm as an out-pouching from the yolk sac (Figure 22-4). It helps form blood cells, the umbilical vessels, and participates in the formation of the urinary bladder. Within the fetus, the allantois forms a tube termed the **urachus** which joins the apex of the urinary bladder to the umbilical cord. Through this tube, urinary wastes produced in late gestation by the fetus are channeled out toward the chorion where they can be absorbed by the maternal circulation and subsequently excreted by the mother. Part of the allantois fuses to the chorion to form the **chorioallantois** to facilitate this exchange. After birth, the intra-fetal part of the allantois (urachus) normally becomes a fibrous cord termed the median umbilical ligament but it may persist as a **urinary umbilical fistula** (also called a patent urachus). This can be surgically corrected. (Note: the unpaired *median* umbilical ligament should not be confused with the left and right *medial* umbilical ligaments which are vestiges of the umbilical arteries).

The term **placenta** refers to the structure by which the fetus is joined to the uterine wall (Figure 22-5). It is formed by the chorion of the fetus and the lining tissues of the uterine wall. In its fully formed state, the placenta is a disc-shaped structure about seven inches in diameter and one inch thick. The fetus is anchored to it by the umbilical cord. Within the placenta, the fetal capillaries lie in close proximity to maternal capillaries from the uterine wall. Most bacteria do not cross this barrier but some viruses can. Although fetal and maternal blood do not mix, *per se*, at the placenta, small "leaks" due to traumatic episodes may allow some fetal blood access to the maternal circulation. This is the mechanism by which an Rh negative mother may be sensitized to an Rh positive fetus. If anti-Rh antibodies produced by the mother diffuse across the placental barrier, they can cause a breakdown of fetal red blood corpuscles resulting in a disease termed **erythroblastosis fetalis**.

Table 22-4 Significant Developmental Events

Time	Event
Day 0	Fertilization (combination of sperm and secondary oocyte)
2-3	Cleavage to form a solid ball of cells (morula)
4-5	Formation of blastocyst
6±	Implantation of blastocyst in uterine wall
Week 2	Gastrulation and formation of the basic tissues
3	Notochord forms, initial organogenesis
4	Heart, head, eyes, lungs, digestive organs form
5	Limbs are initially formed
6	Fingers and toes begin to separate
8	All systems are formed (embryo is 3.5 cm long), fetal brain waves can be detected
12	Fetus is about 9.0 cm long and weighs 50 g
16	Heart beat can be auscultated (first beats at 4 weeks)
20	Crown-rump length: 20.0 cm; weight: 1.0 pound
25	Crown-rump length: 24.0 cm; weight: 2.0 pounds
29	Crown-rump length: 27.5 cm; weight: 2.5 pounds
38	Crown-rump length: 36.0 cm; weight: 7.5 pounds (birth is imminent)

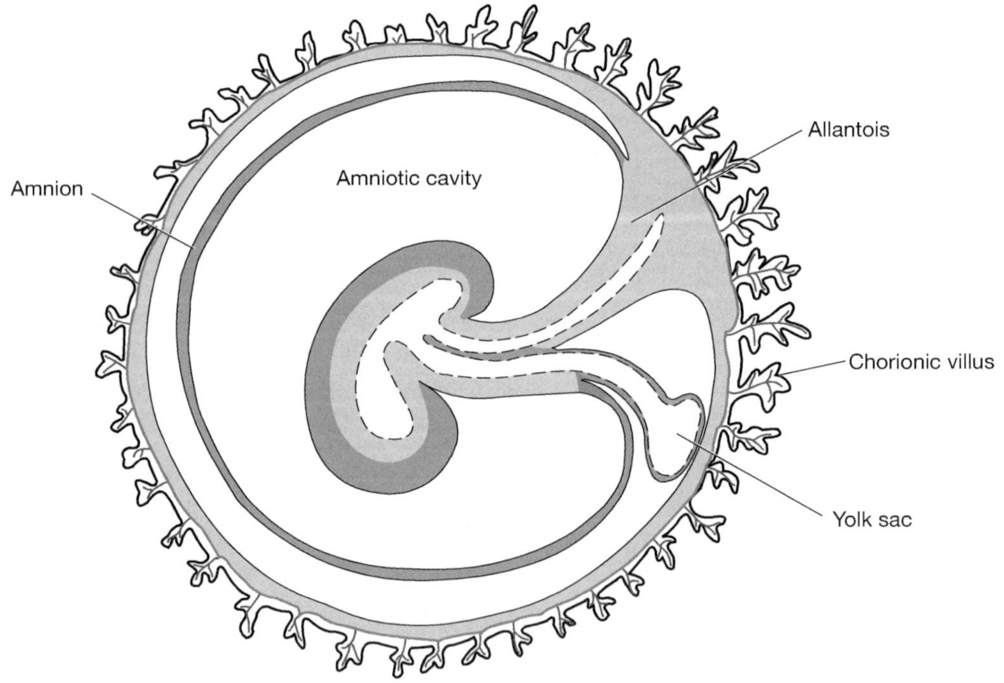

Figure 22-4

Extraembryonic Membranes

In mammals, the yolk sac is vestigal and quickly involutes. The amnion forms a protective, fluid-filled cavity around the developing conceptus. The chorion, and to a lesser extent the amnion, form the fetal component of the placenta. The allantois is connected to the developing urinary bladder by a tubular channel called the urachus. Late in gestation, when the kidneys become functional, this channel carries urinary wastes out to the placenta for transfer to the mother's bloodstream.

Objectives

9. Indicate the basic tissue disposition of each of the three primary germ layers.
10. Name the four extraembryonic membranes and state the function of each one.

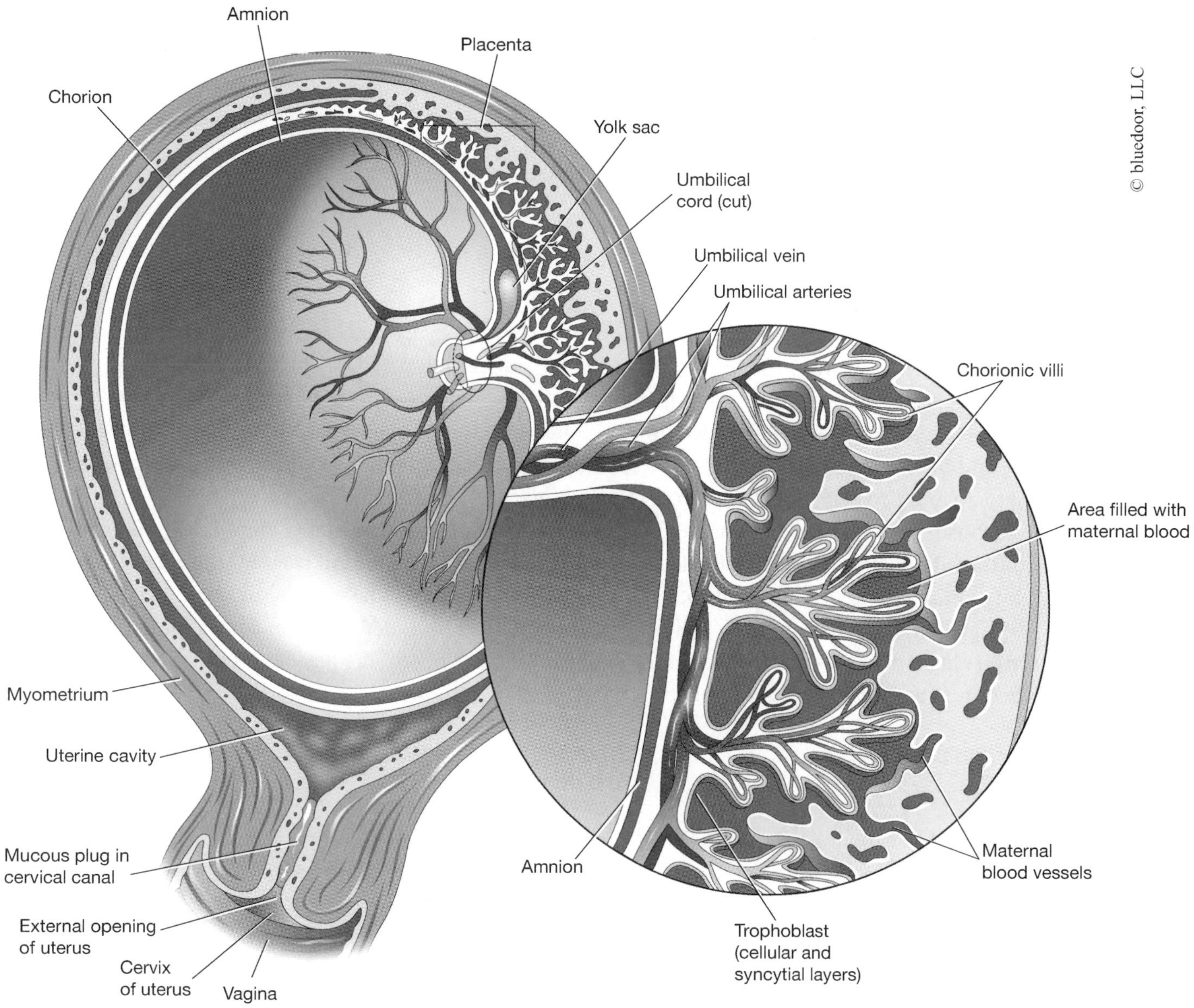

Figure 22-5

Structure of the Placenta

The placenta is formed from some maternal tissue contributed by the endometrium and some fetal tissue contributed by the chorion and allantois. The fetal component forms finger-like projections called chorionic villi that are surrounded by maternal blood to facilitate nutrient/waste exchange. Note that maternal blood and fetal blood remain separate and do not mix.

Organogenesis and Growth

Most organs initially form during the early part of the embryonic period (weeks 3-8 after fertilization). During the remainder of gestation, they undergo refinement and enlargement (*see Developmental discussions in the various chapters*). Significant developmental events during this time are summarized in Table 22-4, 22-5, and 22-6.

Objectives

11. State the time beyond fertilization when each of the following occur: two cell stage, morula, blastocyst, nidation, gastrulation, notochord forms, heart beats, limbs form, brain waves can be detected, heartbeat can be detected, fetus weighs 1.0 pound, birth, lungs exchange O_2/CO_2.

Parturition

The average human gestational period is 266 days ± 2 weeks. Projected delivery dates are usually calculated at 280 days from the beginning of the last menstrual period. The term **labor** is applied to the sequence of events which accompany parturition. The beginning of **true labor** is heralded by painful contractions of the myometrium at regular and frequent intervals. This may be preceded by several bouts of **false labor** with contractions at irregular intervals. Contractions are induced by oxytocin and prostaglandins and serve to expel the fetus from the uterus.

Labor is divided into three stages: dilation, expulsion, and placental (Figure 22-7). During the **dilation stage**, the cervical canal dilates to about 10 cm and the amnion usually ruptures. This stage may require only a few hours or may require more than a day. The **expulsion stage** of labor is the period when the fetus is actually delivered by forceful uterine and abdominal contractions. The **placental stage** includes the period after the expulsion stage wherein the placenta is expelled. This usually occurs within minutes after birth.

Objectives

12. Name the three stages of labor and the major event associated with each one.

Postnatal Development

Postnatal development may be divided into six periods: neonatal period, infancy, childhood, adolescence, adulthood, and senescence. These are the normal stages of maturation and degradation leading to physical death. The **neonatal period** extends from birth to the end of the first month. During this time the neonate does not gain significant weight but undergoes numerous physiological changes related to thermoregulation, hydroregulation, and significant alterations in the functional status of the digestive, respiratory, and urinary systems.

Infancy extends from one month of age until the end of the second year. Growth is very rapid during this time and most two-year olds weigh 3.5-4.0 times as much as they did at birth. Deciduous

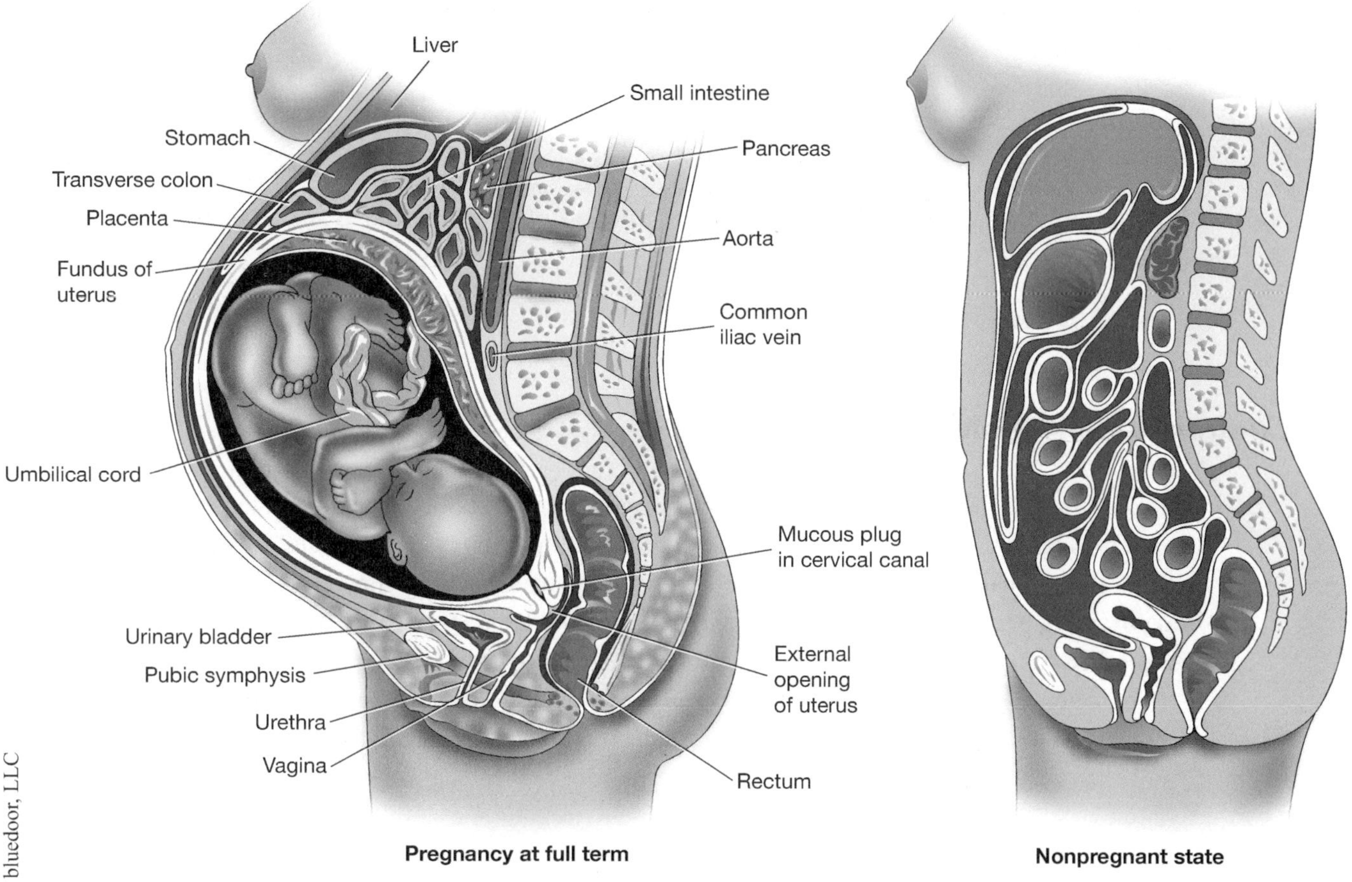

Figure 22-6

Organ Relationships: Pregnant *vs.* Non-pregnant

Tremendous displacement of abdominal organs occurs as the uterus enlarges due to growth of the conceptus. The urinary bladder bears the brunt of the conceptus weight because it remains below the fetus. Most other abdominal organs are displaced superiorly.

teeth begin to erupt at about six months of age and most infants have a full set by the time they are two years of age or shortly thereafter. Most infants can walk unassisted by one year of age.

Childhood begins at two years of age and extends to adolescence. Children gain an average of 7 pounds of weight and 2.5 inches of height per year during childhood. Most deciduous teeth are replaced by permanent ones during this time. Childhood ends and **adolescence** begins at **puberty** (sexual maturity). Menstruation in girls first occurs at 11(±) years and boys begin to produce viable sperm at about 13 years of age. There is considerable individual variation. During adolescence the secondary sex characteristics develop. In boys these include a deepening of the voice, increase in muscularity, and an increase in the density and thickness of body hair. Secondary sex characteristics in girls include development of breasts, redistribution of body fat, higher voice, and smoother, thinner skin. Other anatomic differences which develop between the sexes include greater height and weight in males and broader pelvises in females. There is no clear-cut point at which adolescence ends and **adulthood** begins. Similarly, adulthood blends imperceptibly into **senescence**. With time, virtually all organs in every body system undergo degeneration and loss of function. Several theories have been advanced to explain why this occurs. When vital functions are critically impacted, **death** ensues.

Objectives

13. Name the six postnatal periods and indicate the period of time associated with each one. (It is not possible to be exact on some of them).

Clinical Considerations

Abnormalities detected at birth are termed **congenital** defects. The science involved with the detection and classification of physical abnormalities of neonates and fetuses is termed **teratology**. Couples genetically predisposed to producing defective offspring may elect to have chromosomal **karyotyping** performed on cells collected via amniocentesis. **Heritable** diseases are those which are genetically transmitted and may not manifest themselves until later in life.

The science of aging is termed **gerontology**. Health problems of the aged have gained more notoriety as a larger percentage of the population is surviving into senility.

Objectives

14. Differentiate *congenital* from *hereditary* and define gerontology and teratology.

Clinical Case Studies

Case 1—During a difficult childbirth due to malposition of the fetus, the monitor on the fetal heartbeat suddenly went from 150 to nearly 200 beats per minute and remained there. The attending obstetrician, who had been digitally trying to reposition the fetus, immediately called for the C-section surgical pack and administered local anesthetic to the mother's abdominal region. Why did he suddenly make a decision to perform a C-section?

Case 2—Near the beginning of her seventh month, an expectant mother developed a minor vaginal discharge that was tinged red with blood. After evaluation, her obstetrician immediately ordered her to bedrest for the duration of her pregnancy. Why?

Case 3—Parents of a new baby boy consulted with their pediatrician regarding whether or not to have their child circumcised. After hearing discussion on both sides of the issue, they remained undecided and finally asked the physician (a father of three boys) what had been his decision with his own children. What are the arguments pro and con regarding this procedure?

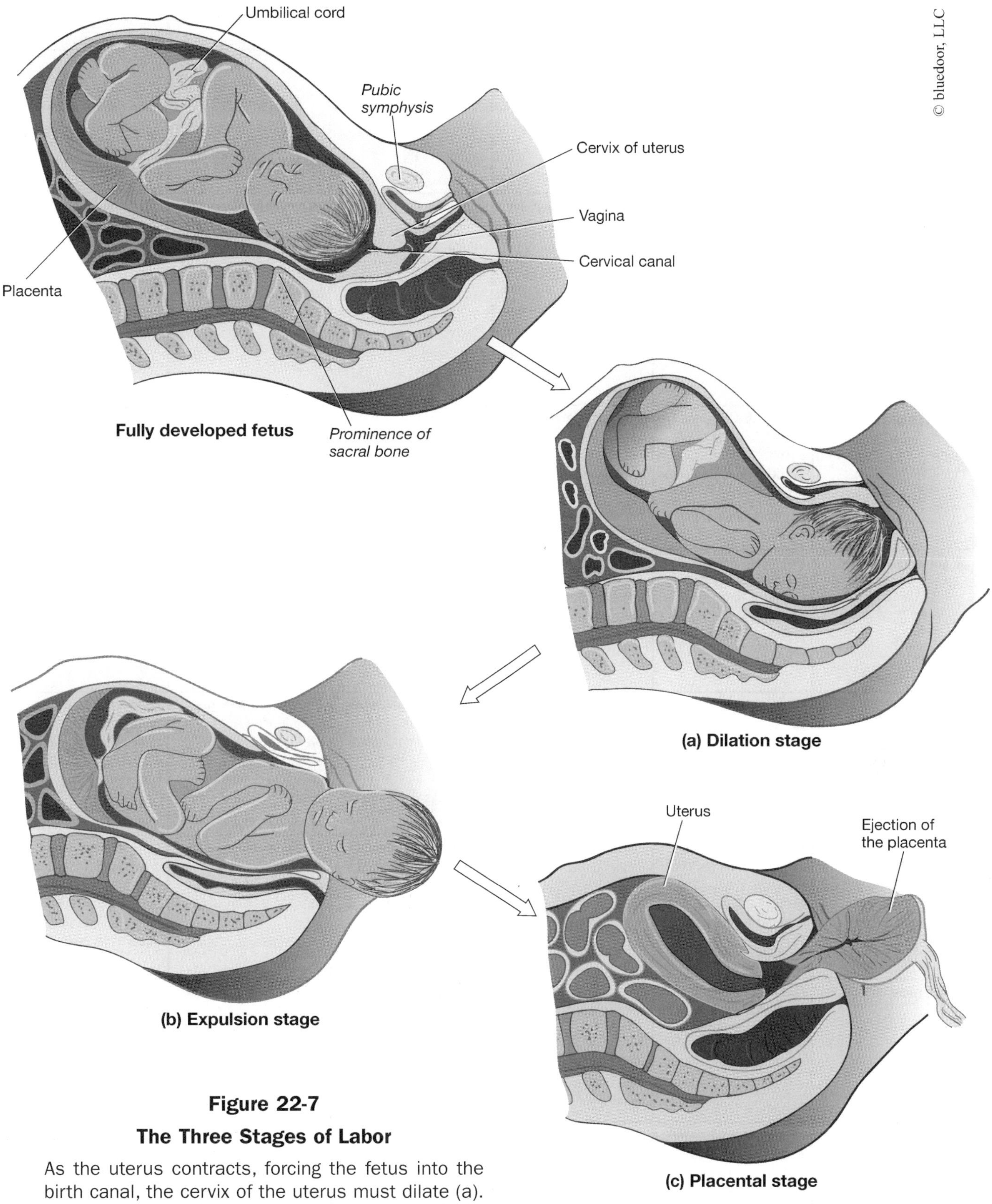

Figure 22-7
The Three Stages of Labor

As the uterus contracts, forcing the fetus into the birth canal, the cervix of the uterus must dilate (a). The amnion usually ruptures toward the end of this stage adding lubricating fluid which facilitates the expulsion stage (b). The placenta is usually expelled within an hour after birth (c).

Table 22-5 Developmental Landmarks Through Week 8

	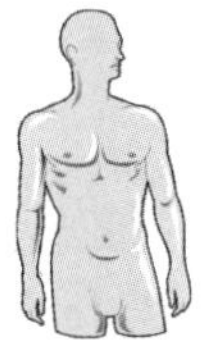	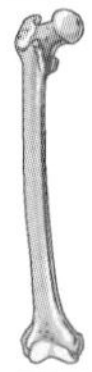	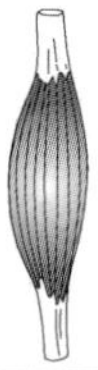	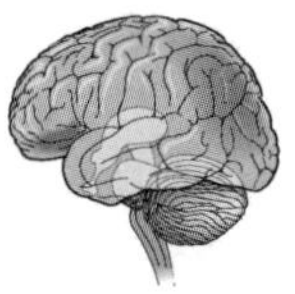	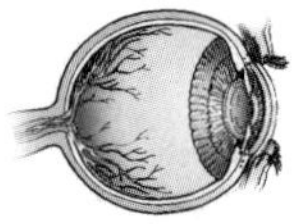
Age	**Body as a Whole**	**Skeletal System**	**Muscular System**	**Nervous System**	**Sensory Organs**
2.5 weeks	Embryonic disc flat, primitive streak prominent, neural groove indicated.	Notochordal plate present.		Neural groove initiates.	
3.5 weeks	Neural groove closes, first several somites present, cylindrical body separating from yolk sac.	Mesodermal segments begin appearing, older somites have sclerotomes, notochord is a cellular rod.	Mesodermal segmentation begins, older somites have myotome plates.	Neural groove closing to form neural tube, neural crest appears.	Optic vesicle and auditory placode present, spiral ganglia appearing.
4 weeks	Branchial arches completed, flexed (S-shaped) heart prominent, all somites present, limb buds present.	All 40 (±) somites present, sclerotomes form primitive vertebrae around notochord.	All 40 (±) somites present.	Neural tube closed, three primary brain vesicles present, nerves and ganglia forming.	Optic cup and lens pit forming, auditory pit detaches to form otocyst, olfactory placodes differentiate.
5 weeks	Nasal pits prominent, tail prominent, liver prominent, umbilical cord organizes.	Condensations of mesenchyme occur where future bones will develop.	Pre-muscle mesodermal masses present in head, trunk, and limbs.	Brain assumes five vesicle stage, cerebral hemispheres bulge, nerves and ganglia better developed.	Lens vesicle is free, vitreous primordium appears, otocyst elongates, olfactory pits deepen.
6 weeks	Head becomes size dominant, limbs recognizable, maxillae remain separate but mandible halves fuse.	Cartilage modeling of future bones begins.	Fused myotomes spread ventrally, segmentation has mostly disappeared.	Three primary brain flexures present, diencephalon large, meninges forming.	Optic disc has nervous/pigmented layers, lens vesicle thickens, three divisions of ear differentiate.
7 weeks	Face/neck forming, digits indicated, back straightens, tail regressing.	Cartilage modeling continues.	Muscles differentiating throughout body and assuming final form.	Enlargement of cerebral hemispheres, hypophysial sac and neurohypophysial bud in contact, choroid plexuses appear.	Nerve fibers invade optic stalk, eyelids forming, fibrous/vascular tunics differentiate, olfactory sacs open into oral cavity.
8 weeks	Nose flat, eyes widely separated, digits well-formed, body rounded, fetal state attained.	First ossification occurs.	Fetus capable of some movement.	Typical cells appear in cerebral cortex, olfactory bulbs appear, meninges become definitive.	Visual axes converging, ear assuming definitive structure, taste buds present, nostrils plugged.

After Arey, L.B., *Developmental Anatomy,* Ed. 7, W. B Saunders, Philadelphia, 1965

Table 22-5 (continued)

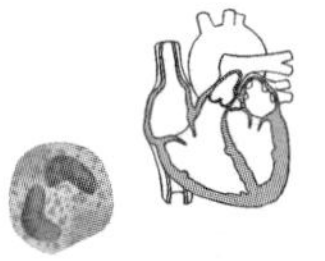	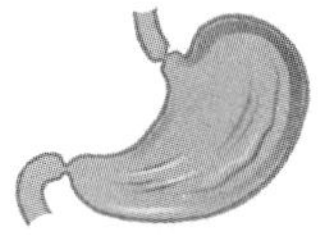	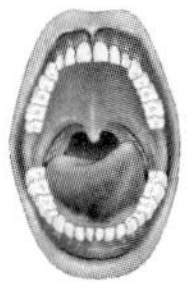	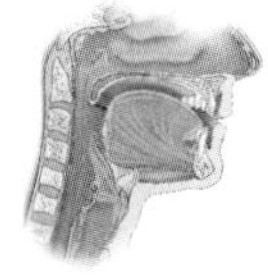	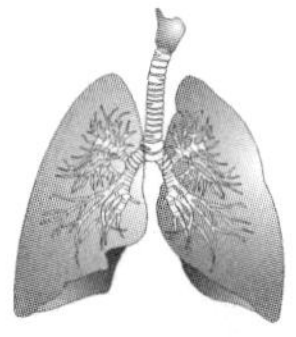	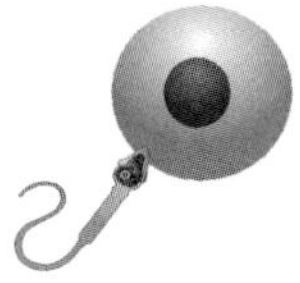
Cardiovascular System	**Digestive System**	**Mouth**	**Pharynx**	**Respiratory System**	**Urogenital Organs**
Blood islands appear on chorion and yolk sac.	Gut not separated from yolk sac.				Allantois present.
Paired embryonic vessels present, primitive heart bends into an "S" shape and begins contracting.	Foregut, hindgut, liver bud, cloaca, cloacal membrane present.	Mandibular arch prominent, stomodeum present as a pit, oral membrane ruptures.	Pharyngeal pouches forming, thyroid gland indicated.	Respiratory primordium appears as a groove on floor of pharynx.	Pronephros forms, pronephric duct grows inferiorly, cloaca and cloacal membrane evident.
Aortic arches and cardinal veins completed, paired aortae fuse, heart has sinus, atrium, ventricle and bulbus.	Simple tubular intestine, pancreatic buds appear, gallbladder and biliary ducts forming.	Maxillary/mandibular processes well developed, lingual primordia appear, hypophysial sac ("Rathke's pouch") indicated.	Five pharyngeal pouches present, pouches 1-4 have closing plates, thyroid gland a stalked sac.	Trachea and lung buds prominent, laryngeal opening is a simple slit.	Pronephros degenerated, its duct (now mesonephric duct) reaches cloaca, mesonephros and metanephros differentiating.
Head and limbs vascularized, vitelline and umbilical veins transforming, cardiac septae appear.	Intestine elongates into a loop and cecum initiates.	Jaws outlined, hypophysial sac elongated.	Pharyngeal pouches develop dorsal and ventral diverticula, thyroid gland bilobed, thyroglossal duct atrophies.	Bronchial buds indicate pulmonary lobes, arytenoid swellings and epiglottis appear.	Mesonephros reaches its caudal limit, ureteric and pelvic primordia distinct, genital ridge bulging.
Hemopoiesis occurs in liver, aortic arches transforming, bulbus absorbed into right ventricle, heart becoming definitive.	Intestinal loop undergoes torsion, stomach rotates, and cloaca subdivides.	Lingual primordia fusing, labio-dental laminae appearing, parotid/submandibular buds appear.	Thymic sacs, ultimobranchial sacs, parathyroid glands well developed and ready to detach.	Pulmonary lobes differentiate, bronchi arborize, larynx temporarily blocked.	Cloaca subdivides, tubules develop, unisexual genital tubercle present, Müllerian duct appears.
Cardinal veins transforming, inferior vena cava appearing, cardiac valves present, primitive spleen appears.	Intestinal loop herniates into umbilical cord, rectum/urinary bladder separate, anal membrane ruptures.	Single tongue present, labial and dental laminae separate, mandibles distinct, palate folds present.	Thymi elongating and losing lumina, parathyroid glands invading thyroid gland, ultimobranchial bodies fuse with thyroid gland.	Larynx well formed, laryngeal and tracheal cartilages developing, conchae appear.	Mesonephros reaches its apex, metanephric duct begins branching, urinary bladder/urethra separates from rectum.
Main vessels established, primitive lymph sacs appear, A-V bundle present.	Small intestine coils within umbilical cord, intestinal villi appear, liver disproportionately large.	Lingual muscles well differentiated, earliest taste buds appear, neurohypophysial bud detaches from mouth, sublingual gland appearing.	Auditory tube and tympanic cavity distinguishable, thymic halves unite, thyroid follicles forming.	Lungs appear gland-like due to bronchial branching, nostrils closed by epithelial plugs.	Testis/ovaries distinguishable, Müllerian ducts ready to unite as utero/vaginal primordium, genital ligaments indicated.

Table 22-6 Developmental Landmarks, 10 Weeks To Term

Age	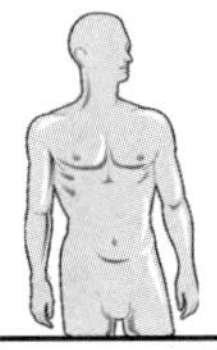 **Body as a Whole**	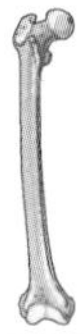 **Skeletal System**	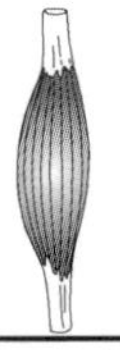 **Muscular System**	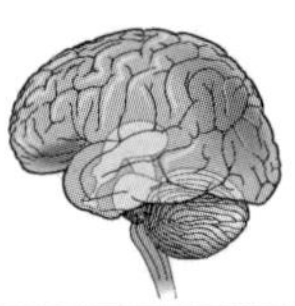 **Nervous System**	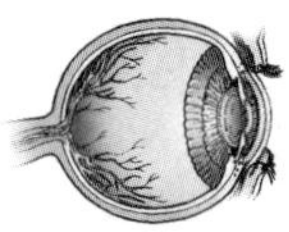 **Sensory Organs**
10 weeks	Head erect, limbs well-formed, nail folds indicated, umbilical hernia reduced.	Ossification continues.	Perineal muscles finally differentiating.	Spinal cord attains definitive internal structure.	Iris and ciliary body differentiating, eyelids fused, lacrimal glands budding, spiral organ developing.
12 weeks	Head remains dominant, nose gains bridge, sex obvious.	Notochord rapidly degenerating, some bones well formed.		Brain becomes definitive, enlargements occur on spinal cord, glial cells differentiate.	Ocular organization generally complete, layering of retina occurring, nasal septum and palate fusions completed.
16 weeks	Face appears humanoid, hair appearing on head, muscles spontaneously contracting.	Most bones well modeled (many not ossified), joint cavities appear	Fetal movements can be detected by mother.	Cerebral lobes obvious, corpora quadrigemina appear, cerebellum becomes prominent.	Eye, ear, and nose appear definitive, general sensory receptors differentiating.
5 months	Lanugo hair appears and vernix caseosa collects.	Some bones partially ossified, some have not yet begun ossification (especially carpal and tarsal bones) *(5 mos. +).*		Myelination of spinal cord begins.	Ossification of nasal bones and auditory ossicles.
6 months			Perineal muscles complete their development.	Definitive strata appear in cerebral cortex.	
7 months	Fetus lean, wrinkled, and red; eyelids re-open.			Cerebral fissures become distinct.	Vascular tunic of eyeball well-developed, retinal layering completed, retina light perceptive. Eyelids re-open *(7-8 mos.).*
8 months	Testes invading scrotum.				Taste perceptive.
Term	Fat collecting, wrinkles smoothing, body rounding.			Myelination of brain begins.	Ear not yet sound perceptive.

After Arey, L.B., *Developmental Anatomy,* Ed. 7, W. B Saunders, Philadelphia, 1965

Table 22-6 (continued)

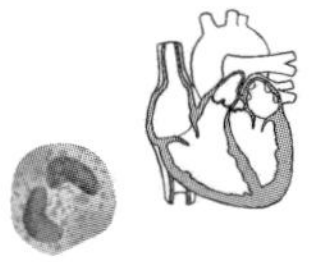	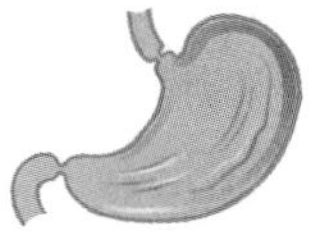	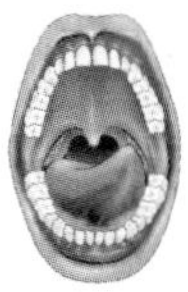	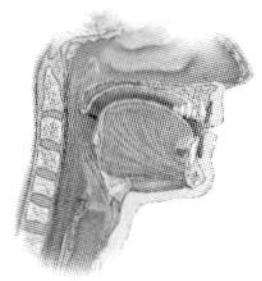	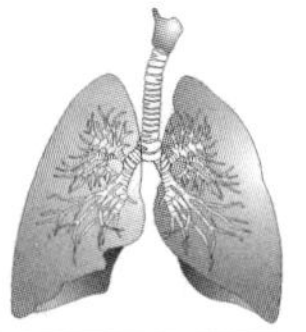	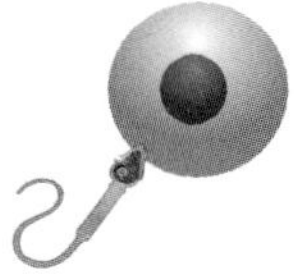
Cardiovascular System	**Digestive System**	**Mouth**	**Pharynx**	**Respiratory System**	**Urogenital Organs**
Thoracic duct and its tributaries developed, lymph nodes appear, anucleate RBC's predominate in blood.	Intestine retracts from umbilical cord, anal canal differentiates, pancreatic alveoli appear.	Fungiform and vallate papillae differentiate, labia separate from substructure, enamel organs and dental papillae forming.	Thymic parenchyma differentiates, ultimobranchial bodies involute.	Nasal septum and nasal cartilages form, vocal folds appear, larynx reopens.	Kidney able to secrete, urinary bladder expands, genital duct of opposing sex degenerating, lubricating glands appear.
Hemopoiesis occurs in bone marrow tissue, blood vessel walls stratify.	Layers of tunica muscularis differentiate, pancreatic islets appear, bile is secreted.	Filiform and foliate papillae differentiate, dental primordia form cups, buccae present, palate fusion complete.	Tonsillar crypts invaginate, thyroid gland attains typical structure.	Conchae prominent, nasal glands form, lungs acquire definitive shape.	External genitalia become distinct, prostate and seminal vesicles appearing.
Hemopoiesis occurs in spleen, myocardium well developed.	Gastric and intestinal glands differentiate, meconium starts to collect.	Hard and soft palates differentiate, hypophysis attaining definitive structure.	Lymphocytes accumulate in tonsils, pharyngeal tonsils develop.	Nasal sinuses begin to develop, tracheal glands appear, elastic fibers formed in lungs.	Kidneys become definitive, testes positioned for later descent, uterus and vagina recognizable.
Hemopoiesis increases in bone marrow tissue and decreases elsewhere. *(5-10 mos.).*	Lymphatic nodules appear in gut wall and muscularis mucosae differentiates.	Enamel and dentine depositing, lingual tonsil forming.		Nasal bones ossify.	Vagina regains lumen.
	Ascending colon becomes distinct.	Primordia for permanent teeth indicated. *(6-8 mo.)*		Nostrils re-open.	Uterine glands appear. Scrotum solid until testes and vaginal tunics descend. *(7-9 mos.).*
Spleen assumes definitive structure.	Esophageal glands differentiate.				
	Plicae circulares present.				
Some fetal blood conduits are discontinued.		Deciduous teeth not yet erupted.		Pulmonary arborization only two-thirds complete, frontal and sphenoidal sinuses incomplete.	

Points to Ponder

Nidation—five to seven days after fertilization. The exponentially growing conceptus is now a hollow (fluid-filled) ball of cells called a blastocyst. Embryologists distinguish a group of cells on the inner aspect of one side of the blastocyst as the definitive formative group (that develops into the individual). Given the name embryoblast or inner cell mass, most of it continues development as the embryo proper *vs.* the rest of the cells (collectively called the trophoblast) that form parts of some of the extraembryonic membranes. As the embryoblast continues to develop, the cells organize themselves into three layered groups: ectoderm (outer group), mesoderm (middle group), endoderm (inner group). Excited embryologists can witness this process called gastrulation under a microscope. It has been studied extensively in *Rana pipens* (leopard frog) and in other vertebrate species—including mankind when embryologists have been able to get hold of an early one. These three layers then begin forming tissues and organ rudiments. What guides this amazing process remains largely unknown. We've learned to send men to the moon, but we can't explain a simple biological process which has been going on since the dawn of time.

Ten lunar (nine calendar) months after conception, the uterus has had enough. Influenced by chemical regulators, some of which it produces itself, the uterus decides to reject its endometrial parasite. Sometimes it makes this decision too early and the fetus isn't fully prepared for life as we know it. Other uteri seem unwilling to expel their cargo and must be chemically encouraged. Childbirth (labor, parturition, travail) is divided into three parts (so we can speak about it in an organized fashion): dilation, expulsion, and the placental stage. The uterus begins practicing for this event by contracting well ahead of schedule. Many a first time mother-to-be has made more than one trip to the local delivery room only to find that the uterus didn't really mean it—yet.

These early, false alarm contractions are mere preparations for the big squeezes yet to come. They shift and tilt the fetus into the proper position for the final luge—usually. Sometimes junior stubbornly refuses to assume the doctrinally correct posture (head first) and must be encouraged with the probing fingers or forceps of Dr. Obgyn. Failing that, an abnormal presentation is sometimes successfully delivered, but just as often, for the sake of mother and offspring, the fetus is spared the bottleneck gauntlet of the birth canal. Canonized under Roman law (and thus indirectly related to the Caesars), the procedure involves two major cuts—one in the abdominal wall and one in the uterine wall.

Regardless of one's vaginal or abdominal entry into the world, postnatal development follows a predictable pattern: suckle, urinate, defecate, grow. Infant, child, adolescent, adult. Doctor, lawyer, teacher, priest, janitor, cashier, criminal, nurse. Along the way we develop our personal rendition of secondary sex characteristics and other factors of individual variation including height, weight, hair color, eye color, *etc.* As an old nursery rhyme indicates, little girls are composed of... "sugar and spice and everything nice" while boys are made of "snakes and snails and puppy-dog tails" as well as a longer list of disgusting habits.

Along life's path we parent children of our own and then...we die. The unifying thread that binds us all together is a common biological history. We share it with each other and we share it with animal life in general. Ontogeny. May life be with you—for a while.

Review Questions

1. Which one of the following stages of ontogeny is the briefest?
   A. cleavage
   B. organogenesis

C. senescence
D. fertilization
E. gastrulation

2. Which two extraembryonic membranes form the fetal portion of the placenta?
A. yolk sac and amnion
B. amnion and chorion
C. chorion and allantois
D. allantois and amnion
E. yolk sac and chorion

3. The shortest portion of maturation is termed ______________________ and the longest is called ______________________.
A. infancy—senescence
B. infancy—adulthood
C. the neonatal period—adulthood
D. the neonatal period—adolescence
E. childhood—senescence

4. Which stage of ontogeny is mismatched with events that occur during that period?
A. gametogenesis—spermatogenesis
B. gastrulation—formation of the morula
C. gametogenesis—oogenesis
D. organogenesis—interactions of various tissues to form body structures
E. cleavage—initial cell divisions of the conceptus terminating in formation of the blastula

5. Which post-fertilization event is mismatched with a time period?
A. nidation—5 to 7 days after ovulation
B. fertilization—within 2 days of ovulation
C. formation of morula—3 days after fertilization
D. first division of zygote—about 8 hours after fertilization
E. birth—38 $\pm$ weeks after ovulation

6. Which method of birth control would not be classified as a " barrier" technique?
A. condom
B. intrauterine device
C. diaphragm
D. tubal ligation
E. vasectomy

7. Which one of the following is the poorest example of "ontogeny recapitulating phylogeny"?
A. sequential development of pronephric, mesonephric, and metanephric kidneys
B. the series of embryonic aortic arches that develop in mammals
C. the presence of vestigial limb bones in some species of snakes
D. the presence of a heart in all higher species of animals
E. the development of non-digit-bearing metacarpal and metatarsal bones ("splint bones") in ungulates

8. Which stages of ontogeny are encompassed by the embryonic period?
   A. organogenesis and part of growth
   B. fertilization, cleavage, and gastrulation
   C. ovulation through organogenesis
   D. gametogenesis and fertilization
   E. fertilization through birth

9. How are sperm and ova transported through the uterine tubes?
   A. sperm swim through the uterine tubes and ova are transported via peristalsis
   B. sperm are transported by peristalsis and ova are transported via ciliary action
   C. ova are transported by ciliary action and sperm swim
   D. both are transported by ciliary action
   E. both are transported by peristalsis

10. Which term is misdefined?
   A. congenital—genetic
   B. teratology—study of physical abnormalities of neonates and fetuses
   C. gerontology—study of aging
   D. amniocentesis—procedure for withdrawing a sample of fluid to check for certain diseases before birth
   E. embryoblast—the portion of a conceptus from which the main part of the individual develops

Thought Questions

1. Can twins have different biological fathers?

2. Is it necessary to tie off the umbilical cord at birth?

3. Why does the major increase in fetal body mass occur during the last trimester of gestation?

4. What is the best defense against sexually transmitted diseases?

5. Why is ultrasonography used instead of radiography to image early fetuses?

6. What structure, when identifiable on a sonogram, indicates that a fetus is a male?

7. How do birth control pills prevent pregnancy?

8. Explain how a fetus can have a different blood type than its mother.

9. Explain why women with large numbers of children tend to ovulate fewer times during their lives than women with no children or only a few children.

10. Is there a male menopause?

11. How do pregnancy tests work?

12. What are the usual consequences of using withdrawal or the rhythm method of birth control?

13. Can a reproductively competent woman experience cessation of menstruation without pregnancy?

14. Why cannot a tubal pregnancy be carried to term?

15. Explain how the uterine tube can simultaneously transport sperm toward the ovary and ova toward the uterus.

16. Which forms of birth control could be viewed as a form of abortion?

17. Why is there a discrepancy between the weight of a pregnant woman at term and the combined weight of the newborn baby and its mother after birth?

18. What two major structures must be incised during a cesarean section?

19. How can amniocentesis be used to detect some forms of genetic disease?

20. Why do the cells continually get smaller as cleavage progresses?

21. Why do amniocentesis needles so rarely strike the placenta?

Answers to Clinical Case Studies

Case 1—The fetal heartbeat indicated stress. Sometimes this occurs when the umbilical cord becomes entangled around the fetus's neck. Immediate C-sections in such cases may be necessary to prevent fetal death or severe hypoxia that can result in mental retardation.

Case 2—Blood-tinged vaginal discharges during pregnancy may indicate a partial tearing of the placenta from the uterine wall. Extreme care in such cases may be required to prevent enough disruption to cause an abortion.

Case 3—In circumcised males, the glans penis is more easily cleaned and wives of circumcised males have been shown, in some studies, to have a lower than average incidence of cervical cancer. There are some religious implications for circumcision. On the other hand, it is a barbaric procedure causing considerable discomfort. Those to whom the procedure is done are rarely asked their opinion because they are too young to have one. The difference in cervical cancer incidence (in wives) is quite small and some have suggested that the studies may be flawed because of the ethnic backgrounds in which the data were collected. There is also an argument that circumcision reduces the sensitivity of the glans penis—not directly, perhaps—but indirectly due to its continued contact with clothing, *etc.* Unfortunately, control study subjects on this point are difficult to find.

Answers to Review Questions

1. D.
2. C. They partially fuse to form the chorioallantois.
3. C.
4. B. The morula is formed during cleavage.
5. D. The first division occurs about 24 hours after fertilization.
6. B. IUD's prevent nidation.
7. D.
8. A.
9. B.
10. A. Some congenital (present at birth) things are hereditary (genetic) and some are not.

Answers to Thought Questions

1. Yes—if two ova were released and they were fertilized by sperm from different men.
2. No—if it were, mammals would have become extinct long ago.
3. Growth (by cellular division) is somewhat exponential. In early development, when the cell numbers are doubling with every division, the total embryonic mass is so small that doubling still does not result in a significantly-sized mass for many cell generations.
4. Abstinence/monogamy.
5. Sonography has not been shown to be harmful. Radiography can alter nucleic acids leading to inborn errors of metabolism and cancer.
6. Penis/scrotum.
7. Oral contraceptives are progesteroids which prevent ovarian follicle maturation and ovulation.
8. Fetal blood is entirely separate from maternal blood during gestation. The ABO blood type is determined by simple Mendelian genetics based on the genotypes of the mother and father.
9. After puberty, women typically ovulate once each month until menopause except when they are pregnant. During gestation, the ovarian cycle is interrupted.

10. No—men are normally fertile until they die.

11. They employ a color-change chemical reaction which detects chorionic gonadotropin in the urine. This hormone is produced by the placenta during pregnancy.

12. Children.

13. Yes—during periods of prolonged emotional or physical stress, the corticosteroid output of the adrenal glands can interrupt the ovarian cycle.

14. The wall of the uterine tube is far too thin and friable to stretch enough to accommodate the growing fetus.

15. The relatively large ova are "swept" down the uterine tube by the cilia of the lining epithelium. The sperm are forced up the tube by peristalsis and are so small that many of them pass between the cilia.

16. Intra-uterine devices (IUD's) and the "morning after" (post-coital) pill. They prevent nidation.

17. The placenta, extraembryonic membranes and their associated fluids account for the difference.

18. Abdominal wall and uterine wall.

19. The amniotic fluid contains cells sloughed off the amnion. These can be examined microscopically and their chromosomes analyzed (karyotyped).

20. Until implantation, the conceptus receives no nutrition from its mother. Consequently, the cells get progressively smaller for the first several generations.

21. Placentation usually occurs on the upper central and posterior wall of the uterine lining. An amniocentesis needle is passed through the lower anterior abdominal wall and then the anterior wall of the uterus.

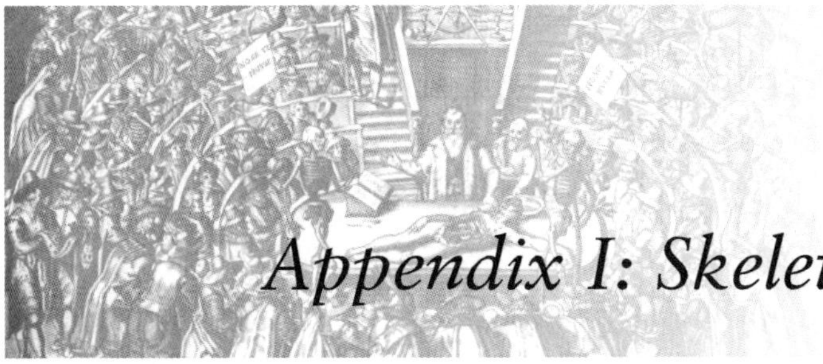

Appendix I: Skeletal Muscles

Part A, Muscles of the Head

Muscles of the Face

m. epicranius—O: (all bellies) epicranial aponeurosis I: (occipital belly) occipital bone, (frontal belly) skin of eyebrow and nose, (lateral, temporoparietal parts, bellies) muscle and cartilage of the auricle A: move the scalp (wrinkle brow, wiggle ears, *etc.*).

m. procerus—O: fascia over nasal bone, lateral nasal cartilage I: skin between eyebrows A: wrinkle nose, depresses medial aspect of eyebrow

m. nasalis—O: maxilla I: into ala and contralateral muscle (over bridge of nose) near corner of mouth A: wrinkle nose, dilate nostrils

m. depressor septi nasi—O: incisive fossa of maxilla I: nasal septum and ala nasi A: constrict nares

m. orbicularis oculi—O: maxilla, frontal and lacrimal bones I: encircles the eyelid and returns to origin A: close the eyelids

m. corrugator supercilii—O: orbicularis oculi m., nasal prominence of frontal bone I: skin of eyebrow A: draw eyebrow inferomedially

m. depressor supercilii—O: lateral part of orbicularis oculi m. I: skin of eyebrow A: depress eyebrow

m. auricularis anterior—O: superficial temporal fascia I: auricular cartilage A: draw auricle forward

m. auricularis superior—O: galea aponeurotica I: cartilage of ear A: elevate auricle

m. auricularis posterior—O: mastoid process of temporal bone I: cartilage of ear A: draw auricle posteriorly

m. orbicularis oris—O: maxilla, nasal septum, mandible I: continuous with other muscles at angle of mouth A: close and purse lips

m. depressor anguli oris—O: anterior aspect of mandible I: tissue near corner of mouth A: depress corner of mouth

m. transversus menti—O: depressor anguli oris m. I: depressor anguli oris m. A: wrinkle chin

m. risorius—O: fascia over masseter m. I: skin at angle of mouth A: draw angle of mouth laterally

m. zygomaticus major—O: zygomatic bone I: orbicularis oris m. near angle of mouth A: draw superior lip up and laterally

m. zygomaticus minor—O: zygomatic bone near maxillary suture I: tissue of superior lip A: draw superior lip superiorly and laterally

m. buccinator—O: mandible, maxilla I: orbicularis oris m. A: compress cheek and retract angle of mouth

m. mentalis—O: incisive fossa of mandible I: skin of chin A: wrinkle skin of chin

m. levator anguli oris—O: canine fossa of maxilla I: orbicularis oris m. and skin at corner of mouth A: elevate corner of mouth

m. levator labii superior—O: maxilla, zygomatic bone I: orbicularis oris m. of superior lip A: elevate upper lip

m. depressor labii inferioris—O: anterior aspect of mandible (between mandibular symphysis and mental foramen) I: orbicularis oris m. (and skin) of lower lip A: depress lower lip

m. levator labii superioris alaeque nasi—O: nasal process of maxilla I: cartilage of the wing of the nose and upper lip A: raise upper lip and dilate nostril

Muscles of the Eye

m. rectus superior—O: upper border of optic canal I: upper aspect of sclera A: rotate eyeball upward (and medially)
m. rectus inferior—O: circumference of optic canal I: underside of sclera A: rotate eyeball downward (and medially)
m. rectus medialis—O: circumference of optic canal I: medial side of sclera A: rotate eyeball medially
m. rectus lateralis—O: lateral margin of optic canal, margin of superior orbital fissure I: lateral side of sclera A: rotate eyeball laterally
m. obliquus superior—O: lesser wing of sphenoid bone above optic canal I: sclera A: rotate eyeball downward and laterally
m. obliquus inferior—O: orbital plate of maxilla I: sclera A: rotate eyeball upward and laterally
m. levator palpebrae superioris—O: upper border of optic canal I: tarsal plate of upper eyelid A: elevate upper eyelid

Muscles of the Auditory Ossicles

m. tensor tympani—O: cartilaginous part of auditory tube I: manubrium of the malleus A: tense tympanic membrane
m. stapedius—O: pyramidal eminence of tympanic cavity I: posterior neck of stapes A: reduce stapedial movement (vibrations)

Muscles of Mastication

m. masseter—O: zygomatic arch of the skull I: coronoid process and ramus of the mandible A: elevate mandible (clench teeth)
m. temporalis—O: temporal fossa of skull I: coronoid process and ramus of the mandible A: elevate mandible (clench teeth)
m. pterygoideus lateralis—O: pterygoid process and adjacent greater wing of sphenoid b. I: condyloid process of mandible and articular disc of temporomandibular joint A: protract mandible, depress mandible (weakly)
m. pterygoideus medialis—O: maxilla, sphenoid and palatine bones I: medial aspect of mandible (near the angle) A: elevate mandible and move it laterally

Extrinsic Muscles of the Tongue

m. genioglossus—O: mental spine of mandible I: hyoid bone and underside of tongue A: protrude and depress tongue
m. hyoglossus—O: body and greater cornu of hyoid bone I: side of tongue A: retract and depress tongue
m. chondroglossus—O: medial side and base of lesser cornu of hyoid bone I: substance of tongue A: retract and depress tongue
m. styloglossus—O: styloid process of temporal bone I: margin of tongue A: elevate and retract tongue

Muscles of Palate and Fauces

m. levator veli palatini—O: apex of petrous portion of temporal bone I: aponeurosis of soft palate A: raise soft palate
m. tensor veli palatini—O: scaphoid fossa of sphenoid bone, wall of auditory tube I: aponeurosis of soft palate, horizontal part of palatine bone A: tense soft palate, open auditory tube
m. uvulae—O: posterior nasal spine of palatine bone, aponeurosis of soft palate I: palatine uvula A: elevate palatine uvula
m. palatoglossus—O: under surface of soft palate I: side of tongue A: elevate tongue, constrict fauces
m. palatopharyngeus—O: soft palate I: aponeurosis of pharynx, dorsal border of thyroid cartilage A: assist deglutition

Part B, Muscles of the Neck

Suboccipital Muscles

m. rectus capitis anterior—O: lateral mass of atlas I: basilar process of occipital bone A: flex and rotate head
m. rectus capitis posterior major—O: spinous process of axis I: occipital bone A: extension of cervical joints, rotation of head
m. rectus capitis posterior minor—O: dorsal arch of atlas I: occipital bone A: extension of cervical joints, rotation of head
m. rectus capitis lateralis—O: upper surface of transverse process of atlas I: jugular process of occipital b. A: flex and rotate head
m. obliquus capitis superior—O: transverse process of atlas I: occipital bone A: extension of cervical joints, rotation of head
m. obliquus capitis inferior—O: spinous process of axis I: transverse process of atlas A: rotation of head

Suprahyoid Muscles

m. digastricus—O: (anterior belly) digastric fossa of mandible, (posterior belly) mastoid notch of temporal bone I: intermediate tendon of hyoid bone A: elevate hyoid bone, depress mandible
m. stylohyoideus—O: styloid process of temporal bone I: body of hyoid bone A: elevate hyoid bone and tongue
m. mylohyoideus—O: mylohyoid line of mandible I: body of hyoid bone A: support floor of oral cavity, elevate hyoid bone
m. geniohyoideus—O: mental spine of mandible I: body of hyoid bone A: elevate and draw hyoid bone anteriorly

Infrahyoid Muscles

m. sternohyoideus—O: manubrium sterni I: body of hyoid bone A: depress hyoid bone and larynx
m. omohyoideus—O: superior border of scapula I: lateral border of hyoid bone A: depress hyoid bone
m. sternothyroideus—O: manubrium sterni I: thyroid cartilage A: depress thyroid cartilage
m. thyrohyoideus—O: thyroid cartilage I: greater cornu of hyoid bone A: elevate and change the form of the larynx

Pharyngeal Muscles

m. constrictor pharyngeus superior—O: medial pterygoid plate of sphenoid bone, pterygomandibular raphe, mylohyoid ridge of mandible, mucous membrane floor of mouth I: median raphe of posterior wall of pharynx A: constrict pharynx

m. constrictor pharyngeus medius—O: cornua of hyoid bone, stylohyoid ligament I: median raphe of posterior wall of pharynx A: constrict pharynx

m. constrictor pharyngeus inferior—O: deep to cricoid and thyroid cartilaginous surfaces I: median raphe of posterior wall of pharynx A: constrict pharynx

m. stylopharyngeus—O: styloid process of temporal bone I: thyroid cartilage, pharyngeal constrictors A: elevate and dilate pharynx

m. salpingopharyngeus—O: pharyngeal opening of auditory tube I: posterior part of palatopharyngeus A: elevate nasopharynx

Laryngeal Muscles

m. cricothyroideus—O: anterior and lateral aspects of cricoid cartilage I: lamina of thyroid cartilage A: tense vocal folds

m. crico-arytenoideus posterior—O: posterior aspect of cricoid cartilage I: muscular process of arytenoid cartilage A: separate vocal folds

m. crico-arytenoideus lateralis—O: lateral surface of cricoid cartilage I: muscular process of arytenoid cartilage A: approximate vocal folds

m. vocalis—O: thyroid cartilage I: vocal process of arytenoid cartilage A: shorten vocal folds

m. thyro-arytenoideus—O: lamina of thyroid cartilage I: muscular process of arytenoid process A: shorten and relax vocal folds

m. arytenoideus obliquus—O: dorsal aspect of muscular process of arytenoid cartilage I: apex of opposite arytenoid cartilage A: close inlet of pharynx

m. arytenoideus transversus—O: dorsal aspect of muscular process of arytenoid cartilage I: continuous with thyroarytenoid, apex of opposite arytenoid cartilage A: approximate arytenoid cartilage

Other Muscles of the Neck

platysma—O: fascia over pectoralis major and deltoideus muscles I: lower mandibular region A: depress lower lip, wrinkle skin of neck and upper chest (as in yelling/screaming)

m. longus colli—O: (superior oblique portion) transverse processes of third to fifth cervical vertebrae; (inferior oblique portion) bodies of first to third thoracic vertebrae; (vertical portion) bodies of cervical vertebrae V-VII and thoracic vertebrae I-III I: (superior oblique portion) tubercle of anterior arch of atlas; (inferior oblique portion) transverse processes of fifth and sixth cervical vertebrae, (vertical portion) bodies of second to fourth cervical vertebrae A: flex joints of cervical vertebral column

m. longus capitis—O: transverse processes of third to sixth cervical vertebrae I: basal portion of occipital bone A: flex cervical vertebral column

m. scalenus anterior—O: transverse processes of third to sixth cervical vertebrae I: tubercle of scalenus anterior muscle of first rib A: elevate first rib

m. scalenus medius—O: transverse processes of second to sixth cervical vertebrae I: tubercle of first rib A: elevate first rib

m. scalenus posterior—O: tubercles of fourth to sixth cervical vertebrae I: second rib A: elevate first and second ribs

m. sternocleidomastoideus—O: manubrium sterni, sternal extremity of clavicle I: mastoid process of temporal bone A: turn head toward opposite side (if contracting unilaterally); flex joints of cervical vertebral column (if contracting bilaterally)

Part C, Muscles of the Thorax

m. pectoralis major:

clavicular part—O: body and sternal extremity of clavicle I: crest of greater tubercle of humerus (lateral lip of intertubercular groove of humerus) A: flex shoulder joint

sternocostal part—O: sternum, first six ribs I: crest of greater tubercle of humerus (lateral lip of intertubercular groove of humerus) A: abduction of superior limb at shoulder joint

abdominal part—O: aponeurosis of external abdominal oblique muscle I: crest of greater tubercle of humerus (lateral lip of intertubercular groove of humerus) A: rotate superior limb medially at shoulder joint

m. pectoralis minor—O: ribs 3-5/6 near costochondral joints. I: coracoid process of scapula A: draw scapula anterior, inferior; elevate ribs

m. subclavius—O: first rib and its costal cartilage I: inferior surface of body of clavicle A: depress acromial extremity of clavicle

m. serratus anterior—O: center of lateral aspects of first 8-9 ribs I: anterior aspect of medial border of scapula (from superior angle to inferior angle of scapula) A: rotate and protract scapula, elevate ribs

mm. levatores costarum:

longi—O: transverse processes of thoracic vertebrae 7/8-10 I: posterior aspects of ribs 9/10-12 near the costal angle (inserts into second rib below vertebra of origin) A: elevates ribs; extends, laterally flexes and rotates thoracic part of vertebral column

breves—O: transverse processes of seventh cervical vertebra and thoracic vertebrae 1-11 I: inserts just medial of the angle of the rib below the vertebra of origin A: elevates ribs; extends, laterally flexes and rotates thoracic part of vertebral column

mm. intercostales externi—O: inferior borders of ribs I: superior borders of ribs (each one inserts into rib inferior to its origin) A: elevate ribs (to increase volume in thoracic cavity), maintain tension in the intercostal spaces

mm. intercostales interni—O: inferior borders of ribs I: superior borders of ribs (each one inserts into rib inferior to its origin) A: depress the ribs (to decrease the volume in the thoracic cavity), maintain tension in the intercostal spaces

mm. intercostales intimi—(separated from internal intercostal mm. by intercostal nn.) O: inferior border of rib, costal cartilage I: superior border of rib, costal cartilage A: depress ribs (to decrease volume in thoracic cavity), maintain tension of intercostal spaces

mm. subcostales—O: inner surface of ribs near angle of rib I: inner surface of first, second, and third rib below A: elevate ribs in inspiration

m. transversus thoracis—O: mediastinal surface of sternum and xiphoid process I: costal cartilages of second to sixth ribs A: narrow chest

diaphragm (thoraco-abdominal diaphragm):

costal part—O: deep surface of last six ribs and their costal cartilages I: central tendon of diaphragm A: draw central tendon of diaphragm down, increase volume of thoracic cavity

lumbar part—O: lumbar vertebrae 1 to 2/3, lateral medial lumbocostal arches I: central tendon of diaphragm A: draw central tendon of diaphragm down, increase volume of thoracic cavity

sternal part—O: deep surface of xiphoid process of sternum I: central tendon of diaphragm A: draw central tendon of diaphragm down, increase volume of thoracic cavity

Part D, Muscles of the Abdomen

Muscles of the Anterior, Lateral, and Posterior Abdominal Wall

m. rectus abdominis—O: pubic crest and pubic symphysis I: xiphoid process of sternum and costal cartilages 5-7 A: draw thorax downward (flexes joints of vertebral column), compress abdomen

m. obliquus externus abdominis—O: ribs 5-12 I: anterior sheath of rectus abdominis muscle (and thence to linea alba), anterior half of iliac crest (lateral aspect), inguinal ligament A: draw thorax downward (flex joints of vertebral column), compress abdomen, rotate vertebral column

m. obliquus internus abdominis—O: anterior half of crest of ilium, lumbar fascia, iliac fascia, inguinal ligament I: ribs 10-12, sheath of rectus abdominis m. (and thence to linea alba) A: draw thorax downward (flex joint of vertebral column), compress abdomen, rotate vertebral column

m. transversus abdominis—O: costal cartilages of rib 7-12, lumbar fascia, iliac crest, inguinal ligament I: xiphoid process of sternum, posterior lamina of sheath of rectus abdominis m. (and thence to linea alba) A: compress abdomen

m. pyramidalis—O: anterior portion of pubis, anterior pubic ligament I: linea alba A: tense abdominal wall

m. quadratus lumborum—O: crest of ilium, thoracolumbar fascia, lumbar vertebrae I: rib 12, transverse process of first four lumbar vertebrae A: bend lumbar vertebral column laterally

Muscles of the Pelvic Diaphragm

m. levator ani:

- **m. pubococcygeus**—O: pubis, anterior to obturator canal I: anococcygeal ligament, lateral aspect of coccyx A: support pelvic viscera and resist increased intra-abdominal pressure
- **m. levator prostatae**—O: anterior part of pubococcygeus muscle I: prostate, tendinous center of perineum A: support and compress prostate, involved in control of micturition
- **m. pubovaginalis**—O: anterior portion of pubococcygeus muscle I: urethra and vagina A: involved in micturition
- **m. puborectalis**—O: lateral aspect of pubic bone I: continuous posteriorly with the corresponding muscle of opposite side A: support pelvic viscera, resist increased intra-abdominal pressure
- **m. iliococcygeus**—O: obturator canal I: lateral aspect of coccyx and anococcygeal body A: support pelvic viscera, resist increased intra-abdominal pressure

m. coccygeus—O: ischial spine I: inferolateral portion of sacral bone A: support and elevate coccyx

m. sphincter ani externus—O: apex of coccyx and surrounding fascia I: tendinous center of perineum A: close anus

Muscles of the Urogenital Diaphragm

Muscles of the Superficial Perineal Space:

- **m. ischiocavernosus**—O: ramus of ischium I: crus of penis (crus clitoridis) A: maintains erection of penis (clitoris)
- **m. bulbospongiosus**—O: central point of perineum, median raphe of bulb I: fascia of penis (clitoris) A: constrict bulb of urethra
- **m. transversus perinei superficialis**—O: ischial tuber I: central tendon of perineum A: tense central point of perineum

Muscles of the Deep Perineal Space:

- **m. sphincter urethrae**—O: inferior ramus of pubis I: median raphe posterior and anterior to urethra A: compress urethra

m. compressor urethrae—O: inferior ramus of pubis I: contralateral muscle and vagina (female), prostate (male) A: compress urethra

m. sphincter urethrovaginalis—O: ischial and inferior pubic rami I: lateral aspect of vagina and periurethral tissue A: compress vagina, greater vestibular glands, and urethra

m. transversus perinea profundus—O: ischial ramus I: median raphe of perineum A: draw back central point of perineum

Part E, Muscles of the Back

m. trapezius—O: occipital bone, nuchal ligament, spinous process of C7 and thoracic vertebrae I: clavicle, spine and acromion of scapula A: draw head laterally or posteriorly, rotate scapula

m. latissimus dorsi—O: spinous processes of lower 5-6 thoracic vertebrae, lumbar vertebrae, median sacral crest I: posterior ridge (medial border) of intertubercular groove of humerus A: extend, adduct, medially rotate the limb at the shoulder joint

m. rhomboideus major—O: spinous process and corresponding supraspinous ligaments of T2-T5 vertebrae I: medial border of scapula below level of spine A: pull (retract) scapula toward vertebral column and slightly superiorly

m. rhomboideus minor—O: spinous process of C7 and T1 vertebrae I: medial border of scapula at the level of its spine A: pull scapula toward vertebral column

m. levator scapulae—O: transverse process of C1-C4 vertebrae I: superior angle of scapula A: elevate scapula

m. serratus posterior:

inferior—O: spinous process of T11-T12 and L1-L3 vertebrae I: inferior border of ribs 9-12 A: lower ribs in expiration

superior—O: ligamentum nuchae, spinous process of upper thoracic vertebrae I: ribs 2-5 A: elevate ribs in inspiration

m. splenius capitis—O: inferior half of ligamentum nuchae, spinous process of C7-T3 vert. I: occipital b. A: rotate head and draws it back

m. splenius cervicis—O: spinous process of T3-T6 vertebrae I: transverse process of C1-2/3 vert. A: rotate head and neck, draws head back

mm. erector spinae:

m. iliocostalis:

lumborum—O: iliac crest I: angle of ribs 6/7-12 A: extend lumbar vertebral column

thoracis—O: superior border of angle of ribs 7-12 I: angle of ribs 1-6, transverse process C7 A: keep thoracic spine erect

cervicis—O: angle of ribs 3-6 I: transverse process of C4-C6 vertebrae A: extend joints of cervical vertebral column

m. longissimus:

thoracis—O: transverse and articular process of lumbar vertebrae, thoracolumbar fascia I: thoracic transverse processes, ribs 2/3-12 A: extend joints of thoracic vertebral column

cervicis—O: transverse process of T1-T4/5 I: transverse process of C2-C6 vert. A: extend joints of cervical vert. column

capitis—O: transverse process of T1-T4/5, articular process of C4/5-C7 vertebrae I: mastoid process of temporal b. A: draw head backward and rotates head

m. spinalis:

thoracis—O: spinous process of T10-L2 vert. I: spinous process of upper thoracic vert. A: extend joints of vertebral column

cervicis—O: spinous process of C5-C7 and T1-T2 vertebrae I: spinous process of axis (sometimes C2-C4) A: extend vertebral joints

capitis—O: spinous process of upper thoracic and lower cervical vertebrae I: occipital bone A: draws head back

mm. interspinales:

cervicis—O/I: between spinous processes of contiguous cervical vertebrae A: extend the cervical vertebral column

lumborum—O/I: between spinous processes of contiguous lumbar vertebrae A: extend the lumbar vertebral column

thoracis—O/I: between spinous processes of contiguous thoracic vertebrae A: extend the thoracic vertebral column

mm. transversospinales:

m. semispinalis:

thoracis—O: transverse processes of T6-T10 vertebrae I: spinous process of C6-T4 vertebrae A: extend and rotate joints of vertebral column

cervicis—O: transverse processes of T1-5/6 vertebrae I: spinous process of C2-C5 vertebrae A: extend and rotate joints of vertebral column

capitis—O: transverse processes of C4-T5/6 vertebrae I: occipital bone A: draw head back

mm. multifidi—O: sacral bone, sacroiliac ligament, mammillary processes of thoracic and articular processes of cervical vertebrae I: spines of contiguous vertebrae above A: extend and rotate vertebral column

mm. rotatores:

cervicis—O: transverse processes of cervical vertebrae I: base of spinous process of superjacent vertebrae A: extend and rotate vertebral column

thoracis—O: transverse processes of thoracic vertebrae I: base of spinous process of superjacent vertebrae A: extend and rotate vertebral column

lumborum—O: transverse processes of lumbar vertebrae I: base of spinous process of superjacent vertebrae A: extend and rotate vertebral column

mm. intertransversarii:

laterales lumborum—O/I: transverse processes of adjacent lumbar vertebrae A: flex vertebral column laterally

mediales lumborum—O/I: accessory process of one lumbar vertebra to mammillary process of the contiguous lumbar vertebra A: flex vertebral column laterally

thoracis—O/I: anterior tubercles of adjacent thoracic vertebrae A: flex vertebral column laterally

posteriores cervicis—O/I: posterior tubercles of adjacent cervical vertebrae A: flex vertebral column laterally

anteriores cervicis—O/I: anterior tubercles of adjacent cervical vertebrae A: flex vertebral column laterally

Part F, Muscles of the Superior Limb

Muscles of the Shoulder (Scapula)

m. supraspinatus—O: supraspinous fossa of scapula I: greater tubercle of humerus A: abduct limb at shoulder joint

m. infraspinatus—O: infraspinous fossa of scapula I: greater tubercle of humerus A: extend shoulder joint, rotate brachium laterally (externally)

m. teres minor—O: lateral border of scapula I: greater tubercle of humerus A: adduct limb at shoulder joint, rotate brachium laterally (externally)

m. teres major—O: inferior angle of scapula I: medial border of the intertubercular groove of the humerus A: extend shoulder joint, adduct limb at shoulder joint, rotate brachium medially (internally)

m. subscapularis—O: subscapular fossa I: lesser tubercle of humerus A: rotate brachium medially (internally)

m. deltoideus—O: acromial extremity of clavicle, acromion and spine of scapula I: deltoid tuberosity of humerus A: flex and extend shoulder joint, rotate brachium (both medially and laterally), abduct limb at shoulder joint

m. coracobrachialis—O: coracoid process of scapula I: medial border of humerus A: flex shoulder joint, adduct limb at shoulder joint

Anterior Muscles of the Brachium

m. biceps brachii—O: (long head) neck of scapula; (short head) coracoid process of scapula I: tuberosity of radius, deep antebrachial fascia A: flex elbow joint, flex shoulder joint, supinate antebrachium

m. brachialis—O: anterior border of humerus I: coronoid process of ulna A: flex elbow joint

m. brachioradialis—O: lateral supracondylar crest of humerus I: base of styloid process of radius A: flex elbow joint, supinate antebrachium (from pronated position), pronate antebrachium (from supinated position)

Posterior Muscles of the Brachium

m. triceps brachii—O: (long head) lateral border of scapula, (lateral head) lateral and posterior aspects of humerus, (medial head) medial and posterior aspects of humerus I: olecranon of ulna A: extend elbow joint, extend shoulder joint (long head), adduct limb at shoulder joint

m. anconeus—O: lateral epicondyle of humerus I: olecranon (and adjacent body) of ulna A: extend cubital joint

Anterior Muscles of the Antebrachium

m. flexor carpi radialis—O: medial epicondyle of humerus I: anterior aspects of bases of second and third metacarpal bones A: flex carpal joint, abduct manus at carpal joint

m. flexor carpi ulnaris—O: (humeral head) medial epicondyle of humerus, (ulnar head) olecranon and body of ulna I: pisiform bone, hamulus of the hamate bone, base of fifth metacarpal bone A: flex carpal joint, adduct manus at carpal joint

m. flexor digitorum superficialis—O: medial epicondyle of humerus, coronoid process of ulna, proximal aspect of radius I: middle phalanges of digits 2-5 A: flex carpal joint, metacarpophalangeal joints, proximal interphalangeal joints.

m. flexor digitorum profundus—O: proximal aspect of ulna I: separate tendons to the distal phalanges of digits 2-5 A: flex carpal joint and digital joints

m. flexor pollicis longus—O: anterior aspect of radial body I: distal phalanx of pollex A: flex digital joints of pollex

m. palmaris longus—O: medial epicondyle of humerus I: flexor retinaculum, carpal ligaments, palmar aponeurosis A: flex carpal joint

m. pronator teres—O: medial epicondyle of humerus and medial side of coronoid process of the ulna I: middle of the lateral side of the body of radius A: pronate the antebrachium and manus

m. pronator quadratus—O: distal, anterior aspect of the body of the ulna I: distal, anterior aspect of the body of the radius A: pronate manus

m. supinator—O: lateral epicondyle of the humerus I: proximal body of radius A: supinate the antebrachium and manus

Posterior Muscles of the Antebrachium

m. extensor carpi radialis longus—O: lateral supracondylar crest of humerus I: dorsal aspect of base of second metacarpal bone A: extend carpal joint, abduct manus at carpal joint
m. extensor carpi radialis brevis—O: lateral epicondyle of humerus I: dorsal aspect of base of third metacarpal bone A: extend carpal joint, abduct manus at carpal joint
m. extensor carpi ulnaris—O: lateral epicondyle of the humerus, proximal, posterior aspect of body of ulna I: base of fifth metacarpal bone A: extend carpal joint, adduct manus at carpal joint
m. extensor digitorum—O: lateral epicondyle of humerus I: middle, dist. phalanges of digits 2-5 A: extend carpal jt., extend 2-5 digital joints.
m. extensor digiti minimi—O: lateral epicondyle of humerus I: fuses with tendon of digital extensor m. distributed to the fifth digit and also attaches to the proximal phalanx A: extend carpal joint, extend digital joints of fifth digit
m. extensor pollicis brevis—O: posterior aspect of body of radius (and antebrachial interosseous membrane) I: dorsal surface of proximal phalanx of thumb A: extend metacarpophalangeal joint of thumb, abduct thumb at metacarpophalangeal joint
m. extensor pollicis longus—O: posterior aspect of body of ulna (antebrachial interosseous membrane) I: dorsal aspect of distal phalanx of thumb A: extend digital joints of thumb, abduct thumb at metacarpophalangeal joint
m. extensor indicis—O: posterior aspect of ulnar body I: dorsal aspect of proximal phalanx of digit 2 A: extend 2nd metacarpophalangeal joint.
m. abductor pollicis longus—O: posterior aspects of radial and ulnar bodies I: lateral side of base of first metacarpal bone A: extend digital joints of thumb, abduct thumb at metacarpophalangeal joint

Intrinsic Muscles of the Manus

Thenar Muscles:

m. abductor pollicis brevis—O: scaphoid bone, ridge of trapezium bone, transverse carpal ligament I: lateral surface of base of proximal phalanx of thumb A: abduct thumb

m. flexor pollicis brevis—O: transverse carpal ligament, ridge of trapezium bone I: base of proximal phalanx of thumb A: flex metacarpophalangeal joint of thumb and adduct thumb

m. opponens pollicis—O: ridge of trapezium bone, transverse carpal ligament I: radial aspect of first metacarpal bone A: flex first carpometacarpal joint, oppose thumb

Hypothenar Muscles:

m. abductor digiti minimi —O: pisiform bone, tendon of flexor carpi ulnaris muscle I: medial surface of base of proximal phalanx of little finger A: abduct little finger

m. flexor digiti minimi brevis—O: hamulus of the hamate bone, transverse carpal ligament I: medial aspect of proximal phalanx of little finger A: flex joints of little finger

m. opponens digiti minimi—O: hamulus of the hamate bone, transverse carpal ligament I: ulnar aspect of fifth metacarpal bone A: rotate, abduct fifth metacarpal bone

m. palmaris brevis—O: palmar aponeurosis I: skin of medial border of hand A: tense skin on palm of hand

Intermediate Muscles of Manus:

m. lumbricales—O: tendon of flexor digitorum profundus muscle I: extensor tendons of four medial fingers A: flex metacarpophalangeal joints, extend interphalangeal joints

m. interossei dorsales—O: by two heads from adjacent sides of metacarpal bones I: extensor tendons of digits 2-4 A: abduct digits 2-4, flex proximal metacarpophalangeal joints of digits 2-4

m. interossei palmares—O: sides of metacarpal bones 2,4,5 I: extensor tendons of digits 2,4,5 A: adduct digits 2,4,5 and flex metacarpophalangeal joints of digits 2,4,5

m. adductor pollicis—O: sheath of flexor carpi radialis m., anterior carpal ligament, bases of second and third metacarpal bones, capitate bone, and distal two-thirds of third metacarpal bone I: proximal, medial surface of base of proximal phalanx of thumb A: adducts and opposes thumb

Part G, Muscles of the Inferior Limb

Anterior Muscles of the Hip

m. iliopsoas:

m. iliacus—O: iliac fossa I: lesser trochanter of femur bone (adjacent body of femur bone) A: flex coxal joint, rotate thigh laterally (externally)

m. psoas major—O: bodies of T12-L5 vertebrae I: lesser trochanter of femur bone (adjacent body of femur bone) A: flex coxal joint, rotate thigh laterally (externally)

Posterior and Lateral Muscles of the Hip

m. gluteus maximus—O: sacral bone, iliac crest, coccyx I: proximal, lateral aspect of femoral body, iliotibial tract (see tensor fascia latae) A: extend coxal joint, rotates thigh laterally (externally), some adduction of limb at coxal joint

m. gluteus medius—O: gluteal surface of ilium I: greater trochanter of femur bone A: abduct limb at coxal joint, rotate thigh laterally (externally)

m. gluteus minimus—O: gluteal surface of ilium (between anterior and inferior gluteal lines) I: greater trochanter of femur bone (anterior surface) A: abduct limb at coxal joint

m. tensor fasciae latae—O: anterior superior iliac spine (and nearby ilium) I: iliotibial tract A: flex coxal joint, abduct limb at coxal joint

Medial Muscles of the Hip

m. piriformis—O: ilium, 2-4 sacral vertebrae I: superior border of greater trochanter of femur bone A: rotate thigh laterally (externally)

m. obturator externus—O: pubis, ischium, superficial surface of obturator membrane I: trochanteric fossa of femur bone A: rotate thigh laterally (externally)

m. obturator internus—O: pelvic surface of os coxae, margin of obturator foramen, ramus of ischium, inferior ramus of pubis, internal surface of obturator membrane I: greater trochanter of femur bone A: rotate thigh laterally (externally)

m. gemellus superior—O: spine of ischium I: greater trochanter of femur bone A: rotate thigh laterally (externally)

m. gemellus inferior—O: tuber of ischium I: greater trochanter of femur bone A: rotate thigh laterally (externally)

m. quadratus femoris—O: upper part of lateral border ischial tuber I: quadrate tubercle of femur bone A: adduct, rotate thigh laterally (externally)

Anterior Muscles of the Thigh

m. sartorius—O: anterior superior iliac spine I: medial aspect of tibial tuberosity A: flex coxal joint, rotate limb laterally (externally), flex genual joint

m. quadriceps femoris:

- **m. rectus femoris**—O: anterior inferior iliac spine (and adjacent ilium) I: tibial tuberosity (via patella and patellar ligament) A: flex coxal joint, extend genual joint
- **m. vastus lateralis**—O: lateral aspect of body of femur bone I: tibial tuberosity (via patella and patellar ligament) A: extend genual joint
- **m. vastus medialis**—O: medial aspect of body of femur bone I: tibial tuberosity (via patella and patellar ligament) A: extend genual joint
- **m. vastus intermedius**—O: anterior aspect of body of femur bone I: tibial tuberosity (via patella and patellarligament) A: extend genual joint

m. articularis genus—O: distal fourth of anterior surface of body of femur bone I: synovial membrane of genual joint A: elevate joint capsule of genual joint

Medial Muscles of the Thigh

m. gracilis—O: inferior ramus of pubis I: medial aspect of proximal aspect of tibial body A: adduct limb at coxal joint, flex genual joint, rotates limb medially (internally)

m. pectineus—O: pecten of pubis I: proximal end of posterior aspect of femoral body (below lesser trochanter) A: adduct limb at coxal joint, flex coxal joint

m. adductor longus—O: pubis symphysis and adjacent body of pubis I: middle third of medial lip of linea aspera of femur bone A: adduct limb at coxal joint

m. adductor brevis—O: inferior ramus of pubis I: medial lip of linea aspera of femur bone (superior part) A: adduct limb at coxal joint

m. adductor magnus—O: ischiatic tuber, inferior ramus of pubis, ramus of ischium I: linea aspera and adductor tubercle of femur bone A: adduct limb at coxal joint, extend coxal joint

m. adductor minimus—O: ischial tuber, inferior ramus of pubis, ramus of ischium I: posterior aspect of femur proximal to linea aspera of femur bone A: adduct limb at coxal joint

Posterior Muscles of the Thigh

m. biceps femoris—O: (long head) ischiatic tuber, (short head) lateral lip of linea aspera of femur bone I: fibular head, lateral condyle of tibia A: extend coxal joint (long head), flex genual joint, rotate limb laterally (externally)

m. semitendinosus—O: ischiatic tuber I: medial aspect of the proximal part of tibial body A: extend coxal joint, flex genual joint, rotate limb medially (internally)

m. semimembranosus—O: ischiatic tuber I: medial condyle of tibia (posterior aspect) A: extend coxal joint, flex genual joint, rotate limb medially (internally)

Anterolateral Muscles of the Crus

m. tibialis anterior—O: proximal, lateral aspect of tibia, crural interosseous membrane I: medial cuneiform bone, first metatarsal bone A: flex (dorsiflex) tarsal joint, invert foot

m. long digital extensor—O: lateral condyle of tibia, proximal fibula, crural interosseous membrane I: distal phalanges of digits 2-5 A: flex (dorsiflex) tarsal joint, extend digital joint of digits 2-5

m. extensor hallucis longus—O: middle of fibula, crural interosseous membrane I: base of distal phalanx of big toe A: extend digital joints of big toe flex (dorsiflex) tarsal joint

m. peroneus longus—O: proximal third of fibula I: medial cuneiform bone, base of first metatarsal bone A: extend (plantar flex) tarsal joint, evert pes

m. peroneus brevis—O: distal half of fibula (lateral aspect) I: base of fifth metatarsal bone A: evert pes, extend (plantar flex) tarsal joint

m. peroneus tertius—O: lower third of body of fibula I: dorsum of base of fifth metatarsal bone A: flex (dorsiflex) tarsal joint, evert pes

Posterior Muscles of the Crus

m. gastrocnemius—O: (medial head) distal posterior femur bone above medial condyle, (lateral head) distal posterior femur bone above lateral condyle I: tuber calcanei A: extend (plantar flex) tarsal joint, flex genual joint

m. soleus—O: proximal, posterior tibia (below line of soleus muscle), and fibula I: tuber calcanei A: extend (plantar flex) tarsal joint

m. plantaris—O: lateral epicondyle of femur bone (posterior edge thereof) I: tuber calcanei A: extend (plantar flex) tarsal joint

m. popliteus—O: lateral epicondyle of femur bone I: posterior aspect of tibia above soleal line of the tibia A: flex genual joint, rotate crus medially (internally)

m. flexor hallucis longus—O: distal two-thirds of fibula, crural interosseous membrane I: base of distal phalanx of first digit A: flex digital joints of first digit, invert pes

m. flexor digitorum longus—O: tibia (middle third of posterior aspect) I: distal phalanges of digits 2-5 A: flex digital joints of minor toes, extend (plantar flex) tarsal joint

m. tibialis posterior—O: posterior aspect of tibia and fibula I: plantar aspect of tarsal bones (except talus) and metatarsal bones 2-4 A: extend (plantar flex) tarsal joint, invert pes

Intrinsic Muscles of the Pes

Special Muscles of the Hallux:

- **m. extensor hallucis brevis**—O: anterior aspect of calcaneus I: base of proximal phalanx of big toe A: extend digital joints of big toe
- **m. flexor hallucis brevis**—O: plantar aspect of cuboid bone, lateral cuneiform bone I: base of proximal phalanx of big toe A: flex joints of big toe
- **m. abductor hallucis**—O: medial tubercle of calcaneus, plantar fascia I: medial surface of base of proximal phalanx of big toe A: flex joints of big toe
- **m. adductor hallucis**—O: (oblique head) bases of metatarsal bones 2-4, tendinous sheath of peroneus longus muscle (transverse head) capsules of metatarsophalangeal joints 3-5 I: lateral aspect of base of proximal phalanx of big toe A: adduct big toe

Special Muscles of Fifth Digit:

- **m. flexor digiti minimi brevis**—O: base of fifth metatarsal bone, plantar fascia I: lateral surface of base of proximal phalanx of little toe A: flex joints of little toe
- **m. abductor digiti minimi**—O: medial and lateral tubercles of calcaneus, plantar fascia I: lateral surface of base of proximal phalanx of little toe A: abduct little toe

Muscles Common to Several Digits:

- **m. extensor digitorum brevis**—O: dorsal surface of calcaneus I: fuses with long digital extensor tendons of digits 1-4 A: extend joints of toes 1-4
- **m. flexor digitorum brevis**—O: medial tuberosity of calcaneus, plantar fascia I: middle phalanges of digits 2-5 A: flex joints of toes 2-5
- **m. quadratus plantae**—O: calcaneus, plantar fascia I: tendons of flexor digitorum longus muscle A: assists in flexion of digital joints

m. lumbricales—O: tendons of flexor digitorum longus muscle I: extensor tendons of digits 2-5 A: flex metatarsophalangeal joints

m. interossei dorsales—O: surface of adjacent metatarsal bones I: extensor tendons of digits 2-4 A: abduct toes, flex digital joints

m. interossei plantares—O: medial surface of metatarsal bone 3-5 I: extensor tendons of digits 3-5 A: adduct toes, flex digital joints

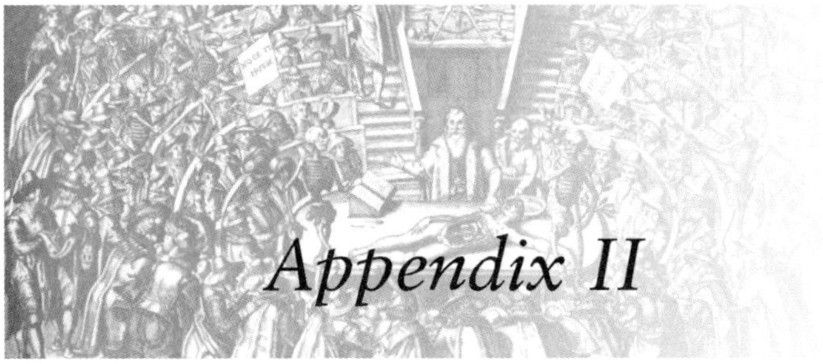

Appendix II

Summary of the Special Muscles of the Digits of the Hand

There are eight different "pollicis" (thumb) muscles:

1.	m. abductor pollicis longus	long and short abductors
2.	m. abductor pollicis brevis	
3.	m. flexor pollicis longus	long and short flexors
4.	m. flexor pollicis brevis	
5.	m. extensor pollicis longus	long and short extensors
6.	m. extensor pollicis brevis	
7.	m. adductor pollicis	two "adductors"
8.	m. opponens pollicis	

These eight muscles give the thumb its remarkable dexterity. With the exception of the opponens pollicis muscle, some part of each one of these muscles can be palpated directly:

a. Three "pollicis" muscles form the thenar eminence (flexor pollicis brevis, abductor pollicis brevis, and opponens pollicis muscles).
b. Three can be distinguished as tendons on the lateral or posterolateral aspect of the carpus (extensor pollicis brevis, extensor pollicis longus, and abductor pollicis longus muscles) where they form the borders of the "anatomic snuffbox."
c. One forms part of the muscular webbing between the first and second metacarpal bones (adductor pollicis).
d. One can be palpated only as a tendon on the anterior aspect of the proximal phalanx of the thumb (flexor pollicis longus). Unlike the fifth digit (which also has several muscles of its "own") the pollex does not receive tendons from the superficial digital flexor, deep digital flexor, or from the digital extensor muscle.

There are four different "digiti minimi" (fifth digit) muscles.

1. m. extensor digiti minimi (lies medial to the digital extensor m. fascicles)
2. m. abductor digiti minimi*
3. m. flexor digiti minimi brevis*
4. m. opponens digiti minimi*

There is only one "special" muscle of the second digit (m. extensor indicis).

* These three muscles form the hypothenar eminence.

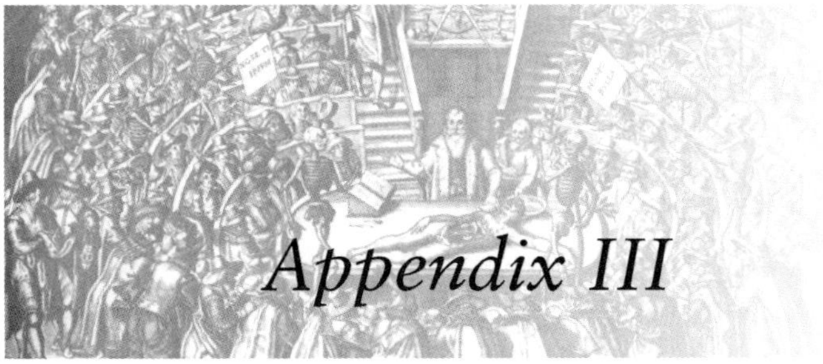

Appendix III

Cranial Nerve Facts and Learning Aids

1. A mnemonic used to help remember the *names* of the cranial nerves is the nonsense... "On Old Olympus' towering top a fat vicious goat vandalized a hat." (There are other more interesting but less socially acceptable versions).
2. A *functional* mnemonic is... "Six sailors made merry, but my brother said bad business, my man!" In this memory aid, "m" indicates motor (mainly), "s" indicates sensory (only) and "b" indicates both motor and sensory. The five cranial nerves which are primarily motor (CN III, IV, VI, XI, XII) do carry proprioceptive fibers but since these are the only sensory fibers present, they are ignored.
3. Most cranial nerves are limited in their distal distribution to the head, but the vagus and accessory nerves are exceptions.
4. Four of the cranial nerves carry some autonomic (visceral efferent fibers) fibers (CN III, VII, IX, X). These are parasympathetic preganglionic fibers whose postganglionics are distributed to the smooth muscle, cardiac muscle, and glands in the head, neck, thorax, and abdomen.
5. Three cranial nerves (CN III, IV, VI) control eye movement by innervating the extrinsic eye muscles. $LR_6SO_4Rest_3$ is an innervation formula where LR= lateral rectus, SO= superior oblique muscle, and Rest= the other muscles of the eye. The other cranial nerves involved with the eye are the optic nerve (vision), the ophthalmic branch of the trigeminal n. (general sensation), and the facial n. (lacrimation and closure of the eye).
6. Taste is carried primarily by two cranial nerves. The facial nerve carries taste fibers from the anterior two-thirds of the tongue and the glossopharyngeal nerve carries taste fibers from the posterior one-third of the tongue. Other cranial nerves distributed to the tongue include the hypoglossal nerve (motor to the muscles of the tongue) and the trigeminal nerve (general sensation from the tongue via the mandibular nerve).
7. The salivary glands are innervated by the facial nerve (sublingual and submandibular glands) and glossopharyngeal nerve (parotid gland).
8. All of the so-called "special" senses are carried by cranial nerves including olfaction (CN I), vision (CN II), taste (CN VII, IX), audition (CN VIII), and balance (CN VIII).
9. The principle cranial nerve carrying general sensation (heat, cold, pressure, pain, touch) from the head is the trigeminal nerve. Its three component nerves are sensory to nearly everything in the anterior half of the head.
10. The longest cranial nerve is the vagus nerve and it is the major nerve supplying motor fibers to the glandular epithelium and smooth muscle tissue of the respiratory and digestive systems. About 80% of its fibers are sensory (visceral afferent) fibers from those same areas.

11. The only cranial nerves that do not emerge from the skull are the vestibulocochlear nerves. They enter the internal acoustic meatus (on the inside of the skull) to innervate the cochlear duct and vestibular apparatus of the inner ear. The other cranial nerves pass through various foramina to reach the organs that they supply (four pairs pass through the supra-orbital fissures and three pairs pass through the jugular foramina).

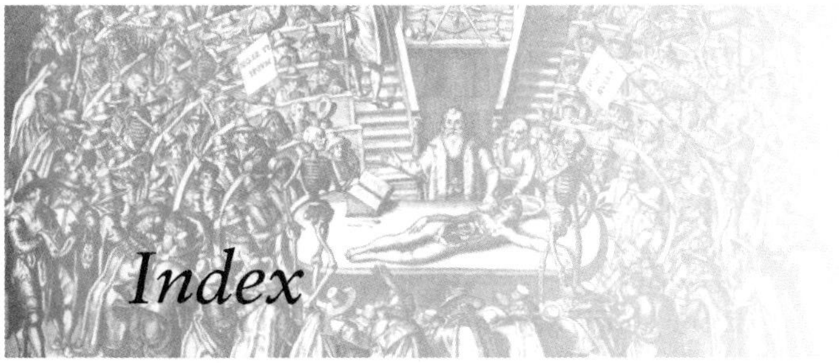

Index

Abdomen, 1, 15, 226, 246, 588, 619
Abdominal cavity, 18, 588, 619
Abdominal press, 229
Abduction, 190, 209, 211
Abrasion, 91, 105
Absorption, 589, 591
Accessory sex gland, 698, 708, 711
Accommodation, 401, 402, 403, 412, 413
Acid, 36
Acid/base balance, 495, 639, 675
Acromegaly, 141, 461, 471, 481
Acromioclavicular joint, 202
Actin, 233
Action of a muscle, 225
Active transport, 31, 32, 39, 40
Acromegaly, 141, 461, 471, 481
Adduction, 190, 209, 211
Adenosine triphosphate, 43
Adipose tissue, 13, 57, 58, 74, 80, 117
Adrenal medulla, 390, 459, 460, 462, 476
Aerobic, 7
Afferent impulses, 288
Agonist, 227, 237
"Air-blood barrier", 636, 650, 652
Albino 93, 97
Albumin 494, 533
Alzheimer's disease, 314
Amelia, 141
Amino acid, 11, 37, 464
Amylase, 613
Anal canal, 589, 610
Anaphase, 33, 47
Anatomic snuffbox, 261
Anatomy, 1, 2, 3, 4, 23
  gross a., 4
  microscopic a., 4, 57, 59
  regional a., 4
  surface a., 4, 92, 101
  systemic a., 4
  topographic a., 4
Anencephaly, 297
Angle
  costal a., 175
  sternal a., 174
Anisotropic band, 226, 234
ANS, 285, 286, 288, 375, 376, 377, 378, 382, 383, 384, 385, 390, 391
Antagonist, 225, 226, 237
Antebrachial interosseous membrane, 202
Anterior, 20
Anterior cruciate ligament, 206
Anterior nasal aperture, 154
Antidiuretic hormone (ADH), 462, 471
Anulus fibrosus, 200
Aorta
  abdominal a., 514
  arch of a., 540, 543, 545
  ascending a., 62
  thoracic a., 514
Apex
  of fibular head, 138
  of hair, 91, 100
  of patella, 134
  of sacrum, 172
Aponeurosis, 76, 227
Appendicular skeleton, 114, 120
Arachnoid granulation, 308
Arachnoid mater, 288, 308
Arbor vitae, 288, 304
Arch
  costal a., 175
  pubic a., 133
  vertebral a., 169
  zygomatic a., 153, 155, 163
Areola, 97
Arrector pili muscle, 93, 100, 390
Arteriole 491, 508
Arthrotomy, 215
Arthritis, 214
Arthrocentesis, 214
Arthrology, 189, 191
Arthroscopy, 215
Articular cartilage, 74, 77, 114, 125, 196
Articular cavity, 191
Articular disc, 77, 189, 190, 197
Articular meniscus, 77
Articulation (see joint)
Ascending (part of the) aorta, 62
Asthma, 637, 662
Astrocyte, 288, 293
Atlanto-axial joint, 200, 202
Atlanto-occipital joint, 189, 200, 202, 217
Atlas (C1), 151, 171
Atom, 11

ATP, 43
Atrophy, 31, 49, 276
Attachment, 225, 231, 237, 330
Auditory ossicle, 151, 153, 154, 156, 240, 431, 432, 437
Auditory tube, 431, 432, 437
Auscultation, 2, 6, 21, 548
Autonomic ganglia, 292, 324, 352, 375, 390
Autonomic nervous system, 285, 286, 288, 375, 377, 378, 379, 380
Avulsion, 92, 93, 105, 178
Axial skeleton, 113, 114, 115, 120, 151, 153, 189, 197, 201, 202
Axilla, 104
Axis (C2), 171
Axon, 286, 294

Ball of foot, 104
Base
  of a bone (see that bone)
  of skull, 152, 160
Basic tissue, 58
Bell's palsy, 239, 324, 360
Belly of a muscle, 226
Bile, 588, 615
Biological macromolecule, 2
Bipolar neuron, 290, 323, 330
Blastocyst, 59, 751, 758, 759
Blood, 13, 57, 58, 74, 79, 115, 117, 491, 492, 494, 507
Blood pressure regulation, 675
Body
  of sternum, 151, 174
  pineal b., 302, 459, 460, 461, 467, 468
Body defense, 491, 495
Bone
  Atlas, 151, 171
  Axis, 171, 179, 186
  Calcaneus, 115, 138
  cancellous b., 115, 117
  capitate b., 128
  carpal b., 114, 127
  clavicle, 114, 115, 125, 128
  coccyx, 134, 151, 171, 173
  compact b., 113, 114
  cortical b., 114, 117
  cuboid b., 138
  dense b., 114, 117
  ethmoid b., 151, 162, 166
  femur b., 114, 133, 137
  fibula, 20, 114, 138, 139
  flat b., 113, 114, 123, 125
  frontal b., 158
  hamate b., 115, 128
  humerus, 114, 115, 126, 130
  hyoid b., 151, 154, 155, 156
  ilium, 114, 133
  incus, 154, 437
Bone — *continued*
  inferior nasal concha, 151, 168
  intermediate cuneiform b., 138
  irregular b., 113, 114, 123
  ischium, 114, 133
  lacrimal b., 151, 168
  lateral cuneiform b., 138
  long b., 113, 114, 123, 126, 177
  lunate b., 115, 127
  malleus, 153, 154, 436, 437
  mandible, 168, 169
  maxilla, 163, 166
  medial cuneiform b., 115
  metarcarpal b., 114, 128
  metatarsal b., 114, 138
  nasal b., 167
  navicular b., 138
  occipital b., 160
  os coxae, 114, 132, 136
  palatine b., 158, 167
  parietal b., 153, 159
  phalanx, 114, 115, 128
  pisiform b., 115, 203
  pubis, 133
  radius, 127, 131
  rib, 151, 153, 174, 175
  sacral b. (sacrum), 151, 171, 172
  scaphoid b., 115, 127
  scapula, 115, 125, 129
  sesamoid b., 113, 114, 115, 123, 125, 233
  short b., 115, 123
  "shoulder blade", 114, 115
  sphenoid b., 153, 158, 161, 165
  spongy b., 113, 115, 117
  stapes, 153, 154, 437
  sternum, 151, 153, 173, 174
  sutural b. (wormian b.), 194
  talus, 138
  tarsal b., 114, 138
  temporal b., 160, 164
  tibia, 114, 134, 139
  trabecular b., 115, 117
  trapezium b., 128
  triquetral b., 115, 128
  ulna, 115, 127, 131
  vertebra, 151, 171
  vomer, 167
  zygomatic b., 158, 163
Bone marrow, 124
Bone marrow tissue, 58, 75, 113, 117
Bone tissue, 57, 58, 71, 75, 113, 114, 115, 116, 117, 118, 119
Bones of the skull, 153
Bony palate, 163
Bony pelvis, 130
Bony sacrum, (see sacral b.)

Border
  blind b. of nail, 91, 101
  free b. of nail, 91, 101
  lateral b. of nail, 91, 101
  of a bone (see that bone)
Brachial plexus, 323, 324, 344, 346, 347
Branch (ramus)
  anterior b. (of spinal n.), 323, 324, 344
  of a bone (see that bone)
  posterior b. (of spinal n.), 323, 324, 344
  r. communicans (of spinal nerve), 323, 324, 325, 344, 376
Breast, 97, 99
Bronchial tree, 635, 636, 644, 645, 646, 648
Bronchioles, 390, 635, 636, 647, 648
Brow, 104
Bruise, 277, 281, 625, 631
Buffer, 37
Bulbopontine sulcus, 334
Bulbourethral gland, 698, 711
Burn, 102
Bursa, 225, 227, 232, 233, 727, 731, 734

C1 (see atlas), 171
C2 (see axis), 171
Calcaneus, 115, 138
Calcitonin, 459, 462, 473
Calvaria, 155
Canal
  anal c., 588, 589, 610
  birth c., 726, 729
  carpal c., 233, 260
  central c. (of osteon), 116, 152
  central c. (of spinal cord), 286, 304
  "haversian" c., 144
  hypoglossal c., 339
  nutrient c., 113, 116, 125
  optic c., 161, 330, 404
  perforating c., 116
  vertebral can., 171
Cancer, 31, 49, 92, 103, 698, 716
Capitate bone, 128
Capsular ligament, 196, 199
Carbohydrate, 32, 38
Cardiac muscle, 11, 57, 62, 380, 498
Carotene, 93, 97
Carpal bones, 114, 127
Carpal canal, 233, 260
Carpal flexor retinaculum, 233
Carpal groove, 128
Carpal joint, 189, 202, 203, 239
Carpometacarpal joint, 197
Cartilage
  articular c., 74, 77, 114, 125, 189, 196
  corniculate c., 644
  costal c., 77, 151, 152, 153, 173
Cartilage — *continued*
  cricoid c., 637, 644
  elastic c., 57, 58, 71, 74, 433
  epiphyseal c., 77, 114, 152, 176
  fibrocartilage, 57, 58, 74, 196
  hyaline c., 57, 58, 59, 74, 194
  nasal c., 77
Cartilaginous joint, 189, 190, 192, 194, 195
Cauda equina, 288, 304
Cavitation, 2, 16, 17, 24
Cavity
  abdominal c., 588, 619
  articular c., 191
  cranial c., 16
  joint c., 189, 196
  nasal c., 168, 635, 637, 640
  oral c., 587, 593, 596
  pelvic c., 588, 619
  pericardial c., 16, 496
  peritoneal c., 16, 588, 619, 620
  thoracic c., 16, 636, 654
  tympanic c., 435
Cecum, 590, 609
Cell (see also specific types), 2, 11, 31, 33, 39, 41, 44, 45, 46, 47
Cell body (of a neuron), 80, 289, 291
Cell cycle, 31, 46, 47
Cell membrane, 31, 39, 41, 44
Cell theory, 31, 33
Cementum, 597
Central canal of spinal cord, 286, 304
Central nervous system, 285, 287, 288, 289, 299
Centriole, 44, 46
Centromere, 33, 47
Cerebellar hemisphere, 304
Cerebellar peduncle, 304
Cerebellar vermis, 304
Cerebellum, 286, 287, 303
Cerebral gyri, 301
Cerebral hemisphere, 286, 301
Cerebral sulci, 301
Cerebrospinal fluid, 286, 287, 308
Cerebrovascular accident, 286, 313
Cerumen, 97, 432, 436
Ceruminous glands, 66, 91, 97, 436
Cervical plexus, 345, 346
Cervical vertebra, 151, 171
Chamber
  of eye, 402, 410
Chemoreceptor, 352, 355
Childhood, 752, 765
Chondroblast, 71
Chondroclast, 59, 74
Chondrocyte, 71, 191
Chorda tympani, 334, 336
Chordata (chordate), 1, 2, 3, 8, 9

Choroid, 308, 403, 405
Choroid plexus, 308
Chromaffin cell, 480
Chromatin, 38, 44, 46
Chromosome, 33, 46
Cilia, 44, 46, 67, 101, 402, 415, 447
Ciliary body, 405
Ciliary muscle, 390, 405
Circulation, 491, 492, 493, 512, 513, 515, 516, 535, 539, 671
  systemic c., 491, 493, 512
Circumduction, 211
Cisterna chyli, 560, 565
Class, 8, 9
Clavicle, 114, 115, 125, 128
Cleft palate, 141, 589, 622
Clinical hyperextension, 215
Clitoris, 738
CN I, 329, 330
CN II, 329, 330
CN III, 330
CN IV, 330, 331
CN V, 330, 331
CN VI, 330, 334
CN VII, 330, 335
CN VIII, 330, 336
CN IX, 330, 337
CN X, 330, 337
CN XI, 330, 338
CN XII, 330, 339
CNS, 285, 286, 287, 288, 289, 295, 308, 378
Coccygeal vertebra, 153, 173
Coccyx, 134, 171, 173
Cochlea, 325, 433, 440, 441
Collagen, 59, 71
Collagenous fiber, 71
Collateral ligament, 196, 206
Colon, 366, 588, 609, 610
Color blindness, 408, 420
Comminuted fracture, 178
Composite joint, 189, 190, 192
Concha
  inferior nasal c., 168
  middle nasal c., 162
Concussion, 286, 312
Condyle (see that bone)
Cone, 288, 402
Conjunctiva, 402, 415
Contralateral, 20
Contusion, 276
Cord
  medial c. (brachial plexus), 346
  posterior c. (brachial plexus), 346
  spermatic c., 698, 699, 711, 712
  spinal c., 286, 288, 289, 304, 305, 306, 310, 343
Cornea, 403, 404
Corpus callosum, 288, 302
Costal arch, 175
Costochondral joint, 200, 202
Costotransverse joint, 200, 202
Cramps, 226, 276
Crena ani, 103
Cribriform foramina, 153, 162
Crista ampullaris, 358, 432, 447
Crural interosseous membrane, 206
CSF, 286, 287, 307, 308
Cuboid bone 138
Curvature
  of vertebral column, 173, 190, 603
Cutaneous receptor, 324, 355
Cuticle, 100, 101
CVA, 286, 313
Cytochemistry, 31, 34
Cytokinesis, 32, 33, 47
Cytology, 31, 33
Cytoplasm, 31, 32, 43, 296

Deep, 20, 247, 252, 267, 269, 335, 673
Deep fascia, 225, 232
Degenerative arthritis, 214
Deglutition, 227, 228, 589, 591, 604
Dehydration synthesis, 32, 36
Delayed union, 152, 179
Dendrite, 59, 80, 287, 289
Dental alveoli, 163, 168
Dental pulp, 76, 597
Dentin, 597
Dentoalveolar joint, 190, 194, 202
Deoxyribonucleic acid (DNA), 31
Depolarization, 287, 294
Dermatitis, 92, 102, 105
Dermatome, 274, 353, 360
Dermis, 76, 91, 92, 94, 96
Desmosome, 43
Development
  bone, 151, 176, 177
  brain, 310
  glandular epithelium, 67
  muscular system, 226, 274
  nervous system, 286, 297, 299
Diaphragm, 16, 246, 636, 655, 757
Diaphragma sellae, 312
Diaphysis of bone, 115, 124, 176
Diencephalon, 286, 288, 297
Diglyceride, 38
Dipeptide, 35, 37
Diploid, 32, 33, 48
Directional terms, 2, 20
Disaccharide, 33, 38
Disc
  articular d., 77, 190, 197
  interpubic d., 77, 205
  intervertebral d., 77, 169, 190, 200, 215

Dislocation, 190, 191, 214
Dissection, 1, 2, 3, 4, 5
Distal, 20, 600
Distal interphalangeal joint, 203, 206
Distal radio-ulnar joint, 202
Disynaptic reflex, 365
DNA, 37, 38
Dorsal, 20
[Dorsal hollow] nerve cord, 8
Dorsiflexion, 209
Duct
  lactiferous d., 97
Dura mater, 286, 288, 308, 312
Dwarfism, 141, 471, 481
Dyslexia, 288, 313

Earlobe, 435
Ectoderm, 59, 60, 759, 761
EEG, 313
Efferent impulses, 289
Ejaculation, 697, 698, 709, 711, 756
Elastic cartilage, 74
Elastin, 71
Elbow joint, 202
Electroencephalogram, 313
Electroencephalography, 286, 313
Electrolyte balance, 675
Electrons, 10
Embryo, 8
Emission, 707, 710
Emulsification, 590, 591
Enamel, 597
Encapsulated receptor, 355
Endochondral ossification, 151, 176
Endocrine gland, 11, 69, 462
Endocytosis, 32
Endoderm, 59, 60, 431, 759, 761
Endomysium, 76, 231
Endoneurium, 76, 326
Endoplasmic reticulum, 32, 43, 44
Endothelium, 496
Ependymal cell, 293
Epicondyle (see that bone)
Epidermis, 91, 92, 94, 95, 96
Epilepsy, 313
Epimere, 274
Epimysium, 226, 231
Epinephrine, 392, 476
Epineurium, 324, 326
Epiphyseal cartilages, 77, 152, 176
Epiphyseal line, 152, 176
Epithalamus, 302
Epithelium
  columnar e., 64, 66, 640
  cuboidal e., 64
  endothelium, 496

Epithelium — *continued*
  glandular e., 57, 58, 66, 67, 68, 69, 375, 380
  membranous e., 57, 59, 63, 64, 65, 67
  mesothelium, 496, 593
  pseudostratified columnar e., 63, 66, 640
  respiratory e., 637, 640
  simple columnar e., 63
  simple cuboidal e., 63
  simple e., 63, 64, 117
  simple squamous e., 63, 117
  squamous e., 63, 95, 117
  stratified columnar e., 63
  stratified cuboidal e., 63
  stratified e., 64
  stratified squamous e., 63, 95
  surface e., 59, 63
  transitional e., 63, 66, 684
ER, 32, 43
Erection, 697, 698, 709
Erythrocyte, 59, 74, 533
Esophagus, 588, 602, 603
Estrogen, 461, 477
Ethmoid bone, 162, 166
Ethmoidal sinus, 153, 162
Eversion, 211
Exocytosis, 32
Expiration, 636, 660
Extension, 190, 207, 209, 211, 239
Extensor angle, 207
External, 20, 91
External acoustic meatus, 77, 160, 431, 436
External anal sphincter muscle, 252, 610
External ear, 431, 432, 433
Exteroceptor, 352, 355
Eye movement, 229
Eyeball, 401, 402, 403, 404, 406, 407, 409, 416

Facial nerve paralysis, 360
Facilitated diffusion, 31, 32, 39
False rib, 151, 152, 175
Falx cerebelli, 312
Falx cerebri, 312
Family, 3, 9
Fascia
  deep f., 225, 232
  f. lata (femoris), 262,
  superficial f., 94, 232
Fascicle, 227, 231, 504
Fasciculus, 227, 325
Fatty acid, 11
Fauces, 240, 242, 587, 593, 595
Femur bone, 114, 133, 137
Fertilization, 729, 751, 754, 755, 756
Fiber
  collagenous f., 71
  elastic f., 71

Fiber — *continued*
muscle f., 60
nerve f., 80, 326, 408
perforating f., 124
reticular f., 71
"Sharpey's" f., 144
Fiber tract, 291, 324, 326
Fiberoptic examination, 21
Fibril, 46
Fibrinogen, 74, 533, 711
Fibroblast, 71
Fibrocartilage, 57, 58, 74, 196
Fibrocartilage joint, 191
Fibrocytes, 71
Fibrous connective tissue, 58, 71
Fibrous joint, 189, 192, 193
Fibrous tunic, 401, 402, 404
Fibula, 114, 138, 139
Fibular, 20, 137, 138
Fibular collateral ligament, 206
Filtrate, 672, 678
First class lever, 212
Fissure
cerebellar f., 304
cerebral f., 312, 315, 770
inferior orbital f., 404
superior orbital f., 330, 331, 335, 404
Fixator, 225, 227, 238
Flagella, 46
Flagellum (tail) of sperm, 44, 707
Flexion, 190, 207, 209, 211
Flexion crease, 104
Flexor angle, 207
Floating rib, 151, 175
Follicle
hair f., 92, 100
Fontanel
anterior f., 156
anterolateral f., 153, 156
posterior f., 156
posterolateral f., 156
Foramen
anterior sacral f., 172
f. magnum, 153, 155, 156, 161, 306
f. of luschka, 316
f. of magendie, 316
f. ovale of sphenoid bone, 334
f. rotundum, 331
infraorbital f. of maxilla, 163
intervertebral f., 152, 171
jugular f., 334
mental f., 168, 334
nutrient f., 125
stylomastoid foror., 161
transverse f., 171
vertebral f., 171
Force, 211
Forebrain, 297
Forehead, 104
Fossa
cranial f., 156
cubital f., 104
lesser supraclavicular f., 104
of a bone (see that bone)
popliteal f., 104, 115
temporal f., 241
Fracture, 152, 178, 179
Free nerve ending, 355, 358
Frontal bone, 158
Frontal sinus, 159
Fulcrum, 211
Function(s)
cardiovascular system, 491, 494, 495
central nervous system, 289, 388
digestive system, 587, 591, 608
endocrine system, 460, 479
female reproductive system, 725, 729
integumentary system, 91, 93, 94,
lymphatic system, 559, 561
male reproductive system, 697, 700
muscular system, 225, 228
nervous system, 285, 288, 289
peripheral nervous system, 289
respiratory system, 635, 639
skeletal system, 113, 118
urinary system, 671, 675

Gallbladder, 588, 615, 616
Ganglia, 285, 291, 292, 323, 324, 325, 336, 337, 338, 351, 352, 378, 383, 388, 390, 391
Ganglion (ganglia)
autonomic g., 292, 324, 352, 390
celiac g., 391
ciliary g., 330, 385, 391
cochlear g., 358
geniculate g., 352
inferior cervical g., 399
inferior g. (CN IX), 337, 338, 352
inferior g. (CN X), 337, 338, 352
inferior mesenteric g., 387, 391
"Meissner's" g., 358
middle cervical g., 391
motor g., 324
named peripheral g., 351
otic g., 337, 388, 391
paravertebral g., 351, 376
sensory g., 291
sublingual g., 354
submandibular g., 338, 354, 390, 393
superior cervical g., 393
superior g. (CN IX), 332, 336, 339, 340, 354, 375, 377, 384, 391, 393, 397, 401

Ganglion (ganglia) — *continued*
superior g. (CN X), 352, 323, 325, 335, 344, 351, 352, 390
superior mesenteric g., 387, 391
sympathetic g., 375, 391
sympathetic trunk g., 377, 383, 390
terminal g., 388
trigeminal g., 331
vestibular g., 337, 352, 358
Ganglion cell, 330
Gap junctions, 43
Gene, 33, 46
Genus, 8, 9
Giantism, 141, 471, 481
Gland
apocrine g., 91, 93, 97, 98
ceruminous g., 66, 91, 93, 97, 98, 436
eccrine g., 91, 93, 97, 98
endocrine g., 11, 69, 462
exocrine g., 11, 57, 66, 68, 69
gastric g., 66, 603
holocrine g., 93, 97
mammary g., 66, 91, 92, 97
merocrine g., 59, 66, 93, 97
sebaceous g., 66, 91, 92, 93, 97, 98
sudoriferous g., 66, 93, 97, 98
sweat g., 91, 390
tubular g., 97, 603, 607, 610, 611
unicellular g., 57, 69, 70, 88, 593
Glandular epithelium, 57, 58, 66, 67, 68, 69, 375, 380
Glial cell, 58, 59, 81, 285, 293, 295
Glucose, 461
Glyceride, 38
Glycerol, 11
Golgi complex, 43, 44
Gomphosis, 190, 191, 194
Gouty arthritis, 214
Gray matter, 287, 304
Groove (sulcus)
bicipital g., 102
bulbopontine s., 334
carpal g., 128
costal g., 175
gluteal g., 104
neural g., 297
posterior median s., 304
posterolateral s., 337
Ground substance, 11, 59, 60, 71
Gullet (fauces), 242, 587, 595
Gustatory cell, 358
H band, 324
Hair, 91, 92, 93, 99, 100, 101
Hair follicle, 92, 100
Hair root ending, 355, 358
Hamate bone, 115, 128
Haploid, 33, 48
Hard palate, 593
Head
of bone (see that bone)
of muscle (see that muscle)
Heat production, 225, 231
Hemiplegia, 313
Hemoglobin, 97, 535
Hemopoiesis, 115, 118, 535
Heritable, 766
Heterotrophic, 7
Hindbrain, 297
Hip joint, 190, 205, 206
Histology, 57, 59
Histopathology, 58, 82
Hominidae, 8, 9
Homo sapiens, 1, 3, 9
Hormone, 35, 59, 69, 459, 460, 461, 462, 463, 464, 465, 466, 467, 471, 472, 474, 476, 495, 700, 737
Humero-radial joint, 202
Humero-ulnar joint, 202
Humerus, 114, 115, 126, 130
Hyaline cartilage, 74
Hyaline cartilage joint, 194
Hydrocephalus, 312
Hydrolysis, 33, 36, 591
Hydroregulation, 94, 675
Hydroxyapatite, 114, 116
Hyoid bone, 154, 155, 156
Hyperextension, 215
Hyperflexion, 209
Hyperplasia, 33, 49
Hypertrophy, 32, 49, 276
Hypodermis, 59, 76, 92, 94, 96, 232
Hypomere, 274
Hyponychium, 101
Hypothalamus, 286, 302, 459, 461, 465, 477
Hypothenar eminence, 104, 227, 261
Hypoxia, 661

I (isotropic) band, 225, 227, 234
Ilium, 133
Incus, 153, 154, 437
Infectious arthritis, 214
Inferior, 2, 15, 20
Inferior colliculus of mesencephalon, 330
Inferior orbital fissure, 404
Inferior pelvic opening, 131
Infertility, 699, 716
Injection/maceration, 6
Inorganic compound, 11
Inspiration, 636, 657
Insulin, 477, 481
Integumentary system, 13, 91, 93
Intercarpal joint, 203
Intercostal spaces, 152, 175
Interdigital web, 104

Intermediate, 20, 43, 138
Intermediate cuneiform bone, 138
Intermediate junctions, 43
Intermetacarpal joint, 203
Intermetatarsal joint, 206, 207
Internal, 20
Internal acoustic meatus, 440
Internal ear, 431, 432, 439, 440
Interneuron, 290, 365
Interphalangeal joint, 203, 206, 207
Intertarsal joint, 206, 207
Interventricular foramina, 308
Intervertebral disc, 77, 169, 190, 200, 215
Intervertebral disc disease, 190, 215
Intervertebral foramina, 152, 171
Intervertebral symphysis, 200, 202
Intracapsular ligament, 196, 199
Intramembranous ossification, 151, 152, 176
Inversion, 211, 410
Ipsilateral, 20
Iris, 403, 405
Ischium, 133
Isotropic band, 227, 234

Joint
- acromioclavicular j., 202
- ankle j., 190
- atlanto-axial j., 200, 202
- atlanto-occipital j., 200, 202
- ball and socket j., 197
- bicondylar j., 197
- carpal j., 189, 202, 203
- carpometacarpal j., 203
- cartilaginous j., 189, 190, 192, 194, 195
- composite j., 190, 192
- costochondral j., 200, 202
- costotransverse j., 200, 202
- coxal j., 205, 206
- cubital j., 202, 203
- dentoalveolar j., 190, 194, 202
- distal interphalangeal j., 203, 206
- distal radio-ulnar j., 202, 203
- elbow j., 189, 202, 203
- femoropatellar j., 205, 206
- femorotibial j., 134, 206
- fibrocartilaginous j., 189
- genual j., 205, 206
- ginglymus, 191, 197
- gomphosis, 190, 191, 194
- hinge j., 191, 197
- hip j., 190, 205, 206
- humeral j., 202
- humero-ulnar j., 202, 203
- hyaline cartilage j., 194
- intercarpal j., 203
- interchondral j., 200, 202

Joint — *continued*
- intermetacarpal j., 203
- intermetatarsal j., 206, 207
- interphalangeal j. of hallux, 206
- interphalangeal j., 203, 206, 207
- interphalangeal j. of thumb, 203
- intertarsal j., 206, 207
- intervertebral symphysis, 200, 202
- knee j., 190, 205, 206
- manubriosternal symphysis, 153, 200, 202
- metacarpophalangeal j., 203, 211
- metatarsophalangeal j., 206, 207, 211
- middle carpal j., 203
- of axial skeleton, 189, 197, 201, 202
- of inferior limb, 190, 205, 206, 208
- of pisiform bone, 115, 203
- of superior limb, 189, 200, 203, 204
- parts (synovial j.), 189, 196, 197, 198, 199
- pivot j., 197
- planar j., 197
- proximal interphalangeal j., 203, 206
- proximal radio-ulnar j., 202, 203
- pubic symphysis, 133, 205, 206
- radiocarpal j., 202, 203
- sacroiliac j., 205, 206
- sellar j., 191, 197
- shoulder jt., 189, 209
- simple jt., 189, 191, 192
- spheroidal j., 197
- sternoclavicular j., 202, 203
- sternocostal j., 200, 202
- suture, 191, 192, 194, 202
- symphysis, 191, 196
- synchondrosis, 191
- syndesmosis, 191, 192
- synovial j., 189, 191, 192, 196, 197, 198, 199
- talocrural j., 206, 207, 211, 214, 217
- tarsal j., 206, 207
- tarsometatarsal j., 206, 207
- temporomandibular j., 197, 202
- tibiofibular j., 206
- tibiofibular syndesmosis, 206
- transverse tarsal j., 206, 207
- trochoid j., 197
- wrist j., 202
- zygapophyseal j., 191, 200, 202

Joint capsule, 76, 196

Keratin, 59, 68, 92, 94
Kidneys, 66, 460, 461, 465, 477, 671, 672, 673, 675, 676, 682
Kinesthetic receptor, 355
Kingdom, 7, 9
Knee joint, 190, 205, 206
Kyphosis, 191, 215

Labor, 752, 764, 767
Laceration, 92, 103
Lacrimal bone, 151, 168
Lacrimal gland, 403, 418
Lacuna, 71, 115, 116
Lamella, 115, 116, 117
Lamellated corpuscle, 355
Lamina of vertebral arch, 169
Lamina propria, 76, 590, 593, 681
Larynx, 635, 637, 642, 643
Lateral, 20
Lateral cuneiform bone, 138
Left atrioventricular valve, 503
Lens, 401, 402, 409, 410, 412, 413, 418
Leucocyte, 59, 74, 535
Leucopoiesis, 115, 535
Lever, 190, 211, 212, 213
Lever arm, 211
Lever system, 190, 211
Ligament
  anterior cruciate l., 206
  collateral l., 196, 206
  cruciate l., 206
  extracapsular l., 196, 199
  fibular collateral l., 206
  glenohumeral l., 199
  iliofemoral l., 199
  intercarpal l., 199
  intertarsal l., 199
  intracapsular l., 196, 199
  ischiofemoral l., 199
  l. of femoral head, 199
  posterior cruciate l. (PCL), 206
  tibial collateral l. (MCL), 199, 217
Linea alba (albicans), 251
Lipid, 11, 31, 32, 33, 36, 38, 561
Lips, 593
Liver, 66, 366, 538, 588, 615, 616, 617, 621
Liver cells, 588, 615
Lobe
  frontal l. (brain), 301
  insular l. (brain), 302
  occipital l. (brain), 302
  of cerebellum, 303, 304
  of cerebral hemisphere, 286, 301
  parietal l. (brain), 302
  temporal l. (brain), 302
Locomotion, 10, 118, 190, 211, 227, 228
Longitudinal, 20, 179, 241
Lordosis, 191, 215
Lumbar plexus, 345, 349
Lumbar vertebra, 151, 170, 172
Lumbosacral intumescence, 304
Lumbosacral plexus, 324, 349
Lunate bone, 115, 127
Lunula, 93, 101
Luxation, 191
Lymph, 559, 560, 561, 563, 565
Lymph node, 559, 560, 567, 572
Lymphatic system, 13, 559, 561, 562, 578
Lysosome, 33, 44, 46

M line, 234
Magnetic resonance imaging, 6
Major parts of body, 1, 15, 16
Malleus, 153, 154, 436, 437
Mammal, 8, 9
Mandible, 168, 169
Mandibular symphysis, 168
Manubrium of sternum, 174
Mastication, 227, 228, 240, 244, 591
Matrix, 11, 58, 59, 71
Matrix of nail, 92, 101
Maxilla, 163, 166
Mechanical advantage, 213
Mechanoreceptor, 352, 355
Medial, 20
Medial cuneiform bone, 115
Medulla
  of lymph node, 75
Medulla oblongata, 286, 288, 304
Medullary cavity, 113, 114, 124
Meiosis, 32, 48
Meissner's corpuscle, 355, 358
Melanin, 92, 96, 100
Melanocyte, 93, 97, 471
Membrane
  antebrachial interosseous m., 202
  basement m., 64
  crural interosseous m., 206
  mucous m., 2, 13
  serous m., 3, 16, 593
Membranous epithelium, 59, 63, 64, 65, 67
Membranous labyrinth, 432, 440
Meninges, 286, 287, 288, 307, 308
Meningitis, 313
Menisci tacti, 355, 358
Mental illness, 313
Mentolabial groove, 104
Mesencephalic aqueduct, 302, 308
Mesencephalon, 286, 297, 302
Mesoderm, 59, 60, 274
Mesomere, 274
Mesothelium, 496, 593
Metacarpophalangeal joint, 203, 211
Metamerism, 2, 3, 16
Metaphase, 33, 47
Metaphysis, 152
Metaplasia, 31, 49
Metatarsal bones 114, 138
Metatarsophalangeal joint, 206, 207, 211
Metencephalon, 288, 297

Microencephaly, 297
Microglia, 293
Micromelia, 141
Microtubule, 44, 46
Microvilli, 44, 59, 68, 608
Midbrain, 297
Middle, 20, 33, 59
Middle carpal joint, 203
Middle ear, 431, 432, 436, 438
Mitochondria, 43, 44
Mitosis, 31, 32, 47, 48
Moment arm equation, 213
Monoglyceride, 38
Monosynaptic reflex, 365
Monosomy, 49
Morphology, 1, 3, 16
Motor impulse, 287, 289
Motor neuron, 13, 378
Motor unit, 225, 226, 227, 238
Mouth, 593, 769, 771
MRI, 6
Mucosa, 2, 13, 587, 589, 593, 681, 684
Mucous membrane, 2, 13, 587, 593
Multipolar neuron, 289
Muscle
  abductor pollicis brevis m., 261
  abductor pollicis longus m., 261
  adductor hallucis m., 227
  adductor longus m., 104
  adductor magnus m., 345
  adductor pollicis m., 261
  anconeus m., 227, 258
  anterior m. of hip, 262
  arrector pili m., 93, 100, 390
  auricularis m., 237, 240
  biceps brachii m., 258
  biceps femoris m., 263
  brachialis m., 258
  brachioradialis m., 258
  buccinator m., 237, 240
  bulbospongiosus m., 252
  ciliary m., 390, 405
  coccygeus m., 252
  corrugator supercilii m., 240
  crico-arytenoideus lateralis m., 243
  deltoideus m., 15, 254
  diaphragm, 16, 246, 636, 655, 757
  digastricus m., 102, 237, 243
  epaxial m., 254
  epicranius m., 237, 240
  extensor carpi radialis brevis m., 261
  extensor carpi radialis longus m., 239, 261
  extensor carpi ulnaris m., 261
  extensor digiti minimi m., 261
  extensor digitorum m., 261
  extensor indicis m., 261
Muscle — *continued*
  extensor pollicis brevis m., 261
  extensor pollicis longus m., 261
  external anal sphincter m., 252, 610
  flexor carpi radialis m., 259
  flexor carpi ulnaris m., 260
  flexor digitorum longus m., 265
  flexor digitorum profundus m., 278
  flexor digitorum superficialis m., 278
  flexor hallucis brevis m., 233
  flexor hallucis m., 233, 265, 268
  flexor pollicis brevis m., 233, 261
  gastrocnemius m., 265
  gemellus superior m., 228
  geniohyoideus m., 237, 243
  gluteus maximus m., 262, 345
  gluteus medius m., 262, 345
  gluteus minimus m., 262, 345
  gracilis m., 262
  hamstring mm., 263
  hypaxial mm., 254
  iliacus m., 262
  iliococcygeus m., 237
  iliocostalis m., 237
  iliopsoas m., 262, 265
  inferior oblique m., 414
  inferior rectus m., 414
  infraspinatus m., 254
  interspinalis m., 254
  ischiocavernosus m., 252
  lateral rectus m., 414
  latissimus dorsi m., 254
  levator ani m., 252
  levator scapulae m., 254
  levatores costarum breves mm., 245
  levatores costarum longi mm., 245
  long digital extensor m., 263, 264
  longissimus m., 237
  longus capitis m., 243
  longus colli m., 243
  masseter m., 240
  medial rectus m., 414
  mentalis m., 237, 240
  multifidi mm., 237
  mylohyoideus m., 243, 334
  nasalis m., 237, 240
  nomenclature of mm., 226, 237, 239
  obliquus externus abdominis m., 278
  obliquus internus abdominis m., 278
  of abdomen, 226, 246
  of anterior antebrachium, 226, 254, 260
  of anterior brachium, 226, 254
  of auditory ossicles, 240
  of back, 226, 251, 252, 254
  of eye, 239, 240, 401, 414, 416
  of facial expression, 239

Muscle — *continued*
of hand, 259, 260, 261
of head, 226, 239, 240, 241, 242
of larynx, 243, 635, 642, 645
of mastication, 240, 244
of neck, 226, 243
of palate and fauces, 242
of perineal region, 250
of pes, 268, 272, 273
of pharynx, 243, 245
of posterior brachium, 226, 254
of shoulder and scapula, 254
of superior limb, 226, 254
of thorax, 226, 245
of tongue, 240, 241, 246
omohyoideus m., 104, 237, 243
opponens pollicis m., 227, 228, 261, 262
orbicularis oculi m., 414
orbicularis oris m., 231, 240
palmaris longus m., 259
pectineus m., 263
pectoralis major m., 97, 104
peroneus brevis m., 264
peroneus longus m., 264
peroneus tertius m., 265
piriformis m., 262, 345
plantaris m., 265, 266
platysma, 227, 243
popliteus m., 266
pronator quadratus m., 261
pronator teres m., 261
psoas major m., 262
puborectalis m., 237
pyramidalis m., 248
quadratus femoris m., 262, 345
quadratus lumborum m., 248, 677
quadriceps femoris m., 262
rectus abdominis m., 248
rectus femoris m., 262
rectus inferior m., 240, 330
rhomboideus major m., 254
risorius m., 240
sartorius m., 262
semimembranosus m., 263
semitendinosus m., 263
serratus anterior m., 245
soleus m., 265, 266
spinalis m., 237
stapedius m., 240, 438
sternohyoideus m., 237, 243
sternothyroideus m., 237, 243
styloglossus m., 240, 595
subclavius m., 245
subcostales m., 245
suboccipital mm., 243
subscapularis m., 254

Muscle — *continued*
superior oblique m., 414
superior rectus m., 414
supinator m., 237, 261
supraspinatus m., 254
temporalis m., 240, 241
tensor fasciae latae m., 262
tensor tympani m., 240, 438
teres major m., 254
teres minor m., 254
thyrohyoideus m., 237, 243
tibialis anterior m., 345
transversus abdominis m., 248
transversus thoracis m., 245
trapezius m., 254
triceps brachii m., 258
vastus intermedius m., 262
vastus lateralis m., 262
vastus medialis m., 262
Muscular dystrophy, 276+
Muscular system, 13, 225, 228, 274
Mutations, 49
Myasthenia gravis, 276
Myelencephalon, 297
Myelin, 287, 288, 293
Myelin sheath, 293
Myoblast, 274
Myocyte, 60, 233
Myofiber, 60, 227, 233
Myofibril, 59, 60, 227, 223, 236
Myofilament, 62, 227, 233
Myomere, 59, 234
Myosin, 233
Myotube, 274

Nail, 91, 92, 101, 102
Nasal bone, 167
Nasal concha, 162, 168
Nasal septum, 640
Natal cleft, 105
Navicular bone, 138
Neck
anatomic n. (humerus), 127
of a bone (see that bone)
surgical n. (humerus), 127
Neoplasia, 33, 49
Nerve
abducens n., 334, 364
accessory n., 338, 364
accessory obturator n., 345
auriculotemporal n., 335
axillary n., 344
buccal n., 335
coccygeal n., 345
cochlear n., 336
common fibular n., 345, 349

Nerve — *continued*
cranial n., 323, 324, 326, 328, 330, 331, 334, 352, 364, 365
deep temporal nn., 335
dorsal scapular n., 334
facial n., 335, 339, 364, 388
femoral n., 345, 349
frontal n., 335
genitofemoral n., 345
glossopharyngeal n., 337, 340, 364, 388
hypoglossal n., 339, 342, 346, 364
iliohypogastric n., 345
ilio-inguinal n., 345
inferior alveolar n., 168, 336, 337, 363
inferior gluteal n., 347
infraorbital n., 334, 335
lacrimal n., 335
lateral cutaneous femoral n., 345
lateral pectoral n., 344
lateral pterygoid n., 335
lingual n., 335
long thoracic n., 334
major palatine n., 335
mandibular n., 334, 335
masseteric n., 335
maxillary n., 162, 331, 335
medial cutaneous antebrachial n., 344
medial cutaneous brachial n., 344
medial pectoral n., 344
medial pterygoid n., 335
median n., 334
mental n., 334, 335
minor palatine nn., 335
mixed n., 326
motor n., 82, 277, 326
musculocutaneous n., 344, 347
n. of the internal obturator muscle, 345
n. of the piriformis muscle, 345
nasociliary n., 335
nasopalatine n., 335
obturator n., 345, 349
oculomotor n., 330, 364, 385
olfactory n., 329, 364
ophthalmic n., 331, 335
optic n., 329, 364, 408
perforating cutaneous femoral n., 345
pharyngeal n., 335
posterior cutaneous femoral n., 345
pudendal n., 345
radial n., 344, 347
sciatic n., 345, 349
sensory n., 326
short ciliary n., 330
spinal n., 289, 304, 323, 324, 325, 326, 343, 344, 345, 352, 354
subclavian n., 344

Nerve — *continued*
subscapular nn., 344
superior alveolar nn., 335
superior gluteal n., 345
suprascapular n., 344
thoracodorsal n., 344
tibial n., 345, 349
trigeminal n., 331, 335, 337, 360, 364
trochlear n., 331
ulnar n., 344, 347
vagus n., 337, 341, 364, 388
vestibular n., 336
vestibulocochlear n., 336, 340, 364
Nerve cell, 59
Nerve fiber, 80, 326, 367, 408
Nerve tracts, 326
Nervous impulse, 288, 295
Neural groove, 297
Neural plate, 297
Neural tube, 8, 297
Neurocranium, 152, 153, 158
Neurogenic shock, 376, 392, 547
Neuroglia, 13, 59, 81, 285, 293
Neurolemmocytes, 293
Neuromuscular spindle, 357, 358
Neuron
afferent n., 291
autonomic n., 297, 594
bipolar n., 290, 330
efferent n., 290, 291
interneuron, 290, 365
motor n., 13, 378
multipolar n., 289
postganglionic n., 291, 376, 378
preganglionic n., 291, 376, 378
pseudounipolar n., 290
sensory n., 378
somatic afferent n., 291
somatic efferent n., 290
visceral afferent n., 291
visceral efferent n., 291
Neurotendinous spindle, 357, 358
Neurotransmitter, 287, 296, 385
Neutron, 10
Nipple, 59, 97
Nociceptor, 325, 352, 355
Nomina Anatomica, 1, 2, 7, 69, 192, 216, 314
Norepinephrine, 296, 376, 383, 476
Normal anatomical position, 18
Nose, 635, 640
Notch
of a bone (see that bone)
vertebral n., 171
Notochord, 3, 8
Nuclear membrane, 46
Nuclear pore, 46

Nucleic acid, 11, 32, 38
Nucleolus, 44, 46
Nucleotide, 38
Nucleus of cell, 43, 466, 291
Nucleus pulposus, 200

Observation, 1, 4
Occipital bone, 160
Occiput, 104
Olfactory bulb, 329
Olfactory cell, 329, 358, 360
Olfactory epithelium, 329
Oligodendrocyte, 288, 293
Ophthalmoscope, 421
Optic canal, 161, 330, 404
Optic chiasm, 302, 330
Oral cavity, 587, 593, 596
Orbit, 154, 158, 401, 404, 405
Order, 8, 9
Organ, 1, 2, 13
Organelle, 2, 11, 33, 44, 45
Organic compound, 11
Orifice closure, 229
Origin of muscle, 225, 227, 231
Osmosis, 39, 40
Ossa coxae (coxarum), 130
Osteoblast, 71, 115, 116
Osteoclast, 59, 71, 115, 116
Osteocyte, 71, 116
Osteoid, 115, 116
Osteology, 113, 115, 116, 151
Osteomalacia, 141
Osteon, 115, 116, 152
Osteoporosis, 115, 141
Ovary, 66, 366, 465, 477, 725, 729
Oxytocin, 461, 468, 471

Pacinian corpuscle, 355, 358
Palate, 240, 242
Palatine bone, 158, 167
Palatine tonsil, 560, 573, 595
Palm of hand, 104, 228
Palmar, 20
Palpation, 3, 5
Palpebra, 401, 403, 415, 417
Pancreas, 66, 366, 465, 477, 478, 588, 590, 616, 618, 619
Pancreatic juice, 619
Papilla
  fungiform p., 259, 595
  of tongue, 595
Papillary layer (of dermis), 96
Paralysis, 59, 276, 313, 325
Paraplegia, 313
Parasympathetic part of the ANS, 375, 385
Parasympathomimetic drug, 392
Parathyroid gland, 462, 474, 482
Parietal bone, 153, 159
Parkinson's disease, 313
Parotid gland, 612
Parturition, 752, 764
Patella, 134, 139
Patellar ligament, 206
Patellar reflex, 365
Pectoral girdle, 120, 125, 203
Pedicle of vertebral arch, 169
Pelvic girdle, 114, 120, 130, 134, 206
Pelvimetry, 178, 179
Pelvis, 15, 130, 131, 135
Penis, 390, 697, 709, 710, 741
Peptide, 32, 33, 43, 465
Percussion, 6
Perforating canal, 116
Perforating fiber, 124
Pericardial cavity, 16, 496
Perimysium, 231
Perineurium, 326
Periodontal membrane, 194
Periodontium, 76, 194, 597
Perionyx, 93, 101
Peripheral nervous system, 287, 288, 323
Peristalsis, 590
Peritoneal cavity, 16, 588, 619, 620
Peritoneum, 588, 589, 590, 608, 619, 620, 621
Peroxisome, 44, 46
PET scan, 6
Phagocytosis, 33, 41
Phase
  G1 p., 31, 47
  G2 p., 31, 47
  interphase, 33, 47
  S p., 47
Phantom pain, 324, 366
Pharyngeal pouch, 8
Pharynx, 325. 587, 590, 601, 635, 642, 769
Phospholipid, 38
Photoreceptor, 352, 355
Phylum, 9
Physiology, 3
Physis, 3, 115
Pia mater, 288, 308
Pinocytosis, 33, 41
Pisiform bone, 115, 203
Pituitary gland, 460, 461, 462, 467, 468, 469, 472
Planar suture, 192
Plane
  coronal p., 2, 18
  frontal p., 18
  median p. (midsagittal p.), 18
  sagittal p., 18
  transverse p., 18
Plasma, 493, 533

Plexus
  brachial p., 324, 344, 346, 347
  cervical p., 345, 346
  choroid p., 308
  lumbar p., 345, 349
  lumbosacral p., 324, 349
PNS, 285, 287, 288
Poliomyelitis, 313
Polypeptide, 38, 464
Polysaccharide, 3, 11, 38
Pons, 302
Posterior, 20
Posterior branch of spinal nerve, 324, 344
Posterior cruciate ligament, 206
Posterior funiculi (of spinal cord), 306
Posterior gray column (of spinal cord), 304
Postganglionic neuron, 291, 376, 378
Posturing, 228
Prehension, 228, 591
Pressure
  blood p., 21, 545, 675
Primary center of ossification, 153, 176
Primary germ layer, 59, 60, 761
Primates, 8, 9
Process
  articular p., 171
  of a bone (see that bone)
  spinous p., 171
  transverse p., 171
  xiphoid p., 77, 153, 174
Prominent vertebra, 171
Pronation, 211
Prophase, 33, 47
Prosencephalon, 297
Prostaglandin, 38, 711
Protein, 11, 32, 35, 37, 38
Protons, 10
Protraction, 211
Proximal, 20, 101
Proximal interphalangeal joint, 203, 206
Proximal radio-ulnar joint, 202
Pseudounipolar neuron, 290
Puberty, 765
Pubic arch, 133
Pubic symphysis, 133, 205, 206
Pubis, 133
Pulmonary alveoli, 637, 650, 652
Puncture wound, 105
Pupil, 405, 415
Purine, 11
Pyrimidine, 11

Quadriplegia, 313

Radial, 20
Radiocarpal joint, 202
Radiography, 6, 21
Radius, 127, 131
Ramus (see branch)
Ramus communicans, 344, 376
Receptor, 324, 325, 467
Rectum, 590, 610
Referred pain, 324, 325, 363, 366
Reflex
  auditory r., 286, 445
  disynaptic r., 365
  knee jerk r., 365
  micturition r., 672
  monosynaptic r., 365
  spinal r., 325, 361
Region
  abdominal r., 104, 609
  epigastric r., 104
  hypochondriac r., 104
  hypogastric r., 104
  inguinal r., 104
  lateral abdominal r., 104
  perineal r., 104, 250
  umbilical r., 104
Renal tubule, 673, 678, 680
Repolarization, 287, 295
RER, 43
Resistance, 211
Respiratory epithelium, 66, 637, 640
Respiratory system, 13, 635, 636, 638, 639, 641, 660, 769, 771
Resting potential, 293
Reticular connective tissue, 75
Reticular fiber, 71
Reticular layer (of dermis), 92, 96
Reticulin, 71
Reticulocyte, 75
Retina, 358, 403, 408
Retinacula, 233
Retraction, 211
Rheumatoid arthritis, 214
Rhombencephalon, 288, 297
Rib, 151, 153, 173, 174, 175
Ribonucleic acid 38
Ribosome, 33, 43, 44
Rickets, 141
Rigor mortis, 276
RNA, 38
Rod, 403
Root
  of brachial plexus, 324
  of hair, 100, 355, 358
  of spinal n., 325
Root ending, 355, 358
Rotation, 190, 211
Rotator cuff, 254
Rough endoplasmic reticulum, 43

Saccule, 432, 440, 443, 447
Sacral plexus, 324, 345, 349
Sacral vertebra, 172
Sacroiliac joint, 205, 206
Sacrum, 172
Saltatory conduction, 296
Satellite cell, 293
Scalp, 104
Scaphoid bone, 115, 127
Scapula, 115, 125, 129
Scarring, 82, 105
Schindylesis, 192
Sclera, 76, 403, 404
Sclerotome, 274
Scrotum, 698, 712, 741
Second class lever, 213
Secondary center of ossification, 176
Secretion, 58, 66, 69, 98, 680
Sella turcica of sphenoid bone, 161
Semipermeable membrane, 39
Sensory ganglia, 291, 344, 351, 352, 390
Sensory impulse, 287, 289
Sensory nerves, 326
Sensory neuron, 13, 378
SER, 43
Serosa, 3, 16, 593, 681
Serous membrane (serosa), 16, 593
Serrated suture, 192
Shock
  anaphylactic sh., 664
Shoulder joint, 189, 199, 204
Sigmoid colon, 610
Simple diffusion, 32, 39, 40
Simple joint, 189, 191, 192
Skeletal myology, 225, 228
Skin, 59, 91, 92, 93, 94, 96, 97, 98, 356
Skin cancer, 103
Skull, 154, 157, 159, 160, 161, 162, 163
Sliding filament mechanism, 233
Small intestine, 366, 465, 477, 588, 590, 606, 608, 611
Smooth endoplasmic reticulum, 43
Smooth muscle, 11, 62, 117, 228, 378
Sodium-potassium pump, 287, 293
Soft palate, 595
Sole of foot, 105
Somatic afferent neuron, 291
Somatic efferent neuron, 290
Somite, 274
Special sense, 289, 352
Species, 8, 9
Spermatic cord, 698, 699, 711, 712
Sphenoid bone, 153, 158, 161, 165
Sphenoidal sinus, 161
Sphygmomanometer, 494, 545
Spina bifida, 141, 297
Spine
  of a bone (see that bone)
  vertebral column, 153, 172, 173
Spinal cord, 286, 288, 289, 304, 305, 306, 310, 343
Spinal nerve, 289, 304, 323, 324, 325, 326, 343, 344, 345, 352, 354
Spiral organ, 358, 433, 446
Spleen, 571, 574
Squamous suture, 192
Stapes, 153, 154, 437
Sternal angle, 174
Sternoclavicular joint, 202
Sternocostal joints, 200, 202
Sternum, 151, 153, 173, 174
Steroid, 38, 464
Stomach, 465, 478, 588, 603, 605, 606, 607
Strabismus, 325, 335, 403, 419
Stratification, 16
Stratum
  s. basale, 93, 94
  s. corneum, 92, 93, 95
  s. germinativum, 92, 95
  s. granulosum, 93, 95
  s. lucidum, 93, 95
  s. spinosum, 93, 94
Stretch mark, 96
Styloid process (see that bone)
Subarachnoid space, 308
Subatomic waves and particles, 10
Subcutaneous tissue, 94, 232
Subluxation, 191, 214
Submandibular ganglion, 388, 391
Submucosa, 76, 590, 593, 608
Subpubic angle, 133
Sugar, 11, 33, 35
Sulcus (cerebral), 301
Sulcus (see groove)
Superficial, 20
Superficial fascia, 94, 232
Superior, 15, 20
Superior colliculus of mesencephalon, 330
Superior orbital fissure, 330, 331, 335, 404
Superior pelvic opening, 131
Supination, 211
Surface (see that structure)
Surface
  of a bone (see that bone)
Surgery, 6
Sutural bone, 194
Suture
  coronal s., 159, 194
  cranial s., 202
  ethmoidolacrimal s., 194
  ethmoidomaxillary s., 194
  frontal s., 194
  fronto-ethmoidal s., 194

Suture — *continued*
frontolacrimal s., 194
frontomaxillary s., 194
frontonasal s., 194
frontozygomatic s., 194
intermaxillary s., 194
internasal s., 194
lacrimoconchal s., 194
lacrimomaxillary s., 192, 194
lambdoid s., 194
median palatine s., 194
metopic s., 194
nasomaxillary s., 194
occipitomastoid s., 194
palatomaxillary s., 194
parietomastoid s., 194
planar s., 192
sagittal s., 194
schindylesis, 192
serrated s., 192
spheno-ethmoidal s., 194
sphenofrontal s., 194
sphenomaxillary s., 194
sphenoparietal s., 194
sphenosquamous s., 194
sphenovomerine s., 194
sphenozygomatic s., 194
squamomastoid s., 194
squamous s., 192, 194
temporozygomatic s., 194
transverse palatine s., 194
zygomaticomaxillary s., 194
Sympathetic part of the ANS, 375, 383
Sympathetic trunk, 344, 351, 383
Sympathetic trunk ganglia, 351, 377, 383, 390
Sympathomimetic drug, 377, 392
Symphysis
intervertebral s., 200, 202
mandibular s., 168
manubriosternal s., 153, 200, 202
Synapse, 287, 288, 296, 298, 352
Synchondrosis, 191
Syndesmosis
radioulnar s., 202, 203
tibiofibular s., 206
tympanostapedial s., 153, 437
Synergist, 227, 237
Synostosis, 191, 196, 215
Synovial (tendon) sheath, 227
Synovial fluid, 191, 196
Synovial joint, 189, 191, 192, 196, 197, 198, 199
Synovial membrane, 196
Syphilis, 313
System
integumentary, 13, 91, 93
muscular, 13, 225, 228, 274

System — *continued*
nervous, 13, 285, 286, 287, 288, 290, 297, 299
skeletal, 13, 768, 770
somatic, 13
visceral, 13
Systemic circulation, 493, 512

Talocrural joint, 206, 207
Talus, 138
Tarsal bone, 114, 138
Tarsal joint, 199, 206-209, 219, 223, 275, 282
Tarsometatarsal joint, 206
Taste bud, 206, 207
Taxonomy, 1, 3, 7, 9, 189, 192
Tay-sachs disease, 313
Telencephalon, 288, 297
Telophase, 33, 47
Temporal bone, 160, 164
Temporomandibular joint, 197, 202
Tendon sheath, 227, 232, 233
Tendon
"Achilles" t., 7, 278
aponeurosis, 227, 231
calcanean t., 266
of insertion, 264, 275, 280, 286
of origin, 76
"patellar" t., 217
Tendons, 227, 231
Tentorium cerebelli, 312
Testis, 66, 465, 478, 697, 698, 701, 703, 714
Testosterone, 478
Thalamus, 288, 302
Thenar eminence, 104, 261
Thermoregulation, 94, 495
Third class lever, 213
Thoracic cavity, 16, 636, 654
Thoracic vertebra, 171
Thoracic wall, 654
Thorax, 15, 226, 245, 529, 636, 637, 653, 654
Threshold, 294, 378
Thyroid gland, 462, 471, 473, 482
Tibia, 114, 134, 139
Tibial, 20
Tibiofibular joint, 206
Tibiofibular syndesmosis, 206
Tight junction, 43
Tissue
adipose t., 13, 57, 58, 74, 80, 117
areolar t., 71, 74
basic t., 58
blood t., 11, 57, 58, 74, 79, 492, 494, 533
bone marrow t., 58, 75, 117
bone t., 58, 71, 75, 113, 114, 115, 116, 117, 118, 119
cardiac muscle t., 62, 380, 498
cartilage t., 58, 71, 78, 117
connective t., 11, 57, 60, 71, 192, 286, 308

Tissue — *continued*
connective t. proper, 11, 58, 71, 73, 76, 117
epithelial t., 11, 57, 60, 63
fibrous connective t., 58, 71
mesenchyme, 59, 75
muscle t., 11, 57, 59, 60, 61, 62
nervous t., 13, 58, 60, 80, 117
primitive connective t., 58, 75
reticular connective t., 75
skeletal muscle t., 62, 235
smooth muscle t., 11, 62, 117, 228, 378
Tongue, 240, 241, 246, 587, 595, 598
Tonsil, 560, 561
Tooth, 590, 597, 598, 599, 600, 601, 624
Trachea, 635, 637, 644, 646
Tracheostomy, 661
Tract
ascending t., 324
descending t., 324
fiber t., 291, 324, 326
nerve t., 326
Transplant technology, 82
Transverse, 18, 20
Transverse tarsal joint, 206, 207
Trapezium bone, 128
Trapezoidal bone, 254
Traumatic arthritis, 214
Triangle
anterior cervical tri., 103-104
carotid t., 104
clavipectoral t., 104
deltopectoral t., 104
femoral t., 105
infraclavicular t., 104
muscular t., 104
occipital t., 104
of neck, 103
omoclavicular t., 104
omotracheal t., 104
posterior cervical t., 104
subclavian t., 104
submandibular t., 104
submental t., 104
suprahyoid t., 104
Trichosiderin, 93, 100
Trigeminal neuralgia, 360
Triglyceride, 38
Triquetral bone, 115, 128
Trisomy, 49
Trochanter (see femur bone)
True rib, 153, 175
Trunk
inferior t. (brachial plexus), 346, 347
middle t. (brachial plexus), 346, 347
superior t. (brachial plexus), 346, 347
sympathetic t., 344, 383
Tubercle of bone (see that bone)
Tuberosity (see that bone)
Tuberosity of a bone (see that bone)
Tubulation, 6
Tympanic membrane, 432, 433, 436, 437, 443

Ulna, 115, 127, 131
Ulnar, 20, 115, 344
Ultrasonography, 3, 6
Umbilicus, 104
Ureter, 671, 673, 681, 688
Urethra, 672, 673, 683, 684, 685, 697, 699, 708
Urinalysis, 22, 689
Urinary bladder, 390, 671, 673, 683, 684
Urinary system, 13, 671, 672, 673, 674, 686, 687
Urine, 671, 673, 675, 678, 680, 683, 753
Uterine tube, 590, 725, 727, 730, 733, 734
Uterus, 725, 727, 730, 734, 735
Utricle, 432, 433, 440, 443, 447

Vacuole, 44, 46
Vagina, 726, 727, 737
Valve, 503, 608
Venous return, 229
Ventral, 20
Ventricle
Fourth v., 302
Lateral v., 302
third v., 302
Vermiform appendix, 590, 609
Vertebra, 151, 169, 170, 171, 172, 173, 202
Vertebral canal, 171
Vertebral column, 153, 172, 173
Vertebral formula, 151, 174
Vertex, 104
Vibrissa, 101, 640
Visceral afferent neuron, 291
Viscerocranium, 153, 163
Vitreous chamber, 410
Vocalization, 229, 640
Vomer, 167

White blood cells, 74
White matter, 287, 304

Xerophthalmia, 325, 360, 403, 421

Z line, 234
Zygapophyseal joint, 191, 200, 202
Zygomatic arch, 153, 155, 163
Zygomatic bone, 158, 163
Zygomorphism, 16
Zygote, 753, 757